COMPREHENSIVE GUIDE TO PRE-HOSPITAL SKILLS: A Skills Manual For—

EMT-BASIC
EMT-INTERMEDIATE
EMT-PARAMEDIC

Alexander M. Butman, BA, D.Sc., REMT-P
Scott W. Martin, BS, REMT-P
Richard W. Vomacka, BA, REMT-P
Norman E. McSwain, Jr., MD, FACS, REMT-P

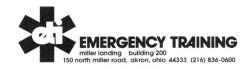

EMERGENCY TRAINING
miller landing   building 200
150 north miller road, akron, ohio 44333 (216) 836-0600

Editor-In-Chief

Alexander M. Butman, B.A., D.Sc., REMT-P

Managing Editor

Richard W. Vomacka, B.A., REMT-P

Graphics Director

Tom Petrich

Senior Photographer

Mike Anthol

WARNING:

Printed in the United States of America ISBN Number: 0-940432-09-9

Authors and General Editors

Alexander M. Butman, B.A., D.Sc., REMT-P

Executive Director
Emergency Training Institute
Akron, Ohio

Coordinator of Graduate Education,
Paramedic Education Program
Akron General Medical Center

Adjunct Professor of Emergency Medical Services
Central Connecticut State University
New Britain, Connecticut

Scott W. Martin, B.S., REMT-P

Director of Paramedic Education
Akron General Medical Center
Akron, Ohio

Immediate Past President
Ohio Instructor/Coordinator Society

Richard W. Vomacka, B.A., REMT-P

Vice-President and Editorial Director
Emergency Training Institute
Akron, Ohio

EMS Training Coordinator
Brimfield Township Fire Department
Kent, Ohio

Advanced EMS Instructor
Robinson Memorial Hospital
Ravenna, Ohio

Norman E. McSwain, Jr., M.D., FACS, REMT-P

Professor of Surgery
Tulane University School of Medicine
New Orleans, Louisiana

Medical Director
Pre-Hospital Trauma Life Support Program
National Association of EMTs

IT IS WITH GREAT HONOR THAT I INTRODUCE THIS COMPREHENSIVE GUIDE TO PRE-HOSPITAL SKILLS to the educators and providers of our Nation's EMS community. In the past we have had to search long and hard to find sound educational materials to cover the essential skills required to manage the variety of patients that challenge our practice of emergency medical care every day.

Finally there is a comprehensive skills text written on a professional level that every EMS provider can use. From a simple reading of the table of contents the EMS educator or EMT can see the value of this book for teaching and learning the skills needed to deliver competent patient care at each level.

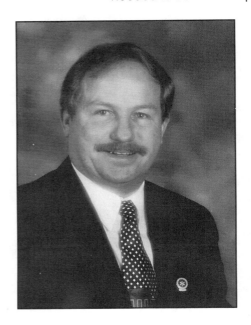

I've been excited about this book since its concept was first introduced to me a number of years ago. As we examined the skills at all levels in developing the EMS "blueprint", and "rolled out" the 1994 EMT-Basic curriculum across the nation, we became acutely aware of the need for *teaching* skill sheets. Sheets which, unlike the brief testing evaluation sheets used to measure performance, include detailed descriptions. This book provides the answer.

It contains a multiple page step-by-step *teaching* skill sheet for each of the more than 190 pre-hospital skills identified for the Basic, Intermediate, and Paramedic levels of training. I'm impressed with the clarity and detail of the descriptions these contain for each task that the EMT must perform when using the skill. The descriptions and corresponding photos for each step are medically correct. Nowhere in our professions literature are the component tasks that make up each skill described so completely.

The detailed *teaching skill sheets* provide a photo for each step that standardizes the presentation. The guesswork is gone. Students can now take a book home and implant a medically correct process of skill delivery in their mind. The instructor will use this section as an aid to demonstrations of skills. It is a slow motion, take the skill apart, break it down to its simplest step, attitude. *WOW!* If only I had had this text when I was teaching. I know the pressure of my first attempts at an error free demonstration would have been relieved. My students could repeat and repeat a skill without constant direct supervision because everyone in the class would have a medically correct written breakdown of each skill.

With all of the present changes in the scope of practice and the curricula (and those anticipated in the future), one thing still remains constant. Even though the levels may alter, there is very little change in the individual interventions and skills that the EMT must be able to competently perform. Accurately, these skills are defined as "psychomotor" skills. The "motor" portion is the observable manual manipulations that are actually performed by the EMT. The "psych" root of the term refers to the cognitive understanding that is also necessary. As students learn a skill they must have a fluent understanding of its underlying general principles, therapeutic objectives and generic components before attempting to perform it. The "motor" manipulations are the easiest parts to teach since they are easily observed and corrected. It is more difficult to teach the proper cognitive "psych" elements. This book, with its detailed introductions and skill sequences, simplifies and includes the proper stable knowledge base for this essential learning ingredient.

Once a student masters the detail in each complex skill, they need a quick short listing of the steps involved. Here it is! Each of the complex skills which is taken apart, examined in detail, and then put back together in the teaching skill sheets is presented again in a precise Summary Skill Sheet at the end of the topic section.

When the class breaks into small groups for individual skills practice, this summary sheet acts as a handy concise reference. The instructor can be confident of the consistency in the hands-on sequences seen repeatedly, as each group uses the summary sheets to ensure that fellow students are correctly performing the individual steps and sequence required. Then, after leaving the class, the same sheets aid the student in reviewing and memorizing the proper sequence of the steps.

I want to thank the Emergency Training Institute for adding the National Registry test instruments to this essential text. The National Registry of Emergency Medical Technicians wants EMTs to deliver safe and effective care. We are not a publisher nor a provider of EMS education. We feel that every textbook should have our testing instruments within the covers. We will not provide teaching sheets which correlate to our examination—it is not our role. However, this textbook fulfills that need in a comprehensive manner.

To my friends Alex Butman, Scott Martin, Rick Vomacka and Norman McSwain, Jr., I want to express my congratulations on this important textbook. I know of no finer team to present the critical concepts for providing the skills needed to resolve the myriad of patient presentations in today's EMS world. Let us hope that through books such as this one we can effectively eliminate the "kills" from skills. We no longer have to "kill" our students over the teaching and testing of skills. With such a resource and reference, each EMT can go forward and deliver the kind of care that the citizens of our nation expect. At the time of an emergency, the patient has a right to expect no less than the excellence that this book promotes.

William E. Brown, Jr., R.N., M.S., CEN
Nationally Registered EMT-Paramedic
Columbus, Ohio
October, 1994

Contents
And Listing Of Individual Skills By Topic

Section 11: Hemorrhage Control And Shock Management Skills **461**

Section 12: Skills For Medication Administration And Establishing An IV **503**

Section13: Spinal Immobilization Skills **627**

Additional Contributors

Richard L. Judd, Ph.D., REMT-I

Vice-President of University Affairs
Central Connecticut State University
New Britain, Connecticut

John W. Mason, EMT-P

EMS Coordinator
Robinson Memorial Hospital
Ravenna, Ohio

President Ohio EMT
Instructors Association

Virginia K. Riedy, RN, REMT-P

Paramedic Coordinator
Providence Hospital
Sandusky, Ohio

Paramedic Coordinator
Medical College Hospitals
Northwest Ohio Paramedic Program
Toledo, Ohio

Patricia Ambrose, REMT-P

Lead Paramedic Instructor
Providence Hospital
Sandusky, Ohio

Paramedic Coordinator
Medical College Hospitals
Northwest Ohio Paramedic Program
Toledo, Ohio

**The National Registry of
Emergency Medical Technicians**

Columbus, Ohio

For inclusion of their
Practical Skill Testing Sheets

Dedication

Unfortunately, there is an increasing trend to discount the learning ability of the EMT and, in an attempt to simplify the training, to increasingly oversimplify the materials. Advocates of this recent trend would have us believe that the EMT only "needs-to-know" *what* to do, and that an understanding of *why* is only "nice-to-know" and even that such enlargement may be a needless distraction. The EMT must learn and retain a vast amount of knowledge. Regardless of recent representations to the contrary, meaningful emergency care requires complex decision-making by the EMT, and the decisions must include both *some assessment* and some *diagnostic* basis. Even though one often provides ventilation to a patient based only upon the assessment that his air exchange is absent or insufficient, if attempts to provide ventilation are unsuccessful the EMT must diagnostically determine whether this is caused by an open wound of the thorax, a tension pneumothorax, a foreign body obstruction, or edema from an allergic reaction. The necessary remediation and interventions for each are vastly different, and can only be decided with some understanding of the mechanisms of normal ventilation and a differentiating diagnosis made from the specific history and presenting signs and symptoms. One cannot determine the appropriate skills to employ without this underlying understanding.

Often skills are introduced with varying and seemingly arbitrary steps and without a comprehensive introduction or clear rationale for their therapeutic physiologic effect, indications and contraindications, the techniques involved, or their sequence. These understandings are *not only* essential to the EMT's determination of which skills are required or will best meet the individual patient's needs, but also to his ability to easily learn and retain the vast number of skills that are required of him.

This book is founded upon the belief that skills must include a clear explanation of why as well as *how* each technique and sequence is performed. In a broader sense it is dedicated to the principle that EMS must be based upon true education and not on simple rote memorization and the uncomprehending delivery of care by a series of knee jerk-like reactions.

It is our considerable combined experience that most of the EMTs throughout this country, regardless of their certification level or State's minimum requirements (although often masked by humility and station-house humor), strive for increased knowledge and excellence. It is our hope that this book will be an essential tool which significantly contributes to these goals.

This book is dedicated to the vast majority of EMTs everywhere who, over the years, have proven that they are intelligent self-directed learners and professionals (whether paid or volunteer), and to the Instructors who strive to provide them with real education.

We join with them in the continued belief that neither the delivery of emergency care nor those who provide it in the field, are simple.

This book is also dedicated to the many individuals whose efforts are recognized in the acknowledgments on the following page.

Acknowledgments

The Publisher and Authors would like to thank each of the individuals listed below for their sustained contribution to this Work over the past three years. Without the outstanding effort of each of these individuals, this book would not have been possible.

Our thanks to Tom Petrich who designed and laid out the pages and cover of this text. His work on the design resulted in a high standard of graphics which aid the reader in comprehending the material and content of the text. We would also like to thank Tom for his illustrations and editorial help, and Mike Anthol of Media Dimensions for the photography. These visual demonstrations provide significant additions to the reader's understanding.

We would like to thank the staff of Book Masters, Inc., of Ashland, Ohio, and JK&L Typesetting of Akron, Ohio, who set the type and made up the prepress files, and the staff of Book Crafters Inc. of Chelsea, Michigan, for their usual high quality of printing and manufacture.

Particular appreciation goes to Patricia Hughes and Jeannie Butman, EMT-A, for encoding the manuscript and for Jeannie's editorial assistance.

Tremendously important to us has been the support and active assistance that we received from the following list of equipment and product manufacturers and distributors. Without their willingness to loan us new equipment to study and use for photographic sessions we would not have been able to provide the richness and diversity of equipment options that is evident throughout this text. We also wish to acknowledge our thanks for their assistance in answering sometimes critical questions about their products, as we probed for the correct or the best or the most effective ways to utilize them.

Ferno, Inc. (Steve Schmidt), Laerdal Medical Corporation (Mike Giancola) and SKEDCO, Inc. (Bud and Catherine Calkin) were simply incredible in making available anything we needed whenever we asked. Physio Control Corporation (Tony Donofrio), Respironics, Inc. (Gene Scarberry), Sheridan Catheter (Vern Erchenbrecher) and Bac Pac (Jim Doherty) were most generous with their time and products in support of this text.

The myriad products and supplies that fill so many of these pages were obtained from Parr Emergency Medical Products (Joel Culp and Tom Parr) and Penn Care Medical Products (Shaun Bryant). We appreciate their quick shipping and extended loans of equipment.

We are also grateful to the Brimfield Fire Department, Robinson Memorial Hospital, and Akron General Medical Center for making available equipment and supplies and, occasionally, backdrops.

Richard L. Judd deserves special thanks because, beyond his direct contribution, he has caused us to repeatedly re-examine the educational processes used in EMS and particularly to evaluate how skills are taught, learned and measured.

Each author would like to also acknowledge
some individuals who made an essential impact, enabling him to make his
key contribution to the book.

My unending thanks for the support and understanding that I enjoy
from my wife Jeannie and young daughter Alexandra—
their love has kept me going when this project was at its bleakest moments
and the tasks seemed never-ending.

— A.M.B. —

I dedicate this book in memory of my grandfather, William P. Kuglar, founding member
and fire chief of the Richmond Volunteer Fire Company and Rescue Squad,
Richmond, Ohio (1945–1962). He instilled in me the importance
of helping those in need, even at the greatest risk to myself if those risks are the
responsibility I have accepted, and to be fair, honest, hard working
and caring to people that I touch because people in need
can only afford for me to do it right the first time.

— S.W.M. —

To my parents, Muriel and Frank, who taught me how important learning is;
to Drs. Don Boyle and Norman McSwain and Alex Butman,
who taught me how much fun it can be;
to my children, Joe and Margaret, who I hope learn the
same lessons; and to my wife Virginia, whom I love.

— R.W.V. —

To my daughter, Merry, whose support and inspiration continue to drive me
to try and improve patient care in the field.

— N.E.M., Jr. —

Preface

This is not a primary EMT or Paramedic textbook. Primary textbooks contain all of the necessary material that is covered in a course. This is also not a topical monograph, a text which covers all of the material on one topic, such as a Trauma or Cardiology text. Rather, this unusual book solely addresses skills. It is a comprehensive detailed guide to the vast number of pre-hospital skills that the EMT is expected to be able to perform.

There are a variety of excellent textbooks available at the First Responder, EMT-Basic, EMT-Intermediate and EMT-Paramedic levels. However, the vast scope of information that each book must contain precludes them from having the space needed to cover the skills pertinent to that level in any depth. At the time of publication of this book, none of the primary texts contained a complete step-by-step presentation of all of the skills identified for that level of care. It is not practical for one book to include all of the didactic knowledge *and* all of the skills. Therefore, this book solely contains skills and information regarding skills. *It has been designed to be used in conjunction with any primary textbook.* The primary text furnishes the reader with the didactic knowledge base. This skills text provides a full comprehensive step-by-step demonstration, using photographs and a detailed text, of every pre-hospital skill.

This book is the culmination of over five years of careful observation and study of pre-hospital skills by the authors. We have observed skills being taught in the classroom, practiced in clinical settings, tested in practical exams and, most importantly, delivered in the field in real emergency situations. These observations, plus our experience in the daily delivery of care as responders and our experience in teaching skills through the years, has been an important basis for this work. We have further been fortunate to serve on a wide range of pre-hospital boards and committees which discuss skills delivery and testing. The members represented expertise from different parts of the country as well as a variety of EMS systems—large and small; paid and volunteer; basic and paramedic; fire department-based, hospital-based, and third service; and urban, suburban, rural, remote and even wilderness settings.

Too often, pre-hospital skills are taught and tested on a rigid, only-one-right-way basis. That basis is generally the instructor's or examiner's preference, with other choices being labelled "wrong". We disagree with this "my-way-or-highway" definition. It is our experience that there are some skills presently being taught or practiced which employ methods that either do not work or do not work adequately, or even produce deleterious side effects to the patient. ***These*** are "wrong", since they either do not meet the patient's needs or are potentially harmful. However, we have also found that for almost every skill there are a variety of methods and variations—each of which will adequately and safely meet the patient's needs. Selecting among these successful methods is either a discretionary preference or is determined by the situation, equipment, or personnel available. It is our strong belief that good skills training cannot be limited to simply learning a sequence of steps. Instead, it must include a generic understanding of the therapy provided as well as the steps involved. Our approach provides the EMT with a basis from which to competently select from among all of the various valid options. To this end, each section of this guide opens with an introduction to that section's skills—discussing the generic concepts that are the underlying principles to be followed when applying them.

Even though this book solely contains skills and information pertinent to their delivery, we still faced severe space limitations. Demonstrating every skill with every possible variation and every brand and model of each piece of equipment would have been extremely confusing and impractical. Therefore, the authors have carefully selected a good way to perform each skill using equipment found to be widely in use.

We have evaluated each skill and have refined steps that are often glossed over in their instruction. We feel strongly that skills instruction must include realistic considerations of the problems encountered by EMTs in their field application.

Even though this is a comprehensive guide and the authors believe that it presents a "best" way to perform a skill, the reader must keep in mind that there is *not* "one best way". It is our hope that no reader will condemn a method or device or variation because it is not included herein. It is NOT the authors' intent to determine or even imply that the included methods are better than options that may not have been included. Granted, some few options have been excluded because they don't work very well—however, most of the options we didn't include were left out to avoid redundancy, because they were not in wide use, or even because we didn't know about them. No distant author can determine which methods and equipment you should use—that determination can only be appropriately made by your medical director, a local or regional medical authority, or your state EMS agency.

Among the fifty states there is no common universal agreement as to which skills are allowable at each level of certification. In some states there are even different definitions from region to region. The EMT-Basic curriculum is presently being revised, and ensuing changes at all three levels can be expected—leading to even more significant differences. To make this text comprehensive and universal we have included all of the skills we found to be commonly included in each level of pre-hospital certification—without any indication of EMT level. Skills commonly thought to be invasive or having vast physiologic effect have been labelled as "ALS" skills. This identification is only included as a guide and the reader must use local and state guidelines to identify which skills are appropriate in his locale for any given level of certification.

In special technical rescue situations some of these skills may have to be altered or abridged or may even be impractical. It is beyond the scope of this book to include such variations or the numerous additional skills that are used by rescuers expert in each dimension of technical rescue.

Nothing presented here should be misconstrued as implying that a skill can be appropriately learned solely from a book. Skills must be practiced, and before any provider can safely apply a skill his level of competence must be demonstrated and approved by the appropriate medical authority under which he operates. This book is solely designed to be used in conjunction with initial courses and continuing education programs for EMTs at all levels, including hands-on practice and remediation by a qualified EMS instructor. It has been designed for use by EMT students as well as experienced EMTs at all levels, and is not intended for the lay public or self-instructional use.

We hope you find it an amazing new resource with which to learn, and we hope that it contributes to your excellence in providing a high quality of patient care.

Notes On Terminology

GENDER

Patients, EMTs, and medical directors may be of either gender. The authors, editors and publisher acknowledge the contributions made to EMS by both male and female responders and by both male and female medical directors. Repetitive dual references to "he/she" or "his/her" are space consuming and often jar the reader's concentration. Therefore, according to the generally accepted standards of grammar, reference to the gender of patients, responders, and medical directors is masculine except where a specific illustration shows it be to the contrary.

PROVIDER REFERENCES

The authors have found the term "provider" to be somewhat awkward as the generic term for the pre-hospital care giver. As previously noted, this book is for recognized pre-hospital providers at all levels—the care giver may be a First Responder, EMT-Basic, EMT-Intermediate, EMT-Paramedic, pre-hospital certified nurse, Physician's Assistant, or even a physician in the field. Regardless of other training, the most common and comfortable generic term representing such providers is "EMT". Accordingly, in the interests of simplicity and consistency, the term "EMT" is used generically to refer to the person delivering the pre-hospital care even when a skill is generally restricted to only certain levels. To avoid the wordiness of "The senior EMT in charge . . ." we have adopted the term "crew chief" to designate the EMT directing the team performing the skill. Our use of the term "EMT" should not be interpreted to imply anything regarding the appropriate certification level for the application of the particular skill.

SECTION
Learning EMS Skills
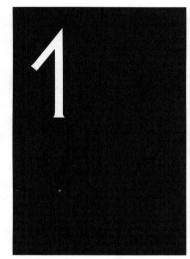

Learning EMS Skills

WHAT IS A SKILL?

EMT education and training encompass three basic categories of learning and knowledge:

- A knowledge base of the material
- Knowledge that enables the providers to differentiate between situations so as to select which actions are appropriate for each patient
- The physical ability to perform all of the skills that might be required.

Skills are physical acts. They are a hands-on examination or treatment done by the EMT to the patient, such as providing ventilations or starting an IV. Some employ equipment, some do not. The key definition of a skill is that—as well as knowledge and thinking—it includes an action or series of actions which are performed. Although the EMT's knowledge is the foundation, it is the sum of the skills performed that is the actual emergency care provided and the essence of EMS.

LEARNING EMS SKILLS

To appropriately perform a skill, an individual must know when it is indicated, when it is contraindicated, and how to examine for both indications and contraindications. He must also know the steps and sequence in the skill, must know how to recognize and select the necessary equipment, and must be able to perform the skill including the preparation and use of any required equipment—all within an appropriate time frame.

Skills—how they should be taught, how they are learned, and tested, the appropriate method to perform a skill, the equipment to be used, and the level of other knowledge needed to safely perform a skill—are widely debated subjects among EMS Educators. It is however universally agreed that you can't learn a skill from a book. If you can't learn a skill from a book, the reader may ask, why should I use one? Although one can not learn a skill solely from a book, one can not learn most skills **without** a book (or another form of printed material).

An understanding of how one learns a skill will be of material benefit, making it easier for you to learn and retain the many required skills and help you to use this book in a valuable manner.

TYPES OF SKILLS

There are two categories of skills, *simple skills* and *compound skills.* The difference is based upon the number and type of steps in each, not on their ease or difficulty to perform.

A Simple Skill is one comprised of a relatively few sequenced steps. As well as individual primary steps, a simple skill may also include one to two steps which describe a sub skill, such as "Do a tongue-jaw lift" or "Attach to supplemental oxygen at 10 to 15 Lpm".

A Compound Skill is one containing a significant number of steps. A skill is also considered a *compound skill* regardless of the number of steps if any of the steps included are a generic description of an entire simple or other entire compound skill. Examples are, "Open the airway", or "Provide CPR."

A skill is also included in the *compound skill* category if, after a given step and based upon the signs and symptoms, the EMT must select from one or another list of different steps to follow. For example, if there is a palpable carotid pulse one list of steps (one branch) is followed; if there is no palpable carotid pulse, a different list of steps (or branch) is followed instead. Skills which include such branching choices are called **Compound Branching Skills.**

The selection of which skill is needed and which of the available alternatives is the best to use is made prior to initiating the skill. This choice—since it precedes the skill—is not included in the categorizing of skills. The categories have little bearing on the performance of a skill but are key learning considerations because each of the three types represent a different learning problem.

HOW SKILLS ARE LEARNED

It is a common belief that a skill is learned simply from seeing it demonstrated and then practicing it until one is proficient. However, due to the vast number of simple skills the EMT must learn and the complex nature of compound skills, the skills learning process must include other steps as well. We learn what we understand, what we see, and what we do. Therefore, skills demonstrations must be exact and in their early presentation must not include confusing arbitrary variables. It is often said that "what we learn first, we learn best". Therefore, if the demonstration we see has errors or if we repeat a mistake while practicing the skill that goes uncorrected, then we learn the error as being correct. When watching a skill's introductory presentation it is hard to establish the sequence or pace, therefore more than one demonstration of a skill is necessary. The presentation of the skills in detailed photographs in this text provides the student with a stable reference and with the ability to easily see the sequence repeatedly.

When learning a skill the following procedure will be beneficial:

1. Prior to class, read the skills that will be covered and familiarize yourself with the steps—*do not attempt to practice it* as this can lead to learning an erroneous procedure

2. Watch the first classroom demonstration carefully without referring to the book.

3. When the demonstration is repeated follow along in the book and add any notes you want to make. The book eliminates the need for copious note taking or sketching since the photos and body of information are already there. Just add your own special comments.

4. Practice the skill while supervised by a qualified instructor. The instructor should correct and remediate errors and problems as soon as they occur to ensure that incorrect practices are not accidently learned.

5. Continue practicing in the lab until you can perform the skill easily and without needing lengthy thought to recall the next step. Periodically repeat the skill with supervision throughout the course.

6. In the case of some skills, once you have been cleared in performing them properly in the controlled classroom situation you will be able to practice them with supervision in an actual clinical environment such as the Emergency Department or in the field. (In such cases it is key that this only be done under direct line-of-sight supervision until you are certified.)

7. As your course continues, new skills will be added. Periodically practice *all* skills learned to date, not just the new ones.

8. In addition to supervised practice, review and practice in small peer groups is recommended. To assure that correct procedures are practiced, prior to performing the skill study the steps in the text and, during practice, one student should follow along in the text.

9. Prior to a practical exam, carefully study those skills in the text that will be covered. Be sure that without referring to the book you can verbalize or write out (reproduce) the steps in proper sequence without omission. One secret to success is practice, practice, and more practice.

10. With a peer group, "test each other" by selecting which skill to do next in random order from those that will be on your test. Identify any skill with which you are having a problem.

11. If the problem is in retaining and recalling the sequence of steps, more study of a short form list of the steps is required. If the problem is in the physical performance of the skill, you should seek help from your instructor.

12. Once you are certified, commonly used skills are reinforced by their repeated performance. However, skills not performed regularly should periodically be reviewed in the text and in supervised practice sessions as part of a continuing education program.

LEARNING COMPOUND SKILLS

As well as the preceding dozen general steps for learning a skill, some additional items are required to learn and retain **compound skills** and **compound branching skills.**

Due to the limited number of steps in a **simple skill** and the fact that most of these have an apparent order, the correct sequence for performing the skill can be learned without a conscious effort from the repeated practice. This is not so with a **compound skill.**

Learning and retaining the sequence of steps in a **compound skill** requires another key step. Due to the larger number of steps, practice alone rarely provides the EMT with the ability to reproduce the proper sequence without omission or error. Instead, once the parts of the skill have been practiced and learned a list of the steps must be studied in order to learn and retain their proper sequence. Due to the detail required to introduce the steps in a new skill the pages in which the procedure is presented are too lengthy to study for easy retention of the correct sequence. Instead, a shorter **Summary Skill Sheet** is required. In the Summary Sheets each step is presented as simply a short phrase or "cue" ("Open the Airway"), and each sub skill is unified into one generic step ("Insert a simple airway adjunct").

A Summary Skill Sheet of each complex compound skill is found at the end of each section of the book.

Even though the steps in the Summary Sheets are presented in a short form, they are still longer than the clues that an individual student could write for himself. It is easiest to remember things we have digested and stated in our own words. Therefore, if you have difficulty in retaining the sequence from the **Summary Skill Sheet,** we heartily recommend that you rewrite the list using your own meaningful terms to describe each step. As well as producing your own personalized list which will make learning easier, the process of forming and writing your own clues for each step will aid retention.

A **Compound Branching Skill** requires yet another process. Even when using a short **Summary Skill Sheet** it is difficult to retain all of the steps in each possible branch or choice. When you have been introduced to one of these skills and have practiced it, stop and think about it. Usually each of the branches represents a separate sub-skill. For example: if the patient is breathing, the steps of the skill for providing supplemental oxygen follow; while if the patient is not breathing the steps for providing ventilation and supplemental oxygen with the BVM follow.

Trying to remember all of the possible steps by rote memory does not work well if at all. However, by understanding and adding the conceptual basis for each branch to the skill sheet, and further by collectively labeling the sub-skills represented by the options, you will find it much easier to retain. Remembering if the patient has a pulse to continue the steps of ventilation with periodic pulse checks and if the pulse is absent to follow the CPR skill steps, is much easier than remembering all of the various steps involved as if they were new. Once a compound branching skill is understood, an algorithm can be very useful in retaining the sequence.

COURSE SKILLS PROGRESSION

Skills are taught in a course so that they are introduced in a meaningful progression. Ventilation skills include steps for managing the airway, therefore the airway management skills are taught first. Similarly airway and ventilation skills are each a part of CPR so these are both taught first and then do not need to be repeated in detail when CPR is taught. This focuses the student's attention solely on the additional items being introduced. This also allows the steps in the presentation to be reduced.

COMMON SKILL RELATIONSHIPS

A skill is rarely an isolated single entity with little or no relationship to other skills. Commonly, a skill has a similar purpose and like elements as a large group of skills. For example, all of the airway management skills have some common items and considerations. Within that large group, each skill also fits into a sub-group with even closer similarities. All of the manual airway skills have a closer similarity with each other than does a manual airway skill and an adjunct airway skill. Skills are presented in this guide in Sections corresponding to the large groups surrounding a topic.

The introduction to each Section includes a discussion of the common factors and criteria that represent the general understandings one must have in applying the skills in that Section. By understanding these, the student will readily recognize the similarities and relationships between a group of skills. This in effect diminishes the number of unique items that must be learned.

To retain a skill one must understand it. To understand it, one must understand **why** each step is done, **why** it is done in a particular way, and **why** it is done **when** it is done. It is easy to retain a series of steps that one has digested and understands. Trying to remember steps you don't understand is similar to trying to remember a random meaningless sequence of numbers is a nearly impossible task. In any level of EMT course there are too many skills for successful rote memorization. Skills must truly be learned, not simply memorized.

TOOLS TO HELP YOU LEARN SKILLS

There are many aids to help you learn a skill. Many instructors first introduce a new skill in the classroom using slide or videotape presentations to demonstrate the steps. Using a media presentation ensures that each step is performed exactly and that it can be clearly seen from the same angle by each student. Some institutions make the videotape available, allowing students the opportunity to review the taped demonstration as often as needed. If available, such a review—particularly of a skill that you are having some difficulty with—will be most useful.

Many institutions offer optional additional supervised practice sessions, as well as the required hands-on skill labs. It is a universal finding that students who elect to attend most of these consistently do better on practical exams and have better skills delivery in the field. You should take advantage of such sessions.

This book can be the key aid in helping you learn, review, and retain skills if you use it meaningfully:

- Prior to a skills lab, study the skills to be introduced carefully
- Read the introduction to the Section to learn the general principles
- During the lab add your own special notes as needed to the printed text
- While practicing in a peer group have one student follow along and check the steps in the text. For compound skills, study the sequence in the **Summary Skill Sheet**
- Prior to a practical test, review each of the skills to be included
- If a test sheet is included, study it! Pay special attention to the **Critical Criteria**
- Periodically review skills that have not been used or practiced lately.

The book format allows you random and repeated access to any item you need, whether in class or at home—anywhere and anytime you need it—without the use of a video player or slide projector.

UNDERSTANDING DEMONSTRATION DIRECTIONS

With the variety of positions in which a patient and his limbs may be found, directions such as "up the arm" are subject to different interpretations which can easily lead to confusion and error. In a patient who has an arm raised over his head, "up" can be interpreted to mean either towards the shoulder or towards the wrist.

Using proper medical terminology provides precise, clear, and concise directions. A basic group of these terms have been used in the skills demonstrations within this book and are commonly used by instructors in their classroom demonstrations. The front half of the patient is designated as *anterior,* the back half of the patient is *posterior.* These terms can also be used in an adjective form to describe direction. Moving an arm **posteriorly** means moving it in the direction that the back of the patient faces, while **anteriorly** is in the direction that his front faces. Inserting a device in an **anterior-to-posterior** direction clearly means from front to back and, **posterior-to-anterior** means back to front. References to the **right side** or **left side** (or to the **right hand,** or **left leg** etc.) when unqualified are always references to the *patient's* right and left, not the EMT's.

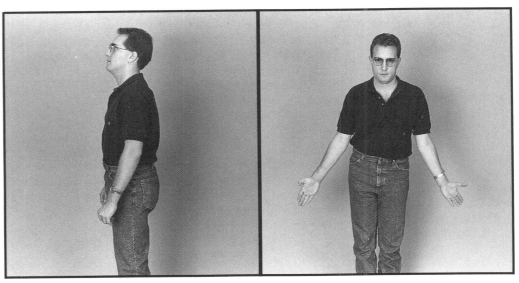

When an instruction is to mean the EMT's right or left instead, it will be qualified such as: "With your left hand" or "the EMT's left hand".

The term **superior** means "up" and **inferior** means "down". Like "up" and "down", they refer to true vertical height and therefore have the potential for confusion because they change as the patient's position is changed. In a standing patient, superiorly would be in a direction towards the patient's head and inferiorly will be in a direction towards his feet *but,* if he is placed in a supine position superiorly would be towards his anterior side and inferiorly towards his posterior side. With the variety of changes in the position of the patient and the variety of movements of his limbs that may be included in a skill, terms that have transient anatomical meaning depending upon his exact position at any one time, can easily be misinterpreted. ***Therefore, within this text the use of superior and inferior are limited to standing patients.***

The terms "cephalad" and "caudad", "medial" and "lateral", "proximal" and "distal", are each based upon specific anatomical references that remain unchanged regardless of the position of the patient or his limbs. Due to their consistent clarity throughout the range of movement of the patient, they are widely used in the skills descriptions in this book. These terms are used to define a direction from a given stated or unstated point of reference. **Cephalad** means towards the head. **Caudad** means towards the tail, however in reference to human anatomy it is universally extended to mean in the direction of the feet. "Move your hand six inches cephalad" means to move your hand from its present position six inches towards the patient's head.

The midline of the body is an imaginary anterior-to-posterior plane dividing the body into mirror-image left and right halves. The terms "medial" and "lateral" refer to this midline. **Medial** means towards the midline and **lateral** means towards the outer side of that half of the body, or away from the midline. Moving your hand **medially** is moving it in the direction towards the patient's midline and moving it **laterally** is moving it in the direction away from the midline.

"Proximal" and "distal" are useful terms in reference to the limbs. **Proximal** means towards, or closer to, the heart. **Distal** means away from, or further from, the heart. This always refers to movement along the normal structure of the body, such as along an arm or leg. "On the leg proximal of the knee" means any point between the knee and the hip, or in the direction from the knee toward the hip. "Distal of the knee" means any point between the knee and the tip of the toes, or in a direction from the knee towards the foot. Additionally the term **"distal circulation"** is used to refer to checking the circulation at a point distant from the heart. Commonly the radial pulse is checked as the **distal pulse** in an arm, and the pedal pulse is checked as the **distal pulse** in a leg.

The terms "abduct" and "adduct" are also useful. To **abduct** a limb is to move it away from the torso or, in the case of a leg, away from the neutral in-line position with the midline lying between the legs. To **adduct** a limb is to move it towards the torso or, in the case of a leg, toward the neutral in-line position.

Some references to the EMT's position relative to the patient are commonly made. Unless a specific reference is made to the EMT's anatomy, the references for location or direction refer to the patient's anatomy. "An EMT kneels at each side of the thorax facing the midline" indicates that one EMT is kneeling on the ground at the *patient's* thorax on the patient's left side and a second EMT does the same at the *patient's* right thorax. Both face each other squarely, perpendicular to the *patient's* midline.

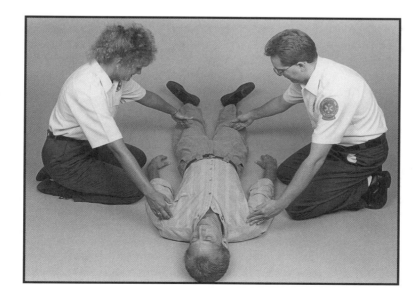

References to the EMT's cephalad arms are to each EMT's arm that is at the *patient's* cephalad direction, and so on. In this way the tedious and unclear concerns over whose right and whose left arm are being referred to are avoided. With a supine patient, reference to "from above the patient's head" means from a position beyond the patient's head facing in a caudad direction rather than being a reference to elevation.

In the section dealing with *Fracture Splinting Skills* and the section on *Spinal Immobilization Skills* the term **neutral in-line position** is used. This should not be confused with the **normal anatomical position** commonly shown in anatomical charts. The **neutral in-line position** is generally supine with the head and neck in natural alignment with the torso (this commonly requires some padding behind the head). The legs are together and in-line so that the midline is exactly between them, and the arms are extended along the torso lying neutrally with the palms in towards the lateral sides of the leg along the thigh. The midline of the head, neck, torso and between the legs are *in-line,* forming a single straight line.

SECTION
Safety Skills
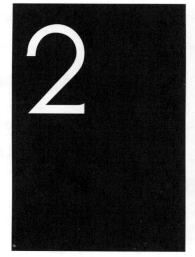

Safe Practices for Infection Control

INTRODUCTION

Until recently the predominant concern among responders in regard to their own safety dealt with physical injury: being involved in a motor vehicle accident during a response; being injured by a violent patient; sustaining injury from fire, hazardous substances or building collapse; or injuring oneself while lifting or carrying a patient. The advent of the Human Immunodeficiency Virus (HIV) and the spread of the Hepatitis B and now C viruses makes it very important that EMS providers consciously and stringently act to protect themselves from these "new" hazards as well. In addition to these diseases, EMTs are also being subjected to resurgences of Meningitis, Influenza, Tuberculosis, Chickenpox, Rubella, Pneumonia, and Measles to degrees that have not been seen in this country for generations.

These are not simply illnesses that come and go—they can affect the EMT to the point where they interfere with his ability to report for duty, they can be spread to members of his household, they can result in long-term if not life-long disability, and they can cause death to the EMT or to those around him. While much attention has been focused on AIDS, it is known that the risk to EMTs is much greater from Hepatitis B (HBV) than from HIV—and the Hepatitis C virus (HCV) is believed to pose an even greater risk to health care workers than HBV.

Federal regulations and laws have been enacted to increase the health care worker's protection from infectious diseases. These are lengthy documents which far exceed the space available in this text, and they continue to be updated at far too rapid a pace for any textbook to follow. Rather, we direct the EMT's attention to some of the basic and fundamental precautionary measures which can and should be taken.

EXPOSURE AND COMMUNICABLE PATHOGENS

The EMT must be constantly alert to anticipate any opportunity of "exposure" to an infectious disease. Exposures primarily occur through direct or indirect contact with contaminated blood or other body fluids. Bloodborne diseases include HIV, HBV, HCV, and syphilis. Airborne diseases are spread by droplets which have been produced by a cough or sneeze. Airborne diseases include Chickenpox, Tuberculosis, Mumps, Rubella, and Meningitis. Disease may also be spread by direct contact with infected non-blood secretions—often known as "other potentially infectious materials" (OPIM). These include any unfixed tissue or organ, semen, vaginal secretions, cerebrospinal fluid, synovial fluid, pleural fluid, pericardial fluid, peritoneal fluid, amniotic fluid, saliva in a dental procedure, and any other body fluid that may be contaminated with blood.

PROTECTION

The EMT's best protection from infectious disease is just that—protection, not attempting or hoping for a cure after incurring the disease. Protection takes two forms: prophylactic immunizations and precautionary practices.

The EMT can be immunized against some of the diseases to which he is vulnerable. Immunizations help to reduce the risk of contracting a disease, but they are not available for every disease. Diseases for which EMTs are commonly vaccinated include HBV, tetanus, diphtheria, measles, mumps, rubella, polio, and influenza. EMTs can be immunized from some diseases by a single dose of vaccine, while others require several doses and/or periodic "boosters". The HBV vaccine, for example, typically requires three injections over a seven month period in order for the necessary immunity to develop. Tetanus and diphtheria "booster shots" are usually recommended every ten years. Federal regulations now require employers to provide HBV immunizations for EMTs at no charge, and many employers have also found that providing other common immunizations at no charge leads to improved employee health records and increased productivity.

UNIVERSAL PRECAUTIONS

Two terms have been adopted to describe precautionary work practices which are designed to protect the EMT from the risk of exposure to blood and other potentially infectious materials: "Universal Precautions" (UP) and "Body Fluid Isolation" (BFI). These practices must become a constant part of the EMT's work life—things that are done on every call, with every patient, regardless of the circumstance or identity of the patient. Some of these practices are simple, very easy to perform, and hopefully have been part of your normal routine already. They include washing your hands with an antiseptic hand cleaner soon after any potential exposure and disposing of all contaminated sharp objects in specially designed and marked containers. Other measures may require additional supplies on the ambulance, detailed preparations for various circumstances, or discontinuing some practices.

After handwashing, the most common form of universal precaution is wearing protective latex gloves—the simplest form of "Personal Protective Equipment" (PPE). Further PPE measures include non-absorbent "barrier" gowns, face masks and eye shields, shoe covers, and various types of patient care equipment which is designed to shield the EMT from the patient's body fluids while permitting treatment or resuscitation to continue. One example of the latter is mouth-to-mask devices equipped with one-way valves which have become standard adjuncts for professionals in circumstances where they would previously have performed mouth-to-mouth resuscitation.

The choice of what PPE to use in a given case is usually best made on the basis of which tasks or procedures are being performed. A patient who is HIV-positive and has suffered a sprained ankle but no open wounds, for example, can properly and safely be cared for with only disposable gloves—there is no need for a gown, face mask and eye shield, shoe covers, etc. (And the gloves are simply a wise precaution with any patient because of the possibility of unnoticed small openings on the patient's or EMT's skin). A routine venipuncture for collecting a blood sample requires only gloves—there is no anticipation of blood or OPIM spraying wildly around the area. By contrast a prehospital childbirth where blood and amniotic fluid are present in significant quantities calls for gloves, mask, eye shield, and barrier gown—regardless of whom the mother may be or her prior health history. We have included a basic PPE task list to illustrate the level of protection that is appropriate in various situations, however the EMT must be familiar with his own agency's protocols and follow them conscientiously.

SHARPS PRACTICES AND DISPOSAL

A key area of concern in preventing the spread of bloodborne diseases is the use and disposal of "sharps"—needles and other sharp objects which can convey blood particles from the patient to the EMT. Previous practices of sticking contaminated IV needles into cot mattresses or squad bench covers must be stopped, along with the practice of two-handed recapping of needles. Infection Control programs call for the total elimination of all needle-stick injuries. New "needle-less" IV systems are being implemented which eliminate the need for all sharp objects beyond the original IV needle catheter which is inserted into the patient's vein.

DECONTAMINATION

A final important part of infection control is the decontamination and "clean up" after a call. Contaminated materials must be properly disposed of in marked containers which meet Federal and local guidelines. The EMS Service may be able to

RECOMMENDED PERSONAL PROTECTION EQUIPMENT ACCORDING TO TASK OR ACTIVITY				
Task/Activity	Gloves	Gown	Mask*	Eyeshield
Bleeding control Spurting Blood	YES	YES	YES	YES
Bleeding Control Minimal Bleeding	YES	OPTION	OPTION	OPTION
Childbirth	YES	YES	YES	YES
Blood Drawing	YES	OPTION	OPTION	OPTION
Starting IV	YES	OPTION	OPTION	OPTION
Giving Injection	YES	OPTION	OPTION	OPTION
Taking Rectal Temperature	YES	OPTION	OPTION	OPTION
Intubation (ET/EOA)	YES	OPTION	YES	YES
Suctioning Oral/Nasal	YES	OPTION	YES	YES
Manual Airway Clearing	YES	OPTION	YES	YES
Handling/Cleaning Soiled Equip/Vehicle	YES	YES	OPTION	OPTION

CONTAGIOUS DISEASES				
Disease	Gloves	Gown	Mask*	Eyeshield
Tuberculosis	OPTION	OPTION	YES	OPTION
Chicken Pox	YES	YES	YES	OPTION
Meningitis	OPTION	OPTION	YES	OPTION
Whooping Cough	OPTION	OPTION	YES	OPTION

* "Mask" means a device covering the mouth and nose and through which fluids cannot be absorbed. The ideal mask is one which includes an approved eye shield as well.

use the disposal facilities of local hospitals, or may have to register itself as a hazardous waste generator and contract with an outside agency to properly dispose of contaminated materials. Preparing the ambulance for the next call also includes disinfecting both the patient compartment and any equipment which came into contact with the patient. Many EMS items are becoming disposable, and are simply discarded after a single use. Again, the EMT must know and follow his agency's regulations and practices in order to provide proper protection for himself, his co-workers, and his patients.

It is important to note that the goal of these newly implemented infection control programs is not to reduce the incidence of exposures or needle sticks—but to **eliminate** them. A sharps control program has an immediate goal of **zero-incidence** needle stick injuries. The term "body fluid isolation" is more dramatic and emphatic than "universal precautions", and it means exactly what it says—to isolate and protect the EMT from the patient's body fluids. An EMT who does not adopt and employ these measures fully can look forward to a short career in EMS—either by becoming ill or injured through poor work practices or as a result of disciplinary measures established to force compliance.

Other Safety Skills

INTRODUCTION

The EMT must be prepared for a variety of dangers that are commonly a part of the provision of emergency medical services in the field. These must be met with alertness, awareness, and training in special safety skills which may be required to keep the EMT and the patient safe. Other than mentioning the most common problems, it is outside the scope of this text and of EMT training courses (Basic, Advanced, or Paramedic) to address the specific training needed for each of the particular hazards.

ATTITUDE

Many EMTs perceive that their humanitarian or official role as care givers provides them with a mystical mantle of protection which will save them from harm. The word "accident" in itself is unfortunate—implying some irrevocable act of Fate outside human control. Most EMS injuries can be avoided with increased awareness and a more cautious attitude. The EMT's mind-set often is a key contributor to placing him in an environment or situation which invites or allows harm to occur.

SAFETY PRE-SET

Although some rapid decisions may have to be made in the face of danger, the EMT's pre-set safety attitude and his **safety skills** are the most important items in consistently minimizing risk. Three axioms form the philosophical basis which must underlie his actions:

- The initial, paramount, and primary concern must be the EMT's safety.
- Although others have some responsibility, the EMT must assume the primary responsibility for his own safety
- The EMT will **not** take uncontrolled risks regardless of the consequences of that decision.

The EMT must understand the limitations of his role. It is a potentially dangerous oversimplification to just say that it is to "save lives". Although the goal is certainly to save lives, it must also include the understanding that some patients will die regardless of the care provided, and that his role does not obligate the EMT to take **undue** risks.

Taking contained, **controlled risks** for which one is properly trained, properly equipped, and for which one has the necessary resources at the scene, is a part of EMS. Taking dangerous **uncontrolled risks,** or attempting maneuvers or actions for which one has not been properly trained or equipped, is neither "heroic" nor a part of the EMT's obligation, duty-to-act, or role. *The EMT who has not come to these understandings is a danger to himself and his fellow responders.*

As with other skills, Safety has a series of key steps that should be performed in a given sequence.

GENERAL SAFETY SKILLS

1. Regardless of the nature of the call, proceed to the scene in a safe manner consistent with the area, traffic, and weather, and using life belts and restraint devices.
2. Take appropriate Universal Precautions and don appropriate PPE before exiting the ambulance.
3. Assume the scene is dangerous: identify all possible dangers (environmental, man-made, interpersonal).
4. Rule-out those dangers which are not present.
5. Mitigate or control (reduce) dangers that are present, as possible. Proceed **only** when the scene is acceptably safe.
6. At no time enter a scene or situation where safe operation requires training or equipment or other resources beyond what is available to you.
7. If an unacceptable risk remains, withdraw to a safe location and arrange for the necessary resources to render the scene safe. Only proceed once the scene is acceptably safe.
8. Once the scene is safe, identify a safety officer to monitor scene safety and provide an alert if circumstances change.
9. Proceed to the patient and provide care with reasonable speed. Excessive haste ultimately causes delay and increases the chances of injury.
10. Use proper techniques to lift and move the patient to safeguard yourself and the patient.
11. Regardless of urgency, transport the patient in a prudent manner, always using proper strapping and immobilization techniques and seat belts.
12. Safely and properly dispose of "sharps", contaminated wastes and linens, and maintain Universal Precautions while cleaning the patient compartment and reusable equipment.

DRIVING SKILLS

Driving an ambulance requires hands-on instruction and practice in an actual ambulance, plus an understanding of safe emergency vehicle operation in a variety of traffic situations. A driver's license and experience in normal motor vehicle operation are not sufficient prerequisites for driving an ambulance, much less operating it under emergency conditions. Safe operation of an ambulance requires completion of a special course of instruction and in many areas requires additional licensure or certification. Assuming that you are entitled to the right-of-way, and that other drivers will yield it to you, will eventually result in a collision.

MVA SCENE SAFETY

The scene of a motor vehicle collision (MVA), whether on local roads or a highway, always contains a high risk of a dangerous secondary crash. Most EMTs are not aware that accidents caused by a second vehicle colliding with the wreckage—or into the ambulance which is parked at the scene with EMTs and patients inside—is one of the major causes of serious injury and death to EMTs. **Flares or a raised hand do NOT stop oncoming vehicles. Barriers do.** Accordingly, a fire truck or other large vehicle should be placed between the oncoming traffic and wherever the EMTs are working. Care must be taken to place the barrier far enough back so that it cannot be pushed into the scene, but not so far back that it fails to prevent vehicles from just driving around it. In addition to the emergency vehicles' flashing lights at the scene, a clearly visible pattern of lighted or reflective warning devices should be placed in both directions from the scene to alert approaching drivers of the danger ahead.

In all MVAs the vehicle electrical and fuel systems present a fire danger. Danger has not been controlled at an MVA scene unless and until a fire engine is present and precautions have been taken against a possible ignition.

FIRE AND STRUCTURAL COLLAPSE SCENE SAFETY

Fire is always unstable and dangerous. Only EMTs who are properly trained in fire fighting should enter the fire scene or be involved in the fire search and rescue mission. Constant practice in the use of self contained breathing apparatus (SCBA), fireground safety, and fire suppression tactics, is required to remain sufficiently proficient to function in such an environment with relative safety. As the firefighters remove the patient(s) from the fire area they should be taken to an EMS staging area for assessment and care. Such an area should be clearly identified and should be established far enough from the actual scene that neither the EMTs nor the patients are subject to flame, heat, smoke, falling debris, structural collapse, or the effects of explosion. An appropriate response should include enough EMS units to provide continuous coverage at the scene for the firefighters and any additional patients as well as for transporting the initial victims. Although traumatic injuries and burns are expected in such circumstances, care must also include attention to the more subtle signs of carbon monoxide (CO) poisoning or other noxious fume inhalation even in the apparently uninjured.

Once a building's structural integrity has been altered, its remaining strength is unpredictable. Therefore, any structure which has suffered significant damage from fire, or any building that has had some structural collapse from any cause, must be considered to be structurally unsafe.

HAZARDOUS MATERIALS SCENE SAFETY

Two items are key to safety at a hazardous materials scene:

1. early recognition, before responders enter the area and become exposed, and

2. proper training, equipment, and procedures for managing the situation once it has been identified.

HAZMAT situations present a danger from toxic substances and/or from the chances of fire and explosion. Treating patients within the contaminated area or immediate scene area unnecessarily increases the danger to them and the EMTs. Instead, the injured should rapidly be removed to a staging area where EMS personnel can assess and treat them in safety. Some patients will need to be decontaminated before being brought to the treatment area. The treatment area should be established in a protected and safe location distant enough from the incident so that if the situation escalates, patients and EMTs will remain safe until they can evacuate to a further location. The treatment area should always be beyond the possible explosion "perimeter" or "drift" or "runoff path" of the substances involved.

SAFETY AT SCENE OF VIOLENCE

Any scene where a patient has been shot, stabbed, or assaulted with any weapon or object is extremely dangerous and should not be entered by the EMT until it is contained (unless the EMT is a trained member of a responding tactical squad). Prior to rushing in to treat the victim, the EMT must assure himself that the police have secured the scene. "Securing the scene" means that the police have the weapon(s) in their possession or that they have assured themselves that any armed perpetrator has fled the scene and is not hidden and still within range.

In cases where violence and assault have occurred without a weapon, it is sometimes assumed that the responders can "handle" anyone. This is an attitude that often results in injury to the EMT. One must always remember that martial arts training or weapons are great equalizers. Regardless of the person's size or apparent strength, anyone trained in hand-to-hand combat or who is armed with a weapon can cause serious injury or kill you. Containing a violent or potentially violent person is a police function. The police have the training, equipment and resources to do combat—the EMT does not.

When a violent or armed person is involved the EMTs should remain in a safe place until the violent person is disarmed and contained. If a patient is violent, he needs to be contained and have his limbs restricted (as with handcuffs) before treatment can safely be begun.

DEALING WITH THE MENTAL PATIENT SAFELY

Even a mental patient's psychiatrist has difficulty in predicting his patient's behavior. The EMT must remember that rational thought rarely predicts the behavior of irrational people. Rapidly assessing the patient's psychological profile in the field simply cannot be done with any reliability. The EMT must always assume that the mental patient—regardless of his calm presentation—is irrational. Irrational behavior, and what can trigger a violent episode, is unpredictable. Therefore, all mental patients are unpredictable and have the potential to suddenly become dangerously violent. Further, they may be stronger than they appear or may be armed.

The safe EMT approach includes police containment and a weapons search of the mental patient whether he appears unruly or not.

CONCLUSION: THE "ABC'S" OF SCENE SAFETY

Always assume that a scene or situation is dangerous.

Be prepared—identify or rule-out, or get out!

Contain, limit, or eliminate each potential danger.

Defensive driving and defensive safety should be practiced at all times.

EMT safety is the paramount priority at all times.

SECTION
**Patient
Assessment
Skills**

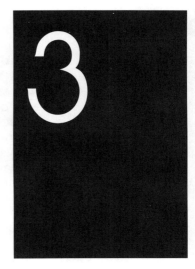

Patient Assessment Skills

INTRODUCTION

The EMT's *Patient Assessment* is the key to the quality of care provided. One will not treat what one does not properly identify as a problem. Patient Assessment, with its:

- various examining sub-skills
- required sequence based upon urgent priorities
- many steps
- large number of possible items to be found
- need to positively rule-out items NOT found

is the most complex of all of the EMT skills at each level of pre-hospital care.

HOW TO USE THE PARTS OF THIS SECTION

If the required subskills were presented within the sequence of the overall assessment it would be difficult to focus on the flow of the overall progression. Therefore each subskill is introduced separately prior to the presentation of the entire sequence of steps. In this way the overall sequence can be presented without interruption, and each subskill appears as a single step in context within the overall assessment.

Once the reader has studied and practiced the overall assessment sequence with the aid of the photos and text, the longer Teaching Skills Sheet will be useful in retaining the sequence of the many steps and the questions to be answered by each. Finally, once the EMT is proficient in performing the assessment, the shorter Summary Skills Sheet will be useful in retaining the correct order of the key parts.

VITAL SIGNS

Classically the *vital signs* are considered to be: Level of Consciousness (LOC), Pulse (P), Blood Pressure (BP), Respiration (R), Skin (as a measure of peripheral perfusion), and Temperature (T). In the pre-hospital arena Temperature is generally only estimated as "hot", "normal", or "cool", and is quantified by use of a thermometer only for specific conditions rather than in all patients. The pulse rate, BP, and respiratory rate are numerical measures of vital function and as such are quantifiable without subjective interpretation that can vary from one EMT to another. Therefore they are a useful and relatively stable comparative index of the patient's condition even when taken by different care givers and when compared with either normal ranges or previously obtained results. This is not to imply that they are more important than LOC or skin or the other unquantifiable measures surrounding circulatory and respiratory status. Any single vital sign may be misleading and if taken alone may be an inaccurate measure of the patient's condition. The vital signs need to be assessed as a group, with each considered in the context of the others in order to be reliable and truly informative. Relying on one without the others is a poor diagnostic practice.

OTHER DIAGNOSTIC SIGNS

In addition to the vital signs, there are other diagnostic signs—and the skills associated with them—that are a key part of the pre-hospital patient examination and assessment. Those that require special introductory understandings or represent a sub-skill containing several steps are presented in detail with the vital signs—preceding the presentation of the overall patient assessment process. Some diagnostic signs do not have identifiable skill steps, being more conceptual than itemized, and are not aided by the use of photographs. These are presented in differing formats for greater clarity.

PART A:

Individual Skills In Obtaining Vital Signs And Other Key Diagnostic Signs

PALPATING A PULSE

A pulse can be palpated at any place where an artery is near the surface of the skin and where the artery can be pushed against a firm surface—either a bone or a well-developed muscle. The surge of blood produced by each ventricular contraction is felt under the EMT's fingers. The pulse reflects the frequency (number) and regularity of heartbeats per minute, and by its presence and strength indicates the quality of circulation at the palpated location. In conscious adults and children the *radial artery* is the most common location palpated. The pulse is evaluated for:

Presence—The presence of a palpable radial pulse indicates that the patient has a functional heartbeat. It also signals that the patient's systolic blood pressure is usually 80 mmHg or greater, although this is not reliable in all cases. The absence of a palpable radial pulse in an unresponsive patient may indicate cardiac arrest. The carotid pulse (brachial pulse in infants) should be immediately checked in such cases. Only by checking other pulses can one determine whether the absence of a peripheral pulse reflects a localized or systemic condition.

Rate—The rate is counted using a watch or clock. The number of heartbeats in 15 seconds is multiplied by 4 to obtain the pulse rate per minute. It is more accurate and may be easier to count the beats for 30 seconds and multiply by 2, therefore this is a recommended option. The pulse rate, stated simply as a number, describes the number of beats per minute at rest. The average adult pulse at rest is about 72. The normal range (*normocardia*) is from 60 to 100, and the patient with such a reading is said to be *normocardic*. *Tachycardia* is an abnormal accelerated rate greater than 100. *Bradycardia* is an abnormally slow rate that is less than 60. The normal rate in children is 60 to 110; in infants from 80 to 160.

Regularity—The normal pulse is *regular,* meaning that the beats occur at a consistent interval. When a pulse is *irregular* it indicates that the heart is beating with varying intervals between beats, or that some beats are being "dropped" due to electrocardial conduction problems and do not result in blood being ejected by the ventricles. Either situation represents a potentially dangerous condition.

Quality—The quality of a pulse refers to its strength when palpated. The pulse can be reported as "strong" or "full", or as "weak" or "thready".

When recording the pulse it is written as "P–76, strong and regular", and the time is also logged. It is **not** necessary to write "per minute" as this is assumed, however the quality and regularity should be included with the rate.

1. To locate the **radial pulse** place the tips of your 1st and 2nd fingers flatly on the palm side of the patient's wrist so that they cover the area from the midline laterally toward the patient's thumb, as shown. Apply mild pressure to palpate the pulse. If necessary move the fingertips slightly until the pulse is felt the strongest. Your thumb should not be used to palpate, as your pulse can be mistaken for the patient's. Determine if the pulse is present (palpable), strong or weak, and regular or irregular.

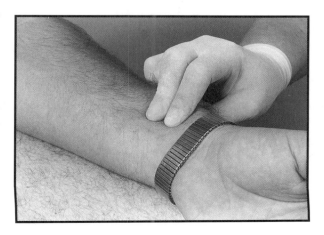

2. To count the pulse rate, look at your watch. Wait until the second hand is at either the 12, 3, 6, or 9 o'clock position and then count the number of heartbeats felt in 15 seconds. Multiply the number of beats in 15 seconds by 4 to obtain the rate per minute. Finally, record the rate, strength, regularity and the time the pulse was taken.

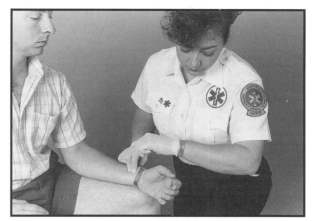

3. In unresponsive adults and children, palpating the **carotid pulse** is considered the most reliable for determining pulselessness since it is easy to locate and may persist when more distal peripheral pulses are no longer palpable. Position yourself next to the patient's neck and locate the larynx with the tips of your first two or three fingers. Then slide the fingers towards you into the groove between the trachea and the large muscles of the neck. You may have to move your fingertips slightly to locate the exact pulse. Palpate gently to avoid occluding the artery or inadvertently producing bradycardia by stimulating the vagus nerve.

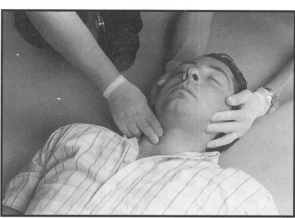

4. The **femoral pulse** may also be used to determine pulselessness, however it can be difficult to locate through clothing or in obese patients. Visualize the crease formed between the leg and the abdomen. Place the tips of your first two or three fingers just proximal to the midpoint of this crease, pointing toward the navel. Gently push posteriorly, moving your fingers ½ to 1 inch towards the navel, slightly indenting the soft anterior abdomen as shown. If the femoral pulse is not found retract your hand and repeat the procedure, advancing the fingertips slightly more to the left or right of the midpoint.

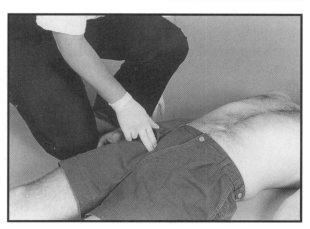

5. In infants, palpation of the **brachial pulse** is recommended since the short, chubby neck makes it difficult to locate the carotid artery. Abduct and rotate the infant's arm as shown so that it is palm-up. Place the tips of your first two or three fingers on the ulnar side of the infant's arm between the elbow and shoulder and press gently. You may have to slightly relocate your fingertips until the strongest point for palpation is found. The apical pulse should never be palpated to determine pulselessness since precordial impulses may be neither visible nor palpable in infants who do have a heartbeat.

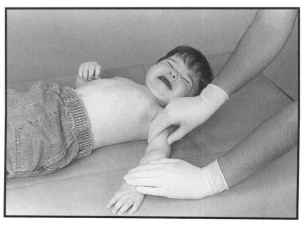

TAKING THE BLOOD PRESSURE—INTRODUCTION

Blood pressure is measured in millimeters of mercury (mm Hg). The **systolic pressure** reflects the higher pressure that occurs during the contractions of the ventricles of the heart. The **diastolic pressure** is the residual pressure that remains while the heart relaxes. The BP is reported as the systolic pressure *over* the diastolic pressure and is written as a fraction. For example, a normal BP of 120 systolic and 78 diastolic is reported as "BP is 120 over 78" and is written as "BP $^{120}/_{78}$". The normal ranges are:

Adult males—Systolic between 90 and 140 mm Hg with a diastolic between 60 and 90 mm Hg.

Adult females—Systolic between 80 and 140 mm Hg with a diastolic between 60 and 90 mm Hg.

Children—Systolic between 70 and 140 mm Hg with a diastolic between 50 and 90 mm Hg. The *expected* systolic pressure for a child can be approximated as: Systolic BP = 80 + (2 × the child's age in years).

Infants—Systolic between 70 and 110 mm Hg with a diastolic between 50 and 70 mm Hg.

Although no single sign is in itself a definitive indicator, it is generally accepted that—with associated signs and symptoms—a systolic pressure of or below 90 in males, 80 in females, and 70 in children must be assumed to indicate **hypotension.** A systolic pressure of or greater than 150 or a diastolic pressure of or greater than 90 in adults must be considered to indicate **hypertension.**

Blood pressure is taken using a sphygmomanometer. Three types of sphygmomanometer are commonly found. The mercuric type has a column of mercury and a long vertical gauge. It is not recommended for the pre-hospital setting since it must be used in a stable position, is cumbersome, and is unreliable if jarred or shaken. Various electronic models are available providing a digital read-out of the BP (and usually also the pulse rate). The aneroid sphygmomanometer is the type most commonly used in EMS. It has a round light-weight durable gauge which can be used accurately in any position.

This type has a cuff containing an inflatable bladder and velcro for securing it to the patient's arm; a circular gauge connected to the bladder by a rubber tube which can be clipped to a strap-holder on the outside of the cuff or be held separately for ease of reading in various positions; and a rubber bulb connected to the bladder by a second rubber tube and containing a one-way stop valve. When the valve is turned to the "closed" position and the bulb is squeezed, air can be pumped into the cuff's bladder but it cannot exit. When the valve is opened, air can exit the bladder deflating the cuff. The valve allows for fine adjustment, letting the EMT determine the speed of deflation with extreme control. The circular aneroid gauge usually has a large darker line marking each 10 mm Hg space with four lighter lines dividing each intervening space into five equal parts each with a 2 mm Hg value.

As well as the normal adult sized cuff, three additional sizes should also be available: a larger cuff for adults with large upper arms; a smaller cuff for adults with small upper arms and children; and an infant cuff. Use of an improperly fitting cuff will result in inaccurate readings.

The blood pressure *should be* taken with the arm positioned at the level of the heart. In the pre-hospital setting this is not always possible. The EMT should be aware that changes in the patient's position, the height of the arm relative to the heart, which arm is used (it is generally higher in the dominant arm), different ambient noise levels, and differences in hearing ability from one EMT to another, can result in as much as a ± 10 mg Hg difference in the perceived BP readings. When taking multiple BP readings these variables should be controlled as much as possible and must be considered in the context of other signs and symptoms in determining their meaning.

TAKING THE BLOOD PRESSURE BY AUSCULTATION

The most common method for taking the blood pressure is by auscultating the brachial artery with a stethoscope while using the sphygmomanometer. The auscultation method is dependent upon hearing and should only be used in places with low ambient noise levels. Although possible, it is extremely difficult to obtain an accurate BP by auscultation in the back of a moving ambulance. In places with high noise levels the palpation method or use of a suitable electronic sphygmomanometer should be selected.

1. Bare the arm to be used and hold the arm with the palm up so that the antecubital fossa faces you. Place the cuff on the upper arm with its lower edge 2 to 3 cm above, and the arrow (denoting the bladder's center) pointing to, the antecubital fossa. Then fasten the velcro so that the cuff is applied snugly. If the cuff's circumference is too great or too small to fasten snugly with the velcro properly attached—exchange the cuff for one of the proper size.

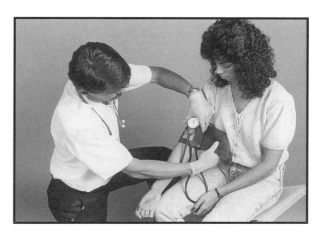

2. With your stethoscope at hand, place the tips of your fingers in the antecubital fossa and move them laterally from the midline until you locate a point where the brachial artery can be clearly palpated under your finger tips. This may be just distal to or under the distal edge of the cuff.

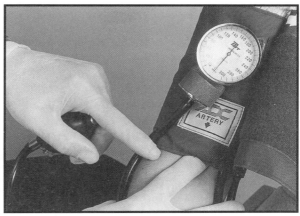

3. Without removing your finger tips, place the stethoscope head (with the diaphragm towards the patient's arm) next to your finger tips. Then, slide it over the pulse location so the diaphragm now replaces the position of your fingertips. Continue holding the diaphragm firmly in place so that it can not move until you are finished taking the BP. Next, place the stethoscope in your ears. Note that at this time no sound should be heard. Be sure you are in a position to see the gauge clearly.

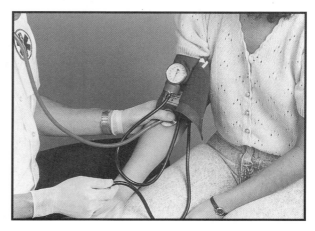

4. While holding the rubber bulb in your available hand, close the one-way valve (usually by turning it clockwise until tight). Now inflate the cuff by repeatedly squeezing and releasing the rubber bulb until the gauge is at 200 mm Hg.

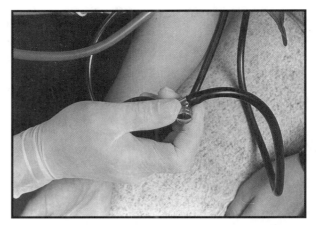

5. Loosen the valve a small amount until the air is slightly passing out of the cuff and the gauge reading is *slowly* lowering at a controlled pace. Letting the air out too fast will result in a missed or inaccurate low reading. If the air is released too slowly, it is unpleasant for the patient and may also result in an artificially high reading. Facility in proper adjustment of the air release comes with practice.

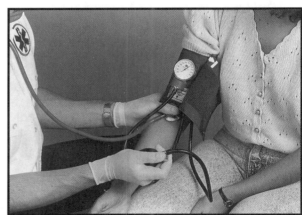

6. At a given point as the gauge's reading lowers the needle commonly starts oscillating (bouncing) with each heart beat. This point is **not** a true indication of the BP. Sometimes the needle will stall at this point, requiring that the valve be opened slightly more to continue the gauge's proper descent. Shortly after this the pulse beat becomes audible through the stethoscope as a faint "tapping" sound which increases in intensity as the cuff deflation is continued. Pre-hospital the point at which the sound of the pulse (tapping) was first heard should be noted as the **systolic pressure.**

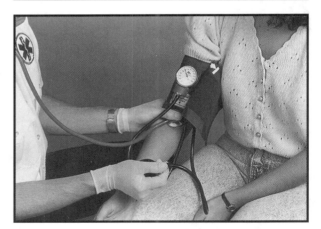

7. Continue the controlled deflation of the cuff while carefully observing the gauge. The pulse sounds may vary in character: become muffled, louder, or even "gap" or continue unchanged. Any finer distinction of these sounds is irrelevant pre-hospital. As the gauge readings continue to lower the pulse sounds will disappear. The gauge reading when the sounds disappear should be noted as the **diastolic pressure.** In some cases of marked hypotension the sounds will continue without disappearing and the diastolic pressure should be recorded as "0".

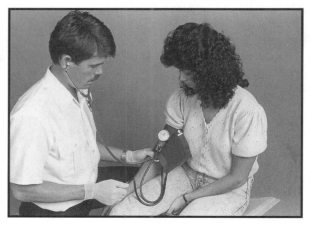

TAKING THE BLOOD PRESSURE BY PALPATION

The palpation method does not include use of a stethoscope or any audible component—making it ideal for use in places with high noise levels. It is the method commonly used in the back of the ambulance if the BP can not be auscultated. By palpation the EMT can only obtain the systolic blood pressure, without any measurement of the diastolic pressure. When using this method the blood pressure is reported as the systolic pressure obtained followed by the words "by palpation". For example, "BP 120 by palpation".

1. Apply the correctly sized cuff to the patient's upper arm in the same manner as previously described for the auscultation method. Hold the rubber bulb in one hand and shut the turn-valve. With your other hand locate the patient's radial pulse in the same arm to which the cuff has been applied. While you continue to palpate this pulse, inflate the cuff until the gauge is at 200 mm Hg. This will occlude the artery causing the radial pulse to disappear and be no longer palpable. *DO NOT move your finger tips from the location at which the pulse was located earlier.*

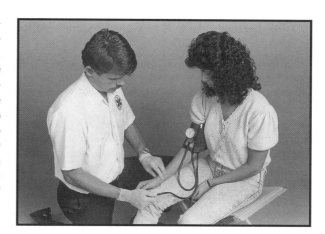

2. Position yourself so that you can clearly read the gauge. Then open the valve slightly allowing air to exit the cuff and the gauge needle to lower at a controlled rate. At a given point in the needle's descent the radial pulse will reappear, again being palpable under the fingertips. Note the gauge reading at which the palpable pulse reappeared, indicating the patient's **systolic pressure** followed by the words "by palpation".

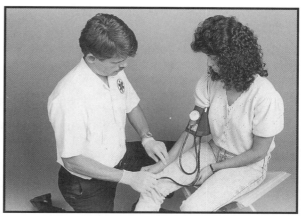

SOME ADDITIONAL TIPS IN THE USE OF THE BP CUFF

- If a reading is missed, do not re-inflate the partially deflated cuff as this will make the ensuing findings inaccurate. Instead, open the valve, fully deflate the cuff, wait a minute or so, and then repeat the process from the beginning.
- If you will be periodically rechecking the patient's BP the cuff can be left on his arm. Care must be taken to fully deflate the cuff by squeezing the remaining air out of it with the valve open to avoid the possibility that it will act as a venous constrictor and impair the distal circulation.

INTRODUCTION TO RESPIRATORY EVALUATION

Determining the patient's respiratory quality involves several elements:

Rate—the number of breaths per minute is counted using a watch or clock with a second hand. It is counted for 15 seconds and multiplied by 4 or 30 seconds and multiplied by 2, to obtain the number of breaths per minute. It is most easily done by counting each peak chest rise. Although these can be observed, it is easier to feel the chest rise under the EMT's hand. The average adult respiratory rate (at rest) is between 16–18 breaths per minute. The normal range in adults is between 12 and 20 breaths per minute. Anyone breathing less than 12 or more than 20 should be suspected of having inadequate minute volume and may require assisted ventilation. Any adult with a rate less than 10 or greater than 30 has an inadequate volume and needs to have assisted or provided ventilations. Children have a faster normal rate than adults. The normal range for children under 13 is between 20 and 30 breaths per minute and for newborns between 30 and 50 breaths per minute. An accelerated rate above the normal range for an age group is called **tachypnea,** a slow rate below the normal range is called **bradypnea,** and a lack of spontaneous ventilation is called **apnea** (such patients are *apneic*).

Depth—The depth of a breath is also a key measure of air exchange. Shallow breaths with limited chest excursion produce less air exchange than deep breaths. Pre-hospital the amount of air exchanged per breath, the **tidal volume,** can not be quantified with a measurement, but can only be estimated as a factor of normalcy. For example, the depth can be described as "normal", "shallow", or "deep" as a subjective judgement from experience. The depth can be seen or felt as the amount of chest rise **(chest excursion)** with each breath. As well as the degree of excursion, the EMT needs to evaluate its symmetry. Normally, chest excursion is equal on both sides. Both chest excursion and breath sounds need to be compared from one side to the other. A lack of bilateral symmetry indicates reduced exchange on one side. Although chest excursion generally indicates the breathing depth it may not in all cases indicate air exchange in the lungs. Therefore, the actual air movement at the nose and mouth should be felt or auscultated to confirm the actual volume exchanged. Both the rate and the amount exchanged per breath (indicated by the depth) are key factors in evaluating the air exchange per minute **(Minute Volume),** which is the actual measure of ventilation.

Effort—Normally breathing is a painless, effortless, noiseless process which does not involve conscious thought or special posture or positioning. Difficult breathing is called **dyspnea.** Dyspnea is witnessed by breathing becoming a conscious, painful, or exaggerated effort. As breathing becomes more labored the patient may require a special posture to breathe and his chest excursion and facial expression will mirror the effort required. In extreme cases the use of collateral muscles of the face and neck can be seen. As well as the rate and depth, patients with difficulty breathing should be reported as having "dyspnea" or "marked dyspnea" and if ventilations require significant effort they should be described as "labored".

Speech—In conscious patients the ability to speak is a readily evident measure of breathing effort and oxygenation. Normally, one can speak fluently without the need for noticeable pauses to breathe. Patients who can only speak *with* noticeable pauses after each sentence have dyspnea. With marked dyspnea patients can only speak 2 or 3 words at a time before they need to "catch their breath". The patient's ability to think, **mentation,** can also be evaluated from his verbal responses.

Level of Consciousness—Patients who are oriented and respond appropriately to questions do not have severe cerebral hypoxia. Disorientation and progressive lowering levels of consciousness occur when inadequate ventilation results in cerebral hypoxia. Increased hypoxia ultimately progresses to unresponsiveness. If a patient is oriented, speaks normally, and is fully conscious, we can conclude that ventilation and oxygenation are adequate at the moment. In patients with lowered levels of consciousness, unconsciousness, or coma, inadequate ventilation and oxygenation should be suspected and carefully evaluated even though the cause may be from a variety of other conditions.

Observation and palpation of the chest—Observing the depth and symmetry of chest excursion; observing the thorax for wounds, sucking chest wounds, bruises indicating possible underlying pulmonary injury, splinting or guarding indicating fractures or other injury to the rib cage or sternum; and checking for paradoxical movement are all important parts of evaluating breathing. Any such injuries or conditions may cause present or ensuing respiratory problems.

Sounds—Normal respiration is a noiseless process to the ear. Bubbling, gurgling, snoring or stridorous sounds heard near the mouth or nose by ear are indicative of an airway problem requiring immediate attention. Although some gross abnormal breathing sounds may be heard by ear, most can only be heard by auscultating the chest with the stethoscope.

Auscultation—Proper auscultation of the lungs with the stethoscope indicates if adequate pulmonary air exchange exists and identifies whether bilateral breath sounds are present or if sounds are diminished or absent on one side (indicating that a pneumothorax, hemothorax or one of many diseases such as pneumonia is present, or that a lung has previously been removed). Auscultation of the lungs also identifies if pathological sounds (called **adventitious** sounds) are present. The presence of such sounds—wheezes, rhonchi, or rales—indicates a pulmonary problem and the EMT must assume that respiration is lessened and a serious problem may exist.

Cyanosis—In patients with adequate circulation, hypoxia commonly results in changes in the color of the red cells which produces a bluish appearing color to the blood vessels which are seen through the skin and mucous membranes. This bluish coloring can most easily be seen in the mucosa (under the tongue) and at the finger nail beds, but may also be seen as a general change in skin color. The presence of cyanosis is a definite indicator of hypoxia; however, the absence of cyanosis does not mean that hypoxia is not present.

SUMMARY—EVALUATING RESPIRATION

The most immediate considerations are: does the patient have a patent airway and spontaneous respirations; does the air exchange appear adequate or inadequate; and is respiration normal or does the patient have dyspnea? Only later in the assessment sequence is it further qualified by obtaining an exact respiratory rate and by observation, palpation, and auscultation of the chest. The part of the evaluation which is considered included in the Vital Signs is the rate, depth if abnormal, and whether it is labored or not. In recording respiration one writes the rate, depth if abnormal, and if effort is abnormal. For example, "R-16, shallow and labored". The absence of any comment regarding depth or labor after the rate indicates that each is normal. If either is abnormal, such comment must not be left out.

EVALUATING RESPIRATORY VITAL SIGNS

Classically the evaluation of respiration includes as part of the *vital signs* the rate, depth, and effort. On initial contact with the patient the assessment of actual air exchange must be included as a priority item to assure that there is a patent airway and that adequate spontaneous respiration is present.

1. In a conscious patient the most rapid method of ascertaining airway patency, air exchange, and the level of oxygenation is from the patient's appearance and verbal response. At a glance the EMT can evaluate if the patient has or has not positioned himself to ease breathing and if breathing requires a significant conscious effort. The fluidity of speech will indicate if the patient has dyspnea and how marked it is. From the verbal response the EMT can also determine the patient's gross LOC and mentation. An oriented patient who responds appropriately does not have any marked cerebral hypoxia, and therefore, may be assumed to have adequate air exchange at present.

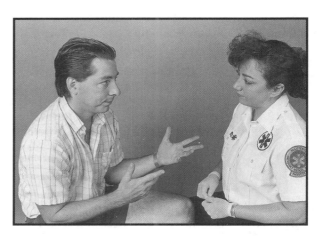

2. In an unconscious patient the EMT must assume that the patient can not properly maintain his airway and does not have adequate air exchange until proven otherwise. After opening the airway with a manual maneuver the EMT should *look, listen,* and *feel* for air exchange and chest excursion. From aside the patient's head, turn your head so you are facing in a caudad direction and bend down until your ear is an inch or two from the patient's mouth and nose. The patient's exhaled air should be plainly felt at the EMT's cheek and ear, and the rhythmic chest rise should be visible with each breath.

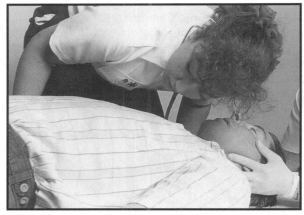

3. At the side of the highway or in other situations where gusty wind conditions are present it may be difficult to reliably discern the patient's regular exhalations by feeling them with your ear. In such cases, auscultation over the trachea with the head of the stethoscope placed at the suprasternal notch, as shown, will provide clearly audible air movement sounds upon inspiration and expiration in breathing patients. The suprasternal notch is selected because it is easily accessed for auscultation without the time needed to bare the chest, and because air movement sounds are easily heard over the trachea.

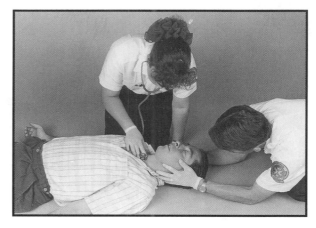

4. In some situations due to lighting, clothing, or individual anatomy, chest excursion can be difficult to see. When chest rise can not readily be visualized the EMT should confirm its presence by feeling the chest excursion. Both depth and symmetry can be readily palpated even through most clothing by resting the hands on the rib cage at the lateral edges of the anterior mid thorax as shown.

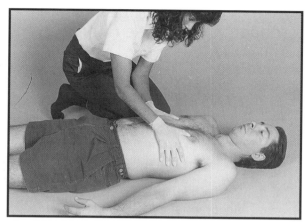

5. The respiratory rate is most easily obtained by counting the breath at the peak of the inspiratory chest rise. This is commonly done by positioning your arm so that the chest rise can be seen directly beyond your watch face. Due to the relative slowness of the average breathing rate it is easy to obtain an inaccurate rate by only counting for 15 seconds. Therefore, it is recommended that the number of peak inspirations be counted for 30 seconds and multiplied by two in order to obtain a reliable per minute rate.

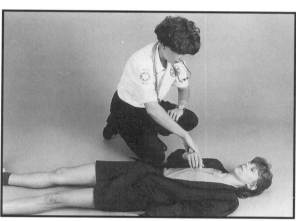

6. Normally breathing is an automatic event which occurs without cognitive thought. When one's attention is directed to it, however, a cerebral override often will alter its depth and rate. Therefore, in alert patients the respiratory rate should by taken without focusing the patient's attention on his breathing. The EMT can achieve this easily be seeming to continue evaluating the pulse. Once you have finished taking the radial pulse, without making reference to respiration, move the arm slightly to where the chest rise can be clearly seen or felt and count it.

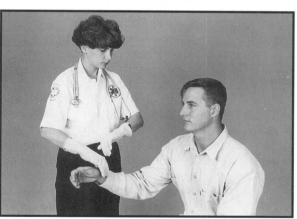

7. In unconscious patients, once other priorities have been met, the respiratory rate can easily be counted by looking at your watch and feeling the chest rise under your other hand. In patients who are being artificially ventilated the record of respiratory rate while being ventilated must be recorded, to include a note of the provided artificial ventilation. For example "R-20 by BVM" (Bag-Valve-Mask). Periodically ventilations should be stopped *for no longer than 30 seconds* to ascertain if spontaneous respiration has returned and its rate.

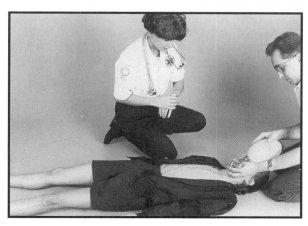

EVALUATING THE LEVEL OF CONSCIOUSNESS (LOC)—
INTRODUCTION TO THE ENLARGED AVPU

Pre-hospital, the patient's level of consciousness (LOC) is evaluated early in the assessment process using the AVPU scale. The EMT reports the *best response* the patient can make and qualifies it with a pertinent description of the quality of the response at that level. AVPU is an acronym representing:

A— *Alert and awake.* Patient spontaneously opens his eyes, speaks and moves spontaneously and is oriented to events around him. In alert and awake patients the EMT needs to evaluate the patient's orientation as well.

V— *Responds to verbal stimulus.* Patient responds when spoken to or to other auditory stimulus. His best response should be noted as should whether the response is appropriate or inappropriate. If inappropriate, describe.

P— *Responds only to painful stimulus.* The patient does *not* respond to verbal stimulus—only to pain. One should note how he responds to pain "withdraws", "moans", etc.), describing the best response elicited.

U— *Unresponsive to any stimulus.* Even with painful stimulus the patient remains flaccid and without movement, uttered sound, or other response.

Upon starting the exam it will be immediately evident whether the patient is conscious or unconscious. Once airway patency, adequacy of ventilation, and a lack of significant external bleeding have been confirmed and any other priority interventions for these have been provided, the EMT will need to further evaluate how conscious or how deeply unconscious the patient is.

In conscious patients, one further evaluates the level of consciousness by the patient's alertness and mentation, spontaneity of eye blink, speech and movement, and orientation.

Mentation is determined from the patient's ability to respond logically and appropriately to the EMT's questions and his ability to follow simple commands. Care must be taken to discern between a lack of understanding caused by language or cultural differences; a lack of hearing either caused by noise distraction or a hearing impairment; unwillingness to answer based upon fear, hostility or legal apprehension; *or* a lack of proper mentation. Also, care must be taken to distinguish between socially inappropriate responses such as hostility or cursing (which may be normal for a given patient) and medically inappropriate responses.

The patient's alertness and orientation to three items—person, place, and time (A & Ox3)—are also evaluated. The patient's alertness includes a judgement of how he responds and how oriented he is to the events around him. His orientation to person is based on whether he clearly knows his first and last name. His orientation to place deals with whether he knows where he is or what type of place he is in (some transient patients may not know the town name). Orientation to time surrounds a general understanding of the time-of-day (morning, afternoon, evening, etc., *not* necessarily the specific hour and minute), and the day of the week and month. The patient who is alert and oriented to person, place, and time is commonly reported as "Patient is A & Ox3".

In unconscious *patients* one further evaluates if and how they react to verbal stimulus; or if only to painful stimulus and how; or if they remain unresponsive regardless of the application of painful stimulus.

As well as the present level of consciousness the EMT should also obtain a careful history from the patient and others present, including noting any changes of LOC or periods of unconsciousness that may have occurred prior to the EMT's arrival. If the patient has chronological or locational gaps ("I don't know how I got out of the car . . .") in his memory, these must be assumed to represent a period of unconsciousness.

DOING THE ENLARGED AVPU

1. On arrival, at a glance, the EMT can determine if the patient appears to be *conscious* or *unconscious*. In **alert awake** patients further evaluation of the quality of consciousness—whether mentation is normal or changed and whether the patient is alert and oriented to the events around him—can be determined from the appropriateness of his responses to questions and simple commands that are a part of the continuing assessment. Next, evaluate if the patient is oriented to person, place and time. If not record the level of alertness, describe the appropriateness of the responses, and indicate his orientation including any pertinent negatives.

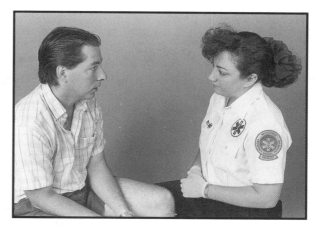

2. In a patient who appears to be stuporous or unconscious the EMT should continue with the ABC assessment and urgent interventions. When these have been provided the neurological evaluation can continue. Moving down the AVPU scale, see if and how the patient reacts to **verbal stimulus.** First, see if the patient is arousable by asking, "If you can hear me, open your eyes." If the patient opens his eyes or otherwise responds, go on to additional questions and simple commands. Note the patient's best motor ("opens eyes only", "makes meaningful movements on command", etc.) and verbal ("speaks when spoken to", "moans") responses.

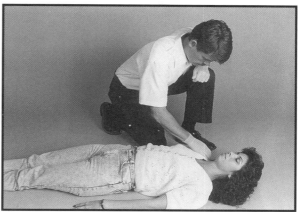

3. If the patient does not respond to normal verbal stimuli, go on to see if he will respond to a **noxious verbal stimulus** by yelling "Open your eyes!" in his ear. Note if and how he responds. If he does, include mention that he only responded to "loud verbal stimulus". Care must be taken to determine if a lack of response is due to the patient's LOC level or possibly impaired hearing.

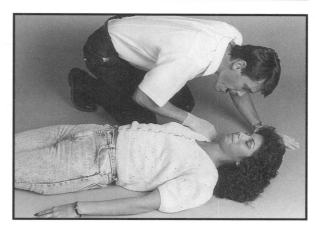

4. If an unconscious patient does *not* respond to verbal stimulus, next (following the AVPU scale) one determines if the patient will respond to a **painful stimulus.** Very strong fingertip pressure applied between the EMT's thumb and fingers to the patient's trapezious muscle (as shown) is recommended. This produces significant pain without a high risk of deleterious side effects. Since the nerves in this area descend directly from the brain, a response can be elicited even if the patient has suffered a high spinal cord injury that leaves the rest of the body paralyzed or insensitive.

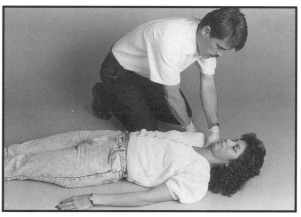

5. The *normal* response to a painful stimulus includes localizing its source (identifying where it hurts) and with an organized movement attempting to push away or withdraw from the source. In patients who no longer localize pain a lesser level of appropriate response to a painful stimulus may be seen as agitation with a general body-wide flailing out to try to remove the source (infants under 6 months are limited to such a response) or as flexion of the body into a fetal position in an attempt to withdraw from the painful stimulus and protect the vital viscera.

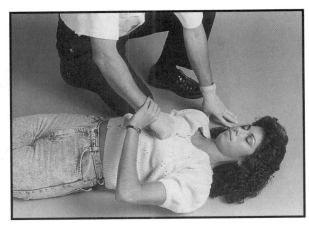

6. Inappropriate pathological responses to a painful stimulus may include arbitrary focal body movements unrelated to the location of the pain, or when insult to the brain stem has occurred two unique pathological posturing responses may result. With **decorticate posturing** the patient's torso and legs are maximally extended and rigid (often resulting in such arching that the middle of the back, buttocks and upper legs are lifted off the ground) while flexion of the upper extremities occurs with the hands rotated inwards so that the fingers point towards the upper torso or head.

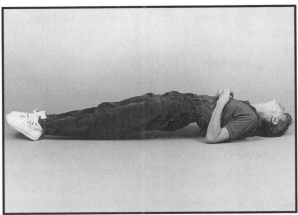

7. Patients who respond to pain with **decerebrate posturing** have even more profound brain stem injury. With decerebrate posturing, the patient's torso and legs are maximally extended and rigid (the same as with decorticate posturing) while the upper extremities are extended with the hands rotated outwards and the hand and fingers are in an unnatural crippled-appearing manner. When noting that a patient *only* responded to painful stimulus, the EMT must include a description of how he responded.

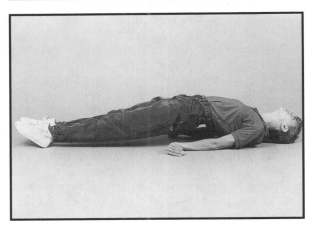

8. If the patient does not respond to a painful stimulus but remains unmoving and **unresponsive** then he is noted as being "Unresponsive".

Using the **AVPU Scale,** the best initial response from A to V is noted: **A**lert and how well he is oriented; or only responds to **V**erbal stimulus and how; or only responds to **P**ainful stimulus and how; or regardless of stimulus remains **U**nresponsive. The EMT should also note any LOC changes that appear to have occurred prior to his arrival and any that occur after the initial AVPU was recorded.

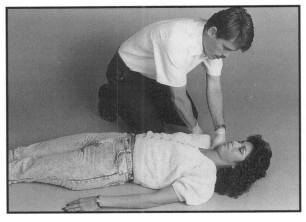

LEVEL OF CONSCIOUSNESS—GLASGOW COMA SCALE

As noted on the preceding pages, the initial pre-hospital LOC should be evaluated and noted using the *AVPU scale.* In some patients, such as those with head trauma or unexplained unconsciousness, once the ABC priorities and AVPU have been completed a more definitive method of LOC measurement may be desirable. The *Glasgow Coma Scale* is used to provide a more detailed set of response criteria as well as a numerical quantification of the patient's LOC based upon his best responses to three categories: eye opening, motor response, and the patient's verbal ability. In many areas, to avoid delay and possible inconsistency, pre-hospital evaluation beyond AVPU only includes the response criteria of the Glasgow Coma Scale, not the point values of their sum. The EMT will have to follow his local protocols.

AVPU is generally considered the Vital Sign measure of LOC with the more definitive Glasgow Coma Scale, examination of the pupils, and motor and sensory checks in the extremities, being considered as additional neurologic diagnostic signs.

GLASGOW COMA SCALE	
Eye Opening	
Spontaneous eye opening	4 points
Eye opening on command	3 points
Eye opening to painful stimulus	2 points
No eye opening	1 point
Best Motor Response	
Follows command	6 points
Localizes painful stimuli	5 points
Withdrawal to pain	4 points
Responds with abnormal flexion to painful stimuli (decorticate)	3 points
Responds with abnormal extension to pain (decerebrate)	2 points
Gives no motor response	1 point
Best Verbal Response	
Answers appropriately (oriented)	5 points
Gives confused answers	4 points
Inappropriate response	3 points
Makes unintelligible noises	2 points
Makes no verbal response	1 point
Total = [ ]	
Note: Lowest possible score = 3; Highest possible score = 15	

EVALUATING THE PATIENT'S TEMPERATURE—INTRODUCTION

Thermometers—A patient's temperature is routinely taken with a thermometer as part of the arrival vital sign work-up in the Emergency Department. Pre-hospital, however, it is commonly only estimated on each patient by feeling and observing the skin. It is usually only taken with a thermometer when the history or exam suggests a condition usually associated with a fever or lowered body core temperature, with seizures, or when the skin feels abnormally hot or cold to the touch. Whether the EMT should routinely take the temperature using a thermometer of patients who present with any *medical emergency,* or in which cases, should be determined by local protocols.

All people have a *temperature.* Those whose temperature is above the normal range are said to have a **fever,** and persons having a fever are said to be **febrile.** The temperature is measured either in degrees Fahrenheit or degrees Centigrade.

Historically, temperature has been taken using a reusable glass thermometer containing a continuous column of mercury. The mercury rises in the calibrated glass tube and stays at the patient's temperature level until it has been read and the thermometer is shaken down—returning it to a sub-normal starting point. Most glass thermometers are calibrated in both Fahrenheit and Centigrade scales. Oral and Rectal glass thermometers are distinguished from each other by the shape of the reservoir bulb (generally silver) at the thermometer's distal end: oral ones having a cylindrical tip about a half inch long and rectal ones having a shorter, more bulbous tip. Either may be used to take an axillary temperature. After each use the thermometer is cleaned by wiping it repeatedly using suitable antiseptic fluid. In addition the glass thermometer is inserted in a single-use thin plastic cover sleeve (which is closed at the distal end) prior to each use. This serves both as an aseptic consideration and to add some safety in the event that the glass should crack or break. The cover is disposed of after each use and a new one is applied just prior to the next use. Glass thermometers are slow to register body temperature, and require between 2 1/2 and 10 minutes of insertion, depending on the specific location being used, to provide an accurate reading.

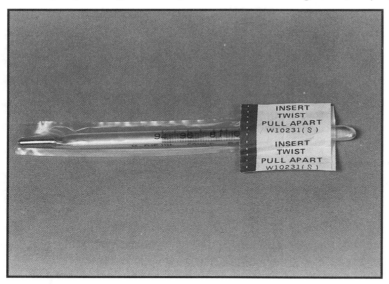

In the past few years electric (electronic) thermometers have become widely used in the hospital setting. The type used in most hospitals has a small box with a display window and a metal probe connected to it by a thin wire. Prior to each use the probe is inserted into a one-use hard plastic tip which narrows to a gently rounded point at its distal end. The tip is designed to be universal for either oral, rectal or axillary use. This tip completely covers the probe and is disposed of immediately after use. Lately a tympanic model has been introduced which uses a disposable ear piece and accurately takes the temperature at the easily accessed ear canal in a few seconds. *Only a tympanic thermometer should ever be inserted in the ear. Insertion of any other type is extremely dangerous.* This type is not demonstrated in this text since it should only be used following the manufacturer's directions which are specific to each different model. Recently, inexpensive one-piece electric thermometers with a distal tip shaped like a glass tube and a 3/4 inch wide flat proximal end containing a digital display window have become commonly used by EMS. These use a disposable film cover slip over the probe end and may be used for either oral, rectal or axillary measurement.

Electric thermometers, regardless of style or brand, generally have an on-and-off switch and reset to "0" when turned off, not requiring "shaking-down". A second switch allows the user to select whether the readout is to be in the Fahrenheit or Centigrade scale. Electric thermometers are recommended for pre-hospital use since they are safer to use than glass ones, the digital readout is easier to read than a column of mercury, and they are faster—generally requiring only about ten seconds rather than several minutes of uninterrupted placement.

Another type of thermometer is a celluloid-like strip that is held on the forehead. A thermo-chemical reaction produces either a visible color bar which appears along a scale, or a large number that denotes the temperature. Such thermometers may provide the EMT with a rapid and easy way of more accurately estimating the temperature.

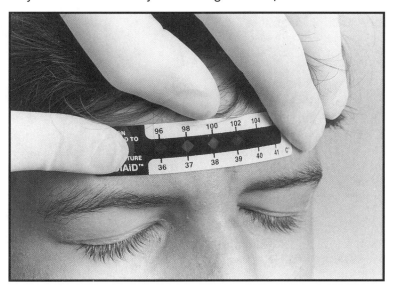

Scales—Body temperature is measured using either the *Fahrenheit* or *Centigrade* (also called Celsius) scales. In the Fahrenheit scale, at sea level, the freezing point of water is 32 degrees and the boiling point is 212 degrees. In Centigrade the freezing point is 0 degrees and the boiling point is 100 degrees. The Centigrade scale is a metric measure widely used internationally. Most people in the United States are more used to the Fahrenheit scale, therefore it is the one used in this text. When recording a temperature the EMT must record the scale used. Temperature is recorded in degrees and tenths of degrees followed by an "F" for Fahrenheit or "C" for Centigrade, and the location at which it was measured. For Example, "T–99°F, oral" or T–37.2°C, oral".

Almost all medical thermometers allow the EMT to read either scale, however if you need to convert one to the other the following formulas are used:

$$\text{F temperature} = \frac{9\ (\textbf{Centigrade temperature} + \textbf{32 degrees})}{5}$$

$$\text{C temperature} = \frac{5\ (\textbf{Fahrenheit temperature} - \textbf{32 degrees})}{9}$$

If the calculated result includes a figure beyond tenths of a degree (37.22°C), round it to tenths "T–37.2°C, oral".

Location for Taking the Temperature—The patient's temperature can be taken with the thermometer placed in the mouth (oral), in the rectum (rectal), in the armpit (axillary) or in the ear (tympanic). Standard glass or electric thermometers can be used for taking the oral, rectal or axillary temperature, however a special tympanic thermometer is required to accurately and safely take the temperature in the ear. *Use of any thermometer in the ear except a tympanic one with a special earpiece is dangerous and contraindicated.*

Oral temperature is the most commonly taken in adults. The thermometer is placed in the mouth and held with the lips closed under the tongue. A glass thermometer should be held under the tongue for at least 3 to 4 minutes; an electric one for a period as described in its directions for use (usually about 10 to 20 seconds). Oral temperature readings may not be accurate for patients who have had hot or cold liquids or who have smoked in the preceding 30 minutes. They are also unreliable in a patient who continues to talk or breathe through his mouth once the thermometer has been inserted under the tongue. Even with the mouth held closed, oral temperatures will vary slightly depending on the patient's respiratory rate.

Rectal temperature better reflects the body's core temperature and is not affected by the previously mentioned variables that may alter an oral temperature. **The rectal temperature will on average be 1 degree higher than the oral temperature.** When taking a temperature is required, rectal (or tympanic) rather than oral temperatures should be taken in:

- Children under 6
- Patients who have seizure activity
- Patients who are confused, disoriented, or incapable
- Patients who are unconscious
- Patients suspected of having hypothermia
- Patients with any tachypnea or dyspnea

Rectal temperature is taken by first lubricating the covered distal tip of the thermometer and then inserting it between 1 and 1 1/2 inches into the anal canal. Once properly inserted, the thermometer must be firmly held in place so that it is not involuntarily drawn in or expelled, and the patient must be restrained from rolling over. **An un-held thermometer inserted in the anal canal presents a serious danger to the patient even if he is unmoving, therefore the EMT should not release his grasp even for an instant.** A glass rectal thermometer should be held in place for at least 3 minutes and an electric one for the period described in the directions. In patients who have a possible acute cardiac problem, one should not take a rectal temperature as this can produce a vagal response resulting in a dangerous bradycardia.

Tympanic temperature reflects the body core temperature and the expected findings and ranges are the same as for a rectal temperature. The earpiece should be inserted in the manner and for the length of time indicated in the directions.

Axillary temperature is the least accurate temperature measurement and its use should be limited to situations where taking an oral or rectal temperature is impractical. When taking an axillary temperature the thermometer is placed at the axilla (the junction between the arm and chest) and held with the upper arm pressed firmly against the lateral thorax. The thermometer's bulb should be in direct contact with both the skin and the arm and thorax at about the mid axillary line. A glass thermometer needs to be held in such a position for approximately ten minutes. When using an electric thermometer follow the directions for its use. **Axillary temperatures average 1 degree less than oral readings.**

Normal Ranges and Fever—Although the temperature taken using a thermometer is exact the normal temperature ranges and identifying which levels indicate a fever are not. Like other signs and symptoms, temperature must be considered in the context of a variety of other signs and symptoms. The following norms will provide a guideline to the EMT:

ADULT TEMPERATURE GUIDELINES

Location	Normal Range	Consider Febrile	Considered Potentially Dangerous
Oral	96.4°F– 99°F	Greater than 99°F	103°F, or greater
Rectal	97.4°F–100°F	Greater than 100°F	104°F, or greater
Axillary	95.4°F– 98°F	(Take oral or rectal temperature)	

PEDIATRIC TEMPERATURE GUIDELINES

Location	Normal Range	Consider Febrile	Considered Potentially Dangerous
Oral	96.4°F–100°F	Greater than 99°F	104°F, or greater
Rectal	97.4°F–101°F	Greater than 100°F	105°F, or greater
Axillary	95.4°F– 99°F	(Take oral or rectal temperature)	

Body temperature can be affected by level of activity, respiratory rate, excessive clothes or bed covers, environmental temperature and humidity, elevation above or below sea level, and a variety of other factors. A person's temperature commonly fluctuates during the course of a day with lower readings in the early morning and higher readings in the evening. An adult's normal oral temperature may be as low as 96.4°F in the early morning and as high as 99°F in the late evening. A child's normal temperature may even fluctuate more within a day, ranging from 97.4°F rectal in the early morning to 101°F rectal in the evening. An Infant's or small child's temperature may also be unnecessarily high if they have been bundled in excessive clothing. The temperature of females in the childbearing years will also fluctuate during each 28 day cycle relative to the dates of ovulation.

Conclusions—The previously shown norms are only guidelines and even a low grade fever may indicate the onset or presence of a serious or even potentially dangerous condition. Any fever that is 2 degrees or more above the normal range should be considered as a significant finding, and any elevation in temperature can produce febrile seizures (more commonly in small children). Febrile seizures may result from a rapid rise in fever at lower levels, being caused by the rate-of-rise rather than its ultimate height. As well as the level, the duration of a fever is a key factor. Any sustained fever beyond a few days should be viewed by the EMT as a significant finding. In elderly patients a well advanced illness may only have a remarkably low fever associated with it due to the lowered immune system response common in that age group. Therefore, in elderly patients even a low grade fever should be considered significant.

When evaluating core temperature for hypothermia, a thermometer which reads as low as 50°F will be needed (below the range of normal medical thermometers). A rectal temperature below 96.8°F must, with the history and other signs and symptoms, be considered as a possible indicator of the onset of moderate hypothermia. Any rectal temperature below 91.4°F is considered indicative of severe hypothermia.

ESTIMATING THE PATIENT'S TEMPERATURE

The temperature of all patients should be estimated by the EMT, seeing whether the skin appears normally warm, abnormally hot, or abnormally cold. Both the environmental temperature and the coldness of the EMT's hand must be considered. If your hands are cold, warm them prior to feeling the patient's skin temperature.

Although the patient's skin is felt while palpating the pulse, since commonly the radial pulse is used this indicates the distal temperature in the limb and may not properly reflect the core body temperature. Temperature is best estimated using the back of the EMT's hand placed against the patient's forehead as shown below.

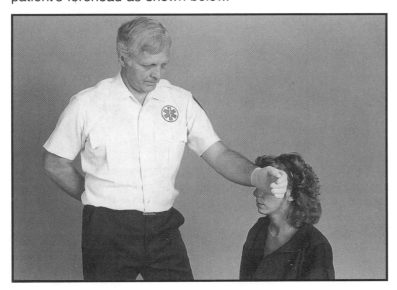

In a cold environment the central body temperature is better estimated by placing the EMT's hand under the clothing at the lateral thorax with the fingers extended into the axilla. This location can easily be accessed even in fully clothed patients by opening one or two buttons at the top of the shirt or blouse or by reaching up from the bottom of an item such as a sweater. The skills for taking the temperature by thermometer are presented in the following pages.

TAKING AN ORAL TEMPERATURE—GLASS THERMOMETER

The temperature in adults and children over six years of age who are alert, oriented, cooperative, capable, and who have not had recent seizure activity is most commonly taken orally. General guidelines for taking and evaluating temperature have been presented in the preceding pages. Since taking an oral temperature involves handling an object which contacted body fluids, the appropriate universal precautions should be observed. The use of a glass oral thermometer will be demonstrated first followed by the pertinent modifications to be made when using an electric thermometer.

1. Remove the glass thermometer from its protective case and first check to be sure it is: an oral thermometer, not cracked or otherwise broken, and that the mercury in the calibrated section is an uninterrupted single column. To check the latter, hold the thermometer up with the calibrated side facing you and slightly roll it until the mercury appears as a wide clear band within the glass tube. Next, check that it has been properly shaken down by checking that the mercury reads below 95°F. If not, shake it down and recheck it.

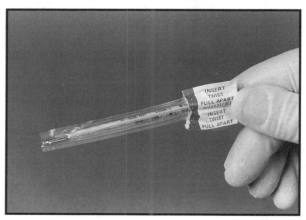

2. Insert the thermometer's distal end into a disposable film cover and advance it until fully inserted. If the type used has a peel-off backing, peel it off and discard it.

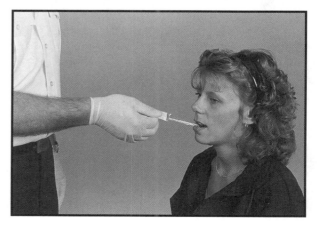

3. Explain what you are going to do and instruct the patient to open his mouth wide and elevate his tongue towards the roof of the mouth. Insert the thermometer until it is under the full length of the tongue.

4. Have the patient close his mouth, holding the thermometer with the underside of the tongue and his closed lips. **Warn him not to hold it with his teeth.** Instruct him not to talk (remember, don't ask him any questions while the thermometer is in his mouth), to keep his lips shut firmly around the thermometer, and to breath normally through his nose. Should the patient be supine or in a lowered semi-sitting position, the EMT should maintain a light grasp on the proximal end of the thermometer.

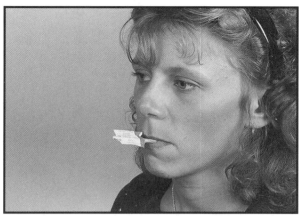

5. Once the thermometer is properly in place, check your watch and note the exact minute displayed. Leave the thermometer in place under the patient's tongue for 3 to 4 minutes. Should the patient attempt to speak or otherwise open his mouth several times, or if the respiratory rate is rapid, the time should be extended to 5 minutes. If the process is interrupted, replace the thermometer in the patient's mouth and start timing the 3 to 4 minutes again.

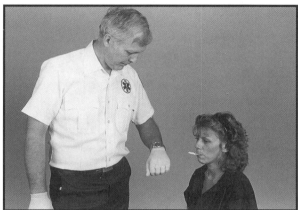

6. Once the proper time has elapsed, remove the thermometer and hold it up with the calibrated side towards you. Rotate it slightly until the mercury appears as a wide band and note the calibrated reading at the highest level of the mercury. Each longer line in the marking signifies one whole degree and each of the four shorter lines in between signifies an additional 2/10ths of a degree (0.2). For example, if the mercury ends at the third short line beyond the long line marked 98°, the temperature is 98.6°. Record the temperature, whether "F" or "C", "oral", and the time taken.

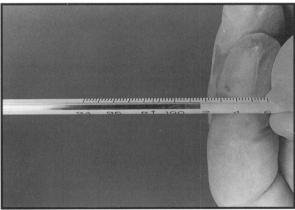

7. Remove the disposable cover and discard it in an appropriate "contaminated" container.

8. Shake the thermometer down until it reads less than 95°F.

9. Vigorously wipe the entire thermometer with a 4X4 containing antiseptic fluid or an antiseptic wipe.

10. Place the clean thermometer into its protective case and put it away.

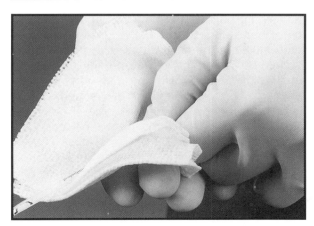

TAKING A RECTAL TEMPERATURE—GLASS THERMOMETER

The temperature should be taken rectally in infants and small children; larger children and adults who are agitated, confused, not capable, or unconscious; any patient with tachypnea or dyspnea; patients who have eaten, had fluids, or have smoked in the last 30 minutes; anyone who has or recently had any seizure activity; or any patient in whom an accurate core body temperature is needed. General guidelines have previously been presented in the introduction to *Evaluating the Temperature.* For aesthetic and safety reasons, the only glass thermometers that should be inserted in the anal canal are those with a short, bulbous rounded tip designed for rectal use.

1. Take the thermometer out of its protective case and check that it is intact and a rectal type. Check that it has been shaken down properly. If not, do so now. Then insert it into a disposable cover film and peel off any backing. Bare the buttocks and have the patient assume or place him in a prone position. Next copiously apply water soluble lubricating jelly on approximately the first inch of the proximal tip of the thermometer.

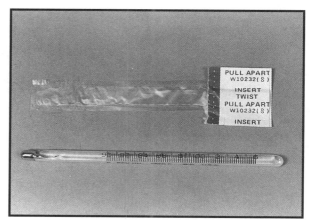

2. Press firmly down on the small of the patient's back with your cephalad forearm so that he can not roll over or suddenly move (or have another EMT or parent do this). While holding the readied thermometer in your caudad hand, spread the cheeks of the buttocks apart with the the thumb and first finger of your cephalad hand until you can clearly visualize the anus.

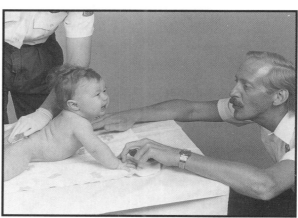

3. While holding the buttocks apart with your other hand insert the proximal end of the thermometer into the anal canal. The thermometer should be inserted into the anus in-line with the midline of the body with the distal end elevated above the proximal end so that the thermometer is held at about a 30 degree angle of elevation. Continue advancing it until between 1 and 1 1/2 inches in an adult or 1/2 to 1 inch in an infant or small child (depending upon size) has been inserted. Continue holding the patient so he cannot move. With the other hand continue to hold the end of the thermometer at all times.

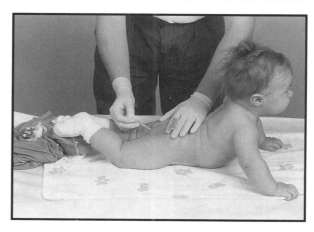

4. Check the exact time. The thermometer should be held in place for between 2 1/2 and 3 minutes. After this time has elapsed, carefully withdraw the thermometer and clean the jelly from the buttocks and anus with a suitable wipe.

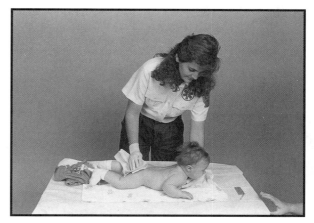

5. Read the thermometer. Remember, rectal temperature norms are 1 degree above those found orally. Next, record the temperature reading, whether "F" or "C", that it is "rectal", and the time taken. Replace (or have someone replace) the patient's clothing.

6. Discard the disposable cover in a suitable "contaminated" container and clean the thermometer with a 4X4 wet with antiseptic fluid or an antiseptic wipe.

7. Shake down the thermometer and replace it in its protective cover.

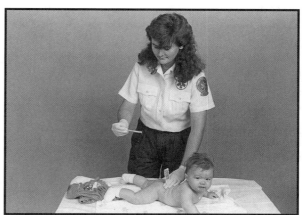

TAKING AN AXILLARY TEMPERATURE

Taking the temperature in the axilla produces the least reliable reading and requires longer insertion time. Therefore, this location should only be used when taking an oral or rectal temperature is impractical. The EMT may find it useful, since it can easily be taken while enroute, to confirm that a fever is *NOT* present in a patient whose skin felt normal upon exam. If a glass thermometer is used it should be in place for at least ten minutes. For a temp-dot or electrical thermometer, follow the manufacturer's direction's. Remember the normal axillary temperature is one degree less than for an oral temperature.

1. Remove the thermometer from its protective case and, if glass, make sure it is intact and shaken down. If electrical, turn on and check that it is working.

2. Insert the end into a disposable cover.

3. Remove the patient's shirt (or open the top 2 or 3 buttons) and insert the thermometer so that the tip is at the mid axillary line and at the highest possible point in the axilla. Have the patient adduct his arm fully, holding the thermometer to the chest wall as shown and note the time.

4. After the appropriate time, read and record the temperature, if "F" or "C", "axillary", and the time taken.

5. Discard the cover properly, clean off the thermometer, shake it down or turn it off, and replace it in the protective case.

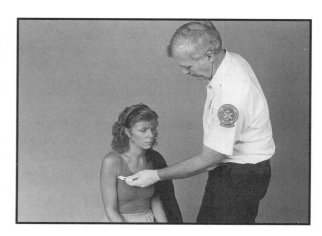

TAKING THE TEMPERATURE—ELECTRIC THERMOMETER

Electric thermometers are safer, faster, and easier to use than glass ones. Unlike glass thermometers, the same electrical thermometer is designed for either oral or rectal (and axillary) use. Larger (IVAC type) models have a portable case connected by a wire to a separate probe which is inserted into a disposable hard plastic—single use tip prior to each use. When not in use, this type is placed onto a re-charger base. A smaller self-contained type resembling a glass thermometer at its distal end with a wide flat proximal end containing a read-out window is commonly used pre-hospital and is the type demonstrated here.

1. Take the thermometer from its protective case, insert its distal tip into a disposable film cover and remove any backing (or if the larger type, remove the probe from its storage place in the case and insert it into a disposable hard plastic tip).

2. Turn the thermometer on/off switch to on (Larger models turn on when the probe is removed from the case) and place the selector switch to either the "F" or "C" setting. Check that either "0", or the lowest reading, or a test pattern appears, indicating that the thermometer is ready for use.

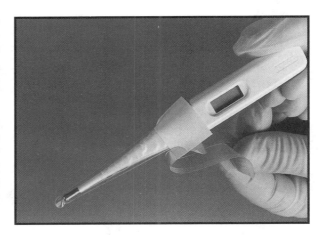

3. If taking an oral temperature, place the distal tip under the tongue and have the patient hold it firmly with the tongue and closed lips. Note the exact time. If taking a rectal temperature, follow the previous directions for lubricating the tip, inserting the probe into the anal canal, and holding the patient and thermometer. Leave the thermometer inserted for the time indicated (usually 10 to 15 seconds), or until an audible signal indicates that the necessary time has elapsed.

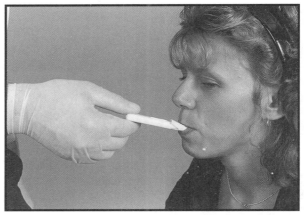

4. Remove the thermometer and read the digital display. Record the temperature whether "F" or "C", whether oral or rectal, and the time at which it was taken.

5. Discard the disposable cover in a "contaminated" container properly and clean the thermometer with a 4X4 wet with antiseptic fluid or an antiseptic wipe. Turn the thermometer off or, in larger models return the uncovered probe into its holder.

6. Replace the thermometer in its protective case or back on its charger as appropriate.

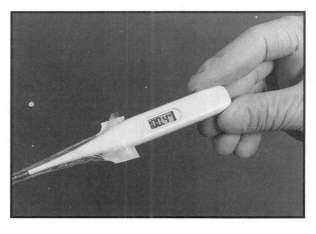

TAKING THE TEMPERATURE—TEMPA-DOT THERMOMETER

Single use, disposable thermometers are available. The most common is made of plastic, is sterile, and comes in a foil sealed sterile wrapper. These have a series of dots, instead of a linear calibration, with a dot representing each 2/10ths of a degree of temperature. A thermochemical reaction changes the color of the dot which represents the patient's temperature and the dots representing all of the temperatures lower than it. The dots retain the color of changes for a sustained period. After use this type of thermometer is discarded. The ones presently available can be used for taking either oral or axillary temperatures but *NOT* rectal.

1. Remove a sheet of foil-wrapped thermometers from the box and tear off an individual thermometer package. Peel back the foil and remove the thermometer by its distal end. Check that all dots are of the same color. Insert the distal end in the patient's mouth as you would any oral thermometer, and have the patient hold it in place with his tongue and closed lips for just over one minute. If used in the axilla, it should be inserted with the dots facing the thoracic wall and the tip at the mid-axillary line as high in the axilla as possible, held squeezed between the upper arm and thorax for three minutes.

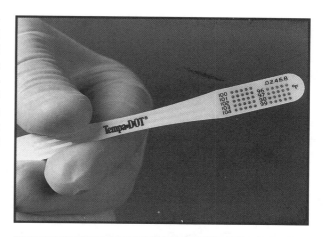

2. After the proper time has elapsed, remove the thermometer and read the temperature. From 96°F to 104°F are printed in sequence in two columns. Next to each there are five dots. The first is marked "0" and each of the others represents an additional 0.2°F. All of the dots from 96.0°F to the patient's actual temperature will change color. If the first dot marked "0" next to a number is the highest to change, then the temperature is that whole number of degrees with "0" tenths. If the changed dots include the 0.2 degree dot it is that whole degree plus 2 tenths, and so on as marked. Record the temperature in the usual manner and discard the thermometer in a proper "contaminated" container.

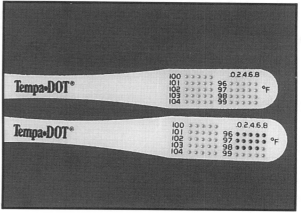

USING A FOREHEAD STRIP TYPE THERMOMETER

This type of thermometer is a celluloid strip which is held on the forehead. A thermochemical reaction produces either a bar in-between a scale or causes numbers to appear, depending on the brand used. The EMT will find this type useful in obtaining a further estimate in small children and agitated adult patients when determining if taking a rectal temperature is indicated. By itself a temperature taken at the forehead is not considered accurate enough to be more than a quantified estimate.

1. Take a strip from the case and place it on the center of the forehead until the bar or a number clearly appears and no longer changes. Care must be taken to hold it only by its edges so that it does not reflect the EMT's temperature. This type should be read while in place on the forehead as most brands do not "hold" a reading once removed.

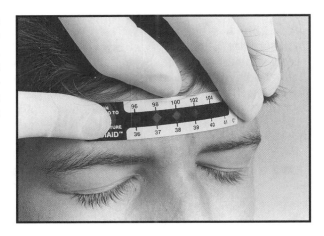

If a reading showing a fever is seen, the EMT may want to obtain a more accurate oral or rectal temperature. If not, record the highest temperature obtained followed by the words "at the forehead".

EVALUATING THE SKIN

Evaluation of the skin, although dependent upon subjective judgments that are not quantifiable, is considered a Vital Sign because changes in the skin that can be easily observed early in the exam often reflect key systemic problems of body temperature, quality of circulation, blood oxygen levels, or an allergic reaction. The **skin** is *one* of the important signs in determining:

- the presence and level of shock (hypoperfusion)
- cardiac or vascular problems
- fever
- other conditions where the body cannot dissipate heat (hyperthermia)
- conditions in which the body cannot produce and maintain an adequate body core temperature (hypothermia)
- hypoxia
- generalized allergic reactions
- others

A difference between the skin body-wide and the skin in only one area or limb may be a key indicator of impaired or absent circulation, presence of an infection, tissue freezing (frostbite), or other injury to that part. Bruises and hematomas indicate areas of injury and raise the question of potential underlying damage. The huge universe of medical conditions that can cause changes in the skin are covered in your primary textbook and are outside of the scope of this book. Some general comments in evaluating the skin, however, are key to doing the assessment.

Overall, the skin is evaluated for *color, temperature, and moisture.* It is also examined to locate areas with different temperature or color, wounds, bites, scars, bruises, hematomas, burns, frostbite, and hives or other rashes.

Color—The skin color in healthy individuals varies greatly from person to person. Based upon inherited characteristics, the amount of pigmentation determines if the skin's underlying coloration is whitish, olive colored, yellowish, brown, or black. Upon careful observation one notes that normal skin color is a complex subtle mixture of colors and hues.

Regardless of the underlying color, the skin includes some pink coloration caused by the red color of the oxygenated blood circulating through the many blood vessels that are located near the skin's translucent surface. Changes in the amount of blood circulating through these vessels, changes in their size (their fullness or if they dilate or constrict), a loss or lack of production of red cells, or a lack of sufficient oxygen in the blood will result in changes in the pink hue of the skin. It is primarily the change in this pink hue that is significant and that is reported as the "skin color". Regardless of the different underlying pigmentation and color, the skin in healthy individuals is recorded as "pink". If due to conditions such as high blood pressure or fever the skin appears flushed and more reddish, it is described as "red". If, as when shock is present, it is less pink than normal it is described as "pale", and as shock advances and no pink hue remains, as "white". Sometimes with advanced shock the skin, which normally appears opaque, appears to become more translucent and then is described as "waxy".

The blood's reddish color results from the bonding of oxygen with the hemoglobin. When blood oxygen levels are inadequate the blood becomes a brownish-blue. If circulation in the surface vessels is adequate this results in the skin and mucous membranes having a greyish-blue tint rather than a pink one. This bluish coloring is called **cyanosis** and the patient or his skin are described as *cyanotic*. Certain conditions result in "pooling" of blood in the veins (generally the inferior ones), called lividity. The pooled blood does not circulate and rapidly becomes hypoxic, causing cyanotic or purplish areas in the otherwise pink or pale skin. This patchy variation of skin colors is described as "mottled".

Changes in liver function can also affect skin color. Certain liver abnormalities can result in a yellow (or in advanced cases brownish-yellow) coloring to the skin called **jaundice.** In such cases the patient or skin are described as *jaundiced.*

Temperature—At room temperature the normal feel of the skin is described as "warm". When a person has been exercising vigorously, is in a hot place for a sustained period or in the sun, or has a fever, the skin feels hotter than usual and is described as "hot". When a person has a circulatory deficit such as in early shock there is a reduction in the surface tissue's metabolic process resulting in the skin feeling cooler than normal. The skin in such cases is described as "cool". As the shock advances the metabolism is reduced even more and involves deeper tissues, causing the skin to become even colder to the touch. This is described as "cold". The EMT must take the situation and other signs and symptoms into consideration when assessing the skin. In patients who are out in a very cold or very hot climate the environmental temperature will cause changes in the skin's temperature.

Moisture—Normally, at rest and room temperature, the skin is dry. When the body overheats the sweat glands open and release fluid onto the skin's surface as needed to aid in cooling the body. When the patient is in shock the reduced perfusion to the sphincters of the sweat glands causes them to open and fluid to be released. Depending upon the amount of perspiration the skin is described as: "dry", or if only damp as "clammy", if more wet as "moist", and if profusely bathed in sweat as "wet". Medically, if the skin is wet the patient is said to have **diaphoresis,** and he and his skin are said to be *diaphoretic*. When this is profuse the patient is said to have *marked diaphoresis*.

Patterns and Norms of Color, Temperature and Moisture—Normally, at rest and room temperature, the skin is pink, warm and dry. When a healthy person is in a hot environment, or exercising the skin will be red, hot, and moist or wet. Patients with a moderate or high fever will also have red, hot, and moist or wet skin. When a healthy person is in a cold environment the skin will be pink or red (ruddy), cool or cold, and dry.

In patients in early compensating shock, as blood is shunted from the skin to more important parts of the body, the skin becomes pale, cool, and clammy. As shock advances the skin becomes white or greyish, possibly waxy, cold, and wet. Marked diaphoresis is common. In some cases, as venous pooling occurs, the skin may become mottled.

Red, hot, and dry skin may result from a variety of causes such as high blood pressure or exposure to the sun. When seen in a patient who has been in a very hot environment, the lack of perspiration witnessed by the dry skin should alert the EMT to the possibility that the patient has heat stroke or has become dehydrated.

Rashes—Localized or body wide rashes may be associated with a variety of diseases and problems. A wide range of types of rashes exist (red petichiae, small pustulates, etc), but only one distinction is key for the EMT to make: hives as opposed to all others. Hives appear generally as white or reddish flat raised splotches. Their size may vary and in extreme cases they may be seen to advance from one area of the body to another. Any hives should be considered as a sign that a systemic allergic (anaphalactic) reaction is progressing. Since other types of rashes may be from a communicable disease, the EMT should take proper precautions. Many rashes are first seen in areas where the skin is more sensitive, therefore, the EMT should examine the skin in the upper arm near the armpit (palm side of the upper arm), on the medial thigh, or on the back for signs of early onset. The EMT should note the location of any rash found.

Turgor—The skin turgor is the normal tension of the skin caused by the outward pressure of the underlying cells and the fluid that surrounds them. Normally the skin is moderately tight, allowing one to pinch and lift it about 1/2 inch (less in healthy infants and more in the elderly). When the patient has lost fluid and is dehydrated the skin is "looser" and one can easily pinch and lift it higher without effort. In extreme cases it will stay raised, this is called "tenting". If excess fluid is retained (hyperhydration) the skin becomes shiny and taut. This may be associated with edema (swelling) particularly in inferior parts of the body. It is common to find edema at the ankles. When one indents the edematous area with a finger and the skin's return is delayed, it is called "pitting edema".

CAPILLARY REFILL TEST

Capillary refill time is one method used to evaluate the quality of the patient's peripheral perfusion as a reflection of his systemic blood pressure and/or to evaluate the quality of the distal circulation in a limb. When firm pressure is exerted upon the patient's nail bed it whitens and, once the pressure is released, remains blanched for a brief period before returning to its normal reddish-pink color. With adequate perfusion the normal color should return in two seconds or under. If longer than two seconds is necessary, capillary refill is said to be "delayed" and peripheral perfusion is considered below normal either due to lowered levels of circulation in that limb or, in the absence of a local problem, reflecting systemic hypotension (from hypovolemia or another cause). In cold temperatures the nail beds may be blanched and have delayed or indeterminable color changes due to the body's response to the cold.

A study done at UCLA published in 1988 (Schriger, D. L., and Baroff, L. J.,: Ann. of Emerg. Med.) suggests that differences in sex, age and temperature affect normal capillary refill times and that normal times which included 95% of the subjects studied would be: 2 seconds or less for children and male adults, 3 seconds or less for female adults, and 4.5 seconds or less for persons 65 years or older.

The same reporters in a 1991 study concluded that capillary refill does not appear to be a useful test for determining mild-to-moderate hypovolemia and that at this time there is no evidence that it is of any value in assessing hypovolemic states in adults (children were not studied). Many, however, still feel capillary refill time has value as an easily obtained measure of general peripheral perfusion, and little if any debate has been raised surrounding its value in evaluating the distal circulation in a given limb.

1. Squeeze the nail bed firmly between your thumb and first finger.

2. Check the time and release your fingers. Continue holding the limb so you can observe the color of the nail bed.

3. Time the number of seconds the blanched white color remains in the nail bed before it returns to the normal reddish-pink (as seen under the other nails). If two seconds or under, note it as "normal". If greater than two seconds, note it as "delayed".

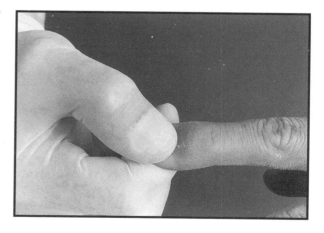

EVALUATING SHOCK

A full discussion of shock, including its complex pathophysiology, progression and resulting changes, varying interactive mechanisms and management is beyond the scope of this book. However, in a discussion of diagnostic signs a brief overview of the signs and symptoms of shock and its levels will be useful.

As the first phase, called *compensated shock,* commences one of the earliest signs is marked anxiety. The skin becomes pale, cool, and moist and capillary refill becomes delayed. The pulse rate elevates, becoming tachycardic. The blood pressure remains in the normal range even though in some cases the diastolic pressure may rise slightly. In small children and some adults there may be some mild tachypnea. Since in the compensated phase the body's defenses maintain adequate blood pressure and vital organ perfusion, no changes in the level of consciousness occur.

When the patient's shock increases to the *decompensated phase* the skin becomes white and cold and there is marked diaphoresis. The pulse rate elevates with increasingly marked tachycardia. The blood pressure drops and some pulses become no longer palpable. The level of consciousness alters, progressing from disorientation to unconsciousness. As decompensation progresses the skin can become waxy, mottled, or grey looking. The tachycardia can progress to over 140 or to a bradycardia. The blood pressure continues to fall. When low enough, only a systolic reading may be obtainable. The patient will progress to coma and usually become incontinent.

The chart presented below is a useful summary:

SHOCK ASSESSMENT		
	Compensated	**Decompensated**
Pulse	⬆ tachycardia	⬆⬆ marked tachycardia can progress to bradycardia
Skin	pale, cool & moist	white, "waxy," cold, marked diaphoresis
Blood Pressure	normal range	⬇ lowered
Level of Consciousness	unaltered	altered, ranging from disoriented ➡ coma

It is important to note that a drop in blood pressure and changes in the level of consciousness are **late** signs of shock and indicate progressing decompensation.

CHECKING THE MOTOR, SENSORY AND DISTAL CIRCULATORY STATUS IN ALL FOUR EXTREMITIES (MSC × 4)

Motor or sensory deficits in the extremities of a responsive patient may result from brain injury, spinal cord injury, or injury to a limb(s). Similarly, a deficit in distal circulation may reflect a reduction in systemic circulation resulting in hypotension and peripheral hypoperfusion, or compromised circulation in that limb. Each of the above represents a serious emergent problem. Some commonly used terms will be useful:

Hemiparesis—weakness on one side of the body

Hemiplegia—paralysis of one side of the body

Hemianesthesia—numbness or tingling on one side of the body

Paraparesis—weakness in both lower extremities

Paraplegia—paralysis of the lower portion of the body including both legs

Para-anesthesia—numbness or tingling in both lower extremities

Quadraplegia—paralysis of all four extremities (commonly the body from the neck down)

Motor or sensory deficits on one side (hemi) of the body indicate injury to (or loss of some functions of) the brain. Bilateral neurological deficit below a given point in the body (but not above it) indicates spinal cord injury. A deficit in only one limb generally indicates injury to that limb or to the nerves that innervate it. It is important to note that a lack of neurological deficit in the extremities does not allow one to rule out brain, spinal column, or limb injury. To avoid unnecessary movement from limb-to-limb, all three—motor ability, sensory response, and distal circulation—are checked consecutively in one limb, then in the next limb, and so on. To evaluate if the strength is bilaterally equal (the same on both sides), one must also check the strength of the hand grasp (or of the feet when pushing) simultaneously on both sides.

Motor ability, sensory response, and distal circulation in all four extremities is abbreviated as "MSC x 4", or simply "MSC". When all are normal they are recorded as "MSC x 4 intact" (or "normal"), or "MSCs intact". If deficits are found the EMT should record them and in which limb they were found, then write "other MSCs intact".

1. To determine if strength is bilaterally equal or if any hemiparesis exists, the EMT should extend both his hands toward the patient with only the first two fingers of each hand extended. Next, instruct the patient to grasp your outstretched fingers with both his hands simultaneously and to squeeze them as hard as he can. Note whether the grasp is bilaterally equal or weaker on one side. If the patient has an injured arm or hand, the same check can be made by having him simultaneously push against your hands with his feet.

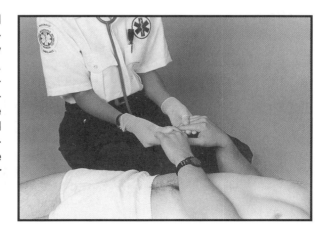

2. In checking the MSCs in all four extremities, start with one arm. In order to check the **motor ability,** instruct the patient to wiggle the fingers of that hand and note if he can or can not move them.

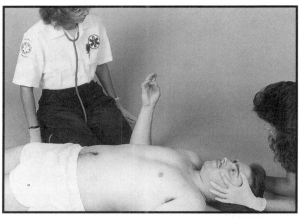

3. To check the **sensory response** in the arm, you will want to use your bandage (EMT) scissors or a similar object. Hold the scissors open by their pivot point and note that one tip is pointed and one tip has a blunt flat end. Explain what you are doing and demonstrate the feel of each by pressing first one and then the other carefully onto the sensitive back of the hand, describing the pointed tip as "sharp" and the flat tip as "blunt". Have the patient look away and instruct him to tell you when he first feels the object touch and whether it feels sharp or dull. Then press one of the tips onto the top of the hand and note his response. Some protocols simply limit the check to feeling the touch.

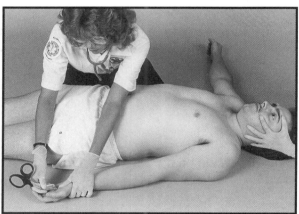

4. To check the **distal circulation** in the arm, palpate the radial pulse. In cases where distal pulses are not palpable, the distal circulation should still be checked using either a capillary refill or by comparing the temperature of the limb to the others. (The reason why the formerly used term "Motor, Sensory and Pulses MSP x 4" has been changed to MSC x 4). Note the result. Next, move to the other arm and repeat the steps.

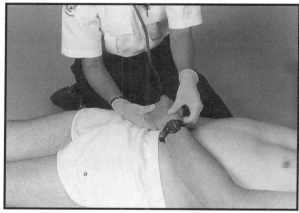

5. Next, check the MSCs in one leg. Have the patient wiggle his toes or, if the patient is wearing shoes, have him move his foot. Check the sensory response on the dorsum of the foot and then check the pedal pulses. If the patient is hypotensive, cold, elderly or has the Pneumatic Anti-Shock Garment applied the pedal pulses may not be palpable. In such cases check the distal circulation in the leg by feeling and comparing the foot's temperature with the other foot and that of the hands, or by using the capillary refill test. Lastly, check the MSCs in the other foot.

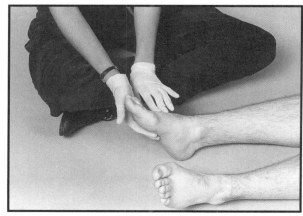

CHECKING THE PUPILS—INTRODUCTION

The eyes are checked as part of the neurological examination since, if uninjured, the pupils and their reactions can reflect altered brain function (and the resulting neurological deficit) from injury to the brain, increased intracranial pressure, or chemical changes. The acronym PEARRL is used. It stands for:

P—Pupils

E—Equal

A—And

R—Round

R—Regular in size

L—React to light

The pupil is normally round in shape. It is a circular hole which appears to be a black dot in the center of the pigmented iris. It serves as an optical diaphragm, varying its size between 1.5mm and 8mm depending on the strength of the available light. At normal levels of light the pupil appears mid-sized. When less light is available the pupil dilates, allowing more of the light to enter the eye and making it possible to see in dim light. When light levels are high or a bright light is suddenly introduced the pupil constricts, allowing less light to enter protecting the sensitive tissue of the retina from damage. Based upon sensory information regarding light levels that the brain receives from the eye, it regulates the pupil's size by sending command messages through the third cranial nerve (called the oculomotor nerve) to the muscles of the iris. Changes in the iris' muscle cells surrounding the pupil result in its rapid dilation or constriction.

Normally both pupils are equal (within 1mm) and remain equal as they change size in response to different light levels. When a bright light is introduced into one eye (or higher levels of light enter one eye than the other), due to a **consensual reaction** both pupils constrict equally to the appropriate size for the pupil receiving the most light. In the total absence of any light no motor commands are issued and the pupils are relaxed and fully dilated. When a little light is introduced they constrict slightly. As the light level rises they constrict more and more. When the pupils are any size other than fully dilated, constant stimuli from the brain along both left and right intact oculomotor nerve pathways are necessary to maintain the pupils' size and equality. Pupillary size normally changes instantly (briskly) when the light changes. In the absence of any eye injury a lack of reaction to light (fixed pupils), abnormal or sluggish reactions to light, significantly unequal pupils, or a lack of consensual reaction when a bright light is introduced into one eye, must be assumed to result from insult to the brain or one of the oculomotor nerves. In some cases with increased intracranial pressure, the oculomotor nerve on one side becomes compressed and stimuli can no longer pass along it. Since the muscles of the iris on the same side (ipsilateral) no longer receive motor commands to constrict, they relax and the pupil becomes fully dilated and fixed—no longer reacting to light. This is called a "blown pupil".

Drugs, both topical or systemic, will also affect the pupils. Central Nervous System depressants can result in sluggish or unreactive pupils. Atropine and other parasympathic drugs will cause the pupils to dilate regardless of light. Opiates cause severe constriction often resulting in "pinpoint" fixed pupils.

EXAMINING THE PUPILS—PEARRL

The pupils are usually examined in normal light levels by first looking at them for shape, size and equality, and then by checking their reactiveness and consensual reflex by introducing and removing a bright light into each eye. The normal size (at regular room light levels) is described as either "normal", "regular", or "mid-sized". If they are considerably larger than normal they are described as "large" or "dilated", and if considerably smaller as "small", "constricted" or (in the extreme) "pinpoint". If normal in every regard they may collectively be described as "Pupils are equal, round and reactive", or "PEARRL normal".

1. Facing the patient, move close and look at each eye for any injury or obvious abnormality. Next look at each pupil in turn, noting whether it is normal and round or otherwise. Move back slightly and look at both pupils simultaneously. Check if they are equal or unequal and if the size appears normal for the light level which is present.

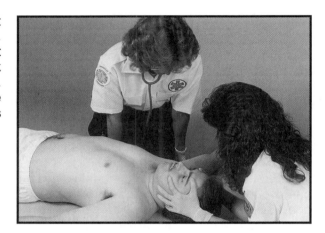

2. Turn on your examining light and hold it anterior to but slightly away from one side of the head so the light is not in the eye. If the patient is conscious tell him what you are going to do. If he is unconscious you will need to hold the eye lids open on both eyes simultaneously while examining the pupils.

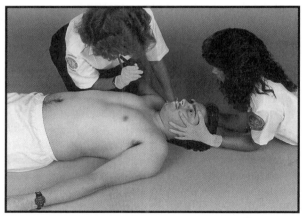

3. While looking at the pupil of the eye on the side of the flashlight, move the flashlight medially until it shines directly into that eye. Note if the pupil's reaction is normal constriction, sluggish, or unresponsive. Next move the flashlight laterally until the light no longer shines in the eye. Once the light is removed, check that the pupil returns briskly to its previous size.

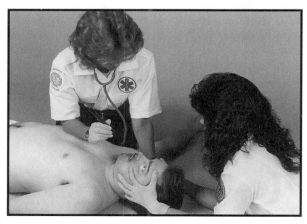

4. After a few seconds, move the flashlight medially and reintroduce the light in the same eye as first, but observe the **other** pupil. Note if this pupil constricts normally when the light is introduced into the initial eye or if the consensual reaction is absent. Then remove the light source from the initial eye while observing if the second pupil returns briskly to its normal size.

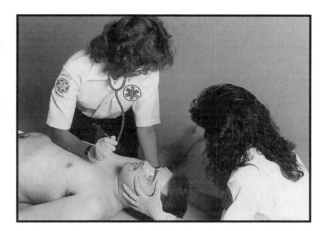

5. Now repeat steps 3 and 4, introducing the light each time into the second eye to evaluate its reactiveness and to determine if an intact consensual reflex causes constriction of the initially examined pupil.

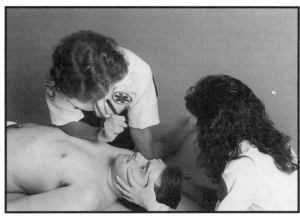

Note: When placed in a sufficiently bright environment even normal pupils will not react to the introduction of additional light since they are already maximally constricted and unable to close any further. To ascertain whether they are reactive or fixed, the EMT should block out rather than introduce light. Cover both of the patient's eyes with your hands to completely block out the light. After a few seconds lift the bottom of one hand just enough to see the pupil and allow indirect light to reach the eye. The shaded pupil should become approximately normal in size. Next, slowly lift that hand and completely remove the shading. If the eye is functioning normally it should again maximally constrict as bright light is reintroduced. Repeat the process in the other eye.

Note: Sometimes the acronym PEARRLA is used. The last "**A**" stands for "accommodation"—an additional examination (not commonly done pre-hospital) which ascertains if the pupil's reaction to accommodation is normal. For this, an object such as a pen is held upright a foot or so from the patient's face and then is moved to almost touching the tip of his nose. Both eyes will normally converge and focus on the object as it gets closer. When it is about 20mm from each pupil, the pupils constrict as a result of *near-point contraction*. These two reactions together are commonly reported (although technically a misnomer) as "normal reaction to accommodation".

EXAMINATION OF THE CHEST—INTRODUCTION

The chest is examined using three methods:

- **Observation**
- **Palpation**
- **Auscultation**

These examinations are commonly performed in the above sequence, but at times priorities may require some changes. They provide the EMT with key information about the patient's respiratory quality and identify significant injuries to or conditions of the thorax.

The chest can not be observed and properly examined through clothing. The common lack of privacy in the pre-hospital setting can make this a problem when examining a female patient. In most cases a female patient's chest can be properly observed and examined by opening or pulling-up the jacket, blouse or sweater without removing the patient's brassiere. If the patient is not wearing a brassiere, the clothing can be partly opened or pulled away at the upper thorax and then partly pulled up from the bottom, allowing for sufficient examination without the need to bare the breasts in the field. Although it is easier to palpate and auscultate the exposed chest it can be palpated through thin clothes and can be auscultated by inserting and moving the head of the stethoscope under the clothing. The EMT will have to determine how best to do this based upon the situation, degree of injury, and the need to maintain body heat.

A book can not teach the various feelings palpated under the hand or the identification of the different breath or heart sounds. The latter can be introduced using audio or video tapes, but are ultimately learned by actual supervised auscultation in a clinical environment. The physiological meaning of the different sounds and their diagnostic implications are presented in the EMT course and in your primary textbook. The approach here is limited to a demonstration of the physical examining steps and a discussion of the items to be examined for at each of them.

To communicate the difference between the presence of constant pain, pain which is only present with the taking of a breath, and a pain which is only produced upon palpation different terms are used. Pain which only comes with inspiration, or otherwise rhythmically with each breath, or with any deep breath, is called **pleuritic pain.** Pain which only occurs when an area is touched, pressed, or firmly pushed against is described as **pain-on-palpation,** or by the common abbreviation **"POP".**

OBSERVATION OF THE CHEST

When initially observing the bared anterior chest the EMT should confirm that the chest rise and rate appear adequate, and in trauma victims the chest should be scanned to make sure that there is no segment of the chest wall that moves paradoxically (moving in and out in the opposite direction to the rise and fall of the rest of the chest), no sucking chest wound, and no wound with any significant external bleeding. If a sucking wound is found the lateral and posterior chest will have to be examined as well to locate or rule-out the possibility of an additional sucking exit wound. If ventilation is inadequate or a flail segment, sucking wound, or any significant external hemorrhage is found, the appropriate intervention should be provided before going any further.

Continue evaluating the chest excursion. Is the patient splinting or guarding any part of the chest? Does the chest excursion appear to have bilateral symmetry or is there less chest rise on one side than on the other? If so, which side? If chest excursion is not equal on both sides, is the chest symmetrical at peak inflation or full deflation? If it is symmetrical at full deflation, when the lungs are basically empty, and less or no rise occurs on the injured side upon inspiration, this indicates limited inspiration on one side (such as would occur with a pneumothorax on that side). If however the chest is only symmetrical at or near peak inspiration, and becomes asymmetrical as the patient exhales, this indicates that inspired air is trapped in one side of the mediastinum and can not be purged by exhalation. The presence of a tension pneumothorax should be suspected. Observe if there is any intercostal (area between the ribs) or sternal retraction with each breath. Is there any intercostal bulging? If yes, does it come and go with each breath, or is it present at all times regardless of the breathing cycle?

Next, scan the chest from top to bottom and look for other wounds, bruised or ecchymotic areas, deformities, subcutaneous emphysema, or burns. Note any that are seen and consider the potential underlying or associated injuries these may indicate. Also note if any surgical scars are present and consider their implications (such as previous removal of a lung or implantation of a cardiac pacer). Lastly, from your findings and consideration of the potential need to protect the spine, evaluate whether the posterior thorax needs to be observed also. Once observation of the chest is completed, proceed to palpation.

PALPATING THE CHEST

The primary palpation of the chest is performed early in the examining sequence to confirm the adequacy and symmetry of chest rise and to identify (or rule-out) closed injuries of the chest beyond those that can be observed.

Palpating along the length of each individual rib in sequence is overly time consuming and missed areas can result from confusion or because the posterior thorax is often not readily available early in the trauma exam. Because the thoracic cage is a contiguous cylindrical structure (except the lowermost pair of "floating" ribs on each side), when the EMT squeezes the antero-lateral aspect of the chest as the patient inhales, any injuries along the entire circumference of the portion of the thoracic cage being palpated (not just the limited part of each rib that lies directly under the EMT's hands) will be identified by pain-on-palpation, untofore pathological movement indicating a lack of normal thoracic continuity, or by crepitus (a grating feeling produced by the rubbing together of broken bone ends). To ensure that every area of the thoracic cage is stressed, the chest will have to be palpated in four areas; the upper thorax, the mid-thorax, the posterior lower thorax, and over the sternum.

1. Rest your hands lightly on the anterior lateral margin of the rib cage. First feel the presence of chest rise and evaluate its adequacy. Next feel if there is bilateral symmetry of chest excursion or if it is diminished on one side. If there is less excursion on one side than the other, determine whether this reflects a lack of chest rise (inflation) or lack of chest fall (ability to purge air) on the injured side.

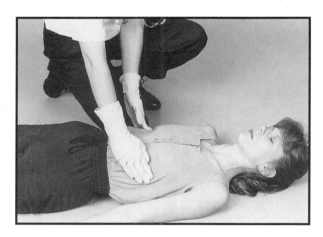

2. Next, place the heel of each hand on the anterior upper thorax so the fingers surround the anterior curve of the chest wall with the fingertips on the mid axillary line and the thumbs extended on the anterior chest pointing towards the suprasternal notch. Spread the fingertips apart so the first finger's tip is in the axilla and the rest cover as large a part of the lateral aspect of the thorax below the axilla as is comfortable. Your hands from the tips of each thumb to the edge of each little finger should contact the upper third of the thorax containing the first five ribs.

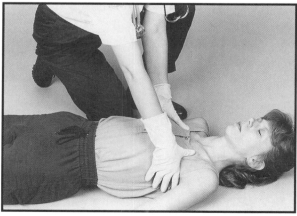

3. Squeeze the thorax by applying pressure medially with the fingers of both hands while simultaneously pushing posteriorly with the extended thumbs, and instruct the patient to take a deep breath. Does he complain of pain, wince, or guard, limiting his degree of inhalation? Any of these would indicate that there is pain-on-palpation. Note if you felt any untofore movement or crepitus. Ask the patient to resume normal breathing and release the pressure.

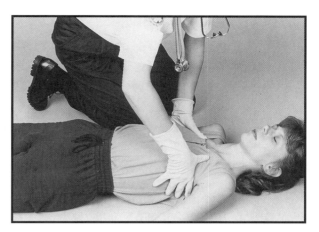

4. Maintaining the exact previous posture of your hands and fingers, move your hands down the thorax until the tip of the little finger is just over the lowest aspect of the ribcage at the mid-axillary line and the anterior part of one (or more) ribs is still felt below each thumb. Your hands contain the mid and part of the lower thorax containing the 5th thru the 10th rib. In the same way as previously described, squeeze producing circumferential pressure and have the patient inhale. Note any POP, untofore movement, or crepitus. Instruct the patient to breathe normally and release your pressure.

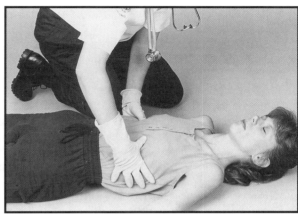

5. The lowermost two "floating" ribs are palpated by placing the heel of each hand on the mid axillary line at the lower thorax with the fingers and thumbs held together under the patient's flanks and then pressing anteriorly, note if there is any POP or crepitus. Since the ribs have no anterior connection, individual movement is expected. Pain-on-palpation in this area may indicate either injury to the lower thorax, diaphragm, flanks, lower spine, kidneys, or other retroperitoneal contents.

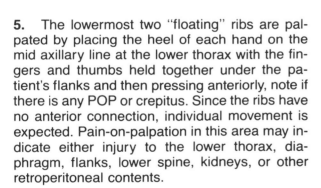

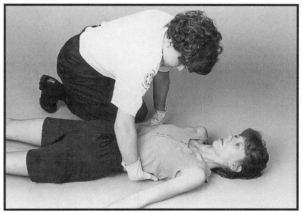

6. Lastly, to check the sternum for injury, place the fingers of one hand on the midline of the sternum—covering it from cephalad of the ziphoid process to the suprasternal notch—and press firmly. Note any deformity, POP, untofore movement, or crepitus.

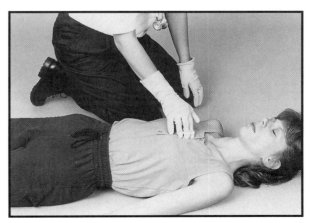

AUSCULTATING THE CHEST

The chest is auscultated to evaluate breath and heart sounds by isolating them using the stethoscope. Breath sounds are evaluated for depth, bilateral symmetry, and to identify any adventitious (abnormal, pathological) sounds that may be present. Heart sounds are evaluated to determine if their character is normal or abnormal, and if they are heard with usual clarity and amplitude or instead appear muffled or distant. The following is limited to a demonstration of the steps employed in auscultating the chest and does not include interpretation of the various breath and heart sounds.

Breath Sounds

Breath sounds are usually initially listened to over the midlung fields where they can be heard the loudest. The midlung can be auscultated anteriorly, laterally, or posteriorly. In the pre-hospital setting it is most commonly auscultated in the readily available anterior chest near the mid-clavicular line. In females a more superior mid-clavicular site, or a more lateral site such as on the anterior axillary line is recommended to avoid the sound reduction caused by the breast tissue and embarrassment.

Breath sounds are auscultated at the same location on both sides to determine if they are absent or diminished on one side, and to identify any adventitious sounds that may only be present on one side. As a lung collapses it retracts towards the mainstem bronchi. Therefore the apices and bases are also auscultated bilaterally since a lung progressively collapsing may result in absent or diminished breath sounds at either of these sites earlier than at the midlung. Sometimes with a hemothorax, as gravity results in blood collecting in the lower lung first, breath sounds may solely be absent or diminished at the bases. Similarly adventitious sounds caused by fluid in the lungs (such as basilar rales) are early often only heard at the bases.

Since the lungs are smaller at the apices and bases than at the midlung, the breath sounds heard in these locations are normally more quiet than those over the midlung field. Their character is different as well. Normal breath sounds are made up of two simultaneously heard elements: rhythmic **bronchial sounds** produced by the movement of air through the bronchi, and the constant low murmur-like **vesicular sounds** believed to come from the alveolar exchanges. Both sounds are said to be balanced at the midlung while the bronchial sounds are more dominant at the apices and quieter at the bases.

1. To auscultate the midlung fields on one side of the anterior thorax, place the head of the stethoscope on the mid clavicular line just above the nipple line (higher in females). Determine if breath sounds are present or absent. If present, estimate if the rate appears normal, too fast, or too slow. Then note the inspiratory and expiratory duration to evaluate the depth. Next, determine if any adventitious sounds are heard and, if present, identify the type and severity.

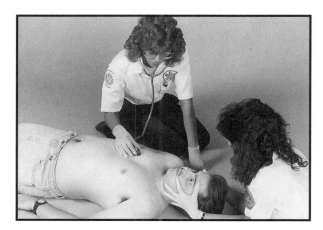

2. Move the stethoscope head to the same location on the opposite side of the anterior thorax and determine whether breath sounds are present on this side. If present you will want to compare the loudness (amplitude) of both sides. Since amplitude is hard to recall, listen while moving the stethoscope head back and forth from one midlung field to the other and note if the sounds are bilaterally equal or if they are diminished on one side.

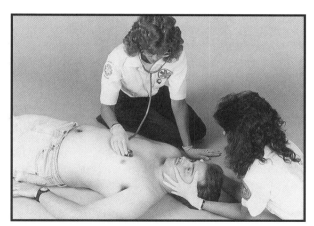

3. Next, auscultate the apices. Place the head of the stethoscope about an inch below the clavicle and just lateral to the outer edge of the sternum on one side. Determine if breath sounds are present. At the apices the sound is more bronchial (air movement) than vesicular (low murmur), and is quieter than over the midlung. Move your stethoscope back and forth from one apex to the other and note if sounds are diminished on one side or if any new adventitious sounds are heard.

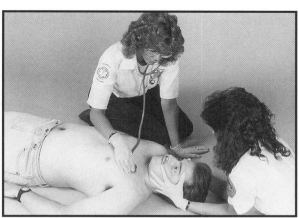

4. Next auscultate the bases. Since the posterior and lateral aspect of the base of the lungs extends three to four inches lower than at the mid-anterior thorax, the bases are auscultated at the mid axillary line between one and two inches cephalad of the palpable lower margin of the lateral rib cage. First auscultate each base for present breath sounds and any newly heard adventitious sounds (such as basilar rales). Then, by moving the stethoscope from one side to the other repeatedly, ascertain if the sounds are bilaterally equal or diminished on one side.

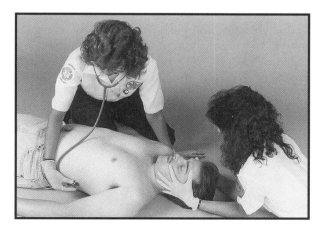

Heart Sounds

Once you have finished auscultating the breath sounds, the initial in-depth respiratory evaluation has been completed. After reviewing your findings and the interventions provided, you are ready to continue the examination of the thorax by auscultating the heart sounds.

Apical heart sounds, although not always taught, should be included in every assessment. Regardless of the EMT's level of training, only gross distinctions should be made in the field. Finer distinctions are difficult to make accurately and delay the assessment's progress in identifying conditions with a greater priority. Heart sounds should overall be categorized as *normal* or *abnormal.* Normal heart sounds (which the EMT needs to become familiar with by actual auscultation), have two distinct separate abutting sounds which are heard without interruption. Phonically they can be represented as **lŭb-dŭb,** sounded as two distinct syllables of a single word. Except with a brady-cardia less than 50, each beat follows the last without apparent pause, resulting in what sounds like a continuous stream of one then the other being heard alternately: lŭb-dŭb, lŭb-dŭb, lŭb-dŭb, and so on. A variety of abnormal sounds may be heard including a lack of distinction between the two sounds so that they are heard as one longer sound. With different abnormalities other sounds (fluid or "murmuring" sounds) may be heard in-between them.

In ascertaining if heart sounds are normal the EMT must also evaluate *how well* they can be heard. Normal heart sounds appear loud and are clearly heard as dominant and "nearby" through the stethoscope. If auscultated through fluid (as in cases with a hemothorax or pericardial tampon-ade), the heart sounds become muffled or "distant" sounding.

5. Heart sounds are auscultated with the head of the stethoscope placed just below and slightly medial to the left nipple. In females the head of the stethoscope is placed caudad of the left breast and moved up under it to place it near the heart's location. Listen and note if the heart sounds are normal or abnormal, and if they are of normal amplitude and clarity or appear muf-fled or distant.

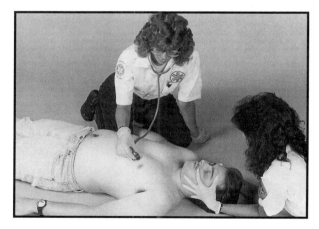

EXAMINATION OF THE ABDOMEN AND PELVIS—INTRODUCTION

Once the EMT has ascertained from the history if there is any abdominal pain, the partially bared abdomen is examined by visualizing it for injuries and to determine whether it appears normal or distended. Next, it is palpated to identify if it feels normal or rigid, if there is pain-on-palpation, and if there are any palpable masses. Lastly, the pelvis is palpated for injury as witnessed by pain-on-palpation, untofore movement, or crepitus.

With patients in shock the presence of a distended or painful abdomen, a palpable mass in the abdomen, signs of an unstable pelvis, or the presence of unexplained levels of shock (even if the abdomen is asymptomatic), must be assumed to be associated with intra-abdominal bleeding. Although intra-abdominal bleeding most commonly results from trauma, the EMT must note that it can also occur *in the absence of trauma* from such conditions as an intra-abdominal aneurysm, GI bleeding, or an ectopic pregnancy.

Abdominal pain is classically identified and reported as being in one or more of the four quadrants of the anterior abdomen. Due to the nature of the abdominal lining (the peritoneum) and its innervation, the fact that many abdominal organs lie in more than a single quadrant, and since blood or spilled caustic contents from an injured organ may cause irritation of the abdominal lining (peritonitis) in areas beyond that in which the organ lies, pain often appears in multiple locations or to be generalized throughout the abdomen. When the large muscles of the anterior abdominal wall are palpated the increased underlying pressure is reflected to an area more vast than that directly under the examiner's hand. This can produce pain in a broad area, making it difficult for the patient to accurately identify its specific location.

The objective of the initial pre-hospital abdominal examination is to identify the presence of any significant injury, external bleeding, intra-abdominal hemorrhage, or signs of a surgical abdomen— not to make a specific diagnosis. Since repeated palpation may result in additional injury to insulted organs, and in order to avoid needless delay, it is recommended that the examination of the abdomen be limited to: visualization, feeling the medial area for a mass, palpation of first one side then the other, and palpating the pelvis. Auscultation of bowel sounds is not recommended. Auscultation over the epigastrium is only recommended in patients who are being ventilated, to identify inadvertent gastric insufflation.

EXAMINING THE ABDOMEN

1. Scan the clothing covering the abdomen for bleeding and then expose the anterior abdomen. Except patients with multi-systems trauma, partially unfastening the covering clothing and lowering the top of the underpants to the upper margin of the genital area will sufficiently expose the abdomen for examination in the field. Observe the anterior abdomen for wounds, eviscerations, bruised or ecchymotic areas, scars, or the presence of a rash, and, note if the abdomen appears normal or distended.

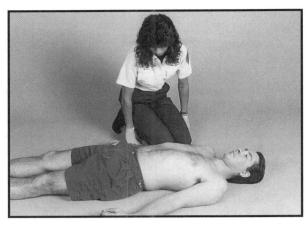

2. Place your hand on the mid-abdomen and feel if it is soft or rigid and distended. A rigid guarded abdomen suggests the presence of peritoneal irritation. When touched the abdomen may reflexively become rigid. If the patient can consciously overcome this guarding, allowing the abdominal muscles to relax, it is considered soft. Next feel if there is any palpable mass. If yes, is it pulsating (pulsatile)?

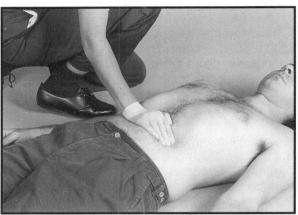

3. Next, rest your hand on one side of the abdomen so that the tips of your extended fingers are about 1½ to 2 inches lateral of the navel (umbilicus). Without moving the heel of the hand, firmly push the abdominal wall inward with the fingertips. From the patient's facial expression, guarding, or comments, note if this produces pain-on-palpation (POP). Without removing your hand slowly diminish the pressure until the abdomen has returned to its original relaxed position. *Do not release the pressure suddenly.*

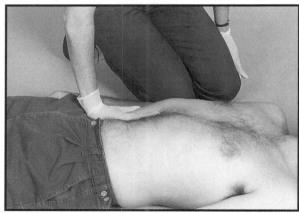

4. Repeat the procedure in Step 3 on the other side of the abdomen. If local protocols require palpation of all four quadrants, press with the fingertips in the center of each quadrant in turn. Additional palpation of the posterior retroperitoneal area for pain-on-palpation is not necessary since this area has already been palpated when checking the lower rib cage in the thoracic exam. Pain or POP in the flanks is commonly associated with the kidneys (or other retroperitoneal contents), but may also result from injury to the lower back.

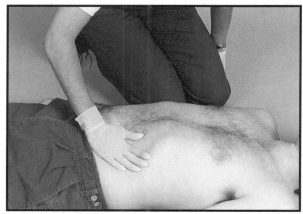

PALPATING THE PELVIS

After examination of the soft anterior abdomen continue by palpating the pelvis. If palpation with strong pressure produces either pain, untofore movement, or crepitus, a pelvic fracture with associated intra-abdominal hemorrhage must be assumed.

The bones of the pelvis are connected by fused, unmovable joints into a single solid ring-like structure. Any part of this structure moving independently is abnormal and is described as *untofore movement.* For any part to move independently one or more fractures or separations of the fused joints must have occurred. The palpation of any such movement, regardless of degree, represents a loss of continuity in the pelvic girdle making it unstable.

An unstable pelvis commonly has intra-abdominal or retroperitoneal hemorrhage associated with it. Based upon the amount of bleeding immediately post insult this may be symptomatic, producing both abdominal signs and signs and symptoms of profound shock, or it may initially be occult (hidden). In either event, progressive internal hemorrhage and shock must be assumed and managed pre-hospital in any patient with an unstable pelvis.

Patients with an unstable pelvis should not be logrolled except when use of an alternate method would result in a life threatening delay in meeting an urgent ABC need **or** in moving the patient out of danger. Timely use of the PASG (inflating all three chambers) will immediately promote tamponading and control of the intra-abdominal hemorrhage, and the inflated garment will support and splint the pelvis when moving the patient onto the longboard. A scoop stretcher or either a proper sliding or lifting method should be used, since even when splinted by the inflated PASG the patient should not be logrolled.

The sacrum is the weight-bearing base of the spinal column and the posterior center portion of the pelvic girdle. Due to the significant force necessary to fracture the pelvis, and because the sacrum is common to both the pelvic girdle and the spinal column, patients who have an unstable pelvis additionally must be considered to have an unstable spine and *require full spinal immobilization.*

1. Initial palpation of the pelvis is done by simultaneously applying bilateral pressure to the pelvis. After locating the iliac crests, place your hands so that they encircle the lateral pelvis with the thumb over the iliac crest on each side. Press strongly with both hands towards the midline and simultaneously rotate the hands slightly so that the thumbs apply firm anterior-to-posterior pressure on the iliac crests. Note if there is any POP, untofore movement, or crepitus.

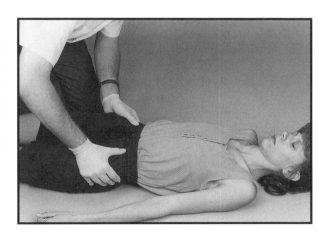

2. With some pelvic fractures, simultaneous bilateral pressure may not produce signs of an unstable pelvis. If the previous step was negative, locate the iliac crest on one side of the anterior pelvis and with the heel of the hand press firmly on it in an anterior-to posterior direction. Then, repeat the procedure, pressing on the other iliac crest. Note any POP, untofore movement, or crepitus. If an unstable spine is suspected, support one side of the pelvis while pushing on the other to avoid undue movement.

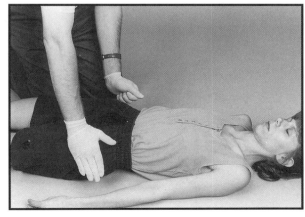

Note: If a hip or upper femur injury or any wounds, bruises, roadrash, etc., are under or very near the EMT's hands when palpating the pelvis, in the absence of untofore movement one can not identify if any POP or crepitus is from the pelvis or the other injury. Additional palpation at other locations on the pelvic girdle away from these injuries will allow one to make a determination. If POP or crepitus no longer results then one concludes the pelvis is stable and that these were from the other injuries. If the POP or crepitus is reproduced when the pelvis is palpated elsewhere, then one must assume the pelvis is the source and that it is unstable. If one can not make a clear determination, then the management must include appropriate treatment for a fractured hip, unstable pelvis, and an unstable spine.

SKILLS FOR OBTAINING THE PRE-HOSPITAL HISTORY

Obtaining a good history that includes all of the pertinent information, and organizing it into a precise meaningful report, is an art. Although some guidelines are included here, the EMT will need practice in a variety of situations in the field in order to become skilled in history taking.

The entire pertinent history is generally not obtained in a single isolated step. Instead, parts of it are elicited at different times during the physical examination. If alert and oriented, the patient should be the primary source of the history along with events that the EMT observes from the situation and scene. Additional useful information may often be obtained from a relative, a meaningful other, persons accompanying the patient, others involved, witnesses, or police officers at the scene. The EMT must be careful to note which information is from the patient and which is from others, and must carefully indicate in recording the history the source when it is other than the patient ("Mother states, no known allergies"; "According to witnesses, no unconscious period occurred post insult").

If the patient is unconscious, a small child, or non-verbal from another cause, the history will have to be obtained from the relative or other care giver at the scene, others involved, or witnesses. In such cases the EMT should also check the patient for any medical alert bracelet or neck medallion and the victim's wallet or purse for a medical information card or hospital identification card. If any such cards are found they should accompany the patient to the emergency department. The receiving emergency department can call the hospital which issued the identification card, regardless of its location, for any key history and even have them FAX items such as previous EKG's.

In an awake and alert patient the majority of information in the history comes from the patient's answers to a series of questions asked by the EMT. The clarity and accuracy of the answers (or the number of additional questions and explanations needed) is dependent upon how carefully the EMT selects the sequence in which the questions are asked and how precisely each question is worded. Clearer answers will be obtained from short simple questions. Complex or compound questions should be avoided. Only ask one question at a time, waiting for its answer to be completed before asking the next one. Use terms the patient is likely to understand, avoiding more technical medical language. For example, asking when the patient urinated last is more likely to be understood than asking when he voided last. Complete all of the questions surrounding one topic before going on to the next one. Jumping from one topic to another, then a third, and then returning to an earlier one will be confusing to both the patient and EMT.

There are two categories of questions: **open** and **directed.** Open questions ("Where do you hurt?", "How would you describe the pain?", Do you have any medical conditions?") cause the patient to answer solely in his own words. Since the question did not contain a variety of possible answers, the patient provides his impression without the chance that the wording of the question "lead" or influenced his answer. It is a good idea to begin each topic with one or more open questions to obtain the patient's uninfluenced response first. However, these often need to be followed by **directed** questions to obtain meaningful further qualification and quantification. Directed questions ("Do you have any chest pain?", "Would you describe the pain as sharp, dull, tearing, throbbing, crushing, burning, achy?") include either stated multiple choices from which the patient selects the most appropriate answer, or are implicitly limited to a "yes" or "no" choice. As well as obtaining more exacting answers, directed questions including numerical choices can help clarify vague descriptions of degree. If a patient says "it hurts lots", his response is unclear and subject to wide interpretation. If asked "On a scale of 1 to 10, how would you rate the pain?" and he responds with "seven", even though his choice is subjective he has communicated precisely without chance for differing interpretations of his impression. Another key use of directed questions is to rule-out specific items in the history. If one asks a patient where they hurt and their response does not include the chest, one is not sure whether they could have overlooked it, or it is overshadowed by worse pain elsewhere, *or* it truly is not present. Therefore, for key areas one specifically asks. For example, "Do you have any chest pain?". If the patient says "no", the EMT is sure it is not an oversight. This is reported as, "Patient denies chest pain".

The short pre-hospital history includes twelve components. Some of these contain information which is essential for the assessment and management of the patient. Others include information which, although not immediately necessary, will be useful for the hospital Emergency Department (especially if the patient's level of consciousness deteriorates).

Overview Of The Pre-hospital History

1. **Patient identification** (name, home address, telephone number).
2. **Name** (and phone or location) **of party to notify of the emergency.**
3. **Hospital and Doctor of record.**
4. **Age and sex.**
5. **Chief complaint** (and if trauma, mechanism of injury)
6. **Location** (type), **activity, and time of onset of incident.**
7. **History of this event or episode.**
8. **Previous medical history.**
9. **Medications, prescribed or taken.**
10. **Allergies.**
11. **Last meal eaten and any oral intake in last four hours.**
12. **Any unusual event in the last hour, day, week or month.**

The following is an amplification of the items included above:

Patient Identification—You will need the patient's name in order to address him or her, and the patient's full name, home address, and phone number are an important part of both the pre-hospital and hospital record.

Name of Party to Notify—Even though notification is commonly made either by the police or the hospital, the name and phone number or location of the person to be notified should be obtained early on by the EMT in case the patient is not able to provide this information later. Although notification usually is more a matter of comfort for the patient rather than a medical issue, in some cases it is pertinent to patient care in the Emergency Department based on additional history or permissions needed from the relative or other key party.

Hospital and Doctor of Record—In some cases this may be a factor in determining which hospital the patient is transported to. In all cases, even when the patient's doctor or hospital of record are not local, it will be useful for the Emergency Department to have should they need to contact either to obtain additional information about the patient's past history.

Age and Sex—These are important factors in the assessment since different problems are more commonly associated with different age groups and sexes. If the patient can not communicate his age to the EMT, it should be estimated and noted as "approximately" followed by the estimated age.

Chief Complaint (CC)—The chief complaint, and in cases of trauma the exact mechanism of injury, should be noted near the beginning of the history since these together with the **type of location, activity and time of onset** are often essential in understanding the rest of the history and the physical exam. For example, if the chief complaint is difficulty breathing, whether this started yesterday while sitting at home watching T.V., or today when mowing the lawn, or immediately after being the unrestrained driver in a motor vehicle accident, provides different frames of reference for the complaint and findings in the exam. When trauma is involved the mechanism should be described exactly, avoiding such vague comments as "fell". Instead, the EMT should be specific, "Patient fell down approximately 12 carpeted steps onto hardwood floor", or "Patient fell in carpeted living room without any apparent physical obstacle". In the case of motor vehicle accidents it is important to note if the patient was wearing restraints or not, and to note exactly what occurred including the degree of damage to the vehicle. Often the addition of a simple diagram will be useful. A chief complaint of "unconsciousness" is used for patients who do not respond to verbal stimuli along with any mechanism of injury and description of how found.

History of this Event or Episode (Hx)—The history of this episode includes information surrounding or leading up to this ambulance call, including events of the past hours and days if they are—or could be—associated with the present illness or injury. For the sake of clarity we have separately identified the chief complaint, mechanism of injury if trauma, the type of location, activity prior to onset, and the time of onset. In obtaining the history of the present illness the EMT should seek additional information, including other complaints and symptoms; whether onset was sudden or gradual; the location; type and severity of any pain; anything that exacerbates or alleviates the pain or condition; the course of events since onset; and any changes in level of consciousness prior to or since onset. Which questions still need additional elaboration, or which other questions should be asked, will vary on a case-by-case basis depending on the answers obtained to the preceding questions and the findings in the physical exam. Do not overlook the patient's environment or "social" events that may be a contributing factor, such as "Onset occurred after a family argument", or "Patient lives alone", etc.

Previous Medical History—Obtaining a complete "doctor's office" medical history is unnecessary and time consuming in the field. Pre-hospital the pertinent past history (PPHX) should be limited to include any previous episodes of a similar nature or same illness, and any past significant illnesses, conditions, injuries, or major surgery. After asking the patient if he has any past medical problems or conditions, the EMT should specifically ask if the patient has any history of:

- Heart problems
- Blood pressure problems
- Respiratory problems
- Diabetes or other sugar problems
- Seizures
- Stroke or repeated loss of consciousness
- Hepatitis, AIDS, tuberculosis, Alzheimer's disease, cancer, or other similar illnesses
- Loss or changes in normal body function
- Significant trauma

These directed questions will either identify an item not previously mentioned by the patient, or by his specific denial will allow the EMT to rule-out a history of each.

In some cases comments regarding the patient's general health add an important dimension to the history. Such comments as, "In a previously healthy child", or "Patient indicates frequent upper respiratory infections in the last year", can be important.

Medications—All medications prescribed for the patient should be listed and noted on the report. Be careful to write each clearly and exactly. Often if the EMT does not recognize a medication it is helpful to ask the patient what he takes it for. Sometimes a prescribed medication will indicate the history of a condition not previously mentioned. It is a surprisingly common occurrence to find a patient who has denied any heart condition and has Lasix or some other diuretic ("water pills") prescribed for him. Of the medications prescribed, ascertain which ones have been taken regularly and which specifically today. If any are prescribed on an "as needed" basis, ascertain if they have been taken and note why. Since often not included, be sure to ask if the patient has taken any non-prescription medications and note which and how frequently.

Allergies—Ascertain if the patient is allergic to any medications or foods. If yes, note "Allergic to . . ." and the name of the medication or food. If they have no history of any allergic reaction, record **"NKA"** (standing for "No known allergies") on your report. If the patient states that he has hay fever, or is allergic to pollen, dust, dog hair, cats, etc., these are included in the past history but are not the same as allergies to any medications or foods. The EMT should follow local guidelines as to whether persons solely allergic to such irritants but not any medications or foods should be noted as "NKA" or not.

Medications and Allergies, although a part of the past medical history, are usually noted separately as shown herein.

Last Meal Eaten and any Oral Intake in last four hours—The EMT should note when the patient ate his last full meal, and anything else that the patient has eaten, drank, or taken orally in the last four hours. Should the patient become unconscious and require surgery this will be key information for the anesthesiologist.

Any Unusual Event—Questioning if anything unusual occurred in the last hour, day, week, or month prior to the onset of illness or the accident often results in identifying an event which the patient does not relate to his condition but which, to trained medical personnel, could be related and may be extremely important. An answer such as:

"He fell and struck his head last month"

or, "I had a tearing pain in my shoulder just before I collapsed"

or, "I went SCUBA diving yesterday"

or, "My BMs have been almost black lately",

suggest possibilities and avenues for further examination that might otherwise not be initially considered.

Once the twelve components of the history have been learned the EMT may find the mnemonic **A M P L E** useful as a reminder of some of the key components. AMPLE stands for:

A — Allergies

M — Medications

P — Previous illnesses or injuries

L — Last meal/oral intake last 4 hours

E — Events preceding/associated with this episode (illness or injury)

Like most mnemonics, AMPLE is not complete. It has been included here since it is commonly found in texts as a guideline. The list presented in the *Overview of the Pre-hospital History* (found on the preceding pages) is more comprehensive and is recommended when initially learning and reviewing the components that should be included in a good pre-hospital history.

SKILLS FOR EVALUATING PAIN

Pain is one of the most common symptoms and chief complaints with which patients with an acute medical emergency or trauma present.

In trauma victims, pain is often a key tool in locating injuries either by its presence or its appearance when an area or part of the body is palpated or moved. It is generally explained by either the injuries found or by other signs of underlying injury and rarely requires further qualification in the field.

Patients with an acute medical emergency often present with pain which, since not associated with any identifiable injury, is initially unexplained. Pain is hard to describe. Initially patients will generally limit their comments to a general location and impression such as, "My stomach hurts a lot". By following a specific sequence of directed questions the EMT can systematically obtain more information. The following list will serve as a good guide for qualifying the pain further:

A Guide To Evaluating Pain
1. **Chief Complaint** (the pain or other problem)
2. **Location** (region and exact place)
3. **Radiation** (or other areas) **of pain**
4. **Severity** (quantification of strength)
5. **Onset** (time and activity when pain started)
6. **Associated signs and symptoms** (if any)
7. **Quality** (description of character)
8. **Persistence** (constant, intermittent, only when _____ ?)
9. **Course since onset** (duration, frequency, changes)
10. **Aggravation or Alleviation** (anything which does either)
11. **Previous History** (same or similar pain prior to this episode?)
12. **Any unusual occurrence** (prior to this episode)

The addition of the questions to be answered and some comments will provide a useful addition to the reader's understanding of this list.

Chief Complaint—The patient's chief complaint and whether it includes or is related to the pain provides a key context for the EMT's further evaluation of the pain.

Location—Where do you hurt? Point with your finger to the exact place where it hurts. Note the pain as "generalized" and the area if the patient can not provide a specific location.

Radiation—Is the pain only exactly where you pointed or does it radiate to or cover a larger area? If a larger area, show me the boundary of the area that hurts with your hand. Does the pain appear to travel from one area to another? Do you have pain anywhere else? If so, where?

Severity—Would you describe the pain as mild, moderate, or severe? On a scale of 1 to 10 (with one being the mildest and ten the strongest) how would you rate the pain?

Onset—Exactly when did the pain first start? What were you doing at the time the pain started? Just prior to it starting?

Associated Signs—and Symptoms—How did you feel otherwise when the pain started? Did you have any other symptoms (such as weakness, nausea, shortness of breath, etc.) Anything that started with or just prior to the pain? Anything that comes and goes with the pain?

Quality—In your own words describe what the pain feels like. Once the patient has described the pain go on to ask—which of the following would you include in describing the pain. Is it Dull? Sharp? Tearing? Throbbing? Burning? Crushing? Grating? Achy?

Persistence—Is the pain constant, intermittent (comes-and-goes seemingly by itself), or only present when provoked by some specific act or action (i.e; when touched, when moved, upon inspiration, with urination, etc.)?

Course since onset—Has it been present since onset? If it comes and goes, how often does it start (frequency) and for how long is it present (duration)? Have there been any periods without pain (relief from pain)? Has there been any change in its strength or quality since onset? Has there been any change in its frequency or duration since onset?

It is important for the EMT to differentiate between the interval in intermittent pain and a period without pain. For example, a patient in labor may have pains starting every five minutes and lasting about 45 seconds, but then may have a 30 minute period where these intermittent pains subside before they commence again.

Similarly, if the pain only occurs when provoked by some act or action (such as moving an arm), a period in which the provoking action has not occurred is not noted as a period without pain. Only a period in which no pain results from the provoking action would be considered as being without pain.

Aggravation or Alleviation—Is there anything which makes the pain worse? Is there anything which makes the pain better? Is there anything which makes the pain go away?

Previous History—Have you ever had the same pain (as present now) before? When was the last time? Was it the same strength, weaker, or stronger than this time? Is anything else different? Have you had it before that? How often? Has it been diagnosed by a physician? Did the physician give you any instructions or prescribe anything in the event that the pain returned?

Any Unusual Occurrence—Have you done any unusual activity, eaten or taken anything new or unusual, or has anything unusual occurred prior to the onset of the pain or in the last few days, weeks or month? Any illness, tiredness, change in body function; any falls or other injuries; any trips or unusual physical activity in the past weeks or months?

Although lengthy when presented in a written form which includes all of the possible questions, the pertinent questions and answers can be obtained from the patient in a few short minutes. It must be noted that in the case of urgent patients the initiation of transportation should not be delayed for lengthy questioning. Instead questions beyond the expanded AMPLE history should be asked in the ambulance while enroute to the hospital.

Once you have learned the 12 areas of questions for evaluating pain found in the preceding discussion, the alphabetical sequence—**O P Q R S T U** (in many texts limited to the "P Q R S T" method) may be useful in remembering the key areas of questions to ask. The letters, O, P, Q, R, S, T, U, stand for:

O—**Onset/Other findings**—When did it start? What activities preceded onset? Other associated signs and symptoms at onset?

P—**Provoking/Palliative**—What brought the pain on? Anything that makes it better or worse?

Q—**Quality**—What does it feel like?

R—**Region located/Radiation**—Where is the pain located? Does it radiate elsewhere? Any other places with pain?

S—**Severity**—On a scale of 1–10 how strong is the pain?

T—**Timing**—Is it constant, intermittent, or felt only when provoked? Frequency and duration? At any time in the past have you had the same or similar pain?

U—**Unusual**—Any unusual occurrence, or unusual signs and symptoms associated with the pain or event.

PART B
Doing The Patient Assessment

AN INTRODUCTION TO PATIENT ASSESSMENT

Patient assessment includes a variety of different components in addition to the hands-on physical examination. Unquestionably a good physical exam is the central and largest element of the assessment; however further details, significant confirmations, and additional vital pieces of information not otherwise available can be obtained from the other components. The components of the pre-hospital assessment are:

- Evaluation of safety
- Evaluation of the scene and situation
- Mechanism of injury or reason EMS was called (nature of the problem)
- Chief complaint(s)
- Physical exam
- History of this episode (or event)
- Pertinent past history
- Evaluation of findings, clinical impression
- Monitoring of patient's condition with periodic rechecking of key indicators

Additional non-assessment items (e.g., interventions, packaging, initiating transport, reporting, etc.) require steps that should occur at specific places within the assessment sequence. Since these need to be learned in the context of the overall assessment they have been integrated into the patient assessment skills presented in the ensuing pages.

CRITERIA FOR SEQUENCING OF ASSESSMENT PARTS

The primary criteria which determine the order in which the individual steps in the assessment are performed are the degree of danger and the urgency for identifying and providing care for each condition or injury that *could be* present. The sequence is established so as to identify the most urgent items first, then items of lesser urgency, and lastly, items which are not urgent. In the order of urgency, the priorities are to identify:

1. *Any dangers* at the scene (evaluate safety, scene, situation, mechanism, spine needs).
2. Overall LOC, respiratory and circulatory status to determine *any need to immediately provide management for:* the airway, ventilation, cardiac arrest, shock, or external hemorrhage (prior to further assessment and identification of the individual conditions causing the deficit).
3. *Immediately* life-threatening conditions/injuries.
4. Any other conditions/injuries whose systemic impact *could become life-threatening.*
5. *Other conditions/injuries with systemic implication.*
6. *If the patient is URGENT,* requiring initiation of transport without further delay, or NON-URGENT indicating additional assessment and care should continue prior to moving and transporting.
7. Any localized individual conditions/injuries which could result in *loss of limb or permanent disability.*
8. *Any other localized conditions/injuries.*

Examining the patient separately for each priority in-turn is unnecessary and would be both redundant and time consuming. By combining those of similar urgency into larger categories a more practical limited number of key parts (with evident priorities) can be identified in the examining sequence. The list suggests three distinct categories of priorities:

1. Identification of *immediately* life-threatening conditions/injuries.
2. Identification of *other* conditions/injuries which could become life-threatening or have a significant systemic impact.
3. Identification of *localized* conditions/injuries having **NO** life-threatening potential).

UNDERSTANDING CURRENT PROBLEMS IN PRE-HOSPITAL ASSESSMENT

To learn and intelligently apply any compound branching skill one must understand the various problems, choices, and rationales for its separate parts and overall sequence. In the case of the pre-hospital assessment it is essential to know its historical evolution in order to fully understand the rationale and application of its contents.

Classically, since the earliest days of EMS, the patient examination has been taught as having two parts: the **Primary Exam** and the **Secondary Exam** (sometimes called the *Primary Survey* and the *Secondary Survey*). Time has shown this to be an oversimplification resulting in confusion over the exact meaning of these terms and which steps each includes.

There is universal agreement that examination steps to identify airway patency, spontaneous respiration, adequate air exchange, appropriate chest excursion, dyspnea, a palpable pulse, pulse quality (strength, estimated rate, and regularity), quality of peripheral perfusion (skin color, temperature, moisture), other major signs and symptoms of shock, external hemorrhage, gross level of consciousness (expanded AVPU), are parts of the Primary Examination. There is also universal agreement that the steps performed in a head-to-toe examination to identify localized individual musculoskeletal and soft tissue injuries are parts of the Secondary Examination.

However, no standard or agreement exists surrounding items such as observation and palpation of the neck; observation and palpation of the abdomen; palpation of the pelvis; quantitative vital signs; PEARRL; evaluation of left and right, inferior and superior motor ability and sensory responses, and determining if oriented to person, place, and time; etc. Some instructors (and texts) include these as part of the Primary Examination. Some include them as part of the Secondary Examination. Others divide the list, including some of the items in each; still others—although including this list as part of the Secondary Exam—teach that different individual items from this group may need to be moved into the Primary exam on a patient-by-patient basis depending upon the initial findings.

As a result of these differing definitions no universal understanding exists of where the Primary Examination ends and Secondary Examination begins. In years past since the Secondary exam was done immediately following the Primary exam in all patients, the overall sequence of individual steps was unchanged regardless of which of the preceding definitions one used. The distinction was solely semantic, and as such did·not impact on the quality of care the EMT provided.

The significant conceptual changes in the past few years, which introduced the need to identify urgent patients early in the assessment process and recognize the different needs and priorities of *urgent* and *non-urgent* patients, have made it essential that students clearly understand the content definitions of each part of the assessment sequence and, which assessment items need to be included and managed prior to initiating transport or making the determination that no urgency exists. A lack of clarity and understanding of these definitions can result in the omission of key steps and interventions prior to initiating transport, or unnecessary delay while steps of little or no value for an urgent patient are completed. Either could have a serious impact on the quality of care and patient outcome.

As the EMT curriculum changes presently in process are introduced and phased in at varying times throughout the country, even more new terms and definitions will be used from one course to another and in the different editions of the available textbooks, resulting in even greater confusion in learning and retaining the many steps included in this complex skill.

The varying definitions of the Primary and Secondary examination contents are a by-product of the number of revisions made in the EMT curriculum since its onset in the 1970's and the way in which they were made. Over this greater than twenty year period, numerous piece meal additions and modifications of previous additions and modifications occurred. In recent years, even the inclusion of the vast conceptual changes surrounding the assessment and management of urgent patients did not result in the authorship of a newly-organized, entirely rewritten, clear assessment presentation which no longer included the terms "Primary Examination" and "Secondary Examination". Unfortunately, these terms' genesis in the earliest EMT training, and their longevity as accepted "cornerstone" assessment terms have made curriculum writers and instructors loathe to discard them even though their lack of universally accepted meaning has rendered them obsolete. Probably nothing proves the extent of the problem or the need for a new approach more strongly than the fact that Patient Assessment continues to be the single most failed practical skill station in tests throughout the country.

Over the past years the authors of this book have constantly struggled with the aforementioned problems in the presentation of the patient assessment sequence as they, singly or in combination, served on a variety of EMS course curriculum development committees, skill testing criteria revision committees, advisory boards, panels and conference faculties and as co-authors of other works. Several of them were charged with the task of developing a newly-organized complete assessment teaching sequence that would present the material in a precise easily learned progression that would be meaningful when used with any of the different individual course or textbook sequences presently taught or previously learned. The new teaching sequence they developed is found in the pages that follow.

NEW COMPREHENSIVE PATIENT ASSESSMENT SKILLS SEQUENCE

The new patient assessment sequence presented here is comprehensive. As well as the steps in the actual physical examination, it contains steps representing the other elements needed for a thorough patient assessment from initial arrival at the scene to transfer of the patient at the hospital. Even places in the sequence where a key cognitive thought process should occur, have been identified as steps (such as, reviewing previous findings and arriving at conclusions).

The sequence has been divided into six major parts with several sub-parts identified within each. Dividing the list of individual steps into titled parts is essential for learning and retention of the numerous steps. The title of each part is an important collective term, clearly identifying the purpose and priority of the group of steps involved. Similarly, the labels of sub-parts signal a change of focus or specific activity within a part. Because of the variety of meanings and the confusion surrounding terms commonly used, new labels for the parts and sub-parts have been developed. To avoid the potential for even greater confusion by the introduction of new terms, titles for the sub-parts were selected which describe the nature of the activity in self-evident or (when once introduced), clear language (ie. "Safety", "Global Survey", "In-depth A, B, C, D, Examination", "Review Findings", "Additional Localized Item Examination", etc.) For ease of understanding and learning, the titles selected for the parts are either a self explanatory collective term (PART V—Monitor) or are compounded from the elements contained (PART I—Safety, Scene, Situation, and Spine).

The six parts into which the assessment sequence is divided are:

PART I—Safety, Scene, Situation, and Spine (Size-up)

PART II—Initial Systemic Examination

PART III—Review, Re-evaluate, Rule-Out and Rank

PART IV—Additional Localized Item Exam, Packaging, and Transport

PART V—Monitor

PART VI—Radio, Report, and Record

PART I—Safety, Scene, Situation and Spine: This earliest part of the assessment occurs from receipt of the call information from the dispatcher to the time the EMT is at the patient's side. The "size-up" includes three sub-parts, each with a different key focus. Upon arrival the EMT should assess the scene and situation. The first consideration is to evaluate and assure that the scene is safe. The second is to identify generally what happened (the nature of the call) and the number of patients involved. Any additional EMS units or other rescue resources that may be needed should be summoned at this time. The third is to obtain more specific information about the event.

In the case of a trauma victim, as the EMT approaches the victim he should determine the specific mechanism of injury involved (type of collision and damage to the vehicle, or height and nature of a fall etc.) The exact mechanism of injury increases the EMT's suspicions that certain injuries may be present, and is the predominant factor in determining if the potential of spine trauma and the need for immediate and thereafter continuous spinal immobilization exists.

In a medical emergency, information about what events precipitated the calling of an emergency ambulance (why called) provide key information analogous to that provided by the mechanism of injury in trauma. Generally, while the person who greets the EMT is leading him to the patient's location he provides information about the patient's complaints or problems, their duration, the events preceding the episode, and if there are previous episodes or any known medical history. Additional information is observed from the social situation and where and how the patient initially presents. One can generalize this part of the assessment as being the considerations and information one obtains prior to being at the patient's immediate side.

PART II—Initial Systemic Examination: When examining a patient, vast general information can be obtained in a few seconds. As greater depths of detailed information are sought for each area of investigation, more and more time is required. Therefore, the initial physical examination is limited to finding (and intervening in) or ruling out any items with systemic impact or which experience shows commonly have a significant systemic implication. Additional examination and the time required to identify and manage individual localized items is deferred to a later time in the assessment sequence after all systemic conditions have been identified and resolved.

The impact commonly associated with items which have a systemic implication varies depending on the different nature and resulting pathophysiology of each. Some, which have vast impact on the neurological, respiratory, circulatory or bio-chemical status of the body, produce critical systemic deficits immediately post insult, or have the potential for producing rapid deterioration while the patient is in the EMT's care. Others have a slower course and do not commonly progress to an acute emergency. Although there are different levels of urgency, the EMT must consider any patient with a condition associated with systemic impact as potentially unstable until further examination at the hospital. Two *pessimistic* pre-conceptions are essential when initiating the physical examination. The EMT must assume that:

- **The patient has several conditions/injuries which require immediate identification and intervention if imminent death is to be avoided.**

- **The patient also has every other life threatening (or potentially life-threatening) condition or injury that could exist, until proven otherwise.**

The sequencing of the Initial Systemic Examination reflects these assumptions and the priorities and scope they imply. The examination has two identifiable sub-parts.

First, a 15 to 30 second **Global Survey** is performed to identify any critical interventions that need to be initiated immediately. (It must be noted that in trauma victims the need for spine protection has been previously evaluated from the mechanism of injury. If indicated, a second EMT would provide manual immobilization immediately). After noting the patient's age group, sex, and how he presents, the EMT determines if the patient: is conscious or unconscious, has a patent airway or requires airway management, has adequate spontaneous respiration or needs assisted or provided ventilation, has normal breathing or requires supplemental oxygen, has a pulse (heart beat) or requires CPR, has normal perfusion or shock requiring initiation of BLS shock care, has a normal temperature or appears either too hot or too cold, and has any significant external hemorrhage requiring bleeding control. Additional information is gained from the patient's general appearance, his ventilatory pattern and effort, the pulse quality, skin, the patient's ability to move spontaneously, how he moves, his verbal responses, and his complaints. As well as identifying immediate critical intervention needs, the Global Survey provides the EMT with a rapid gross evaluation of the patient's neurological, respiratory and circulatory functions which together are the key indications of his general condition. The gross evident nature of the indicators included in the Global Survey allow for the simultaneous gathering of a multiplicity of information rather than requiring organization into a prioritized series of separate steps. Once the EMT has obtained a general impression of the patient's condition, and the need for critical immediate interventions has been met or ruled out, it is safe to move on to a more in-depth and time consuming examination of key areas.

The second phase (sub-part) of the Initial Systemic Examination is the rapid **In Depth A, B, C, D Examination.** Its purpose is to examine vital parts and functions of the body in greater detail and depth to identify the presence or absence of specific conditions/injuries with systemic implication, and to further qualify and quantify the level of the patient's vital functions. By a designed progression of examining steps which include observing, feeling, listening and measuring, it identifies the presence or absence of signs and symptoms which, not being immediately apparent, require additional specific examining steps. For example, readily apparent items such as the presence of a patent airway, spontaneous respiration, and whether breathing appeared normal or labored, were evaluated in the global survey. The additional respiratory information one needs requires a number of additional specific steps and more time. Therefore, examining the mouth and mucosa; observing and palpating the neck; observing, palpating and auscultating the chest; counting the exact respiratory rate; (and from these, qualifying the respiratory quality and identifying conditions/injuries of the neck, thorax and entire respiratory system) are done in the In-Depth A, B, C, D Examination.

Although gross deficits with an immediate need for intervention were identified and needed interventions were started during the Global Survey, not all urgent items have been identified without the more in-depth examination done in this phase. Therefore, this further in-depth examination generally follows the priorities of:

A—Airway

B—Breathing

C—Circulation

D—Disability (neurological—CNS)

so that the systemic conditions/injuries found are identified in the order of urgency of their need for intervention. Fortunately, by doing the In-Depth Systemic Examination following a logical topographic geography—with anatomically adjacent steps from the mouth down to the groin; then returning to the head to check the eyes, ears, and nose; and lastly, to the extremities to complete the neurological evaluation—the EMT will obtain information in the A, B, C, D sequence of priorities. If one jumps back and forth from one part of the body to another when examining, regardless of one's ability or experience, it is easy to become confused and omit key items. By examining in the easily remembered anatomical progression of mouth-to-groin, then back to the head, then completing the neuro exam at the extremities, the EMT will obtain the necessary information in the desired sequence with minimal chance of omission and will avoid unnecessary time-consuming movement. In some cases such as when the PASG is to be used, examining the abdomen, pelvis and legs may need to be done earlier in the sequence since once enclosed in the PASG they are no longer available for examination.

The Initial Systemic Examination (both the Global Survey and the In-Depth A, B, C, D Examination including obtaining the enlarged AMPLE history) should take the EMT no longer than 3 to 5 minutes to complete. It should, except for the quantitative vital signs, be performed by a single EMT to assure that consistent findings and impressions occur without introducing the subtle variable interpretations found from one person to another. Since the vital signs are numerically quantified they are not subject to such differences. By having a second EMT take them, while the primary EMT is completing his in-depth A, B, C, D examination, these important indicators can be obtained without any additional time being spent in the field (zero time lapse).

Care must be taken to avoid being distracted from the main items in the Initial Systemic Examination. In trauma victims it is easy to be misdirected by injuries that appear with gross deformity or significant pain but have little or no systemic implication. Similarly, in some medical cases it is easy to be misdirected from more significant items by the patient's focus on items which produce the greatest discomfort, or by a long-standing diagnosis associated with similar episodes. The EMT must never assume that the current episode is limited to the same course, degree, or diagnosis as past episodes. An asthmatic may also be having a heart attack, a trauma victim may also have an underlying medical problem, and patients with a medical problem may also have some pertinent past trauma or trauma secondary to their collapse.

The Initial Systemic Examination should be performed essentially in the same detail and sequence in all patients, whether they are victims of trauma or patients with an acute medical problem and whether the patient's condition/injuries appear minor or significant. Even when the patient is unconscious, the sequence is basically unaltered, and only the method by which one obtains some of the information needs to be modified. This consistency of examination protects the patient (and EMT) from allowing initial impressions to cause an unwise abridgement in the assessment steps resulting in missed systemic conditions. As well, the repeated performance of one general sequence (rather than several differing ones) reinforces the EMT's ability to reproduce the sequence without omission and will promote a progressive increase in his rapid examining skills.

Throughout the Initial Systemic Examination, urgent interventions are initiated as their need is identified and less urgent ones are initiated at logical points as each area of consideration (A-B-C-D) or anatomical area (chest, abdomen, etc.) is completed. Interventions are provided by *the other* EMTs at the scene at the direction of the lead EMT performing the assessment. He should not interrupt his examination, delaying the identification of other items, to actually provide time consuming interventions himself unless limited resources at the scene provide no other choice.

Some intervention items are better (or need to be) deferred to a later part of the assessment. Some may not be possible or practical until after the patient has been extricated or moved. Some may require the completion of the entire Initial Systemic Examination before the EMT can properly determine the best method to meet this specific need within the context of the other systemic injuries or conditions present. In some cases the need for the continuation of time-consuming higher priorities of care may even require the decision to provide little or no care for other relatively non-urgent systemic items. Other time-consuming items (such as IV's for fluid replacement or the establishment of a "lifeline" in the absence of an advanced cardiac care capability) should be deferred in urgent patients until enroute to the hospital, to avoid unnecessary delay at the scene. In some cases the early identification of an urgent critical need that can not be provided in the field will necessitate immediate packaging and initiation of transport, and the remaining Initial Systemic Exam will have to be completed enroute. It must be noted, however, that even in cases with multiple-system trauma or a critical medical problem, this is singularly rarely indicated. In almost all cases, the lead EMT can complete the rest of the Initial Systemic Examination in a minute or two while the other EMTs at the scene are preparing and packaging the patient for transport. The few seconds of delay that may result from his temporary unavailability to help them, is easily offset by the assurance that no other critical items requiring urgent intervention are missed.

PART III—Review, Re-evaluate, Rule-Out, and Rank: After completing the Initial Systemic Examination a series of key evaluating steps involving a specific series of thought processes are required. First, take a few seconds to *review the individual conditions, injuries,* and overall vital systems' indicators that were separately found in the exam to this point, and form a clinical impression of the patient's overall problems and condition. Next, *re-evaluate the interventions* system-by-system that were provided so far, determining which if any need to be increased or changed. Then, in a detailed review, *rule-out each key systemic condition **not found*** by identifying positive findings and pertinent negative findings which deny the presence of that given condition. For example, one can provisionally rule-out the presence of a pneumothorax if the patient has no marked dyspnea, has good air exchange with bilaterally symmetry of chest excursion, and bilaterally equal breath sounds are clearly heard upon auscultation of the midlungs, apices and bases. It must be noted that besides not being able to make a definite diagnosis in the field, one can not definitely rule-out a condition's presence. A number of hidden (occult) conditions may exist which appear asymptomatic because they have either not as yet progressed far enough or because they require diagnostic ability (laboratory studies, X-Rays, etc.) beyond those available in the field. However, the EMT should provisionally rule-out those key conditions/injuries which were not found but which if present could require additional intervention or could result in systemic deterioration. The checklist of items to be considered and ruled-out (since it need not include ones that are grossly apparent) is considerably shorter than one would imagine. The experienced EMT can evaluate each area of items and his findings to effectively do the entire rule-out process in less than a minute. As with other assessment activities, the thought process in reviewing and ruling-out items should follow a logical sequence to avoid confusion and omission. Some EMTs find it helpful to review items with a system-by-system (A, B, C, D) approach followed by those items (such as poisoning or anaphylaxis) whose impact is often not identified in one system. Others prefer to review items topographically from head to groin followed by items not associated with any specific area. Each EMT should select the one with which he is the most comfortable.

The last step in this part of the assessment is to rank the patient's urgency based upon the conditions previously found or ruled-out. The choice is limited to only two possibilities, the patient is either ranked as **URGENT** or **NON-URGENT.** As well as those with obvious critical urgency, patients with any level of urgency—regardless of how slight—are also classified as urgent.

Even patients with systemic conditions that now appear stable or even appear to be improving as a result of the interventions provided must still be considered urgent. This group includes patients with conditions that at any time immediately preceding or during this episode have produced any significant changes in LOC, difficulty breathing, chest pain, blood loss, any level of shock, vital signs outside of the normal range, seizure activity, or motor or sensory deficits (except in an isolated limb injury). This group also includes any patient with a cardiac problem, poisoning, respiratory disease, allergic reaction, diabetic problem, TIA or CVA, or any other condition commonly associated with a potential for sudden deterioration. Regardless of the "goodness" of their present signs and symptoms, all of these patients continue to have the potential for rapid deterioration and therefore must be considered unstable until further examination at the hospital. If the EMT has difficulty in making determination or is left with unresolved questions surrounding the systemic implications of his findings, the uncertainty provides the answer. **If in doubt, *the patient is urgent.*** Patients are only classified as **Non-Urgent** if their conditions/injuries are limited to localized items which do not commonly have any significant systemic implication.

In courses whose focus is limited to trauma care, the terms **multiple systems trauma** and **simple isolated trauma** are often used to define urgent and non-urgent patients respectively. To avoid different terms for trauma, and to clearly identify the need to include the patient's age, general health, and existing medical conditions as well as the injuries in determining urgency, the broader terms **Urgent** and **Non-Urgent** provide a more meaningful and universal (trauma or medical patients) description. The patient's past history rather than current findings may indicate the potential for instability and cause an otherwise non-urgent patient to be considered urgent. For example, an elderly trauma victim with a history of frequent episodes of unstable angina the past few months, regardless of how minor his injuries, must be considered urgent.

The EMT needs to differentiate between patients who urgently need to be moved and patients who are urgent. Sometimes, due to dangers at the scene or such severe weather that continued exposure represents a severe systemic threat, patients need to be moved almost immediately upon arrival by the EMTs. Once the need for other immediate interventions has been eliminated (or is overridden by the imminent danger present) the patient may need to be moved into the ambulance (the ambulance may even need to be moved to a safer location). Once it has been assured that the ambulance is in a safe place, the EMT should complete the Initial systemic Assessment sequence as previously discussed in the parked ambulance, prior to initiating transport to the hospital.

In summary, patients who are found to be critical, have (or might have) conditions commonly associated with systemic impact and potential deterioration, or who have an active history of an unstable critical condition—should be categorized as urgent. It is important to note that although the list of items that would cause a patient to be considered *urgent* is lengthy, experience has shown that the vast majority of patients that the EMT will see will be *non-urgent*.

PART IV—Localized Item Exam, Packaging, and Transport: The assessment sequence to this point has been the same for all patients. From this point a different sequence will be followed for urgent and non-urgent patients to meet the differing needs and priorities of each of the two categories.

In the past years, it has been clearly recognized that increased delay in the field of urgent patients results in increased morbidity and mortality. The longer it takes from insult to the time such patients receive definitive care at the hospital, the less likely their survival. As a result, initiating transport within ten minutes after arrival at the scene has been recognized as an essential life-saving pre-hospital treatment for such patients. Because it is so essential to these patient's survival, this rule needs to be followed almost without exception. Sometimes the time required to effect a rescue, extricate the patient, or carry the patient to the ambulance from a remote location, or by a similar practical problem, will result in unavoidable delay in the field. Voluntary delay, however, is only justifiable when it is required to complete an immediately needed intervention or when definitive care analogous to that provided in the hospital is provided in the field (such as A.C.L.S., a cricothyrotomy, or starting blood replacement, etc.) Even in such a situation, the EMT must carefully weigh the benefit produced by each intervention against the increased delay it will cause and be careful not to extend field time for non essential items. Neither extremely short nor extremely long run times obviate the need to initiate transport of urgent patient without delay. If the hospital is only a few minutes away, other key care except for immediate needs can be provided more efficiently and more definitively with the greater resources available in the emergency department. When the hospital's location necessitates long travel time (and no reduction in it, such as going to a nearer appropriate facility or use of a helicopter is possible) delay in the field simply adds to this problem and significantly further reduces the patient's chance for survival. Deferring further examination and care of items of lesser or no priority until they can be done while enroute to the hospital represents the key way to reduce field time and best meet the urgent patient's care priorities. For such patients any potential increased danger to less significant conditions or injuries that results from rapidly packaging and initiating transport is clearly offset by the greater mortal danger that would be caused by the additional delay in the field required to identify and provide care for each localized item.

To reflect the previously discussed priorities with an **Urgent Patient,** the steps contained in this part of the assessment are sequenced so that the patient is first rapidly packaged and placed in the ambulance with transport being initiated without delay. Then, once enroute, the next priority of steps includes the maintenance of key interventions which were started earlier that require continuous or periodic attention (providing ventilation or CPR, suctioning, etc.), and the initiation of key deferred items such as starting IV's or EKG monitoring. Lastly, if priorities and resources allow, the detailed Localized Item Examination should be performed and additional minor items identified should be cared for. If the patient has critical labor-intensive needs, the Localized Item Examination should only be performed if it will not interfere with the continuance of treatments with higher priorities.

The EMT should not mistakenly interpret the **Urgent** patient's need for definitive care at the hospital as justification for careless haste in rescue procedures, field care, or when leaving the field, or for driving at high speeds or in an otherwise unsafe manner. Such practices are *never* justifiable due to the increased danger they represent to the patient, all of the rescuers, others at the scene, and those on the road.

The steps in this part of the assessment are performed in a different sequence for **Non-Urgent** patients. Since the presence of any conditions for which a need to urgently package and initiate transport has been carefully ruled-out, these patients have different priorities and needs. In the absence of any urgency, the danger of moving the patient and producing additional harm to localized items that have not as yet been identified or cared for makes a "haul-and-run" approach inappropriate. Therefore, all of the detailed steps included in the Localized Item Examination are completed first. Then the chief complaint and additional items identified are each properly cared for (wounds are dressed and bandaged, fractures splinted, etc.). Lastly, the patient is carefully packaged, moved into the ambulance, and transport to the hospital is initiated. Although careful additional examination and itemized care prior to transporting are desired, the EMT should not misinterpret the term **Non-Urgent** to mean "stay-and-play". The time required for these additional steps should only extend the field time by about five to ten minutes. Although it will vary on a case-by-case basis and no exact time frame can be identified for maximum time in the field with a non-urgent patient (compared to ten minutes for an urgent patient), the EMT must take care to avoid unnecessary lingering caused by irrelevant steps. Although no urgency exists, it must be remembered that unnecessary delay extends the patient's discomfort and, by reducing local EMS resources, may result in extended response times for other, possibly urgent calls.

One can summarize this part of the assessment by noting that its three tasks are sequenced inversely for urgent and non-urgent patients. For urgent patients, since time is the key factor, the patient is first packaged and transport is initiated, then once enroute key care items are continued along with those deferred from an earlier time, and the Localized Item Examination is performed last. For non-urgent patients, since thoroughness rather than time is the key factor, the Localized Item Examination is done first, then the chief complaint and other individual items are cared for, and packaging and initiating transport is last.

As well as the aforementioned differences in where and when the Localized Item Examination is done in urgent and non-urgent patients, it also needs to be performed in a different manner for trauma victims and patients with an acute medical emergency. In all patients, the Initial Systemic Examination and the ensuing review and evaluation of its findings will have resulted in any urgency being resolved or ruled-out, safely allowing for more detailed examination at this time. Although the Initial Systemic Examination is the same for patients with trauma and patients with a medical problem, its perspective is different for each.

In trauma victims, in order to avoid distraction or delay from higher priorities, the Initial Systemic Examination—except for a rapid head-to-toe scan for signs of external hemorrhage—was limited to vital body areas and indicators of vital function quality. Purposely, it does not include all of the body or any examination of localized items that were identified by the chief complaints, or coincidentally found. The first objective of the Localized Item Examination is to examine the entire body by firmly palpating each area's anterior, posterior and lateral aspects from head-to-toe, including the palpation of each joint while it is moved, to identify injuries by locating areas with:

- **Pain-on-palpation**
- **Deformity**
- **Sensory deficit**
- **Pain upon movement**
- **Motor deficit, or**
- **Abnormal range of motion**

Experience has shown that pain-on-palpation or pain upon movement are the most valuable of these in locating hidden or less apparent localized injuries. In unconscious trauma victims (or those with significant sensory deficits) clothing should have been removed earlier and the EMT will have to rely on careful visual inspection and palpation for deformity as the key guides in locating such injuries. Since areas included in the Initial Systemic Examination were not examined in such completeness or manner, they should not be omitted from this head-to-toe exam.

The second objective of the Localized Item Examination in trauma victims, once all of the localized injuries have been identified, is to examine each injury in further detail as required in order to determine and furnish the appropriate individual item care and packaging (bandaging, splinting, etc.) needed. Urgent patients, regardless of a lack of indication for spinal immobilization, when previously moved into the ambulance were immobilized in a neutral in-line longbone position on the longboard. This splinted and supported every bone and joint in the body simultaneously, to protect any fractures (both found and not yet identified) when moving the patient prior to performing a detailed head-to-toe examination. This full body splinting should reduce the individual item care needed in such cases, and even provides an adequate margin of safety should other care priorities enroute cause the Localized Item Examination to be omitted.

In *non-urgent patients,* once each individual item has been properly identified, cared for, and packaged, the patient is packaged in keeping with the sum of the conditions and injuries found. Since quite a few minutes have elapsed since the vital signs were taken in the Initial Systemic Examination, in non-urgent patients, they should be repeated while the individual item care and packaging is performed prior to leaving for the hospital. In urgent patients, delay to obtain additional vital signs in the field is unjustified since it will not alter care, and vital signs should only be re-checked once enroute.

Patients with an acute medical problem commonly have a previously diagnosed history of "like" episodes, or complaints that imply an apparently limited group of possible conditions. The EMT must be careful not to jump to limiting conclusions from such early information. Only after completion of the Initial Systemic Examination, and the ensuing review, re-evaluation and ruling-out based upon its findings, can one be sure that no different or second (simultaneous) significant condition is present and that it is safe to proceed to a further assessment which is focused on the limited areas and probabilities suggested. Even when no other conditions have been found, findings in the initial examination commonly modify or enlarge upon the possibilities suggested by the patient's complaints. In urgent patients, items which require any additional depth of examination surrounding further determination of care prior to leaving the scene should have been performed as part of the review and re-evaluation of the initial systemic findings. As in trauma, the additional Localized Item Examination is performed in urgent patients only once higher priorities have been managed and while enroute to the hospital, and in non-urgent patients only after any urgency has been ruled-out.

The first objectives of this exam are to perform any additional examination of areas associated with the chief complaints or previously obtained clinical impression needed, and to ask additional questions to further qualify and quantify the conditions, pain associated with this episode. and the patient's previous medical history.

Once issues surrounding the patient's main condition are resolved, the next objective is to identify or rule out any possibility of hidden or previous trauma. In patients who have a lowered level of consciousness, or who are disoriented, unclear, or otherwise appear incapable, the complete head-to-toe survey (previously described for trauma patients) will need to be done. In alert, oriented patients who are reliable history givers this can be rapidly achieved by inquiries put to the patient ("Have you fallen or been hurt in any way in the last few days? Weeks? Month?" etc.). Experience has shown that often the patient or others at the call may be unclear, or do not recall or know of a fall at night, or for a variety of reasons withhold this information. To be sure that nothing is missed, on medical patients regardless of their apparent reliability it is recommended that at least an abbreviated head-to-toe survey including areas not previously examined also be performed. Lastly, since several minutes have passed since the initial vital signs were taken, they should now be rechecked.

PART V—Monitor: The term "stable" when used in the context of emergency medicine is a relative term. "Stable" patients are those not presently demonstrating (or having conditions commonly associated with) changing vital function status, or vital function measurements outside of the normal range. However, the EMT must understand that no patient is "stable" in an absolute sense implying that change is improbable or impossible. Rather, in stable patients significant rapid change is less likely than in unstable ones but always remains as a possibility. Especially in the immediate post insult pre-hospital environment the patient's condition must always be considered dynamic and potentially changing. The only safe assumption is that periodic sudden deterioration will occur every few minutes, until proven otherwise.

Two different types of activities are required to monitor the patient's condition pre-hospital. Some apparent key indicators such as the appearance of the skin, respiratory effort and profound changes in rate, chest excursion, eye opening, and level of consciousness (spontaneity of speech and movement) in awake patients, can be observed and therefore monitored continuously. Others, such as the pulse rate and quality, respiratory rate, blood pressure, reactiveness in a patient with a lowered level of consciousness, require periodic rechecking with a specific examining procedure performed by the EMT. Some additional key indicators can be continuously monitored if the specialized equipment required is available. The pulse rate and blood oxygen levels can be monitored with a pulse oximeter, and the pulse rate and cardiac rhythm can be monitored if the squad has EKG monitoring capability.

Once enroute, or if field time is necessarily extended, the EMT should continuously monitor the visible indicators of the patient's condition. If any slight deterioration, change in cardiac rhythm, or significant improvement is seen, the vital signs should be rechecked and noted. Even in the absence of such a change, the vital signs should be rechecked and noted periodically. How frequently this should be done, and if any additional items should also be periodically rechecked, is dependent upon the patient's condition, other priorities of ongoing care, and local protocols. In the most stable alert patient who appears unchanging, at a minimum the pulse rate and quality; skin color, temperature, and moisture; and respiratory status (beyond casual observation) should be checked at least every 15 minutes. In cases where rechecking the blood pressure is indicated during transport, but is difficult to do because of vibration or road noise, this should be done using the palpation method rather than by auscultation or it being omitted. Although the importance of repeated vital signs in quantifying the patient's continued stability can not be overemphasized, the authors would be remiss if they did not point out that in cases where periodic rechecking would delay transport or detract from ongoing priorities of care in an urgent patient, the patient's well being rather than its measurement must be paramount. In such cases, once the initial baselines have been established, necessity and common sense may limit items to be rechecked solely to those which could result in a change in the EMT's ensuing care.

PART VI—Radio, Report, and Record: The first five parts of the assessment process and their objectives have been presented in the chronological sequence in which they are performed. The items in PART VI have been presented last because of the different type of activity they represent rather than as any indication of their chronological occurrence within the assessment sequence. Although the verbal report on arrival at the Emergency Department has a fixed place in the sequence, when and to whom the radio report is given and when different information is recorded on the written run report will vary.

Radio Report—Local protocols based upon hospital resources, EMS system design, and medical control philosophy in a given area, will determine to whom and when in the assessment sequence the EMT gives his radio report. Some systems have a centralized medical control (either at one hospital or in a separate location) to whom the radio report is given and which furnishes on-line medical direction, regardless of the hospital to which the patient will be transported. In such systems once the report and the initial medical direction is complete the medical control physician (or his designate) notifies the receiving hospital. More commonly, EMS units give report and receive on-line medical direction from the hospital to which they will be transporting.

In some systems, due to limited in-house emergency resources, EMTs are required to make a radio report immediately after they have treated any urgent patient needs (and before assessing further) to indicate the nature of the call, the number of patients, and the destination hospital. In this way, the hospital has the maximum lead time to assemble the necessary staff before the ambulance arrives at the hospital. Usually in such a system a second radio call is made when leaving the scene to furnish additional patient information, the estimated time of arrival (ETA), and for the medical control physician to review the information and give any additional orders he determines necessary.

In systems where adequate staffing is generally within the hospital on a 24 hour basis, EMTs typically give their radio report just prior to packaging the patient and leaving the scene, or once enroute. In systems where there is no need for the hospital to have early warning, this system avoids unnecessary delay in the field and results in a more organized meaningful radio report.

The local medical control philosophy will also determine when radio contact is made. Some systems require on-line physician concurrence for key procedures, often requiring early radio contact followed by one or more additional contacts thereafter. Other systems operate on a "standing order" basis in which BLS and ALS personnel follow pre-authorized medical control protocols instead of on-line physician orders, and only contact the hospital once the initial assessment and care have been completed.

Each of the previously mentioned systems has its merits and disadvantages. **The EMT must be familiar with and follow his local radio protocols.** All systems should provide the availability for the EMT to obtain on-line physician consultation and direction at any time that the EMT has a problem or is unsure of the best course of action.

Giving a precise radio report (neither too abbreviated nor too inclusive) which is organized in a meaningful sequence for the listener (who has not seen the patient), is an art that can not be taught in a book. Like other skills however, it can be practiced using simulated patient information and non-emergency communication equipment.

Terms such as "radio report" or "radio the hospital" are used generically in this book to represent such communication regardless of whether such contact is by radio, cellular phone, or landline telephone. The EMT must remember that any form of radio transmission (including cellular phones) is not private and others may hear the information being transmitted. Therefore, names or addresses which could identify the patient and violate his right to privacy should not be included.

Verbal Report—The EMT is medically and legally required to give a full verbal report to the healthcare professional at the hospital to whom he is transferring responsibility for the patient. This need remains regardless of the thoroughness of the radio report or the fact that a fully completed written report is left at the hospital. It is a medical safeguard to avoid dangerous confusion or omission. This requirement can not be fulfilled by giving the report to anyone who is not a health care professional or to a health care professional other than the one to whom the patient is being transferred. Even if the EMT has given an abbreviated report to the emergency physician or triage nurse greeting the squad on arrival, he should give a full verbal report to the nurse who will be involved in the patient's primary care in the emergency department.

Record—A complete written record of the situation, patient assessment findings, care given, and any additional pertinent information is established on the run report (sometimes called a "call report"). The term "run report" should be interpreted to mean "patient pre-hospital record" since when more than one patient is involved in a single call a separate run report is made for each patient cared for (or refusing care).

Run reports have identified areas in which to write the information standard to any call such as the patient's name, address, telephone number, age, sex, physician of record, date, times, known allergies, call location, nature of call, unit responding, EMT's names, patient disposition, etc. Also a grid-like series of boxes is usually provided for repeated sets of vital signs and their times to be recorded in one location. Beyond these universal items a wide variety of formats are used for the remaining information to be recorded. These fall into two major types, *discursive* or *check-off*.

Discursive run reports predominantly have blank lines to write on, divided only into major sections by headings such as "Chief Complaint", "History", "Physical Exam", "Clinical Impression", "Treatment", "Patient Meds", etc. The headings simply provide a consistent and easily identified place for each major category of information. The lack of any pre-determined structure within each heading allows the EMT to precisely present only pertinent information (including pertinent negatives), choosing wording that best reflects his exact findings or impressions in the most meaningful sequence for the reader.

Check-off run reports are organized into major sections with the same headings as discursive ones. Additionally, each section is further divided into an area for each item that should be included. For each individual item there are multiple choices each with a box to check. Some choices provide one box for "yes" and another for "no", others have a box for "normal" and another for "abnormal", others provide a box for each of two opposing possibilities such as "equal" and "unequal", and still others provide a box for each of several descriptive terms from which to select the most appropriate. As well, to allow for clarification some items may have a box marked "other" followed by a space in which to identify the specific variation not included in the list of choices. Some items such as "patient medications" have write-in spaces. Similarly this style of report commonly contains a section labeled "Additional Comments" followed by blank lines to allow any required comment or clarification not provided for by the given choices. Run reports mixing these two formats in varying degrees are also commonly in use.

When individual items are recorded and when the run report is completed will depend upon the number of EMTs available and the patient's condition. Ideally, key items and findings are recorded as identified throughout the assessment and treatment process, and ensuing vital signs and times are recorded enroute as taken. When this is possible the run report is completed by the time the ambulance arrives at the hospital (except for dispatch details regarding time back in service and time back in quarters which are not needed on the hospital copy). In non-urgent patients it is a common practice once the assessment is finished for the lead EMT to finish recording while the other EMTs package the patient. Then, being essentially completed except for any additional vitals taken enroute, the run report can be referred to as a basis for the radio report. In urgent patients it is not uncommon for only the patient identification and numerical vital sign findings to be recorded in the field, with the remaining information being recorded enroute or after transfer of the patient at the hospital. Controversy exists surrounding whether run reports should be written while enroute since this commonly results in a lack of legibility and may distract the often single EMT in the back of the ambulance from the patient. Many squads find that this problem can be easily resolved by the use of a separate draft form or blank paper to jot down vital signs and abbreviated notes in the field and enroute. The actual run report is organized and filled out once at the hospital. The desire to have the report completed upon arrival does not excuse a poor quality, incomplete, or illegible run-report regardless of the system used. Vital signs and any other quantified findings need to be written down as obtained or they will not be accurately remembered later.

The run report becomes a part of the patient's permanent hospital record. All items must be clearly and legibly noted and it must be complete. In a discoursive report, care must be taken to record all items found or done. Classically, abnormal findings, items outside of the normal range, and injuries are discussed first. Pertinent negatives, items different than expected or whose absence clarifies a condition found should be included ("Patient complains of chest pain. No shortness of breath, no diaphoresis found). For key areas, to provide a complete record, normal items should also then be noted ("Breath sounds are bilaterally equal and normal. Abdomen soft and normal, pelvis normal"). When using a check-off type, every set of multiple choice questions must be answered. If an examination item is not filled in the reader can not tell if the step was not performed, the findings were thought to be irrelevant, or it was performed and simply not recorded. The medical and legal assumption made is that if any item is left blank, the examining step was not performed. **The universal rule is: if it isn't documented it wasn't done.**

As well as being legible and complete the run report needs to be exact, clear, and well organized. Effective communication should be the objective rather than good literary style. In lieu of long complex sentences, use of short phrases and proper medical abbreviations provide rapidly and easily read information.
For example:

> **"LOC normal and alert; A&O × 3; moves/speaks spontaneously; reacts appropriately to verbal stimuli; PEARRL; MSC × 4 normal; patient denies any altered LOC post-insult".**

Care must be taken to avoid seemingly vague or contradictory comments such as "LOC normal, but appears disoriented." Judgmental and perjorative comments such as "Patient is filthy" should be avoided, being replaced by more tempered and neutral statements such as "Patient appeared disheveled and with poor personal hygiene." Baseless judgments such as "Patient is drunk" or even "appears drunk" are legally dangerous and should not be used until the blood alcohol level has been established at the hospital. Instead, the EMT should note the patient's appearance, any odor of alcoholic beverages, actions and the patient's (or witness') description of the amount of drink consumed.

Run forms are usually self-carbonized and have two (one to be left with the hospital and one to be retained by the squad) or more copies. They should be filled out by writing firmly on a hard surface using a ball point pen (pencil is not acceptable for a permanent legal record) to assure each copy is dark enough to be legible. If an error occurs when filling it out, draw a straight single line through the item you wish to delete, then rewrite it correctly and initial the change. Do not erase items.

In cases where it was not possible to complete the run report before arrival at the hospital, once the EMTs have transferred the patient to the Emergency Department bed and have given their verbal report the lead EMT should complete the written report without further delay. Regardless of where the final entries are recorded, it is required that the EMTs hand a copy of the completed run form to an appropriate member of the emergency department staff before they leave the hospital. In the rare event that the need for the ambulance at another call interrupts completion of the run form, the involved emergency department staff should be notified and given an unfinished copy in the interim. After the second call is completed the EMTs should replace the unfinished copy left at the hospital with a fully completed one.

DOING THE PATIENT ASSESSMENT—STEP BY STEP

Each of the many steps performed in the pre-hospital patient assessment sequence is presented without interruption on the following pages. To allow each identifiable sub-skill to be presented as a single step without the distraction of further explanation, a detailed discussion of the considerations and steps included in each sub-skill has previously been presented in Part A of this section. Similarly to avoid the need to interrupt the sequence, an overview and discussion of each of the major parts into which the assessment is divided, has been presented in the preceding introduction to Part B. The ability to perform these sub-skills and an understanding of the purpose and rationale of each major part of the assessment, are necessary pre-requisites to learning and retaining the many steps and the necessary sequential order of the complete patient assessment process.

The presentation of each step includes discussion of the method used in examining or otherwise obtaining information, and details the questions to be answered by performing that particular step.

PART I—SAFETY, SCENE, SITUATION AND SPINE

1. While enroute to the scene, review the information given to the dispatcher by the caller (remembering that it may not accurately describe the problem). Plan and clearly define the role and responsibilities to be assumed by each EMT when first arriving at the scene.

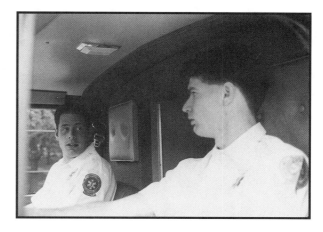

2. As you arrive, size up the overall situation and make sure that it is safe for the ambulance to enter the area. If not, stop at a safe distance from the scene and wait for other responders (fire or police) to indicate that it is now safe to proceed. Then, from the nature of the problem, type of road, traffic flow and position of other vehicles, identify a safe location for the ambulance as near to the patient(s) as possible.

3. Before leaving the ambulance, put on the items needed for body fluid protection and any other protective clothing dictated by the nature of the call or local protocols. From the scene and situation (the scene commander, if present) make sure that the location of the ambulance, the pathway to the patients, and the immediate patient area are safe.

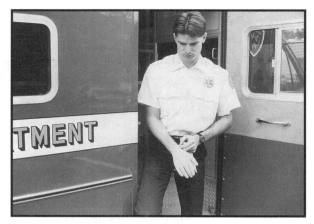

4. Determine what happened (nature of call), and identify the number of patients involved. "Eyeball" each patient, determining whether they appear seriously compromised or not, and whether they are trapped or not. Evaluate EMT resources at the scene and call for any additional EMS units or special medical responders such as a "Life Flight" helicopter that may be needed.

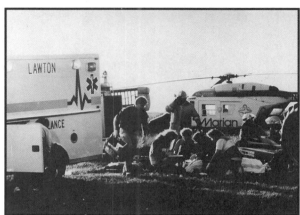

5. Based upon the scene and situation, identify and call for any additional rescue resources that may be needed such as Fire, Police, Heavy Rescue, Technical Rescue, etc. If a scene commander is present, maintain the proper chain of command and notify him of your needs and have him summon them.

Note: The assessment demonstration beyond this step will be limited to a single patient.

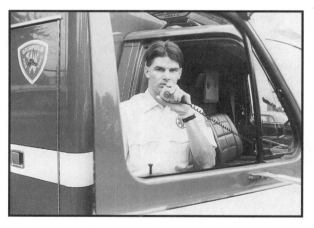

6. Determine the underlying nature of the call—whether it appears to be trauma or an acute medical emergency. Note the nature of the scene: home, office, factory, school, pool, highway, field, etc., and any other apparent factors that may enlarge the possibilities, such as signs of an earlier fire, smoke, etc.

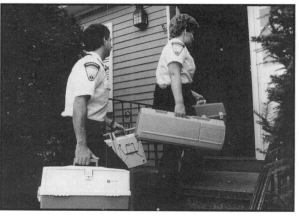

7. (a) **If trauma,** evaluate the specific mechanism of injury and forces which acted upon the patient. Note the nature of the trauma (fall, motor vehicle accident, shooting, etc.) and details such as direction of travel, apparent speed, type of collision, damage to the vehicle, etc. Note the possible injuries these imply. **From the mechanism of injury, determine if suspicion of spine trauma (indicating the need for immobilization) exists or not.**

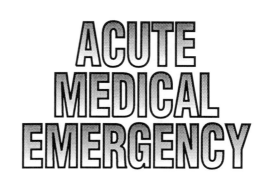

7. (b) **If a medical problem,** from the person greeting you determine the events or nature of the problem that predicated calling EMS. Ask when the problem started and note if onset was sudden or took several hours or days. Note any other information or previous history the person furnishes. Observe and note the implied situation, relationships, appearance of the house (neat or unkempt, etc.), the location (upstairs or ground floor) that you are being taken to, and the room in which the patient is located.

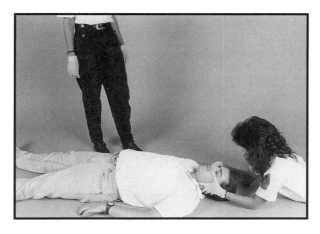

PART II—INITIAL SYSTEMIC EXAMINATION

8. **The Global Survey** starts as you near the patient's side. Throughout the Initial Systemic Examination, any urgent interventions are provided as their need is identified. As you approach, note the patient's sex and approximate age. Observe how he presents (sitting by himself, etc.), whether he appears conscious or unconscious, whether he is supporting himself, moves spontaneously, appears to be breathing, if respiration appears normal or labored, and note any apparent gross injuries or deformities. *If the mechanism suggested spine trauma, direct a second EMT to provide manual neutral in-line immobilization).*

9. Look at the patient's face and note his skin color and general appearance, and if his eyes appear to move, focus, and blink normally. Identify yourself and ask the patient to describe what seems to be the problem and where he has pain. From his responses note whether he responds to verbal stimulus and whether he appears to be normally alert or has an altered mental status (mentation). From his speech determine if he appears to be breathing normally or the level of dyspnea it suggests. Also note if he localizes pain, appears oriented to events around him, and his chief complaints.

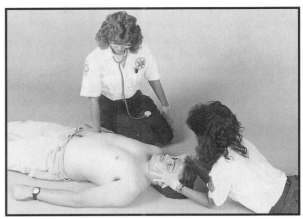

9. (continued) Simultaneously, feel for a radial pulse and note the skin temperature and moisture. Note if a radial pulse is palpable, its quality, and regularity. Estimate if the patient's pulse rate is normal, bradycardic, or tachycardic. From the presence or absence of a palpable radial pulse (in a conscious patient) estimate the Systolic Blood Pressure to be greater or less than 80mmHg respectively. From your findings, obtain an overall impression of the patient's LOC, respiratory status, and circulatory status.

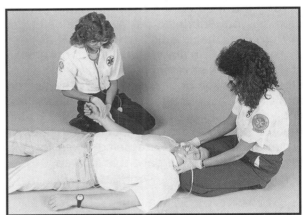

9. (alternate for unconscious patient) If the patient does not respond to your questions, ask more loudly several times if he can hear you. Simultaneously, look at his face noting the skin color and moisture, and feel for a radial pulse and the skin temperature under your hand. If he remains unresponsive, open the airway (protecting the spine if indicated) and look, listen and feel for adequate spontaneous respiration.

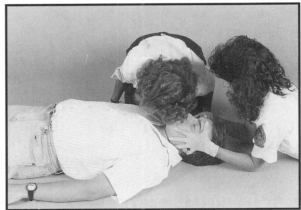

9. (alternate continued) Do not delay or interrupt the A,B,C sequence for any further neurological assessment at this time. If adequate ventilation is present, continue. If it is not, add an airway adjunct and direct another EMT to provide ventilation. If the radial pulse was *NOT* palpable, once adequate ventilation has been confirmed or provided, check for the presence of a carotid pulse. If absent, start CPR. If present, continue your survey.

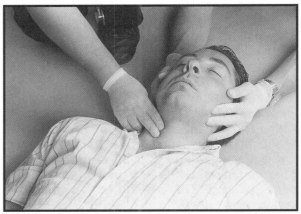

10. Whether the patient is responsive or unresponsive, finish the global survey by scanning the patient's body and area adjacent to it from head to foot for signs of any significant external bleeding. Any wet appearing areas on dark clothing need to be evaluated to determine if they are caused by blood. Any fluid impervious clothing (such as foul-weather gear) needs to be removed at this time to assure that it does not mask any hemorrhage, and any areas that can still not be seen should be felt for the presence of blood. Stop any significant external bleeding found.

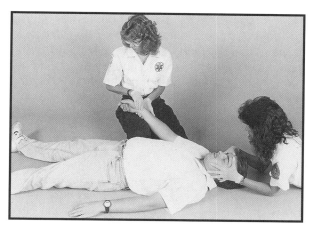

11. Once any immediate needs have been identified and provided for or ruled-out by the completion of the simultaneous Global Survey, the EMT can safely go on to do a more in-depth A,B,C,D Examination. Move your ear near the patient's mouth and listen for any stridor, bubbling, gurgling, snoring, or gross wheezing. Look in the mouth for foreign objects, debris, loose teeth, blood, or anything that could ensuingly block the airway. Evaluate the adequacy of air exchange felt with each breath. Ask the patient to place the tip of his tongue on the roof of his mouth and observe the color of its underside. Is it normal, blanched, or cyanotic?

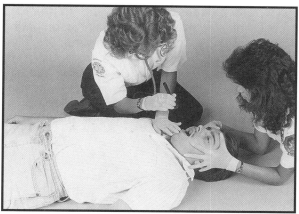

12. Visualize the patient's neck for wounds, bruises or deformities. Observe if the jugular veins are distended in a sitting patient. In a supine patient, observe if they are only normally distended or are pathologically engorged. Palpate the trachea to determine if it is midline or deviated. Palpate the neck and supraclavicular area for the presence of any subcutaneous emphysema.

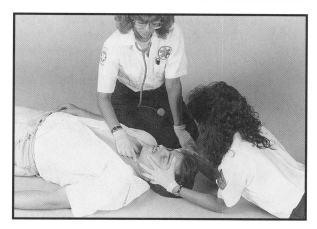

13. Bare the chest to the degree indicated and visualize the anterior thorax. Initially look for any sucking chest wound or paradoxical motion. Note any other wounds or bruises. Observe the chest excursion through several breaths. Note if the depth of excursion appears ample and if it is bilaterally symmetrical, or if the patient is splinting or guarding on one side. Ask the patient if there is any pain on breathing and if so, when it occurs (constant, on inspiration, only at peak inspiration etc.).

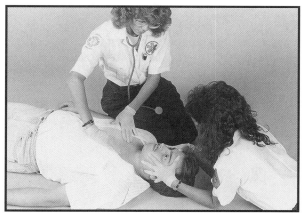

14. In some cases, particularly small children and infants, chest excursion may be difficult to to visualize. In such cases the EMT can better evaluate it for depth and symmetry by feeling the chest rise and fall by resting his hands on the lateral anterior margins of the rib cage.

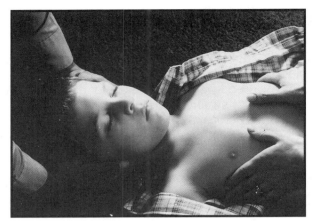

15. Next, palpate the chest with firm pressure to determine if there is any pain-on-palpation (POP), untofore movement, or crepitus. First place pressure on the upper thorax (ribs 1–5) and while observing the patient's face have him take a deep breath. Note if this is painless or results in any grimace or limited inspiration due to pain. Repeat this at the mid thorax (ribs 5–10).

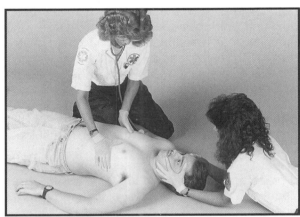

16. Palpate the lower thorax by pressing firmly on the posterior area over the retroperitoneal area with firm posterior-to anterior pressure. POP in this area may either relate to injury to the 11th and 12th "floating" ribs or to the underlying retroperitoneal area (lower back, kidney, etc.). Lastly, palpate the sternum by placing firm pressure over the upper two thirds of the sternum.

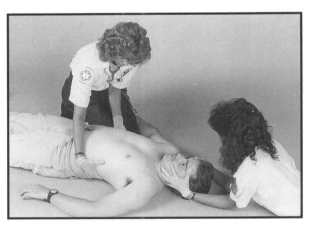

17. Although the adequacy of air exchange has been previously estimated, it can only be ascertained by auscultation. Start by auscultating the right mid-lung field and evaluate the inspiratory and expiratory depth and duration. Comparing an adult's rate and inspiratory/expiratory durations to your own provides a helpful measure. Also note if breathing is regular or irregular, and if any adventitious sounds (wheezing, rhonchi, or rales) are present.

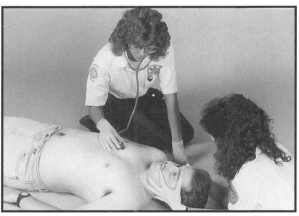

18.   Next compare the breath sounds over both mid-lung fields to ascertain whether they are bi-laterally equal or appear diminished or absent on one side. This can best be done by listening to one or two breaths on one side, then one or two on the other side, moving back and forth several times. Also note if any adventitious sounds not previously heard on the first side are present on the second.

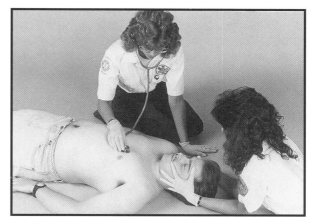

19.   In cases where a lung is progressively col-lapsing, it collapses towards the mainstem bron-chus resulting in diminished or absent breath sounds heard earliest at the apices and bases. Therefore, next auscultate the apices moving the stethoscope back and forth from one side to the other to determine if breath sounds are ab-sent or diminished on either side. If they are, as-sume a partial collapse has occurred and will progress.

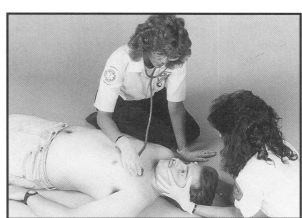

20.   Due to gravity, diminished or absent breath sounds caused by blood or other fluids may early on only be auscultatable at the inferior aspect of the injured side. Similarly, early signs of pulmonary edema may only be heard as basi-lar rales in a sitting patient. Auscultate the bases, moving the stethoscope from one side to the other to determine if breath sounds at either base are diminished or absent, and if any basilar rales are present. This completes the initial in-depth respiratory evaluation (A—airway and B—breathing), except for counting the exact respiratory rate which is deferred until later in the exam.

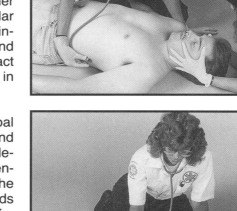

21.   Review your previously obtained global impression of the patient's circulatory status and the implied level of shock, and whether your de-tailed thoracic examination indicated the poten-tial presence of a hemothorax. Next, while at the bared chest, auscultate the apical heart sounds by placing the stethoscope just medial and infe-rior to the left nipple. Determine if they are nor-mal or abnormal, and whether they are heard at normal amplitude or appear distant or muffled.

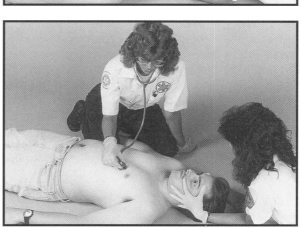

22. Direct another EMT, if available, to obtain an initial set of quantitative vital signs at this time. Waiting to have these taken until you have completed auscultation of the thorax minimizes the chance that the second EMT will interfere with your ability to hear the breath or heart sounds. Without delay, continue your examination by moving down the torso to the anterior abdomen.

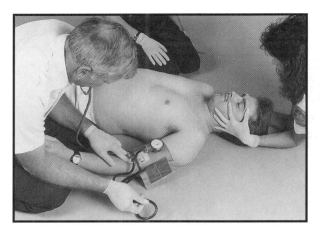

23. Bare the abdomen as needed, and note if it appears normal or distended. Visualize the anterior portion for any bruises, wounds or evisceration(s). Also note if there is any visible vaginal or penile bleeding and, in males, priapism.

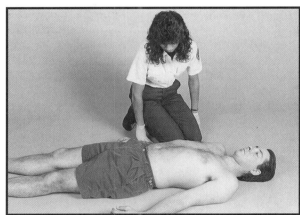

24. Ask the patient if he has any abdominal pain. If yes, have him identify the location by pointing. Then, palpate the mid-abdomen gently to determine if the abdomen is normally soft and pliable, or rigid and distended. The patient may instinctively guard his abdomen, making it rigid when touched. If it is initially soft, or if when asked the patient can relax it, it should be considered soft. Also note if there is any palpable mass and if so, its location and if it is pulsatile (pulsating).

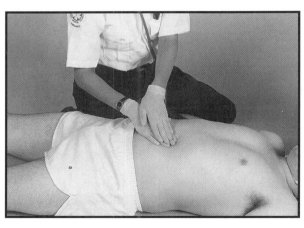

25. Next, palpate the left and right halves of the abdomen (or per local protocol, or if indicated, each of the four quadrants) respectively by pressing firmly into the abdomen with the finger tips. Note if this produces any pain-on-palpation and, if so, where. Pressure should be slowly withdrawn to avoid any sudden rebound which could produce additional injury to aggravated or friable organs. Continue the abdominal examination by next palpating the pelvis.

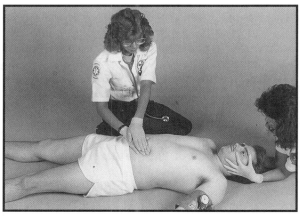

26.   Place the hands over the pelvis as shown. Press firmly towards the midline on each iliac crest simultaneously and note any POP, untofore movement, or crepitus indicating an unstable pelvis and assumed associated intra-abdominal bleeding. If only pain-on-palpation results (without either untofore movement or crepitus) you will have to re-apply opposing bilateral pressure elsewhere along the pelvic girdle. If the POP is reproduced at these different locations on the pelvic girdle, an unstable pelvis must be assumed. If not, a hip or other injury underlying the initial hand position must be assumed instead.

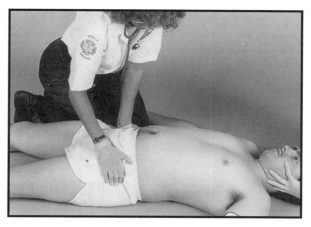

27.   If the opposing bilateral pressure on the pelvis did not identify any abnormality, additional palpation is recommended. Palpating one at a time, place the heel of the hand on each iliac crest, apply firmer anterior-to-posterior pressure, and note any POP, untofore movement or crepitus. Care must be taken when applying such pressure to keep the pelvis from rotating, causing undesirable movement of the spine. (By this time the second EMT should have completed the quantitative vital signs.)

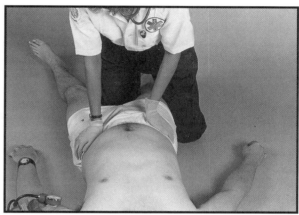

28.   This concludes the in-depth evaluation of the patient's C–Circulatory status except for the final identification or ruling out of the presence of intracranial hemorrhage, and additional evaluation of the quality of the the peripheral circulation (beyond the overall skin evaluation) in each extremity. Therefore, to avoid unnecessarily moving from one part of the patient to another, these have been deferred to the neurological evaluation which follows.

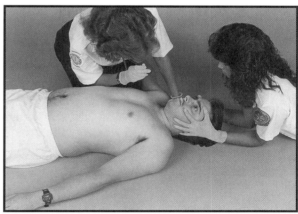

29.   Start the in-depth neurological evaluation (D-disability, neurological) by reviewing the patient's LOC, reactions to verbal stimuli, alertness and mentation (if conscious) found to this point. Move to the patient's head. Check the nose and mouth for signs of blood or cerebrospinal fluid. Check each ear for any blood or cerebrospinal fluid coming from within the ears. Also check just below and slightly posterior to the bottom of each ear for any "Battle's sign".

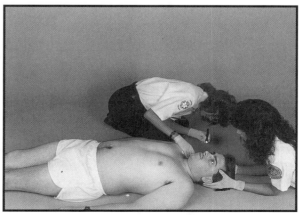

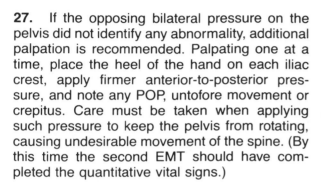
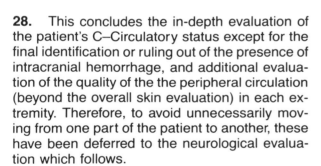
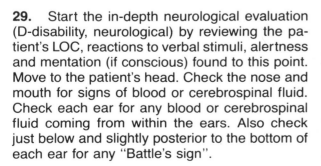

30. Next look at the patient's eyes. Note if there is any periorbital ecchymosis ("Raccoon's Eyes"). Have the patient open his eyes (or hold them open if necessary) and look at each eye to identify any apparent injuries. As part of the PEARRL exam, note if the pupils are round or have another shape, and if the pupils appear equal or unequal. Note if either pupil appears "blown".

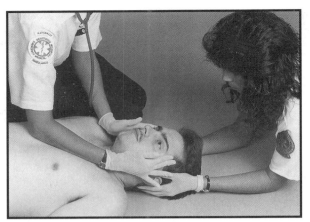

31. Continue the PEARRL exam by shining a light into one eye. Determine if the pupil reacts to light by constricting or not, and if the constriction was normally brisk or pathologically sluggish. Then remove the bright light source. While looking at the other pupil, reintroduce the bright light into the first eye and note if the other pupil constricts equally, demonstrating an intact consensual reflex. Now repeat this entire procedure in the second eye.

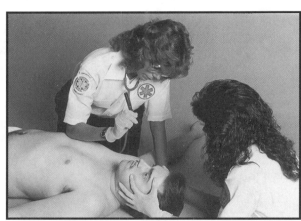

32. In *a conscious patient* you have by now ascertained that he responds to verbal stimulus, whether his responses are appropriate or inappropriate, if he moves spontaneously or only when directed, if he localizes pain, and if he is oriented to the events around him. In order to further evaluate his orientation and mentation, ask him his full name, where he is, and the approximate time (or day of the week) to determine if he is oriented to person, place, and time (A & O x 3).

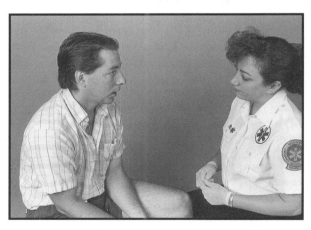

33. Ask the patient and any witnesses if there was any period of unconsciousness, confused or otherwise altered LOC, or any seizure activity preceding or since onset. Next, have the patient recount the exact sequence of events of the accident or medical emergency in his own words. Any apparent lack of continuity in time or movement from one place to another must be assumed to represent a period of unconsciousness. From his response, also evaluate if his mental process (mentation) appears normal or reduced.

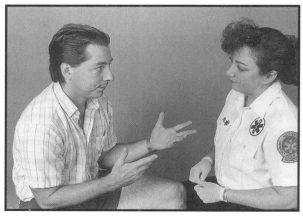

34. Next, check the motor ability and sensory responses in each extremity to identify any neurological deficit on one side or the other, or inferior to a given point, indicating either brain or spine injury respectively. Start by evaluating the patient's strength on each side. Have the patient grasp and firmly squeeze the extended first two fingers of both your hands simultaneously. Note if he can move each of his arms, and if the grasp appears equal or is reduced (weaker) on one side or the other.

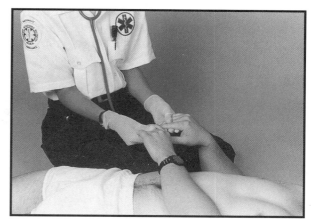

35. Continue by checking the sensory status in each hand and note any deficit found. Sensory ability is best checked by assuring that the patient can discern between pointed and dull objects. While at each arm, also check the peripheral circulation by checking the distal pulse, skin temperature, or capillary refill. Note the quality of the peripheral circulation and if circulation appears to be compromised in either upper extremity.

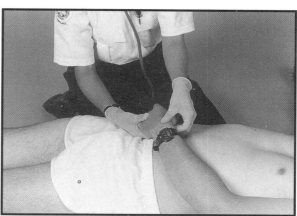

36. Then check the motor ability, sensory responses and distal circulation in each of the lower extremities and note any neurological deficits or compromised distal circulation found. If injury to either arm made it unwise to compare bilateral motor strength at the upper extremities, it can be compared instead at the lower extremities by having the patient push against the EMT's hands with both feet simultaneously. Checking the MSC's in all four extremities (MSCx4) completes the initial in-depth neurological evaluation of the conscious patient.

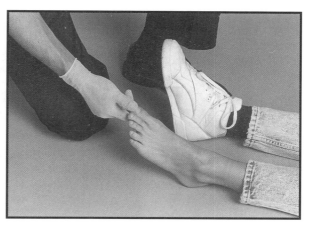

37. In the case of *an unconscious patient,* rather than the further evaluation of alertness, mentation, orientation, and motor and sensory responses indicated in Steps 32–36, the EMT will need to proceed with additional parts of the AVPU exam. It is important to note that in a patient who does not respond to verbal stimulus by awakening, the in-depth ABC examination, checking for signs of a basilar skull fracture, and PEARRL, should be completed without interruption before returning to the continuation of the AVPU exam.

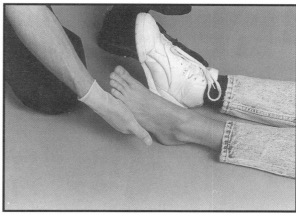

38. In patients who do not respond to verbal stimulus, note if during the PEARRL exam the patient attempted to withdraw from the stimulus caused when a bright light was shown into his eyes. Next, check for a response to a "noxious" loud verbal command. If the patient is still unresponsive, you will need to see if he responds to a painful stimulus. Grasp the trapezius muscle between your thumb and fingers and squeeze extremely strongly to produce pain (this central location and method is recommended although others may be used).

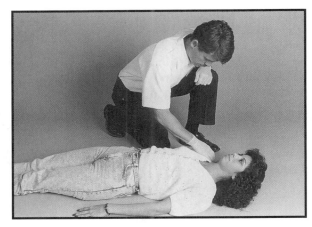

39. Note if he responds to pain (A,V,P,U). Note if he responds normally by attempting to withdraw or remove the painful stimulus, or abnormally with a pathological movement such as decorticate or decerebrate posturing. If he does not respond (normally or abnormally) note that he is "unresponsive to pain (A,V,P,U)".

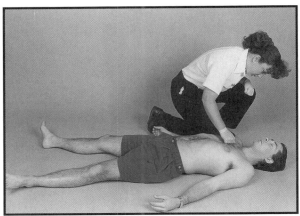

40. If the patient only responds to pain, note which limbs moved as part of his response. Further motor and sensory testing by applying pain at each limb is not recommended. In trauma patients this could result in additional reflex movement which can cause damage to the spine, and in a medical patient it results in unproductive delay. Also, in a patient who does not respond to a painful central stimulus it is without benefit since he will not respond to stimuli at the extremities either. In both cases, simply check the distal circulation in each extremity.

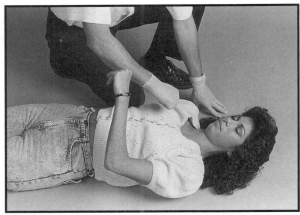

41. In patients who remain unconscious, after you have determined the patient's best response ascertain from witnesses how long the patient has been unconscious. Check if the patient has been incontinent. Check for any medical alert identification at the neck or wrists, and in the presence of a witness check the wallet or handbag for any medical alert card. Evaluate if you can identify the probable cause of the continued unconsciousness.

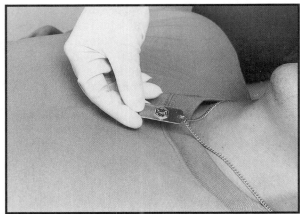

42. In both conscious and unconscious patients, after finishing the in-depth neurological examination you have completed the *Initial Systemic Evaluation.* ***Interventions should have been provided as each need was identified.*** Also, the history of this episode and the key pertinent past history (expanded AMPLE history) should have been obtained during this exam from the patient and anyone accompanying him. Any additional history needed should be obtained at this time.

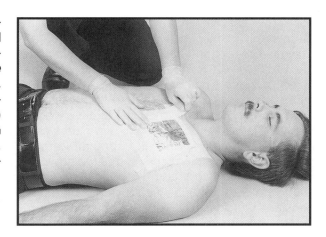

PART III—REVIEW, RE-EVALUATE, RULE-OUT, AND RANK

43. The Initial Systemic Evaluation should have identified all injuries/conditions with any significant systemic implication, the history of this episode and any pertinent past history, and the patient's A,B,C,D status including initial quantitative vital signs measurement. Carefully **review your findings** and form a provisional pre-hospital diagnosis, called the *Clinical Impression.*

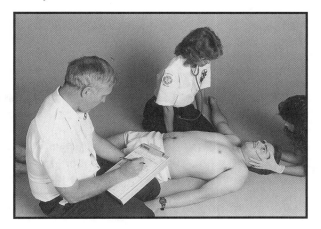

44. Urgently needed interventions have been provided as each need was identified during the exam. **Re-evaluate the interventions** provided based upon their effect on the patient and your Clinical Impression. Re-assess as needed to determine the effectiveness of the interventions provided and to determine if any need to be increased, or if any additional ones are indicated at this time or once enroute.

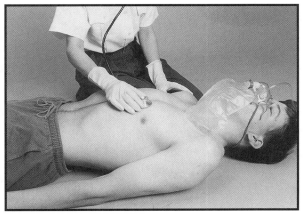

45. To assure that any potentially life-threatening items which were not identified are truly not present and have not just been missed, the EMT needs to consider them in an organized itemized manner, and **rule-out each**. An injury or condition (except those that are totally asymptomatic) can be ruled out relatively accurately by recalling the signs and symptoms commonly associated with it, and comparing these with the initial examination findings (positive and negative), the history and the patient's A,B,C,D status. In less than a minute one can rapidly consider the possibilities (Could he have: intracranial bleeding? Intrathoracic bleeding? A pneumothorax? Heart attack? etc.) and eliminate each.

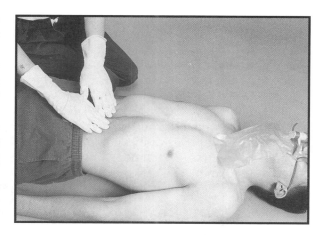

46. All of the initial assessment steps described to this point usually take less than five minutes to complete—possibly several minutes more if time-consuming interventions require interruptions. Based upon his review of the findings of the Initial Systemic Examination and items ruled out, the EMT can now **rank the patient** as either URGENT or NON-URGENT. The divergent needs of these two categories require that a different sequence for each should be followed from this point forward.

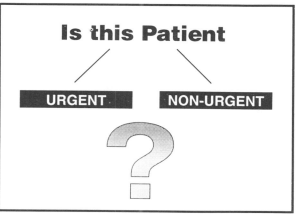

PART IV—LOCALIZED ITEM EXAM, PACKAGING, AND TRANSPORT
URGENT PATIENT

Patients in this category have injuries/conditions which, regardless of the interventions provided in the field, continue to be potentially life threatening and require definitive hospital care (i.e.: blood replacement, surgical intervention, etc.) in order to be stabilized. The elapsed time between onset and definitive care is a paramount factor affecting these patients' morbidity and survival. *Therefore, at this juncture in the assessment sequence, initiating transport to an appropriate facility without delay becomes the key treatment priority in such patients.*

47. Once the findings in the Initial Systemic Examination have been reviewed and any immediately needed interventions have been provided, URGENT PATIENTS should be rapidly packaged as indicated, loaded into the ambulance, and the cot and other equipment should be secured. Transport to the nearest appropriate hospital should be initiated without further delay.

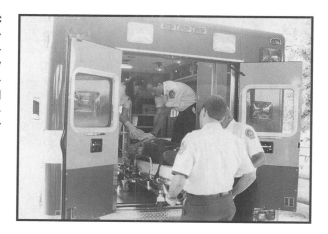

48. Once enroute, the EMTs should transfer the oxygen, if in use, to the on board oxygen source and continue to provide any key interventions indicated. Any key items which were deferred until enroute (i.e.: initiating IVs, cardiac monitoring, etc.,) should be initiated at this time.

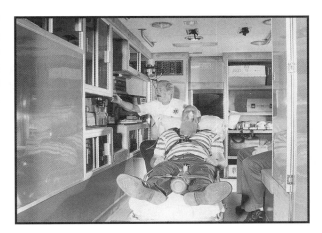

49. If time and EMT resources allow, once key items of care enroute have been established, the **Localized Item Exam** (found in the following pages) should be performed and any additional care indicated should be provided. It is important to note that if EMT resources are limited this *must not* interfere with the proper continuance of higher priorities of care. Such needs or an extremely short run time may preclude the EMT's ability to perform any further pre-hospital examination.

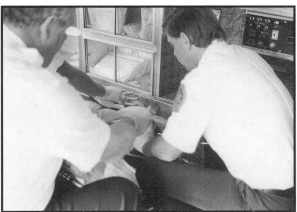

NON-URGENT PATIENTS

Patients in this category have **NO** life threatening injuries/conditions, or any commonly associated with significant systemic impact, and the presence of any such conditions has by this point been ruled out. In the absence of any urgency, further examination to identify all of the localized injuries/conditions present, and care for each, should be done prior to packaging and moving the patient. The reader should note that the items described in steps 47–49 are in an opposite order for URGENT and NON-URGENT patients.

47. Once the patient is determined to be NON-URGENT, the EMT should continue his assessment by performing the *Localized Item Exam* to identify all localized injuries/conditions and obtain any additional history needed. (The steps in this exam are presented in further detail in the following pages).

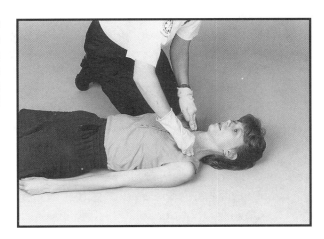

48. Next, each individual injury/condition found should be cared for (i.e.: dressed and bandaged, splinted, etc.) as indicated. In patients who collapsed, or who have simple trauma, based upon the sum of the injuries and areas of pain, the need for spinal immobilization (if not previously found necessary) should again be evaluated.

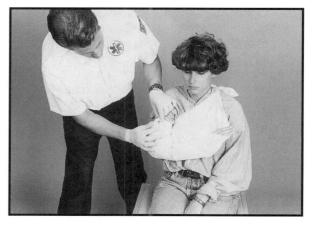

49. After each individual item has been cared for the patient should be placed in the position indicated, carefully packaged, loaded into the ambulance, and transport to the hospital should be initiated.

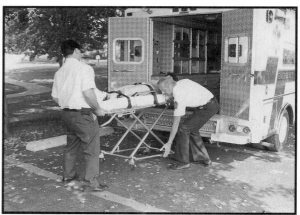

THE LOCALIZED ITEM EXAM

To this point, the patient assessment has been performed essentially in the same manner in all patients regardless of the extent or nature of their problems (with only variations in how one obtains certain information in conscious or unconscious patients), in order to provide a single consistent rapid examination to include all of the elements and areas necessary to identify or rule-out each item with any significant systemic impact or implication. Even the content of the last three steps is basically the same, only differing in when and where (at the scene or once enroute) the **Localized Item Exam** is performed in URGENT and NON-URGENT patients.

As well as other key information surrounding the patient's condition, the previously completed systemic examination will have identified whether the patient is suffering from trauma or a medical problem. Because of the differing nature of these, the questions raised and the further assessment required is different for each.

Trauma Patients—The steps included are:
   a. Do a complete head-to-toe hands-on survey to identify any localized injuries not previously identified.
   b. Obtain any additional history needed.
   c. Re-check vital signs.
   d. Review and determine if these suggest the need to change the care being given and, in the case of NON-URGENT patients, a need to change them to the URGENT category.

Medical Patients—The assessment to this point will have determined whether the findings are limited to the Chief Complaint and conditions associated with it, or if other key conditions must also be considered. The steps included are:
   a. Examine areas related to "Chief Complaint/Conditions Found" in more detail
   b. Obtain a more detailed history and further qualify conditions/pain (O,P,Q,R,S,T,U)

    c. Re-check vital signs

    d. On a head-to-toe basis confirm that there is no hidden trauma

DOING THE HEAD-TO-TOE SURVEY

The purpose of the head-to-toe survey in the *Localized Item Exam* is always the same: to do an organized and complete survey from head-to-toe to locate any items not previously found and to assure that none have been missed. In trauma patients it is a logical continuation after completing the Initial Systemic Examination to examine the entire body (including areas not yet examined) in increased detail in order to locate all of the localized injuries. In the medical patient it assures the EMT that no item has been overlooked because the patient did not remember it, feel it was significant, or purposely withheld the information. It is not uncommon in medical patients that this survey may provide the first indication of trauma which occurred days or weeks earlier, or of injuries which may have resulted from a collapse or fall associated with the present medical condition.

Depending upon earlier assessment findings, the way in which, when, and where the head-to-toe survey is done will vary. In urgent patients it is deferred until enroute whereas in non-urgent patients is it performed prior to moving the patient. In both trauma and medical patients who have any lowered level of consciousness, reduced mental capacity, disorientation, lowered alertness, language barrier, or in whom any question exists regarding their ability to identify and localize pain throughout the body, this exam should include observing and palpating from head-to-toe. In such patients only such thoroughness can assure the EMT that no isolated localized condition or hidden trauma has been missed.

Some instructors and medical directors recommend that this be done as a safe practice in every patient regardless of alertness and reliability. Most, however, believe that in the alert, well oriented, verbal, and reliable patient this can be abridged to having the patient move his head and neck, move each limb in turn against resistance, take a deep breath, bend at the waist, etc., while questioning if any of these produce pain. The EMT will have to follow his local protocols and, if they allow differentiation, use common sense in determining the extent that removing clothes, detailed itemized visualization and palpation of each area is required in the fully alert well oriented reliable patient.

The following demonstrates the complete detailed head-to-toe survey. It must be noted that in supine patients the back and buttocks may need to be examined out of sequence since the patient will need to be moved to obtain access to his back, and this should only be done once. Although a consistent head-to-toe method is advocated, the reader should note that some sequence variations are a matter of personal preference.

a. Observe and palpate the top of the head. Then move on to each side and the back of the head. Continue by examining the facial bones, palpating the forehead, supraorbital ridge, inferior orbital ridge, the cheek bones, the maxilla and mandible. Complete your examination of the head by having the patient articulate his mandible to check if movement produces pain or a loss of continuity at each joint.

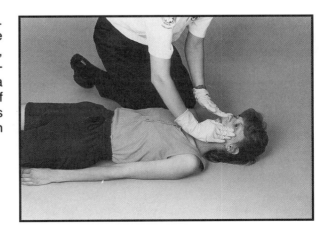

b. Moving down the body, observe the neck and palpate the posterior cervical spine to determine if any significant deformity can be felt or if any pain-on-palpation (POP) is produced. Next, check the superior aspect of the shoulders and each clavicle in turn. Then move around and check each scapula.

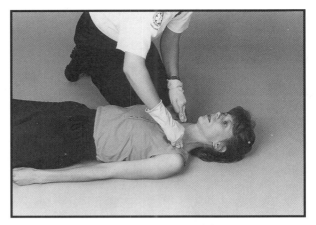

c. Now, starting at one shoulder, move down one of the patient's arms. Check the upper arm, palpate the shoulder joint, and palpate over the humerus. Then palpate over the radius and ulna in turn. Palpate the wrist, hand, and fingers. If no potential fractures are found, next you will want to check the joints for pain-on-movement. Have the patient elevate his arm, then move his elbow, then his wrist, and lastly open and close his hand, and note any painful movements.

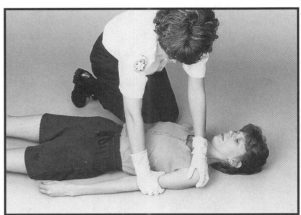

d. Next, repeat this examination in the patient's other arm.

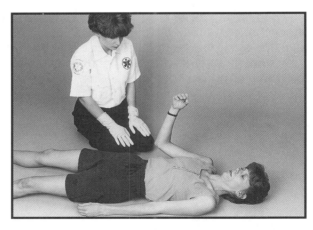

e. Continuing down the body, check the thorax next. Palpate the upper and middle sternum, then palpate along each rib in turn. Do not, in this examining step, palpate the ribs bilaterally at the same time as previously done. Each side should be palpated separately to clearly identify the location of any pain produced.

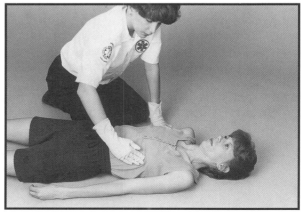

f. Continue the examination of the torso by palpating the rest of the spine. Starting at the neck, palpate over the spine, slowly moving in a caudad direction until you have reached the lower margin of the sacrum.
(Note: palpation of the lower end of the sacrum will generally produce pain if coccygeal injury exists. No additional pre-hospital palpation of the coccyx is necessary.)

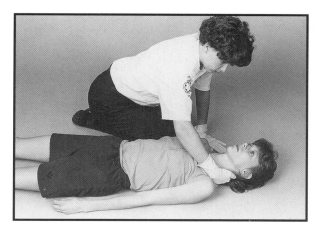

g. Complete the torso exam by palpating each flank (over the kidneys) in turn and then along the circumference of the pelvis on one side and then the other.

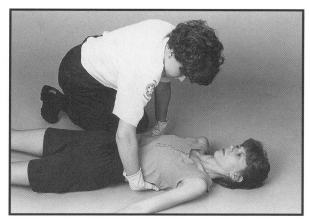

Note: When examining a significantly ill or injured patient who is in a supine position, repeated movement in order to examine each adjacent posterior area of the head and each section of the torso in turn would be unwise or even harmful. In such cases the EMT should first examine the patient from head to toe, limiting his examination of the head and torso to the anterior and lateral aspects which are available without moving the patient. Then, in an appropriate manner, the patient should be rolled onto his side (once) and the entire posterior checked from the upper head to the lower buttocks.

h. Next, continue down the body by examining one leg. First palpate over the hip and the head of the femur. Continue moving distally, palpating along the femur, the knee joint laterally and posteriorly, the patella, along the tibia and then the fibula, the ankle, the dorsal foot, and the toes. If no fracture has been found, check the joints by moving each in turn. Elevate the patient's leg to flex the hip, then bend the knee, then move the ankle, move the foot from flexion to extension, and finally move the toes.

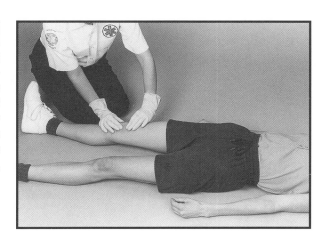

i. After completing the detailed exam of one leg, repeat it in the other leg.

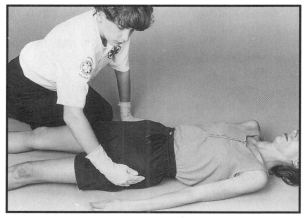

j. An optional step that may be useful in locating occult musculoskeletal injuries (strains or hairline fractures) in limbs where no injury was found can easily be performed by having the patient move each limb against pressure. For each limb, in turn, firmly grasp the patient's hand or foot in your hand and move it (with the patient's cooperation) to a partially flexed position. While you try to maintain the limb's present position, have the patient pull and then push as strongly as possible against your hand.

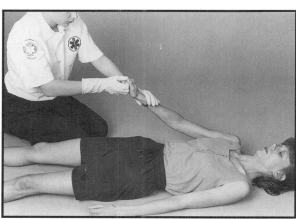

k. Once you have completed the head-to-toe *Localized Item Exam,* note each injury, area of pain, or other abnormality found, and *provide any individual item care* that was found to be needed (if resources and the patient's other conditions allow).

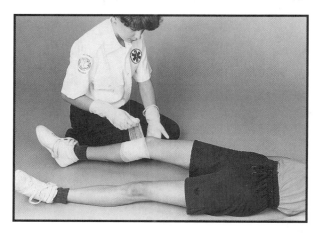

PART V—MONITOR

50. Once enroute, continuously monitor the gross ABC indicators for any changes. LOC, airway patency, and respiratory status can be monitored by maintaining a fairly continuous dialogue with the patient and noting any changes in his alertness and orientation or ease of speech. Any deterioration in circulatory status can be identified by monitoring the patient's LOC, skin color, and skin moisture. If pulse oximetry is available, continuous monitoring is recommended. When indicated, EKG monitoring should also be established and/or maintained during transport.

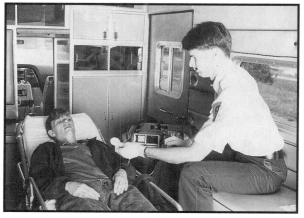

51. Quantitative (exact numerical) *vital signs* cannot usually be continuously monitored pre-hospital. They need, therefore, to be periodically rechecked and to be re-evaluated any time that a significant change in the patient's LOC, respiratory or circulatory status is observed. In a moving ambulance the blood pressure may have to be taken by palpation. In unconscious patients the adequacy of air exchange needs to be confirmed each time that the vital signs are re-checked.

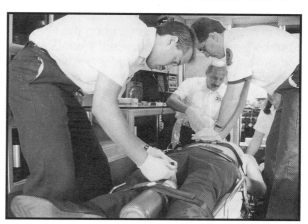

52. From the continuous monitoring of the patient and the comparable numerical quantification supplied by each set of vital signs, the EMT should (after each periodic re-check) evaluate if any increased, changed, or added interventions are indicated—and provide them.

PART VI—RADIO, REPORT, AND RECORD

53. When, how often and to whom **radio reports** are to be given varies from place to place. The EMT must be familiar with and follow his local protocols. Regardless of other differences, two key elements are universal. Upon completion of key assessment steps and interventions, a well organized radio report is transmitted. Second, the hospital to which the patient will be transported is notified, including the estimated time of arrival (ETA).

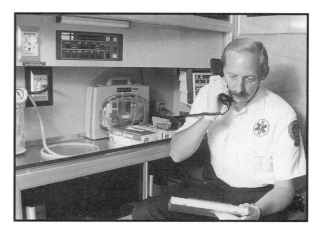

54. Medical practice requires that any health care professional give a full **verbal report** when transferring the primary responsibility for a patient's care directly to the health care professional assuming it, regardless of any previous report or written records. When transferring the patient at the hospital, the EMT must "give report" to the primary nurse assuming the responsibility for the patient. Other reports or transfer of the completed run report do not fulfill or mitigate this responsibility.

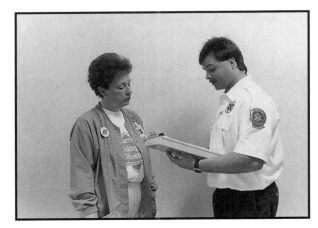

55. When in the ambulance call the **run report** is completed will depend upon the EMT resources available and the patient's condition. In non-urgent calls, it can usually be written as items occur and will have been completed upon arrival. In more serious cases a minimum of quantitative vital signs can be noted during the call, leaving the careful completion of the report to be done at the hospital after the patient has been transferred.

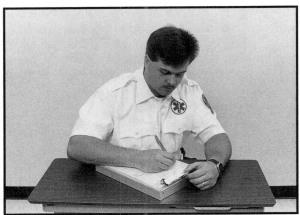

The patient pre-hospital record (or "run report") serves as the medical and legal documentation of the situation, patient data, assessment and care which occurred pre-hospital. It must be legible, clear, accurate and—although precise—complete. Remember the rule: ***If it isn't documented, it didn't happen.*** When writing the run report the EMT should remember that it is the sole remaining source of information about the pre-hospital events that the physician will have once the EMTs leave the emergency department, and that it will become a permanent part of the patient's and service's medical records should any future questions arise surrounding the quality or propriety of the EMT's assessment and care.

PART C:
Patient Assessment Skill Sheets

Detailed Summary Skill Sheet

PRE-HOSPITAL PATIENT ASSESSMENT

PART I—SAFETY, SCENE, SITUATION, AND SPINE

1. Assure SAFETY of scene and situation
2. Take UNIVERSAL PRECAUTIONS at level indicated
3. Ascertain NUMBER OF PATIENTS and general situations of each
4. Call for EMS and OTHER RESOURCES that may be needed.
5. Determine essential NATURE OF PROBLEM precipitating call for EMS
6. IF TRAUMA—determine MECHANISM OF INJURY
   IF MEDICAL—determine CHIEF COMPLAINT(S) and whether it is new or has probably been previously diagnosed.
7. Evaluate potential of SPINE TRAUMA from mechanism/situation

PART II—INITIAL SYSTEMIC EXAMINATION
(Note: provide needed interventions as identified)

GLOBAL SURVEY (Initial Size-Up)

8. OBSERVE patient as approaching and note: age, sex, conscious/unconscious, movement, is respiration spontaneous, and if labored, and how presents.
9. Simultaneously:
   - DIRECT Second EMT to provide manual immobilization if indicated
   - LOOK at patient's face
   - FEEL for radial pulse
   - ASK patient, "Where does it hurt?" and "What happened?"
10. DETERMINE:
    - Gross LOC, orientation and mentation, cerebral perfusion and oxygenation
    - Airway patency
    - Gross Respiratory Status
    - Gross Circulatory Status and Shock Level
    - Chief Complaint(s)
11. Scan head-to-toe for significant BLEEDING and remove any fluid-occlusive clothing.
12. CONTROL any significant external BLEEDING.

IN-DEPTH A,B,C,D, EXAMINATION

A—Airway

13. Listen at mouth for sounds of AIRWAY PROBLEM.
14. Look in mouth for items which could become an AIRWAY PROBLEM

B—Breathing

15. At mouth, evaluate amount of AIR EXCHANGE
16. Look at underside of tongue and evaluate COLOR OF MUCOSA
17. Observe NECK for injuries, stoma, JVD.
18. Palpate NECK for subcutaneous emphysema and tracheal deviation
19. Bare and VISUALIZE CHEST for sucking wounds and other injuries, and to evaluate excursion for depth, bilateral symmetry, or any paradoxical movement.
20. PALPATE CHEST for POP, deformity, or crepitus.
21. AUSCULTATE BREATH sounds for depth, bilateral equality, adventitious sounds, differences at bases or apices.

C—Circulation

22. Re-evaluate for any signs of SIGNIFICANT BLEEDING
23. Auscultate APICAL HEART sounds for character and to determine if amplitude is normal or appears distant or muffled.
24. Direct Second EMT to obtain VITAL SIGNS
25. Bare (as indicated) and VISUALIZE ABDOMEN for distention, wounds or bruises, and note any vaginal/penile bleeding or signs of incontinence.
26. Palpate the ABDOMEN for rigidity, palpable masses, or POP.
27. Palpate the PELVIS for POP, untofore movement, or crepitus.
28. Consider INTERNAL BLEEDING in head, chest or abdomen and decide if the level of shock present is explained by your findings.

(continued)

D—Disability, Neurological Deficit
29. Check the NOSE AND MOUTH for cerebrospinal fluids and/or blood.
30. Check the EARS for cerebrospinal fluid and/or blood, and posteriorly for any Battle's sign.
31. Check the EYES for any injuries, blown pupil, or periorbital ecchymosis (Raccoon's eyes)
32. Check EYES for PEARRL and consensual reflex.
33. Continue NEUROLOGICAL Evaluation

Note: If **CONSCIOUS** evaluate alertness, orientation, and distal, MSCs—if **UNCONSCIOUS** continue enlarged AVPU.

CONSCIOUS PATIENT	**UNCONSCIOUS PATIENT**
a. Evaluate spontaneity and appropriateness of MOVEMENT (to direction) and if localizes pain.	a. Continue AVPU. Determine if patient responds to NOXIOUS VERBAL stimulus and how. If responds, check MSCx4.
b. Note if patient appears awake and ALERT and appears ORIENTED TO EVENTS around him.	b. If doesn't respond to verbal stimulus, apply appropriate PAINFUL STIMULUS.
c. Check A & O x 3	c. Evaluate best response to pain. • Awakens • Responds by moans and attempts to withdraw • Responds by posturing • Other responses • Remains UNRESPONSIVE
d. Check MSCx4 to identify any one sided or inferior neuro deficit or compromised peripheral circulation.	d. Regardless of response, note any eye opening or other SPONTANEOUS MOVEMENT that has been/is seen, and check distal circulation.
e. Inquire about any pre/post insult period of unconsciousness or seizure activity	e. Check for MED ALERT jewelry or cards and check with witnesses for onset and duration of unconsciousness and any unusual motor activity (seizures)

34. During the preceding steps (or at this time) obtain an expanded A–M–P–L–E HISTORY from the patient and/or those accompanying him.

PART III—REVIEW, RE-EVALUATE, RULE-OUT AND RANK

35. Review OVERALL A,B,C,D STATUS and CONDITIONS/INJURIES found.
36. Form an overall CLINICAL IMPRESSION (provisional pre-hospital diagnosis).
37. RE-EVALUATE INTERVENTIONS provided and their effect, and change any as indicated.
38. In a systematic way, RULE-OUT each potential systemic condition not found to be present.
39. RULE-OUT the need for any additional available interventions not presently being provided.
40. RANK patient as either URGENT or NON-URGENT

(continued)

PART IV—LOCALIZED ITEM EXAM, PACKAGING AND TRANSPORT

URGENT PATIENT

41. Package and INITIATE TRANSPORT to nearest appropriate facility without delay

42. Provide any continued, deferred, and ADDITIONAL KEY CARE NEEDED enroute (IVs, ventilation, CPR, Pulse oximetry, EKG monitoring, etc.).

43. If time and resources allow, perform the LOCALIZED ITEM EXAM

NON-URGENT PATIENT

41. Perform the LOCALIZED ITEM EXAM.

42. When completed, provide INDIVIDUAL ITEM CARE indicated for each injury/condition found.

43. Package and INITIATE TRANSPORT

Note: The LOCALIZED ITEM EXAM (Step 43 URGENT PATIENT and Step 41 NON-URGENT PATIENT) is done differently for victims of TRAUMA and patients with a MEDICAL EMERGENCY.

TRAUMA PATIENTS
a. Do a head-to-toe survey.

b. Obtain any additional history needed.

c. Re-check vital signs.

d. Review and determine if vital signs suggest change in care being given, and in NON-URGENT patients do they suggest changing patient to the URGENT CATEGORY

MEDICAL PATIENTS
a. Examine areas related to Chief/Complaint/Conditions found in more detail.

b. Obtain a more detailed history and further qualify conditions/pain (OPQRSTU).

c. Re-check vital signs.

d. On a head-to-toe basis confirm that there is no hidden trauma.

PART V—MONITOR

44. Continuously MONITOR Gross LOC, speech, alertness, mentation, breathing, skin color and moisture.
45. Re-check VITAL SIGNS periodically or if there is any apparent change in the patient.
46. If changes occur in the patient's condition or periodic vital signs, EVALUATE need for increased or additional INTERVENTIONS.

PART VI—RADIO, REPORT, AND RECORD

47. As directed by local protocols, at the proper time in the previous sequence—provide a precise RADIO REPORT to appropriate Medical Control.
48. When leaving scene, NOTIFY HOSPITAL to which you are proceeding and give ETA.
49. Upon transfer of patient at the hospital, give proper VERBAL REPORT to health care professional assuming care of the patient.
50. Prior to leaving hospital, complete the RUN REPORT and leave copy with proper individual at hospital.

SECTION

Airway Management Skills

4

Airway Management

INTRODUCTION

Airway management and breathing are the highest priorities in the management of any patient, whether they are suffering from an acute medical emergency or from trauma. The EMT's mastery of individual airway and ventilation skills, including selecting the best method(s) to meet the patient's needs, is therefore a paramount responsibility in providing proper patient care.

Normally, conscious healthy people maintain and defend a clear open airway spontaneously without conscious thought or effort. Should an item such as a food particle or fluid invade the airway, the **gag reflex** is stimulated—resulting in repeated coughing which provides forceful high velocity expelled air to "blow" the airway clear. When unconsciousness progresses, the patient loses this gag reflex defense and can no longer keep his own airway clear. Additionally, as unconsciousness progresses and muscle tension is lost, in supine patients (the common resuscitation position) the mandible sags and moves posteriorly and the tongue—which is fastened at the posterior lower palate—becomes flaccid. The flaccid tongue can then also move posteriorly and obstruct the airway. Further, once the gag reflex has been lost the patient in this position cannot clear any foreign items or fluids from the airway and they can be readily aspirated into the lungs.

When the patient can no longer maintain his own airway, the EMT must immediately provide airway management if adequate ventilation (spontaneous or provided) and oxygenation are to be continued. The airway can be maintained using a variety of manual methods or adjuncts. Regardless of which method the EMT selects, they each provide the four key elements necessary to maintain a maximum patent airway:

- Keep the mouth open
- Keep the mandible in a normal or anterior-of-normal position (not letting it sag posteriorly)
- Keep the tongue elevated out of the airway
- Keep the head tilted to anatomically provide the maximum and most direct pathway for air exchange (unless contraindicated by possible spine trauma).

Manual maneuvers and simple adjuncts, although furnishing the above mentioned elements, *DO NOT* isolate the lower airway from the oropharynx, nasopharynx and laryngopharynx (which are common and open to regurgitated gastric contents). Therefore in addition to the use of such methods the EMT must continuously remove any debris, fluids, or gastric contents which compromise the airway or could be aspirated into the lungs.

The advanced airway adjuncts protect the airway from gastric contents by either obstructing the esophagus to keep gastric contents from entering the oral cavity or by providing a tube which seals off the trachea and connects it directly to outside the body.

If the airway is obstructed by a foreign body, this will first need to be dislodged and removed before any airway adjunct is inserted or any of the aforementioned airway management techniques will be effective. If all attempts to clear a foreign body fail or the upper airway is so injured or edematous that ventilation through the normal oronasal pathways remains impossible, and if properly trained and certified personnel are available, an emergency tracheostomy should be performed to permit ventilation directly into the trachea through the use of percutaneous transtracheal ventilation (PTV). In the prehospital setting this procedure is only performed when other methods to obtain a patent airway have proven unsuccessful.

AIRWAY MANAGEMENT TECHNIQUES

The various airway management techniques are generally grouped into the following categories:

Basic

- Manual maneuvers—with and without spinal immobilization
- Simple adjuncts—oropharyngeal (OPA) and nasopharyngeal (NPA) airways

Advanced

- Obturator or dual-lumen airways (EOA, EGTA, Combitube, PTL) which isolate the airway from gastric regurgitation
- Definitive management—endotracheal tube (ETT) airway
- Emergency tracheostomy—establishing an alternate transtracheal airway

Special Techniques

- Suctioning
- Vomitus extraction—special positioning or suctioning techniques to evacuate copious amounts of vomitus to avoid life-threatening aspiration or airway obstruction
- Foreign body obstruction removal

Generally, manual maneuvers are most immediately initiated to avoid delay for equipment. Since experience has shown that these are difficult (if not impossible) to sustain for any extended period, as soon as possible they should be replaced with a suitable airway adjunct. Use of an oropharyngeal or nasopharyngeal airway as the initial adjunct used expedites purchase of the airway and proper immediate hyperventilation. Once this has been established and ventilation has occurred for several minutes, when indicated and properly trained personnel are available, a more advanced airway device should replace the simple adjunct to isolate the airway from gastric contents and to protect against aspiration. Except in patients in cardiac arrest, hyperventilation with a high percentage of supplemental oxygen using a simple adjunct should be sustained for several minutes before an advanced (more deeply invasive) airway is inserted not only as an expedient for oxygenation but also to avoid the chance of producing an undesirable bradycardia. In an hypoxic patient (except those in cardiac arrest) contact between the distal tip of an advanced airway and the laryngopharynx can stimulate a vagal reflex and produce a dangerous bradycardia (pulse rate below 60) as a result.

The presence or absence of a gag reflex is also a key consideration in the selection of an airway adjunct. In the prehospital setting only the nasopharyngeal airway and "blind" nasotracheal intubation are the commonly available airway adjunct methods for patients that have a present gag reflex. Use of other adjuncts or methods of intubation, since they can produce vomiting in patients with a gag reflex, are contraindicated in cases where the gag reflex is still intact.

Since all airway maneuvers result in or can result in contact with the patient's bodily fluids, proper universal precautions must be taken prior to their initiation by the EMT. These should always include use of examining gloves and, on a case-by-case basis, should include such other items (face shield, gown, etc.) as are indicated.

Most common airway and ventilation methods (such as the head tilt/chin lift, head tilt/jaw thrust, use of simple adjuncts, endotracheal intubation, etc.) include moving the patient's head and/or neck—hyperextending the neck by rotating the head while advancing its lower third anteriorly into a forward "sniffing" position in order to maximize the airway. The act of maintaining a mask seal while ventilating with a bag-valve-mask device usually produces alternating movement of the head when pressure is applied in a posterior direction. In trauma patients who have suspected spine trauma, any airway method which results in movement of the head or neck is contraindicated. Therefore, in such cases the common airway managements methods need to be altered.

SPECIAL MODIFICATIONS IN THE AIRWAY MANAGEMENT OF PATIENTS WITH POTENTIAL SPINE TRAUMA

In trauma patients these methods must be modified in two ways since movement of the head—and particularly hyperextension of the neck—are contraindicated. First, the EMT must be able to perform airway management procedures in trauma patients with the patient's head and spine maintained in the neutral in-line position. Second, manual immobilization must be continuously provided throughout to avoid unwanted movement. With trauma patients, most airway management and ventilation procedures are best done with at least two EMTs working together whenever possible.

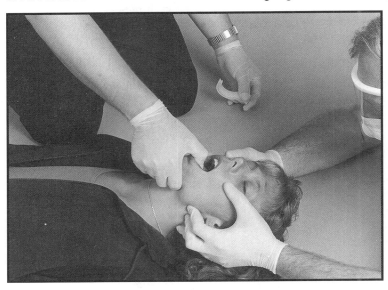

When such maneuvers are required after the patient has been mechanically immobilized to a longboard or other rigid immobilization device, manual immobilization should be provided to protect against the movement which is implicit in such airway maneuvers as inserting an airway or maintaining a mask seal.

Airway management and ventilation skills for trauma patients are best done with at least two EMT's: one to maintain the neutral in-line immobilization of the neck and head, one to actually perform the airway or ventilation skill, and when possible a third to assemble and prepare equipment. Some of the skills shown can be modified to allow a single EMT to maintain in-line immobilization and simultaneously manage the airway and/or provide ventilation, however when performed by only one EMT they generally provide far less stability in maintaining the immobilization. Therefore, when spinal immobilization is part of the patient's overall treatment, the use of single-operator techniques should be limited to those situations when only one EMT is present.

Manual in-line immobilization during airway and ventilation maneuvers can best be provided from one of two positions: kneeling or lying beyond the patient's head (facing down along the patient's body), or from a kneeling position next to the patient's torso (facing his head). The EMT providing the immobilization should be positioned to cause the least interference to the EMT who is performing the airway or ventilation procedure.

When providing manual immobilization to a patient who is on the ground, while lying beyond the patient's head, the EMT first positions himself as shown below. When necessary this can also be done in a kneeling position, however more stable immobilization can be provided from the prone position with both elbows on the ground.

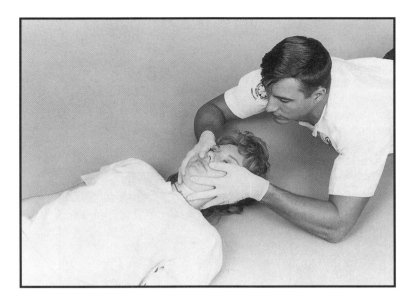

The Patient's head is held between the EMT's hands and brought into the in-line position. The thumbs are placed in the maxillary notch on each side of the nose, and the little finger (or last two fingers) are placed under the posterior lower head. The remaining fingers are spread (pointing in a generally caudad direction) on the flat planes at each side of the head. Pressure between the thumbs and the finger(s) under the posterior lower head prevents flexion or extension, and pressure between the other fingers helps to prevent lateral movement or sideways rotation.

When mask ventilation is to be done, a slight change in hand position will allow the EMT providing immobilization from above the patient's head to also hold the mask. In this way he can provide a good mask seal, properly elevate the chin, and maintain the head immobilization at the same time. This frees the second EMT to concentrate on assuring that adequate ventilations are provided.

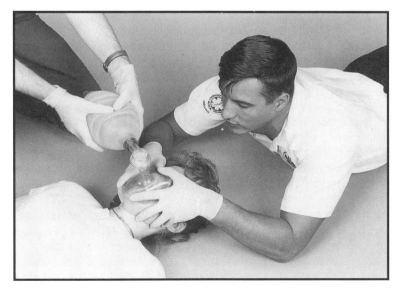

In patients where neutral in-line positioning produces a significant space between the back of the head and the ground, suitable padding should be inserted as early as possible. This makes the task of the EMT at the head easier and reduces the chance that inserting an airway or obtaining a mask seal will cause unwanted movement of the head. When the patient is elevated on the cot the same method of immobilization can be used by standing above the head end of the cot.

In small children with trauma, padding under the posterior torso (as well as immobilization) is required to maintain the neutral in-line position. This is discussed further later in this section under special pediatric airway considerations.

Manual immobilization from alongside the patient is similar to immobilization from above the patient's head. When done from the patient's side, however, the fingers point cephalad instead of caudad. The EMT kneels at the patient's side, angled so that he faces the patient's head. The thumbs are placed on each side of the patient's nose, below the zygoma in the maxillary notch. The little fingers (or last two fingers of each hand) are placed under the back of the caudad third of the head. The remaining fingers are spread on the flat planes at the sides of the head. Lastly the EMT brings his elbows in against his own torso to provide additional support.

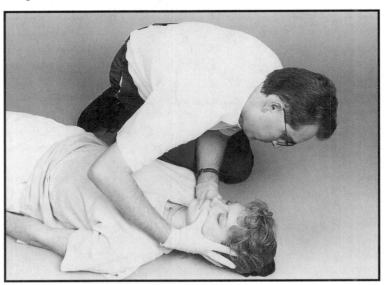

Whenever needed, padding behind the patient's head should be inserted as soon as possible. Providing immobilization from the side leaves the area above the patient's head free for airway management and ventilation procedures. The same technique can easily be used with patients who have been placed on an ambulance cot.

SPECIAL CONSIDERATIONS IN AIRWAY MANAGEMENT OF THE PEDIATRIC PATIENT

The smaller size of pediatric patients obviously necessitates the use of smaller sized airway adjuncts, and the greater variation in body sizes commonly found in the pediatric population requires the availability of a larger variety of airway sizes than is required to meet the common variations found in adults. As well as differences in size, children are not just "little adults" but have some significant anatomical differences which require modification of the adult airway management principles and skills for small children and infants.

In infants and small children (generally a body size normal for a 7 year old or younger) the ratio of the head size to the size of the torso is significantly greater than in adults, and the musculature covering the scapulae has not yet developed the same proportional mass as in an adult. Almost all of the greater proportional head size is in the part of the skull which is posterior to the first cervical vertebrae of the spinal column. Since the increase in cranial size is posterior to the posterior flat plane of the torso, when an infant or small child is placed on a rigid flat surface such as the ground or a backboard, their head is moved to a flexed position that could result in obstructing their airway.

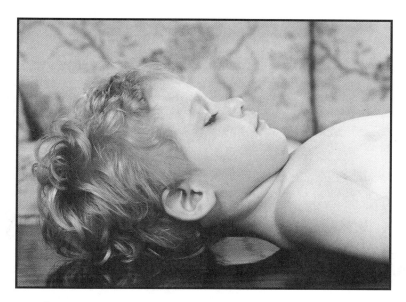

Such movement and ultimate position *is obviously contraindicated in children with possible spine trauma.* It is also **contraindicated in any child,** regardless of the presence or absence of trauma, based upon airway considerations. In adults or children, extensive flexion of the head may readily produce closure or lessening of the airway.

In small children, the cartilaginous rings which protect and maintain the open round shape of the trachea in adults have as yet not become rigid. Therefore either significant flexion or extension of the head and neck in infants or small children can collapse the immature trachea and produce severe or complete airway obstruction.

To avoid the flexion that anatomically results if an infant or small child is placed directly on a rigid flat surface, a folded blanket or similar firm item which is approximately two inches thick should be inserted under their posterior torso.

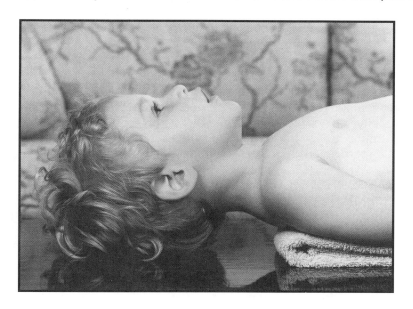

The resulting elevation of the torso above the rigid surface provides space for the larger posterior cranium and allows the head to remain in the neutral in-line position. In cases of trauma, care must be taken to assure that the folded blanket produces a continuous semi-rigid flat surface (without voids, creases, or thicker areas). This must be from the upper margin of the shoulders to the lower margin of the buttocks or mid-thigh and must be of sufficient width to underlie the shoulders and arms on each side as well as the entire width of the torso in order to provide a stable platform upon which to immobilize the thoracic, lumbar and sacral sections of the spine in the proper neutral in-line position.

In cases (with or without trauma) where the potential for CPR exists, the padding must be firm and as extensive as described above to provide a proper platform for chest compressions to be performed.

In any of the above cases the amount of elevation of the torso (thickness of the padding) necessary to produce neutral alignment of the head on a rigid surface varies from child to child. Experience has shown that obtaining the exact amount of padding needed under the torso of a given child is hard to approximate and results in multiple movements of the patient and undue delays. Therefore it is recommended that the EMT over-elevate the torso with two inches of padding and then (as in adults) fill any voids with padding behind the head to achieve the desired neutral alignment or degree of head tilt.

In infants and small children the immature development of the tracheal rings could easily result in airway obstruction through tracheal collapse if an adult-type head tilt was attempted. *Therefore, when managing the airway in infants and small children (when no suspicion of a potentially unstable spine exists), the head should only be slightly tilted into mild hyperextension. Maximal hyperextension or maximal elevation into a forward "sniffing" position are contraindicated.*

Due to the many varying individual pediatric sizes and the fact that no accurate method of determining the length of a patient's airway from the mouth to the carina exists, there are no pediatric versions of either the obturator or dual-lumen type airway devices. Inflation of a large cuff in the esophagus at a point above the carina could produce pressure on the trachea and cause an airway obstruction. Therefore, use of such devices is contraindicated in any patient below a given height—including all pediatric patients except larger adolescents.

Endotracheal intubation, as in adults, is the method of choice for providing protected definitive airway management in infants and small children. Due to the small size and normal narrowing of the upper end of the trachea in infants and small children, the endotracheal tubes in these sizes do not have an inflatable distal cuff. Once inserted and properly in place, the narrow area of the trachea in these patients provides a natural seal around the ET tube. The EMT, when intubating an infant, will find that the vocal cords are more anterior and often more difficult to visualize than those of an adult.

SELECTION OF THE PROPER TECHNIQUE

The EMT should select a particular airway maneuver or airway adjunct based upon that patient's level of consciousness, the patient's condition and needs, consideration of time required (often resulting in the need of a simpler interim adjunct prior to more protected definitive airway care), and his level of training. Some general guidelines, however, may be helpful in this selection:

- The EMT's selection must be keyed to the **patient's immediate** airway problem. (The immediate airway need in a "choking" victim is to clear the foreign object; in an apneic or unconscious supine patient to open the airway, take control of the tongue, and suction as needed; in a newborn to suction the fluid from the nose and mouth; etc.)

In patients who *DO NOT* have a foreign body obstruction:

- Any patient with a significantly lowered level of consciousness needs airway management.

- Consideration of the potential for spine trauma must be given early on. Employing manual maneuvers and using airway adjuncts with patients who have a potentially unstable spine still requires continuous immobilization in the neutral in-line position. In all other cases, airway management should include positioning the patient's head and neck in such a way as to maximize air exchange.

- Manual maneuvers should be used *first* to avoid delay in assuring a patent airway while equipment is located and assembled.

- Since it is difficult (if not impossible) to sustain manual maneuvers (except in cases of cardiac arrest where endotracheal intubation equipment is readied), they should be replaced as rapidly as possible by the appropriate simple adjunct.

In patients with an **INTACT gag reflex** but a significantly lowered level of consciousness:

- A nasopharyngeal airway should be inserted to protect against a later restriction or loss of the airway.

- Once a nasopharyngeal airway is in place, more protected definitive management with nasotracheal intubation should be considered if properly trained and certified personnel are present and if vomiting, fluid management problems, or further lowering of the level of consciousness (as in overdose patients) is anticipated.

In unconscious patients with an **ABSENT gag reflex:**

- An oropharyngeal airway should be inserted and, as soon as practicable, initial suctioning should be performed.

- If properly trained personnel are present, once the airway is managed with an oropharyngeal airway and other immediate A, B, C priorities have been met (including the addition of supplemental high FiO_2 oxygen), the EMT should provide more definitive protected airway management to avoid the potential of airway compromise or aspiration from gastric regurgitation.

- Periodic suctioning and additional suctioning as needed should be provided.

In cases where repeated airway management attempts have failed to provide a patent airway, and when properly trained and certified personnel in keeping with local protocols are available, an alternate airway through the neck should be created by performing an emergency tracheostomy and the patient should be ventilated transtracheally.

Manual Airway Maneuvers—Introduction

The manual airway maneuvers open or maintain the patient's airway as a result of specific positioning of the head, neck, and mandible, without the need of an airway adjunct. Since they do not require any equipment (or loss of time to locate and ready) they are the method of choice for initial management and situations where no airway adjuncts are available (e.g., when an off-duty EMT needs to provide airway management). Four separate manual maneuvers are commonly included in this category:

- **Head Tilt/Chin Lift**
- **Head Tilt/Jaw Thrust**
- **Trauma Chin Lift**
- **Trauma Jaw Thrust**

Both the **Head Tilt/Chin Lift** and the **Head Tilt/Jaw Thrust** involve a simultaneous *triple* maneuver; the head is hyperextended: the mandible is elevated anteriorly beyond its normal position (*pulled* in the case of the chin lift and *pushed* in the case of the jaw thrust); and the mandible is moved slightly caudad to open the mouth.

In the Trauma Chin Lift and the Trauma Jaw Thrust the head is **NOT hyperextended.** Instead, the head is placed (or maintained) in the neutral in-line position and manually immobilized to prevent unwanted movement of the vertebrae while the mandible is elevated (lifted or pushed) and moved slightly caudad. It should be noted that the **Trauma Jaw Thrust** is the only manual maneuver which allows a single EMT to maintain neutral in-line immobilization, an open airway, and even a mask seal, alone. The **Trauma Chin Lift** requires two EMTs in order to be stable and without chance of inadvertent movement of the head.

HEAD TILT/CHIN LIFT

This is one of the two manual airway maneuvers recommended for initial use in patients with a need for airway management who ***do not*** have a potentially unstable spine. As in all airway maneuvers, first assure that the appropriate level of universal precautions have been taken. Should the patient be other than supine, he will first have to be moved into the supine position on his back. Then:

1. The EMT should take a position alongside the patient's head. Place your cephalad hand on the patient's forehead and tilt the head backward to fully hyperextend the neck. In infants and small children the head should only be slightly tilted, as more significant hyperextension can result in collapse of the trachea.

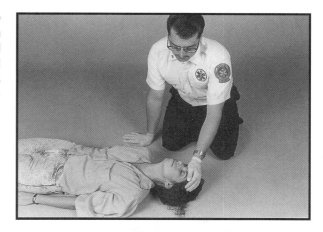

2. Without removing your cephalad hand from the forehead, grasp the patient's chin with your caudad hand. Hold the chin firmly between your thumb on top and the tips of your first two fingers hooked underneath it.

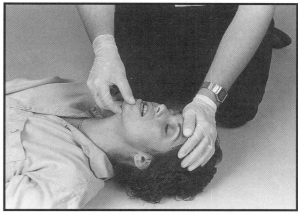

3. While maintaining the head tilt with uninterrupted pressure on the forehead with your cephalad hand, elevate the patient's mandible by firmly pulling it in an anterior direction to lift the tongue from the airway, and also move it slightly caudad to open the mouth.

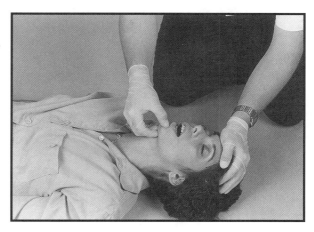

TRAUMA CHIN LIFT

When the potential for spinal trauma is suspected the EMT should employ this "trauma" version of the chin lift maneuver. This is the same maneuver as the "head tilt/chin lift" with three important differences: the head and neck are not hyperextended, the head is immobilized in the neutral in-line position, and an additional rescuer is necessary in most cases. Prior to beginning this maneuver, assure that the appropriate level of universal precautions have been taken and that the patient is in the supine position on his back. Then:

1. One EMT positioned above the patient's head should place his hands on the sides of the patient's head with his thumbs extended over the patient's cheekbones. Next he should move the patient's head into the neutral in-line position and maintain manual immobilization.

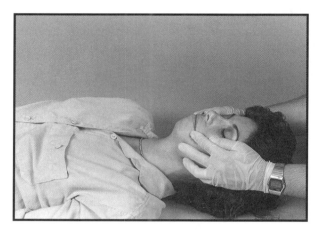

2. A second EMT positioned alongside the patient's head firmly grasps the patient's chin with his caudad hand. The chin is grasped between the thumb placed over the mandible and the first two fingers hooked under it.

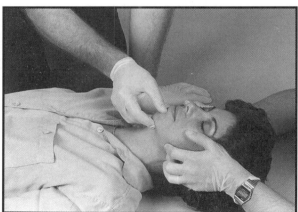

3. While the first EMT keeps the head from moving, the second EMT lifts the chin anteriorly and slightly caudad. This elevates the mandible (pulling the tongue from the airway) and opens the mouth, as shown. If this maneuver must be performed by only one rescuer he should position himself so that his knees and/or thighs can vise-grip the patient's head, leaving his hands free to perform the chin lift.

Note: How manual airway maneuvers and ventilation can be provided simultaneously by a single EMT will be discussed in the *Ventilation Section* of this text.

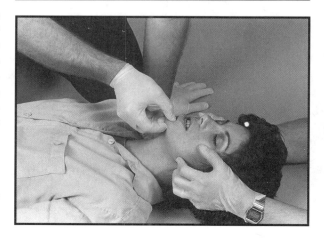

HEAD TILT/JAW THRUST

As noted earlier, the jaw thrust maneuver produces the same movement of the mandible as the chin lift—it is simply the manner of moving the mandible which is different. However with the head tilt/jaw thrust maneuver *both* of the rescuer's hands are involved in *both* tilting the head and moving the jaw anteriorly and caudad. Once the adequate level of universal precautions have been taken and the patient, if needed, has been moved into the supine position:

1. An EMT positioned above the patient's head places his hands on each side of the head and tilts the head and neck to hyperextension. His thumbs are placed on the patient's cheekbones and his third and fourth fingers are extended to grasp the angle of the mandible.

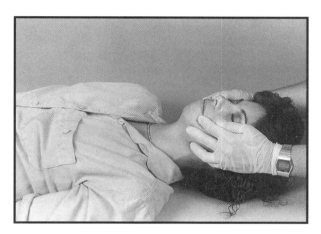

2. While maintaining the head tilt, the EMT causes the mandible to move by pushing anteriorly on the angle of the mandible with his third and fourth fingers—using the thumb-holds on the cheekbones for leverage. The resulting elevation of the mandible pulls the tongue forward from the airway.

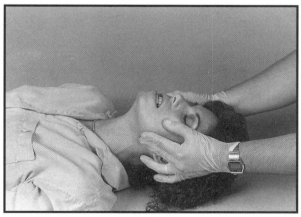

3. Finally, the EMT should place the first fingers of each hand on the patient's anterior chin (over the ridge where the lower teeth are inserted in the gums), and move the mandible slightly caudad to hold the mouth open.

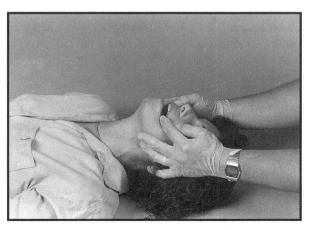

TRAUMA JAW THRUST

The Trauma Jaw Thrust produces the same mandibular movement as the head tilt/jaw thrust but does not include hyperextending the head and neck. It represents the most practical way for a single EMT to maintain an open airway and head immobilization simultaneously without the use of an airway adjunct in patients with suspected spinal trauma. Once the proper level of universal precautions has been taken, and if needed the patient has been moved into the supine position:

1. From above the patient's head, the EMT places his fingers on the sides of the patient's head with the thumbs over the zygoma and moves the patient's neck and head into the neutral in-line position.

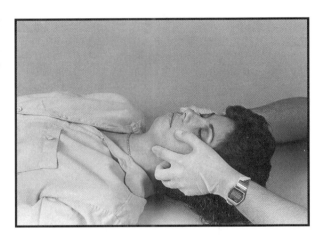

2. While maintaining the immobilization, the angle of the mandible at each side is pushed anteriorly with the 3rd & 4th fingers until the lower jaw is elevated, and the mouth is opened by mild caudad pressure with the EMT's first fingers on the patient's chin.

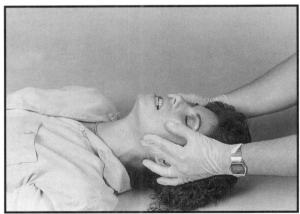

3. The Trauma Jaw Thrust can also be performed from alongside the patient. In this position the EMT's fingers point cephalad rather than caudad and the mandible is elevated by anterior pressure on the angle of the mandible with the EMT's thumbs.

Note: The Trauma Jaw Thrust represents the most practical way for a single EMT to maintain an open airway and head immobilization simultaneously without the use of an airway adjunct. Additional information on how a single EMT can maintain a mask seal while simultaneously providing ventilations will be discussed in the *Ventilation Section* of this text.

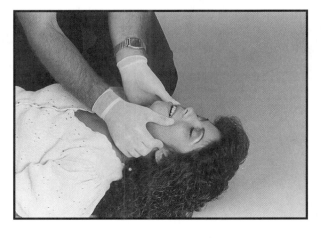

Simple Airway Adjuncts—Introduction

In cases requiring airway management by the EMT, the initial manual maneuvers in almost all cases should as quickly as practical be replaced by the use of a *simple airway adjunct,* since the manual maneuvers can not be easily or reliably sustained for any extended period of time beyond the first few minutes.

The oropharyngeal airway is the simple adjunct of choice in patients with an absent gag reflex. Insertion of an oropharyngeal airway when the gag reflex is intact can result in regurgitation and aspiration of gastric contents, and is therefore contraindicated. The nasopharyngeal airway will be tolerated by most patients with an intact gag reflex and is the simple adjunct of choice in such cases. Therefore, in conscious responsive patients, the nasopharyngeal airway is indicated and use of an oropharyngeal airway should *NOT* be attempted. In unconscious patients, the oropharyngeal airway is the first adjunct selected. If the attempt to insert it results in coughing, gagging, or other signs that the gag reflex is intact, halt the insertion process and rapidly remove the airway from the patient's mouth. In such cases, since the unconscious patient has demonstrated an intact gag reflex, the nasopharyngeal airway should be used instead. If the unconscious patient tolerates the insertion of an oropharyngeal airway, his gag reflex is absent. As soon as the airway is in place and ventilation (if required) has been initiated, his oropharynx should be suctioned.

When the correct oropharyngeal airway is immediately available to the EMT it should be inserted initially, employing only such manual maneuvers as are needed for its insertion. This precludes the need for any manual maneuvers for initial ventilations. Once a simple adjunct is in place and ventilation with a high FiO_2 is established, the EMT (depending upon available resources and his level of training) should replace the simple adjunct with a more definitive and protected airway if possible as soon as practical.

Oropharyngeal airways come in two basic types, which can be used interchangeably. One style is tube-like with a large central lumen running from its distal to its proximal tip and through which air can pass. The second style ("Berman-type") has a narrow rigid center septum with channels open at their outer sides extended from distal to proximal tips.

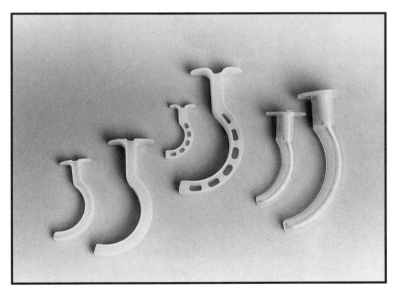

Oropharyngeal airways have a flange at their (outer) proximal end to assure maintenance of the proximal end outside the mouth, then a straight section which passes through the lips and teeth, and finally a curved distal section which is intended to purchase the tongue. This curved segment is designed to match the natural anatomical curvature of the lower oral airway. Oropharyngeal airways come in a variety of sizes and are measured and selected based upon their length. Rather than requiring unnecessary additional choices for the outside diameter, only one girth (properly proportioned to the oral cavity size based upon the selected airway's length) is available.

With nasopharyngeal airways the outside diameter is the key factor for size, since providing the largest pathway for air exchange requires the largest diameter airway that can be inserted through the nostril. If too small a diameter is selected the air exchange may be insufficient, if too large an outside diameter is selected the EMT will either be unable to insert it or may produce nasal trauma while attempting to do so. The length of the airway is also a key sizing consideration since if it is too short it will not be inserted far enough to keep the tongue out of the airway, and if too long it can stimulate the gag reflex.

Two styles of nasopharyngeal airway are presently available. The most common style has a long single-lumen tubular shaft which is slightly curved (to conform to the nasal airway's anatomy), with a bevelled distal end with round edges to minimize injury to the septum during insertion, and a flared "trumpet-like" proximal end which cannot enter the anterior nare due to its larger shape. This first style of nasopharyngeal airway varies from 5mm to 9mm in width, with the length of each being proportional to the width—that is, all 5mm wide airways are the same length, all 7mm wide airways are the same length but different from those that are 5mm wide, etc. If the length is too long for the patient, resulting in stimulating the gag reflex, the airway can simply be withdrawn slightly and taped to hold it in place. This style comes in a flexible rubber-like material or in a rigid hard plastic. To minimize damage to the septum the softer type is recommended for general use pre-hospital. The hard plastic type is only recommended in limited cases where its rigid nature is needed to protect against collapse of the inserted airway in cases where such maxillofacial swelling is anticipated and only by EMTs specially trained in its specific insertion.

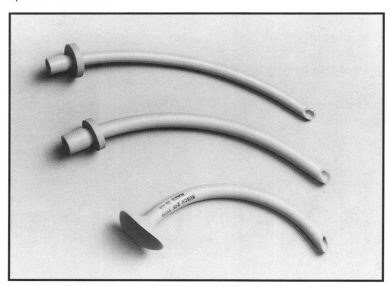

In recent years a second style of "soft" nasopharyngeal airway has become available. In this style, each available diameter has a longer curved single-lumen tube and, instead of the flared "trumpet-like" outer end, has a rubber collet surrounding the long tube which can be moved with firm pressure thereby allowing the EMT to measure and adjust it to the exact insertion length desired for that patient. Although more expensive, this type provides for selection of the exact diameter and placement of a stop at the exact length needed for an individual patient.

OROPHARYNGEAL AIRWAY—TONGUE-JAW LIFT METHOD

An oropharyngeal airway is the initial airway of choice for patients who have an **ABSENT** gag reflex. It is contraindicated in patients who have a present gag reflex. Two methods of insertion are widely used. The most common employs the tongue-jaw lift to secure the tongue against the lower palate to ensure proper insertion over the tongue. Once you are sure the proper level of universal precautions have been taken:

1. "Eyeball" the various sizes and select the length you estimate to be correct for the patient. Measure it as shown, changing it for a longer or shorter one as needed. The correct size oropharyngeal airway should match the distance from the lower edge of the patient's ear lobe to the corner of his mouth.

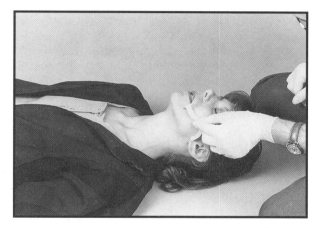

2. While holding the airway just below the flange with a pencil-like grip, insert the thumb of your other hand into the patient's mouth as shown and hold the tongue against the lower palate. Grasp the mandible and tongue between your thumb and your first two fingers and simultaneously elevate the lower jaw and hold the mouth open widely. This is called a Tongue-Jaw Lift. This maneuver is helpful when inserting any airway into the mouth as it assures that the device passes superior to the tongue and does not push the tongue into the pharynx, obstructing the airway.

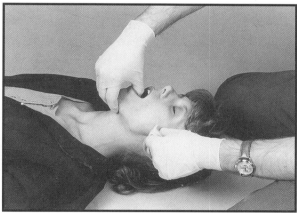

3. While maintaining the tongue-jaw lift, position the oropharyngeal airway so that it is turned at a 90 degree angle to the patient's midline and is held *horizontally* with the distal tip pointing posteriorly, directly into the patient's mouth, as shown.

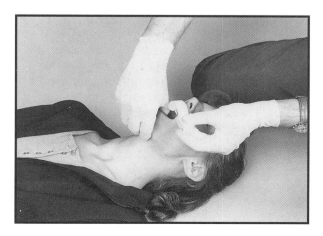

4. Continue maintaining the tongue-jaw lift and insert the tip into the mouth superior to the tongue. Advance the airway into the oropharynx *while gently rotating the flanged end 90 degrees caudally in the horizontal plane to the mid-line of the patient's body. As the airway is rotated, also insert the tip deeper into the mouth, following the normal anatomical curve of the patient's airway. If he gags* at any time during insertion, stop and immediately withdraw it. When inserting an oropharyngeal airway in an infant *it should NOT be rotated into place. Rather, hold it parallel to the infant's midline and use a tongue blade to elevate the tongue, as shown in the following pages.*

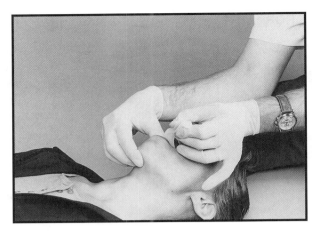

5. Continue inserting the airway until the flange is just anterior to the lips. If the tongue has been properly lifted out of the way the airway should rest easily in this position. Look into the mouth and visualize that the airway is properly placed and that it surrounds the tongue—holding it against the lower palate.

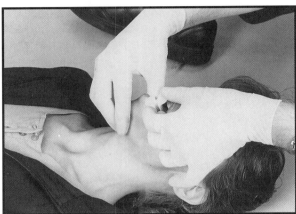

6. Check for air exchange, or in cases where ventilation is to be provided, assure that several breaths are successfully given without any undue resistance or other indication of an airway problem to confirm that the oropharyngeal airway is properly placed. As soon as practical, suction any fluids from the oropharynx.

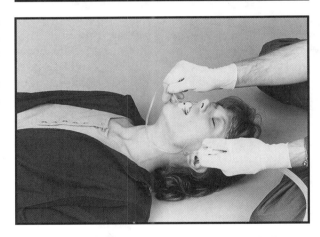

7. If you have any reason to suspect that the patient has an unstable spine, a second EMT will be required to maintain neutral in-line stabilization of the patient's head and neck throughout the insertion procedure. In this photograph the EMT above the patient's head is providing manual immobilization while the EMT alongside the patient is inserting the airway.

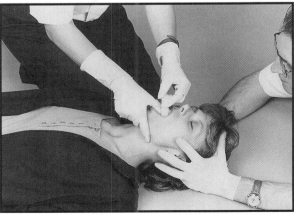

OROPHARYNGEAL AIRWAY—TONGUE BLADE INSERTION METHOD

An oropharyngeal airway can be inserted using a tongue blade instead of using the previously described method employing the tongue-jaw lift. The tongue blade insertion method is safer for the EMT since it eliminates the possibility of accidental tearing or puncture of gloves (or the skin) by sharp, pointed or broken teeth, and it eliminates the possibility of being bitten if the patient's level of unconsciousness is not as deep as previously assessed or if any seizure activity occurs. This method requires that tongue blades be kept readily available with the airways. Once you are sure the proper universal precautions have been taken:

1. To insert an oropharyngeal airway using a tongue blade, hold the airway with a pencil-like grip just below the flange in one hand and the tongue blade in the other. While visualizing the mouth, carefully insert the tongue blade on an angle (about 45° to 60° from vertical) with the distal end more cephalad than the end which you are holding. Keep the tongue blade superior to the tongue and insert it until it is about halfway along the tongue's length. Do not insert the airway yet.

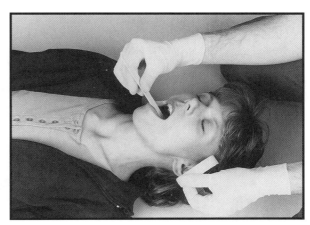

2. Rotate the distal tip of the tongue blade caudally and elevate the tongue against the lower palate. Hold the airway about horizontal, aligning it with the midline of the patient's body as shown. The distal end of the airway should point directly posteriorly into the patient's mouth. Next, extend the arm holding the tongue blade slightly—elevating the tongue and mandible and further opening the mouth.

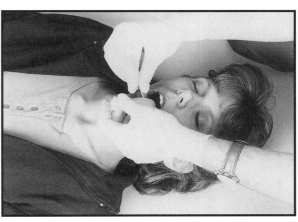

3. When using a tongue blade, the oropharyngeal airway is inserted in the midline of the mouth and is held so that the curve of the device naturally follows the anatomical curvature of the upper airway. (It is *NOT* inserted perpendicular to the midline as discussed for the tongue-jaw lift method). Continue inserting the airway following the curvature of the upper airway. Once the airway is fully inserted (so the flange is just anterior of the upper lip), release the tension on the tongue blade and remove it. Visualize the mouth and check the air exchange to confirm that the oropharyngeal airway has been properly placed.

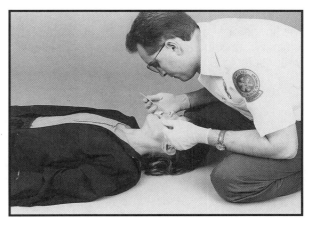

NASOPHARYNGEAL AIRWAY

This simple airway adjunct provides an effective way to maintain a patent airway in patients who still have an intact gag reflex. If properly sized it will be tolerated by most such patients. This airway is placed gently in the nostril, following the floor of the nasal cavity directly posterior to the nasopharynx. If significant resistance is encountered in one nostril, the procedure should be halted and insertion in the other nostril attempted. One possible complication resulting from this device is nasal trauma. Once you have assured that the proper universal precautions have been taken:

1. Kneel at the patient's side and examine the nostrils with a light. Select the largest and least deviated or obstructed nostril (usually the right). Measure the outer diameter of several nasopharyngeal airways against the size of the anterior nostril or the diameter of the patient's little finger. Select a nasopharyngeal airway that is just smaller than the size of the nostril or the same width as the fingernail of the patient's little finger.

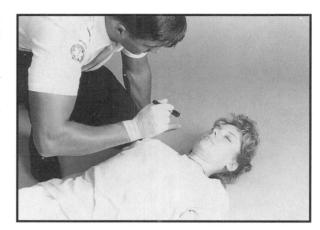

2. Measure the selected airway for proper length by comparing it to the distance from the patient's earlobe to the corner of his nose. If the airway has an adjustable slide on it, position the slide at the correct length. If the airway does not have this feature and you do not have an airway of the proper length available, you will have to keep your fingers at this point throughout the insertion process to identify the correct depth.

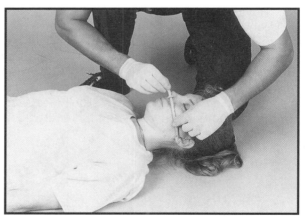

3. Hold the airway in a "pencil-grip" fashion near the flange or at the point at which you wish to stop insertion, and lubricate the distal tip liberally with water soluble jelly.

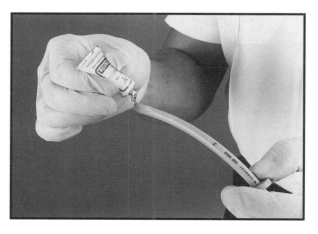

4. While continuing to hold the airway in a "pencil-grip" fashion and with the patient's head tilted back, insert the airway into the selected nostril. Insertion should be in an anterior-to-posterior direction—it should **NOT** be inserted superiorly. If resistance is met a gentle back-and-forth rotation of the airway between the fingers will usually help. Should you continue to meet an obstruction *DO NOT USE FORCE*. Instead, withdraw the airway, re-lubricate it, and attempt to insert it through the other nostril.

   If the EMT suspects that the patient's spine may be unstable, a second EMT will be needed to maintain neutral in-line immobilization manually throughout the procedure.

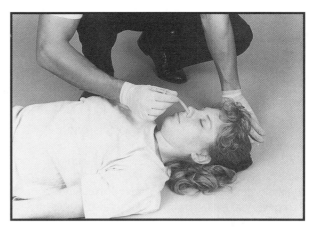

5. When approximately two-thirds of the correct measured length has been inserted, stop. Provide (or have another EMT provide) either a chin lift or jaw thrust to move the mandible anteriorly and to elevate the tongue so that the nasopharyngeal airway passes beyond the posterior margin of the tongue.

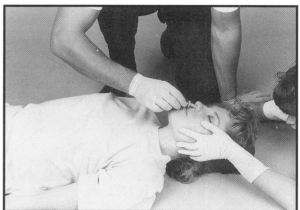

6. Continue insertion until the flange or marker is next to the anterior nare, or until the patient gags. The distal tip of the airway should pass slightly into the posterior pharynx behind the posterior tongue to avoid the possibility of obstruction by the tongue should it fall back. Once the airway is fully inserted, the mandible can be released. If the patient gags in the final stages of insertion, the airway may be too long. Have the patient swallow several times to suppress his gag reflex and withdraw the airway slightly. In such cases the EMT must secure it in place with tape fastened gently around the airway (so as not to crimp it shut) and wrapped around the patient's head, or with the adjustable type, move the collet to the correct position.

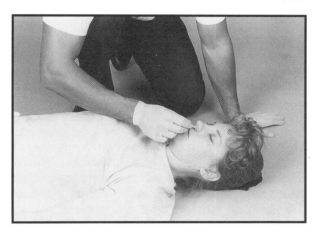

7. Check the patient's air exchange to ensure that the nasopharyngeal airway is properly placed and a patent airway has been secured.

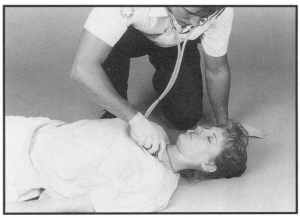

ALS

Esophageal Obturator/Gastric Tube and Dual Lumen Airways—Introduction

The four airway adjuncts in this group have been designed primarily for use by EMTs who are not authorized to perform endotracheal intubation, or for use by trained intubators after attempts at endotracheal intubation have been unsuccessful in apneic patients with an absent gag reflex who require sustained airway management. Although across the country these may be in use at all EMT levels, due to their significantly invasive nature they are considered an Advanced skill in some regions and, due to this potential, have been so indicated in this text.

The EOA® and EGTA® are designed for blind insertion into the esophagus to isolate it and the stomach from continued communication with the airway, and to hold the tongue elevated—allowing for ventilation through the mask and normal air passages without the airway being invaded by gastric contents or the flaccid tongue.

The Combitube® and PTL® airways have overcome the difficulty of maintaining a mask seal by eliminating the mask and instead producing a seal between the mouth/nose and the outside by use of a second cuff which is inflated in the pharynx. These airways have dual lumens and are "blindly" inserted—becoming placed outside the EMT's vision and control—either in the esophagus or trachea. If the tube has been placed in the esophagus it obturates it and, by selecting the correct lumen, ventilation is provided through the normal airway such as with an EOA® or EGTA®. If the tube has been placed in the trachea, ventilation through the alternate lumen provides a direct connection between the outside and the trachea—such as with any endotracheal tube.

To date, published studies evaluating these four adjuncts have failed to clearly prove their effectiveness and are either limited in scope or contradictory. The esophageal obturator airways have become the subject of controversy for a variety of reasons. The American Heart Association has classified them as "IIb"—meaning that their use should be **CONDITIONAL** as they have not been definitely shown to be beneficial. Ventilation volumes achieved are often less then desired and, although they vary from study to study, in some cases may be 50% less than usually found with an endotracheal tube. Difficulty in maintaining a proper mask seal has been identified as a major problem with these devices. Another problem is a lack of positive isolation of the trachea, leaving the possibility of aspiration. The major complication of these devices is unrecognized endotracheal mis-placement, producing total airway obstruction and insufflation of the stomach. While this is a case of "operator error" and not one of mechanical design, its all too frequent occurrence signals that some different approach should be considered. Endotracheal intubation is the preferred definitive method of airway control. Esophageal obturator airways should only be considered when attempts at endotracheal intubation have failed or when endotracheal intubation is not an available option. The Combi-Tube® and PTL® devices suffer from not enough studies having been published to date to make either a clearly beneficial and desirable choice. Further, the studies which have been published to date do demonstrate the critical dependence of these devices upon properly determining through which lumen ventilation is to be performed. Despite their alternative design, there remains the continuing "operator error" problem cited above with the esophageal obturator devices. Therefore, the pre-hospital use of any of these devices is neither endorsed nor discouraged until further study can provide a stronger factual basis upon which to make a decision. Use of these adjuncts remains a matter of regional and local medical judgement, and one should only be used by the EMT if his medical director has included it in the local protocols.

ALS

ESOPHAGEAL OBTURATOR AIRWAY (EOA)®

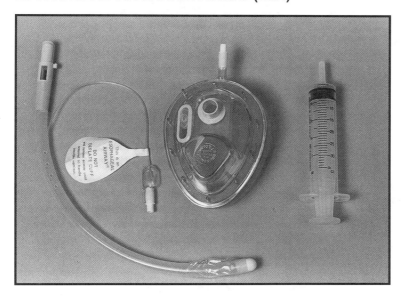

The Esophageal Obturator Airway (EOA) consists of three main parts: the mask, the tube, and a 35cc syringe. The mask is fitted with an inflatable cuff which aids in gaining the necessary seal around the patient's mouth and nose. The syringe provides air to inflate the mask cuff and also the cuff around the distal tip of the tube which seals the esophagus when it is inflated. The tube is closed at its distal end but has sixteen holes along the upper half of the tube through which air passes from the open proximal end of the tube. The tube is designed to be placed in the patient's esophagus and to seal the esophagus from the pharynx when the tube cuff is inflated. When air is then blown into the open end of the tube it passes through the holes in the tube into the pharynx and on into the patient's trachea.

Contraindications For Using The Esophageal Obturator Airway (EOA)®

1. Since only one size of esophageal airway is available, it should not be used in patients under 5'0" or over 6'7" in height

2. Patients with known esophageal disease

3. Patients with severe facial injuries

4. Patients who have ingested caustic agents

5. Are not beneficial in laryngectomy patients who breathe through a tracheostomy

---

1. Prior to inserting the EOA the patient should be hyperventilated and hyperoxygenated to overcome any oxygen deficit that already exists and to establish a reserve against the brief apneic period that will occur during insertion. After assuring that the proper Universal Precaution protective measures have been taken, the patient's lungs should be auscultated for baseline breath sounds against which to compare the breath sounds after insertion.

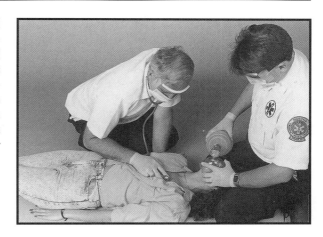

2. Insert the tube into mask until a definite "click" is heard, signifying that it is properly locked in place. The tube should naturally extend down from the mask and then curve away from the direction of the mask's nosepiece. The suction port on the mask must be closed, and the inflatable cuff around the mask should be about half full—not too soft yet not rigid. Experience indicates that on most patients a soft mask cuff provides a better seal than a stiff, rigid cuff.

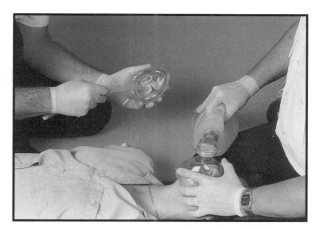

3. Draw back the plunger on the syringe and fill it with 35cc of air, then attach the syringe to the one-way valve at the end of the small feeder tube which branches from the main tube. Depress the plunger to inflate the tube cuff at the distal end of the tube and, while holding the plunger in, verify that the cuff is full and does not leak. Withdraw the plunger and completely deflate the tube cuff in preparation for inserting the tube into the patient. Check to be sure that the suction port on the side of the mask is closed.

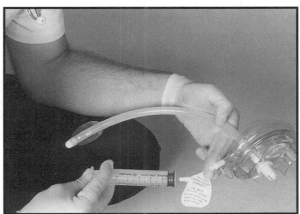

4. With the EOA completely assembled and the tube cuff checked and then fully deflated, continue the insertion preparations by applying a water-soluble lubricant to the distal end of the tube. The syringe, containing 35cc of air, should be firmly attached to the one-way valve.

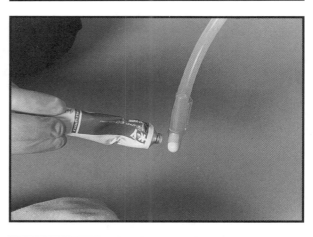

5. The EMT who is to insert the EOA should be positioned directly above the patient's head. This may necessitate changing the position of the EMT who has been ventilating the patient, or may involve changing duties among the EMTs present. Re-gardless, ventilation (and CPR when indicated) should be continued until insertion of the EOA is imminent. Hold the EOA in one hand with the mask upward and with the nosepiece pointing toward you. The distal end of the tube should curve down and out in front of you, pointing toward the patient's feet.

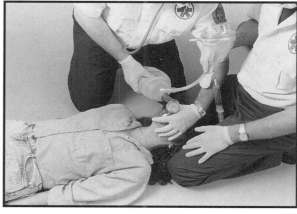

6. Discontinue ventilating and remove any oropharyngeal airway that was in place. Perform a tongue-jaw lift with the hand that is not holding the EOA, lifting the tongue and mandible anteriorly. The patient's head should be slightly flexed to help guide the tip into the esophagus. In trauma patients maintain the head in the neutral in-line position. Insert the distal end of the EOA into the patient's mouth along the midline, with the curve of the tube following the curve of the patient's airway.

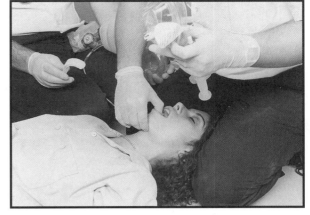

7. Continue advancing the tube into the patient's pharynx and esophagus. It should not be necessary to use force to insert the tube. If difficulty or obstruction is felt while inserting the tube, either redirect it or withdraw it and (after re-ventilating the patient) start again. It may be helpful to increase the extent of tongue-jaw lift.

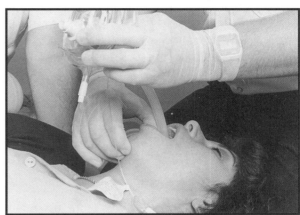

8. Advance the tube until the mask is seated firmly on the patient's face. Hold the mask by placing both thumbs on the sides of the mask with your fingers extending around the mask and the patient's mandible. With your third fingers under the mandible *OR* your little fingers under the angles of the patient's mandible, keep the mandible from sagging posteriorly in order to maintain the mask seal.

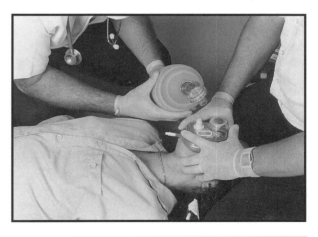

9. Using a bag-valve device or demand valve, ventilate the patient through the tube port on the mask and watch for chest rise. Although recommended in the manufacturer's instructions, *DO NOT* take a deep breath and blow into the tube! Infection Control guidelines and Universal Precautions prohibit any deliberate contact between your skin and the patient's exhaled air. If the tube has been correctly placed into the esophagus the chest should rise with each ventilation. If the tube has been misplaced into the trachea, chest rise will be absent and inflation of the abdomen may be noticed.

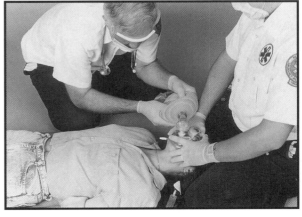

10. Simultaneously with observing for chest rise, auscultate the chest to further confirm the placement of the tube in the esophagus. If breath sounds are clearly audible and the chest rises with each ventilation, the tube is considered to be correctly placed in the esophagus. Continue to maintain the mask seal while ventilating the patient.

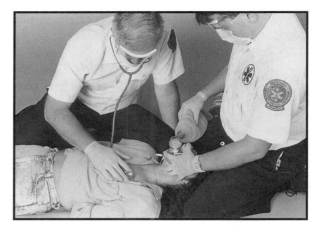

11. Now inflate the tube cuff with 35ml of air to seal the esophagus and help hold the tube in place. You must remove the syringe from the one-way valve in order for the valve to seal and keep the tube cuff inflated. Re-confirm breath sounds by auscultating the mid-lung fields.

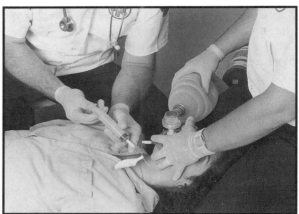

12. Also auscultate over the epigastrium for the *absence* of sounds of air passing through the esophagus and into the stomach. If such sounds are absent this is further confirmation of proper tube placement. If at any time lung sounds **cannot** be heard with each ventilation, or auscultation over the stomach reveals air sounds with each ventilation, immediately remove the EOA and resume ventilation with manual techniques until the patient has been re-oxygenated and re-insertion can be attempted. Periodically recheck by auscultating the lungs and epigastrium for proper placement, and make sure that the pilot balloon remains distended.

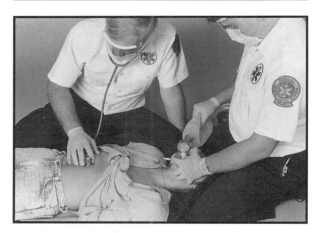

13. If any fluids or foreign material become visible through the mask, suctioning can be performed through the small sliding port on the mask without removing the tube. Remember that the air you are suctioning is the air the patient needs to breathe, so limit the time of each suctioning and resume ventilation promptly!

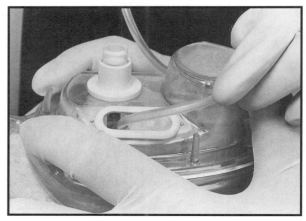

ALS

ESOPHAGEAL GASTRIC TUBE AIRWAY (EGTA)®

The EGTA has four parts. Three of these—the mask, tube, and syringe—although slightly different in specific design are analogous to the same parts in the EOA. The EGTA mask has two circular ports. The esophageal tube snaps into the lower port in the same manner as an EOA, but unlike the EOA no ventilation or air exchange occurs through this port or the EGTA tube.

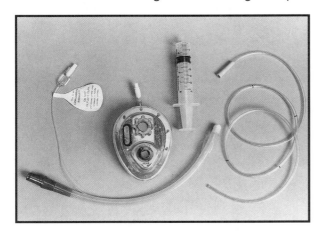

Instead, the BVM or Demand Valve are connected to the other circular port, which is labeled "Ventilate Here", and air passes through that port into the mask and thence into the mouth, pharynx, trachea, and lungs. The esophageal tube is constructed in such a way that it can only be connected to the proper opening in the mask.

The tube of the EGTA has a closed valve in the end that snaps into the mask, an opening at the distal tip, and an inflatable cuff surrounding the distal end. Unlike the EOA, the length of the tube is continuous without any holes or other openings through its side. All air exchange occurs outside of the tube and is completely isolated from the inside of the EGTA tube.

Contraindications For Using The Esophageal Gastric Tube Airway (EGTA)®

1. Since only one size of esophageal airway is available, it should not be used in patients under 5'0" or over 6'7" in height
2. Patients with known esophageal disease
3. Patients with severe facial injuries
4. Patients who have ingested caustic agents
5. Are not beneficial in laryngectomy patients who breathe through a tracheostomy

---

1. Once you have assured that the proper universal precautions have been taken, assemble the mask, tube and syringe of the EGTA, check the mask and cuff, then lubricate the distal tip of the. tube in the same manner as with an EOA. After auscultating the lungs bilaterally, insert the EGTA, confirm proper placement, inflate the cuff and remove the syringe, and reconfirm placement following the same steps as previously described for an EOA (except that ventilation is provided at the port marked "Ventilate Here.")

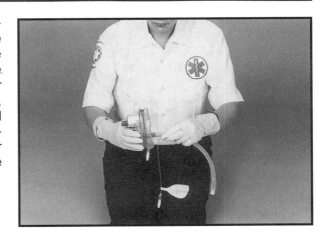

2. Once proper placement and air exchange have been confirmed, and while a second EMT continues ventilation without interruption, the primary EMT should insert the 18 French soft gastric tube which is supplied as part of the EGTA kit. Hold the gastric tube with your dominant hand about two inches above its distal tip, and place your other hand near the other end of the tube. Insert the tip into the opening of the EGTA tube. In the event that local protocols or legal restraints do not allow the EMT to pass a gastric tube or to suction gastric contents, unless also prohibited it is recommended that the gastric tube at least be inserted about two inches into the valve at the proximal end of the EGTA tube in order to open it and allow gastric decompression and communication to the outside.

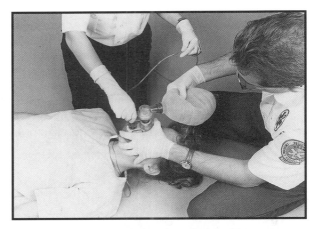

3. With firm pressure push the tip of the gastric tube through the valve in the proximal end of the EGTA tube and continue inserting it. When the tip of the gastric tube is at the distal end of the EGTA tube, it may have to be turned or moved up and down slightly to align it with the small opening in the tip.

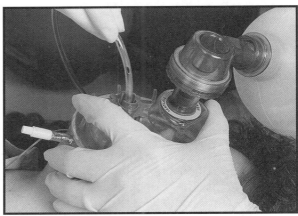

4. Continue passing it down to the second black line on the gastric tube. This places the distal end of the gastric tube approximately six inches beyond the distal tip of the EGTA tube. If any gastric air or fluid pressure has built up, placement of the gastric tube should relieve it. This also enables evacuation of gastric fluid contents by suctioning through the gastric tube, prior to removal of the EGTA.

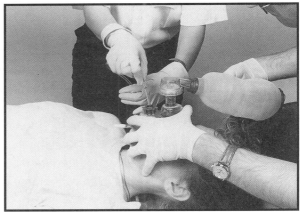

5. Periodically reconfirm proper placement and alveolar ventilation by checking chest rise and by auscultating the lungs and epigastrium, and recheck the condition of the pilot balloon to verify that the distal cuff remains inflated.

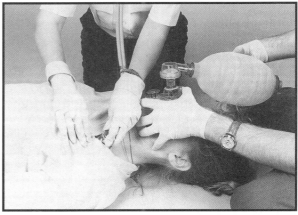

ALS

ESOPHAGEAL TRACHEAL DOUBLE-LUMEN AIRWAY (Combitube)®

The Combitube is similar to the EOA and EGTA in that it involves blind insertion of a device and is promoted for use by EMS responders who are not trained or certified to perform visualized orotracheal intubation, or for use by trained intubators when they are unable to successfully intubate a patient. Unlike the EOA, EGTA, and endotracheal tube, however, its placement in either the esophagus or trachea is not critical to ventilating the patient. Regardless of which location results from the blind insertion, the patient's lungs can be properly ventilated by the EMT's subsequent (correct) choice of ventilating port.

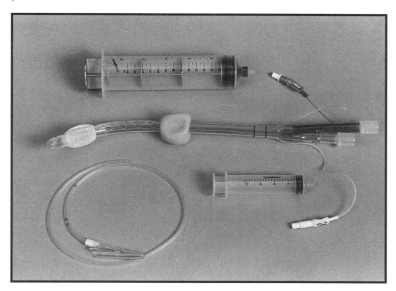

To eliminate the common problems in maintaining a mask seal, instead of a mask the Combitube incorporates a balloon which inflates in the lower pharynx to seal off the airway and trachea distal to it, preventing air from escaping through the mouth and nose. A tube extends through the balloon and, when inserted blindly by the EMT, enters either the trachea or the esophagus. The tube has two lumens, or interior paths. One lumen ends in holes along the side of the tube as is found in an EOA, while the other passes the length of the tube and terminates with several openings at the distal end of the tube—much like an endotracheal tube. The device also employs a distal tube cuff. The proximal end of the tube consists of two smaller tubes which are each connected to a lumen. These two smaller tubes are used in turn to identify which lumen should be used to provide ventilation—e.g., through which path air is able to pass to the lungs.

If the Combitube has been placed in the esophagus then the blue proximal tube (marked "No. 1"), which serves the lumen that terminates in the holes in the pharyngeal section of the tube, is used and the patient is ventilated according to the same principle as the EOA. In this case, as with an EGTA, gastric suctioning can be performed through the Combitube when the tube has been placed in the esophagus and ventilation is being provided through the blue "No. 1" tube. In such cases, a soft suction catheter can be inserted through the clear proximal tube into the esophagus and stomach.

If the Combitube has been placed in the trachea the clear ("White") proximal tube (marked "No. 2"), which connects to the lumen that opens at the distal tip, is used for direct ventilation of the trachea in the same manner as with an ET tube.

As with any advanced airway adjunct, accurate assessment during ventilation of chest rise and auscultation of the lungs and epigastrium is essential to the proper and safe use of this device. Although whether the distal end of the Combitube is placed in the trachea or esophagus is not critical to the ability to ventilate the lungs with this device, determining which proximal tube and lumen has the exclusive pathway to the trachea and lungs is critical. It must be noted that ***unrecognized continued ventilation through the wrong proximal tube (for whichever blind placement of the distal end of the Combitube has occurred) will produce gastric insufflation without any ventilation of the lungs and will result in increasing hypoxia and death.***

The Combitube Is *Contraindicated* In Patients:

- Less than 16 years of age
- Under five feet in height
- Who have an intact gag reflex
- With known esophageal disease
- Who have ingested a caustic substance

Although the Combitube's large pharyngeal cuff tends to overcome the mask seal problem, it is not foolproof. Any balloon can leak, and sharp objects inside the patient's mouth such as dentures, traumatized teeth or foreign objects can produce tears in the pharyngeal cuff. If the cuff fails when the Combitube is placed in the esophagus, air exiting the holes in the tube will more likely return through the mouth to the outside rather than proceed through the trachea to the lungs.

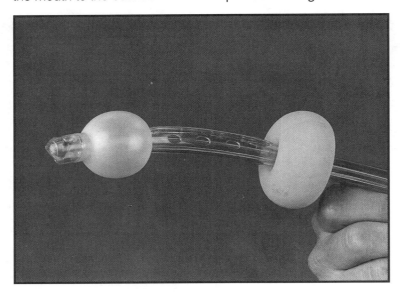

The Combitube package includes the tube itself, two syringes (140ml and 20ml), and a soft suction catheter. The syringes are packaged with the appropriate amount of air already drawn up in each. The tips of the syringes are color-coded to match the color of the one-way valves to which they are to be connected—blue to blue and white to white.

1. Prior to inserting the Combitube the patient should be hyperventilated and hyperoxygenated to overcome any oxygen deficit that already exists and to establish a reserve against the brief apneic period that will occur during insertion. During this ventilation the patient's lungs should be auscultated for baseline breath sounds against which to compare the breath sounds after insertion. The EMT should be wearing protective latex gloves and should additionally consider the use of a face mask and eye shield.

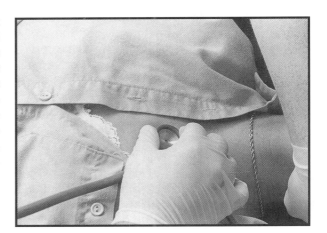

2. Verify that the large blue-tipped 140ml syringe has at least 100ml of air drawn up in it, and connect it to the blue-colored one-way valve and pilot balloon attached to the tube marked "No. 1."

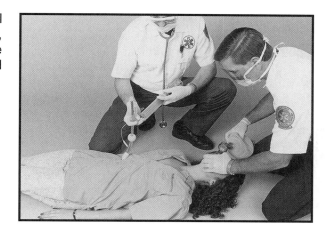

3. Verify that the smaller white-tipped 20ml syringe has at least 15ml of air drawn up in it, and connect it to the white-colored one-way valve and pilot balloon attached to the tube marked "No. 2."

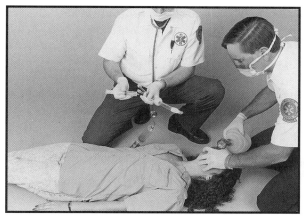

4. Lubricate the distal end of the tube with a water-soluble lubricant such as K-Y jelly. Since with the Combitube the patient *may be* ventilated through the hole at the end of the tube, take care to not occlude the openings with the lubricant.

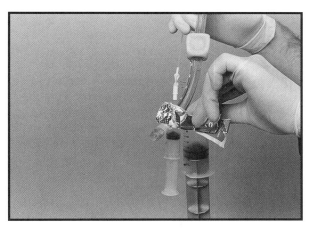

5. The EMT who is to insert the Combitube should be positioned directly above the patient's head. This may necessitate changing the position of the EMT who has been ventilating the patient, or may involve changing duties among the EMTs present. Regardless, ventilation (and CPR when indicated) should be continued until insertion is imminent. Hold the Combitube in one hand so that the distal end curves down and out in front of you pointing toward the patient's feet, following the natural curvature of the patient's pharynx.

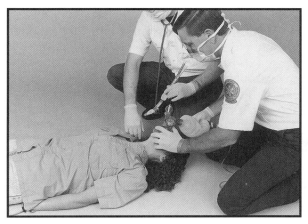

6. Discontinue ventilating and remove any oropharyngeal airway that was in place. Perform a tongue-jaw lift with the hand that is not holding the Combitube, lifting the tongue and mandible upward (anteriorly). Although the manufacturer's directions state that the patient's head can be in any position, it is recommended that the neck be at least slightly extended except in trauma patients. Remember, unlike the EOA, EGTA, or ET tube, the Combitube is designed so that the ability to ventilate the patient occurs regardless of whether the tube ends up in the trachea or the esophagus.

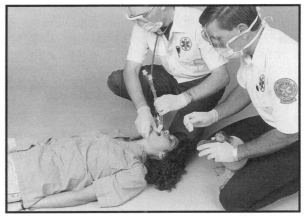

7. Begin inserting the tube into the patient's mouth along the midline, with the curve of the tube following the curve of the patient's airway. This involves directing the tube caudally through the pharynx—*NOT* inserting it at a 90 degree angle to the posterior pharyngeal wall. The importance of maintaining the tube in the midline cannot be overstated—it is key to successful placement.

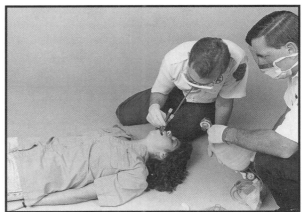

8. Continue gently inserting the tube until the printed ring on the tube is at the level of the patient's teeth (or gumline in edentulous patients). Exercise caution especially in advancing the latex pharyngeal cuff past the patient's teeth. Do not use force, the tube should pass easily. If resistance or obstruction is encountered, withdraw the tube slightly, redirect it, or re-insert it. **Be sure to observe for proper depth insertion**—failure to match the printed rings on the tube with the appropriate landmark has been shown to be a major cause of placement failure.

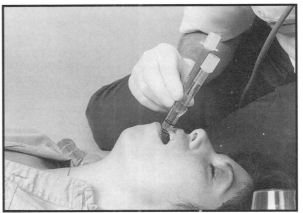

9. With the printed ring at the level of the teeth, inject 100ml of air from the large blue-tipped syringe into the blue colored one-way valve. This inflates the large pharyngeal cuff and seals the patient's pharynx, limiting the flow of air that passes through the Combitube to the lungs without allowing any to escape through the mouth or nose. Remove the 140ml syringe from the blue colored valve, allowing it to close and seal. The blue pilot balloon should be somewhat distended.

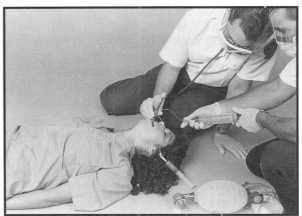

10. ***After the pharyngeal cuff has been inflated,*** inject 15ml of air into the white valve using the smaller white-tipped 20ml syringe. This inflates the distal tube cuff and helps to hold the tube in position, whether it is in the trachea or esophagus. Remove the 20ml syringe from the white one-way valve, allowing it to close and seal. The white pilot balloon should be somewhat distended. Inflation of the distal cuff before the pharyngeal cuff has been shown to prevent the pharyngeal cuff from obtaining proper sealing placement in the lower pharynx.

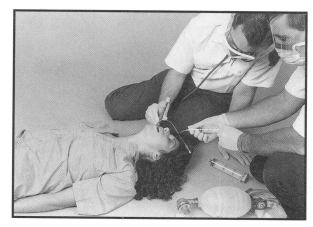

11. Attach the bag-valve or demand valve device to the *blue* tube ("No. 1") and begin ventilations. While observing the thorax for chest rise, auscultate over the epigastrium to confirm the *absence* of air sounds.

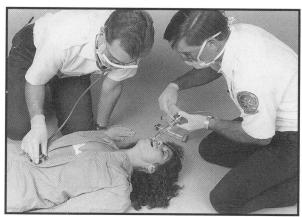

12. If chest rise is seen with each ventilation and no air sounds are heard over the epigastrium, the Combitube has been placed in the esophagus and the patient is being ventilated through the holes in the distal segment of the tube when ventilation is provided through the blue "No. 1" tube.

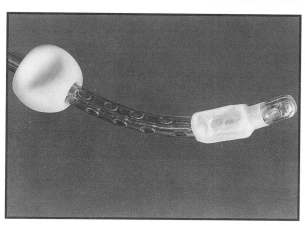

13. If air sounds are heard over the stomach with each ventilation and apparent chest rise is not present, then the Combitube is in the trachea and ventilating through the blue "No. 1" tube is causing air to flow through the esophagus to the stomach. In this situation ***the patient is in mortal danger*** as no oxygen is reaching the lungs. Immediately disconnect the ventilation device from the blue "No. 1" tube, attach it to the clear tube ("No. 2"), and continue ventilations.

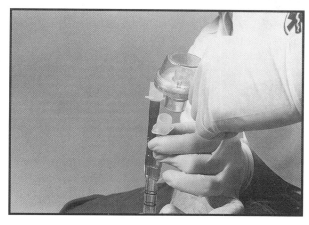

14. Again observe for chest rise and auscultate for the air sounds over the epigastrium. If chest rise is seen and no air sounds are heard over the epigastrium, this signifies that the Combitube has been placed in the patient's trachea and that the air entering the clear "No. 2" tube is continuing the full length of the tube and exiting into the trachea and then proceeding on to properly ventilate the lungs.

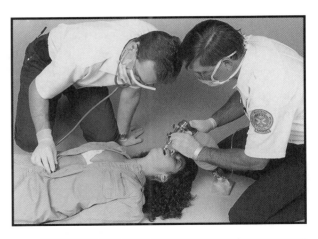

15. Regardless of whether ventilation of the lungs occurred when initially ventilating through the blue "No. 1" or through the clear "No. 2" tube, once it has been verified by witnessing the chest rise and the absence of air sounds over the epigastrium with each ventilation, it is necessary to confirm that proper ventilation of the lungs has in fact been achieved. For confirmation, auscultate over the midlung fields for the *presence* of breath sounds with each ventilation. This should be done immediately after initial insertion, and then periodically to verify continued proper placement. Also re-check the status of the pilot balloons to verify continued inflation of the oral and distal cuffs.

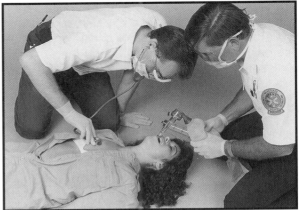

16. When the patient is suspected of having cervical spine trauma, the procedure can be performed with the patient's head maintained in the neutral in-line position. If necessary a single EMT can immobilize the patient's head between his knees while inserting the device, however the procedure is more safely performed with a second EMT immobilizing the head throughout.

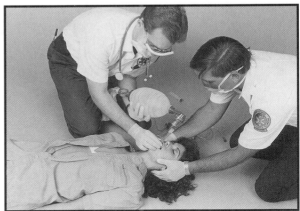

17. When effective ventilation is being provided through the blue ("No. 1") tube, gastric fluids and air can be suctioned from the esophagus and stomach by passing the Combitube's soft suction catheter through the clear ("No. 2") tube. Due to the double-lumen design of the Combitube, this can be performed without concern for the oxygen ventilation process being carried out through the blue tube.

Warning: If the distal end is in the trachea as witnessed by the need to ventilate through the clear "No. 2" tube, tracheal suctioning should only be attempted by an EMT trained in the use of the Combitube *and* in the proper techniques of suctioning an endotracheal tube.

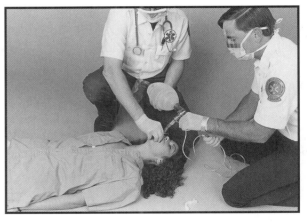

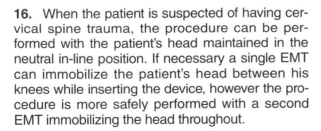

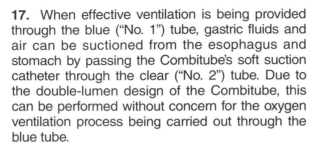

ALS

PHARYNGEAL TRACHEAL LUMEN AIRWAY (PTL)®

The PTL airway consists of the device itself, without any additional parts, accessories, syringes, etc.

The PTL is similar to the Combitube in that it involves blind insertion of a dual lumen device which may be used to properly ventilate the patient regardless of whether the tube ends up inserted in either the esophagus or the trachea. It is similarly promoted for use by EMS responders who have not been trained in visualized orotracheal intubation or for use by trained intubators when attempts at visualized orotracheal placement of an ET tube have been unsuccessful.

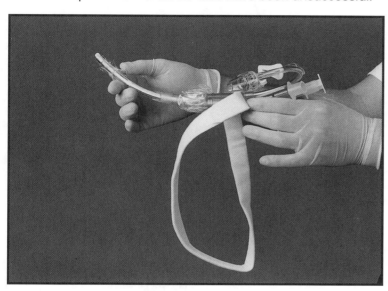

The PTL consists of two balloon-like cuffs which inflate simultaneously when the operator blows into the inflation port by mouth or with a BVM. One balloon-like cuff inflates in the oral cavity and the other at the distal end of the tube. The cuff which inflates inside the mouth provides a seal to prevent the air which is blown in during ventilations from escaping back out through the mouth and nose. The cuff at the distal end of the tube provides a seal around the end of the tube and helps to anchor it in either the esophagus or trachea, into whichever one it is inserted. The tube extends through both cuffs and has two lumens (interior pathways). One lumen ends abruptly just below the oral balloon, while the other passes the length of the tube and terminates beyond the distal cuff with an opening at the distal end of the tube—much like an endotradheal tube. At the proximal end of the tube there are two tubes, each connecting exclusively with one of the two lumens. If the distal tip of the tube ends up inserted in the esophagus, then the BVM or demand valve resuscitator is attached to the green proximal tube to provide ventilation through the pharynx to the lower airway and lungs. If the distal end of the tube ends up inserted in the trachea, the stylet provided by the manufacturer is removed from the clear proximal tube and the BVM or demand valve is attached to the clear tube and used to provide direct tracheal ventilation. Although proper ventilation of the lungs can be performed regardless of whether the distal tip of the PTL has been inserted in either the esophagus or the trachea (as with a Combitube), identification of in which the tube has been inserted and therefore through which proximal tube ventilations should be delivered, is critical. Proper use of this device, as with any advanced airway, is dependent upon the EMT's ability to assess chest rise, breath sounds, and absent air sounds over the epigastrium, with each ventilation. The EMT must be able to establish whether or not ventilation through the selected proximal tube results in successful ventilation of the lungs, or whether the other proximal tube should be used instead. ***Unrecognized continued ventilation through the wrong proximal tube will produce gastric insufflation without any ventilation of the lungs and will result in increasing hypoxia and death.***

The PTL Airway Is *Contraindicated* In Patients:

- Less than 16 years of age
- Under five feet in height
- Who have an intact gag reflex
- With known esophageal disease
- Who have ingested a caustic substance

The PTL's balloon-like oral cavity cuff has been reported to "travel" out of the patient's mouth if it is not properly positioned and seated when inflated and if the head strap is not securely attached to the patient. Care must be taken when inserting the device to avoid contact with sharp objects (such as dentures, broken teeth, or orthodontic devices or wires) to prevent piercing or tearing of the oral balloon or distal cuff. This could result in leaking and loss of the seal needed for adequate ventilation with the device.

1. Prior to inserting the PTL the patient should be hyperventilated and hyperoxygenated to overcome any oxygen deficit that already exists and to establish a reserve against the brief apneic period that will occur during insertion. During this time the patient's lungs should be auscultated for baseline breath sounds against which to compare the breath sounds after insertion. Auscultation at the mid-lung fields is recommended. The EMT should be wearing protective latex gloves and should additionally consider the use of a face mask and eye shield.

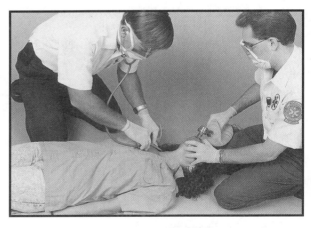

2. The proximal and distal cuffs are checked for proper operation by blowing air into the inflation valve. Because this valve serves only the cuffs and does not connect with the patient's esophagus or airway, this can be done orally. Alternately, a bag-valve or demand valve device can be used to inflate the cuffs. The relief port under the inflation valve must be closed with the small white cap, and the slide clamp must be open, in order for the cuffs to inflate. Inspect the cuffs for any sign of leaking.

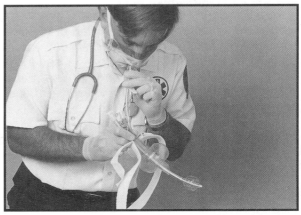

3. When the check is completed, remove the white cap and squeeze both of the cuffs simultaneously to deflate them fully. This must be done manually since the PTL does not employ any syringes as the other devices previously discussed. Then replace the white cap on the relief port. Lubricate the distal end of the long tube (#2) with a water-soluble lubricant.

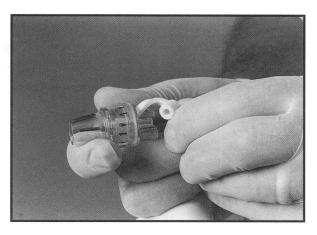

4. The EMT who is to insert the PTL should be positioned directly above the patient's head. This may necessitate changing the position of the EMT who has been ventilating the patient, or may involve changing duties among the EMTs present. Regardless, ventilation (and CPR when indicated) should be continued until insertion is imminent. Hold the PTL below the flange in one hand so that the distal end curves down and out in front of you pointing toward the patient's feet, following the natural curvature of the patient's pharynx. Make sure that the white strap that will encircle the patient's head is hanging free and untangled so that it can be quickly placed around the head once the PTL has been inserted.

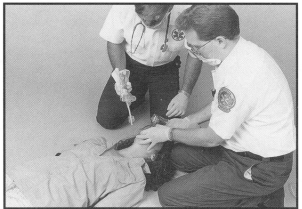

5. The patient's head and neck should be hyperextended if there is no indication of spinal injury, however the PTL can be inserted with the head maintained in the neutral in-line position if so required. With your other hand, perform a tongue-jaw lift, opening the mouth wide and moving the mandible anteriorly. As with the EOA/EGTA and Combitube, advance the tube into the patient's airway but do not force it in. The tube should pass through the mouth and pharynx easily. If resistance is encountered, withdraw the tube slightly, redirect it, and re-insert.

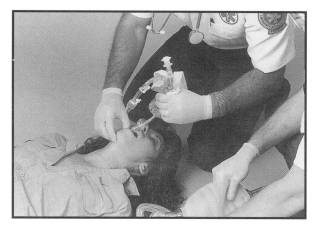

6. Continue insertion until the plastic bite-block flange rests against the patient's teeth. When the plastic bite block flange is at the level of the patient's teeth, the PTL's large proximal balloon will be in the oropharynx and the distal cuff at the end of tube #3 will be in either the esophagus or trachea.

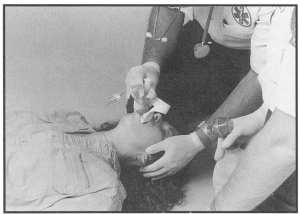

7. Quickly loop the white strap around the patient's head and fasten it with the Velcro® closures. This helps to prevent the tube from "travelling" out of the mouth when the proximal balloon is inflated.

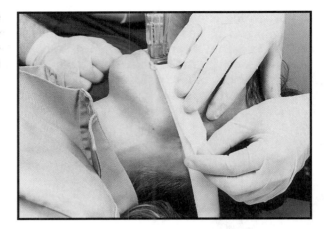

8. It is important that the correct depth be maintained so that each balloon can function properly. Blow into tube #1 to inflate the proximal and distal cuffs. Use the pilot balloon to gauge the degree of inflation and continue to blow into tube #1 until the pilot balloon is noticeably inflated without going to excess.

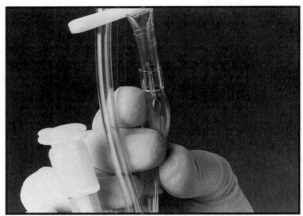

9. With the balloon cuffs inflated, attach a BVM (or other suitable ventilator) to the shorter green tube (#2) and ventilate. Observe for chest rise with each ventilation and simultaneously auscultate over the epigastrium for sounds of air entering the stomach (they should be *absent*).

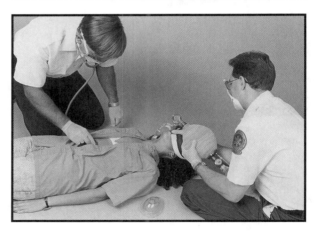

10. If chest rise is visible and no air sounds are heard over the epigastrium with each ventilation it is probable that the distal end of tube #3 is in the esophagus, thereby allowing ventilation through tube #2. Auscultate the midlung fields to confirm the presence of proper breath sounds with each ventilation. Continue ventilating through tube #2, continually monitoring chest rise, and periodically reconfirming proper ventilation by auscultation of the midlung breath sounds and absent epigastric air sounds.

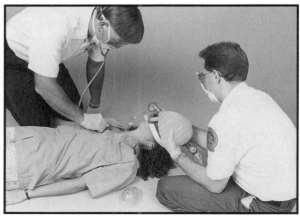

11. When proper ventilation of the lungs through tube #2 is confirmed by auscultation of good mid-lung breath sounds and absent epigastric air sounds with each ventilation, the absence of air sounds over the epigastrium also confirms that the distal end of tube #3 and the distal cuff are placed in the esophagus, sealing it from the air pathway. With such placement, the stylet in tube #3 can be removed and gastric contents can be evacuated by passing an 18 French gastric tube into the esophagus or stomach through tube #3 and applying suction.

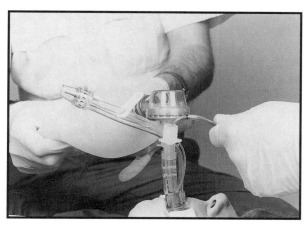

12. If adequate chest rise is *NOT* noticeable and air sounds *ARE* heard over the epigastrium with each ventilation, it is probable that the distal end of tube #3 has been placed in the trachea. The patient is in mortal danger, since no air is reaching the lungs. Immediately stop ventilating through tube #2 and remove the plastic stylet from tube #3.

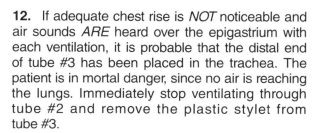

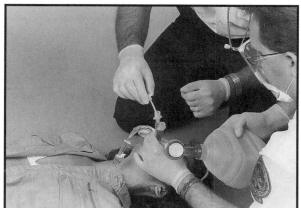

13. Attach the ventilation device to the proximal end of tube #3 and again attempt to ventilate the patient. With the stylet removed, ventilations through tube #3 will cause air to travel through the long tube and exit in the trachea as in any endo-tracheal intubation. Although accomplished blindly as a secondary possibility with the PTL, this inad-vertent endotracheal placement is actually more secure and beneficial than when the distal end of tube #3 has been placed in the esophagus.

14. While ventilating through tube #3, confirm correct placement by observing for chest rise and auscultating over the epigastrium for absent air sounds.

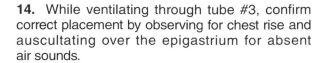

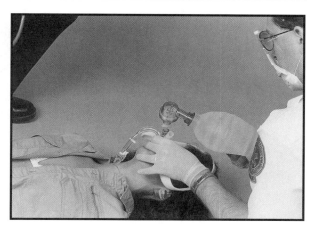

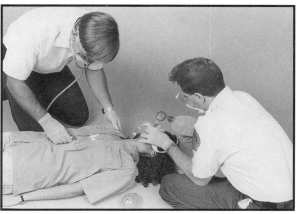

15. Then auscultate the midlung fields while ventilating to confirm the presence of air passing into the lungs with each ventilation. Continue ventilating through tube #3, continually monitoring chest rise and periodically reconfirming proper ventilation by auscultation of midlung breath sounds and absent epigastric air sounds.

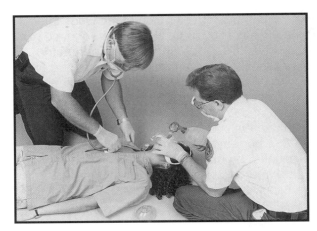

16. Regardless if proper ventilation of the lungs occurred and was confirmed when ventilating through tube #2 or tube #3, continued proper ventilation through the device requires that the cuffs remain properly inflated and the device remains placed at the proper depth. To ensure this, the EMT should periodically squeeze the pilot bulb to confirm continued inflation of the cuffs, should guard and maintain the tight placement of the strap around the patient's head, and check that the plastic bite block flange remains at the correct level immediately above and adjacent to the level of the teeth.

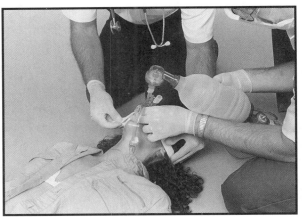

EMERGENCY EXTUBATION OF ADVANCED AIRWAY DEVICES

In cases when the patient begins to revive and to regain his gag reflex, any of the advanced airway devices discussed above **which have been placed in the patient's esophagus** should be removed as quickly as possible to minimize patient discomfort, limit possible trauma from vomiting while the esophagus is obturated, and to limit the chance of aspiration. None of these devices can absolutely prevent vomiting around the distal esophageal cuff, and the wiser course should the patient revive is to remove the device as quickly as possible in a controlled process.

Neither the EOA, EGTA, Combitube nor PTL devices should be used in patients whose lowered level of consciousness and depressed gag reflex is thought to be transient. The presence of a palpable carotid pulse or a history of periods of regaining consciousness, moaning, or movement just prior to the EMT's arrival should alert the EMT that the patient's condition may change and become more responsive in the immediate future. Where an early return of the gag reflex can be anticipated, insertion of an esophageal device may produce more risk than benefit and should be carefully considered before proceeding.

However, if the device has served to tracheally intubate the patient, then it should be left in place until the patient can reach the hospital. This is discussed in more detail at the end of the endotracheal intubation section.

1. As the patient arouses and it is clear that the device will have to be removed, the paramount fear is that the patient will dangerously extubate himself. Direct the ventilating EMT to stop ventilating, remove the BVM from the proximal end of the device, and have him grab the patient's hands.

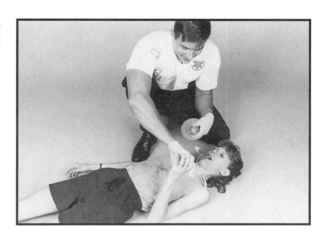

2. Talk to the patient to calm him, telling him **NOT** to touch the tube or attempt to pull it out— that this is dangerous and can hurt him. Tell him that you will remove it but that he must cooperate with you. Tell him to breathe rapidly and to swallow repeatedly (swallowing tends to lessen the gag reflex). **Only with the Combitube** do you need to evacuate the air from the oral cuff before proceeding further. Using the 140 ml syringe, insert it into the one-way valve at the blue #1 pilot bulb and withdraw air until the pilot bulb is flat. Then remove the syringe from the valve.

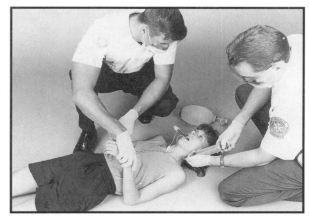

3. Roll the patient onto his side (or roll the long-board onto its side with the patient immobilized to it). Have a suction unit with large bore tubing or a V-VAC® device readily available. If three EMTs are present, one should be holding the patient on his side and securing his hands, one should be responsible for removing the device, and one should be supporting the upper torso and be ready to suction the patient as soon as the device is removed.

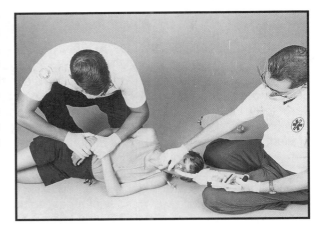

4. Evacuate air from the distal cuff(s).

EOA & EGTA: Make sure that the plunger is all the way into the barrel of the 35 ml syringe (at 0 ml). Insert the tip of the syringe into the one-way valve and withdraw air until it is all evacuated from the distal cuff.

COMBITUBE: Do the same as above with the 20 ml syringe inserted in the one way valve of tube #2.

PTL AIRWAY: Remove the white cap from the nipple found on the underside of the #1 inflation valve. If you have previously closed the slide clamp to isolate the distal cuff you will have to release it as well. You may need to suck air out of the nipple to fully empty both of the cuffs. When empty the pilot bulb should be flat. Unlike the other devices, this procedure will deflate both PTL cuffs simultaneously.

5. Once you are sure that all the air is out of the distal cuff, and with one EMT ready to suction the patient's mouth, pull the device from the patient's mouth following its anatomical curve.

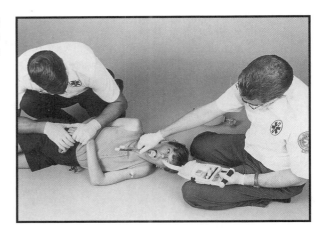

6. Fully suction any gastric contents regurgitated into the mouth and nose before returning the patient to a supine position. Even though suctioning is usually only performed for five seconds at a time, the copious amount of material that may be generated by this event may necessitate suctioning for as long as 20–25 seconds at a time to lessen the chance of aspiration. The EMT should be ready for ensuing nausea and vomiting, and be prepared to again roll the patient onto his side and to repeat the suctioning as needed.

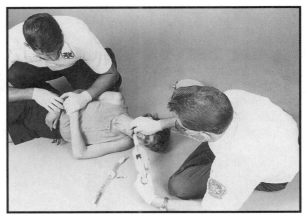

7. As the nausea and vomiting subside and the patient becomes more stable, the EMT should provide supplemental oxygen, assist with ventilations as needed, and consider inserting a nasopharyngeal airway.

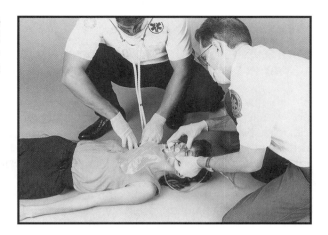

ALS

OROTRACHEAL INTUBATION OF PATIENTS WITH AN EOA®, EGTA®, COMBITUBE®, OR PTL® AIRWAY IN PLACE, AND THEIR REMOVAL AT THE HOSPITAL

Removal of any of these advanced airways, especially from placement in the esophagus, is commonly associated with copious regurgitation of stomach contents. In order to avoid or reduce the possibility of aspiration, except in cases when emergency immediate removal is necessitated by the patient's awakening, prior to removal of any airway device whose distal tip is inserted into the esophagus the patient should be endotracheally intubated "around" that device.

The placement of an endotracheal tube (ETT), prior to removing the other advanced airway from the esophagus, provides a protected airway from the trachea to outside of the mouth, as well as possibly sealing and isolating the airway and lungs from vomitus that is regurgitated into the oral and nasal cavities. Many protocols require that EMTs who are trained in visualized orotracheal intubation be able to intubate "around" these other airways (placed in the esophagus). This is primarily done so that the intubation-qualified EMT can provide a more definitive protected airway than is provided by isolation and obturation of the esophagus. A very important second reason for such training is that the EMT can then assist hospital personnel—if they are not as familiar with these other devices—in their removal in the Emergency Department. Since increased use of the Combitube and PTL airways is a recent event, **the EMT who has inserted either of these devices—*regardless of whether or not he can perform visualized orotracheal intubation*—needs to know the following procedures. He should remain with the patient in the Emergency Department until he has confirmed that the hospital staff is familiar with the device or until an ET tube has been placed and this device has been properly removed.** In the case of EMTs who can not intubate, they may be needed to perform the unique steps relating to removal of the device even though the orotracheal intubation (which does not require familiarity with the EOA, EGTA, PTL or Combitube) is performed by a member of the hospital staff.

Additionally, in order to minimize or eliminate regurgitation with the EGTA (and with the PTL or Combitube when they are placed in the esophagus), a gastric suction tube should be inserted through the device into the esophagus or stomach to relieve gastric pressure and to evacuate stomach contents by suctioning prior to removal of the device. The exact method of passing the gastric tube for each of these devices (each being slightly different in specific detail) has been described in the previous pages as part of the steps for the proper insertion and use of each device.

It must be pointed out that with such a device placed in the esophagus—even when a gastric tube has been inserted, stomach contents evacuated, and the patient endotracheally intubated "around" the device—**removal of the initial advanced airway placed in the esophagus is considered *contraindicated* pre-hospital** except when necessitated by the return of the patient's gag reflex and improved level of consciousness. In most protocols (except for cases of emergent immediate need), removal of any airway which has been placed in the esophagus is limited to being performed in the hospital **only.**

*If with either the Combitube or PTL airway, proper ventilation of the lungs only occurred after the BVM was moved to the secondary ("clear" or "white") proximal tube, then the distal end of the device is in the trachea (the patient has been blindly orotracheally intubated) and **the procedure of intubating "around" the device is contraindicated.** Instead, in such cases, if once at the hospital the physician wants to replace the device with an ET tube, both cuffs must be fully deflated and the device withdrawn prior to any attempt at re-intubating with an endotracheal tube.*

The steps for orotracheally intubating a patient who has any of these advanced airways in the esophagus, then replacing ventilation through them with ventilation through an ET tube, evacuating gastric contents, and finally removing the device at the hospital, all follow the same general method regardless of which device has been used (except that the EOA does not allow for use of a gastric tube or evacuation of gastric contents.) There are only a few minor variations due to design differences. With either the Combitube or PTL airway, the distal tip has been placed in the esophagus if proper ventilation of the lungs has been confirmed when providing ventilation through the *initial* proximal tube (blue #1 for Combitube or shorter green tube of the PTL).

Intubation "around" the device should only be attempted after the patient has been ventilated at a high FiO$_2$ level with a BVM and oxygen reservoir or a demand valve.

Note: The following steps relate the technique for an EMT certified in visualized orotracheal intubation. If the EMT is not so trained but is assisting another health care professional who is, the EMT should follow the instructions relating to the airway device that is in place while the other health care professional performs the visualized orotracheal intubation. Because of the redundancy that would be involved in showing the same step with each of the devices, we have elected rather to avoid all photos and illustrations here.

To intubate patients who have an EOA, EGTA, Combitube or PTL Airway placed in the esophagus:

1. Instruct another EMT to hyperventilate the patient through the device. Prepare and check the laryngoscope and ET tube in the prescribed manner. (See the following pages for VISUALIZED ORO-TRACHEAL INTUBATION.)

2. Have the EMT providing ventilation move alongside the patient's head and, with the laryngoscope and ET tube readily at hand, position yourself beyond the patient's head. When fully ready, direct the other EMT to stop ventilating and to remove the BVM from the airway device.

3. Obtain access to the mouth by rapidly removing the mask (EOA or EGTA) or by deflating the oral cuff *only* (PTL or Combitube). **It is critical that care be taken to ensure that when performing this step the airway device is *NOT* displaced and the distal cuff is *NOT* inadvertently deflated.** This step is performed by:

EOA and EGTA—Squeeze the two locking tabs which hold the tube to the mask to release them and carefully remove the mask.

Combitube—Insert the tip of the 140ml syringe into the blue #1 one-way valve and pull back on the plunger to evacuate all of the air from the oral cuff. The blue pilot bulb should be flat and empty. Remove the syringe from the one-way valve.

PTL—Adjust the white slide clamp on the inflation tube assembly until the tubing that it surrounds is pinched completely shut. (This step is critical in isolating the oral balloon cuff from the distal cuff, and occluding the connection to the distal cuff to prevent its deflation at this time.) Then open the white cap on the underside of the #1 inflation valve. To fully deflate the oral cuff it may be necessary to suck air out through the uncapped port of the #1 valve. Since as long as the distal cuff is still inflated the pilot bulb will remain firm and full of air, visual inspection is necessary to ensure that the oral cuff is deflated.

4. Reach into the patient's mouth with your first and second fingers and move the airway device to the far left margin of the oral cavity and mouth, being careful not to displace its distal end.

5. Insert the laryngoscope blade into the mouth (as well as elevating the tongue and jaw, it is used to hold the airway device to the left) and when the vocal cords are properly visualized insert the ET tube to the proper depth. Remove the laryngoscope and inflate the ET tube's distal cuff.

6. Once the orotracheal intubation has been successfully completed, direct the second EMT to attach the BVM to the proximal end of the ET tube and to reinstitute ventilation. It is important that no more than 30 seconds elapse from the time ventilation was stopped in step 2 until it is reinstituted now. If these steps have not been successfully completed within 30 seconds you will have to stop, rapidly reposition the advanced airway device correctly in the oral cavity, and re-establish the mouth and nose seal. With the EOA and EGTA, refasten the mask to the proximal end of the tube. With the Combitube and PTL, re-inflate the oral cavity cuff properly. (**Note:** With the Combitube this is done with the 140ml syringe. With the PTL you must replace the white cap over the nipple on the underside of the #1 inflation valve *without releasing the slide clamp* and blow into the mouthpiece of the valve until the oral balloon cuff is properly re-inflated. As soon as the device is properly positioned and the seal has been re-established, ventilate the patient for at least 30 to 60 seconds before again attempting to intubate around the device.

7. When orotracheal intubation with the ET tube has been completed and ventilation through it has been initiated, you must assure that the tube is properly placed in the trachea and that proper ventilation of the lungs is occurring. This is equally true if you have reinstituted ventilation through an advanced airway device, as you must verify that it has not become displaced during the intubation attempts. With each ventilation chest rise should be clearly visible and *NO* air sounds should be heard when auscultating over the epigastrium. To further confirm proper ventilation, auscultate the midlung fields where good bilateral breath sounds should be audible.

Note: If the endotracheal intubation around the advanced airway device has been successfully completed in the pre-hospital setting, the now superceded device *should be left in place.* Removal pre-hospital serves no purpose and simply invites a variety of unnecessary complications. It is, therefore, *STRONGLY NOT RECOMMENDED.*

ONCE AT THE HOSPITAL

After arrival at the hospital, if intubation around the advanced airway device has not already been performed, it should be done prior to removal of such a device. Follow the preceding steps or assist hospital personnel in their performance if they are not experienced in the removal of the specific device that has been used.

Although gastric decompression and some exodus of stomach fluids may occur through the tube of a Combitube or PTL which has been placed in the esophagus even before passing a gastric tube through it (or through the tube of an EGTA once the gastric tube is inserted past the valve in the proximal end of the tube), an appropriate gastric tube must be inserted into the lower esophagus or stomach in order to evacuate the stomach's fluid contents.

8. Once the intubation around the device has been completed and ventilation of the lungs through the ET tube has been confirmed, if the appropriate gastric tube has as yet not been inserted through the EGTA, PTL, or Combitube (not possible with an EOA), a gastric tube should be inserted into the esophagus and/or stomach at this point (see previous pages for details for each different device). *Remember, if the Combitube or PTL has required ventilation through the secondary port then the distal end of the tube is in the TRACHEA and passing a gastric tube through it serves no purpose, is dangerous, and contraindicated.*

9. The effective placement of the gastric tube is usually confirmed by the exodus of gastric gasses and fluids through it. When a gastric tube is passed through one of these cuffed devices which is in the esophagus, its misplacement into the trachea is almost impossible. However, if further confirmation of its placement is desired, air from a large syringe which is attached to the proximal end of the gastric tube can be injected through the tube while auscultating over the epigastrium. Definite, positive air sounds should then be heard over the stomach.

Once the gastric tube has been inserted to the proper depth, the stomach's fluid contents should be evacuated by suctioning through the gastric tube. Due to the small diameter of the gastric tube (necessary for it to fit through the lumen) its distal end can easily become obstructed by solid stomach contents during suctioning. This blockage can usually be displaced by injecting air or a sterile fluid (water or saline) into the proximal end of the gastric tube and then reinstituting the suctioning.

10. Throughout these steps care must be taken not to interrupt the ventilation through the ET tube and also to assure that none of the manipulations inadvertently displace it. Proper continued ventilation of the lungs should periodically be confirmed by the patient's appearance, observed chest rise, and auscultation of good breath sounds.

11. After ET tube intubation around the advanced airway device has been accomplished and evacuation of stomach fluid contents through the gastric tube has been performed, the device can be removed. Although the ET tube provides a protected airway, some stomach contents will remain and regurgitation upon removal is common, therefore the patient (or patient and longboard) should be positioned on his side to minimize the risk of aspiration and a staff member positioned at the patient's head should have large-bore suction or a V-VAC ready to rapidly evacuate any vomitus that is regurgitated during or after removal.

12. Check that the pilot bulb of the ET tube is full of air to confirm that the seal around the distal end of the ET tube in the trachea is being maintained. Then, in the specific manner appropriate for the particular advanced airway device used, deflate the distal esophageal cuff. When the distal cuff has been purged of air the pilot bulb for that cuff should be empty and flat—confirming that no air remains in the cuff.

13. Without delay now withdraw the device while large bore suction is held in the oral cavity. During withdrawal of the EOA, EGTA PTL or Combitube the person ventilating the patient should safeguard the ET tube from accidental displacement. Continue withdrawing the device until it and the gastric tube have been fully removed. In some cases, once the distal end of the device is out of the mouth, hospital personnel can hold the gastric tube—allowing its proximal end to be drawn through the device—and then reposition it to the proper depth.

14. Return the patient to a supine position. Continue suctioning the oral cavity as needed and check that the ET tube has not been displaced. The advanced airway device should be properly disposed of in a suitable biohazard container since the use of any of these is limited to a single patient.

ALS
Endotracheal Intubation — Introduction

Placement of an endotracheal tube (ET tube) remains the method of choice for sustained airway management. Endotracheal intubation has remained the standard for definitive airway management because, although requiring practiced skill it nonetheless employs a reliable and uncomplicated adjunct which provides a direct isolated pathway communicating from the outside into the trachea for ventilation. Further, once the ET tube has been inserted and the cuff surrounding its distal end has been inflated to seal the trachea from otherwise communicating with the upper airway, this procedure protects the trachea and lungs from invasion and aspiration of regurgitated gastric contents, blood, or other items which may enter the upper airway.

The seal provided between the outside of the tube and the walls of the trachea also allows for a mechanical ventilator (BVM or other device) to be connected directly to the proximal end of the ET tube without the need for a mask. Since it is difficult (if not impossible) to consistently maintain a mask seal in the field or when moving or transporting the patient, the lack of this need with an ET tube significantly contributes to improved ventilation and oxygenation.

Endotracheal intubation can be performed by passing a tube through either the oropharynx or the nasopharynx and on into the trachea. In patients without a gag reflex it is most commonly achieved by visualized orotracheal intubation — using a laryngoscope to elevate the tongue and provide well lighted, clear observation of the ET tube's insertion through the vocal cords and into the trachea. In unconscious patients without gag reflexes when visualization has not been achievable, "digital intubation" using the EMT's tactile rather than visual senses has proven to be a viable alternative method for insertion.

Although patients with a gag reflex do not well tolerate orotrachael intubation, most will tolerate nasotracheal intubation. "Blind" nasotracheal intubation is the technique of choice in conscious patients and in those unconscious patients who still have a gag reflex. This method does require that the patient maintain spontaneous ventilation, as the patient's air exchange is a key element in assuring proper placement of the tube.

Due to anatomical differences, the techniques and equipment used for orotracheal intubation are slightly different for infants than for adults. Intubation techniques also need to be modified in a trauma victim who is suspected of having a potentially unstable spine. Since the "forward sniffing position" is contraindicated in such patients and the head must instead be immobilized in the neutral in-line position throughout, intubation techniques must be modified accordingly.

ALS

VISUALIZED OROTRACHEAL INTUBATION

In hypoxic patients *who are not in cardiac arrest,* intubation should not be the initial airway maneuver. It should only be performed after the patient has first been hyperventilated with a high FiO_2 using a manual airway maneuver or a simple airway adjunct. Contact with the deep pharynx when intubating a severely hypoxic patient without previous hyperoxygenation can easily produce vagal stimulation resulting in a dangerous bradycardia.

Intubation should be able to be accomplished without interrupting ventilations for more than 20 seconds. Ventilation should *NOT* be interrupted for more than 30 seconds for any reason. Visualized orotracheal intubation is contraindicated in conscious patients or patients with a present gag reflex. *Pre-hospital use of topical anesthesia in such patients is not recommended.*

Visualized orotracheal intubation is best performed with the patient's head hyperextended and slightly elevated anteriorly into what is commonly called a "forward sniffing position."

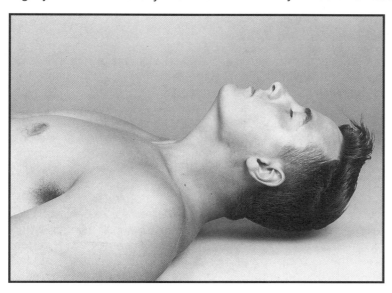

This position brings the different angles of the airway into alignment. It allows the intubator (from beyond the patient's head) the most unobstructed visual pathway to the vocal cords once the tongue and mandible have been elevated with the laryngoscope, as well as the best pathway for inserting the ET tube through the cords. ***Hyperextension of the head and/or use of the forward sniffing position are contraindicated for patients with suspected spine trauma.*** Therefore, visualized orotracheal intubation of trauma patients is performed with the patient's head immobilized in the neutral in-line position.

Intubation while maintaining manual immobilization requires additional training and practice beyond that for intubation of non-trauma patients. This technique is described in the pages immediately following this demonstration of the general steps in visualized orotracheal intubation for patients in whom spine trauma is not a concern.

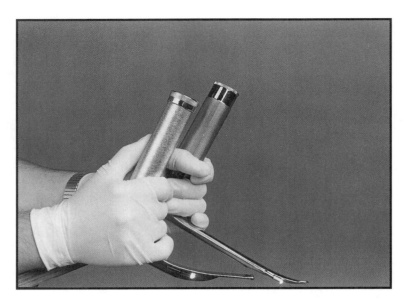

The essential equipment required for visualized orotracheal intubation includes a laryngoscope handle (which contains the batteries that power the light at the end of the blade), an appropriately sized laryngoscope blade, the endotracheal tube itself, and usually a 10cc syringe.

Laryngoscope blades come in a wide range of different specific designs. These can be categorized as being, in essence, "straight" or "curved." Use of a straight blade tends to produce less rotary force (pull towards a "sniffing" position) than is anatomically produced by the shape and method of use of a curved blade. However, since the success rate is often related to individual preference and comfort, selection of blade style must remain a matter of individual choice. Blades are sized according to length, and may range from 0 for newborns to 4 for large adults.

There is a variety of types and styles of laryngoscope equipment available, ranging from single-use disposable plastic handles and blades which are priced economically to extremely expensive gold-plated fiber-optic models which are usually the exclusive province of successful anesthesiologists. As noted above, the most important selection criteria for laryngoscope equipment is whatever works best for the operator performing the intubation. If the tube can be properly placed in the allotted period of time, whatever equipment was used was the right equipment.

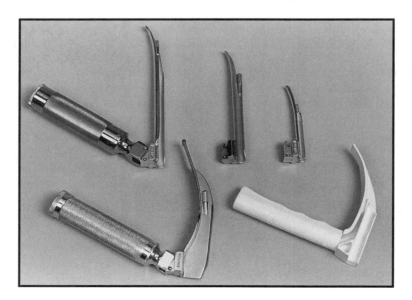

Laryngoscope blades are inserted and clip into place at the end of the handle. Handles and blades are part of a system, and must be compatible in order to work with each other. A fiber-optic handle will-not work with a conventional blade, and vice verse. In the types of laryngoscopes most commonly used by prehospital personnel, a small light bulb screws into a socket near the distal end of the blade.An electric wire built into the blade extends back to the handle end of the blade, where a connection is made to the battery power source from the handle. When a blade that has been clipped into place is snapped into a position perpendicular to the handle, it is firmly locked in that position of use and the electrical connection is completed and the light illuminates. To turn the laryngoscope light off the tip of the blade is folded toward the proximal end of the handle—unlocking the blade and breaking the electrical connection.

Endotracheal tubes come in a variety of diameters and lengths, ranging from 2.5 or 3.0 for newborns to 7.5 or 8.0 for most adults. These measurements are in millimeters (mm) and indicate the internal diameter of the tube, (i.e., the diameter of the lumen). While the larger tubes are typically 35–37 centimeters long, tubes for newborn and pediatric patients can vary widely in length.

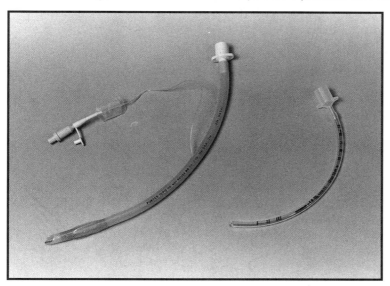

A major difference between adult tubes and those for small pediatric patients is the presence of a distal balloon cuff. Tubes for newborns and pediatric patients under eight years of age are typically uncuffed to avoid damage to tracheal tissue caused by the pressure from the balloon cuff. The upper end of the trachea in these patients is so small that the tube virtually fills the airway, obstructing air leakage without the need of a cuff. In adult patients, the larger size of the trachea requires the use of an inflatable cuff to both hold the tube's distal tip in place and also to prevent air from leaking past the tube. ET tubes are slightly curved (from tip to tip) to match the normal anatomical curvature of the airway from the mouth to the trachea. Cuffed tubes have a thin filler tube attached to the outside of the distal half of the ET tube and hanging freely on the proximal half. This filler tube connects the cuff with a one-way valve into which air can be injected or withdrawn by syringe to inflate and deflate the cuff. Insertion of a syringe into the one-way valve opens it, allowing air to move between the syringe and the cuff. Once the cuff has been properly inflated *the syringe must be removed from the one-way valve to seal it* and avoid an unwanted escape of air and deflation of the cuff. A pilot bulb is included in the filler line, just distal to the one-way valve, to allow the operator to ascertain the level of inflation of the cuff after it passes from view following insertion.

It is mandatory in preparation for performing an intubation that the EMT check the condition and tightness of the tiny bulb at the end of the blade which he has selected to use. Over time, bulbs can become loose or wear out and no longer provide a bright light. Regular preventive maintenance of laryngoscope equipment includes checking the batteries, bulbs, and the status of the electrical contacts at the end of the handles and blades.

One other piece of helpful equipment for use in performing visualized orotracheal intubation is the flexible stylet. Stylets are made of malleable metal or plastic, and are inserted into the endotracheal tube in order to allow the operator to better control the placement of the distal tip. They are particularly helpful in patients with unusual laryngeal anatomy and whenever the ambient temperature is warm enough to make the plastic endotracheal tubes uncontrollably flexible.

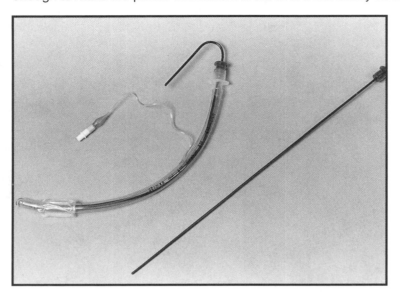

The stylet should be inserted into the tube and carefully measured so that the distal tip of the stylet does not protrude from the distal end of the endotracheal tube. Once this measurement has been made, a helpful trick is to simply bend the proximal end of the stylet markedly at the proximal end of the endotracheal tube so that it cannot slip further into the tube. Once this has been done, mold the ET tube and stylet back into the tube's original slightly curved shape (it will usually have been straightened by the insertion of the stylet). With the stylet in place the ET tube can now be molded slightly before insertion begins, and manipulated with considerable ease during the intubation attempt. Once the tube has been placed in the trachea, the stylet is removed before ventilation is attempted. Some stylets have a sliding "marker" at their proximal end which can also be used to insure that they do not protrude beyond the distal end of the ET tube.

ALS

VISUALIZED OROTRACHEAL INTUBATION

1. Endotracheal intubation is not included in the initial airway and ventilation maneuvers that should be performed in non-breathing patients. Rather, manually opening the airway, inserting a simple adjunct, and providing initial ventilation and oxygenation with a bag-valve-mask or similar device should be the EMT's initial approach. Only when this has been accomplished should plans be made to proceed to intubation. Ascertain that the proper level of Universal Precautions remain in place, and increase any as indicated. Next, confirm that the patient is being ventilated and obtain baseline breath sound information by auscultating the mid-lung fields bilaterally.

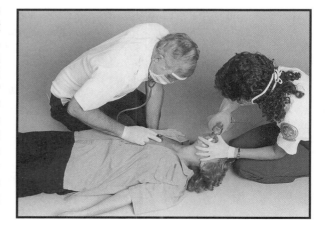

2. Check that the endotracheal tube's distal cuff is intact and holds air properly. With the plunger at the 10ml marker in the barrel of the syringe, attach it to the one-way valve on the thin filler tube or pilot bulb by inserting it firmly into the valve. Inject 10 ml of air and, while holding the plunger from moving in the barrel, check the tautness of the distal cuff and pilot balloon. When you have determined that the cuff does not leak, withdraw the air from the cuff by pulling the syringe plunger slowly back to its original position and leave the syringe securely attached to the one-way valve.

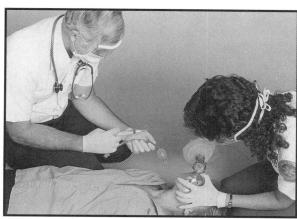

3. Select and assemble the correct size and preferred style laryngoscope blade and attach it to the appropriate handle. Check the light bulb at the end of the blade to make sure that it is bright when lit and that it is fastened tightly.

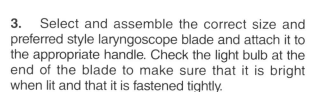

4. Insert a stylet into the endotracheal tube until its distal tip is just short of the ET tube's distal opening, and bend the stylet over the proximal end of the tube to assure that its distal end will not advance beyond the end of the ET tube. Bend the ET tube-stylet combination into a curve (resembling the curve of the tube before the stylet was inserted) to facilitate passage into the trachea.

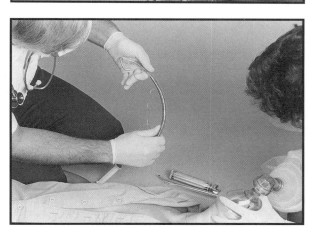

5. Position the patient's head and neck into a hyperextended and "forward sniffing" position. Placing a towel under the patient's head can be helpful in maintaining the head and neck in this position.

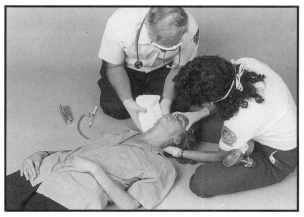

6. The EMT who is to insert the endotracheal tube should be positioned directly above the patient's head. This may necessitate changing the position of the EMT who has been ventilating the patient, or may involve changing duties among the EMTs present. Regardless, ventilation (and CPR when indicated) should be continued until insertion is imminent. Place the endotracheal tube with syringe attached on the patient's chest or in some easily found and properly clean location. Although the EMT will need the thumb and first one or two fingers of his right hand to perform a tongue-jaw lift at the beginning of the maneuver, some EMTs prefer to thread the ET tube through the other fingers of their right hand so that it is never out of their grasp.

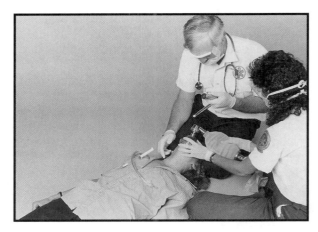

7. Hold the laryngoscope in your left hand (regardless of which of your hands is dominant) and perform a tongue-jaw lift with the right hand, holding the tongue against the lower palate while moving the patient's mandible anteriorly and opening the mouth. Insert the laryngoscope blade into the patient's mouth to the correct depth (about half to two-thirds of the way down the tongue).

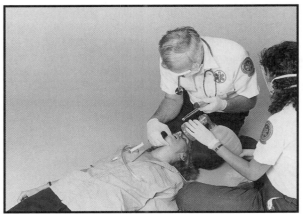

8. Classically, the straight blade is inserted in the right side of the mouth and swept to the left until it is at the midline to purchase the tongue when the tongue-jaw lift is released, and then is advanced under direct visualization until the tip of the epiglottis can be seen underlying the tip of the blade.

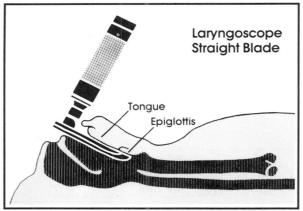

Laryngoscope Straight Blade

Tongue
Epiglottis

9. If a curved blade is used it is inserted directly along the midline, however unlike the straight blade it is only advanced until the tip rests in the vallecula (the indentation at the junction of the base of the tongue and the epiglottis).

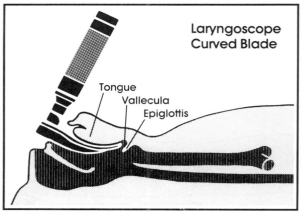

Laryngoscope Curved Blade

Tongue
Vallecula
Epiglottis

10. To reduce the possibility of aspiration, the esophagus may be compressed between the larynx and the cervical spine (Sellick's Maneuver). This is accomplished by having another EMT push the larynx with his thumb and first finger directly posterior toward the cervical spine. A second benefit of this maneuver may be to more readily provide visualization of the vocal cords.

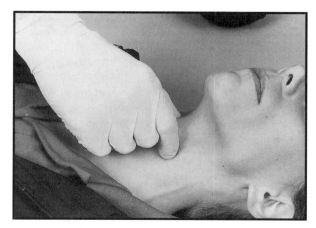

11. With the blade in position, extend your left arm to lift (elevating) against the patient's tongue and jaw with the laryngoscope. The wrist should be kept locked and the line of force should be along a straight line that points up and away from the patient's face at about a 45° angle. Contact along the length of the laryngoscope blade should be made only with the patient's tongue and pharynx—*NOT* with the teeth or gums. This helps to avoid damage to the patient's teeth and facilitates visualizing the vocal cords. As the patient's lower pharynx is exposed, begin to insert the endotracheal tube into the mouth with the right hand.

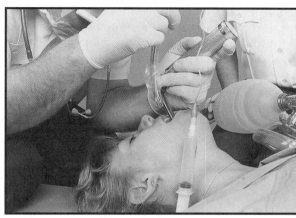

12. Once the vocal cords are clearly visualized, advance the tube between the cords and slightly beyond (not more than an inch). Remove the stylet, inflate the distal cuff with air, and remove the syringe from the one-way valve.

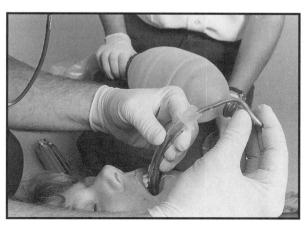

13. Direct the second EMT to attach the BVM or other ventilation resuscitator to the proximal end of the tube and resume ventilation, hyperventilating the patient. Visually check for adequate chest rise with each ventilation. Also auscultate over the episgastrium to confirm the absence of air flow sounds when the patient is ventilated. With the endotracheal tube successfully placed in the trachea and the cuff inflated, no air sound should be heard moving through the esophagus or into the stomach when the patient is ventilated.

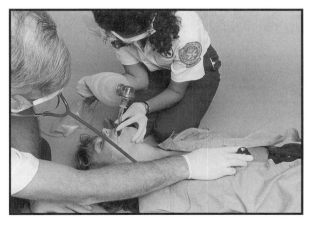

14. If chest rise is *NOT* seen and if air sounds *ARE HEARD* upon auscultation over the epigastrium, immediately stop ventilations and disconnect the BVM or demand valve from the proximal end of the ET tube. The tube may be either bent over outside the patient's mouth and mask ventilations resumed over it, or the tube may be removed by first deflating the distal cuff. In any event, mask ventilations must be immediately resumed for at least 30 seconds before another intubation attempt is made.

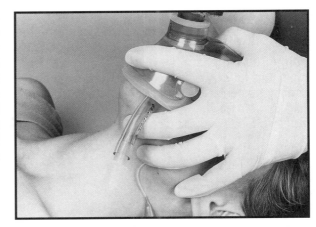

15. If the unsuccessful first tube is left in place, the next intubation attempt should include checking and preparing a second ET tube, and then moving the first tube to the left side of the patient's mouth when the laryngoscope is re-inserted. Following insertion, again observe for chest rise and auscultate over the epigastrium for the absence of air sounds with each ventilation.

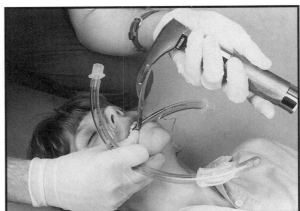

16. From the time of insertion until now the ET tube should be carefully held in place without interruption to assure that it does not move or become displaced. Once the tube's placement has been confirmed by auscultation, secure it in place with tape or a commerical ET tube holder. When using tape be sure to fasten it to the tube at the level of the patient's teeth. This not only secures the tube but also provides a visual reminder of the correct placement depth. Taping around the neck, not just the face, is recommended to better secure the tube.

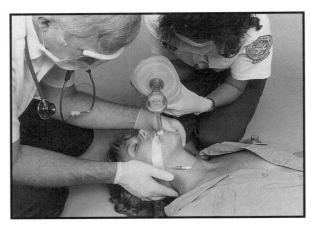

17. Even though the tape marker can be seen, the maintenance of proper positioning and continued adequate ventilation should be periodically confirmed by checking chest rise and the patient's overall appearance. Periodic re-auscultation of the mid-lung fields to ensure the presence of good bilateral breath sounds should also be performed.

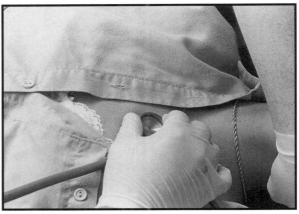

ALS

ALTERNATE METHOD FOR USE OF LARYNGOSCOPE
(For EMTs who have difficulty with the straight-arm method).

During intubation, some operators have difficulty in performing the straight-arm extension necessary to lift the tongue and mandible and allow visualization of the vocal cords. Following is an alternate method which has proven to be helpful for some in overcoming this problem. We are indebted to Sheila Spaid, RN, formerly the Paramedic Training Coordinator at Akron General Medical Center, Akron, Ohio, for sharing this technique with us. Instructors may also find this a useful technique to use when personally trying to maintain a clear sight path for a sustained period in mannikins or cadavers while multiple students visualize the anatomy. The previously described steps for intubation should be followed except that the following steps replace steps 7 through 11 in the previous sequence.

7. (alt) Grasp the laryngoscope handle in your left hand. Your hand should be closer to the "bottom" of the handle—i.e., the end where the blade and handle connect—than would be usual. Bend your wrist as far as possible toward a 90° angle to the right of the midline of your forearm.

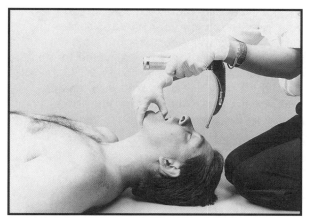

8. (alt) While performing a tongue-jaw lift with your right hand, insert the blade to the correct depth into the patient's mouth, release the tongue-jaw lift, and rest your left forearm on the patient's forehead. (This both keeps the head in the correct position and serves to maintain your left arm's position.) A useful marker is to align the wrinkles in the skin at your wrist with the patient's lower lip.

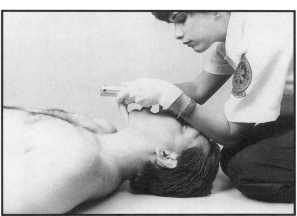

9. (alt) While visualizing the mouth move the tip of the blade to the midline of the oral cavity and to the correct depth (at the vallecula for a curved blade or just beyond the epiglottis for a straight blade).

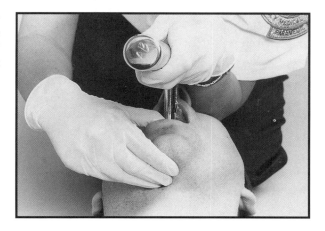

10. (alt) To reduce the possibility of aspiration, the esophagus may be compressed between the larynx and the cervical spine (Sellick's maneuver). This is accomplished by having another EMT push the larynx (held between his thumb and first finger) directly posterior towards the cervical spine.

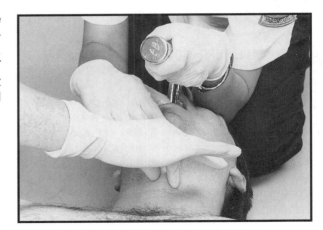

11. (alt) Now without moving your forearm, extend your wrist, returning your hand to a zero-degree in-line position with your forearm. Note the extent of blade movement that has elevated the tongue and mandible without any movement of the arm. This should permit visualization of the pharynx and vocal cords, without bringing the laryngoscope blade to bear against the patient's teeth.

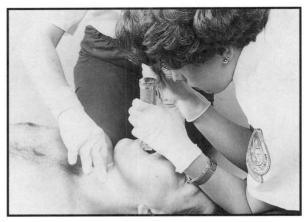

VISUALIZED OROTRACHEAL INTUBATION FOR INFANTS

Visualized orotracheal intubation can be successfully performed on patients of all ages, however the EMT should be aware of some modifications which occur when the patient is an infant. First, only a straight laryngoscope blade is used. The infant's vocal cords are located more anteriorly than an adult's, and a curved blade is both harder to use and more likely to traumatize the infant's oropharynx. Second, only **uncuffed** endotracheal tubes are used. The infant's trachea narrows at its proximal end, providing a close enough margin to effectively hold air below the vocal cords without the need for a pressurized cuff on the tube. A cuff could also be an additional agent for traumatizing the infant's trachea when it is inflated. Finally, whereas an adult's head and next are hyperextended (except in trauma patients) in preparation for visualized orotracheal intubation, the infant's cervical alignment must remain in no more than mild extension due to the potential for crimping and collapsing the immature tracheal cartilaginous rings.

It should also be noted that due to the incomplete formation of the cranium in infants and small children (particularly of the cribriform plate), the "blind nasal" intubation procedure is not attempted in such patients. Similarly, due to the child's small mouth size and the anterior positioning of the vocal cords, the digital-tactile technique is also not employed in infants and small children.

ALS

VISUALIZED OROTRACHEAL INTUBATION OF TRAUMA PATIENTS
(With Neutral In-Line Immobilization)

Hyperextension and elevation of the head into a forward sniffing position, or continued movement of the head and neck, are contraindicated in patients with suspected spine trauma. Therefore, visualized orotracheal intubation of trauma patients is performed with the patient's head immobilized in the neutral in-line position. Intubating with the patient in such a position requires additional training and practice beyond that for conventional intubation. It should only be attempted by persons already qualified in endotracheal intubation who have demonstrated this ability to their medical director's satisfaction.

In hypoxic patients intubation should not be the initial airway maneuver. It should only be performed after the patient has been hyperventilated with a high FiO_2 using manual airway maneuvers and a simple airway adjunct. Contact with the deep pharynx when intubating a severely hypoxic patient without first hyperoxygenating him can stimulate the vagus nerve and produce a dangerous bradycardia.

The EMT should be able to intubate a patient without interrupting ventilation for more than 20 seconds. Ventilation should *NOT* be interrupted for more than 30 seconds for any reason. Visualized orotracheal intubation, as with any patient, is contraindicated in conscious trauma patients or those with a present gag reflex.

1. While manual in-line imobilization, airway control using a simple airway adjunct, and ventilation with a high FiO_2 are being provided, provide care for other immediate urgent "ABC" priorities. Once all such other immediate needs have been met, replacement of the simple airway with a more definitive, protected airway should be instituted. Auscultate the left and right mid-lung fields for the presence/absence of bilateral breath sounds to establish a baseline.

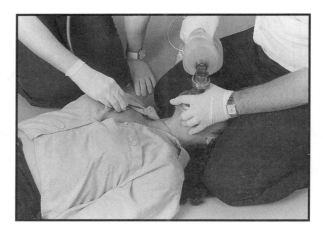

2. Without interrupting the manual immobilization or ventilation, one EMT takes over the manual immobilization from the patient's side. If the neutral in-line positioning results in a void between the back of the patient's head and the ground, a towel or other padding should be placed under the head at this time as this additional support will be an important aid in maintaining neutral alignment during intubation.

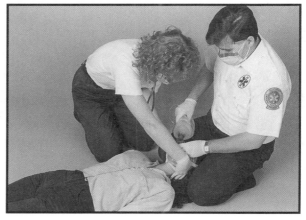

3. The correct size ET tube is selected and all of the additional equipment required is assembled. Use of a stylet has proven to be helpful—but remains a matter of personal preference except when due to climate the ET tube is warm and fluid. The laryngoscope and ET tube are prepared and tested in the usual manner. When ready, the EMT who will intubate instructs the EMT providing ventilation to move to the patient's side opposite from the EMT providing the immobilization, and instructs him to hyperventilate the patient.

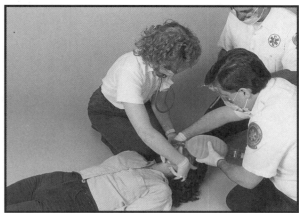

4. The EMT who will do the intubation sits on the ground with one leg over each of the patient's arms and gently moves forward until the patient's head can be secured between his thighs (as shown). Firm pressure is applied with the thighs to the side of the head. The grip of both EMT's will keep the head from moving (including rotation to hyperextension) during intubation.

OR

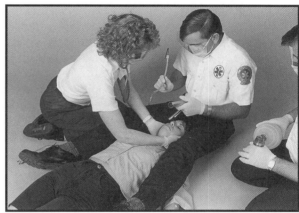

An alternative method is for the EMT performing the intubation to lie prone at the patient's head. When using this technique, however, the second EMT alone has the task of maintaining the head in a neutral in-line position during intubation. Experience has shown that it is often difficult for one EMT, alone, to keep the head from rotating to extension when the tongue and mandible are elevated with the laryngoscope, therefore this variation is only recommended when resources are limited.

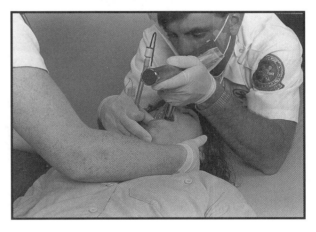

5. When ready, the EMT doing the intubation instructs the EMT hyperventilating the patient to stop. If suctioning is necessary it should be provided and ventilation reinstated for a short period before the instruction to stop is repeated. If an orotracheal airway is in place, remove it. While visualizing the mouth, insert the laryngoscope into it in the usual manner.

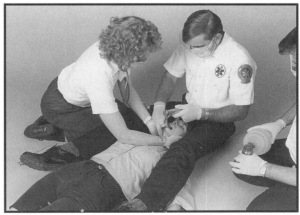

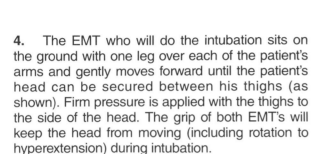

6. Once the blade is properly placed, elevate the tongue and apply gentle traction in a caudad and upward direction (about a 45 degree angle) by extending the left arm. Care must be taken to avoid touching the teeth or using them as a fulcrum.

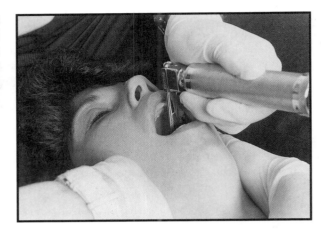

7. In the sitting position it may be necessary for the EMT to tilt his upper torso back in order to visualize the vocal cords. Once the vocal cords can be clearly seen, the endotracheal tube is advanced between the cords. It should be noted that when the head is maintained in the neutral in-line position (dictated by trauma), the intubator may be limited to being able to see the arytenoid cartilage and only the lower half of the cords. Experience has shown this to be ample to provide for proper visualized placement of the ET tube.

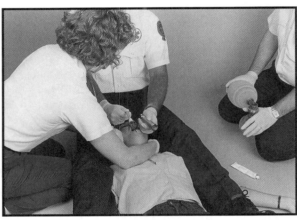

8. After the distal cuff has been seen to pass through the vocal cords (or their lower half), advance the tube slightly further (not more than one inch), remove the stylet (if used), inflate the cuff and remove the syringe from the one-way valve. Attach the Bag Valve device to the end of the ET tube and re-institute ventilation, hyperventilating the patient.

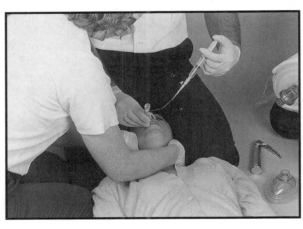

9. Before securing the tube, visually check for adequate chest rise and auscultate over the epigastrium. NO "rushing air" or "bubbling" sounds should be heard. If air sounds are heard over the epigastrium when the bag is squeezed— or chest rise is not seen—the EMT must assume misplacement of the ET tube has occurred. Immediately deflate the cuff and remove the ET tube. Hyperventilate the patient for 2 to 3 minutes and then attempt to intubate him again, following the preceding steps.

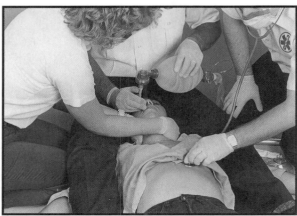

10. When chest rise is seen and air sounds are absent upon auscultation over the epigastrium, to further confirm proper placement and ventilation of the lungs, auscultate for good breath sounds at the mid-lung field on each side. If sounds are present on the right side but absent on the left (unless a left pneumothorax was found when auscultating the initial baselines prior to intubation), the ET tube has been inserted too far and has intubated the right mainstem bronchus. To correct this situation withdraw the ET tube a few centimeters and re-auscultate both mid-lung fields.

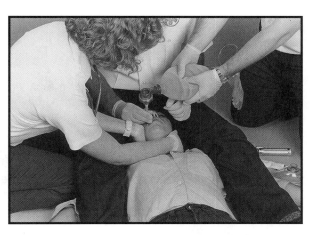

11. Once proper placement has been confirmed, secure the endotracheal tube using a commerical ET tube holder or with tape anchored to the tube at the level of the teeth, then wrapped around the back of the neck and again around the tube.

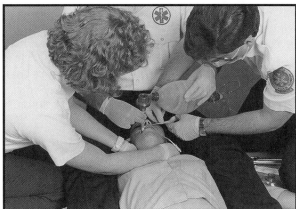

12. Continue ventilations and periodically re-auscultate for good breath sounds over each mid-lung field to confirm that the endotracheal tube remains properly placed and that good alveolar ventilation is occurring bilaterally.

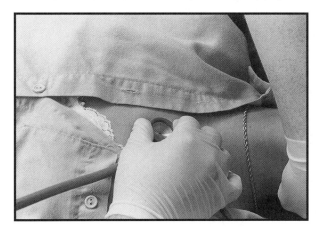

ALS

"BLIND" DIGITAL TACTILE OROTRACHEAL INTUBATION

Inserting an ET tube blindly through the patient's mouth with this technique should only be attempted after attempts at VISUALIZED intubation have failed. This method involves guiding the distal end of the tube with the EMT's fingertips which have been placed deeply into the patient's pharynx. It is especially useful in patients whose airway anatomy makes visualization extremely difficult, trauma victims with copious bleeding in the mouth or nose or when mandibular injury makes use of a laryngoscope unwise or dysfunctional. In view of the fact that the EMT's gloved fingers will be significantly exposed to the patient's oral secretions and that a glove and the skin may be torn by contact with the patient's teeth this technique should be weighed against the choice of a transtracheal cricothyroid procedure, and either should be selected as a last option when other methods of obtaining a protected airway have proven unsuccessful.

1.   The patient is first ventilated with a high FiO_2 using an appropriate device. As other techniques have already been attempted, the patient should be hyper-ventilated and re-oxygenated while the equipment is prepared and checked. Assure that the patient has no gag reflex and is fully unresponsive by applying a central painful stimulus (i.e. pinching the trapezius muscle).

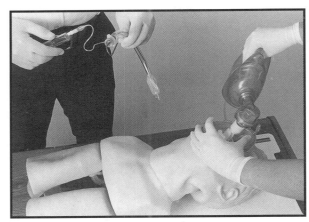

2.   A stylet must be used with this technique. Insert the stylet to the appropriate length into the ET tube, and bend it at a right angle at the proximal end to keep it from advancing further into the tube. Next bend the endotracheal tube and stylet into a curved "hockey stick" shape to facilitate guiding the distal end of the tube into the correct location with the EMT's fingertips. Make sure that your gloves are properly fitting and intact.

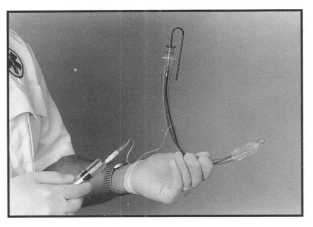

3.   The patient's head should be maintained in a forward "sniffing" position during the insertion. Place a folded towel under the patient's head to assist the second EMT in accomplishing this. In cases where spine trauma is suspected, the second EMT will have to keep the patient's head securely immobilized in the neutral in-line position, making the digital intubation more difficult. The EMT performing the intubation, while holding the readied ET tube with the air-filled syringe attatched in one hand, should position himself at the patient's chest facing the patient. When ready, he directs the EMT providing ventilations to stop and withdraw the oropharyngeal airway. He then inserts two fingers into the patient's mouth, reaching for the epiglottis.

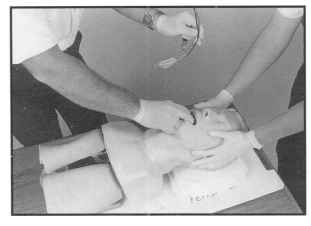

4. The EMT's two first fingers are held together and advanced until they are fully inserted into the patient's mouth and oropharynx, so that the tips of the first two fingers can feel the epiglottis and are just beyond it. Flex the fingers a little way, so that the tips can be felt to slightly elevate the epiglottis, and stop.

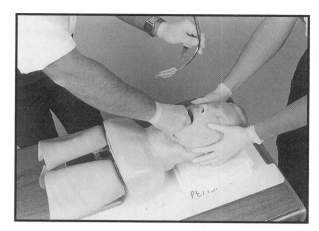

5. Without allowing *ANY* movement of the inserted fingers, insert the bent endotracheal tube into the patient's mouth, guiding its bent distal tip between the first two fingers. These should only be parted enough to let the tube pass between them while still touching them. The technique is sometimes called "Digital Tactile Intubation" because the exact location can be clearly felt by the lateral aspects and tips of the fingers.

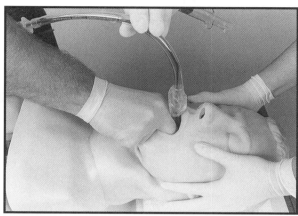

6. Continue to advance the tube between the two fingers until its bent distal tip can be felt at the ends of the fingertips. When the fingertips are slightly flexed, elevating the epiglottis, the very space between the fingertips points directly into the opening of the vocal cords. With the hand holding the proximal end, push the ET tube in a caudad direction while using the fingertips if necessary to "walk" the distal tip into the trachea.

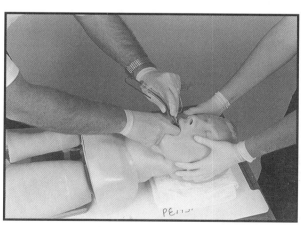

7. With the tube inserted into the trachea, grasp it securely with the still-inserted fingers and withdraw the stylet with the other. While continuing to guide it with the inserted fingers, advance the tube fully to the proper depth with the other hand.

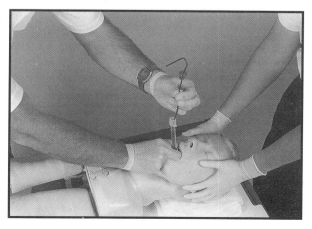

8. While continuing to hold the tube securely, inflate the distal cuff with the syringe. The second EMT should have the bag-valve or other ventilation device ready to attach to the proximal end of the tube as soon as the cuff is inflated.

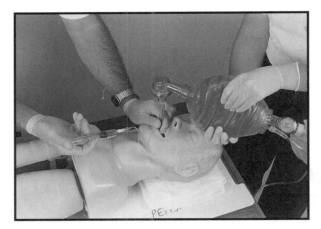

9. The EMT who performed the intubation should confirm correct tube placement by observing for chest rise and auscultating over the epigastrium while the second EMT ventilates the patient. As always, if positive chest rise is not seen or if air sounds are heard over the stomach with each ventilation, the tube has been misplaced in the esophagus. It should be immediately removed and the patient reventilated for at least one minute before intubation is re-attempted.

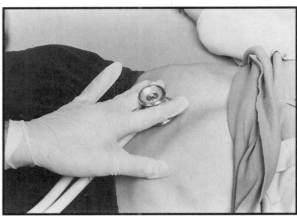

10. Once chest rise and absent breath sounds over the epigastrium have been noted, additional confirmation of proper placement and ventilation of both lungs should be obtained by auscultating over the mid-lung fields bilaterally while the second EMT continues to ventilate the patient. If the tube has been advanced too far, intubating the right mainstem bronchus, it should be slightly withdrawn until bilateral breath sounds are auscultatable. The tube must be manually held in place throughout this process.

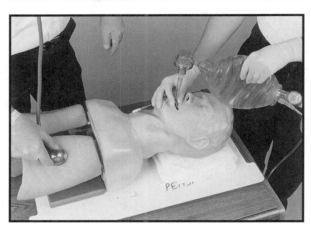

11. When correct placement and depth in the trachea have been confirmed the tube can be fastened in place with tape or an ET tube holder, and manual support can be released. The patient should be periodically re-assessed not only for adequacy of ventilation but also for maintenance of proper tube placement.

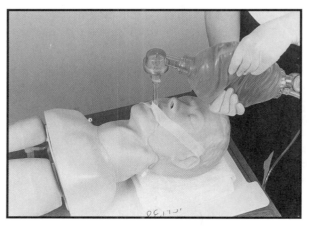

BLIND NASOTRACHEAL INTUBATION

Blind nasotracheal intubation provides the EMT with a method of intubating a patient who is conscious or who has a lowered LOC but retains a present gag reflex. The technique is dependent upon the patient's spontaneous ventilations to assure proper alignment when passing through the vocal cords and into the trachea, and is therefore limited to use in spontaneously breathing patients. Further, it requires a cooperative or subdued patient, and an environment in which the EMT can hear and feel air exchange at the external end of the ET tube.

This technique should be used as the initial method of intubation for breathing patients who have a presnet gag reflex *or* who have sub-maxillary injuries (such as fractured mandible) which preclude, or make undesirable, the use of an orotracheal approach. In other breathing patients who do not have a gag reflex it is only chosen after unsuccessful visualized orotracheal attempts, either when visualization has proven a problem (necessitating a "blind" method) or after several visualized attempts have been unsuccessful.

Contraindications for use of blind nasotracheal intubation include:

- Apnea
- Injury to the maxilla, zygoma, inferior orbit, nose, or cribriform plate
- Suspicion of an anterior basilar skull fracture.

This technique should only be attempted by personnel qualified in endotracheal intubation who have demonstrated their ability to perform this additional intubation skill to their medical director's satisfaction.

Blind nasotracheal intubation is commonly performed with the patient first positioned with his head hyperextended and elevated (on a folded towel) anteriorly into a forward sniffing position. This position aligns the posterior nasopharynx most fortunately with the trachea to provide for tracheal rather than esophageal blind intubation.

In trauma victims with suspected spine trauma, movement to this position and continued movement are contraindicated. Therefore, in trauma victims the patient's head is moved and immobilized throughout in the neutral in-line position by a second EMT. Although this increases the chance of misplacement, it is necessary to protect the spine.

1. While the patient is provided with a high FiO_2 and, if needed, assisted or provided ventilation depending on the level of the patient's need (and manual in-line immobilization if indicated), the EMT who will perform the intubation should kneel at the patient's upper torso, turned slightly towards the patient's face. Auscultate the mid-lung fields bilaterally to establish a baseline.

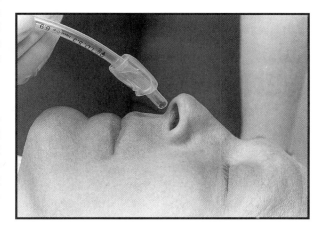

2. Briefly interrupt oxygenation to inspect the nostrils with a penlight. Select the largest and least deviated or obstructed (commonly the right one). Compare several sizes of ET tube to the size of the anterior nostril and select the tube that has an outside diameter just smaller than the diameter of the chosen nostril.

3. While oxygenation is continued, gather and check the equipment needed. A key check to be made is that the distal cuff is intact and holds air. **Note:** A Stylet should *NEVER* be used when performing a nasotracheal intubation since it would impair proper insertion and could easily result in producing additional significant injury. When ready to proceed, lubricate the distal tip and cuff of the ET tube liberally with a water soluble lubricating jelly.

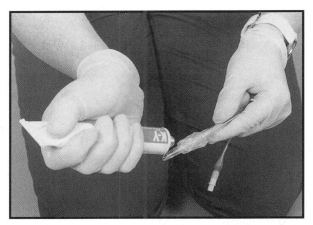

4. The assisting EMT who is positioned above the patient's head should hold the head in extension, tilted to the "forward sniffing" position, to facilitate entry of the tube into the nostril and along the nasal air passage. Placing a towel under the patient's head may help with this maneuver. In patients with suspected spine trauma for whom such a position is contraindicated, the assisting EMT should firmly hold the head immobilized in the neutral in-line position instead.

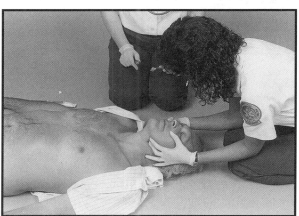

5. Hold the ET tube between the thumb and first two fingers with the distal tip pointing posteriorly into the selected nostril and the other end (with the adaptor) pointing anteriorly and caudally as shown. Advance the tube into the nostril, guiding it in an anterior-to-posterior direction—*NOT* superiorly. Advancing it superiorly will commonly result in resistance and potential injury at the turbinates. A slight back-and-forth rotation of the tube between the fingers may be useful in aiding its passage through the nostril and into the pharynx.

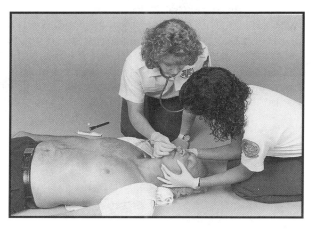

6. Once the tube has been advanced through the nose and into the pharynx, listen closely to the breath sounds at the external (proximal) end of the tube. Slightly rotate the tube back and forth while listening. When breath sounds are the loudest and the greatest misting of the tube occurs when the patient exhales, stop any further rotation. The distal end of the tube should be lined up with the opening in the vocal cords and the trachea beyond it. If the patient is conscious ask him to take a deep breath, then gently pass the tube into the trachea while he does.

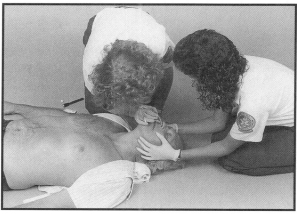

7. If the patient is unconscious or has a noticeably lowered level of consciousness, the assisting EMT should be directed to perform a jaw thrust when the ET tube has been passed through the nose and is in the oropharynx. This ensures that the tongue is elevated and will not block the ET tube's advancement. Once successfully in the trachea advance the tube to the correct depth to ensure that the cuff is beyond the vocal cords. Inflate the cuff with the syringe and remove the syringe from the one-way valve.

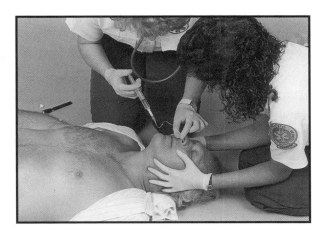

8. Since the patient is breathing spontaneously (or blind nasal intubation would *NOT* have been performed), the initial check for proper placement is different than when an apneic patient has been intubated. Check and note whether upon exhalation the misting continues and note if air is felt and heard exhausting *from the proximal end of the tube,* or instead *from the mouth and nose* around the outside of the tube (but *NOT* out of its proximal end), or *both*. If air movement is felt both from the proximal end and around the tube, additional inflation of the cuff is required to provide a seal at the distal end.

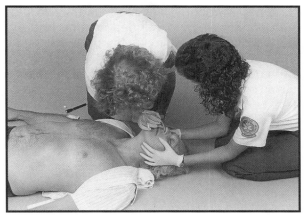

9. *If continued misting and air with each exhalation are clearly felt exclusively at the promixal end of the ET tube,* it is properly placed in the trachea. Further confirm good ventilation of the lungs by observing chest rise and by auscultation of good bilateral breath sounds over the mid-lung fields. If baseline breath sounds were auscultated bilaterally and now are only heard on the right side, the ET tube is inserted too far—intubating the right mainstem bronchus. Withdraw it slightly and re-auscultate for the return of good bilateral breath sounds.

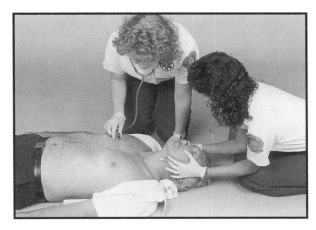

10. If air exchange is felt upon exhalation exclusively around the outside of the tube from the mouth (and nose) rather than at the proximal end, the distal tip is misplaced in the esophagus. In a breathing patient, when an ET tube has been misplaced in the esophagus, air exchange can continue through the oral and nasal pharynx around the outside of the misplaced ET tube. However, this produces a **dangerous situation** since if the patient's air exchange becomes reduced or he becomes apneic, any needed ventilation could not be mechanically provided around the tube and any air ventilated into the tube will exclusively be directed into the esophagus and stomach without any ventilation of the lungs.

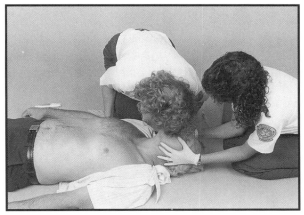

11. In such cases, the distal cuff should immediately be deflated and the tube withdrawn (completely or from the trachea and posterior pharynx—leaving it in the nose). After the patient has breathed air with a high FiO_2, the preceding steps should be repeated to nasally intubate the trachea.

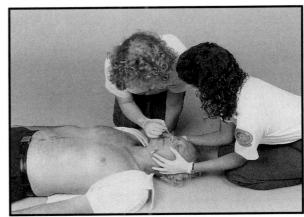

12. Once correct placement in the trachea has been confirmed by continued misting and air exchange exclusively through the proximal end of the ET tube, and continued ventilation of the lungs assured by auscultation of good bilateral breath sounds over the mid-lung fields, secure the tube in place with tape. Connect the BVM (complete with collector and high flow O_2) or a demand valve to the proximal end of the ET tube and provide ventilations appropriate to the patient's needs. If the patient is conscious, the procedure should be explained to him.

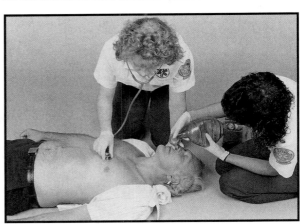

13. Once assisted ventilation has been successfully initiated, confirm proper placement by the absence of air sounds when auscultating over the epigastrium during several provided breaths. Periodically discontinue the assisted ventilation and immediately remove the BVM from the ET tube to allow unencumbered spontaneous ventilation. Evaluate the unassisted ventilation to determine if continued assisted (or provided) ventilation is still required.

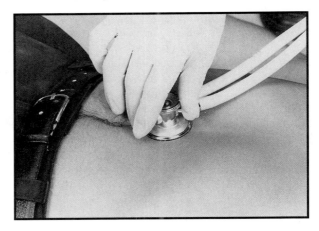

NOTE: If spontaneous ventilation is restored to an acceptable rate and depth (adequate Minute volume) the ET tube should be left in place and supplemental oxygen enrichment should be supplied. This can be achieved by holding an oxygen mask with high flow O_2 near the proximal end of the ET tube (but *NOT ON* it). **WARNING:** *Care must be taken to assure that neither mask, tape, nor any other item* occludes the free movement of air in and out of the ET tube's proximal end.

Periodically check the chest rise and bilateral breath sounds over the midlung fields to confirm that proper air exchange is continuing or to identify the need for reinstituting assisted or provided ventilations with the BVM or demand valve.

Suctioning — Introduction

In patients who, due to lowered levels of consciousness with an associated impaired or absent gag reflex, can no longer maintain a patent airway for themselves, airway management not only involves management of the tongue by *insertion* of an airway adjunct, but must also include *removal* of any fluids, vomitus, debris (i.e., broken teeth) and pieces of partially digested food by use of a suction device. Suctioning is a critical EMT skill when any of the above items are present in the mouth, nose, pharynx, trachea or airway adjunct and:

- Threaten to occlude or partially block the airway,
- Deter or make impossible the placing of an airway adjunct,
- Or could be aspirated into the trachea and lungs.

It must be noted that blockage of the airway (or airway adjunct) by any of these which is not recognized and alleviated by suctioning will result in hypoxia, cell death, and irreversible biological death of the patient in just a few short minutes.

Aspiration of any significant amount of vomitus or other gastric contents (about one-half cup or more) is generally fatal. In such cases, regardless of successful resuscitation in the field and the ensuing treatment at the hospital, these patients usually die within days or weeks of the occurrence.

A suction machine works by imposing a vacuum against the fluid or small objects to be removed. With most suction units the material is drawn by the vacuum through a suction catheter and a connecting tube into a jar-like suction cannister. The vacuum source is connected (generally through a separate connecting hose) to a port at the top of the suction cannister. These cannisters have a sealed (airtight) cover to prevent air leakage resulting in a loss of vacuum pressure. A special safety valve placed between the suction cannister and the vacuum source keeps fluid from going beyond the cannister and into the mechanism which produces the vacuum, protecting its continued operation from becoming fouled. Many of the more sophisticated suction units also contain a *purging button* which — when temporarily pressed — reverses the function, converting the vacuum to positive pressure and allowing (once the suction tip has been removed from the patient) for any materials which may be obstructing the suction tip or connecting tube to be "blown out." In units without this feature the line can be "flushed" to clear it by suctioning sterile water or normal saline.

The vacuum necessary for suctioning can be created in a variety of ways. The source can be:

- An electric motor which powers an attached compressor
- An attachment to a motor vehicle engine manifold which accesses the vacuum produced by the engine's normal operation
- An attachment to a permanently installed vacuum line (pipes connecting to a central motor, compressor, and vacuum bank at another location)
- A manually powered "pump"
- Negative pressure produced in a syringe (plunger or rubber bulb type).

Although the operation of a suction device does not include the need to perform any operation on the usually sealed components of the vacuum pump source, it may be helpful for the EMT to understand that:

- Air compressors are simply complex air pumps
- Air pumps provide increased air pressure by compressing air (usually by use of a piston or bellows-type device) within a container, which is allowed to exit through a one-way valve while outside air is drawn in through another (the way a BVM works).
- Positive pressure (greater than room air) is produced at the *discharge end* of an air pump and negative pressure (a vacuum) by the pump's refilling at the *intake end.*
- Suction devices simply connect to the intake end of the pump, where its action (and the nature of the one-way valves) results in producing a substantial vacuum.

Although suction units may have a variety of different specific arrangements and designs, the following components are necessary for suctioning:

- A pump (manual or powered vacuum source)
- A suction hose connecting the pump and the top of the collecting cannister, usually including a safety valve to protect from invasion of the pump by cannister contents
- An airtight cannister for the collection of suctioned materials
- A suction connecting hose between the cannister and the suction catheter or tip to be used, allowing flexibility in the distance and direction it is used from the cannister
- An appropriate suction catheter or tip
- Sterile water or normal saline to suction in order to "flush" the tip and connecting tubing as needed.

Hand-powered units may have a connector directly inserted between the pump and cannister or between the cannister and tip, instead of separate connecting suction tubing. Regardless of specific design, the components from the pump to the distal tip of the catheter must be connected and sealed without any leakage to the outside in order to maintain the vacuum pressure. Even the smallest "pinhole" leak will severely reduce the vacuum available for suctioning and an opening of only two to three millimeters in diameter will result in no suction at all beyond that opening.

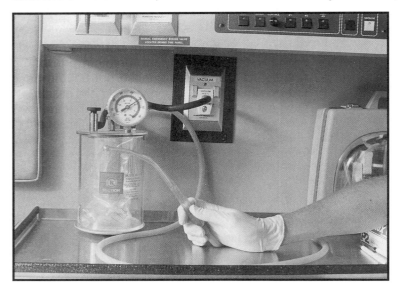

Suction devices can be broadly classified as either *fixed or portable* units. Fixed units include hospital and ambulance in-wall "piped" systems as well as wall-hung ambulance units that cannot be moved from place to place. These typically feature larger collection cannisters than do portable units, and due to their lack of mobility, require longer suction connecting tubing in order to reach a patient who cannot be placed immediately close to the machine. These also usually provide for the availability of more suction and have finer controls. While they tend to be more reliable in operation (or sustained use) than portable units, they are dependent upon their continued sealed integrity and supporting power systems. Failure of the ambulance electrical system or loss of power to the hospital building housing the compressor, will cause the wall suction to be inoperable.

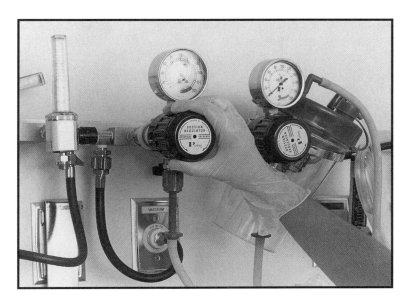

The EMT frequently only sees the "front" or "face" of a fixed suction system—the suction pressure gauge, on/off controls, collection cannister, and tubing connection point. The device which generates the vacuum, and the hoses or pipes which link the visible portions of the device with the more distant ones, is concealed behind the vehicle or building walls and may, in the case of a hospital, be quite some distance away.

Portable suction units, although containing basically the same components, are smaller and lighter than fixed units and are self-contained, providing everything required (except the catheter or tip) for suctioning in a single unit which is not dependent upon being attached to central vacuum pipes or a power source. The same catheters or tips are used with both fixed and portable suction units. Due to their portability, the latter generally have shorter suction connecting tubes and smaller collection cannisters.

Portable suction units are either manually or battery powered. Battery powered units use either disposable or rechargeable batteries and, to provide for a minimum of additional weight, the batteries are relatively small.

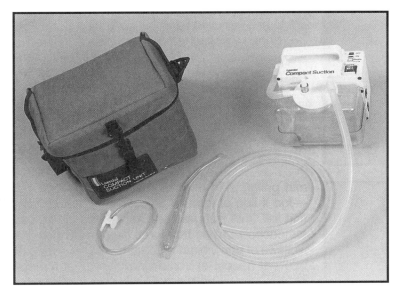

This, along with relatively small collection containers, represents the biggest drawback or area of potential problems with portable units. As with fixed units, if the power supply fails so does the suction.

EMS services should have a preventive maintenance program for both the suction machines and the power supplies. As many devices use rechargeable batteries, a regular program of battery maintenance and conditioning is essential. Most battery-powered portable units include a built-in battery charger so that when not in use they can simply be plugged in to an electrical outlet—keeping the batteries at full charge. Some units require a separate charger, and it is recommended with such units that a spare set of batteries be purchased and kept in the charger. After each use the batteries in the portable unit should be rotated with the recharged ones in the charger.

Fixed or portable powered suction devices generally have an "on/off" control and the more sophisticated ones have a second control which regulates the amount of vacuum being applied. Wall units generally have a variable strength control, whereas in portable units the strength control is generally limited to just "high" or "low." To assure that suction is available the instant it is needed, the suction device should have a suction catheter or tip connected and be turned "on" and running whenever the need for suction is anticipated. Since the vacuum is constantly applied once the device has been turned on, but

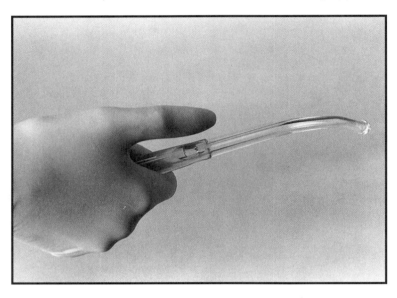

prehospital use involves the need for intermittent rather than continuous suction, a catheter or tip containing a "whistle stop" should be used. The "whistle stop" is an opening (2mm to 4mm in diameter) at the proximal end of the catheter which, even when the suction unit is "on" and operating, causes the vacuum to draw air in through this opening to the outside rather than producing suction at the distal end of the catheter or tip. Only while the machine is operating and this hole is covered (occluded) with a finger will the vacuum produce suction at the distal end of the catheter or suction tip. In this way the machine can be operating constantly yet the EMT has immediate patient-side control of when it does and does not provide suction.

All powered "non manual" suction devices are expected to produce a vacuum of at least 300mm Hg within seconds after being applied (that is, within seconds after being turned on and then having the suction catheter obstructed by a foreign body or by kinking the tube). Fixed units typically display a gauge which shows the amount of vacuum being produced, however these are rare on portable devices and non-existent on manual units.

There is a wide array of devices which fall under the heading of "manual" suction units. These range from commercially manufactured devices such as the "Res-Q-Vac" pictured here to a rubber bulb syringe or an assembly consisting of a barrel syringe and catheter. These could also be titled "rescuer powered," as they require the direct continuous effort of the EMT to operate them. They have three

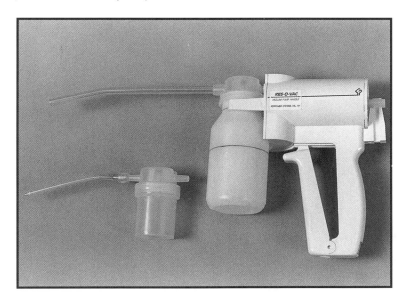

distinct advantages over all of the other devices: they are the most lightweight and portable, they are not dependent upon an outside electrical or battery source, and they provide the EMT with an immediate feeling of compliance and feedback as to the effectiveness of his efforts. Their disadvantages are that they typically have the smallest collection cannisters and that they require the EMT's continuous physical effort to operate (pump) while simultaneously inserting the tip correctly into the patient's mouth—it is not the same as turning on a switch or pushing a button.

One manually operated suction device, the "V-VAC," has unique capabilities from other customary suction units—fixed or portable. Generally, even the most powerful suction units can not remove large amounts of vomitus rapidly enough to keep up with the need caused by copious regurgitation. Even though other units can suction vast volumes of fluid rapidly, due to their limited openings undigested or partially digested pieces of food obstruct the tip, requiring "clearing" before suctioning can be continued.

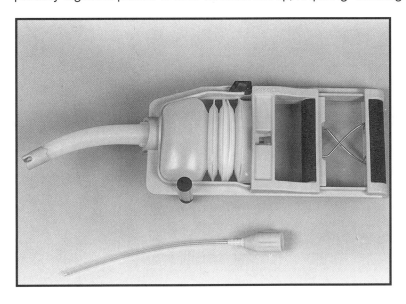

The V-VAC, by eliminating the limited size of the opening of normal tips and connecting tubes, *is the most effective device presently available for extracting vomitus*. By adding the adaptor and suction tip provided with the V-Vac, it can also be used to suction fluids from the mouth and nose in the customary manner. In the authors' opinions, however, this secondary ability of the V-VAC for suctioning other than vomitus is less desirable than the use of a powered portable or fixed unit for such purpose. Due to its unique ability to remove large amounts of vomitus rapidly, the additional availability of a V-VAC as well as (rather than instead of) any other standard powered suction unit is recommended in the field, in the ambulance, and in the Emergency Department. Its secondary ability (with the adaptor) to meet suctioning needs other than the removal of vomitus, although not the first choice, is useful because it allows the V-VAC to *serve as a back-up unit* for such other uses in the event that the powered unit fails. It also allows the V-VAC to be the **best** choice—providing for both the removal of vomitus and other suction needs—in cross-field or wilderness situations when practical considerations necessitate the carrying of only a single small manually powered lightweight unit for any suction need.

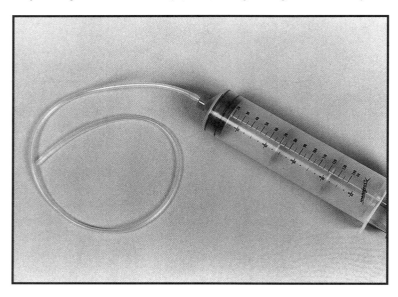

When a bulb syringe or barrel-type syringe is used to produce manual suction, the bulb or barrel acts as both the "pump" and the collection container simultaneously. Since it has a limited capacity for

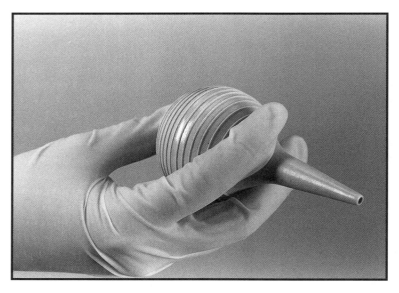

suctioned material (without valves or a separate container in which to store the material drawn into it) after each "draft" to suction material into it has been completed, the tip must be removed from the patient's mouth or nose and the bulb or barrel depressed to empty the syringe's contents before reinserting it. In the case of a barrel syringe this resets it so that the plunger is all the way into the barrel,

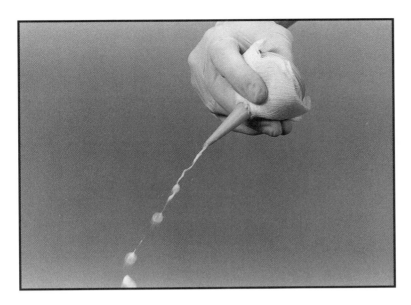

ready to be withdrawn again to produce suction once it has been reinserted. In the case of a bulb syringe, once it has been emptied by repeatedly squeezing it with the tip outside of the patient's nose and mouth, the bulb is fully depressed (squeezed) to prime it and is then inserted again while it is held depressed. When it is properly reinserted in place the bulb is released and the suction vacuum is produced.

Before suctioning, the patient should be hyperventilated. Suctioning should not take longer than five to ten seconds except to remove copious amounts of vomitus to avoid aspiration. High-flow suction will remove highly oxygenated air from the pharynx as well as fluids and foreign matter, and replace it with comparatively low oxygen concentration air from the outside environment. During suctioning, ventilation of the alveoli is minimal or may be totally interrupted. As well as lowering the oxygen level in the pharynx, suctioning interrupts the EMT's provided ventilations and, for any reason, ventilation should never be interrupted for more than thirty seconds at most.

Although many specialized types of suction catheters and tips exist, two are most common in prehospital care. The first is a soft catheter with a point on the proximal end, often called a French catheter, which is designed primarily for nasal suctioning and for suctioning through an ET tube. As previously noted, one with a "whistle stop" added should be used.

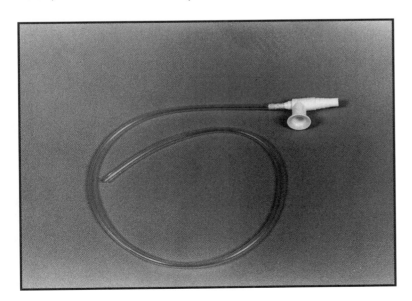

The second common type of prehospital suction catheter is called a "tonsil-tip" or Yankauer tip, and is designed for the rapid evacuation of large amounts of vomitus, blood, and debris from the mouth and pharynx to avoid aspiration.

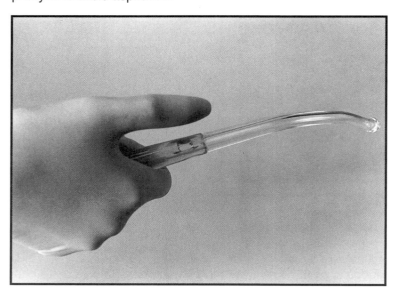

The soft catheter is of little use for suctioning copious quantities of foreign materials, blood, or vomit out of the mouth, nose, and pharynx, or for effectively dealing with large-sized particles. In most cases where prehospital suctioning is indicated, the "tonsil-tip" or Yankauer tip is probably the device of choice except in the case of vomitus when a V-VAC is also available. Allowing an airway to remain blocked while trying to suction large particles or large quantities of vomit or blood is tantamount to suffocating the patient. Using a small diameter flexible French catheter also invites aspiraton of gastric contents into the patient's lungs. This can be catastrophic, as the tremendously acidic materials from the digestive system permanently destroy alveoli and other lung tissue necessary for the respiratory process.

The major hazards of suctioning are hypoxia (usually caused by prolonged suctioning), delay in ventilating, precipitating dysrhythmias through vagal stimulation, and inducing vomiting and aspiration when the gag reflex is present. The EMT must be aware of these problems and be ready to correct them.

The EMT must approach suctioning with consideration for the patient's condition. On occasion the patient will be conscious and able to assist in the process, while in most circumstances the patient will be unresponsive or have such a lowered level of consciousness that he has *NO* control of his airway. Each situation will dictate different approaches and techniques for the EMT, just as the severity of the problem will prescribe what type of equipment is needed and how much suctioning must be performed. Regardless of the need for suctioning, the EMT must always be mindful of the need for *ventilation* as well—no suctioning attempt should last more than five seconds, and every suctioning attempt should be followed by at least twenty seconds of breathing or hyperventilation before more suctioning is performed.

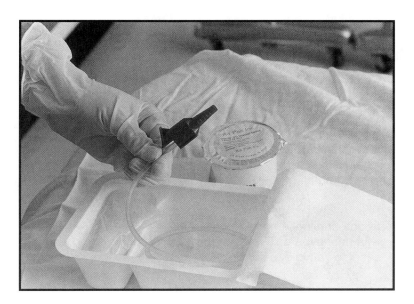

Although the items necessary beyond the suction unit itself can be separately assembled, most hospitals utilize disposable suction kits which contain all of the various items that are needed or helpful when suctioning a patient. These may include lubricant for nasal suctioning and a rinsing bowl or container for cleaning the catheter tip between suctioning attempts. Either sterile water or Normal Saline can be used.

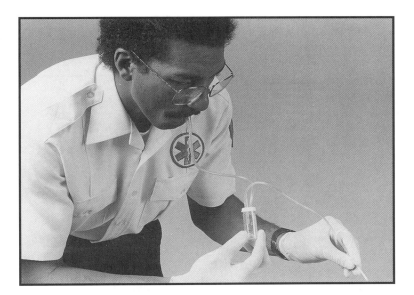

The DeLee suction trap shown here was previously widely used for suctioning newborns and neonates. With the flexible suction tip inserted into the baby's mouth or nose, the operator orally sucked on the other tube, creating a vacuum inside the cannister which drew secretions into the device. The potential for the EMT to aspirate highly contagious bodily fluids into his own mouth has lead to the virtual elimination of this device in the face of current infection control practices. This photo is included here to point out the hazard of this device, rather than to illustrate or recommend its use.

NASAL SUCTIONING

1. A soft flexible suction catheter is indicated for nasal suctioning. After donning gloves and other appropriate protective apparel, connect the catheter to the suction tube. Check that suction is present by applying the catheter tip to the palm of one hand while covering the whistle-stop port. You should be able to feel the suction against your gloved hand.

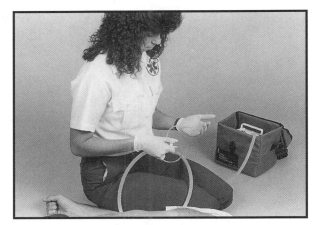

2. Determine the correct length of the catheter by holding it against the patient's face. Measure from the tip of the patient's nose to the tip of his ear lobe, and mark this length by grasping the tube between your fingers at the measured point. This is an easy way to know when you have inserted the catheter deeply enough. Examine both nostrils and select the one which appears largest and is not deviated or deformed.

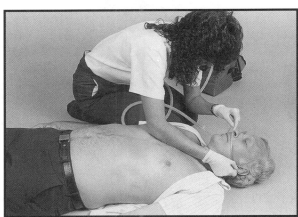

3. Lubricate the end of the catheter and begin inserting it into the select nostril. Keep the whistle-stop port open to avoid creating any suction while the catheter is being inserted. Use a gently rotating twist on the catheter as you insert it, and do not force the catheter if you encounter resistance. Instead, withdraw the catheter slightly, rotate, and attempt to continue insertion. If this cannot be accomplished, attempt insertion in the other nostril.

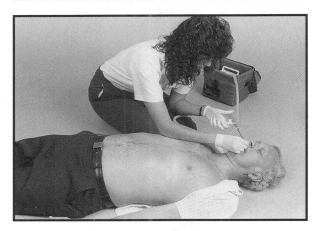

4. When the catheter has been inserted to the pre-determined depth, cover the whistle-stop opening with your thumb or finger. This causes a vacuum to be created at the distal end of the catheter and you should begin to see fluids and other material moving up the catheter.

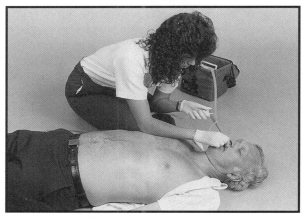

5. With the whistle-stop port still covered, begin to withdraw the catheter. Continue to gently rotate the catheter between your fingers as you withdraw it. Because suctioning evacuates oxygen from the patient's lungs as well as fluids and other materials, it is essential that each application of vacuum not be maintained for more than five seconds, and that the patient be allowed to breathe or be ventilated for 15 to 30 seconds after each suctioning attempt before the suction is again imposed.

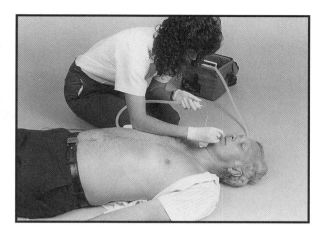

6. Clean out the catheter, flushing it by inserting the patient end into a container of sterile water or saline and, by covering the "whistle stop," apply the vacuum to draw the clean liquid through the tube.

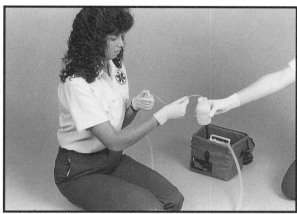

ORAL SUCTIONING

1. A soft flexible suction catheter can also be used for oral suctioning. After donning gloves and other appropriate protective apparel, connect the catheter to the suction tube. Check that suction is present by applying the catheter tip to the palm of one hand while covering the whistle-stop port. Determine the correct length of the catheter by holding it against the patient's face. Measure from the edge of the patient's mouth to the tip of his ear lobe, and mark this length by grasping the tube between your fingers at the measured point.

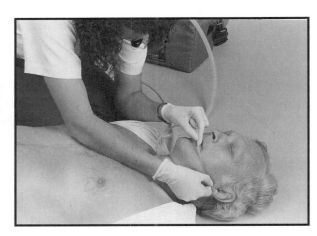

2. Insert the catheter into the patient's mouth along the medial plane and cover the whistle stop port to create a suction vacuum.

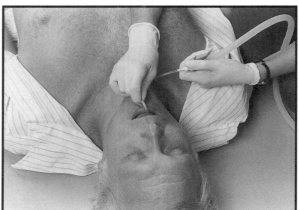

3. While applying the suction, move the catheter around inside the mouth in order to best locate any materials to be removed. After no more than 5–10 seconds, and while still applying suction, withdraw the catheter from the patient's mouth.

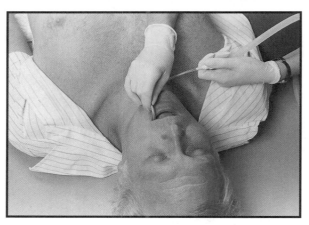

4. Each time that the catheter is removed from the patient's mouth it should be flushed with sterile water or saline to remove any material that could clog the suction ports. Insert the catheter into the rinsing fluid and cover the whistle stop port to draw the fluid through the catheter.

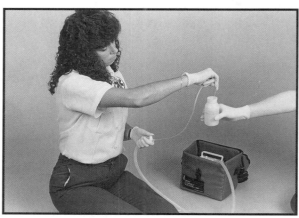

5. If the vomitus or other material to be removed with the use of a standard fixed or portable suction unit is particularly voluminous, or consists of some solid pieces, a "tonsil tip" or Yankauer suction tip having a greater capacity (due to larger openings) should be used rather than a soft flexible catheter. These also have a whistle stop port which must be covered to create a vacuum. Like the catheter, the tonsil tip device should be moved about inside the mouth to reach all of the material to be removed. When a patient who is supine regurgitates, the patient (or the patient and backboard) should be placed on his side immediately, and then his mouth should be suctioned, to avoid aspiration.

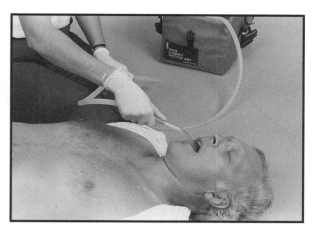

6. Tonsil tip devices also need to be rinsed between suction attempts. Insert the tip into the sterile water or saline and cover the whistle stop port to create a vacuum, drawing the rinsing fluid through the tip.

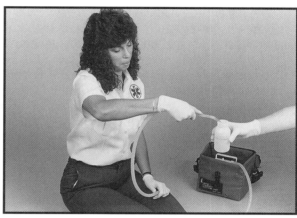

VOMITUS EXTRACTION (V-VAC® Suction Unit)

The V-VAC suction device is more appropriately termed a "vomitus extractor" due to its ability to suction a large volume of vomitus including considerable partially digested pieces of food. The V-VAC allows more rapid suctioning of vomitus, including solids, than conventional suction units and, due to the frequent need for this in the field, is recommended as an additional piece of equipment. The V-VAC is hand-powered and draws material through the large bore tip which is part of the replaceable single-use cannister when the operator squeezes the sliding handle.

1. The patient should be placed in a "jowl down" position on his side. In immobilized trauma patients in whom spinal trauma is also a concern, the patient and backboard should be turned onto the side as a unit. The EMT should be positioned so as to allow full easy access to the patient's face and mouth.

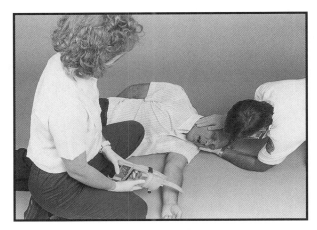

2. Insert the V-VAC into the patient's mouth and create the vacuum by repeatedly squeezing the handle. It is important that the flip-open exhaust valve on the collection cannister be maintained in the upright position during suctioning so that it does not inadvertently pop open during use.

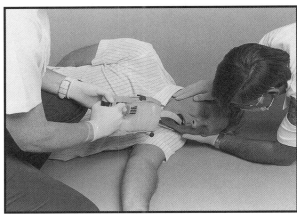

3. When suctioning is completed or if the collection cannister should become full, the cannister is removed and replaced with a new empty cannister. The full cannister should be handled in accordance with biological hazard procedures, however in overdose and poisoning cases there may be value in preserving the cannister so that it can be examined and analyzed at the hospital.

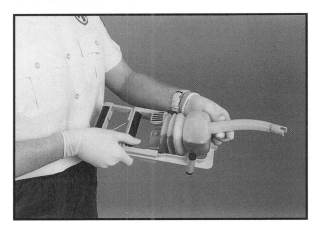

HAND OPERATED PORTABLE SUCTION (Res-Q-Vac® Suction Unit)

The Res-Q-Vac suction unit is a small self-contained manually operated suction unit that, due to its reliable manual operation, light weight, and extremely small storage size, has proven to be extremely useful in cross-field and wilderness medical packs where, due to considerations of space and weight, portable powered units have often been omitted in the past. Although the V-VAC affords more flexibility, the Res-Q-Vac's ability to rapidly empty the cannister without the need for a replacement cannister provides a space advantage. It—as with the V-VAC—is also a useful adjunct for Mass Casualty situations or as a "stand-by" unit for power failure situations when a shortage of powered units occurs.

1. The Res-Q-Vac suction unit consists of a pistol-grip type handle assembly to which is attached a single-use collection cannister and suction tip. The device uses different sized cannisters for adults and pediatric patients, and can accommodate suction tips ranging from very small flexible tubes to Yankauer tips.

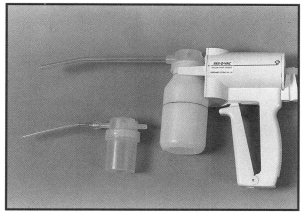

2. The unit is assembled by attaching the selected collection cannister with its permanently connected suction tip to the pistol-grip handle. When the pediatric cannister is used it attaches directly to the handle, while an adaptor yoke is used for the larger adult cannister. The handle and yoke can be cleaned and disinfected between patients. The cannister (with tip) is an expendable single-patient use item.

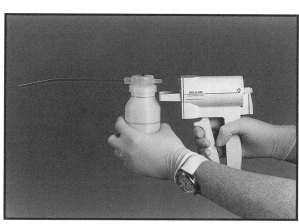

3. As with other hand-held suction devices the EMT performing the suctioning should be positioned for best access to the patient's mouth and nose. The suction tip should be inserted into the patient's mouth and moved about while suction is applied to remove the largest amount of material. Between suctioning attempts the tip can be cleared by applying suction while inserting the tip into a sterile water or saline rinse solution.

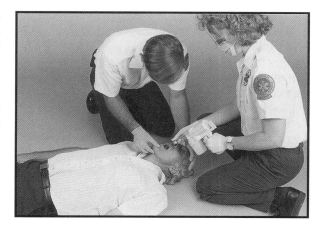

SUCTIONING AN ENDOTRACHEAL TUBE

Endotracheal tubes, although providing a protected airway from gastric contents, may require suctioning to remove fluids accumulating in the ET tube, trachea, or mainstem bronchi. Suctioning through an ET tube should only be performed by (or under the supervision of) EMTs qualified in endotracheal intubation.

1. Begin the process of suctioning the patient through an in-place endotracheal tube by assuring ventilation while selecting and measuring a flexible suction catheter. Establish the length of the suction catheter by rough approximation or by actually comparing it to the length of another ET tube of the same size. When suctioning through a pediatric sized ET tube, direct comparison is recommended since the length of such tubes vary much more than do adult tubes.

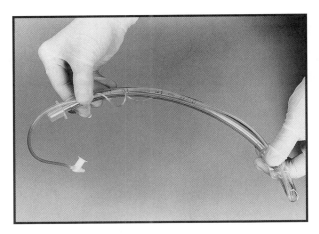

2. Using the thumb and index finger of one hand to mark the maximum insertion length of the catheter, feed the catheter into the ET tube with the other hand. The whistle stop port is open during this time and suction is not being applied. Insertion should be accomplished as promptly as possible—remember, *the patient is not being ventilated while you are doing this!*

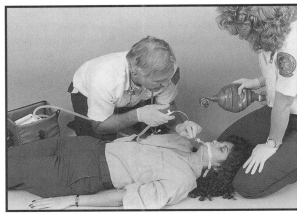

3. As soon as the catheter has been inserted to the proper depth, cover the whistle stop port with the thumb or first finger of the hand that was used to insert the tube. This allows you to maintain the length marker with the other hand. With the "whistle stop" occluded and suction applied, withdraw the catheter from the ET tube slowly and steadily until it is fully removed. Immediately reinstitute ventilations for at least twenty seconds while flushing the suction catheter with sterile water or saline before again suctioning the patient.

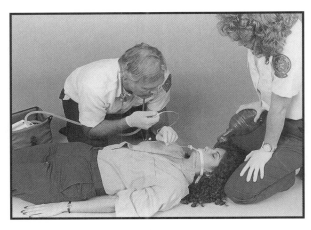

INFANT SUCTIONING WITH RUBBER BULB SYRINGE

Due to their small delicate tissues, except when specially trained neonatal or infant care personnel are available with specialized equipment, newborn and infant suctioning of the mouth and nose should only be performed using a rubber bulb syringe. Use of other suction devices in such patients by the EMT is considered dangerous and is *NOT* recommended.

1. For neonates and infants, the preferred suction device for oral and nasal suctioning is a rubber bulb syringe. Two important early steps are key to successful use of this device: first, cut a hole in the center of a 4x4 gauze pad and insert the tip of the bulb syringe through the hole. This allows a firm grip on the otherwise smooth surface of the bulb which will become very slippery when it gets wet. Next, squeeze the bulb fully *BEFORE* inserting it into the baby's nostril. This expels air from the bulb and allows suction to occur when the bulb refills.

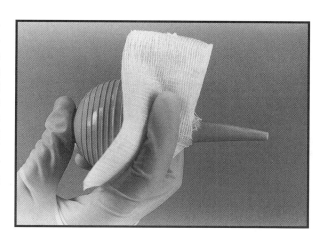

2. Now insert the tip of the bulb syringe into one of the child's nostrils and release the bulb. This creates a suction which not only refills the bulb with air but also draws fluids and foreign materials from the nostril and nasal pharynx into the bulb. Be very careful to not again squeeze the bulb while the tip is in the baby's nostril, as this would expel the bulb's contents back into the baby's nose! *The syringe bulb must never, while inserted in the patient, be squeezed*—this will eject previously suctioned material back into the infant's mouth with considerable pressure.

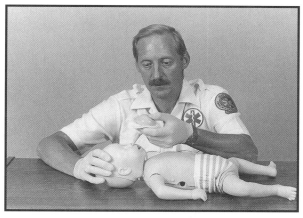

3. Withdraw the syringe tip from the baby's nostril, point it away from the child and again squeeze the bulb completely several times. This will expel the fluids and material from the bulb and ready it for the next suctioning attempt. If time allows beforehand, a suitable container should be provided into which the suctioned fluids and material can be expelled. Keep the bulb squeezed after expelling the material, in preparation for the next suctioning attempt.

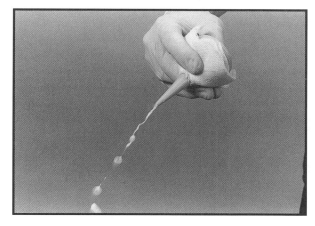

4. Now insert the tip of the bulb syringe into the other nostril and again release the bulb to create a vacuum and remove fluids and other materials from the baby's nose.

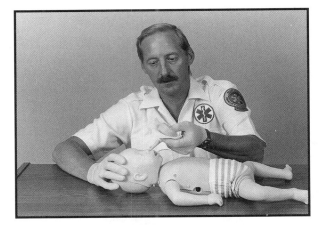

5. Withdraw the syringe tip from the baby's nostril, point it away from the child and again squeeze the bulb completely several times to expel the fluids and other materials from the bulb.

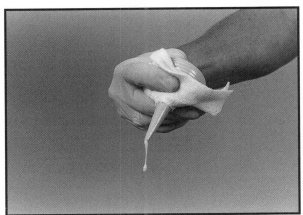

6. With the bulb still depressed, insert the syringe tip into the baby's mouth and release the bulb to suction material from the oral cavity. Withdraw the bulb syringe from the mouth and again expel the collected material into a cannister by squeezing the bulb. Repeat the suctioning process as needed until the baby is able to breathe clearly without any signs of upper airway obstruction caused by fluids or material in the oral or nasal cavities.

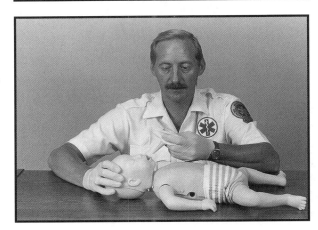

ALS

ETI SUMMARY SKILL SHEET
Esophageal Obturator Airway (EOA)®

1. TAKE/maintain appropriate UNIVERSAL PRECAUTIONS.

2. CONFIRM that the patient is being VENTILATED PROPERLY and with a high oxygen concentration.

3. AUSCULTATE bilateral BREATH SOUNDS to establish a baseline.

4. DIRECT that patient be HYPERVENTILATED.

5. CONNECT EOA TUBE to EOA MASK.

6. CHECK MASK cuff INFLATION.

7. CHECK that SUCTION PORT on mask is CLOSED.

8. CHECK distal TUBE CUFF for leaks. Leave 35ml syringe attached to one-way valve.

9. LUBRICATE distal end of TUBE.

10. DIRECT VENTILATOR TO MOVE to side of patient's head and POSITION YOURSELF above patient.

11. HOLD EOA by TUBE and direct STOP of VENTILATIONS.

12. REMOVE oropharyngeal AIRWAY and PERFORM TONGUE-JAW LIFT.

13. MOVE patient's HEAD INTO SLIGHT FLEXION unless spine trauma is suspected. If spine trauma is suspected, direct maintenance of neutral in-line immobilization.

14. INSERT EOA tube into patient's mouth along mid-line.

15. ADVANCE TUBE until mask is seated firmly on patient's face.

16. DIRECT RESUMPTION OF VENTILATIONS with BVM or demand valve.

17. OBSERVE for CHEST RISE and AUSCULTATE CHEST for bilateral breath sounds with each ventilation to confirm proper tube placement.

18. IF PROPER PLACEMENT is NOT CONFIRMED, immediately REMOVE the EOA and direct RESUMPTION OF HYPERVENTILATION with a manual airway technique. After 30 seconds or more, re-attempt insertion of EOA.

19. If PROPER PLACEMENT in the esophagus is CONFIRMED by proper ventilation of the lungs, INFLATE the distal TUBE CUFF with the 35ml syringe.

20. REMOVE SYRINGE from the one-way valve after inflating cuff.

21. AUSCULTATE over MID-LUNG FIELDS to re-confirm presence of bilateral breath sounds and AUSCULTATE over the EPIGASTRIUM to confirm the ***absence*** of air sounds with ventilations.

22. SUCTION oral cavity as necessary.

ALS

ETI SUMMARY SKILL SHEET
Esophageal Gastric Tube Airway (EGTA)®

1. TAKE/maintain appropriate UNIVERSAL PRECAUTIONS.

2. CONFIRM that patient is being VENTILATED PROPERLY and with a high oxygen concentration.

3. AUSCULTATE bilateral BREATH SOUNDS to establish a baseline.

4. DIRECT that patient be HYPERVENTILATED.

5. CONNECT EGTA TUBE to EGTA MASK.

6. CHECK MASK cuff INFLATION.

7. CHECK that SUCTION PORT on mask is CLOSED.

8. CHECK distal TUBE CUFF for leaks. Leave 35ml syringe attached to one-way valve.

9. LUBRICATE distal end of TUBE.

10. DIRECT VENTILATOR TO MOVE to side of patient's head and POSITION YOURSELF above patient.

11. HOLD EGTA by TUBE and direct STOP of VENTILATIONS.

12. REMOVE oropharyngeal AIRWAY and PERFORM TONGUE-JAW LIFT.

13. MOVE patient's HEAD INTO SLIGHT FLEXION unless spine trauma is suspected. If spine trauma is suspected, direct maintenance of neutral in-line immobilization.

14. INSERT EGTA tube into patient's mouth along mid-line.

15. ADVANCE TUBE until mask is seated firmly on patient's face.

16. DIRECT RESUMPTION OF VENTILATIONS with BVM or demand valve through port marked "Ventilate Here."

17. OBSERVE for CHEST RISE and AUSCULTATE CHEST for bilateral breath sounds to confirm proper tube placement.

18. IF PROPER PLACEMENT is NOT CONFIRMED, immediately REMOVE the EGTA and DIRECT RESUMPTION of HYPERVENTILATION with a manual airway technique. After 30 seconds or more, re-attempt insertion of EGTA.

19. If PROPER PLACEMENT in the esophagus is CONFIRMED by proper ventilation of the lungs, INFLATE the distal TUBE CUFF with the 35ml syringe.

20. REMOVE SYRINGE from one-way valve after inflating cuff.

21. AUSCULTATE MID-LUNG FIELDS to re-confirm presence of bilateral breath sounds and AUSCULTATE over the EPIGASTRIUM to confirm ***absence*** of air sounds with ventilations.

22. After confirming proper placement and with ventilations underway, INSERT GASTRIC SUCTION TUBE through valve in proximal opening on EGTA tube.

23. ADVANCE GASTRIC TUBE until its tip is approximately 6" past the distal end of the EGTA tube.

24. If your protocol allows, use suction to evacuate fluid stomach contents through gastric tube.

25. PERIODICALLY RE-CHECK CHEST RISE and AUSCULTATE over the MID-LUNG FIELDS and over the EPIGASTRIUM with delivered breaths to verify continued proper placement and ventilation of the lungs.

26. SUCTION the oral cavity as necessary.

ALS

ETI SUMMARY SKILL SHEET
Esophageal Tracheal Double-Lumen Airway (Combitube®)

1. TAKE/maintain appropriate UNIVERSAL PRECAUTIONS.

2. CONFIRM that the patient is being PROPERLY VENTILATED with a high oxygen concentration.

3. AUSCULTATE bilateral BREATH SOUNDS to establish a baseline.

4. DIRECT that patient be HYPERVENTILATED.

5. VERIFY that the BLUE-TIPPED 140ml SYRINGE HAS at least 100ml of air drawn up, and CONNECT it TO the BLUE ONE-WAY VALVE and pilot balloon marked tube "No. 1."

6. VERIFY that the WHITE-TIPPED 20ml SYRINGE HAS at least 15ml of air drawn up, and CONNECT it TO the WHITE ONE-WAY VALVE and pilot balloon marked tube "No. 2."

7. LUBRICATE the distal end of the tube WITHOUT OCCLUDING the distal OPENINGS.

8. DIRECT VENTILATOR TO MOVE to side of patient's head and POSITION YOURSELF above the patient. HOLD the COMBITUBE by its tube.

9. Direct STOP of VENTILATIONS.

10. REMOVE oropharyngeal AIRWAY and PERFORM TONGUE-JAW LIFT.

11. SLIGHTLY EXTEND the PATIENT'S HEAD unless spine trauma is suspected. If spine trauma is suspected, direct maintenance of neutral in-line immobilization.

12. INSERT TUBE into patient's mouth along mid-line.

13. ADVANCE TUBE until the printed ring on the tube is at the level of the patient's teeth.

14. INJECT 100ml of AIR FROM the large BLUE-TIPPED SYRINGE into the blue one-way valve to inflate the large pharyngeal cuff.

15. REMOVE the 140ml SYRINGE from the BLUE ONE-WAY VALVE.

16. CHECK for proper distension of the BLUE PILOT BALLOON.

17. INJECT 15ml of AIR INTO the WHITE ONE-WAY VALVE from the small white-tipped syringe to inflate the distal tube cuff.

18. REMOVE the 20ml SYRINGE from the WHITE ONE-WAY VALVE.

19. CHECK for proper distension of the WHITE PILOT BALLOON.

20. ATTACH the BVM or demand valve to the blue tube and DIRECT RESUMPTION OF VENTILATION.

21. OBSERVE for CHEST RISE with each ventilation and AUSCULTATE over the EPIGASTRIUM to confirm *absence* of air sounds with ventilations.

22. IF CHEST RISE is *NOT* seen and AIR SOUNDS *ARE* heard over the EPIGASTRIUM, immediately DISCONNECT the BVM or demand valve FROM the BLUE TUBE and CONNECT IT TO the clear "No. 2" TUBE.

23. RESUME VENTILATIONS THROUGH the clear "NO. 2" tube and again OBSERVE for CHEST RISE with each ventilation and AUSCULTATE over the EPIGASTRIUM to confirm *absence* of air sounds with ventilations.

24. WHEN CHEST RISE IS SEEN and AIR SOUNDS *ARE NOT* HEARD over the EPIGASTRIUM (regardless of which tube is being used), proper VENTILATION of the lungs must still be CONFIRMED by AUSCULTATING over the MID-LUNG FIELDS for the presence of breath sounds with delivered ventilations.

25. PERIODICALLY RE-CHECK for continued proper distention of BOTH PILOT BALLOONS.

26. PERIODICALLY RE-CHECK by bilateral CHEST AUSCULTATION for continued proper ventilation of the lungs.

27. IF effective VENTILATION *THROUGH the BLUE "NO. 1" TUBE* was confirmed, PASS the Combitube's SOFT GASTRIC SUCTION CATHETER through the clear "No. 2" tube TO ALLOW SUCTIONING of gastric fluids and air from the patient's esophagus and stomach.

ALS

ETI SUMMARY SKILL SHEET
Pharyngeal Tracheal Lumen Airway (PTL®)

1. TAKE/maintain appropriate UNIVERSAL PRECAUTIONS.

2. CONFIRM that the patient is being VENTILATED PROPERLY and with a high oxygen concentration.

3. AUSCULTATE bilateral BREATH SOUNDS to establish a baseline.

4. Close the relief port with the small white cap, open the slide clamp, and blow air into the inflation valve to CHECK the PROXIMAL AND DISTAL CUFFS for proper operation.

5. Remove the small white cap and DEFLATE BOTH CUFFS FULLY. Replace the white cap on the relief port.

6. DIRECT that patient be HYPERVENTILATED.

7. LUBRICATE distal end of the long TUBE.

8. DIRECT VENTILATOR TO MOVE to side of patient's head and POSITION YOURSELF above patient.

9. HOLD the PTL TUBE below the flange and direct STOP of VENTILATIONS.

10. REMOVE oropharyngeal AIRWAY and PERFORM TONGUE-JAW LIFT.

11. SLIGHTLY EXTEND the PATIENT'S HEAD unless spine trauma is suspected. If spine trauma is suspected, direct maintenance of neutral in-line immobilization.

12. INSERT PTL TUBE into patient's mouth along mid-line.

13. ADVANCE TUBE until flange rests against patient's teeth.

14. LOOP white STRAP AROUND patient's HEAD AND SECURE IT in place.

15. BLOW INTO TUBE NO. 1 to inflate the proximal and distal cuffs. Use pilot balloon distention to gauge degree of inflation.

16. DIRECT RESUMPTION of VENTILATIONS with BVM or demand valve attached to SHORT GREEN NO. 2 TUBE.

17. OBSERVE for CHEST RISE with each delivered breath and AUSCULTATE over EPIGASTRIUM for the *absence* of air sounds to confirm proper tube placement.

18. IF CHEST RISE is *NOT* SEEN and AIR SOUNDS *ARE* HEARD over the EPIGASTRIUM, immediately DISCONNECT the BVM or demand valve FROM the GREEN NO. 2 TUBE, REMOVE the STYLET FROM TUBE NO. 3, and CONNECT the BVM or demand valve TO TUBE NO. 3.

19. RESUME VENTILATIONS THROUGH TUBE NO. 3 and again OBSERVE for CHEST RISE with each ventilation AND AUSCULTATE OVER THE EPIGASTRIUM to confirm *absence* of air sounds with ventilations.

20. REGARDLESS OF THROUGH WHICH TUBE VENTILATIONS ARE BEING DELIVERED, when proper ventilation of the lungs is indicated by observed chest rise and the absence of air sounds at the epigastrium when breaths are delivered, CONFIRM that AIR IS PASSING INTO THE LUNGS BY AUSCULTATING over the MID-LUNG FIELDS.

21. IF proper VENTILATION of the lungs is being PERFORMED THROUGH TUBE NO. 2, REMOVE the STYLET FROM TUBE NO. 3 and PASS a soft GASTRIC SUCTION TUBE THROUGH TUBE NO. 3 to allow suctioning of gastruc fluids and air from the patient's esophagus and stomach.

22. PERIODICALLY RE-CHECK by bilateral CHEST AUSCULTATION for continued proper ventilation of the lungs. Also RE-CHECK for continued PROPER DISTENTION of the PILOT BULB, make sure that the WHITE HEAD STRAP remains SECURE, and assure that the PLASTIC FLANGE REMAINS AT the LEVEL OF the patient's TEETH.

ALS

ETI SUMMARY SKILL SHEET
Visualized Orotracheal Intubation

1. TAKE/maintain appropriate UNIVERSAL PRECAUTIONS.

2. CONFIRM that the patient is being VENTIALTED PROPERLY and with a high oxygen concentration.

3. AUSCULTATE bilateral BREATH SOUNDS to establish a baseline.

4. SELECT correct size ET TUBE.

5. ATTACH 10–20cc SYRINGE TO one-way valve on filler tube and inject 10cc of air to inflate distal TUBE CUFF and CHECK it FOR LEAKS. Confirm tautness of pilot bulb.

6. WITHDRAW AIR FROM CUFF with syringe and LEAVE SYRINGE securely ATTACHED to one-way valve. Pilot bulb should be flat.

7. SELECT appropriate laryngoscope BLADE and ATTACH it TO HANDLE. CHECK that LIGHT BULB is tightly SECURED and that it ILLUMINATES when blade is snapped into position.

8. INSERT STYLET into ET tube until distal end of stylet is just short of the ET tube's distal opening, and bend proximal end of stylet over the proximal end of ET tube to keep it from advancing further through the tube.

9. SHAPE the ET TUBE/STYLET combination appropriately to facilitate passage into the trachea.

10. UNLESS SPINE TRAUMA is suspected, HYPEREXTEND the PATIENT'S HEAD and POSITION IT IN the "FORWARD SNIFFING POSITION." If spine trauma is suspected, direct that the head be maintained in the neutral in-line position. Appropriate padding under the patient's head can be helpful in maintaining the desired alignment.

11. DIRECT that patient be HYPERVENTILATED.

12. LUBRICATE distal end of the ET TUBE.

13. DIRECT VENTILATOR TO MOVE to side of patient's head and POSITION YOURSELF above patient. If spine trauma is suspected, assume one of the postures that permit you to work while still maintaining the neutral alignment of the patient's head and spine.

14. HOLD the laryngoscope HANDLE and blade IN your LEFT HAND. DIRECT that VENTILATIONS BE STOPPED and with your right hand REMOVE the oropharyngeal AIRWAY and PERFORM a TONGUE-JAW LIFT.

15. INSERT laryngoscope BLADE into right side of patient's mouth and gently advance blade to correct depth while sweeping blade to the left and observing landmarks.

16. DIRECT assisting EMT to apply ANTERIOR-TO-POSTERIOR PRESSURE ON the patient's LARYNX.

17. EXTEND your LEFT ARM to LIFT against patient's tongue and jaw with LARYNGOSCOPE.

18. WHEN VOCAL CORDS are VISUALIZED, BEGIN INSERTION of ET TUBE into patient's mouth.

19. ADVANCE TUBE between the vocal cords and slightly beyond. REMOVE STYLET.

20. INFLATE distal CUFF by injecting 10cc of air through filler tube. Remove syringe from one-way valve. Throughout, MAINTAIN firm GRASP ON proximal end of TUBE where it exits the patient's mouth.

21. DIRECT RESUMPTION of VENTILATIONS with BVM or demand valve connected to proximal end of ET tube. Direct HYPERVENTILATION.

22. OBSERVE for CHEST RISE with each delivered breath and AUSCULTATE OVER THE EPIGASTRIUM for *absence* of air sounds with ventilations.

23. IF CHEST RISE is **NOT** SEEN and if AIR SOUNDS **ARE HEARD** upon auscultation over the EPIGASTRIUM with each breath, immediately stop ventilations and disconnect the BVM or demand valve from the proximal end of the tube. The tube may either be bent over outside the patient's mouth and mask ventilations resumed, or the tube may be removed by first deflating the distal cuff by withdrawing air through the filler tube with the 10cc syringe. In either case, MASK VENTILATIONS MUST BE IMMEDIATELY RESUMED.

24. AFTER at least THIRTY SECONDS OF VENTILATION, RE-ATTEMPT to INTUBATE the patient. If the tube has been left in place (in the esophagus), move the first tube to the left side of the patient's mouth, again visualizing for the vocal cords, **and using a second ET tube to intubate the patient.**

25. Again OBSERVE for CHEST RISE with each delivered breath and AUSCULTATE over the EPIGASTRIUM for *absence* of air sounds with ventilations.

26. IF CHEST RISE IS SEEN and AIR SOUNDS **ARE NOT HEARD** upon AUSCULTATION over the EPIGASTRIUM with each breath, CONFIRM proper VENTILATION of the lungs by AUSCULTATING over the MID-LUNG FIELDS for the **presence** of air sounds with each delivered breath.

27. IF baseline breath sounds were bilaterally equal but BREATH SOUNDS are now HEARD ONLY ON RIGHT side, WITHDRAW ET TUBE 1–2cm and RE-AUSCULTATE. Continue this process until equal bilateral sounds are again heard.

28. ONCE PROPER VENTILATION of the lungs has been CONFIRMED by chest auscultation, SECURE ET TUBE in place with tape wrapped around the head/neck or with a commerical ET tube holder.

29. PERIODICALLY RE-CONFIRM adequate VENTILATION by observing for CHEST RISE and AUSCULTATING over the MID-LUNG FIELDS for bilateral breath sounds.

30. DISPOSE of any SINGLE-USE ITEMS and properly CLEAN REUSABLE EQUIPMENT according to infection control guidelines.

ALS

ETI SUMMARY SKILL SHEET
Blind Nasotracheal Intubation

1. TAKE/maintain appropriate UNIVERSAL PRECAUTIONS.

2. CONFIRM that the patient is being provided with a high FiO$_2$ and that ADEQUATE spontaneous VENTILATION EXISTS or is provided by assisted ventilation.

3. AUSCULTATE bilateral BREATH SOUNDS to establish a baseline.

4. Examine nostrils and SELECT correct size ET TUBE.

5. ATTACH 10–20cc SYRINGE to one-way valve on filler tube and inject 10cc of air to INFLATE DISTAL TUBE CUFF and CHECK it FOR LEAKS. Confirm tautness of pilot bulb.

6. WITHDRAW AIR FROM CUFF with syringe and LEAVE SYRINGE securely ATTACHED to one-way valve. Pilot bulb should be flat.

7. LUBRICATE distal end and cuff of the ET tube.

8. POSITION YOURSELF at the patient's upper torso, turned slightly toward the patient's face.

9. A SECOND EMT above the patient's head SHOULD HOLD THE HEAD IN EXTENSION, tilted to the FORWARD SNIFFING POSITION unless spinal trauma is suspected. If spinal trauma is suspected, the head and neck should be immobilized in the neutral in-line position.

10. HOLD the ET TUBE between the thumb and first two fingers, with the distal tip pointing posteriorly into the selected nostril.

11. ADVANCE the TUBE INTO the NOSTRIL, guiding it in an anterior-to-posterior direction. A slight back-and-forth rotation of the tube may be helpful.

12. IF the patient is NOT CONSCIOUS the ASSISTING EMT should PERFORM a JAW THRUST while the tube is being advanced through the nose and pharynx.

13. As the tube is advanced, LISTEN closely FOR BREATH SOUNDS AT THE PROXIMAL END of the tube AND SLIGHTLY ROTATE THE TUBE back and forth WHILE LISTENING. WHEN the BREATH SOUNDS ARE LOUDEST AND the GREATEST MISTING of the tube OCCURS with exhalation, STOP rotating.

14. IF the patient is CONSCIOUS, have him take a deep breath and gently ADVANCE the TUBE FURTHER WHILE he is INHALING. IF the patient is NOT CONSCIOUS, try to TIME ADVANCING the TUBE WITH one of the patient's INHALATIONS.

15. ADVANCE the TUBE to the CORRECT DEPTH to ensure that the DISTAL CUFF is BEYOND the VOCAL CORDS. INFLATE the CUFF with the syringe and REMOVE the SYRINGE from the one-way valve.

16. CHECK that MISTING CONTINUES and WHETHER AIR can be FELT EXITING the proximal end of the ET TUBE, OR from the MOUTH AND NOSE around the tube, or both. If air movement is detected both through the tube and also from around the outside of the tube, the distal cuff needs additional inflation.

17. IF AIR MOVEMENT is detected ONLY AROUND the OUTSIDE OF THE TUBE and NOT THROUGH the PROXIMAL END, IMMEDIATELY DEFLATE the distal CUFF and WITHDRAW the TUBE from the esophagus (it may remain in the nose). Have the patient breathe a high FiO2 for a few moments, then repeat the steps to nasally intubate the trachea.

18. IF AIR MOVEMENT IS DETECTED ONLY THROUGH the proximal END OF the ET TUBE, further CONFIRM GOOD pulmonary VENTILATION by OBSERVING for CHEST RISE and by AUSCULTATING GOOD BILATERAL BREATH SOUNDS over the mid-lung fields.

19. IF baseline breath sounds were bilaterally equal but BREATH SOUNDS ARE NOW HEARD ONLY ON RIGHT SIDE, WITHDRAW the ET TUBE 1–2cm AND RE-AUSCULTATE. Continue this process until equal bilateral sounds are again heard.

20. ONCE PROPER VENTILATION of the lungs HAS BEEN CONFIRMED by chest auscultation, SECURE ET TUBE in place with tape wrapped around the head/neck or with a commercial ET tube holder.

21. IF the breathing PATIENT CANNOT PROVIDE SUFFICIENT AIR EXCHANGE for himself, CONNECT a BVM (with collector and high-flow O2) or demand valve to the proximal end of the ET tube and PROVIDE ASSISTED VENTILATIONS appropriate to the patient's needs.

22. PERIODICALLY RE-CONFIRM ADEQUATE VENTILATION by observing for CHEST RISE and AUSCULTATING over the MID-LUNG FIELDS for bilateral breath sounds.

23. IF VENTILATIONS ARE BEING ASSISTED, PERIODICALLY DISCONTINUE ASSISTED VENTILATIONS and disconnect the BVM or demand valve to DETERMINE IF CONTINUED ASSISTED OR PROVIDED VENTILATION is REQUIRED.

24. DISPOSE of any SINGLE-USE ITEMS and properly CLEAN REUSABLE EQUIPMENT according to infection control guidelines.

ALS

ETI SUMMARY SKILL SHEET
Blind Digital—Tactile Orotracheal Intubation

1. TAKE/maintain appropriate UNIVERSAL PRECAUTIONS.

2. CONFIRM that the patient is BEING VENTILATED with a high FiO2.

3. APPLY a central PAINFUL STIMULUS (i.e. trapezius muscle pinch) to CONFIRM that the patient is FULLY UNRESPONSIVE (and has a LOC less than that associated with a continued gag reflex.).

4. AUSCULTATE bilateral BREATH SOUNDS to establish a baseline.

5. ATTACH 10–20cc SYRINGE to one-way valve on filler tube and INJECT 10cc of AIR to inflate distal TUBE CUFF and CHECK it FOR LEAKS. Confirm tautness of pilot bulb.

6. WITHDRAW AIR FROM CUFF with syringe and LEAVE SYRINGE securely ATTACHED to one-way valve. Pilot bulb should be flat.

7. INSERT STYLET into ET tube until distal end of stylet is just short of the ET tube's distal opening, and bend proximal end of stylet over the proximal end of ET tube to keep it from advancing further through the tube.

8. SHAPE the ET TUBE/STYLET combination into a curved "HOCKEY STICK" shape.

9. LUBRICATE distal end and cuff of the ET TUBE.

10. POSITION YOURSELF at the patient's upper torso, facing the patient.

11. UNLESS SPINE TRAUMA is suspected, the ASSISTING EMT SHOULD HYPEREXTEND the patient's HEAD and position it IN THE "FORWARD SNIFFING POSITION." If spine trauma is suspected, direct that the head be maintained in the neutral in-line position. Appropriate padding under the patient's head can be helpful in maintaining the desired alignment.

12. WHEN READY to insert the ET tube, DIRECT that VENTILATIONS BE STOPPED. WITHDRAW the oropharyngeal AIRWAY and INSERT THE FIRST TWO FINGERS INTO the patient's MOUTH, and FEEL FOR the EPIGLOTTIS.

13. ONCE THE EPIGLOTTIS IS FELT, ELEVATE IT by lifting the fingertips slightly, THEN INSERT THE BENT ET TUBE into the patient's mouth and GUIDE ITS bent DISTAL TIP BETWEEN THE FIRST TWO FINGERS.

14. ADVANCE THE TUBE UNTIL its bent distal TIP can be felt AT THE FINGERTIPS. With the hand holding the tube's proximal end, PUSH THE TUBE CAUDALLY while using the fingertips to "WALK" THE distal TIP INTO THE TRACHEA.

15. With the tube inserted into the trachea, grasp it firmly with the still-inserted fingers and WITHDRAW THE STYLET with the other hand. As soon as the stylet is removed, ADVANCE the TUBE FULLY to the DESIRED DEPTH.

16. INFLATE the distal CUFF by injecting air through the one-way valve on the filler tube with the syringe.

17. ATTACH the BVM or demand valve to the proximal end of the ET TUBE and DIRECT RESUMPTION OF VENTILATIONS. Direct hyperventilation.

18. OBSERVE for CHEST RISE with each delivered breath and AUSCULTATE over the EPIGASTRIUM for *absence* of air sounds with ventilations.

19. IF CHEST RISE IS *NOT* SEEN and if AIR SOUNDS *ARE HEARD* upon auscultation OVER THE EPIGASTRIUM with each breath, immediately STOP VENTILATIONS and disconnect the BVM or demand valve from the proximal end of the tube, DEFLATE the DISTAL CUFF by withdrawing air through the filler tube with the 10cc syringe, and WITHDRAW THE TUBE. Mask VENTILATIONS must be IMMEDIATELY RESUMED for at least thirty seconds before another intubation attempt is made.

20. IF CHEST RISE *IS* SEEN AND AIR SOUNDS *ARE NOT HEARD* upon auscultation over the EPIGASTRIUM with each breath, CONFIRM proper VENTILATION of the lungs by AUSCULTATING over the MID-LUNG FIELDS for the *presence* of air sounds with each delivered breath.

21. IF baseline breath sounds were bilaterally equal but BREATH SOUNDS ARE NOW HEARD ONLY ON RIGHT SIDE, WITHDRAW ET TUBE 1–2cm and re-auscultate. Continue this process until equal bilateral sounds are again heard.

22. ONCE proper VENTILATION of the lungs has been CONFIRMED by chest auscultation, SECURE ET TUBE in place with tape wrapped around the head/neck or with a commercial ET tube holder.

23. PERIODICALLY RE-CONFIRM ADEQUATE VENTILATION by observing for CHEST RISE and AUSCULTATING over the MID-LUNG FIELDS for bilateral breath sounds.

24. DISPOSE of any SINGLE-USE ITEMS and properly CLEAN REUSABLE EQUIPMENT according to infection control guidelines.

SECTION

Positive Pressure Ventilation and Assisted Ventilation Skills

5

Introduction

Respiration is the entire complex process which takes oxygen from the outside air, transports it to each of the body cells, uses it through metabolism within the cell, and transports and eliminates the CO_2 produced as a by-product of metabolism to the outside. Respiration involves a variety of complex chemical processes involving almost all of the major body systems. Ventilation describes the initial component of respiration—the proper exchange of air from the outside (through the airway) into the alveoli of the lungs. All of the other components required to produce proper oxygenation and CO_2 elimination at the cellular level, and life itself, are dependent upon the maintenance of proper ventilation.

In healthy humans, this is a spontaneous process which occurs properly without conscious thought or effort. When increased activity or other physiologic changes require increased oxygen, or when CO_2 builds up in the body, chemoreceptors detect the problem and the respiratory center in the medulla automatically increases ventilation to resolve the imbalance by changing the rate and/or depth of breathing. Although ventilation is automatic, the individual can also consciously affect his ventilation.

When a patient is apneic, or can not provide adequate ventilation for himself, ventilation must be provided or increased (by assisted ventilations) by the EMT in order to ensure sufficient air exchange and oxygenation. In patients with inadequate air exchange, its restoration including airway control and provided positive pressure ventilation becomes the EMT's first priority of care.

Absent or inadequate ventilation is commonly the result of *chest trauma* or *pulmonary medical problems*. It also results from:

- Loss of a patent airway.
- Brain injury and a loss of the neurological stimulus to breathe.
- Spinal cord disruption (or disruption of key nerves of the thorax and diaphragm) interrupting the neurological pathway from the brain to the muscles needed for respiration.
- Mechanical restriction of necessary chest excursion.
- Abdominal distention from insufflation.
- Hemorrhage producing significant blood loss.
- Congestive heart failure resulting in pulmonary edema.
- Cardiac arrest.
- Profound shock from any cause.
- Chemical imbalance.
- Toxins or drugs which cause respiratory depression or cessation.
- Near drowning or other external obstructions (plastic bag, etc.) resulting in suffocation.
- Containment in an anoxic (or prolonged containment in a hypoxic) environment.
- Advanced sepsis.
- Respiratory impact of any degenerative disease or vital organ failure.
- Significant hypo or hyperthermia.
- In children, exhaustion.

Apnea, agonal breathing, or marked hypoventilation should be recognized immediately upon the initiation of the Global Examination and prior to the identification of its specific etiology. Regardless of its etiology, the primary immediate treatment for inadequate or absent ventilation is to restore adequate air exchange by providing positive pressure ventilation using a suitable device. The maintenance of a patent airway must always be a consideration in ventilation, and has been discussed as a separate detail in the preceding section of this text.

APNEA, AGONAL BREATHING, OR DYSFUNCTIONAL VENTILATION

Since irreversible brain cell death commences in only four to six minutes after a lapse in oxygenation (and significant other vital organ cell death soon follows), no delay for additional assessment or other reasons—regardless of how brief—should occur in providing ventilation once it has been identified as being absent or so dysfunctional as to essentially be absent. Additional problems relating to the specific etiology of the apnea or gross hypoventilation are secondary to providing ventilation, and with only several exceptions do not impact upon the EMT's ability to ventilate the patient properly. When a patient is apneic or has agonal ventilations, only the following take priority over and justify a delay in initiating ventilation:

- Mitigation of danger to the EMT and/or patient at the scene.
- Initiation of proper Universal Precautions.
- Removal of a foreign body obstructing the airway.
- Suctioning of vomitus, debris or other copious fluids from the upper airway before they are "blown down" and aspirated.
- Manual closing of a recognized sucking chest wound.
- Removal of enough weight (or debris) to allow for some chest excursion where an object or cave-in prohibits chest rise.
- Performing a manual airway maneuver or rapid insertion of a single adjunct to maintain an open airway.

Even when there is a flail chest with paradoxical movement of the flail segment, the essential immediate treatment is to initiate positive pressure ventilation. Stabilization of the flail segment is not a pre-requisite for effective positive pressure ventilation, but is only a secondary value in improving the effectiveness of the continued provided ventilations.

Airway obstruction (when unwitnessed), a tension pneumothorax, extreme gastric distention, and sucking chest wounds that do not bleed significantly, are only generally first discovered when ventilation of the patient has been initiated and the presence of one of these conditions defeats the EMT's ability to obtain air exchange or significant chest rise with each positive pressure inspiratory attempt.

When the EMT fails to be able to properly ventilate the patient after re-checking airway patency, if any air is being exchanged the ventilations should be continued and a further rapid respiratory assessment done to identify the specific problem encumbering the EMT's ability to provide fully adequate ventilation. Once it has been identified, the proper steps (closing the sucking wound, decompressing the tension pneumothorax, relieving the gastric distention, etc.) should if possible be taken to ameliorate the problem. In order not to distract from the basic presentation of the steps providing positive pressure ventilation (using several methods and types of equipment), the skills necessary to overcome each of the specific additional problems that could interfere with the EMT's ability to provide ventilation are presented in detail in a separate Section following this one, rather than being included here.

Since the onset of EMS, initial ventilations have been immediately provided using the mouth-to-mouth or mouth-to-nose method in conjunction with a manual airway maneuver since neither required the presence nor preparation of any special equipment. Present day knowledge of the possibility of transmitting Hepatitis, the HIV virus, and other infectious diseases by body substance contact, and the present accepted standards of universal body substance precautions, clearly define unprotected ventilation as an unreasonable and uncontrolled risk for health care professionals that lies outside of any need-to-act obligation.

Given present day standards it is an unnecessary risk for EMTs on or off duty to perform unprotected mouth-to-mouth or mouth-to-nose ventilation. The use of either of these unprotected methods may represent a significant risk to the EMT's health, even his life, and therefore are no longer accepted practices in the treatment of the public, regardless of the expediencies present, nor are they included in this text. Airway First Responder or off duty personal kits should include a bag-valve-mask or a mask with a one-way valve (or at minimum an effective shield or barrier device) and at least rubber gloves to protect the EMT from any contact with airborne exhaled sputum droplets, sputum collection, blood or other body fluids. Such equipment should always be a part of the initial equipment carried in by on-duty responders. In off-duty situations there is universal agreement that a short delay in retrieving the personal kit containing this equipment prior to initiating ventilation is justified by the risk to the responder that would otherwise occur, and that it does not constitute "abandonment." The situation is analogous to needing to perform a cliff rescue without a suitable rope or other equipment present, and going to get the nearest proper rescue equipment prior to attempting a rappel.

Ventilation can be provided using six different types of equipment. Although the many brands of each type have some differences, within each type (category) they are basically the same in overall design and use. The six categories are:

1. Mouth-to-Face Shield (Barrier)
2. Mouth-to-Mask (with one-way valve)
3. Bag Valve Mask Resuscitator (BVM)
4. Demand-Valve Resuscitator
5. Automated Transport Ventilator (ATV)
6. (ALS) Percutaneous Transtracheal Ventilation (PTV)

Each of these must be used in conjunction with a manual airway maneuver or airway adjunct in unconscious patients or those with a significantly lowered level of consciousness.

Although a further description of the components and about the use of each type of device will be presented in the introduction of each skill, a short description of each will be useful at this time.

Mouth-to-Face Shield Ventilation—describes the provision of ventilation similar to earlier taught mouth-to-mouth methods but through a barrier or "filter shield" which separates the EMT and the patient as an infection control consideration solely. Presently there is only limited proof of the effectiveness of such barriers.

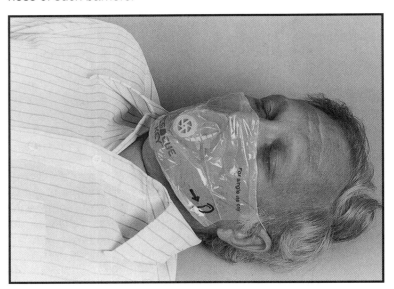

Mouth-to-Mask Ventilation—employs a mask (similar to that used with other ventilators) connected to a one-way valve through which the operator's exhaled air passes to ventilate the patient. The term "mouth-to-mask ventilation" when used in this and most text refers to such a mask and one-way valve combination. Even though the one-way valve may not be separately mentioned, this is simply a form of editorial brevity. A mask without such a valve for infection control should not be utilized. Some models include a port for the attachment of supplemental oxygen to increase the oxygen level of the provided breaths.

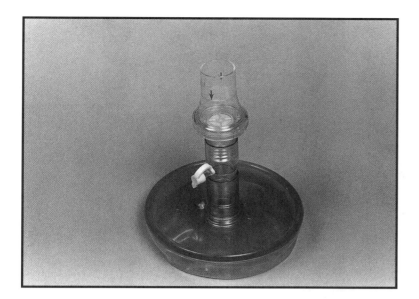

Bag Valve Mask Resuscitator (BVM) — describes an oval or cylindrical self-filling rubber bag with one-way valves at either end. The valve at the patient end has an opening that is of a universal size allowing attachment to either a mask or directly to an advanced airway tube (i.e.: endotracheal tube). When the bag is squeezed the increased pressure in the bag closes the valve at the non-patient end and opens the one at the patient end — allowing air to be "blown" into the patient. When the depressed bag is released the negative pressure in the bag seals the valve at the patient end and opens the one at the other end — allowing the bag to refill. The valve at the patient end has an additional communication to the outside through which the patient's exhaled air is eliminated (since it cannot enter the bag). The valve at the non-patient end communicates with the outside allowing the bag to either refill with ambient room air or, when an oxygen reservoir (sometimes called an "accumulator" or "collector") and supplemental oxygen are connected, with oxygen enriched air.

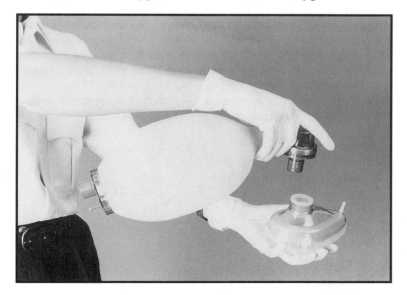

Demand-Valve Resuscitators — have an oxygen source and regulator, a flexible high pressure hose and a "head" (which further reduces the oxygen tank's pressure). The mask connects to a universal fitting on the head and a trigger (or button) on the head controls the delivery of positive pressure oxygen. When the trigger or button is pressed, oxygen under pressure is "blown" into the patient. When it is released, the pressure stops and the patient's exhaled air is blown-out through a second valve and port common to the outside. Should the patient commence breathing on his own, a separate "demand" valve allows him to obtain oxygen (without positive pressure triggered by the EMT) with each inspiration. This feature is the source of the device's name. These resuscitators also include a pressure relief valve which releases in the event that a dangerous increase in the airway and alveolar pressure is caused by too much volume being delivered.

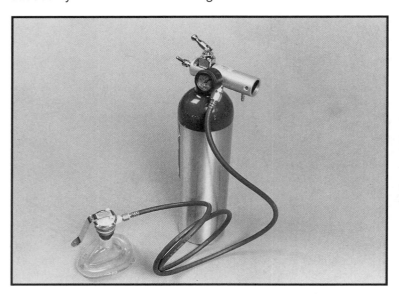

Automated Transport Ventilators (ATV)—are small portable units similar in function to larger hospital ventilators. When properly connected to a high pressure outlet of an oxygen regulator, it will automatically deliver a given volume of positive pressure ventilation at a set interval and rate to the patient without any action required by the EMT to provide each positive pressure breath. Most models have two controls: one allows the EMT to set the number of breaths per minute (actually setting the time of the interval between breaths), and the second allows the EMT to regulate the volume delivered with each inspiration. Like the Demand Valve Resuscitator there is a head to which the mask attaches and which contains a one way valve and port common to the outside to allow for the elimination of the patient's exhaled air, plus a "demand" feature should spontaneous ventilation be restored. Almost all models have a high pressure relief valve and most have a variety of alarms.

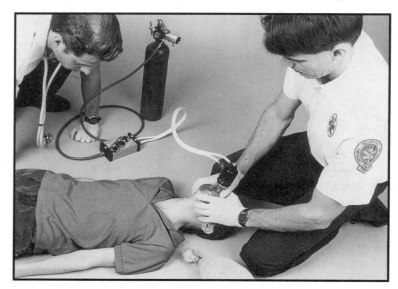

ALS Percutaneous Transtracheal Ventilation (PTV)—describes a procedure requiring a special assembly of commonly available equipment rather than a specific commercially available ventilator. PTV is an ALS procedure and is used only when all other methods of obtaining a patent airway have proven unsuccessful in clearing an obstructed airway or when injuries or conditions do not allow for ventilation through an oral and/or nasal pathway. In such cases a tracheostomy is performed and, using the PTV equipment, ventilation is provided by oxygen insufflation through a needle/catheter inserted into the trachea through the anterior lower neck. The PTV equipment, an oxygen tank and regulator are connected by tubes with a whistle-stop opening to the needle or catheter inserted in the patient's trachea. Oxygen from the regulator is alternately provided for inspiration and stopped for expiration by the EMT covering and uncovering the whistle-stop. This assembly is analogous to, and should be thought of as, a ventilator.

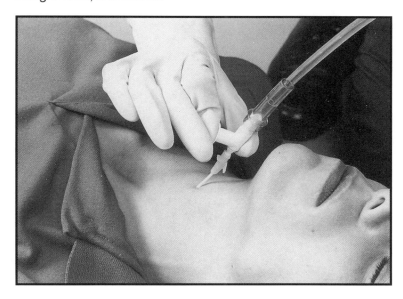

Any patient who has been apneic or has only a dysfunctional breathing rate or pattern has marked hypoxia. Hypoxic patients need to be ventilated with a high flow and a high percentage of oxygen. The oxygen delivered to the patient varies depending on the percentage of oxygen in the delivered "air." This is described as the FiO_2. FiO_2 is the abbreviation standing for the "fraction" of oxygen in the inspired air or, more simply stated, the percentage of oxygen in the air being delivered to the patient stated as a decimal fraction. Ambient room air contains approximately 21% oxygen, therefore the FiO_2 of room air = 0.21. In almost all cases hypoxic patients should, by use of supplemental oxygen, have a delivered FiO_2 of 0.85 to 1.00.

With most devices, the FiO_2 is only directly affected by the liter-flow of the supplemental oxygen delivered when the liter-flow is *insufficient.* Instead, when an adequate liter flow exists, FiO_2 is mostly determined by the design of the delivery device. The design of each specific device determines the amount of ambient air which mixes with the supplemental oxygen at each inspiration and therefore affects the ultimate percentage of oxygen in the inspired air. For example, if the design of the device is such that an equal mixing of ambient room air (considered as an FiO_2 of 0.20 or 20% for calculations) with the supplemental oxygen connected to it at an FiO_2 of 1.00 or 100% occurs, then the FiO_2 delivered by that device will be 0.60, or 60%. The EMT does not need to do such calculations, but should understand this "mixing principle." As well he should be familiar with the FiO_2 that is generally ascribed to each device. These have been included in the following description of the devices.

As a consideration of the situation and urgent need to immediately initiate ventilation in such patients, initial ventilation is often supplied with the EMT's exhaled air (FiO_2 = 0.16 or 16% oxygen) or unenriched ambient air (FiO_2 = 0.21 or 21% oxygen). In such cases, once a patent airway is obtained and ventilation has been started, and other key priorities have been met, the equipment being used should be added to or replaced in order to provide an FiO_2 of between 0.85 and 1.00. ***Sustained ventilation for any extended period with a low FiO_2 should not occur. As soon as the situation and resources allow, this should be increased to providing an FiO_2 of 0.85–1.00.*** Although some recent studies indicate that the actual percentage of oxygen supplied by some of the different ventilators or ventilation methods used may actually be somewhat lower than is commonly ascribed to them, the presently accepted figures will provide the EMT with a useful comparison. Although these may not be exactly accurate, the vast relative differences clearly indicate which should only be used to initiate ventilation as rapidly as possible, and which should be added to or replaced for sustained ventilation once time and resources allow. The following chart assumes an adequate liter flow and a proper seal where supplemental oxygen is included, and that a proper volume is furnished for each breath.

APPROXIMATE OXYGEN CONCENTRATIONS DELIVERED BY DIFFERENT VENTILATION METHODS AND EQUIPMENT			
Device/Method	FiO$_2$	–	Oxygen Concentration
Normal Spontaneous Ventilation	FiO$_2$ = 0.21	or	21%
Mouth-to-Face Shield	FiO$_2$ = 0.16	or	16%
Mouth-to-Mask, exhaled air *only*	FiO$_2$ = 0.16	or	16%
Mouth-to-Mask, O$_2$ attached	FiO$_2$ = 0.38–0.50	or	38–50%
BVM, ambient air *only*	FiO$_2$ = 0.21	or	21%
BVM with supplemental O$_2$ attached *without* an accumulator	FiO$_2$ = 0.40–0.60	or	40–60%
BVM with both an accumulator and supplemental oxygen attached	FiO$_2$ = 0.85–1.00	or	85–100%
Demand Valve Resuscitator	FiO$_2$ = 0.85–1.00	or	85–100%
Automated Transport Ventilator	FiO$_2$ = 0.85–1.00	or	85–100%
Percutaneous Transtracheal Ventilation	FiO$_2$ = 0.85–1.00	or	85–100%*

*Although the concentration of oxygen delivered with PTV is 85–100 percent, due to the limited volume that can be exchanged, the alveolar oxygen concentration will inherently remain significantly less. In the other methods above, this only occurs if the EMT fails to provide proper volume for each inspiration.

KEY CONSIDERATIONS IN PROVIDING VENTILATION

Regardless of the device used to provide ventilation to the apneic patient, several key considerations are universal.

A Patent Airway—Any unconscious patient, or patient with an absent or failing gag reflex can not (or must be assumed to be unable to) maintain his own airway. Therefore, the first priority is to open the airway with a manual maneuver and then to initially maintain a patent airway with the use of a simple adjunct. When the simple adjunct is at hand it can be used initially without delay. More definitive airways should only be used once hyperventilation with a high FiO$_2$ has been provided for several minutes—both to guard against delay and to avoid (except in patients in full arrest) the chance of a vagal response common when the laryngopharynx is stimulated during insertion of these "deeper" airways. In some cases, opening the airway will be sufficient to cause a return of spontaneous ventilation.

Mask Seal—Maintaining a complex mask seal is key to providing a proper volume with positive pressure ventilation of (except when advanced airway devices with an inflatable cuff to provide a seal are used).

Failure to maintain a good mask seal will result in air leaking around the mask and a loss of proper volume with each delivered breath. Many recent studies and experience have shown that a continuous mask seal is difficult to maintain, particularly in a moving ambulance, and that a loss of mask seal is a common cause of inadequate air exchange with provided ventilation. The maintenance of a good mask seal requires both the application of firm anterior-to-posterior pressure around the entire outer anterior circumference of the mask against the face and firm pressure with several fingers placed under the chin (or angle of the mandible bilaterally) to keep the mandible elevated anteriorly into the mask. If the mandible is allowed to "sag" posteriorly it will make it impossible to seal the caudad part of the mask to the face. Keeping the mask sealed and the mandible elevated simultaneously is a physically difficult maneuver which, if it is to be continuously maintained under field and transport conditions, generally requires two hands. With a Mouth-to-Mask Device, Demand Valve Resuscitator, or Automated Transport Ventilator, a single EMT will have both hands available to maintain the mask seal. With the Bag-Valve-Mask device, however, at least one hand is required to deflate the bag. Although sealing the mask with one hand and squeezing the bag with the other is possible, it is extremely difficult for a single operator to consistently keep the mask seal and depress the bag to provide adequate inhalations with only one hand available for each task. Therefore, when using a BVM, two EMTs are recommended as quickly as resources allow. With two EMTs providing BVM ventilation, one maintains the airway and mask seal with both hands while the second provides ventilations by depressing the bag (depending on the operator's hand size, with one or both hands, to ensure that an adequate volume is delivered from the bag).

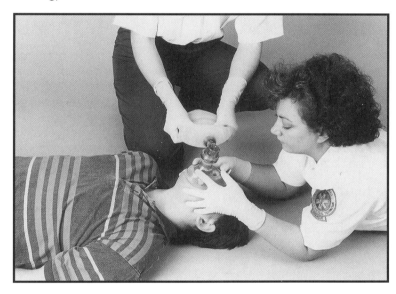

It is recommended that the two operator use of the BVM be the normal standard when a mask is used (prior to intubation), and single operator use be limited only to times when resources and other patient priorities allow for the availability of solely one EMT. Further advantages of the use of two EMTs in any method of ventilation include allowing for the setting-up and adding of the collector and oxygen by one while the other continues to ventilate, and for one to suction as needed with a minimum of interruption in ventilation.

The directions in the skill demonstration found in this section assume that a standard firm see-through mask with a inflatable cuff at its circumference is being used.

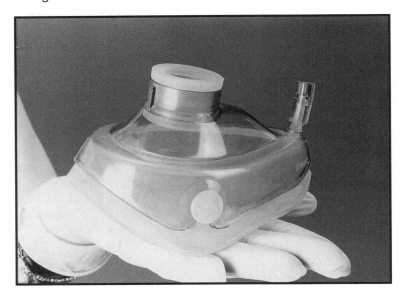

With such masks, a common error is over-inflation of the cuff so that it becomes distended and firm, therefore not readily conforming to the face. These cuffs should only be inflated to between 75 and 80% of their capacity, leaving them malleable so that they will shape and conform to the face with only moderate anterior-to-posterior hand pressure needed to produce a seal. If when the mask is selected for attachment to the ventilator it is found to be too inflated, the few seconds required to remedy this problem will cause less delay than that resulting from ensuing mask seal problems. Care must be taken not to release so much air that they become underinflated as this will also result in an inability to obtain a seal, and face injury from the edge of the hard center section of the mask can occur.

When a mask is used with any ventilator, the EMT may find it easier to obtain a mask seal with the soft round Respironics "blob" mask than the more conventionally shaped ones. Although which mask is used is a matter of preference, most providers have found that the larger inflatable circle allows one to maintain a mask seal with less anterior-to-posterior pressure than required with conventional designs, and that the mask conforms to many sizes and face shapes allowing for easy provision of a seal even when this is difficult or impossible with other masks.

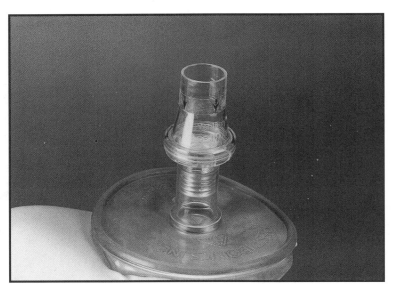

The mask has a standard size opening allowing connection to any standard BVM or "head" part of other ventilators. Due to its design the same mask can be used for children or adults. When this mask is to be used for Mouth-to-Mask Ventilation, the one-way valve used with it *must* be of the same brand to ensure a proper fit.

Volume of Delivered Breaths—For provided ventilations to be beneficial each breath must provide a proper volume (tidal volume) of air. The amount necessary is primarily a factor determined by the patient's size. The current American Heart Association "JAMA" guideline is each breath provided for an adult should be between 800ml and 1200ml. Obviously it is less for smaller adults, children and infants. The delivered volume can not be measured in the field but is instead determined by visualization of the chest (and periodic auscultation).

At each breath the EMT continues to provide volume until the patient's chest has clearly been seen to rise. Care must be taken not to continue to maximum chest rise or beyond as this will provide an excessive volume. For an individual patient the EMT will often first provide too little volume and then too much with the initial few breaths, until he finds the correct level for ensuing breaths. One of the major advantages of the BVM is the feel of the increasing resistance in the bag. As more air is forced in, the pressure rises and the EMT can feel the pulmonary *compliance* in the bag. This provides an additional indicator of when the proper volume has been achieved (or if the mask seal has been lost). If the EMT has small hands, the size and shape of many models of BVM make it difficult to squeeze enough of the contents out of the bag when squeezing it with one hand. Since most models contain about 1600mls of air, one must squeeze the bag so that more than one half of all of the air it contains is forced out in order to provide 800ml with a breath. As well as to assure easy maintenance of a mask seal, two-operator use of the BVM is recommended since this allows one operator to squeeze the bag with either one or both hands to ensure that a proper volume of air is delivered.

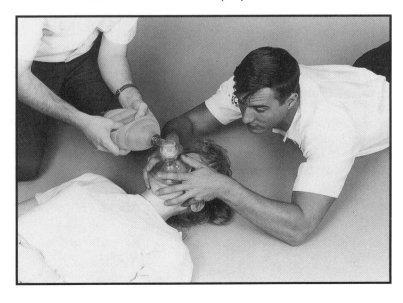

When only one EMT is available, requiring that he maintain the mask seal with one hand while squeezing the bag with the other, squeezing the bag against his forearm, thigh (if kneeling), or chest (if standing) will prove easier and more consistently provide an adequate volume than when it is simply squeezed between his thumb and fingers. An earlier taught method of "rolling-up" the bag has been found to be cumbersome and often results in inadvertently disconnecting the bag from the mask, and is not recommended.

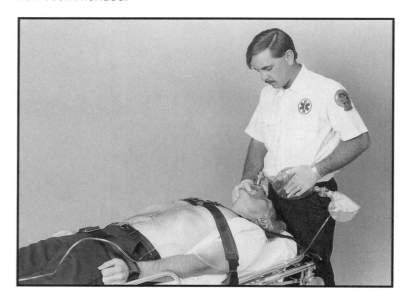

With any device, too little volume at each breath will result in hypoventilation and continued hypoxia. However, too much volume at each breath will also result in a problem that eventually can obstruct the EMT's ability to ventilate the patient. The esophagus, which is a soft pliable tube, is normally held closed by the adhesion of its soft moist wall to itself. Even when fluid or a bolus of food passes through it to the stomach, only the immediate portion containing the food is pushed open while the part above it re-closes. This keeps air and digestive gasses from freely communicating between the pharynx and the stomach. When a good mask seal exists and an excessive volume of air is delivered with a breath, the air compresses and the *pharyngeal pressure increases*. When this pressure exceeds the *esophageal adhesion pressure,* the esophagus is blown open and any additional air delivered is blown into the stomach. The esophagus is normally held closed with a pressure equal to 55−60psi. The pressure needed to properly expand the lungs is only between 35−45psi under normal circumstances. After repeated breaths resulting in such *gastric insufflation* have been delivered, the abdomen fills with air and becomes increasingly distended. When the abdomen becomes distended enough, it pushes the diaphragm upwards interfering with the ability of the lungs to expand—thereby reducing their capacity to less than that required for adequate air exchange.

Regurgitation is commonly associated with the purging of air when reducing abdominal distention. Since the aspiration of sufficient gastric contents is fatal, this unnecessary complication from the delivery of too high a volume of air at each breath is best avoided.

Either insufficient volume or excessive volume with each provided breath can be dangerous, and if continued may result in death.

Sudden surges of excess pressure can similarly result in gastric insufflation. Current models of Demand Valves and Automatic Transport Ventilators are designed to avoid such surges at the initiation of each positive pressure breath. When a Bag-Valve-Mask device is used, it is important that the bag should be squeezed with a steady continuous pressure at each breath instead of a sudden overly forceful "puff" to avoid such a surge.

Rate and Interval—When ventilating a patient, two considerations of timing are key to providing proper air exchange:

- The rate, since the number of breaths per minute together with the tidal volume determines the minute volume, and

- The interval between provided inspirations, since adequate time must occur between each provided inspiration to allow for the patient's exhalation to be completed to provide for sufficient expiration of air.

The normal respiratory rate in adults is between 12 and 20 breaths per minute with an average rate somewhere between 16 and 18 (with 350 to 500ml of air exchanged at each breath). When providing ventilations to an apneic patient to counter the hypoxia and buildup of CO_2, generally an equal level of ventilation is recommended. By ventilating the patient at a similar or slightly higher rate, 12 to 24 times per minute, this will be achieved due to the generally increased tidal volume (500–800ml) provided with each breath. Whenever a respiratory rate is given, unless otherwise indicated, it is assumed to be approximately equal in its interval over a minute's time rather than to have an irregular rhythm. To avoid hyperoxygenation of the provider when Mouth-to-Face Shield or Mouth-to-Mask ventilation using exhaled air is furnished, or in order to synchronize one breath in between each cycle of chest compressions when giving CPR, the respiratory rate may need to be limited to 10 to 12 breaths per minute. As long as each provided breath equals or exceeds 800ml, adequate air exchange (minute volume) will be provided even at this slower rate.

With CPR, when the EMT is assisting in an in-hospital Emergency Department resuscitation, he may find a ventilation provided after each 3 or 4 compressions, rather than the common standard of 1 breath after each cycle of 5 chest compressions, in order to provide more ventilation and oxygenation. This increased ratio of ventilations to chest compressions should only be done in the field after BVM or other mechanical ventilation with a high FiO_2 has been instituted, and when local protocols recommend it. **Ventilations should be provided at a rate of 10 to 20 per minute.**

Even when ventilation is provided by the EMT at a proper rate and volume, hyperinflation and inadequate air exchange can occur if the necessary interval to allow for adequate exhalation is not provided between each delivered inspiration. Adequate exhalation is necessary to eliminate CO_2 and to avoid its increased concentration in the lungs and blood. Excessive levels of CO_2 in the blood can cause undesirable vasodilatation. With the mask seal (or seal provided by the inflatable cuffs in advanced airways), and the operation of the valves in the BVM and other mechanical ventilators, when positive pressure is supplied the airway and lungs are a closed system. The valves only open, allowing communication and exhausting of air to the outside, when the positive pressure is interrupted between each provided inspiration. With each breath an equal volume must be allowed to be exhaled as is supplied. If less is exhaled than furnished, after several breaths the retained volume increases, the air is compressed, and the resulting pressure increase will cause the esophagus to be blown open and air will enter the stomach. If this gastric insufflation continues, the abdomen will become distended and interfere with the EMT's ability to ventilate, and may produce regurgitation and possibly aspiration. To avoid this the EMT must allow proper time for exhalation.

In a healthy person who is breathing spontaneously the active process of the chest rising and the diaphragm flattening which causes inhalation requires less time than the passive process (due to primarily atmospheric pressure and gravity) which results in exhalation. When providing ventilation, approximately two to three times as much time is needed for exhalation as for positive pressure inspiration.

Although the EMT does not apply this ratio as a measured time when ventilating, he should be aware of the ratio to avoid increasing the ventilation to so high a rate that there is no longer enough time between the provided inspirations to allow for full exhalation.

When ventilations are provided in conjunction with CPR, the exhalation time is less and not a factor requiring continuous attention by the EMT. With CPR, forced exhalation results from the chest compression following the provided inspiration rather than through the usual passive process.

The Bag-Valve-Mask device has an analogous factor to the needed exhalation time in its design. Inspiration can be rapidly provided by the active process of squeezing the bag, however when the pressure is released it requires a longer period of time for the bag to passively refill. Generally this is not an additional problem since the time required for the patient to exhale exceeds the "refill time" required by most brands of BVM. Care must be taken when attempting rates of over 16 breaths per minute not to ventilate faster than required for complete refilling of the bag. If the bag is not allowed to completely refill between provided inspirations an inadequate volume can result at each breath, and even with a faster rate the minute volume will be reduced or insufficient.

Hyperventilation—Due to the patient's hypoxia (and often hypoperfusion) the goal of provided ventilation is to provide greater oxygenation than that normally achieved by spontaneous ventilation. In patients who have had inadequate air exchange (due to apnea or a reduced minute volume or when provided ventilations have had to be interrupted) CO_2 retention occurs. Excessive levels of retained CO_2 interfere with the complex process of respiration, produce acidosis and an increasing metabolic imbalance, and can result in vasodilation which contributes to shock. Therefore, a second objective of provided ventilations is to eliminate ("blow-off") excess retained CO_2.

When ventilating a patient, both goals—increasing oxygenation and reducing CO_2 levels—are achieved by providing an increased minute volume. In textbooks and other medical literature, the instruction to provide an increased minute volume is generally stated as **"hyperventilate the patient."** Commonly the instruction to hyperventilate the patient is erroneously followed by significantly increasing the rate of provided ventilations.

With Mouth-to-Mask devices and Demand Valve Resuscitators, too fast a rate generally reduces the inspiratory time and therefore the amount of air provided at each breath (tidal volume). Instead of increasing the minute volume these numerous small "puffs" will actually reduce it. Also, when too little air is provided with each breath—even though oxygen and CO_2 exchange will occur in the mask, pharynx, and remaining airway (the dead space)—little or no exchange will occur in the more distant alveoli.

With a Bag-Valve Mask device the same problem will occur if the volume delivered at each breath is too little. More commonly, with the BVM the operator increases the force and speed with which each inspiration is provided. Even though this increases the volume, it results in an initial pressure surge and a continued too high pressure throughout the inspiratory phase which results in gastric insufflation and progressing abdominal distention. With a BVM, the proper volume for inspiration should be provided by consistent sustained gentle progressive squeezing of the bag over a two second duration. Attempts to increase the number of breaths per minute that result in "mashing" the bag actually produce less air exchange in the alveoli (and also produce abdominal distention) than when a sufficient duration for proper positive pressure inspiration is allowed.

As well as the problems associated with higher rates of provided positive pressure ventilations, increasing the rate invites an inadvertent shortening of the duration required for completed exhalation.

In attempting to hyperventilate the patient, care must be taken not to exceed the patient's tidal capacity. Too great a volume with each breath, as has previously been discussed, will produce an undesirably high increase in pharyngeal pressure.

When providing ventilation: too great a volume with each breath, too much pressure or pressure surges, or too fast a rate will each result in poor air exchange, gastric insufflation, and abdominal distention.

It is important to note that the normal minute volume provided by spontaneous ventilation is between 6500 and 8500ml/minute. Therefore when ventilation is provided at 15 breaths/min at 800ml each, or 20 breaths/min at 600ml each, the Minute Volume is increased to one and a half times normal—"hyperventilating" the patient—whereas faster rates generally provide less.

Initiation and Interruption—Once the patient's apnea or dysfunctional breathing is identified, ventilation should be immediately initiated by the EMTs and should be continued until adequate spontaneous ventilation returns, the ventilating responsibility is transferred to another health care professional, or the patient is pronounced dead. It is generally accepted (and commonly a testing requirement) **that the time from identification of the problem to the provision of the first ventilation should not be greater than 30 seconds.**

Once started, ventilation should only be interrupted when absolutely necessary. When other needs (suctioning, intubation, moving the patient onto a longboard or down stairs, etc) require such an interruption, the time between the peak inspiration provided in the last breath before interruption and the peak inspiration of the first breath when ventilation is resumed, is preferably 20 seconds or less and should not exceed 30 seconds. Simply stated, **provided ventilation should not be interrupted for more than 30 seconds at any one time.**

When a necessary interruption is anticipated the patient should be hyperventilated for 5 to 10 breaths prior to it, and again for a similar number of breaths when ventilation is reinstituted. This maximizes the oxygen concentration in the lungs prior to interruption and rapidly restores it after. If ventilations need to be interrupted more than once in a short time period, or if 30 seconds elapses while attempting a procedure and ventilation was reinstituted but again needs to be interrupted, the patient should be hyperventilated for at least 5 to 10 breaths between interruptions.

Sequence—Due to the urgency in initiating ventilation, the EMT will need to institute ventilation without the delay of preparing and assembling complex equipment or the time required for the insertion of an advanced airway. Even though, ultimately, ventilation in the field should include definitive airway management and ventilation with a high FiO$_2$, since these are time consuming to effect and initially time is the key concern, they are generally not included when initiating ventilation. Only once airway management using a manual method or a simple adjunct and ventilation with exhaled or room air has been established and other urgent patient priorities (such as suctioning and hemorrhage control, if needed) have been met, should time be taken for supplemental oxygen to be added or for another ventilation device to be introduced so that ventilation is provided with a high FiO$_2$. Similarly, only after the patient has been hyperventilated with a high FiO$_2$ should more definitive airway management be attempted. Obviously if ample resources allow, supplemental oxygen can be added almost immediately after initiation of ventilation and more definitive airway equipment can be simultaneously readied. *It is important to note that the initiation of ventilation should not be even slightly delayed by the time needed to locate, open, prepare and connect supplemental oxygen to provide a high FiO$_2$.* Instead, this should be considered as a second phase of ventilation, which is only performed once initial airway management and ventilation have been initiated and are successfully in progress.

It is key to understand that the length of time required to initiate ventilation is dependent upon the usual carry-in equipment policy of the squad. Since the information given to the dispatcher is often unreliable to the situation that the EMTs find upon arrival, *the need for airway adjuncts and the need to immediately initiate ventilation must be anticipated on every call.* To provide for this immediate potential need, carry-in equipment must include a rapidly usable ventilator both for adults and small children. Therefore regardless of the squad's preference in equipment for sustained ventilation with a high FiO$_2$ or other ventilation equipment separately carried on the ambulance, it is recommended that Mouth-to-Mask and/or BVM ventilators (adult and pediatric) together with basic airway adjuncts be included in all primary carry-in kits. Due to their small cost, size and weight this is a practical and effective way to assure their immediate availability and to avoid the delay implicit in the lengthened time needed to open and adjust oxygen equipment which can be set up once the patient's more immediate priorities have been met.

Selection of Ventilation Equipment—A variety of studies have been published comparing the effectiveness of the different types of ventilators used in the field. Several have concluded that Mouth-to-Mask ventilation is the most reliable method of consistently providing proper ventilation by the largest sample of practicing EMTs, however Mouth-to-Mask devices do not answer the physical problems of needed positioning by the EMT, the progressive fatigue inherent in providing ventilation with exhaled air for a sustained period, and the FiO$_2$ limited to 0.38−0.50 which is provided with this method when connected to supplemental oxygen.

Other studies have concluded that the Demand Valve-Mask is superior to the Bag-Valve-Mask since the mask seal is easier to maintain with these rather than when the need to squeeze a bag is involved. These studies however, have only dealt with perceived user-ease and have not adequately addressed the difficulty in timing the inspiratory duration correctly to avoid furnishing too great a volume with each breath. With this type of ventilator the practice and skill required in "regulating" the amount of air provided with each breath is greater than is generally recognized, and gastric insufflation and abdominal distention are commonly associated with its use.

Some studies conclude that Automated Transport Ventilators are the easiest and best to use since, once the device has been properly adjusted, it is automated and the EMT needs only to focus on the maintenance of the mask seal or proper placement of an advanced airway adjunct. These studies assume that the "airway high pressure" alarm will warn the EMT if the volume has been set too high and his ensuing re-adjustment will avoid a progression to abdominal distention.

A review of the current literature leaves the reader with a variety of conclusions. Most of the studies do not include all of the variables that should be considered such as: size, weight, portability, rate of oxygen use, ease of use, skill maintenance needed to ventilate properly without resulting deleterious side effects, cost, time needed for set up, mechanical reliability, disposability versus the effort and effectiveness of cleaning, etc.

The studies presently available have not provided any clear scientific recognition of one presently acceptable type of ventilator being either clearly superior or clearly inferior for providing sustained ventilation than are the others. This leaves the choice then as one of preference for each squad.

The quality of the EMT's initial training, continued skills maintenance (either by frequent call use or periodic supervised practice sessions), and good quantitative measurement (pulse oximetry during the call and blood gases upon arrival at the hospital) are probably more important to ensuring that proper ventilation is provided than which type of high FiO_2 ventilating equipment is used.

The major equipment factor affecting the EMT's ability to sustain proper ventilation is which type of airway adjunct is used, rather than which type of ventilator. The difficulty in consistently maintaining a mask seal is universally reported as one of the major causes of inadequate provided ventilation. For even the most experienced EMT, the consistent maintenance of the mask seal in the back of a moving ambulance is extremely difficult. Use of airway adjuncts that do not include the need to maintain a mask seal can be a significant factor in ensuring better ventilation and oxygenation. As a reflection of this, curriculum changes presently under study include consideration of enlarging the current pre-hospital practice of endotracheal intubation performed by only EMT Paramedics to include this skill also as a requirement at the EMT-Intermediate level and as an option at the EMT-Basic level.

For EMS squads that operate where local recreational activities or terrain make sustained portaging of patients on trails or across open fields a common occurrence, inclusion of an Automated Transport Ventilator (ATV) is highly recommended—regardless of cost. It is improbable that both an adequate mask seal and proper inspiratory volume can be sustained with any other type of ventilator when the EMTs have to carry a patient any significant distance in a basket litter, or transport him on an all-terrain vehicle, Sno-Cat, or rescue sled. When personnel who can intubate are not available preceding such a carry-out, use of an ATV reduces the EMT's ventilation task while transporting the patient to the ambulance solely to maintenance of the mask seal.

Endotracheal intubation (or use of another non-mask dependent advanced airway) in such situations is almost a requirement if a proper provided minute volume is to be maintained at all times without fail. In such environments, even when the patient has been intubated, it is difficult to sustain a good minute volume with a ventilating device that requires consistent timed intermittent actions by the EMT to provide proper inspiratory volume and frequency. For such transports, use of a portable automated device is beyond doubt easier and more reliable and may—once further studies are completed—prove to be the only reliable method.

Assisted Ventilation (Increasing Minute Volume)—Apnea or agonal dysfunctional breathing are so obvious that they are almost always immediately identified and managed as the EMT starts his assessment. In other more subtle cases of hypoventilation and hypoxia this is unfortunately not so.

Although the hypoxia is generally recognized and treated, the hypoventilation is not. ***When a patient has an inadequate air exchange, furnishing a high FiO_2 with a 100% non-rebreather reservoir mask is of little or no benefit and, until the required intervention is provided, hypoxia and morbidity will progress.***

Even with an FiO_2 of 0.85–100%, without adequate air exchange the oxygen levels in the alveoli and bloodstream will remain inadequate and CO_2 will continue to be retained.

The measure used for air exchange in the lungs is **Minute Volume**, the amount of air exchanged in a minute. The minute volume is determined by the amount of air exchanged at each breath (Tidal Volume) times the number of breaths per minute (Respiratory Rate). This can be stated as:

Minute Volume = (Volume of air exchanged per breath) x (number of breaths per minute)

—OR—

Minute Volume = Tidal Volume x Rate

As previously indicated, adults breathe at an average rate of 16–18 breaths per minute and exchange a Tidal Volume of between 375 and 500ml per breath. This produces an average Minute Volume of between 6,500 and 8,500ml. If the Minute Volume drops significantly below this range, hypoxia will occur even when supplemental oxygen enrichment is provided and will progress until an adequate minute volume is either reinstated spontaneously or is provided by the EMT.

It is important to note that both an adequate rate and depth (depth being a major factor in Tidal Volume) are necessary to produce an adequate Minute Volume. Obviously, if the patient's breathing rate is significantly below the normal range of respiratory rates (bradypnea) the minute volume will be inadequate. Less obviously however, if the patient's rate is greater than the normal range (tachypnea) the minute volume is also usually inadequate. When (usually due to a reduced tidal volume) the chemoreceptors identify a build-up of CO_2 (above 40 torr) in the blood, they signal the brain's respiratory center to increase the rate. This first line of compensation results in an increased rate of between 20–30 breaths per minute. If this compensation is not sufficient, or for any reason analogous chemoreceptors in the medullary respiratory center detect that the blood oxygen levels have fallen below 60 torr (40% less than the normal level of 100 torr) the brain's respiratory center directly compensates by increasing the rate. If the hypoxia continues the rate will continue to increase and, as a result of this form of compensation, can exceed 30 breaths per minute. Any rate over 30 per minute must be assumed to be associated with severe hypoxia secondary to an inadequate minute volume.

Therefore such patients need to have an adequate minute volume provided (by BVM or other ventilator).

One can summarize this in three simple statements:

1. Patients with a rate below 12 or above 20 should be suspected of having an inadequate minute volume—assess further to determine if provided ventilations or solely supplemental oxygen is needed.

2. Patients with a rate below 10 or above 30 almost certainly have an inadequate minute volume—provide ventilation with a high FiO_2.

3. Even patients with a respiratory rate between 12 and 20 can have an inadequate minute volume if the air exchanged per breath (tidal volume) is not adequate, therefore the EMT must assess all of the indicators of the respiratory condition in all patients regardless of the presence of a rate in the normal range.

Any patient who cannot provide an adequate minute volume for himself should have it provided for him by the EMT, using a BVM or other mechanical ventilator to assist his ventilations.

Providing assisted ventilations to an unconscious patient or a patient with a markedly lowered level of consciousness can generally be achieved without a problem. When the patient is alert, however, it requires the EMT to obtain the patient's cooperation. Because such patients are often frightened or combative, this can be considerably more difficult than in unconscious patients. The specific additional techniques needed to provide an adequate minute volume to such patients are discussed in the skill section for *Providing Assisted Ventilations* found near the end of this section.

SPECIAL CONSIDERATIONS IN THE PEDIATRIC PATIENT

The term "pediatric" covers a population spanning a vast range from the newborn to the older adolescent years. The differences in size and development, except for adolescents who have a body size near that of an adult, necessitate some special ventilation considerations in children. These primarily surround differences from adults in:

- Normal range of respiratory rate and volume.
- Airway anatomy and size.
- Mask size needed.
- Volume to be delivered at each breath.
- In small children, pathophysiology of respiratory arrest.
- In smaller children (generally 7 years or under), padding needed to maintain a proper position for ventilation.

Obviously, in children having a significantly smaller size than an adult the tidal volume capacity is smaller, and the amount delivered at each breath needs to be less, in order to avoid excessive volume and pressure. In smaller children, the normal rate of ventilation is higher than for adults and therefore the range of normal rates is higher. Whereas a rate of 44 breaths a minute would represent an alarming tachypnea in an adult, it is normal in a newborn. Similarly, even though 16 breaths per minute is normal for an adult, it represents a significant bradypnea in newborns, infants and even toddlers, and probably indicates that an inadequate minute volume exists.

Particularly in pre-school years, since children normally grow and develop at different rates (often in growth spurts), there may be substantial normal differences in size and weight between children of identical age. Due to this, anatomically and medically, the child's weight or height (length) will serve as more accurate indicators than does his exact chronological age. Therefore, when providing ventilation, the EMT should use these measures, rather than the child's age as a guide. If the patient's body looks like that of an average eight year old, the normal eight year old parameters should be used even if he is actually only six years old and large for his age. In this text, to be consistent, pediatric patients have been categorized into six "age" groups. The following chart describes the average height and weight ranges generally ascribed to patients in each of these.

EXPECTED FINDINGS (Range of Mean Norms)			
Group	Age	Average Height	Average Weight
Newborn	Birth to 6 wks.	51−63 cm	4−5 kgs
Infant	7 wks. to 1 year	56−80 cm	4−11 kgs
Toddler	1−2 years	77−91 cm	11−15 kgs
Preschool	2−6 years	91−122 cm	14−25 kgs
School Age	6−13 years	122−165 cm	25−63 kgs
Adolescent	13−16 years	165−182 cm	62−80 kgs

The normal range of spontaneous ventilation rates expected for each group is important in determining rates (bradypnea or tachypnea) that may indicate the presence of an inadequate minute volume requiring ventilatory assistance. As previously discussed, in evaluating ventilation both *rate* and *depth* (indicative of the tidal volume exchanged with each breath) are key factors in evaluating the Minute Volume. In small children particularly, *effort* must also be considered as a key factor in determining which patients require assisted provided ventilations. In small children a significantly increased effort can rapidly result in exhaustion and, if sustained, in respiratory arrest which will shortly include cardiac arrest.

PEDIATRIC RESPIRATORY RATES			
Group	Age commonly associated with patient's developmental size	Normal range of breaths/min	Suspect inadequate MV & need for ventilatory assist
Newborn	Birth to 6 wks.	30−50	<30 or >50
Infant	7 wks. to 1 year	20−30	<20 or >30
Toddler	1−2 years	20−30	
Preschool	2−6 years	20−30	
School Age	6−13 years	(12−20)−30	
Adolescent	13−16 years	12−20	<12 or >20

Therefore, in small children who have a significantly increased respiratory effort, even when adequate air exchange remains, assisted ventilation should be provided before the child becomes further exhausted and diminished exchange or respiratory arrest develops.

When ventilations are provided or assisted to a patient of any age group, adult or child (and except where a lower rate is necessitated by Mouth-to-Mask, Mouth-to-Shield, or CPR), it should be provided at approximately the average normal rate of spontaneous ventilation or just slightly higher. In small children, therefore, the recommended rate at which ventilations should be provided is higher than the 16–20 breaths/minute recommended for adults, adolescents, and older children. Although the accepted pediatric references vary slightly, a general guideline is a recommended rate of 20–24 ventilations/minute in small children, and 24–30 ventilations/minute in infants. In the presence of lung disease a slightly higher rate may be required to achieve adequate ventilation, with an important exception. When the patient has asthma, bronchitis, or other conditions causing "air trapping" an even more extended time than is required for inhalation is needed for completing exhalation. A slower rate will be required to allow enough time for adequate exhalation to avoid "stacking" some of the volume of several provided breaths which can result in excessive pulmonary volume and pressure.

As well as the many sizes of each airway adjunct that must be stocked to accommodate the large range from infant to the largest adult, both carry-in and in ambulance equipment should at least include one infant size, one child size, and one adult size mask—and preferably several sizes for each of the three categories. As well, having a Respironics Seal-Easy mask to use with patients on whom another size or style may not provide a good mask seal is also highly recommended. If Bag Valve Mask ventilators are used by a service, then an adult size bag, a neonatal bag and a pediatric bag should be included in the carry-in and on-board equipment. Although infants and small children can be ventilated with an adult bag using the correct size mask, this is not a good practice since the higher rates used in children require a bag with more rapid refill capability, and when ventilating small children with an adult bag it is more difficult to avoid delivering an excessive volume with each breath. Adult size bags should not be used with infants and small children as a routine EMS procedure just to avoid the need to carry the proper two additional sizes. Using an adult bag on infants and small children is only justified in remote rescue situations where space limitations and low likelihood of need do not allow for their inclusion, or when the proper size equipment fails.

The lack of properly sized pediatric airway and ventilation equipment on an emergency ambulance is unjustifiable, even regardless of a low frequency of need, since the appropriately sized equipment is required to provide the highest quality of care within the EMTs capability for any child who needs airway and ventilation management.

Providing ventilation with neither too small nor too great a volume at each breath can be even more difficult in infants and small children than in adults, particularly for the EMT who is rarely called upon to ventilate such patients. Careful observation of the bared chest and abdomen while providing each ventilation is needed. The proper volume produces clearly observable chest rise but not so much that the chest excursion is exaggerated or maximal. If after excursion of the chest is seen, the EMT continues to provide additional volume until the chest excursion is at its maximum capacity, an excessive volume will be delivered and gastric insufflation will result.

Frequent periodic auscultation over the midlung field and over the epigastrium is particularly helpful in children, along with continuous observation of chest excursion, in ascertaining that the volume provided with each breath is neither too small nor too great. This also aids in identifying when exhalation has ended, signalling the time for the provision of the next positive pressure inspiration.

As was discussed in the preceding section on *Airway Management Skills,* in children seven years or under (due to the larger head size relative to the torso and the fact that most of the additional size is posterior to the point where the cranium attaches to the spinal column) padding is required under the torso to elevate it about two inches so that severe flexion does not occur when the child is placed supine on a rigid surface. In these children, such padding and elevation of the torso must be considered a key adjunct needed to provide proper ventilation and should be provided early on when ventilation is initiated.

Due to the soft nature of the immature trachea in infants and very small children, care must be taken to avoid inadvertent placement of the fingers and pressure over the trachea when elevating the mandible in order to maintain the mask seal. Unless this is carefully guarded against it can easily occur due to the child's small size relative to the EMT's hands. Firm pressure at the outside of the lower palate or over the trachea in small children can result in a diminished or occluded airway—either by pushing the tongue into the airway or by collapsing the trachea, respectively.

SPECIAL CONSIDERATIONS WHEN VENTILATING TRAUMA VICTIMS WITH SUSPECTED SPINE INJURY

In patients with potential spine trauma the forward sniffing or hyperextended head position that is normally used to maximize the airway must be avoided, and instead airway management and ventilation must be performed while the patient is maintained in the neutral in-line position. To achieve this, ventilation efforts must include manual immobilization of the head in the neutral in-line position, usually by a second EMT, or if one is not available for this task then simultaneously by the EMT providing the ventilations. When two EMTs are available, this can most easily be achieved by one EMT positioned beyond the head who provides the head immobilization and the mask seal while the second EMT (positioned at the side of the patient's head) provides the ventilations.

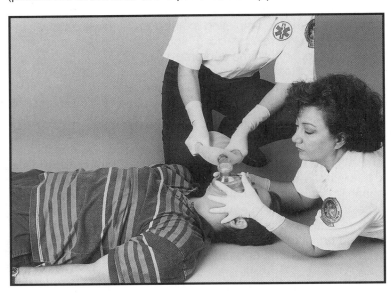

Alternately, in cases where the need to perform other items which requires the EMT to be positioned above the patient's head are anticipated (such as a trauma intubation), the manual head immobilization and mask seal can be provided by one EMT positioned at the patient's lower thorax facing his head, thereby allowing the second EMT to perform ventilations from a position above the patient's head. From this position the head is immobilized by placing the thumb anteriorly on the notch where the maxillary teeth meet the zygoma, spreading the first and second fingers at the sides of the head and placing the third and fourth fingers just under the posterior curvature of the head at its lateral edges.

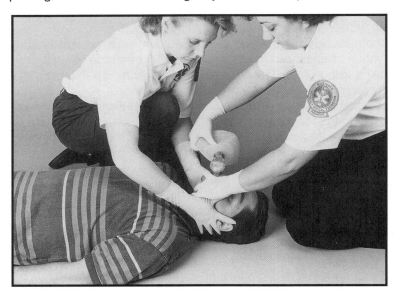

Although it is more difficult to sustain the manual immobilization from the side of the patient's thorax than from beyond his head, this positioning allows an EMT to maintain the manual immobilization from its initiation until it is replaced by mechanical immobilization, without the need to transfer it from one EMT to another, when a procedure requires the EMT providing treatment to be positioned beyond the patient's head. Regardless of how carefully such transfers are done, they usually have some inadvertent loss of immobilization and slight movement associated with them.

When the EMT providing the immobilization from alongside the patient's thorax must also maintain the mask seal, his hand position will have to be slightly different than when he is solely holding the head if he is to produce pressure around the entire perimeter of the mask and also prevent the mandible from sagging posteriorly resulting in a loss of the mask seal. To produce a seal the thumb and first finger are placed around the anterior circumference of the mask at each side and anterior-to-posterior pressure is applied to the mask. The mandible is kept from sagging posteriorly either by holding it with the third finger placed under it (elevating it from both sides), or by placing the tips of the fourth finger (or fourth and fifth) under the angle of the mandible at each side. With either method the remaining fingers are extended, pointing posteriorly, along the flat lateral planes of the head and moderate medial pressure is applied to maintain the immobilization.

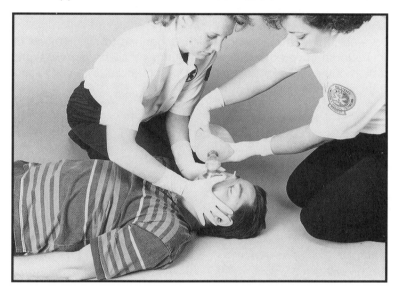

When a single EMT must immobilize the head, maintain a mask seal, and provide ventilation, the procedure required differs for different types of ventilators.

With Mouth-to-Mask, Demand Valve Resuscitators, and Automated Transport Ventilators, the EMT can most effectively maintain manual head immobilization and mask seal with his hands while positioned beyond (above) the patient's head. Lying with the elbows on the ground provides a more secure base when immobilizing the head than does kneeling, and is recommended when possible. When a single EMT provides Mouth-to-Mask ventilation and immobilization he will have to kneel, however, in order to be able to bend down to blow into the one-way valve.

With a **Bag-Valve Mask** the EMT kneels so that his knees are just immediately beyond the patient's shoulders with one flexed leg next to each side of the head. The head is immobilized by firmly squeezing it between the EMT's thighs leaving both hands free to provide the mask seal, keep the mandible elevated, and squeeze the bag.

Single operator use while immobilizing the head will be demonstrated and discussed further as skills for using each device are presented.

Since—when 98% of all adults are placed supine on a rigid surface (the ground or a longboard) and the head is in the neutral in-line position—a space of between one-half and three and one-half inches occurs between the occiput and the firm surface, the padding needed to fill this void must be considered an essential part of initiating ventilation in patients with suspected spine trauma. If padding has not been placed to fill the void under the occiput, the EMT providing the manual immobilization (regardless of his positioning) will find it difficult to maintain the neutral in-line position of the head due to the anterior-to-posterior pressure required to provide a mask seal, and hyperextension (which is contraindicated in such cases) generally results.

ADDITIONAL KEY ELEMENTS

As well as the aforementioned essential elements in ventilating the patient, periodic assessment of the provided ventilations including auscultation and the other signs and symptoms associated with pulmonary ventilation and cellular oxygenation must be performed to assure the effectiveness of the EMT's care. Provided ventilations should periodically be interrupted to ascertain if adequate spontaneous ventilation has resumed. It is hoped that the use of pulse oximetry to provide continuous quantitative measurement of the blood's oxygenation will shortly become a required part of pre-hospital care at all levels. The skills employed for pulse oximetry are presented in a later section of this text which deals with *Measurement Of Patient Ventilation And Oxygenation.*

An understanding of the material covered in this introduction, which is generic to all methods of provided or assisted ventilation, and the material covered in Section 4—*Airway Management*—are necessary (and assumed) in the presentation of the skills for using each type of ventilator or ventilation method found in the remaining pages in this section.

MOUTH-TO-SHIELD (BARRIER) VENTILATION

This general discussion (to provide some reference) is included, rather than specific step-by-step directions as for the other skills in this book, because *Mouth-To-Shield Ventilation* is not a recommended EMT skill.

A variety of ventilation barrier shields are presently available. These are generally an air and fluid impervious plastic sheet which is placed over the patient's face. In its center is an opening with a "filter" made of material through which air—but not airborne sputum droplets—can pass.

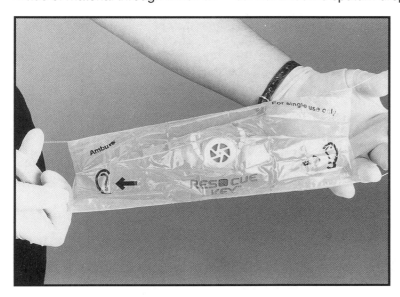

Most of these also have a short (approximately 1/2 inch) tube on the operator's side of the shield over the filter to keep the EMT's mouth from coming into contact with the filter material which, after several breaths, will become wet and contain sputum from both the EMT and the patient's exhaled air. Therefore, brands that do not have such a tube to keep the EMT from contact with the contaminated filter must be considered even less safe than those that do.

At present, studies surrounding the effectiveness of the infection protection provided by these shields (with or without a tube) provide insufficient proof to scientifically state that they provide effective safety for the EMT. Therefore, they should not be considered for on-duty use by EMTs at this time since a variety of safer alternatives exist. ***If an individual EMT elects to use such a device when off-duty, he should understand the possible remaining exposure risk.***

Even with a barrier shield, examining gloves should be worn by the EMT prior to any direct patient contact. Next, the shield should be unfolded and placed over the patient's face so that the opening containing the filter, or filter and tube, is directly over the patient's mouth—and in some models is secured at the patient's ears to keep it from moving. Ventilation with such a shield is performed in the same way as mouth-to-mouth ventilation, except that it is through the filter in the shield between the operator and the patient's face.

While kneeling beside the patient's face and perpendicular to his midline the operator places the heel of his cephalad hand on the patient's forehead and pinches the nostrils shut (through the barrier) between his thumb and first finger. Then, with his caudad hand, he performs a head tilt/chin lift.

Next, while bending down, he seals his mouth over the patient's mouth with the shield between them and provides a breath by blowing his exhaled air through the filter and into the patient. The chest should be observed to rise when each breath is provided. Lastly, the operator removes his mouth after each breath to allow the patient to exhale.

This procedure is repeated at a rate of 12 per minute (markedly higher rates can result in operator hyperventilation and inability to continue) until this method can be replaced with a simple adjunct and a better ventilation device.

MOUTH-TO-MASK VENTILATION

Mouth-to-Mask Ventilation is primarily used to replace Mouth-to-Mouth Ventilation which, due to infectious disease concerns, is no longer considered a safe or appropriate procedure. As well as providing isolation between the patient and the rescuer, these devices also provide for easier delivery of exhaled air ventilations than other methods.

Many enlightened EMS services, (or other public service agencies) provide its members with a Mouth-to-Mask device to be kept in their personal car so that if they arrive at a scene where ventilation is required prior to an ambulance, they have the infection control benefit it provides. This allows them to avoid the difficult decision between taking an undue personal risk or delaying the start of ventilations— neither of which represents a desirable choice. Similarly Mouth-to-Mask devices—due to their small size and cost, and the simplicity and rapidity with which they can be deployed to safely initiate ventilation—are carried in First-Responder vehicles (such as Police, Fire and Rescue vehicles) and in First-Responder packs (such as those carried by Park Rangers, Ski Patrol members, etc.) to protect such individuals when the need for ventilation or CPR exists prior to the arrival of the EMS unit.

A variety of Mouth-to-Mask "Pocket Masks" are available. These commonly include two or three parts: The parts are; a mask with a center port; a one-way valve, one end of which inserts into the port in the mask and the other end that has a short tube in which to blow; and lastly an oxygen connection nipple which in some models is a fixed part of the mask and in others is part of a short extension tube which, when supplemental oxygen is to be added, is connected between the one way valve and the mask. Models that do not have the option for attaching supplemental oxygen are not recommended for on-duty use.

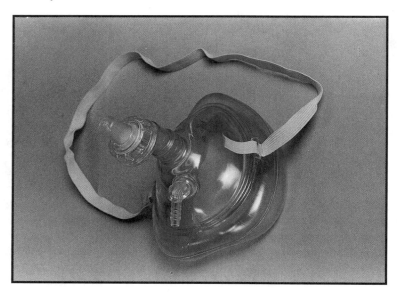

References in this or other texts to Mouth-to-Mask Ventilation without specific mention of a one-way valve simply represent editorial brevity and should not be misinterpreted to imply that such a valve is not needed. A mask without a one-way valve to protect the EMT should not be used.

The one-way valves are sealed and, since they cannot be opened and cleaned, are single-use disposable items. The mask, after cleaning, can be re-used with the addition of a replacement one-way valve. The size and style of the tube at the end of the one way valve (that connects to the mask and the mask-port) are unique to each brand and therefore *only parts of the same exact model and brand should be used together.*

The small size, weight and cost of Mouth-to-Mask or Bag Valve Mask Ventilators allows the inclusion of either in every carry-in kit ensuring their immediate presence at any time on all calls. This— together with their unique ability to be readied in one or two seconds to initiate ventilation without the delay required to assemble, turn-on, and adjust other ventilators—makes them desirable adjuncts for the timely initiation of ventilation of the apneic patient.

Mouth-to-Mask ventilation, due to the effort required and low FiO_2 furnished with exhaled air, is a temporary method—replacing Mouth-to-Mouth ventilation to ensure the immediate initiation of safe provided ventilation. Even when supplemental oxygen is later added, since the FiO_2 is only increased to 0.38–0.50, it should be viewed as an interim method and be replaced as soon as practical with a mechanical ventilator that with less effort provides an FiO_2 of between 0.85 and 1.00.

Once the initial rapid size up has identified that the patient is unresponsive and apnea continues, unresolved by opening of the airway:

1. After assuring that the necessary universal precautions have been taken, remove the mask and one-way valve from their container and insert the correct end of the one-way valve into the port in the mask. Blowing through it once is recommended so that if any difficulty in providing breaths ensues, faulty equipment can be eliminated as a potential cause.

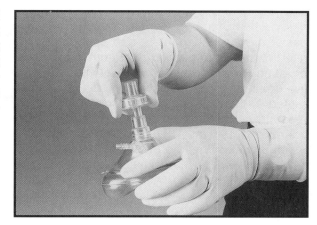

2. From a kneeling position beyond the patient's head orient the assembled unit so that the narrower part of the mask is towards you, and spread the mask and place it over the patient's nose and mouth onto the patient's face. Place the thumb and first finger of each hand around the anterior circumference of the mask, and place the fourth (or 3rd and 4th) fingers under the angle of the mandible as shown.

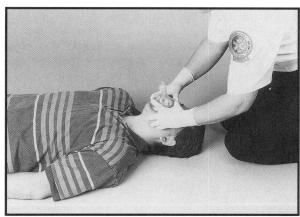

3. While performing a head tilt/jaw thrust and maintaining the mask seal, bend over and place your mouth over the proximal end of the one-way valve. While viewing the chest using your peripheral vision, provide a sustained breath until the chest is seen to rise sufficiently.

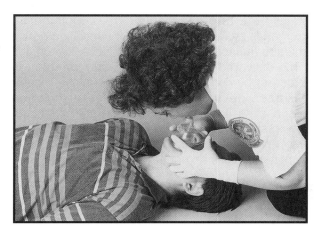

4. While maintaining the jaw-thrust, remove your mouth from the one-way valve to allow the patient to exhale. Observe the chest fall and be sure that enough time is allowed between each provided breath, for the completion of exhalation. Repeat steps 3 and 4 at a rate of 12 breaths per minute. After delivering 2 breaths (or simultaneously, when two EMTs are available) check for a palpable carotid pulse to determine whether airway management and ventilation, or full CPR, are needed.

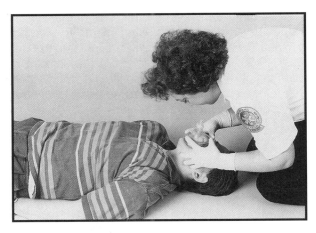

5. Often the immediate availability of an oropharyngeal airway allows for its insertion without delay when initiating ventilation. This provides easier airway management and supercedes the need of a manual method right from the onset of provided ventilation. If this was not possible, after five or six ventilations, ventilation should be interrupted and the EMT (or a second EMT) should measure and insert an oropharyngeal or nasopharangeal airway. Then, ventilation should be resumed. After insertion of a simple airway adjunct, to provide a mask seal the mandible must be kept from sagging by firm anterior pressure with the fourth fingers under the anterior mandible or under the angles of the mandible as before.

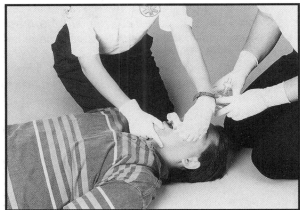

6. Due to rescuer fatigue and the low FiO_2 inherent in exhaled air mouth-to-mask ventilation, once ventilation has been established and other urgent priorities have been met, this method should be replaced by another ventilation device that is less tiring and provides an FiO_2 of 0.85–1.00. As soon as practical, a second EMT should set up and ready such equipment and it should be substituted without significant interruption in ventilation.

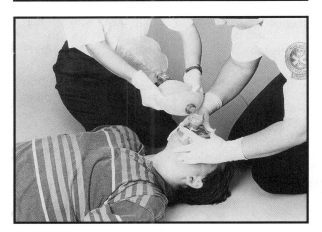

7. In the rare situation where, supplemental oxygen is available but not other ventilating equipment to replace the mouth-to-mask ventilation, the FiO_2 delivered should be increased as soon as practical by connecting the nipple on the mouth-to-mask device, using a Universal Oxygen Connecting Tube, to the portable oxygen regulator which should be set at 15 LPM (or its highest setting). When replacement with another ventilator is imminent, this is an unnecessary added task.

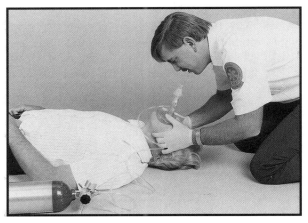

8. In cases where spine trauma is suspected, mouth-to-mask ventilation can be performed using the same general steps as have been previously described, except that a trauma jaw thrust should be used (instead of the head tilt/jaw thrust) and the EMT must maintain immobilization of the head in the neutral in-line position as well as providing ventilations throughout.

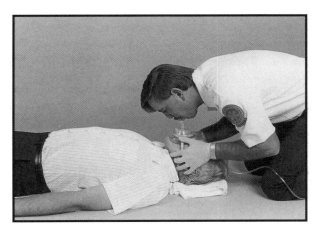

9. With Mouth-to-Mask devices a single EMT can readily maintain the head tilt (or in cases of spine trauma, neutral in-line immobilization, elevation of the mandible, mask seal, and provide ventilation while a second EMT readies other equipment or provides for other patient needs. Although no benefit is provided by two EMTs ventilating the patient with a mouth-to-mask device, should this be desired, the airway and mask seal (and if indicated immobilization of the head and neck) are provided by the EMT above the patient's head and breaths are provided by the second EMT from a position alongside the patient's head and perpendicular to his midline.

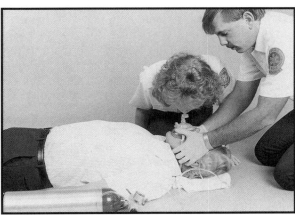

USING A BAG VALVE MASK VENTILATOR (BVM)

The Bag Valve Mask Ventilator is the most universally used device for providing ventilation pre-hospital and in the hospital emergency setting. Regardless of local preferences for ventilation equipment, all EMTs are expected to be proficient in its use. Presently it is the only ventilator which is immediately ready without supplemental oxygen equipment to provide initial ventilation, and which then later allows for the addition of oxygen to provide ventilation with an FiO_2 of 0.85–1.00.

This device uniquely provides the operator with constant positive feedback by the feel of the bag. This *compliance* assures the operator of successful inspirations, and changes in compliance warn the EMT when either a loss of mask seal or pathological airway or thoracic problems interfere with air delivery. This "feel" and the control it provides represent a key additional guide when providing ventilations and is of particular benefit with assisted ventilation.

Bag Valve Masks are available in a variety of models (brands) including both multi-use and disposable single-use models. With the advent of inexpensive disposable single-use models, the BVM has gained a key additional feature. Cleaning the "heads" and contaminated parts of the one-way valve, a task inherent to all ventilators, has always represented a pre-hospital problem surrounding both the skill and effort it requires, and in the question of how successfully the cleaning provides assurance that no chance of contamination from one patient to another is possible. With disposable single-use BVMs these problems, and the dangers of improper reassembly, are simply avoided.

The Bag Valve Mask Ventilator, although it contains a variety of valves, is reliable and has only two separate parts that the EMT needs to deal with when initiating ventilation—the bag and the mask.

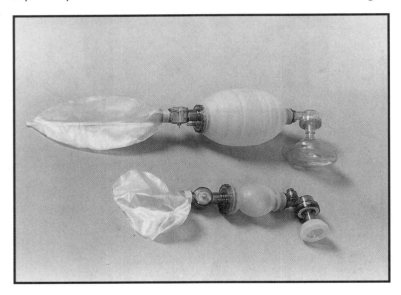

When attaching supplemental oxygen a third part, the reservoir or accumulator, is added and a standard low pressure Universal Connecting Tube and a high flow supplemental oxygen source (portable or on-board oxygen units) are required.

The bag has a one-way outlet valve at one end and a one-way inlet valve at the other. The bag is malleable (flexible) generally being made of rubber or plastic material which allows its shape to change to diminish its size when squeezed and automatically return to its original size and shape when it is released.

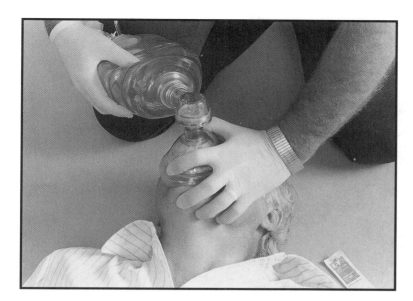

When the bag is squeezed its volume is reduced, increasing the pressure in the bag. This closes the inlet valve and provides positive pressure to open the outlet valve and "blow" the air into the patient's lungs. When the bag is released it returns to its original larger size and the negative pressure that results closes the outlet valve, opens the inlet valve, and results in the self-filling of the bag from the outside air. Although the capacity and specific shape of each individual model varies, most bags have a capacity of approximately 1600ml and are either cylindrical or football-like in shape. The volume that the bag is diminished by when squeezed is almost directly reflected by the volume of air delivered to the patient. Similarly the pressure applied to the outside of the bag is almost equally translated to the positive pressure with which the air is delivered (except when excessive volumes result in undesirable higher pressures).

A one-way outlet valve is attached to and protrudes from one end of the bag. It allows air to pass from the bag into the patient when the bag is squeezed, but directs exhaled air to the outside without allowing it to re-enter the bag. The plastic housing surrounding the outlet valve has a tube extending from its side which has the 22mm outside diameter and 15mm inside diameter which is universally used for providing a pressure fit connection with standard masks, endotracheal tubes, or other advanced airway adjuncts. Experience has caused the present American Heart Association guidelines to specify that these valves not contain any pop-off or other high pressure release mechanism.

The second one-way valve, generally found at the BVM's other end, is the inlet valve through which air enters to refill the bag when the squeezed bag is released. Generally the accumulator connects to the outer case of that valve (or a tube part of it) however, no standard exists for this connection. Only the accumulator for a given model can be attached to it. A standard low pressure nipple is also generally a part of the inlet valve (or a part of the outlet valve in some models) to allow for connection of a Universal Oxygen Connecting Tubing without using an accumulator.

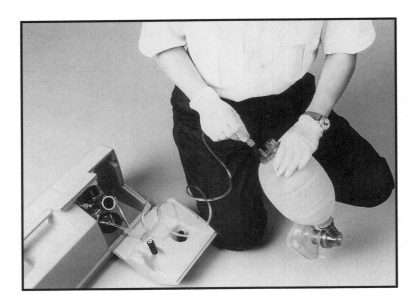

When the connecting tubing from the supplemental oxygen is attached to this nipple without an accumulator, even a 15 LPM flow rate is not great enough to provide the necessary volume to refill the bag in its short refill phase, and ambient air is also drawn in through the inlet valve. This mixing of 100% oxygen and room air results in an FiO_2 limited to 0.50 and therefore does not represent the recommended method for adding supplemental oxygen.

The accumulator is either a closed second bag (larger but similar to the bag on a reservoir oxygen mask) or a large flexible tube (similar to a length of automobile radiator hose) and open at its proximal end. Either style attaches to the inlet valve of the bag valve device.

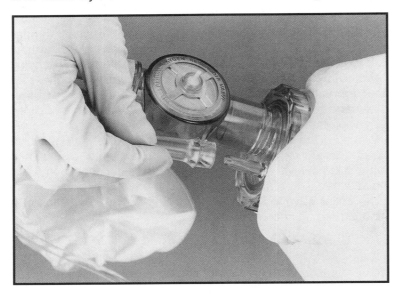

When attached, the bag valve's inlet valve communicates solely with the accumulator—allowing the bag to refill exclusively from the accumulator's contents rather than ambient air (or a mixture of oxygen and ambient air). At its other end the accumulator has a nipple for connection to the high flow oxygen source.

With all BVMs the approximately 800ml delivered with a breath is entirely replaced in the few seconds between releasing the hand pressure on the bag and the bag's return to its original size and shape. Contrary to a common misconception, no additional filling or increase in the oxygen concentration occurs between that time and when the bag is again released after the next positive pressure inspiration has been delivered. When the accumulator and a 15 LPM oxygen source are connected to the intake valve of the bag-valve device, oxygen flows into the accumulator throughout the respiratory cycle. It acts as a reservoir which accumulates enough oxygen between cycles that the primary bag can adequately refill exclusively with the oxygen in the accumulator in spite of its short refill time. Since no ambient air is drawn in to mix with the oxygen, when an accumulator is used the FiO_2 delivered by the BVM is 0.85–1.00.

Individual models may have some mechanical and design variations in the previously discussed general arrangement—one even has an optional demand-valve head that can be used instead of an accumulator. The preceding general principles of operation however, are important to know when using a BVM since regardless of whether or not they are exactly mechanically accurate to the model being used, they provide an understanding of key factors involved in the steps in using any such device.

WARNING: *All of the parts used (except the mask) should be of the same brand and model since, usually, these parts are NOT safely interchangeable.*

Once the initial rapid size-up has identified that the patient is unresponsive and that apnea continues, unresolved by opening of the airway:

1. While maintaining the airway attach the correct size mask to the BVM and place the assembled unit so that the mask is properly oriented over the patient's nose and mouth. The immediate initiation of ventilation should not be delayed by the additional time required to add an accumulator and supplemental oxygen at this point.

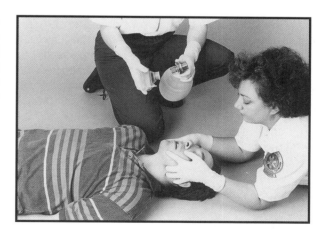

2. While the EMT positioned beyond the patient's head provides a mask seal by pressing firmly on the anterior circumference of the mask with his thumbs and first fingers and performs a head tilt/jaw thrust, the second EMT takes a position at the side of the patient's head and carefully positions the bag valve device in relationship to the mask until it is properly oriented for easy use.

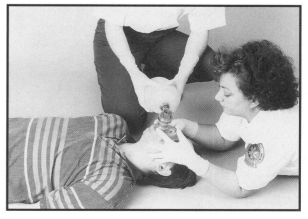

3. While visualizing the chest, the EMT at the side of the patient's head provides a breath by slowly progressively squeezing the bag between the thumb and opposing fingers of both hands (if his hands are large enough, a single hand can be used instead). Care must be taken to make this a slow continuous gentle process without any initial or ensuing sudden surges.

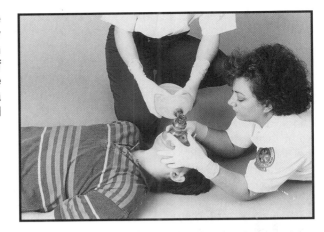

4. The bag is slowly squeezed until the chest has been seen to rise a similar distance as with normal inspiration, but is not yet near the maximum limit of the chest excursion. As well as carefully visualizing the chest rise at each breath, the experienced EMT will also be guided by the "feel" of the bag in confirming when a sufficient volume has been successfully delivered. Inspirations should be provided so that the inspiratory phase takes approximately between one and two seconds in adults.

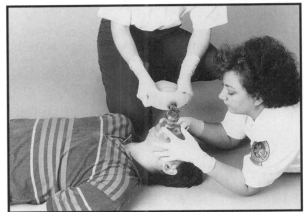

5. If the bag will not deflate when squeezed and air cannot be "blown" into the patient, the airway is not patent. Reposition the head and re-attempt to ventilate, If the problem remains unresolved by repositioning, a foreign body obstruction must be assumed and resolved. If the air enters but too little compliant resistance is felt, further assessment to identify the presence of a thoracic problem is required.

CAN'T VENTILATE:
- Repositon Head
- Manage Foreign Body Obstruction
- Consider Other Causes

VENTILATES BUT NO CHEST RISE:
- Mask Seal
- Open Pneumothorax
- Neck Breather
- Airway Misplacement

6. Once an adequate inspiratory volume has been delivered, while continuing to support the bag the operator releases his pressure on the bag—allowing it to refill and for the patient to exhale. Remember, exhalation requires a longer time than that needed for positive pressure inspiration. Careful observation of the chest is needed to identify when exhalation has been fully completed.

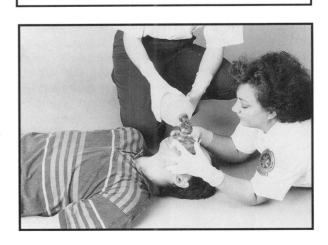

7. After providing a second breath, ventilation should be interrupted for 5–10 seconds to palpate the carotid pulse in order to determine whether continued ventilation alone or full CPR is required. After palpating the pulse, ventilation should be reinstituted.

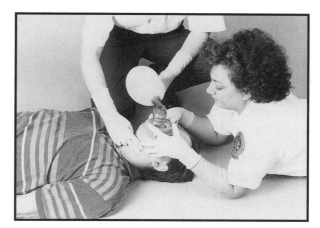

8. Often the immediate availability of an oropharyngeal airway allows for its insertion without a delay when initiating ventilation. When possible, this provides easier airway management, and supercedes the need for a manual method right from onset. If this was not possible ventilation should be interrupted after providing 5 or 6 breaths and either an oropharyngeal or nasopharyngeal airway should be inserted.

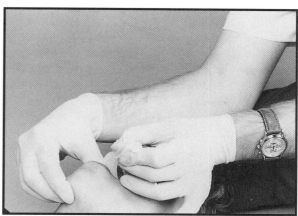

9. Except when sufficient resources allow for the preferred 2 operator use of the BVM to be continued, commonly at this point ventilation will have to be temporarily transferred to a single operator—returning to 2 operators as soon as other priorities have been met. After a simple airway adjunct has been inserted and ventilation resumed, the lungs should be auscultated bilaterally to confirm that proper pulmonary air exchange is present and to establish a baseline.

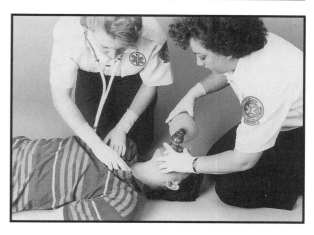

10. Once auscultation confirms that adequate air exchange is being provided, adding supplemental oxygen to provide a high FiO_2 should next be addressed. While ventilation is continued, another EMT should connect Universal Oxygen Connecting Tubing to the portable oxygen unit, open the tank, set the flow rate at 15 LPM, attach the oxygen connecting tube to the accumulator and—without interrupting the ventilation—connect the accumulator to the bag (in accordance with the specific design of that model).

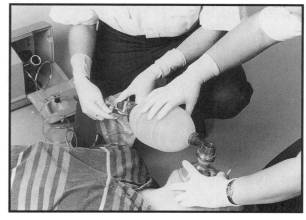

The specific method that an accumulator and supplemental oxygen attaches to the BVM varies from model to model. With most models, one end of the accumulator is designed to fasten with a pressure fit to the bag while the other end of the accumulator has a nipple to which the Universal Oxygen Supply Tubing from the oxygen source is connected. To use the accumulator of one popular model, the oxygen connecting tubing is connected directly to the BVM's oxygen nipple and the collector is attached elsewhere to the proximal end of the bag (with no externally visible connection between them). Such a separate connection in other models would result in the oxygen being connected only to the BVM—bypassing the accumulator—and would limit the FiO_2 to 0.50. To avoid the possibility that only limited or no oxygen enrichment occurs (or worse, that the BVM is rendered inoperable) due to incorrect connection, *the connections between the supply tubing and the accumulator with the BVM must be done using only the parts and in the manner prescribed for that specific model.*

The preceding demonstration has shown the correct sequence when *initiating* ventilation with a BVM in an apneic patient. Supplemental oxygen (including an accumulator) was only added after ventilation with room air and a simple airway adjunct had been established to avoid the unwarranted brief delay implicit in readying and connecting this ancillary equipment. In cases when someone at the scene is already providing Mouth-to-Mouth, Mouth-to-Shield, or Mouth-to-Mask ventilation, once the EMT has conformed that good air exchange is being effected and that a palpable pulse is present—a *slight* delay in taking over ventilation is not a problem. In such cases only, the EMT should select the correct size oropharyngeal airway, set-up the supplemental oxygen, and pre-connect it and the accumulator to the BVM so that ventilation with a high FiO_2 is immediately available when the EMT takes over the ventilations.

11. Once BVM ventilation including a simple airway adjunct, accumulator and supplemental oxygen has been provided for several minutes, if properly trained/certified personnel are present, the patient should be intubated. The EMT providing ventilations should hyperventilate the patient while the EMT who will intubate prepares the necessary equipment. When the EMT who will intubate is ready, the ventilating EMT should move to the side of the patient's head to make the area beyond the head available.

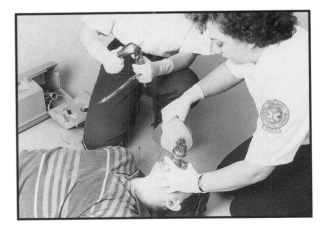

12. When so directed, the EMT providing ventilation should stop and remove the BVM from the patient's face. The mask should be left connected to the bag-valve so that ventilations can be rapidly reinstituted if the intubation attempt must be halted or if several attempts are required. The ventilating EMT should keep track of the time since the last ventilation was provided and warn the intubator if it approaches 30 seconds.

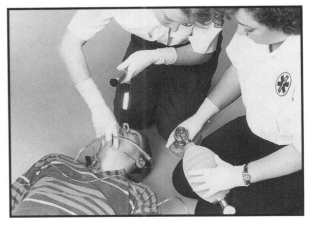

13. Once the ET tube has been inserted, the mask should rapidly be removed from the BVM and the output valve of the BVM connected to the proximal end of the ET tube. Ventilation should immediately be reinstituted. Care must be taken not to push posteriorly on the ET tube at any time, and especially while the intubator is simply holding it prior to taping it in place.

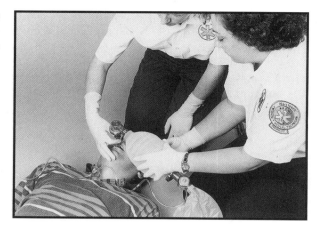

14. Whether the patient is being ventilated by use of the BVM with a mask or with it directly connected to the proximal end of an ET tube (or other advanced airway device), chest rise should be continuously visualized in order to gauge the proper provided inspiratory volume delivered. Further, the midlung fields should be periodically auscultated during ventilation to confirm that proper pulmonary air exchange continues.

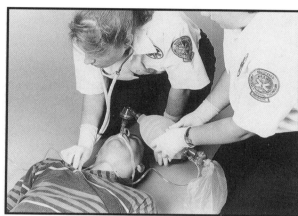

15. When ventilating **patients with suspected spine trauma** with the BVM, the same general sequence as has been demonstrated is followed except that the head needs to be carefully placed in the neutral in-line position rather than hyperextended. Manual immobilization in the neutral in-line position must be maintained without interruption throughout.

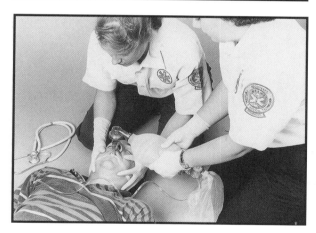

16. When it is necessary to ventilate a patient with a BVM who is being moved from bed to a cot, onto a longboard, moved down stairs, or around or through an obstacle, it is recommended that ventilation be interrupted (for not more than 30 seconds at a time) and reinstituted rather than attempting to continue ventilating during the move. Attempts to continue to ventilate during such moves usually result in a lost of mask seal and inadequate air exchange. In intubated patients maintaining the connection between the ET tube and bag-valve is difficult and can easily result in undue pressure on the ET tube which can result in its displacement. Generally such attempts cause unnecessary delay and danger, and the minute volume delivered is less than if ventilation had been interrupted by design and the patient had been hyperventilated before and after each interruption.

17. When ventilating a patient with the BVM who is on a rolling cot, the cot should be in an elevated position and wheeled so that the foot end of the cot is in front. The EMT providing BVM ventilation should be beyond the patient's head at the rear of the cot, and should direct the rate at which the cot is moved.

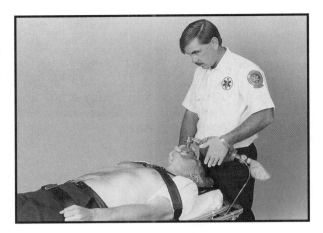

MODIFICATIONS FOR ONE-OPERATOR BAG VALVE MASK VENTILATION

Because two-operator BVM ventilation of unintubated patients can be provided with such increased reliability, it is recommended that one-operator use in such patients be limited to only those times when it is dictated by limited resources and other priorities. When initiating ventilation requires that one EMT provides airway management, BVM ventilation, and manual immobilization of the head (if indicated), a second EMT must still assume the responsibility for providing a simple airway adjunct, timely set-up and connection of the accumulator and supplement O_2, and (when indicated) intubation. The preceding sequence for *BVM Ventilation* should be used in such cases with the following modifications:

1. Due to the difficulty of attempting to do a manual airway maneuver and provide a mask seal with only one hand, a simple airway adjunct should be included from the onset. When providing a mask seal with only one hand, the thumb and first finger need to almost encircle the anterior mask completely to distribute sufficient pressure to the entire circumference of the mask. The last, or last one or two fingers must be placed around the chin so that when their tips are pressed firmly immediately below the mandible they will prevent it from sagging.

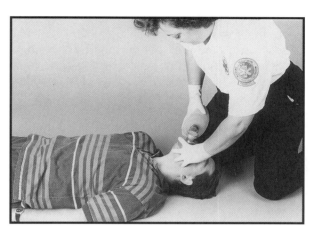

2. Depending upon the EMT's hand size, agility, and the shape and size of the bag, a sufficient inspiratory volume may not always be achieved by squeezing the bag between the thumb and the opposing fingers of one hand. Holding and squeezing it with the flat of the hand against the EMT's other forearm, rib cage, or (when kneeling) anterior thigh will provide better control and ensure a sufficient delivered volume regardless of hand size.

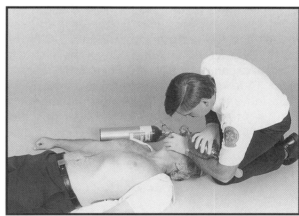

3. In such cases, when the patient is suspected of having possible *spinal trauma* as well, the single EMT providing ventilation must also maintain the head in the neutral in-line position throughout. In order to hold the head when ventilating with a BVM he will have to kneel with his knees just beyond the patient's shoulders and hold the head from moving between his lower legs and thighs. If a void exists between the occiput and the ground (or backboard) it must be filled with padding so hyperextension is not produced by the pressure needed to maintain the mask seal.

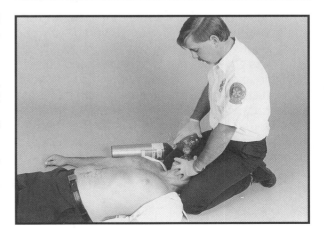

MODIFICATIONS FOR INFANT BAG VALVE MASK VENTILATION

When ventilating an infant with the BVM, an infant mask is required to produce a seal and, to assure that an excessive volume is not inadvertently delivered, an infant-sized bag should be used. When ventilating infants or small children with the BVM, the previously described method must be altered to include the generic modification necessary when providing ventilation to this age group (with any device) that have been discussed in this section's introduction. As well, the following modifications should be made when a BVM is used:

1. Due to the relatively larger head size (posterior to the spine), if a small child or infant is placed directly on a rigid surface, the head will become hyperflexed inhibiting or obstructing proper ventilation. To avoid this about 2 inches of flat padding (such as a folded blanket) needs to be placed under the entire torso to maintain the head in the neutral or mildly extended recommended position *(see Introduction).*

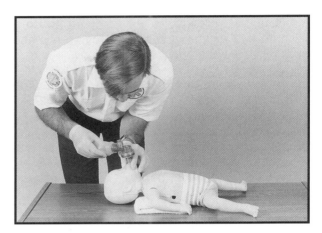

2. Infant masks are generally round and unlike adult masks, do not usually have a particular "nose" end requiring special orientation of the mask. Due to the smaller size of the mask, a mask seal can generally be obtained with a single hand. Care must be taken to avoid inadvertently pressing upon the soft palate or trachea when keeping the mandible elevated as this can obstruct the airway.

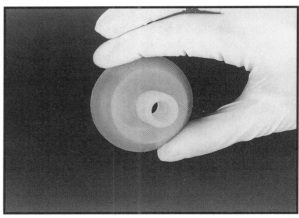

3. Due to the smaller size of the bag, an adequate volume can easily be delivered with one hand. Depressing the bag with two hands invites delivery of an excessive volume with each breath in infants and small children and should be avoided. In such patients, the volume should be less to avoid gastric insufflation, and the number of breaths per minute should be greater than for adults. Due to the smaller size of the bronchi and bronchioles the resistance felt when providing a breath will generally be greater than in an adult.

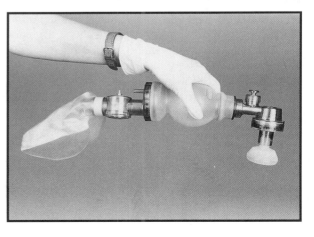

VENTILATION SKILLS **243**

MODIFICATIONS FOR PROVIDING ASSISTED VENTILATIONS WITH THE BVM

When the spontaneously breathing patient, due to an insufficient rate *or* tidal volume (usually having a too fast rate associated with it), cannot provide adequate air exchange for himself or, in the case of a small child, when the effort is producing progressive exhaustion, the EMT will have to provide "assisted ventilations" to produce an adequate minute volume. *Providing a high FiO₂ by non-rebreather reservoir mask and high flow oxygen, without intervening to restore an adequate minute volume in such cases, will result in continued hypoxia and systemic deterioration.*

1. The "feel" and control it provides makes the BVM particularly suitable for providing assisted ventilations. So that the Minute Volume produced by assisted ventilations has a high FiO₂, an accumulator and high flow oxygen should be included. When such patients are *unconscious* the same method as for ventilating an apneic patient should be followed except, if a gag reflex is present, the airway adjuncts used will have to be limited to either nasopharyngeal airway or nasotracheal intubation.

2. When such a patient is conscious and somewhat alert the procedure needs modification to minimize his fears. In such cases, unless otherwise dictated, the patient should be placed in a semi-sitting position and use of an airway adjunct avoided (until a lowered level of consciousness requires one and his tolerance increases). Volunteering to remove the BVM from the patient's face if he periodically needs this (and keeping that commitment), together with continuous assurance, will significantly allay his initial fears.

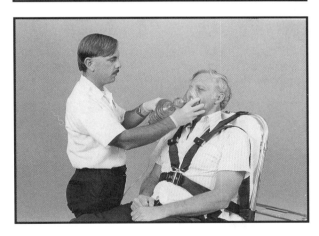

3. After explaining what you are going to do, place the mask of the assembled BVM (with an accumulator and supplemental O₂) over the patient's nose and mouth and start ventilating him with it starting at the rate and depth (even though inadequate) at which he has been breathing. Then over the next 5–10 breaths slowly incrementally adjust the rate and delivered tidal volume until an adequate minute volume has been achieved. In a conscious patient, increasing the minute volume even further to hyperventilate the patient should *NOT* be attempted. This will only contribute to his anxiety and resistance, and is unnecessary since with the high FiO₂ supplied he will be properly hyperoxygenated at a normal minute volume.

USING A DEMAND VALVE RESUSCITATOR (Oxygen-Powered, Manually Triggered Ventilators)

Demand Valve Resuscitators are oxygen-powered and, therefore, are generally found pre-connected to the regulator of a portable oxygen unit or onboard oxygen. Demand valve resuscitators emply a two stage pressure reduction system, one at the regulator and the second at the control head. The head is connected by a high pressure hose to the 50 psi Diameter Index Safety System (DISS) screw-on coupling of the regulator. The head contains a trigger button which must be depressed to activate the positive pressure inspirations and is released to allow for exhalations. Most units, have a handle which extends from the trigger button down the side of the control head which enables the operator to easily squeeze and release it while maintaining the mask seal.

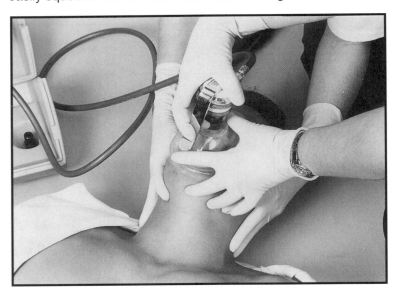

This is achieved by depressing the button located on the top of the control head with the thumb of one hand in models that do not have the preferred extension handle. At one end the plastic case of the control head is formed into an output tube providing a standard 15mm/22mm coupling for connection to a mask or to an ET tube or other advanced airway device.

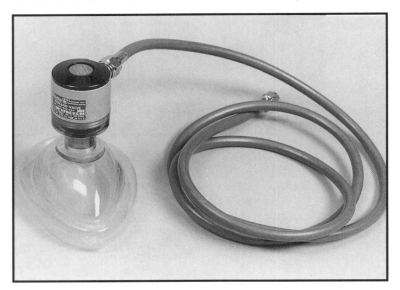

Once the oxygen source has been opened, constant supply of 100 percent oxygen at a designed flow rate of approximately 40 LPM is available at the head to provide positive pressure inspirations whenever the trigger is activated. The head also contains a one-way exhaust valve so that the patient's exhaled air is directly vented to the outside. A high pressure relief valve which opens if pressure reaches or exceeds either 60 or 80 cm H_2O is usually incorporated into the design of the head unit.

These devices also contain a demand flow system (from which their name is derived). Should spontaneous respiration return, whenever the patient's inspiration effort places negative pressure against the demand valve it opens and provides a low pressure oxygen flow even though the positive pressure trigger is not activated by the EMT. Other than when the trigger is activated to provide a positive pressure inspiration or the patient causes the opening of the demand valve by a spontaneous inspiration, no oxygen flows from the device. This conserves oxygen and prolongs the time that a single tank can be used. Many of the models currently available require an unacceptably high inspiratory pressure to open the standard valve (drawn by the patient against the valve) when they are used in a demand mode. Therefore the continued sustained use of the device in patients once spontaneous ventilation is reinstituted is not recommended.

The connection of the resuscitator's head to the high pressure outlet of the regulator separates it from any relationship to the regulator's liter flow adjustment valve (which solely controls the liter flow to the low pressure oxygen nipple). Therefore, this valve should be closed unless its simultaneous use with another patient is required.

Since the lower portion of the demand valve's head contains the exhaust valve which becomes contaminated by the patient's exhaled air, the head needs to be partially disassembled and cleaned after each use, following the manufacturers directions for that specific model. Extreme care must be taken to correctly reassemble the unit or it may not operate properly on its next use.

Most recent models, in keeping with the 1986 AHA recommendations (repeated in 1992), have a "dampening system" so that when the trigger is activated there is not an instantaneous surge of pressure. This avoids an overly rapid flow and excessive volume delivery by limiting the flow to 40L/min or less. Models without these features, provide an excessively high instantaneous flow. With the surge pressure and high flow rate that these older designs provide, gastric distention is likely and has consistently been reported as a problem associated with this device. Also, unfortunately, in most of these devices the flow rate is back pressure dependent. Either due to this (or to aging of the pressure relief system if not properly periodically serviced) they may prematurely cease to deliver oxygen as the back-pressure increases in the inspiratory phase resulting in an inadequate tidal volume being supplied.

To avoid these problems, EMTs using Demand Valve Resuscitators should be sure that all models in present use comply with the 1982 AHA recommendations and should replace those that do not. Further, there should be a regularly scheduled preventive maintenance servicing and testing program by a factory certified repair technician.

Demand Valve Resuscitators presently manufactured are solely designed for use in adults. ***These devices should NOT be used on pediatric patients (infants and children whose body has not yet reached full maturity).***

Manually triggered Demand Valve Resuscitators have been widely used in pre-hospital care for over 20 years due to their believed ease of use compared to the Bag Valve Mask Ventilator. Although activating and releasing a trigger handle while maintaining a mask seal is undeniably far easier than squeezing and releasing a bag, *providing an adequate but not excessive tidal volume* and detecting when a ventilating problem occurs is much more difficult (in the absence of the "feel" provided with a bag).

Proper ventilation with any manually activated ventilating device requires close observation of chest excursion and is an extremely difficult skill. With Demand Valve Resuscitators, an almost universal underestimation of the skill needed has resulted in a lack of sufficient initial training and a lack of sufficient supervised practice time. Proper training must include adequate emphasis on the key indications signaling the operator when timely changes between the inspiratory and expiratory phases should occur. Probably the resulting lack of proficiency has been as key a contributor to the problems associated with manually triggered devices as has the design shortcomings common to earlier models.

Safe use of a Demand Valve Resuscitator (as with any ventilating device) requires the individual to have careful initial supervised practice and a reproducible demonstrated proper level of competence, prior to using it on an actual patient. As well, it requires continued skills maintenance. Personnel who do not frequently ventilate patients should practice the skill and periodically confirm their competence with such equipment as part of a regularly scheduled continuing education program.

Safety requires that when any oxygen-powered ventilator is in use, a Bag Valve Mask (or other manually powered ventilator not requiring oxygen) be immediately available for continuing ventilation to avoid interruption to replace an empty oxygen tank or in the rare event that the ventilator or oxygen supply fails to operate properly.

Once the Universal Precautions have been taken and the decision to use the Demand Valve Resuscitator has been made:

1. Place the unit near the patient's head, open the carrying case, and remove the pre-attached head (some units also require removal of the entire regulator/tank assembly for use). Open the valve of the oxygen tank fully and check the pressure gauge on the regulator to ensure that a sufficient oxygen supply is available. Should oxygen be flowing from the low pressure nipple, turn the liter flow valve to the "off" position.

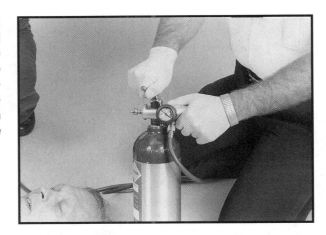

2. Next check the unit. Depress the trigger handle and confirm that a significant gas flow comes out of the unit head's outlet tube. Then, while continuing to depress the trigger, completely occlude the port at the distal end of the outlet tube. If the pressure relief valve is operating the excessive pressure caused by blocking the outlet tube will result in the gas being released from elsewhere on the unit's head. If the pressure relief valve is *NOT* operating properly, the operator's finger will be "blown" off of the port and the unit is unsafe to use.

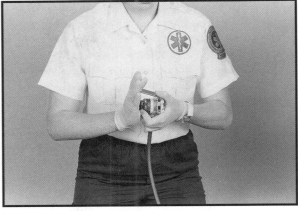

3. Once the unit has been set up and checked, select and attach a correct size mask to the output tube at the distal end of the unit's head. Next, turn the head until the trigger faces the distal half of the fingers of your dominant hand. Then rotate the mask until the nose part is properly oriented to the patient's face. From a position beyond the patient's head, place the assembled mask-head unit so that the mask properly covers the patient's mouth and nose.

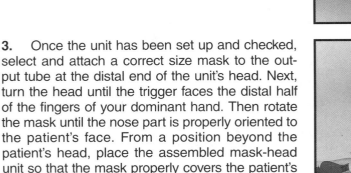

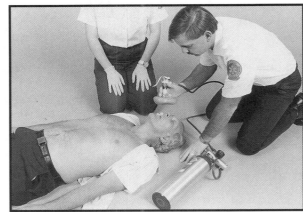

4. Obtain a mask seal by placing the thumbs and fingers of each hand so that together they cover and press against the entire outer one-half to three-quarters of an inch of the mask's anterior circumference. Hook the tips of the third (or third and fourth) fingers under the mandible to keep it elevated. Next, tilt the head (unless spine trauma is suspected) until it is hyperextended or in the forward sniffing position, and place the first finger of your dominant hand on the trigger handle.

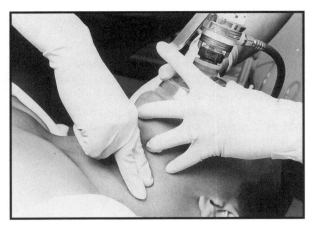

5. To provide a positive pressure inspiration depress the trigger handle (or button) with your finger. Carefully observe the chest and continue squeezing the handle until the chest is seen to rise significantly. Care must be taken to avoid delivering an excessive volume, therefore be sure you release the handle before the chest approaches it's maximum excursion capacity.

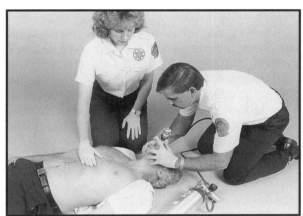

6. If the positive pressure oxygen can not enter the patient's lungs, the airway is not patent. In this case the high limit pressure valve will release, as witnessed by the rushing of oxygen from elsewhere on the unit's head and a lack of chest rise. Reposition the head and repeat the attempt to deliver a breath. If this does not work a foreign body airway obstruction must be assumed and managed. Instead, if—when the handle was pressed—the oxygen flowed normally from the unit but no or minimal chest rise was seen, a failure in the mask seal, an open pneumothorax, or a partial neckbreather must be considered and managed.

CAN'T VENTILATE:
- Repositon Head
- Manage Foreign Body Obstruction
- Consider Other Causes

VENTILATES BUT NO CHEST RISE:
- Mask Seal
- Open Pneumothorax
- Neck Breather
- Airway Misplacement

7. Once an adequate inspiratory volume has been successfully delivered, release the trigger handle. When released it automatically returns to its original "off" position and the positive pressure oxygen flow stops, allowing for exhalation. Remember that exhalation takes longer than inspiration. If proper air exchange is to occur and gastric distention avoided, the EMT must allow sufficient time for complete exhalation before the next positive pressure inspiration.

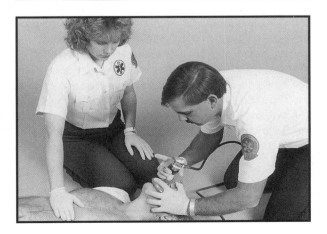

8. After exhalation has been completed again depress the trigger handle and, once the chest has been seen to rise sufficiently, release it to provide the next breath. Continue at a rate of 12 to 20 breaths/minute. While one EMT continues to ventilate the patient a second EMT should simultaneously palpate the carotid pulse. If another EMT is not available, ventilation should be interrupted after the second breath to do this. Then ventilation should be resumed and if the carotid pulse was not palpable the second EMT will have to institute chest compressions.

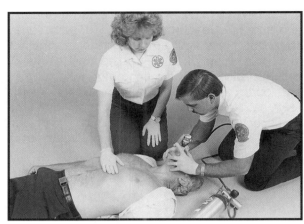

9. The immediate availability of an oropharyngeal airway usually allows for its insertion while the Demand Valve Resuscitator is readied for use, avoiding the need of manual airway maneuvers from onset. If this was not possible, ventilation should be interrupted after five or six ventilations have been successfully delivered, a properly sized oropharyngeal airway should be inserted, and then ventilation should be resumed.

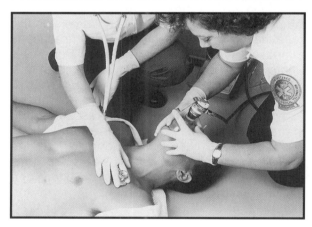

10. After a simple airway adjunct has been inserted and ventilation with the Demand Valve Resuscitator has been resumed, the patient's chest should be auscultated bilaterally to assure that proper pulmonary air exchange is indeed being effected, and to establish a baseline.

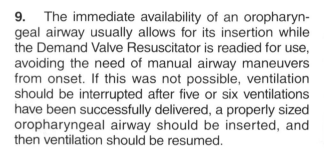

11. Once successful ventilations have been provided for several minutes, and if properly trained/certified EMTs are present and available, the patient should be intubated. While one EMT prepares the necessary intubation equipment the EMT providing ventilations should hyperventilate the patient. When the second EMT is ready, the ventilating EMT should move to the side of the head making the area beyond the head available while continuing to ventilate the patient.

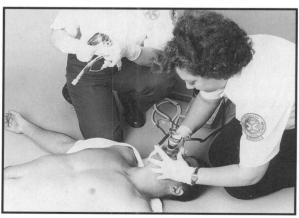

12. When the ventilator is directed to stop, he should remove the mask/head unit from the patient's face and keep track of the time from the last inspiration delivered. The mask should be left on the unit's head so that ventilation can be reinstituted if needed prior to successful intubation. Once the patient has been intubated the mask should be rapidly removed, the outlet tube of the unit's head connected directly to the adaptor at the proximal end of the ET tube, and ventilation resumed.

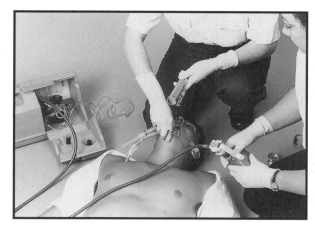

13. Once chest rise is observed and the ET cuff inflated, proper placement should be confirmed by auscultation over the epigastrum and each midlung field. During the continued ventilation of any patient the chest excursion should be continuously visualized to evaluate whether proper inspiratory and expiratory exchange is occurring, and the midlung fields should be periodically auscultated to confirm the maintenance of good pulmonary air exchange. The addition of pulse oximetry as well is highly recommended.

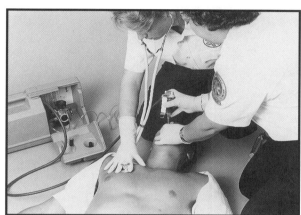

14. When ventilating suspected spine trauma patients with a Demand Valve Resuscitator the same general sequence as has been shown should be followed, except that the patient's head should initially be placed in the neutral in-line position and then immobilized in that position throughout.
Ventilating patients when moving them onto a backboard or cot, and when moving the cot, should follow the same guidelines as presented in steps 16 and 17 for use of the BVM.

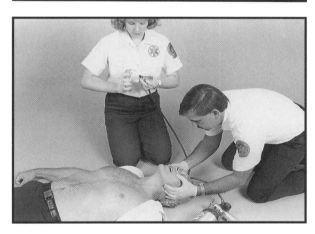

15. If at any time spontaneous ventilation resumes, remove your finger from the trigger handle and carefully maintain the mask seal. A proper seal is necessary for the patient's inspiratory effort to produce the negative pressure needed to open the demand valve and provide a low pressure oxygen flow during spontaneous inspiration. Due to the increased inspiratory effort and continued maintenance of a mask seal required in the demand mode, such use should be replaced with high flow oxygen by non-rebreather reservoir mask as rapidly as possible.

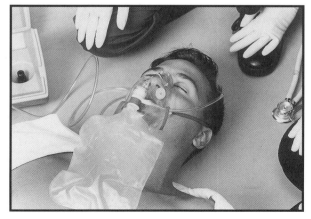

16. After each use, since the mask, one-way valve and distal portion of the unit's head have been contaminated by the patient's exhaled air, they need to be cleaned, sterilized, and properly re-assembled. As needed the other parts should be cleaned and the oxygen pressure checked. Tanks with less than 500 psi remaining (or with a higher pressure if so dictated by local protocals) should be replaced with a full tank. Lastly, before storing the unit, the EMT should make sure that the tank has been properly closed, that any pressure has been bled off, and that the unit is ready for its next use.

USING AN AUTOMATIC TRANSPORT VENTILATOR (ATV)

Automatic Transport Ventilators are small portable oxygen or electric powered ventilators which function similarly to larger in-hospital respirators. Once properly set an ATV automatically delivers a selected tidal volume with an FiO_2 of $0.85-1.00$ over a set inspiratory time, at a given number of breaths per minute and with a given expiratory time in between, without any manual action required by the EMT to produce inspirations or to change from the inspiratory to the expiratory phase. When used with a standard mask an ATV allows the EMT to focus his efforts solely upon continued maintenance of the airway and mask seal, and when used with an intubated patient it frees the EMT to provide for other urgent care priorities.

As with any ventilator (manual or automatic, whether used with a mask, ET tube, or other advanced airway device), chest rise should be continuously monitored and proper pulmonary air exchange confirmed by periodic auscultation over the midlung fields and epigastrium.

A common concern with a time-cycled device surrounds the integration of chest compressions with the ventilations when giving CPR. This concern is unwarranted as, with practice, one can interpose compressions between the delivered breaths without a problem.

The design, operation, and safety mechanisms of each ATV model are different, and only factory matched components can be safely used together. With most brands the control box and patient valve head have been carefully adjusted to work properly as a pair. EMS services with more than one unit of the same model should not interchange these, as this can result in improper or unsafe operation. Due to the differences in operation from one model to the next, the following skills presentation should solely be interpreted as a general guideline. ***For safety, the set up and use of any specific ATV should only be attempted by properly trained and qualified personnel following the manufacturer's specific instructions strictly.*** Any elections left to individual medical judgment should follow local protocols or specific direction from the squad's Medical Director.

Most ATVs are made up of 5 separable parts:

- 1 Control Module (generally a small rectangular box)
- 1 Patient Valve Head
- 2 High pressure oxygen supply hoses with DISS screw-on couplings
- 1 Specially threaded oxygen power hose (or electrical power cord)

The Control Module of the ATV is connected to the high pressure (50psi) outlet of a standard approved medical oxygen regulator by a high pressure oxygen line with Diameter Indexed Safety System (DISS) screw couplings at each end. When the ATV is to be connected to a quick-connect wall unit, a hose with such a connection at one end and a male DISS screw coupling at the other is used instead. The Control Module is generally attached to the Patient Valve head with two connecting hoses. The line supplying oxygen for patient use to the head is a standard high pressure oxygen hose with DISS couplings. The second hose provides oxygen to activate the head and is uniquely threaded to assure proper assembly.

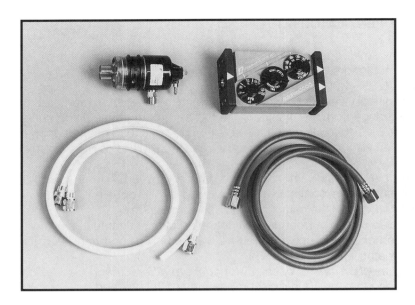

All connections should only be firmly hand tightened since the use of wrenches may result in damage to the parts. Parts can only be safely connected or disconnected when the oxygen tank is closed and all pressure has been bled off. All parts should be pre-connected and the Control Module and Patient Valve Head stored fully assembled to the regulator and oxygen tank so that the ATV is ready for immediate use.

In order to avoid contaminating the one-way valve in the distal end of the Patient Valve Head, an optional additional short flexible hose which is connected to a one-way valve can be added to the output tube of the head (in models allowing this), eliminating the need and danger of disassembling the lower head for proper cleaning after use.

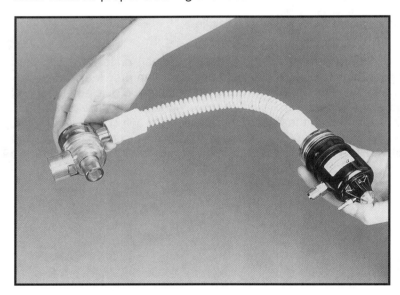

The Control Module, as the name implies, contains the control knobs used to set the devices functions. One control sets the number of breaths per minute (rate). Although different models have a different variety of possible settings, this generally ranges from 8 to 28 breaths per minute. A "0" or off setting is also included and when the device is set to it, no automatic time-cycling or ventilation occurs.

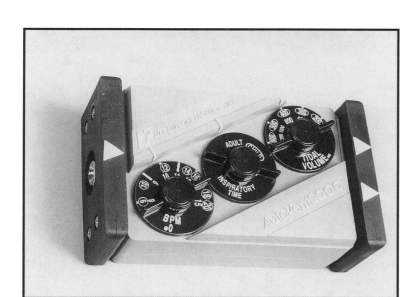

A second control determines the tidal volume to be delivered at each inspiration. Although different models have a variety of possible settings, this generally ranges from 200 to 1200 ml/breath. In some models the inspiratory time (time over which the inspiratory tidal volume is delivered) is pre-set to an average time compatible to adults and larger children (approximately 1.5−2 seconds). Some models contain a third control for setting the inspiratory time either to "adult" (1.5−2 seconds) or to "child" (0.75−1 second). On most models with such a control, when set at "adult" the maximum inspiratory flow rate is limited to about 30 LPM and when it is set to "child" this is lowered to a maximum of about 15 LPM.

In units with such a third control, the inspiratory time should always be set before the tidal volume and rate are set on the other control knobs. If the inspiratory time knob is adjusted after the initial set-up, in most such models it will alter the delivered Breaths Per Minute and Tidal Volume, which may be dangerous.

Because some models do not allow for the shorter inspiratory times or lowered maximum flow rates necessary for small children, *many currently available models should not be used in children under 5 years of age or those with a kilogram weight less than that specified for that particular model.* If the EMT is uncertain as to the specific age/weight under which the model he is using cannot be safely used, he should use a BVM instead when ventilating any child who appears to have a body size less than that of a ten year old.

The Patient Valve head connects to the two oxygen hoses coming from the Control Module, and has an outlet tube with the standard 15mm/22mm diameters at its distal end which allows for connection to a mask, ET tube, or other advanced airway. (If an optional extension tube and second one-way valve are to be used the extension tube is connected to the port of this outlet tube, and the mask to the second one-way valve at the distal end of the extension tube.) The Patient Valve head contains a high pressure audible alarm and, in its lower end, a one-way valve which provides direct communication to the outside for the patient's exhaled air.

With most ATVs the build-up of excessive pharyngeal pressure is guarded against by two or three progressively drastic safeguards. In the event that too high a tidal volume is being delivered or that oxygen entrapment (due to insufficient exhalation) occurs when the patient's airway pressure meets or exceeds about 50cm H_2O, an audible pressure limit alarm located in the Patient Valve head will sound until the pressure decreases or the machine cycles into the expiratory phase.

In most models a high pressure valve which is set when the unit is initially put in service limits the pressure to either 60cm or 80cm H_2O. Most models also contain a back-up device which, should this valve fail to limit the pressure to the 60cm or 80cm H_2O, will blow-off at a pressure of between 90−100cm H_2O—relieving the pressure to the outside and making the unit thereafter inoperable (or at best unreliable) until it has been serviced and checked by a factory authorized service center.

The Patient Valve Head of most ATVs also contain a "demand" feature like that previously described with Demand Valve Resuscitators. Should spontaneous ventilation return the patient can obtain a sufficient liter flow of low pressure oxygen when he produces negative pressure against the valve by "drawing in" air during inspiration as long as the mask seal is maintained. Should spontaneous ventilation resume, the time-cycled positive pressure is stopped by turning the Breaths/Minute control to the "off" or "0" setting. This will stop the automatic cycling but (in models which include it) will not turn off the demand flow feature. Due to the additional inspiratory effort required and the need to maintain a mask seal, this feature should not be used for a sustained period. Instead, it should be replaced by delivery of high flow supplemental oxygen using a non-rebreather reservoir mask.

The correct setting for the Tidal Volume Control will vary from patient to patient based upon the individual's lung capacity—which is mainly determined by his body size. If the tidal volume setting is inadequate at a normal number of breaths/minute, it will result in an inadequate minute volume and continued hypoxia. Regardless of rate, if the tidal volume setting is excessive it will result in increased airway pressure and gastric insufflation.

Although a Tidal Volume setting of 80ml will be appropriate for most adults, a setting calculated for the size of the individual adult is preferred (and for children is required). The correct tidal volume recommended by the AHA to maintain proper lung inflation is between 10ml and 15ml for each kg of body weight. By multiplying the patient's weight by each of these rapidly, the range of appropriate tidal volume can be calculated. (Adding a zero after the patient's kilogram weight produces the number of milliliters at 10 ml/kg, and adding half again as much to it, the number of milliliters at 15 ml/kg.) For example, if the patient weights 75kg, the tidal volume needed will be between 750ml and 1075ml. The highest setting options which falls between these should be selected as the initial setting for the Tidal Volume Control. If this calculated setting results in delivery of too high a tidal volume for the patient, excessive chest rise will be seen and the audible high pressure alarm will sound at the end part of the inspiratory cycle. In such cases the Tidal Volume Control should be set to the next lower setting (and so on if necessary). When lowering the tidal volume setting, care must be taken to avoid moving it below the low end of the range for the patient's weight so that, at the number of breaths selected on the other Control, a sufficient minute volume is still provided.

Since the minute volume is determined by both the number of breaths per minute and the tidal volume, in setting these separate controls the EMT must keep this relationship in mind. Once the patient's tidal volume has been calculated and that control set, then the desired rate needs to be determined and the Breaths Per Minute (BPM) Control set accordingly. The number of breaths per minute selected must be of a sufficient number that when the set tidal volume is multiplied by it, a minute volume equal or greater than that required to provide adequate blood gases is provided.

Because the ATV is used with patients who are apneic and have had sustained hypoxia, a minute volume in the high end of the normal range or moderately higher (greater than 8,000ml/min in adults) is desired. It must be noted that no additional benefit has been demonstrated by providing extremely high minute volumes when compared to those only at the high end of the normal range or moderately higher, and that rates over 20/minute which commonly do not allow sufficient exhalation time) and maximal tidal volumes commonly cause increased airway pressure and gastric insufflation. Therefore a moderate rather than extreme increase in minute volume is recommended. Since the ATV provides an FiO_2 of 0.85 to 1.00 in either its time-cycled ventilator or demand mode, the patient will be desirably hyperoxygenated when an adequate minute volume is present.

Unless otherwise dictated by a special need, the Breaths Per Minute (BPM) Control should be set between 10 and 16 breaths/minute in adults, and (as indicated by the child's size/age) slightly higher for children. Once ventilation with the ATV has been initiated, the EMT should confirm that enough time is allowed to complete exhalation by observing chest excursion and by auscultating during several full cycles.

Since the inspiratory duration remains constant regardless of other settings (except that in some models one constant duration can be set for adults and another for children), the greater the number of breaths per minute selected the shorter the time available for exhalation (the time between the end of one inspiratory cycle and the commencement of the next). Therefore, if a rate is selected which does not allow adequate time to complete exhalation, the Breaths Per Minute setting will have to be reduced to a lower setting which will still provide for a sufficient minute volume. If this fails to correct the problem recheck the tidal volume to ensure that it is not too high for the patient's needs—needlessly increasing the expiratory volume and time required to complete exhalation.

When the ATV is to be used in conjunction with CPR, the ventilatory rate is dictated by the need to coordinate ventilations with chest compressions delivered at a proper number per minute. For adult CPR, the Breaths Per Minute Control should be set at 12/minute, and for children under 8 at 20/minute. When chest compressions are being performed, exhalation is "actively" produced with the first compression after each breath, and leaving sufficient time for full exhalation is no longer a factor.

Although the ATV's oxygen consumption is dependent upon the number of Breaths Per Minute and the Tidal Volume settings selected, the ATV should run on a full "E" tank for about 45 minutes. When used with an ATV, partially depleted "D" or "E" tanks should be replaced with completely full ones after each use regardless of the remaining tank pressure.

As a consideration of weight, most portable EMS oxygen equipment is only designed to include a single tank. With an ATV (particularly in areas where longer than usual sustained use before reaching the ambulance is often dictated by the rescue situation) double-yoked two tank portable equipment is recommended. If the rescue environment prohibits such weight for a single rescuer, the weight of the oxygen tanks can be distributed by having one EMT carry the ATV with only a single tank connected to the two-yoke regulator, an empty tank can be removed and replaced while the ATV continues its operation on the second tank without interruption.

The ATV, being an automated machine, will provide ventilations with more consistent volumes and timing than could a human operator using a non-automated ventilator as long as a proper mask-seal or other airway seal is maintained and a proper oxygen supply is available.

If airway patency is lost, or if the ATV is set at too high a Tidal Volume or at a rate not allowing for sufficient exhalation, the audible alarm will alert the EMT when the airway pressure builds, so that he can rectify the problem. If the machine is set at a combination of Tidal Volume and Breaths Per Minute that is adequate or if the mask or airway seal are lost (repeatedly or for any sustained period), the machine will methodically continue its time-cycled operation without alarm or adjustment—resulting in continuing inadequate ventilation of the patient. Similarly, regardless of its settings even when it is initially operating properly, a loss of adequate oxygen supply or a mechanical failure can result in the delivery of an inadequate rate or volume without any obvious malfunction or notice by the machine.

Without either the "feel" provided with the BVM, or the constant attention required with manually triggered ventilators, the continuance of proper automated ventilation must never be assumed. Chest excursion must be continuously observed without fail to ensure the maintenance of an adequate rate and delivered volume and periodically the chest should be auscultated to ensure proper pulmonary air exchange continues. The addition of pulse oximetry to confirm adequate oxygenation cannot be too highly recommended. *Reliance on the continued provision of adequate proper ventilation without continuous monitoring of chest excursion and periodic checking of bilateral breath sounds and signs of adequate cellular oxygenation is dangerous and can result in the patient's death.*

When initiating the use of the ATV (opening the oxygen tank, setting the ATV's controls carefully, and checking that the machine's gas delivery and high pressure alarm are functioning properly) requires more than 30 seconds. *Therefore, when an ATV is to be used, ventilation should first be initiated using a Bag Valve Mask or Mouth-to-Mask device until the ATV is properly set up and ready for use.* Safety also requires that either a BVM or Mouth-to-Mask device be immediately available at all times should the ATV, oxygen source, or electrical power (in electric models) fail.

Once the proper Universal Precautions have been taken and the initial Global "size-up" of the patient has shown him to be apneic:

1. Immediately direct the initiation of ventilation with a BVM or Mouth-to-Mask device. Insert a properly sized oropharyngeal airway and check for a palpable carotid pulse to identify or rule-out the need for chest compressions. To ensure that proper ventilation is being provided and to establish a baseline, auscultate each midlung field during several provided ventilations.

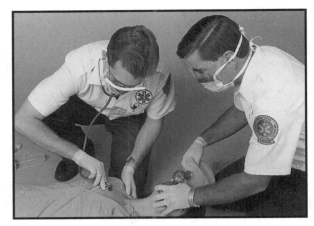

2. Once assured that proper ventilation is being provided and that any other immediate priority has been provided for or ruled out, place the portable oxygen/ATV case near the patient's head. Open it and remove the ATV Control Module and Patient Valve Head. Check that they have been properly preassembled to the regulator/oxygen source and that none of the connecting hoses are loose or kinked.

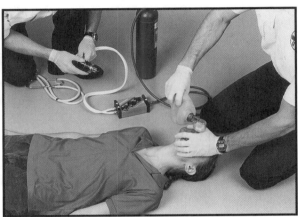

3. Slowly open the oxygen tank with the key and check that the reading on the pressure gauge reflects a full or near full tank. Check that the Liter Flow Control on the regulator is at the "off" or "0" setting to avoid any wasted oxygen flow through the low pressure nipple—which will not be used at this point. This valve does not control or effect the oxygen flow from the regulator's high pressure DISS connection to which the ATV's supply hose is connected.

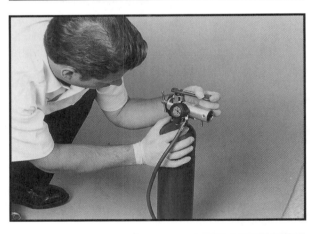

4. If the model is so equipped, set the *Inspiratory Time Control* knob to the appropriate "adult" or "child" setting (or 1.5–2 seconds for an adult or 0.75–1 second for a child). In models that have such a control this will determine the duration and maximum Liter flow delivered at each inspiration. Models without such a control are pre-set to an average for use with either a child or adult. This increases as the minimum size of child below which the unit should not be used.

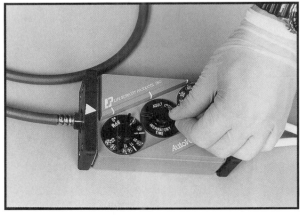

5. Estimate/obtain the patient's weight. Multiply it both by 10 and 15 ml/kg to calculate the appropriate range of tidal volume for that patient. Set the *Tidal Volume Control* knob at the highest or near highest setting available on that model within this calculated tidal volume range.

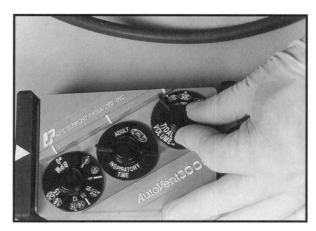

6. Next, set the *Breaths Per Minute Control* knob at the desired rate for the patient's category (adult or child) and situation (the rate for CPR if indicated, or the rate selected for ventilation without CPR). Multiply the selected number of breaths/minute by the selected Tidal Volume to be sure that the resulting minute volume delivered will be in the upper range or just moderately higher than the normal minute volume required for proper ventilation of a patient of this size/age.

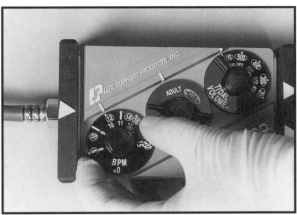

7. Once each of the unit's controls has been set and the ATV has started its cycled operation, place your hand near the Patient Valve Head's outlet tube for several cycles. Confirm that a positive pressure flow of gas can be felt during the inspiratory phase and that it stops flowing during the expiratory phase. This should indicate that proper time-cycled operation appears to be occurring.

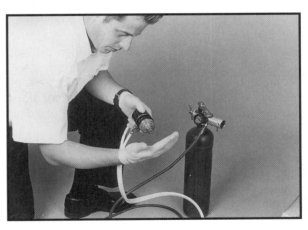

8. Next, move your hand so that you occlude the port at the distal end of the Patient Valve Head's outlet tube. With it completely occluded the audible Pressure Limit Alarm should sound continuously throughout the inspiratory phase, stopping only when the ATV cycles to the expiratory phase. Continue this for a small part of the next inspiratory cycle. The audible alarm should stop sounding immediately when the high pressure in the inspiratory cycle is relieved by the removal of your hand from the output tube.

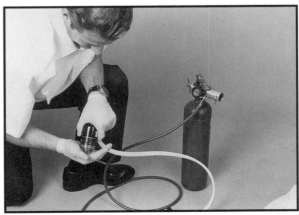

9.   After checking that the ATV's time-cycled positive pressure and high pressure alarm functions are operating properly, install a proper size mask onto the Patient Valve Head's outlet tube. Direct the EMT providing ventilation to stop and remove the BVM. After checking that apnea is still present, place the mask attached to the ATV's Patient Valve Head over the patient's nose and mouth, and have the EMT positioned beyond the patient's head provide a mask seal, head-tilt (unless spine trauma) and elevation of the mandible with both of his hands.

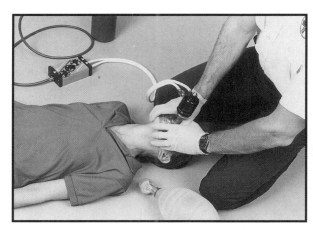

10.   As the machine automatically time-cycles, alternating between providing positive pressure inspirations and stopping to allow for exhalations, carefully observe chest excursion to check that the inspiratory chest rise is adequate but not maximal and that exhalation appears complete before the start of the next inspiratory cycle.

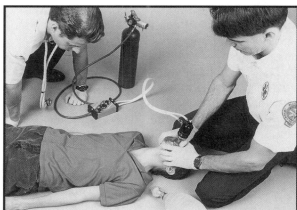

11.   *If the Pressure Limit Alarm sounds at or near the commencement of the* inspiratory phase, the airway is not patent. Reposition the head so that there is slightly more hyperextension and see if the problem is alleviated or if the audible alarm sounds again during the next cycle's inspiratory phase—indicating that it has not been resolved.

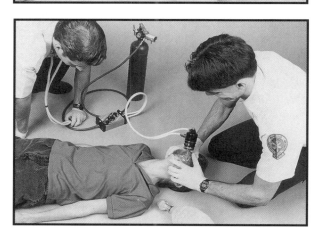

12.   If you are unable to clear the problem, and because the success of the previous BVM ventilation *denies a pre-existing airway obstruction,* revert back to use of the BVM. If the problem persists follow the obstructed airway procedures and, once cleared, reinstitute use of the ATV. If it only occurs when using the ATV, assume that there is a mechanical problem with the ATV and continue ventilation with the BVM adding the accumulator and high flow oxygen as time allows. In such rare cases, the ATV in question should be checked by a properly authorized mechanic after the call, before being placed back in service.

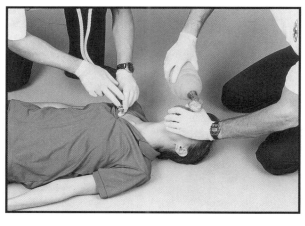

13. *If the Pressure Limit Alarm sounds ONLY near the end peak of the inspiratory phase,* the Tidal Volume setting is too high and an excessive inspiratory volume is being provided. Reset the Tidal Volume Control knob to the next lower setting (then the one beyond that, if necessary, etc.) until the alarm no longer sounds at any time during the inspiratory phase. In the rare case that the Tidal Volume Setting had to be reduced 2 or 3 settings, the EMT may have to increase the number of Breaths Per Minute setting in order to still provide an adequate Minute Volume.

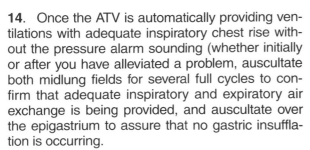

14. Once the ATV is automatically providing ventilations with adequate inspiratory chest rise without the pressure alarm sounding (whether initially or after you have alleviated a problem, auscultate both midlung fields for several full cycles to confirm that adequate inspiratory and expiratory air exchange is being provided, and auscultate over the epigastrium to assure that no gastric insufflation is occurring.

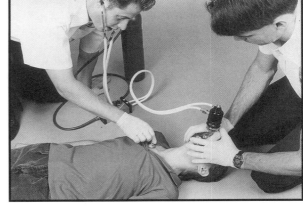

15. Once you have confirmed that the ATV is properly ventilating the patient, the machine's automatic timing should be checked. Using your watch, time the inspiratory phase's duration. It should equal the manufacturer's pre-set inspiration time (ie: 1.5 to 2.0 seconds) or, in models that have an Inspiratory Time setting, between 1.5 and 2.0 seconds if set at "adult," or, if set at "child" between 0.75 and 1.0 second. Next, *time the number of breaths delivered in one minute* to assure that this matches the rate at which the ATV/BPM Control has been set.

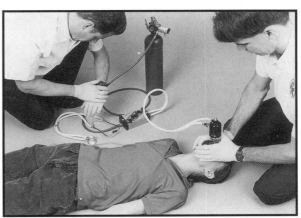

16. After ventilations have been provided for several minutes and properly trained/certified personnel are present and available, ventilation should be interrupted and the patient intubated. Once the ET tube has been successfully inserted the mask should be removed from the ATV's Patient Valve Head, and the Head attached directly to the universal adaptor at the ET tube's proximal end. Confirm proper placement and continued ventilation by observing chest rise and by auscultating over the epigastrium and each midlung field. Finally, secure the ET tube.

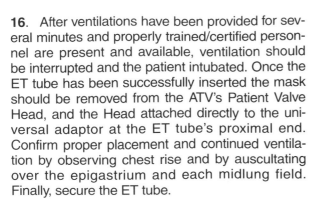

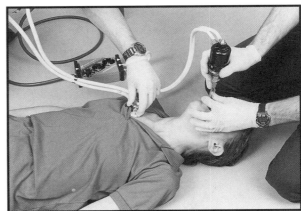

17. Continually monitor chest excursion and periodically re-auscultate to confirm that proper ventilation continues. Periodically check the oxygen regulator's pressure gauge to determine the remaining available oxygen. *Change tanks before the pressure is below the minimum safe pressure indicated by the manufacturer.* With a single-yoke unit, ventilation with a BVM is required while the tank is shut off and changed. Once ATV ventilation with the new tank is resumed, recheck all ATV settings and clinically reconfirm adequate patient ventilation.

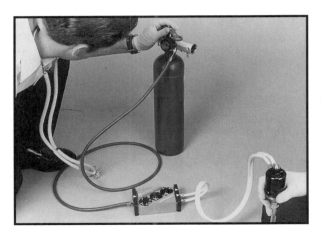

18. *When ventilating a patient with suspected spine trauma,* the preceding sequence for use of the ATV should be followed, except the head should first be immediately placed into the neutral in-line position and manually immobilized without lapse until it is mechanically immobilized to a rigid device. Early on, any padding needed to fill a void between the posterior head and the rigid surface on which the patient is lying should be inserted to avoid inadvertent hyperextension from the pressure required to maintain the mask seal.

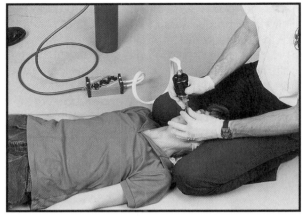

19. After each use, if a disposable one way valve and extension tube have been used, they should be discarded in a proper bio-waste container. If not, the one-way valve and distal portion of the head need to be disassembled, cleaned, sterilized, and carefully and properly re-assembled. As needed, the other parts of the ATV should be cleaned and the tank, regardless of the amount used, replaced with a completely full one. After replacing the tank, set the Tidal Volume Control at 800ml and the Breaths Per Minute Control at 12 (and if controllable, the Inspiratory Time at "adult" or "2 seconds"). Then check the ATV's function for several cycles. Lastly, close the tank, bleed-off any line pressure and set all of the controls to "0" or off before putting the unit away—ready to use.

VENTILATING PATIENTS WHO HAVE HAD A TRACHEOSTOMY

Some patients have had a tracheostomy—a surgical procedure which creates a stoma —that provides an alternate airway through the neck and into the trachea through which they breathe. In most of these, the trachea no longer communicates with the pharynx—making the patient a *complete neck breather.* In some cases some communication has been left resulting in the patient only being a *partial neck breather.* Regardless, patients who have had a tracheostomy, when indicated, need to be ventilated through a stoma in their neck rather than through their mouth or nose. The stoma is found generally just cephalad of the supra sternal notch. It may or may not have a flanged short metal or plastic airway in place through it. To ventilate:

1. Place the patient supine on a firm surface and remove any neck cravat or other garment which may be worn over the stoma as a dust filter. Place a folded towel under the neck and shoulders to cause maximal hyperextension of the head in order to produce as straight a line between the chest and the anterior neck as possible, and to move the chin out of the way. With either a child or Seal-Easy Mask mounted on the BVM, place the unit so that the mask is centered over the stoma. When a child mask is used the flat (chin) end of the mask should be on the uppermost chest and the more tented nose end of the mask over the anterior neck—pointing towards the patient's head.

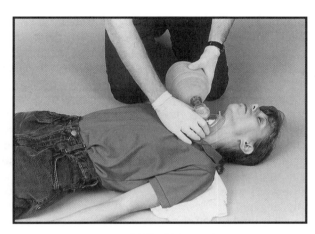

2. From aside the patient's neck, hold the mask with one hand so that your thumb is over one side of the mask and two fingers are over the other. If two operators are available, one provides a seal with one hand on each side of the mask, instead. Finally, press posteriorly until the cuff sides are pushed down onto the anterior lateral sides of the neck and a seal is obtained against the neck and chest. Then institute ventilation and, as soon as resources allow, add the accumulator and high flow oxygen to the BVM.

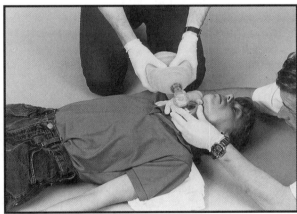

3. In partial neck breathers, since the trachea still communicates with the pharynx, some of the air provided at inspiration will escape through the mouth and nose unless they are sealed. In such cases one EMT is needed to maintain the mask seal and provide ventilation and a second, to seal the mouth and nose. The second EMT positioned alongside the upper thorax should pinch the nostril shut between his thumb and fingers while sealing the mouth with the palm of his other hand during each inspiratory phase. The nostrils should be released and the mouth uncovered during exhalation to facilitate the expiration of a proper volume to avoid air entrapment.

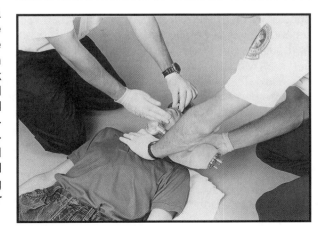

ALS

EMERGENCY "NEEDLE" TRACHEOSTOMY AND PERCUTANEOUS TRANSTRACHEAL VENTILATION (PTV)

Patients who have a fully obstructed airway that cannot be cleared after sustained efforts (including both abdominal thrusts and direct laryngoscopy), *or* who have such extensive maxiofacial or upper airway injury that ventilation by mask or endotracheal intubation is impossible, require ventilation through an alternate pathway. In such cases an emergency tracheostomy must be rapidly performed to provide an opening through the neck into the trachea and provide direct communication between the trachea and the outside. A tracheostomy can be performed by surgical methods, making an incision through the outside of the neck and tracheal wall and inserting a transtracheal airway tube—or more rapidly and easily—by the insertion of a large bore needle or catheter.

A tracheostomy and transtracheal ventilation should only be elected pre-hospital when all other methods of providing a patent airway and ventilation have proven unsuccessful. Transtracheal procedures should only be performed by advanced EMTs who have practiced the procedure in a controlled supervised laboratory environment, have demonstrated their ability to perform it to a proper level of competence to their Medical Director, and when their certificaion and protocols allow.

Performing a *surgical* tracheostomy requires considerably more time than does a *needle* tracheostomy. Since a pre-hospital tracheostomy is only indicated in patients after all other attempts to obtain a patent airway and successful ventilation have failed, a significant delay has already occurred and the additional time required to do this procedure and initiate ventilation is a significant factor in determining outcome. The safe performance of a surgical tracheostomy requires a relatively clean environment, significant training and skill, and a continued high frequency of practice. Even an EMT in an area with a high call rate will rarely need to perform a tracheostomy more than once a year (if that often).

It must be noted however that surgical tracheostomies provide a true airway analagous to the size provided by an endotracheal tube, whereas needle tracheostomies provide only a very limited opening and a significantly lower than normal air exchange even with the largest bore needle. It was earlier believed that ventilation through a needle only provided the minimum oxygenation required to sustain life, and that the restricted expiratory ability through such a small opening would result in CO_2 retention and—over 30 to 45 minutes—a significant build up in blood CO_2 levels. Recent studies have shown that—contrary to the reduced gas exchange and CO_2 retention implied by the diminutive airway furnished through the small lumen of a large bore needle—when this procedure incorporates the proper ventilation method, near normal blood oxygen and CO_2 levels can be maintained even for several hours if necessary.

In the interest of minimizing the delay until ventilation is provided and assuring safe levels of skills maintenance, *the pre-hospital use of needle rather than surgical tracheostomies is recommended.* Since the use of surgical methods is limited to a very small number of advanced EMTs, the skills for performing a surgical tracheostomy have not been included in this text. Neither the previous recommendation nor this exclusion should be misinterpreted as implying that the pre-hospital performance of a surgical tracheostomy is inherently unsafe or contraindicated and without benefit. Rather, it reflects a consideration of the risk-to-benefit associated with frequency of use and the maintenance of skills competency levels generally practical for most advanced EMS services. in areas where not excluded by law or regulation, whether needle or surgical tracheostomies are to be performed remains a decision for the service's Medical Director.

Similarly, whether or not a commercial tracheostomy kit which requires some incision is to be used must be determined by local regulations and the service's Medical Director. Instead of a needle, these kits generally contain a larger needle-like tube through which a sharp pointed shaft called a trocar is placed to facilitate its insertion through the tracheal wall without any surgical opening into the trachea first being provided. Once the tube is inserted into the trachea and the trocar is removed, a ventilator can be fastened to the tube's proximal end. The opening provided by this tube is of a sufficiently large diameter, to allow for ventilation as with any other endotracheal airway. If such a device is to be used, training and use of the device should follow the directions for that specific kit and not the following guidelines for a needle tracheostomy.

When performing a needle tracheostomy the needle is either inserted into the trachea through the crychothyroid membrane (why it is often referred to as a crychothyrotomy) or through the anterior wall of the trachea near its midline. A short 10 gauge emergency tracheal needle, or the more usually available large bore (12, 14, or 16 gauge) over-the-needle IV catheter can be used. The hub found at the proximal end of these IV catheters does not match a common standard for connection to ventilating equipment (since these are primarily designed for another use). Therefore, some form of tubing will be needed that will fit snugly to avoid leakage in or over the hub and whose other end can be readily connected to the ventilation source.

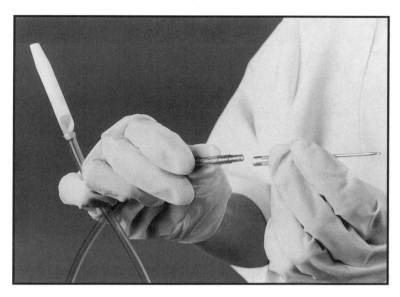

In some protocols, once the over-the-needle catheter has been inserted into the trachea and the needle removed from it, or alternately a 10g. tracheal needle has been inserted, it is connected by tubing to a Bag Valve Mask ventilator. This connection is most easily made by removing the plunger of a 10–30 ml syringe and inserting a #6 to #8 cuffed ET tube two-thirds of the way into the barrel. When the ET tube cuff is inflated it will produce a seal with the syringe barrel, and the BVM can be connected to the ET tube's proximal end.

Although a greater inspiratory and even more extended expiratory time is needed, ventilation is provided with the BVM in the otherwise normal manner.

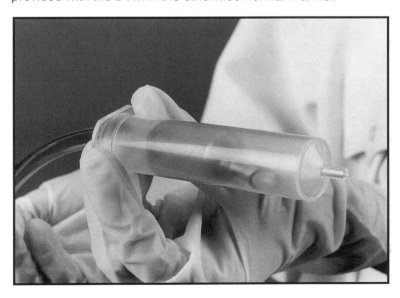

If this method is used, a slow gentle squeezing of the bag will produce a greater inspiratory volume than would result from attempts to force oxygen through the needle with high pressure. Due to the lack of study and scientific proof that this method of ventilation through a needle/catheter provides adequate air exchange to maintain normal or near normal blood gases, until further study, it cannot be recommended except in situations where no other alternative is readily available.

Instead ventilation through a needle is recommended using equipment that allows for alternating delivery of oxygen at 15 LPM directly from the low pressure supplemental oxygen nipple for inspiration with stoppage of the oxygen flow to allow for exhalation. Recent studies have shown that when patients with a needle tracheostomy are ventilated using this method, adequate oxygenation without CO_2 build-up has been provided for an hour or more, (exceeding even the longest run-times common to most EMS systems) and normal blood gases have been maintained.

Although it would seem that a greater volume would be provided through a narrow aperture with a higher rather than lower pressure, this is not ture. As any trained firefighter can attest, raising the pump pressure beyond a given level results in reduced rather than an increased volume being delivered through the small opening in the nozzle. The same principles apply when forcing a gas through a narrow opening such as the relatively small lumen of a tracheal needle or catheter. At a 15 LPM flow rate through a needle, a pressure of about 20–30 psi is produced which maximizes the volume that is delivered through so small an opening, and which, based upon blood gas measurement, appears to be greater than the volume that would be provided by use of a BVM or other ventilator which produces a higher inspiratory pressure. *Even though it would seem that the Minute Volume so delivered would be significantly below normal, there is irrefutable scientific evidence that when this method is properly provided, normal or near normal blood gases can be temporarily maintained.*

Even with the shortest run times and most efficient immediate attempts to otherwise ventilate the patient, apnea and hypoxia will have been present for a considerable time when this procedure is needed and even a few short seconds of delay may result in irreversible death. At the time of publication of this book, no commercially assembled kit containing all of the compatible parts needed to ventilate the patient in whom a needle tracheostomy has been performed was known by the authors to be available. Only a flowmeter with a valve designed for intermittent delivery was found in a catalog of anesthesiology respiratory equipment. Therefore, all of the compatible equipment needed to perform the needle tracheostomy and provide ventilation through it should be pre-assembled, and routinely carried on each advanced unit. Except for the connections to the needle or catheter hub at one end and the regulator nipple at the other, all parts should be modified and pre-connected ready for immediate use without the unnecessary delay that this would require in the field. Such pre-assembly also assures that all of the selected parts are compatible and fit together without leaks, and allows for their proper packaging and sterilization (at the hospital) prior to these home-assembled kits being stored on each vehicle. Since a problem can occur with any equipment, it is recommended that two of these made-up kits be carried on each ambulance and that additional ones be made up and stored at the station to immediately provide for replacement if one is used on a call. For each pre-assembled kit you will need:

- Several 10g. emergency tracheal needles *or* large-bore (12g. or 14g.) over-the-needle IV catheters.
- Two 10–30 ml syringes (one must fit into an IV cannula).
- A standard universal oxygen connecting tube (low pressure gas supply tubing)
- A #6, #7, or #8 (cuffed) ET tube.
- A plastic "Y" or "T" of a size that will allow for connection to a universal oxygen connecting tube's end and a #6, #7, or #8 ET tube when the 15/22mm adaptor is removed from its proximal end (A "Y" with a standard low presure oxygen nipple at each of its open ends is manufactured but hard to locate).
- Two short plastic connecting tubes.
- A suction catheter with a hard plastic whistle-stop opening.

To prepare the Percutanteous Transtracheal Ventilating unit, start by cutting the low pressure universal oxygen supply tubing into two pieces about 12 to 15 inches from one end. Then remove the hard plastic whistle-stop from the catheter end (or if it is in-line, cut the catheter so that one inch of the catheter remains on each side of the whistle stop). With the plastic connecting tubes (if needed) connect each cut end of the oxygen supply tubing to one side of the whistle stop so that the whistle stop is in-line in the reconnected oxygen supply tubing.

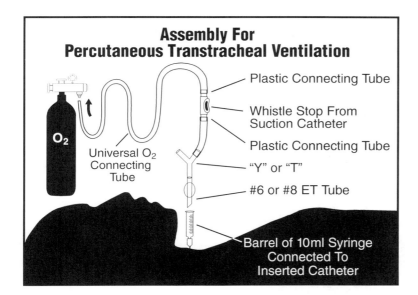

**Assembly For
Percutaneous Transtracheal Ventilation**

O₂

Universal O₂ Connecting Tube

Plastic Connecting Tube

Whistle Stop From Suction Catheter

Plastic Connecting Tube

"Y" or "T"

#6 or #8 ET Tube

Barrel of 10ml Syringe Connected To Inserted Catheter

Next connect the end of the oxygen supply tubing (that has the whistle stop near it) over one side of the "Y" or "T". Then remove the 15/22ml adaptor from the proximal end of the #6, #7 or #8 ET tube and connect it to the distal end of the "Y" or "T". The finished assembly should match the drawing above. To make sure that each connection is secure and without leaks, and to make sure that nothing in the assembly has restricted the flow of oxygen, connect one end to the low pressure nipple of an oxygen source and check that a proper flow occurs out of the tip of the ET tube when the whistle stop and the open port on the "Y" or "T" is covered with your fingers. After it has been checked, this assembly together with the needles (each in its own puncture proof container) and the 2 syringes can be packaged and sterilized.

When such a unit needs to be used, the available end of the oxygen supply tubing is attached to the normal supplemental oxygen nipple of a portable regulator or wall source which has been set at 15 LPM, and the ET tube at the distal end of the assembly is inserted into the barrel of the 10–30 ml syringe attached to the IV cannula inserted into the patient's trachea. Then the cuff of the ET tube is inflated to provide a seal.

Attaching the barrel of a 10ml syringe to the catheter which has been inserted into the trachea provides a secure way to hold the catheter to prevent its kinking, and when used with the ET tube produces an easy and reliable connection without the need to manipulate the catheter—as would be involved if a connection directly to the hub with a piece of tubing was required (as with earlier designs for such assembled equipment).

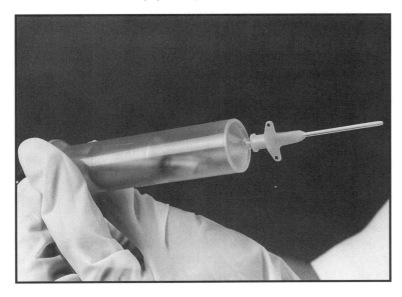

The ET tube (with its cuff not yet inflated) will easily slide into the syringe's barrel and a secure mechanical connection and seal result when the ET cuff is inflated. We have found one brand (Bard-Parker) and size suction catheter which has a hard plastic whistle-stop inserted in its proximal end, which when removed from the catheter allows for a firm direct connection to the end of the oxygen supply tubing and a perfect tight fit into the hub of the IV catheter as shown below:

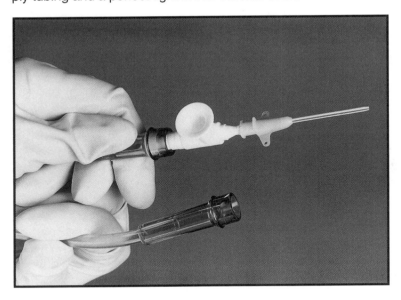

If this particular whistle-stop can be obtained and used the need for the "Y" or "T", the ET tube, and the syringe barrel is eliminated—making pre-assembly and the use of the unit much simpler.

Once the unit has been properly connected to the 15 LPM oxygen flow and to the patient, oxygen will flow out of the whistle-stop hole and the open branch of the "Y" or "T". When the EMT simultaneously occludes both of these openings, a closed tubing system is produced between the oxygen source and the needle or catheter inserted into the patient's trachea. The oxygen's pressure will cause it to flow through the catheter and provide the inspiratory volume. When the EMT releases his fingers—opening both to the outside—the oxygen will flow out of the whistle-stop hole and the patient's exhaled air will be vented to the outside through the open part of the "Y".

Due to the restriction caused by the narrow lumen of the catheter, the times required for adequate inspiration and expiration of an equal volume will each be longer than with other methods of ventilating patients. Chest excursion—with enough time for significant but not maximal chest rise and for proper complete chest fall—must guide the EMT rather than any pre-set concept or a number of breaths required per minute. The EMT must remember that with ventilation through a needle, the steady regular provision of good inspiratory volumes with adequate time for exhalation between them will produce a better minute volume than those which would result from too rapidly alternating between phases. The time allowed for exhalation must be even longer than the extended time required to provide a sufficient inspiratory volume with this method, if an equal amount is to be expired and air entrapment and CO_2 retention are to be avoided. As with any form of ventilation, proper air exchange should be confirmed by auscultation.

If the previously shown pre-assembly is not available when PTV is indicated, while one advanced EMT is doing the needle tracheostomy an alternate immediate substitute can be rapidly prepared by a second EMT using oxygen supply tubing. Using a pair of scissors, carefully cut a small oval hole (about 2mm long and 1mm wide) through the surface of the tube about 6 inches from the connector at one end. Care must be taken that the width of this hole does not extend too far around the circumference of the tube destroying its tubular integrity. A second similar hole is made on a straight line from the first—approximately 12 to 15 inches proximal (toward the other end) of the first one. When using this modified oxygen tube to provide PTV, the end without the two holes is connected to the low pressure oxygen nipple of the regulator or wall unit which is providing the 15 LPM flow, and the connector at the end with the holes is attached directly over the hub of the catheter that has been inserted into the trachea. Both holes are occluded with the thumbs (or a finger) to provide inspiration and are released to divert the oxygen flow and allow for exhalation to the outside.

Equipment has been described and used with only a single hole (or a single whistle-stop opening without a second opening provided by the use of a "Y" or "T" or second whistle-stop) to provide for both the delivery of oxygen and venting of the patient's expired air to the outside during exhalation. The physics of gas flow suggests that at the flow rate and pressure at which the oxygen is supplied, some inbound oxygen may still flow beyond the opening through which the oxygen and exhaled air is exiting, resulting in some continuing positive pressure against which the patient must exhale. This in fact may be a major contributor to the CO_2 retention that has often previously been reported with this method of ventilation. One can only be sure that no continued oxygen pressure exists against which the patient must exhale, and that exhaled air is not reintroduced into the lungs, by having two holes in the system. When during exhalation these are open, the one nearer the oxygen source provides for the diversion of the oxygen flow from the source, and the second, near to the catheter, allows for the venting of the exhaled air to the outside.

Percutaneous Transtracheal Ventilation can be further complicated in patients who could not be ventilated through the nose and mouth but still have some communication between their trachea and pharynx which allows a part of the provided oxygen to escape out of the mouth and nose. To prevent this and maintain delivery of the inspiratory volume to the lungs in such patients, the nostrils must be squeezed shut and the mouth occluded by a second EMT during the inhalation phase. He should remove his hand, allowing the mouth and nose to be open, during the exhalation phase.

Any patient being ventilated by Percutaneous Transtracheal Ventilation must be assumed to have only marginal air exchange and must be considered to be highly unstable. Once the PTV has been established, such patients URGENTLY need more definitive airway management and increased ventilation surgically provided at the hospital. Therefore, transport to a suitable facility should be initiated without delay.

When performing a needle tracheostomy, although the needle can be inserted elsewhere into the trachea, inserting it through the cricothyroid membrane is considered safest. Two favorable anatomical features recommend selection of a cricothyrotomy. First, there are no vital structures between the skin and the airway in the region of the cricothyroid membrane. Second, the cricoid cartilage, although narrow anteriorly, broadens posteriorly to articulate with the thyroid cartilage. This tough posterior cartilagenous wall prevent inadvertent puncture of the back wall of the larynx.

If you are an advanced EMT, properly trained/certified in the procedure, once the patient has been found to be apenic, Universal Precautions have been taken and all other attempts to ventilate him have proven unsuccessful, *or* the extent of his maxiofacial injuries has obviated the need for an alternate transtracheal airway:

1. Direct a second EMT to set up (or prepare) the special ventilating equipment and oxygen unit. Next, connect the syringe to the large bore Over-the needle IV catheter (or 10g tracheal needle, if available). Place the patient on his back with his head held slightly extended (or if spine trauma is suspected, immobilized in the neutral in-line position). Next, put on a pair of sterile gloves (if readily available). Locate the larynx and hold it between the thumb and second finger of your caudad hand to prevent the trachea from moving laterally.

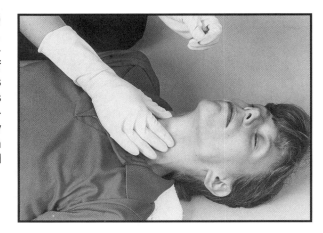

2. While continuing to stabilize the trachea, rapidly clean the area of the trachea below your fingers with an antiseptic swab or wipe, and place your first finger on the center of the larynx. Slide the finger in a caudad direction down the midline of the trachea until the cricothyroid membrane is felt under your fingertip. Remove your finger and, holding the syringe in your cephalad hand, insert the needle at the angle shown through the skin at the midline at the exact level where you located the cricothyroid membrane.

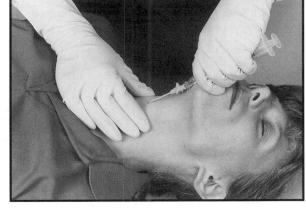

3. Once the tip of the needle is fully under the skin's surface and in the thin underlying muscle, pull up on the plunger of the syringe with your thumb. While maintaining negative pressure in the syringe in this way, continue to advance the needle through the cricothyroid membrane (or the midline of the anterior wall of the trachea between its rings if another site is used).

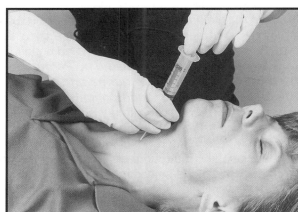

4. Once the tip of the needle has entered the trachea, the upward pressure applied to the syringe plunger will result in air being sucked into the syringe. This serves to confirm the needle's proper location. The syringe and needle should be advanced an additional centimeter or two beyond the point at which air first entered the syringe to assure that it is sufficiently advanced to secure it within the trachea. Care must be taken *NOT* to insert it further in order to avoid contact with the posterior wall.

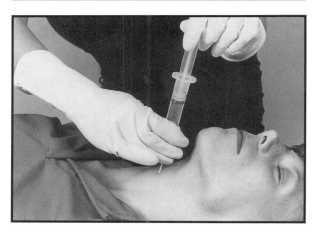

5. While securely holding the hub of the catheter with one hand, remove the syringe and withdraw the needle from within the catheter. Care must be taken to avoid any movement and kinking of the catheter once the rigid needle has been withdrawn. After confirming that the assembly has been properly connected to the oxygen source and a 15 LPM or greater flow exists, carefully connect the distal end to the hub of the catheter in the manner dictated by the specific equipment assembly.

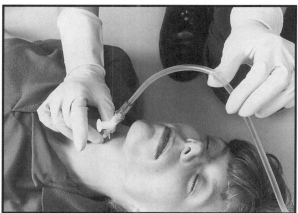

6. To ventilate the patient, while holding the assembly with both hands, occlude the two openings with your thumbs. (The whistle-stop and open end of the "Y" or the two holes made in the tubing). This closes the system to the outside and directs the 15 LPM oxygen flow through the catheter and into the trachea—delivering the inspiratory volume required. The duration required for the inspiratory phase will be greater than two seconds and should be determined by careful observation of the chest rise.

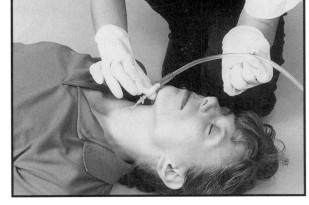

7. Once the chest has been seen to rise adequately (but not maximally), release your thumbs from *both* openings and allow exhalation to occur. Opening both of these ports or holes relieves the positive pressure by diverting the oxygen flow to the outside through the proximal opening and allows the patient's expired air to readily exit through the distal one. Remember that significantly more time is needed to allow for adequate exhalation than for the extended inspiratory time.

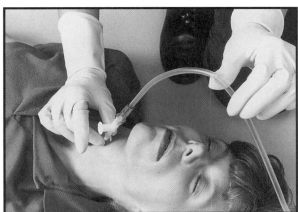

8. Once the chest has been seen to fall fully, occlude both ports (holes) with your thumbs to provide the next inspiration. When adequate chest rise has occurred remove your thumbs, opening the two ports for exhalation, and so on. After the PTV ventilation has been established for several breaths direct a second EMT to re-check the carotid pulse to determine if chest compressions are also needed and continue to ventilate the patient in the manner described. Transport should be initiated to the nearest appropriate facility without delay.

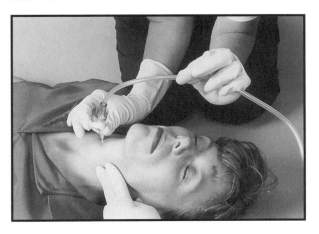

If upon closing both ports to provide inspiration, some oxygen escapes from the patient's mouth and nose, partial communication between the trachea and pharynx exists. When this occurs, the mouth and nose must be sealed during each provided inspiration by having a second EMT squeeze the nostrils shut while simultaneously occluding the mouth with the palm of his hand. He should remove his hand, opening the mouth and nose during the exhalation phase, and alternately re-seal them for each inspiration.

When CPR is indicated and PTV is to be used in association with chest compressions, the restricted slow exodus of air dictated by the small lumen of the catheter presents a problem when the first chest compression is properly rapidly delivered. Although a search of the literature on PTV fails to identify any discussion pertaining to this, the thoracic anatomy and physiology of air exchange strongly suggests that with the airflow so restricted, a normal rapid first compression could result in dislodging the catheter and also producing pulmonary damage. Until further study exists, to avoid these indesirable dangers it is suggested that a slower less forceful single compression solely to expel air be added after each provided inspiration, prior to each cycle of five regularly applied chest compressions. The need to include this step versus the potential danger without it will, in the absence of scientific proof, need to be determined by the squad's Medical Director and should be addressed in the local protocols for needle tracheostomy. Regardless of whether this step is included or not, when CPR is given in association with PTV chest compressions should be delivered at a high enough rate to ensure that between 80–100 compressions occur per minute in spite of the longer time needed to ventilate the patient in between each cycle of five compressions.

ETI SUMMARY SKILL SHEET
Bag Valve Mask Ventilation (BVM)

1. TAKE/Maintain appropriate UNIVERSAL PRECAUTIONS.

2. Perform MANUAL AIRWAY MANEUVER, and CONFIRM continued APNEA.

3. ATTACH proper size MASK to BVM outlet valve.

4. While maintaining the manual airway maneuver, PROVIDE A MASK SEAL over the patient's mouth and nose, and slowly SQUEEZE THE BAG UNTIL a sufficient inspiratory volume is delivered (about 1.5 to 2 seconds in most adults) and ADEQUATE CHEST RISE IS SEEN.

5. Once the chest has been observed to adequately rise, RELEASE THE SQUEEZE on the bag TO ALLOW FOR EXHALATION AND automatic REFILLING OF THE BAG.

6. PROVIDE A SECOND VENTILATOIN (repeating steps 4 and 5).

7. Direct/check for a PALPABLE CAROTID PULSE. CONTINUE VENTILATION.

8. After several ventilations, MEASURE, SELECT and, after interrupting ventilation, INSERT a properly sized SIMPLE AIRWAY ADJUNCT (OPA or, if not tolerated, a NPA).

9. Resume and CONTINUE VENTIALTIONS while observing chest excursion.

10. AUSCULTATE both MIDLUNG FIELDS to confirm proper pulmonary air exchange and to establish a BASELINE.

11. DIRECT another EMT, when he can, TO SET UP the 15L/min OXYGEN SUPPLY and, CONNECT the ACCUMULATOR to the BVM.

12. After several minutes of ventilation with a high FiO_2, when properly trained/certified EMTs are present, PREPARE equipment FOR INTUBATION.

13. INTUBATE THE PATIENT.

14. CONFIRM PROPER PLACEMENT by observing chest rise, auscultating over the epigastrium (no breath sounds) and over each midlung field (present breath sounds) during continued ventilation.

15. IF available, ATTACH PULSE OXIMETER and monitor oxygenation.

16. CONTINUOUSLY MONITOR chest excursion and signs of oxygenation, and PERIODICALLY AUSCULTATE both midlung fields to CONFIRM continued proper ET tube placement and PULMONARY VENTILATION.

ETI SUMMARY SKILL SHEET
Demand Valve Resuscitator (Oxygen Powered, Manually Triggered Ventilators)

1. TAKE/Maintain appropriate UNIVERSAL PRECAUTIONS.

2. PLACE patient IN A SUPINE POSITION, Perform MANUAL AIRWAY MANEUVER, and CONFIRM continued APNEA.

3. OPEN UNIT and take out the unit's head. OPEN OXYGEN tank and check pressure gauge.

4. Press trigger. CHECK THAT OXYGEN FLOWS from the head's outlet port. While depressing the trigger, occlude the outlet port to CHECK that the HIGH PRESSURE RELIEF VALVE releases properly.

5. Select, INSTALL, AND PROPERLY ORIENT the correct size MASK.

6. While maintaining the manual airway maneuver, PROVIDE A MASK SEAL over the patient's mouth and nose, and DEPRESS THE TRIGGER UNTIL a sufficient inspiratory volume is delivered (about 1.5 to 2 seconds in most adults) and ADEQUATE CHEST RISE IS SEEN.

7. Once the chest has been observed to adequately rise, RELEASE the TRIGGER (button or handle) to ALLOW FOR EXHALATION.

8. Once the chest has been observed to fall fully, PROVIDE A SENCOND VENTILATION (repeating steps 6 and 7).

9. Direct/Check for a PALPABLE CAROTID PULSE. CONTINUE VENTILATION.

10. After several ventilations, MEASURE, SELECT and, after interrupting ventilation, INSERT a properly sized SIMPLE AIRWAY ADJUNCT (OPA or if not tolerated, a NPA).

11. Resume and CONTINUE VENTILATIONS while observing chest excursion.

12. AUSCULTATE both MIDLUNG FIELDS to confirm proper pulmonary air exchange and to establish a BASELINE.

13. After several minutes of ventilation, if properly trained/certified EMTs are present, PREPARE equipment FOR INTUBATION.

14. INTUBATE the PATIENT.

15. CONFIRM PROPER PLACEMENT by observing chest rise, auscultating over the epigastrium (no breath sounds) and over each midlung field during continued ventilation.

16. If available, ATTACH PULSE OXIMETER and monitor oxygenation.

17. CONTINUOUSLY MONITOR chest excursion and signs of oxygenation, and PERIODICALLY AUSCULTATE both midlung fields to CONFIRM continued proper placement and PULMONARY VENTILATION.

ETI SUMMARY SKILL SHEET
Automatic Transport Ventilator (ATV)

Note: The following steps should only be used as sequence guidelines. Due to the differences in individual brands and models of ATVs available, the actual mechanical preparation and setting of the controls should follow the specific instructions furnished by the manufacturer.

1. TAKE/Maintain UNIVERSAL PRECAUTIONS.

2. INITIATE VENTILATION with BVM (or Mouth-to-Mask) and INSERT A SIMPLE AIRWAY ADJUNCT.

3. OBSERVE CHEST RISE to confirm airway patency and adequate air exchange.

4. After several breaths, CHECK CAROTID PULSE.

5. AUSCULTATE BILATERAL MIDLUNG FIELDS to confirm pulmonary air exchange and ESTABLISH A BASELINE.

6. OPEN ATV CASE, remove components, CHECK that CONNECTIONS are proper and HOSES are NOT KINKED.

7. OPEN OXYGEN tank and CHECK THAT THE PRESSURE gauge reflects a full or near-full tank.

8. On the Control Module, if so equipped, SET the INSPIRATORY TIME Control.

9. CALCULATE TIDAL VOLUME RANGE, SET the Tidal Volume CONTROL.

10. SET the BREATHS PER MINUTE Control.

11. CHECK that the combined control SETTINGS PROVIDE PROPER MINUTE VOLUME.

12. Place hand near outlet tube, CHECK for proper OXYGEN FLOW during the inspiratory phase and for proper machine CYCLING.

13. Occlude the outlet port, CHECK that the AUDIBLE PRESSURE LIMIT ALARM sounds during the inspiratory phase.

14. ATTACH proper size MASK to patient valve head.

15. Direct STOP of BVM VENTILATION, CONFIRM APNEA continues.

16. PLACE UNIT HEAD/MASK over patient's nose and mouth, have EMT provide MASK SEAL.

17. OBSERVE CHEST EXCURSION for several cycles. Confirm chest rise is clearly adequate but not maximal.

18. IF the Pressure Limit ALARM SOUNDS FROM COMMENCEMENT OF INSPIRATION, reposition the head and otherwise CLEAR THE AIRWAY as needed.

19. IF the Pressure Limit ALARM SOUNDS ONLY AT END PEAK of the INSPIRATORY PHASE, the tidal volume setting is too high. SET TIDAL VOLUME Control to a LOWER setting.

20. Once automatic ventilation is being properly provided by the ATV, AUSCULTATE BOTH MIDLUNG FIELDS to confirm adequate inspiratory and expiratory air exchange is being provided.

21. AUSCULTATE over the EPIGASTRIUM for several cycles to confirm that excessive tidal volume is not resulting in gastric insufflation.

22. Once proper ventilation is confirmed, WITH A WATCH, CONFIRM that the machine's INSPIRATORY TIME and BREATHS PER MINUTE match the control settings (or on models with an Inspiratory Time Setting, the pre-set time).

23. After these confirmations, if properly trained/certified personnel are available, PREPARE and CHECK the INTUBATION EQUIPMENT.

24. When ready, INTUBATE the PATIENT.

25. Once the ET tube has been successfully placed, DISCARD the MASK and CONNECT the Patient Valve Head's OUTLET TUBE DIRECTLY to the proximal end of the ET TUBE.

26. CONFIRM PROPER ET TUBE PLACEMENT by observing chest rise and auscultating over the episgastrium and both midlung fields.

27. Continue to MONITOR CHEST EXCURSION AND PERIODICALLY, CONFIRM continuing proper ET TUBE PLACEMENT AND PULMONARY VENTILATION by auscultation of the midlung fields. Also PERIODICALLY CHECK the OXYGEN pressure gauge.

28. At the completion of use, PROPERLY DISPOSE of SINGLE-USE ITEMS, CLEAN the UNIT, and REPLACE the OXYGEN cylinder with a full one.

ALS

ETI SUMMARY SKILL SHEET

ALS Needle Tracheostomy and Percutaneous Transtracheal Ventilation

1. TAKE/Maintain UNIVERSAL PRECAUTIONS.

2. CONFIRM OTHER VENTILATION attempts though the normal airway have proven IMPOSSIBLE.

3. DIRECT another EMT to SET UP (or prepare) the SPECIAL VENTILATING EQUIPMENT required AND the OXYGEN.

4. CONNECT the SYRINGE to the Large bore IV CATHETER (or 10g. tracheal needle).

5. PLACE PATIENT SUPINE and, unless spine trauma, WITH HIS HEAD slightly HYPEREXTENDED.

6. Put on STERILE GLOVES.

7. LOCATE and HOLD THE LARYNX between the thumb and second finger of your caudad hand.

8. Place the 1st finger on the same hand on the larynx and slide it in a caudad direction until you LOCATE THE CRICOTHYROID MEMBRANE.

9. Remove your fingertip and with your hand CLEAN THE AREA with an antiseptic, then INSERT THE NEEDLE THROUGH THE SKIN over the exact place that the cricothyroid membrane was palpated.

10. While exerting UPWARD PRESSURE on the PLUNGER OF THE SYRINGE, ADVANCE the NEEDLE through the anterior wall of the membrane until it is INTO THE TRACHEA and air enters the syringe.

11. ADVANCE THE NEEDLE 1 to 2cm FURTHER.

12. While securely holding the hub of the catheter, REMOVE THE SYRINGE AND NEEDLE.

13. CONNECT THE PRE-ASSEMBLED VENTILATING SET-UP with 15L/min flow coming through it, TO THE hub of the CATHETER (inserted into the trachea).

14. OCCLUDE BOTH OPENINGS in the assembly with your thumbs, TO PROVIDE THE INSPIRATORY VOLUME, until the chest is seen to rise sufficiently.

15. IF AIR escapes from the patient's mouth and nose, DIRECT a second EMT to OCCLUDE THEM during the inspiratory phase and repeat step 14.

16. Release your thumbs to OPEN BOTH HOLES TO ALLOW FOR EXHALATION until the chest is seen to fully fall.

17. CONTINUE VENTILATION (following steps 14–16).

18. After several ventilations, DIRECT the 2nd EMT to CHECK for a palpable CAROTID PULSE. Initiate chest compressions if indicated.

19. INITIATE TRANSPORT without delay.

SECTION

Problems of Ventilation

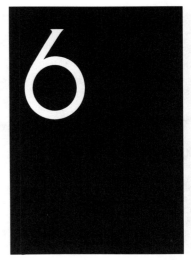

6

Introduction

*NOTE: Classically, the management of "Foreign Body Airway Obstruction" is taught as a part of CPR. In most EMT texts it is included as one of the skills of "Airway Management". Such sequencing would seem to imply that the EMTs discovery of the obstruction occurs during airway manipulation and **before** ventilation is attempted. In reality an airway obstruction is the primary presenting problem only in cases of conscious witnessed obstruction. The EMT is much more likely to identify a foreign body obstruction only through his inability to ventilate an unconscious apneic patient — that is, **after** beginning/attempting ventilation. We have, therefore, placed the discussion of foreign body airway obstruction in this Section dealing with Special Problems of Ventilation rather than in the earlier Section on Airway Management.*

This Section deals with a variety of problems and circumstances that work to defeat effective ventilation. Some, however, are not addressed except in this introduction — generally because their recognition and remediation is either patently obvious, unskilled, and/or outside the scope of this text. Some examples of such situations are near drowning or a structural collapse or cave-in which results in ventilatory embarrassment due to the forceful external restriction on the chest wall that makes expansion of the thoracic cage impossible. Recognition of such a problem is quite elementary for any level of responder, and the treatment must obviously include the elimination of the external item or problem which is interfering with ventilation. The special rescue procedures for such events are beyond the scope of this text. Other etiologies (Foreign Body Airway Obstruction, open wounds of the chest wall, and gastric distention) are addressed in this Section and represent problems whose prompt resolution by the EMT is necessary if the patient is to survive.

The most common cause of airway obstruction in unconscious supine patients is their own tongue. Basic airway maneuvers are used to correct this type of obstruction and have been presented earlier in the airway management skills portion of this text. Airway obstruction from a foreign object can occur to anyone capable of placing objects into their mouth. This could be food, chewing gum, toys, bottle tops, balloons, buttons — just about anything that will fit into the oral cavity and is capable of lodging at the top of the trachea or in the trachea itself.

Generally, conscious patients with a foreign body obstruction will display the "universal choking sign" — a reflex act in which the choking patient automatically grabs at his throat (as if choking himself with his own hands) and violently attempts to cough forcefully with the residual air in his lungs to push the obstruction outward. Unconscious patients may be cyanotic around the face, and there may be signs of struggling from attempting to relieve the obstruction prior to having lost consciousness.

As you approach a conscious patient with a foreign body airway obstruction they may be standing, walking around, or sitting — all while attempting to relieve the obstruction. Your initial assessment should be to determine if the choking patient is moving any air past the obstruction as they attempt to breathe. If the obstruction is only partial, **stridor** (a high-pitched sound) may be heard on inhalation and the patient may be coughing or may even be able to speak if asked "Are you choking?" or "Can you speak or cough?" If vocal sounds can be heard, and while the patient appears to be making progress in clearing the obstruction himself, the EMT should stay with the patient but *NOT* actively interfere. At this stage the patient himself is probably best able to clear the obstruction. However, the EMT should be prepared to rapidly intervene if the patient is making no sounds, cannot speak, or appears to be unable to clear the obstruction and is about to lose consciousness. The recommended BLS level intervention is some version of the "Heimlich Maneuver" based on the patient's body size — subdiaphragmatic abdominal thrusts in adults and children or back blows and chest thrusts in infants.

If you are unable to relieve the obstruction while the adult or child patient is conscious, he may become unconscious in your arms and need to be supported and protected as he collapses to the ground. Further attempts to dislodge the obstruction should continue with the patient in a supine position. An obstruction that could not be previously cleared is often successfully dislodged once the patient is unconscious and his muscles become flaccid.

An obstructed airway in an unconscious patient when no one witnessed the collapse may not be discovered until ventilation attempts prove ineffective.

Each of the foreign body obstruction scenarios will be covered in this Section. Regardless of the patient's status (conscious or unconscious) when the obstruction is relieved, all such patients should still be examined by a physician. Although the obstruction may be gone, laryngeal and tracheal damage and irritation may result. The highly sensitive tissues of the throat and upper airway may react to it's brief presence by becoming inflamed and even swelling shut — creating an equally serious and much more complex to resolve condition than originally existed. The forceful cavitation and displacement of the abdominal contents that repeatedly occurs with the delivery of sub-diaphragmatic thrusts can easily produce damage to the underlying organs and intra-abdominal bleeding. Rib fractures and pulmonary contusions are commonly associated with the repeated compression of the chest that is produced by the delivery of chest thrusts. After having either chest or sub-diaphragmatic abdominal thrusts applied, and regardless of their recovery and the absence of any immediate signs or symptoms of underlying injury, these possibilities must be carefully ruled out at the emergency department before any patient can safely return to normal activities.

PARTIAL FOREIGN BODY OBSTRUCTION

A foreign body can produce a full or partial airway obstruction. If the patient can still move air in and out of his lungs and remains conscious, the obstruction is only partial and the key is to allow him to attempt to relieve the obstruction himself while you encourage him to repeatedly cough. Such patients will be extremely anxious and will benefit from the EMT's presence and reassurance that despite their discomfort they are still exchanging a sufficient volume of air. Stridor and other sounds associated with airway restriction will commonly be present in such cases, and the patient's voice may sound hoarse. As long as the patient's overall condition remains stable and he can pass sufficient air to cough or speak, abdominal thrusts should NOT be provided. It is best to have him continue to attempt to dislodge the foreign body himself by forceful coughing after each few breaths. Moving the patient to a sitting position is safer than trying to maintain him standing and is recommended if the patient will tolerate it. In either case the EMT should support the patient without interfering with his efforts, guarding against the patient's sudden collapse and any resulting injury. Increasing the patient's oxygenation by providing as high an FiO_2 as possible is recommended to lessen or prevent hypoxia, however the extreme anxiety common in such patients makes fastening a mask-type delivery device over the patient's face impractical. Conventional use of a non-rebreather reservoir mask should be reserved until the airway has been cleared and the patient has adequate spontaneous air exchange. Interim alternatives include holding a high FiO_2 mask near the patient's face or using a nasal cannula. While neither will provide an FiO_2 of 0.85–1.00, they represent a more realistic approach and will provide some increase in the oxygen concentration of the air being breathed by the patient.

The patient should be transported without delay in a sitting position — often fully upright or leaning slightly forward will be the most comfortable and easiest positions in which to breathe. While the obstruction is in place, laryngeal abrasion and edema commonly develop. When the foreign body is removed, the patient continues to feel that some airway restriction is present even when air exchange is near or at normal volume. In such cases, unless the foreign object has been expelled the EMT will usually not be able to determine whether the object is still in place or has been swallowed or aspirated. The patient's air exchange and level of consciousness must be continuously monitored for any changes — and deterioration should be anticipated. If the patient becomes too weak to speak or cough, no longer moves air, or becomes unconscious, the appropriate sequence of intervention for unconscious obstructed patients (found on the following pages) should immediately be initiated.

FOREIGN BODY AIRWAY OBSTRUCTION—ADULT FOUND CONSCIOUS

A complete airway obstruction is the ultimate emergency—the functional equivalent of a patient with an open airway who has stopped breathing. The EMT has only a few brief minutes to overcome the obstruction or the patient will begin to suffer irreparable brain cell damage and deteriorate irreversibly toward death.

As noted in the preceding Introduction, the EMT must closely monitor a choking patient with a *partial* obstruction for any signs of general weakening so that active intervention can begin before the patient's condition deteriorates too far.

The technique of choice for conscious adult choking victims was devised in the early 1970's by Dr. Henry Heimlich of Cincinnati, and bears his name. Very simply put, the Heimlich maneuver causes a sudden reduction in the size of the thorax—thereby increasing the pressure of the residual volume of air that is always present in the lungs. The rapid increase in pressure produces a forceful flow of air from the lungs through the bronchi and up the trachea—hopefully "blowing out" the foreign body which is causing the obstruction.

There are several ways of causing the sudden reduction in chest size, among them pushing directly on the chest wall or alternately by compressing the abdomen and directing its contents cephalad against the diaphragm from below. While "chest thrusts"—squeezing compressions of the rib cage itself—are recommended for pregnant patients or individuals who are so large that the EMT cannot get his arms around the patient's abdomen, the EMT's first choice with others should be "sub-diaphragmatic abdominal thrusts". These can be delivered to standing, sitting, or supine patients. As these thrusts should be quite forceful in order to be effective, the EMT must use care to deliver the thrusts along the midline of the patient's abdomen and without making contact with the patient's ribs. The ideal location is on the midline and between the xiphoid and umbilicus, but closer to the umbilicus.

1. When assessing a conscious patient who is choking, you must first determine if the patient is adequately moving air in and out of his lungs. One way to do this is to ask the patient, "Are you choking?", or "Can you speak?" If no vocal sounds are heard the EMT should presume that the airway is completely obstructed. If at any point the patient with a partial obstruction appears to be getting worse, the EMT must immediately intervene and attempt to force the obstruction out of the patient's trachea. Move behind the patient and place both of your arms around the patient's waist.

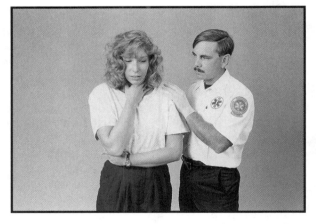

2. Form a fist with one hand and place the thumb over your fingers. Place the flat side of your fist (formed by the first finger and thumb) against the patient's abdominal wall between the navel and xiphoid process.

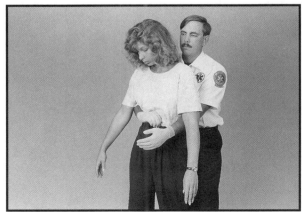

3. With your other hand grasp the outside of your fist (or the wrist of the hand that you previously placed on the patient's abdomen). As you will be pulling inward (toward yourself) with some force, you should be in contact with and brace the patient with your own body from behind.

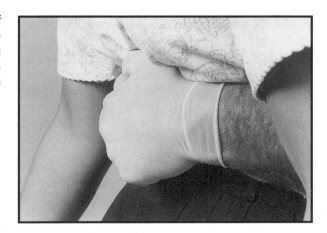

4. To perform the subdiaphragmatic thrusts, pull inward and upward into the patient's abdomen quickly and sharply. Remember, your goal is to depress the abdominal wall and then, with the upward part of the motion, to compress the abdominal contents so that they in turn distend the patient's diaphragm superiorly into his thorax and produce a sudden increase in his intrathoracic pressure. (Sub-diaphragmatic thrusts are contra-indicated in pregnant patients. The procedures to be used in such cases are presented later in this Section.)

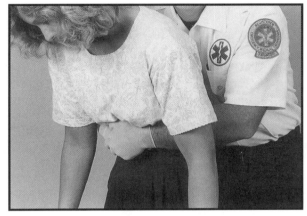

5. Release the pressure of your hands on the abdomen, but be prepared to support the patient if he "rebounds" forward from the effects of your thrust.

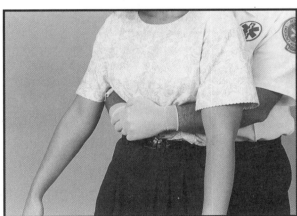

6. Repeat the thrusts continuously until the foreign body is expelled or dislodged sufficiently to allow adequate air exchange, or until the patient becomes so weak that he can no longer stand, or becomes unconscious. Be careful to maintain the correct hand location on the patient's abdomen so that your thrusts do not overlap the patient's ribs or xiphoid process.

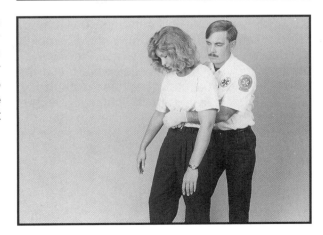

If The Obstructed Adult Becomes Too Weak To Stand:

7. If the patient becomes too weak to continue supporting himself in a standing position, you will have to support him while helping him to the ground in order to help prevent any injury from occurring during his collapse. A useful technique is to insert one of your legs between the patient's legs and, while supporting him with your arms under his armpits and surrounding his chest, let him slowly slide down your leg until he is on the ground. *In attempting to prevent the patient from falling, DO NOT become so entangled or over-reached that you injure yourself or fall.*

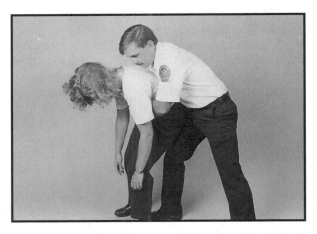

8. Place the patient in a supine position and, if he remains conscious, reinstitute abdominal thrusts. To provide these to a supine patient, first straddle his legs (or kneel immediately next to them facing the patient's head) so that your hands can easily reach the patient's mid-abdomen. Place the heel of one hand against the patient's anterior abdomen between the navel and the xiphoid, with the fingers pointing cephalad. Place your other hand either on top of the first, or grip the wrist of your first hand with the second.

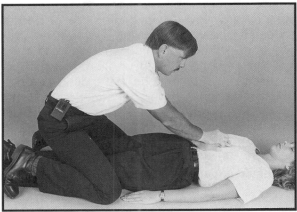

9. With your arms straight and your elbows locked, push both cephalad and posteriorly into the patient's abdomen. As with the standing abdominal thrusts, your goal is to use the abdominal contents to distend the diaphragm and produce a sudden increase in intrathoracic pressure. Your thrust should be "in and up" — into the abdomen first then upward under the diaphragm — for best results.

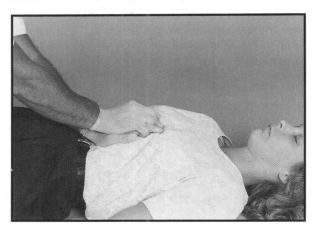

10. After delivering the compression, release the pressure of your hands until the abdominal wall returns to its original position, however do not remove your hands from contact with the patient. Each thrust should be forceful and even, but should not be a stab-like chopping stroke. Continue to deliver abdominal thrusts until the foreign body is expelled or the patient becomes unconscious.

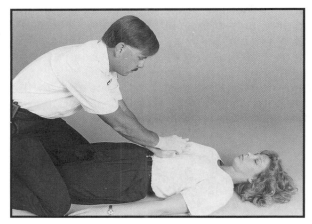

If The Obstructed Adult Becomes Unconscious:

11. If the patient becomes unconscious, stop delivering abdominal thrusts. Conscious obstructed patients who become too weak to continue standing are commonly placed in a supine position on the ground and have abdominal thrusts continued before they become unconscious. In the event that a patient becomes unconscious while still standing, they first need to be lowered into a supine position before continuing with the following steps. Next, immediately open the patient's airway using a tongue-jaw lift. Insert one or two fingers into the patient's mouth and sweep the inside of the mouth in an attempt to extract the obstruction. **Note:** In infants and small children a blind finger sweep is *NOT* performed. Instead the EMT opens and looks into the patient's mouth, and only inserts his fingers to remove a foreign object if it can be seen.

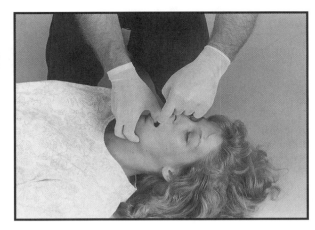

12. After the finger sweep direct another EMT to initiate and maintain a manual airway maneuver while you attempt to ventilate the patient. If the first ventilation attempt is unsuccessful, have him reposition the patient's head while maintaining the manual airway maneuver and again attempt to ventilate.

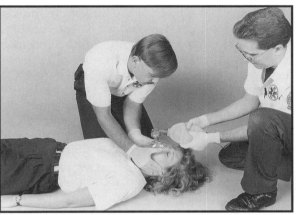

13. If both ventilation attempts are unsuccessful, straddle the patient's legs (or kneel beside them) and, with your hands positioned between the patient's xiphoid process and umbilicus as previously described in steps 9 and 10, resume abdominal thrusts. Count the number delivered.

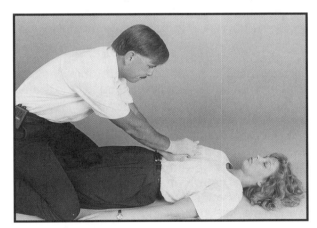

14. After completing five abdominal thrusts, again perform a tongue-jaw lift and a finger sweep of the mouth in an attempt to remove the obstruction.

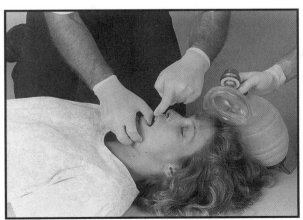

15. Following the finger sweep, and regardless of whether anything was removed from the mouth, again institute a manual airway maneuver and attempt to ventilate the patient. If the ventilation is unsuccessful, re-position the patient's head and attempt another ventilation. If both attempts are unsuccessful, resume the abdominal thrust position and deliver five more subdiaphragmatic compressions.

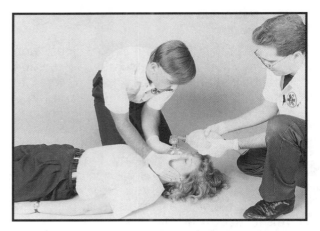

16. Continue the cycle of five abdominal thrusts, finger sweep, and attempted ventilation, until the obstruction is cleared or other advanced care has been instituted. Even after the obstruction has been cleared the patient may still need to be ventilated by the EMT. In the best of cases, when spontaneous ventilation resumes after the object has been removed, a high FiO_2 should still be provided. In the worst cases, even though the airway obstruction has been relieved, CPR will be needed. Even in cases where the obstruction was rapidly cleared and the patient appears to be fully recovered without any signs of damage, the patient should be transported to the hospital to be checked for any resulting laryngeal-tracheal, thoracic, or abdominal injury.

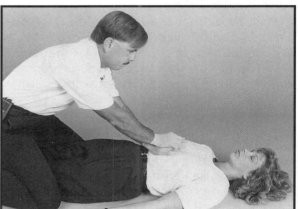

17. If you are unsuccessful after performing these cycles of steps for several minutes, the patient should be rapidly packaged and transported while the steps are continued. If ALS personnel are available, laryngoscopy and removal with McGill forceps or a Kelly clamp should be attempted. If all attempts to clear the airway have failed after 3 or 4 minutes, consideration of a transtracheal procedure will be essential to the patient's survival. If this capability is not available in the field, the patient must be urgently transported to the nearest facility or personnel that can provide it.

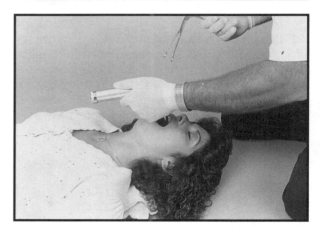

ADULT FOUND UNCONSCIOUS — FOREIGN BODY OBSTRUCTION

When a patient does not respond to your approach and initial greeting, there are many unknowns that must be immediately considered. In some cases, "choking" will have been witnessed prior to the patient's collapse, or may be suggested by the history provided by onlookers or simply by the patient's presence in a dining setting. In other cases a foreign body airway obstruction will only be determined when the EMT is unable to ventilate a non-breathing patient. Regardless of the history presented upon his arrival, the EMT should not jump to conclusions as to the patient's degree of responsiveness or the presence of a foreign body obstruction. Instead, the EMT should follow the step-by-step method recommended by the American Heart Association for assessing any apparently unresponsive patient.

1. First assess responsiveness by speaking to the patient and gently shaking him in an attempt to elicit a response.

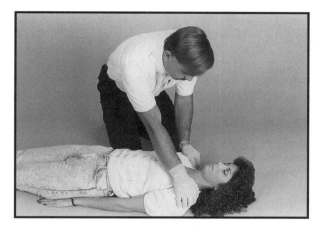

2. If there is no response, open the airway with a manual airway maneuver (with or without spine protection, as indicated) and assess the patient's airway and ventilatory status by looking, listening, and feeling for air exchange.

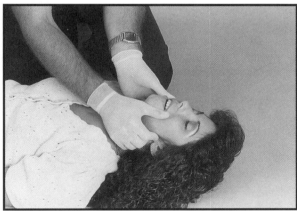

3. If there is no detectable air exchange, attempt to ventilate the patient using a BVM or other ventilator. Do not delay to add supplemental oxygen and a reservoir if you select a BVM — all you want to do at this time is to rapidly initiate ventilation or to identify that there is a problem which defeats your attempt.

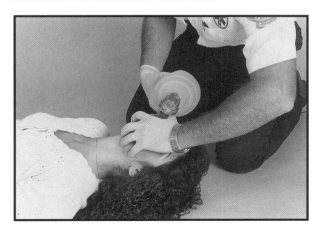

4. If the bag is difficult to compress and there is a lot of air leaking from around the mask, reposition the patient's head by tilting it back further. Ensure that the mandible is elevated and that you have a good mask seal.

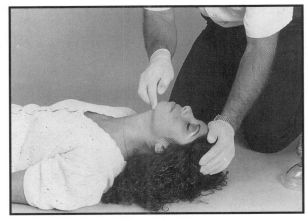

5. Re-attempt ventilating the patient. If no air moves into the patient and there is air leakage from around the mask seal, you must assume that there is a foreign body obstructing the airway. If a BVM is being used it will be very difficult to squeeze. If a Demand Valve or ATV was selected, the high pressure limit valve will release and oxygen will issue from the escape port as well as from around the mask. The ATV's excess pressure alarm will also sound an audible warning.

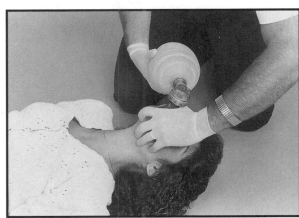

6. Immediately move from the patient's head and straddle his legs. Place the heel of one hand on the midline of the patient's abdomen, between the xiphoid and the umbilicus (but closer to the umbilicus) with the fingers pointing cephalad. Place your other hand on top of the first, and deliver 5 abdominal thrusts as previously described.

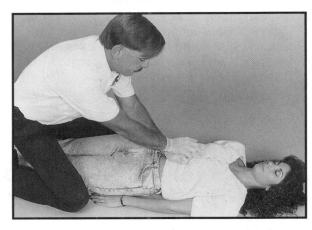

7. Return to the patient's head, perform a tongue-jaw lift and insert the index or middle finger of your other hand into one corner of the patient's mouth and sweep it deeply across the inside of the mouth in an attempt to grasp any foreign objects that may have been dislodged from the trachea into the mouth.

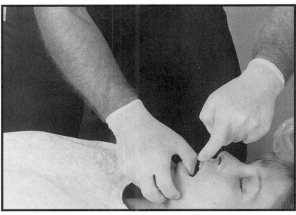

8. Following the finger sweep, and regardless of whether anything was removed from the mouth, again institute a manual airway maneuver and attempt to ventilate the patient. If the ventilation is unsuccessful, re-position the patient's head and attempt another ventilation. If both attempts are unsuccessful, resume the abdominal thrust position and deliver five more subdiaphragmatic compressions.

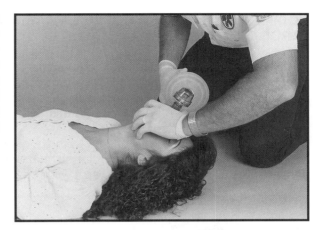

9. Continue the cycle of five abdominal thrusts, finger sweep, and attempted ventilation, until the obstruction is cleared or other advanced care has been instituted. Even after the obstruction has been cleared the patient may still need to be ventilated by the EMT. In the best of cases, when spontaneous ventilation resumes after the object has been removed, a high FiO$_2$ should be provided. The patient should be packaged and transported without delay for definitive evaluation at a hospital prior to discharge. In the worst cases, even though the airway obstruction has been relieved, CPR will be needed.

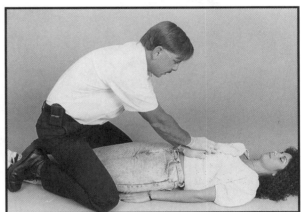

10. If you are unsuccessful after performing these cycles of steps for several minutes, the patient should be rapidly packaged and transported with only minimum interruptions while the steps are continued. If ALS personnel are available, laryngoscopy and visualized removal with a Kelly clamp or McGill forceps should be attempted. If all attempts to clear the airway have failed after 3–4 minutes, consideration must be given to performing a transtracheal procedure if the patient is to survive. If this capability is not available in the field, the patient requires urgent transport to the nearest facility or personnel who can perform it.

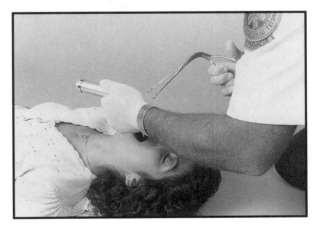

MODIFICATIONS IN OBSTRUCTED AIRWAY MANEUVERS IN CONSCIOUS EXCEPTIONALLY LARGE OR OBESE ADULTS

If the size of a conscious fully obstructed adult is exceedingly larger than that of the EMT, or if the patient is exceptionally large or very obese, it may be impossible for the EMT — while standing behind the patient — to fully encircle the abdomen or to properly place his grasped hands between the patient's xiphoid and umbilicus. In this event the EMT must modify the abdominal thrust technique previously described.

First, attempt to have the patient (with your help) lie down on the floor in a supine position. Kneel beside the patient's thighs at a point so that you can easily reach his abdomen. (Straddling the patient's legs is not recommended as it will increase his anxiety and may be dangerous for the EMT.)

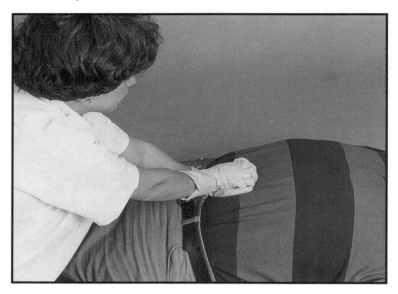

After rapidly explaining what you are going to do, position your hands properly and provide repeated abdominal thrusts using the same techniques as was previously described for patients who can no longer stand by themselves.

In the event that such a patient appears to be too hysterical to cooperate in rapidly being placed supine, the EMT (not being able to encircle the patient's abdomen when standing) will have to use chest thrusts instead of sub-diaphragmatic abdominal thrusts. Chest thrusts are performed repeatedly to forcefully reduce the size of the thoracic cavity.

To provide chest thrusts to a sitting or standing patient, stand immediately behind him and pass your arms under his armpits and around his anterior thorax. With the fingers of one hand palpate and locate the xiphoid process. Form the other hand into a fist and place the side of your first on the lower third of the patient's sternum — superior to and not touching the xiphoid.

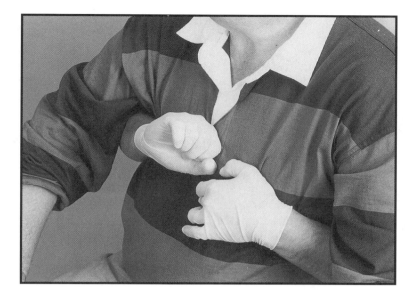

Next, place your other hand over the first and pull directly backward to compress the chest wall posteriorly.

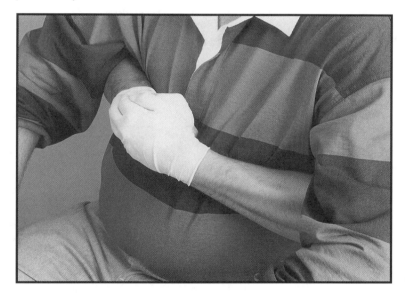

Perform chests thrusts until the obstruction is relieved or the patient becomes too weak to continue standing or becomes unconscious. If, due to weakness or unconsciousness, the patient becomes supine, continue your attempts to clear the obstruction by using the abdominal thrusts described previously.

MODIFICATIONS IN OBSTRUCTED AIRWAY MANEUVERS REQUIRED WITH PREGNANT PATIENTS

Although wide anecdotal experience and several trauma studies have demonstrated that the fetus is well protected in the womb and can withstand considerable blunt compression, there is an absence of good scientific proof that sub-diaphragmatic abdominal thrusts can safely be used without causing injury to the baby or increasing the incidence of spontaneous abortion—or, perhaps, in which trimester(s) they can and in which they cannot. The limited available literature prohibits the use of abdominal thrusts in the third trimester but fails to clearly demonstrate a lack of increased risk in the first two. Experience would certainly suggest that abdominal thrusts may not be appropriate at any time in a troubled or high risk pregnancy. There is also no scientific evidence that abdominal thrusts remain effective in referring pressure up into the diaphragm in pregnant patients.

Since patients needing abdominal thrusts are fully obstructed and cannot speak, determining whether or not a woman is pregnant and—if so—her due date, trimester, and whether or not there have been any problems with the pregnancy or even if this is a high-risk pregnancy, cannot be reliably obtained. In unaccompanied females the lack of ability to speak may even result in the EMT's inability to ascertain whether abdominal protrusion is due to pregnancy, normal post-partum enlargement, or obesity.

Therefore, as a consideration of the potential risks, the question of effectiveness and the difficulty in providing abdominal thrusts when the anterior abdomen is greatly enlarged, *sub-diaphragmatic abdominal thrusts should NOT be attempted in conscious or unconscious females who have been identified as or who appear to be pregnant.* In such cases the appropriate steps previously described for conscious or unconscious patients should be followed with alteration, but whenever abdominal thrusts are called for they should be replaced without chest thrusts.

To perform chest thrusts on a conscious patient:

1. Stand behind the patient and encircle her chest by placing your arms through her armpits. With one hand locate the xiphoid process.

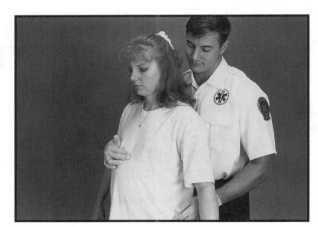

2. Form the other hand into a fist just as you would when performing abdominal thrusts, and place the flat side of your fist on the patient's lower sternum, superior to and not touching the xiphoid process.

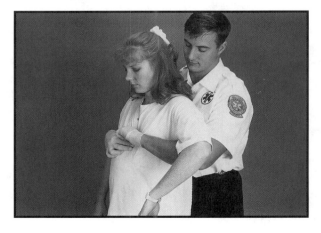

3. Place your first hand over the outside of the fist and pull directly backward to compress the chest wall posteriorly. Perform chest thrusts until the obstruction is relieved or the patient becomes too weak to continue standing or unconscious.

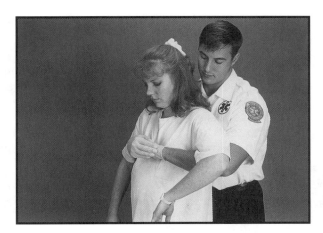

4. Chest thrusts can also be used with the patient in a supine position. The hand placement landmark is the same as that for CPR. Each compression should be delivered directly downward in an attempt to produce a rapid increase in intrathoracic pressure in order to expel the obstruction from the trachea. If the supine patient is conscious the chest thrusts should be continued until the obstruction is relieved or the patient lapses into unconsciousness. If unconscious, five chest thrusts should be delivered followed by a blind finger sweep and an attempt to ventilate the patient. Repeated cycles of thrusts, sweeps, and attempts to ventilate should be made until the obstruction is relieved. As discussed earlier, consideration should be given to beginning transport or to initiating ALS procedures when qualified personnel are available if the initial attempts to relieve the obstruction are unsuccessful.

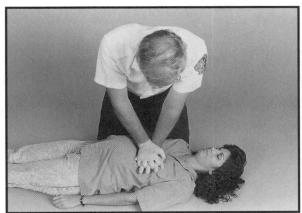

MODIFICATIONS FOR FOREIGN BODY AIRWAY OBSTRUCTION IN CHILDREN (1 – 8 Years Old)

To relieve a foreign body obstruction in a child, with one exception, the EMT should use the same techniques and sequences as would be used for either a conscious or unconscious adult, but with some allowance when performing thrusts or delivering ventilations for the smaller body size and ventilatory capacity of the child.

The exception to the adult procedure relates to the "blind" finger sweep that is performed in adult patients. In children and infants the EMT should first open and look into the patient's mouth for any sign of a foreign body, and only insert his fingers into the mouth if there is something identifiable to reach for.

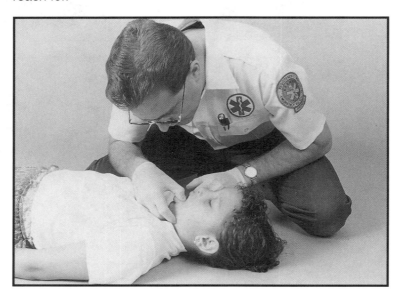

One note of caution in children below 8 years of age relates to **epiglottitis,** a bacterial infection which inflames the epiglottis. This is a serious form of airway obstruction which may mimic a foreign body obstruction. A conscious child may present with signs and symptoms of obstruction but a history that usually includes a rapid onset of fever, inability or lack of desire to swallow, drooling, and an anxious appearance. In this situation minimal aggravation of the child by the EMT is imperative. Calm but rapid transport of the child in the parent's arms without oxygen masks or any other activity that would upset the child is key. Never look into the child's mouth if you suspect that epiglottitis may be present, as this can cause the swollen epiglottis to lodge in the trachea and produce a complete airway obstruction.

FOREIGN BODY AIRWAY OBSTRUCTION IN INFANTS (Birth To 1 Year)

The majority (65%) of all deaths due to foreign body airway obstruction occur in infants less than one year of age. Although the methods and steps employed are quite different from those used for adults and children above one year of age, *they are identical for both conscious and unconscious infants.*

An infant's small size may prompt the EMT to jump immediately to back blows and other obstructed airway maneuvers when presented with an unresponsive infant and a vague history of missing small toys or other objects which could have been swallowed. The propensity for an infant to develop respiratory arrest due to muscle fatigue from fighting a partial obstruction makes it difficult to determine whether the apnea is the result of a full or partial foreign object obstruction, or even from another cause. The EMT should *NOT* immediately assume that apnea is secondary to airway obstruction and should instead follow the normal protocol of determining responsiveness, opening the airway, assessing for breathing, attempting ventilations, etc. Only when diligently following this protocol leads the EMT to the reality of a full foreign body airway obstruction should he undertake the following procedures.

1. Once a complete airway obstruction is recognized, you should immediately pick up the infant and hold him face down along your forearm with his face cupped in the palm of your hand, with his legs straddling your forearm, and with his head held lower than the rest of his body. Support your arm on your thigh or on a firm object to prevent it from moving.

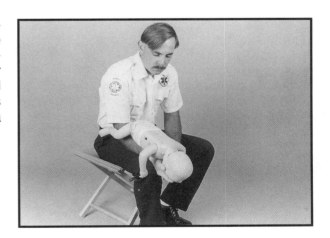

2. Using the heel of your other hand, deliver five firm blows to the infant's back between his shoulder blades. Deliver each blow forcefully enough to compress the thorax and cause an increase in intrathoracic pressure, in hopes that it will dislodge the obstruction. Pause long enough between blows to allow the thorax to "uncompress" and resume its normal shape. Be sure to firmly support the infant's body with your arm while delivering the back blows.

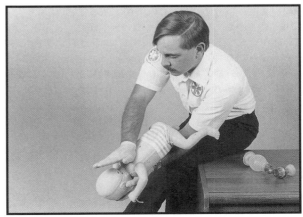

3. After the five back blows, immediately turn the infant over and place him supine on a firm flat surface or on your supported arm. It is desirable to keep the infant's head lower than the rest of his body, but this may not be possible. Turn the infant by placing your free hand on his back, holding his head. This effectively sandwiches the infant between your two hands and arms — one supporting the head, neck, jaw and chest while the other supports the back. Carefully support the head and neck while turning the infant to the supine position.

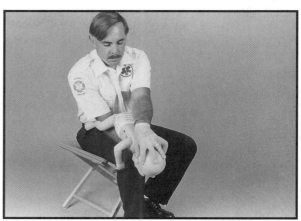

4. With the infant lying on his back, place the tips of your first two fingers on his sternum one finger-width below an imaginary line drawn from one nipple to the other. Your fingers should be side-by-side and in line with the long axis of the sternum, as shown.

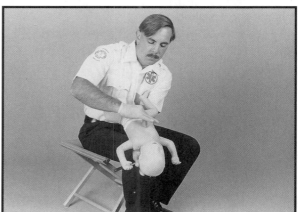

5. While assuring that the infant is firmly supported from behind by your arm and thigh, or by the firm, flat surface, push directly downward with your fingers and compress the infant's sternum approximately one-third to one-half the depth of the chest (usually about 1/2 to 1 inch). Perform five of these chest thrusts.

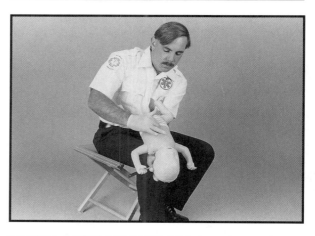

6. After completing the five chest thrusts, open the infant's mouth with a tongue-jaw lift and attempt to visualize the obstruction. If you can see it, try to remove it with your fingers. ***Do NOT perform a blind finger sweep or manually attempt to remove a foreign body from an infant's mouth unless you can actually see it.*** Blind finger sweeps are recommended in adults *BUT NOT WITH INFANTS* and children as they may push the foreign body back into the airway — causing even greater obstruction.

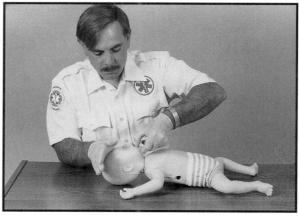

7. After performing 5 back blows and 5 chest thrusts and looking in the infant's mouth, if you do not see the obstruction open the airway and attempt to ventilate the infant with the BVM. If there is no chest rise and no other indication that the ventilation has been delivered, reposition the head and try again. If the second attempt also fails, turn the infant back up on your arm and repeat the earlier cycle of 5 back blows followed immediately by turning the patient over and delivering 5 chest thrusts, then opening the mouth and looking for a foreign body, then re-attempting ventilations, etc.

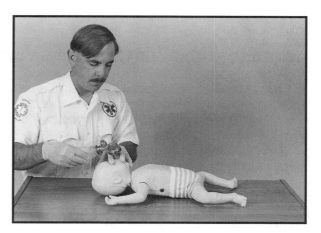

8. If the obstruction persists after a few of these cycles, consider initiating transport while you continue to repeat the cycle of back blows, chest thrusts, visualizing, ventilating, etc. If Advanced Life Support personnel are present, they may attempt a visualized removal with Magill forceps — or if all else fails, a needle cricothyroidotomy to create an alternate air pathway below the level of the obstruction.

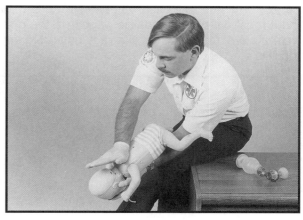

ALS

VISUALIZED REMOVAL OF FOREIGN BODY OBSTRUCTION

The procedures discussed to this point are performed "blindly"—that is, the EMT is not able to see the object he is trying to dislodge while delivering sub-diaphragmatic abdominal thrusts, chest thrusts, or (in infants) back blows. Only in children and infants has visualizing the object been included in the preceding sequences.

However, foreign objects may be able to be removed from the mouth and upper airway under direct visualization by trained advanced personnel using a laryngoscope (or flashlight with tongue depressors) and either Magill forceps or a Kelly clamp. The "blind" procedures already discussed should be initially attempted while the necessary equipment for a visualized attempt is being assembled. Visualized removal will be virtually impossible in a patient who is still conscious or has a gag reflex—the introduction of the laryngoscope blade or tongue depressors, to say nothing of the forceps or clamp, will usually cause so much gagging and motion in such patients that the EMT will find it most difficult to visualize or secure the object. Although the choice of equipment is left to the preference of the operator, it is recommended that a laryngoscope and straight blade be used when possible.

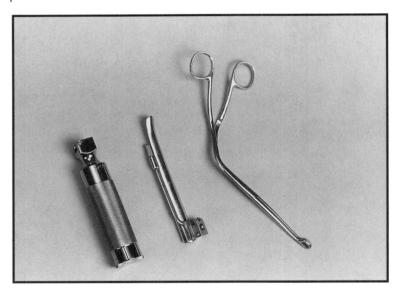

Once appropriate body substance isolation precautions have been taken, the necessary equipment has been assembled and readied, and the patient is lying on his back, position yourself above the patient's head much as you would to perform visualized orotracheal intubation.

1. Hold the laryngoscope in your left hand and insert the blade into the patient's mouth while holding the Magill forceps or Kelly clamp in your right hand. Unlike endotracheal intubation, do not immediately advance the tip of the blade deeply into the patient's oropharynx. Rather, use the lighted tip to visually explore the mouth and anterior pharynx for any foreign objects before moving deeper into the pharynx and toward the trachea.

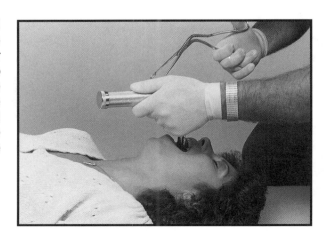

2. Slowly move the blade deeper into the pharynx until you can visualize the foreign object. Again, be cautious that you do not move too quickly and push the obstruction even further into the airway.

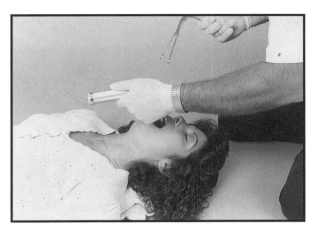

3. Once you have visualized the object, insert the Magill forceps or Kelly clamp into the patient's mouth and grasp the obstruction. With a steady firm motion, withdrawn the obstruction from the patient's mouth.

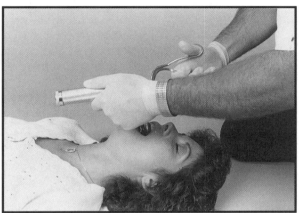

4. If you are unable to grasp the object initially, have a second EMT continue to perform abdominal thrusts to try and advance the object further toward you. After a few attempts, if you are still unsuccessful in removing the obstruction, you should consider performing a cricothyroidotomy if you are trained and authorized to do so.

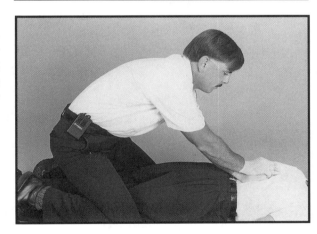

AN INTRODUCTION TO MANAGEMENT OF OPEN AND TENSION PNEUMOTHORACES

An **open pneumothorax** ("sucking chest wound") occurs when an opening is created through the chest wall, thereby allowing a direct flow of air between the thoracic cavity and outside atmosphere. Knife wounds, gunshot wounds and piercing types of injuries can all cause an open pneumothorax, which disrupts the patient's ability to inflate his lungs normally and to draw air into the alveoli. Recognizing and sealing these open wounds can be life-saving in itself.

An open chest wound allows air to enter the chest cavity through the injury site and affects the lung's ability to expand during inhalation. As the patient's chest wall moves outward during inhalation, the negative pressure normally created in the lung on the injured side is lost as outside air is sucked through the hole in the chest wall and into the pleural space outside of the lung—from whence comes the name "sucking chest wound". Only minimal air/oxygen is drawn through the patient's mouth, nose, and trachea into the alveoli of that lung and the lung remains deflated. It is very possible that the first signs that you discover of an open chest wound may be the sound of air passing in and out of the open wound. By quickly recognizing and sealing the open wound you can allow the lung to resume normal inflation. If possible, seal the hole when the patient exhales as there will be less air volume in the thorax at that moment than during the peak inhalation phase of breathing.

The classic occlusive dressing of choice has been Vaseline®—impregnated gauze pads, desirable both for the impermeability of the soaked pad and also of the foil wrapper in which the gauze is packaged. Both are frequently used to seal an open chest wound. Bulky "multi-trauma" gauze dressings, sterilized aluminum foil and flexible plastic films such as Saran Wrap® are other commonly used materials for sealing open chest wounds.

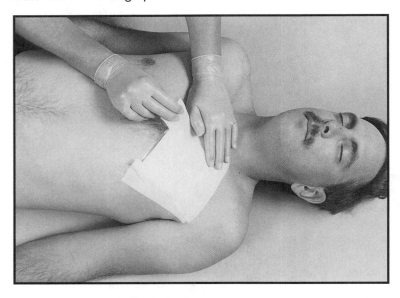

An important adjunct is three inch wide adhesive tape for firmly holding the occlusive dressing in place over the wound. When vaseline gauze is used, the EMT must be careful to wipe the skin around the dressing to remove any of the vaseline which may become placed on the skin and interfere with the tape's adherence to it. If available, the application of benzoin swabs in the area where the tape will lie should be considered to promote greater adhesion to the skin.

If there is an impaled object still in the chest cavity when you examine the patient, you must occlude the wound while leaving the object in place. The occlusive dressing, such as the vaseline gauze pad and foil wrapper, can be cut to fit around the object and then taped to the patient's skin. You must also securely immobilize the protruding object in place so that it cannot move and cause further injury.

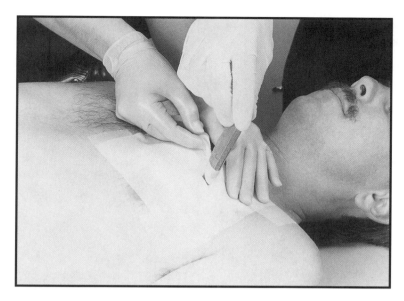

With any penetrating trauma, especially gunshot wounds, be sure to check for the presence of exit wounds or other open wounds on the anterior, posterior and lateral chest wall. Sealing one open chest wound will not overcome the problem if a second open wound remains undiscovered.

Tension Pneumothorax (Develops After Closing An Open Pneumothorax)

Occluding an open chest wound solves the problem of air moving through the chest wall rather than through the intended (anatomic) airway, however it creates the opportunity for an even more dangerous condition to develop — a **tension pneumothorax.** With the chest wall opening sealed, air entering the thorax must again exclusively pass through the trachea and bronchi to reach the lungs. However, when the open chest wound was caused by a penetration it is likely that an opening was also produced in the lung itself and not just the external chest wall. Sealing the chest wall does not seal the wound in the lung, and air entering the injured lung through the bronchus is able to pass through the lung into the pleural space. If the lung inflates during inhalation but collapses sufficiently to cause the opening in the lung to close, a one-way valve is produced and air will accumulate in the pleural space — building the intrathoracic pressure to the point where it not only compresses the injured lung but also causes a shift in the mediastinum and initiates collapse of the lung on the opposite side of the thorax. Further, pressure on the heart and great vessels compromises the patient's cardiac output.

The resolution of this condition is to vent the increased pressure from within the injured side of the chest without recreating the problems of the open pneumothorax. With an open pneumothorax this may be done passively by any level of EMT by applying a dressing and bandage that incorporates a one-way valve effect, or by opening or removing the occlusive dressing to allow the built-up air to escape. When a tension pneumothorax results from a closed pneumothorax, the problem may also be addressed invasively with a needle thoracostomy by those EMTs who have been trained and certified in such advanced life support procedures.

Some protocols call for the use of very flexible material — such as Saran Wrap® — as an occlusive dressing for open chest wounds. In such cases the plastic film is placed over the wound but is not taped to the skin around its complete perimeter—one side or corner is deliberately left untaped. The intention is to create a self-venting one-way valve or "flutter" valve which will allow any air

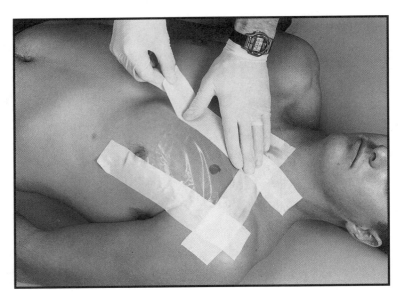

pressure that is building up in the thorax to escape through the untaped portion of the dressing when the patient exhales. When the patient's chest expands with inhalation the film is drawn tightly across the open wound and the negative pressure seals it so that ambient air cannot enter the pleural space. Use of this technique is not an automatic cure-all; a suitable lightweight and flexible material must be available (the vaseline gauze pad and its foil wrapper will *NOT* work for this procedure!), and there is no assurance that air will not leak into the wound or that it will not clot shut despite the plastic dressing's designed ability to vent.

A simpler approach is to initially bandage all the edges of the occlusive dressing completely shut. As time passes, if the patient's ventilatory condition deteriorates and the EMT suspects the development of a tension pneumothorax, the bandage and dressing should be partially removed to expose the wound. If it has not clotted shut, "burping" the wound in this way should allow any pressurized air to escape and thus relieve the developing tension pneumothorax. As with the "self-venting" bandage, the success of this measure in relieving a developing tension pneumothorax is contingent upon the wound remaining open under the dressing so that air can escape when the bandage is removed.

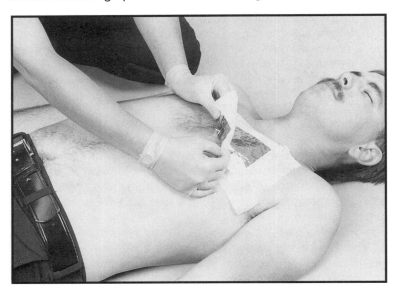

There have been anecdotal reports of protocols which permit the insertion of oxygen connecting tubing or a suction catheter *into* an open chest wound before the occlusive bandage is applied. The proximal end of the tube extends out from under the bandage and ends in some type of one-way valve which permits excess pressure in the thorax to be relieved but does not allow outside air to enter the pleural space. Another suggestion has been to pierce the occlusive bandage with a large bore IV needle/catheter before applying it to the chest. The metal needle is then withdrawn from the catheter and the occlusive bandage is applied over the wound with the distal end of the IV catheter being placed as close as possible to the wound—but not actually inserted into it. A one-way flutter valve or other venting device can then be attached to the hub of the catheter. Each of these methods has some pragmatic value, and some mirror more formal and well-proven surgical procedures that are commonly performed in the hospital such as the insertion of "chest tubes". Their widespread use and successfulness as prehospital procedures, however, is hard to document, and we do not recommend their adoption until sufficient scientific study indicates that they can be effectively and safely used.

Tension Pneumothorax (Develops With A Closed Pneumothorax)

A tension pneumothorax can develop from a closed pneumothorax as well as from an open one. A closed pneumothorax can result from blunt trauma or can occur spontaneously from a lung defect. A tension pneumothorax that develops from a closed pneumothorax can not be resolved by simply opening a dressing—yet relieving the excessive intrathoracic pressure on the injured side remains a true emergency if the patient is to be able to continue to breathe or be ventilated, or if a reduction in cardiac output which could result in marked cellular hypoxia and cardiac arrest is to be avoided.

When personnel trained to decompress a closed tension pneumothorax are not present, the patient must be immediately transported to the nearest personnel or facility with this capability if he is to survive. Advanced Life Support EMTs have the option of inserting a large-bore IV needle/catheter through the patient's chest wall to decompress a tension pneumothorax. After the needle is withdrawn from the catheter a one-way valve is attached that allows air which is accumulating in the pleural space to vent out of the chest but prevents outside air from entering. If a commercial one-way valve is not available, one long-standing method is to tape a finger from a powder-free latex glove to the catheter hub, and to cut a small opening in the other end of the finger. The latex will collapse on itself to prevent ambient air from entering the hub of the catheter, but will readily open to allow air exiting the thorax through the catheter to pass to the outside. Slightly moistening the inside of the latex finger before attaching it to the catheter hub increases its adhesive tendencies and may seal it better against the chance of ambient air entering the thorax through this route.

Another technique to provide a one-way valve is to attach standard IV tubing to the catheter hub. Cut off the drip chamber and "bag spike", fully open the flow valve, and insert the end of the tubing below the water level of a bottle of sterile water or saline which is positioned lower than the patient's chest. As pressurized air escapes from the thorax through the IV catheter it will move along the IV tubing and eventually bubble up through the water or saline. The water keeps any ambient air from entering the tubing and chest, and the negative pressure in the thorax at inspiration is not sufficient to lift any of the sterile water or saline up the tubing as long as the bottle is kept below the level of the IV catheter in the patient's chest.

Even when a needle thoracostomy has been performed, the EMT must still remember that the IV catheter can become kinked in the intercostal muscles or become clotted with blood and the tension pneumothorax can be re-established. The ultimate measure of the treatment's effectiveness in relieving a tension pneumothorax remains the air rushing out of the wound as it is burped or from the needle as it is inserted into the chest. Most important is to see immediate improvement in the patient's ventilatory and circulatory status. Whether relieved by "burping" an occluded open pneumothorax or by decompressing a closed pneumothorax with a needle thoracostomy, the patient's ventilatory and circulatory status must be continuously checked to detect any re-occurrence of the tension pneumothorax that would require that the wound again be "burped" or decompressed.

With any simple pneumothorax, the patient must be continuously monitored to identify if it progresses into a tension pneumothorax that requires steps to relieve the excessive intrathoracic pressure that has developed.

MANAGING AN OPEN PNEUMOTHORAX (And A Developing Tension Pneumothorax)

When an open wound of the thorax allows outside air to freely pass through the chest wall, it defeats the differential pressure-based system which allows our lungs to inhale air and oxygen when the thoracic cage expands. This can be a life-threatening problem which is best resolved in the field by sealing the open wound with an air-tight "occlusive" dressing and bandage. A variety of different techniques and materials can be used to seal the opening, however regardless of which is chosen the EMT must remain vigilant that the patient does not subsequently develop a tension pneumothorax.

1. Having taken appropriate body substance isolation procedures, place your gloved hand over the wound to seal the hole while a second EMT obtains the necessary supplies and equipment.

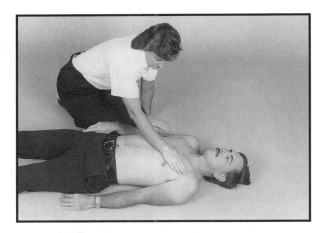

2. You will need at least some Vaseline® gauze, additional gauze pads, adhesive tape, and bandage scissors. If your squad carries any other type of occlusive materials which can be used as a dressing (such as sterile aluminum foil or Saran Wrap®), they should be procured also. Place the vaseline gauze over the wound during the exhalation phase of the patient's breathing cycle, as you remove your hand from the hole. The dressing should amply overlap the edges of the wound. Do not hesitate to add more dressings to the area to assure an occlusive seal if needed.

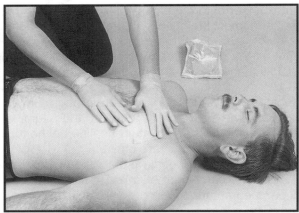

3. With the vaseline gauze in place, use a towel or other material to wipe the skin around the gauze pad to remove any vaseline that has leaked from the pad and which may interfere with taping the bandage in place.

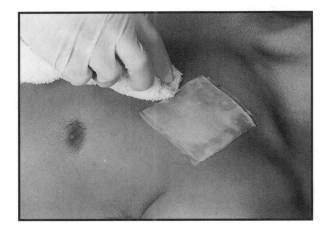

4. Take the foil package in which the gauze was supplied and place that over the gauze pad on the chest. Tape the foil package securely to the patient's skin to make the bandage air tight. If conscious, the patient should report some relief once the hole is sealed.

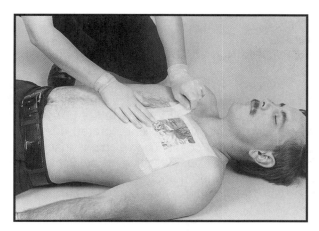

5. An alternative to the use of vaseline gauze is to employ a plastic film to create a self-venting bandage. Place the film directly over the wound with its edges extending beyond the wound by at least 3 or 4 inches in at least one section. Securely tape the film in place, leaving one area of the edge of the film untaped (this should extend at least 3 or 4 inches beyond the edge of the wound). As long as the wound does not close due to clotting, pressurized air should be able to escape from within the chest through the open channel in the plastic film during exhalation while outside air is prevented from entering the chest during inhalation as the film collapses over the hole.

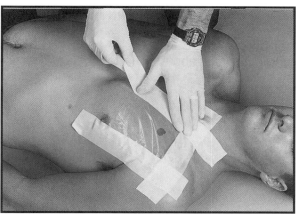

6. Regardless of the materials and methods used, the EMT must continuously observe the patient for any signs of deterioration or increased ventilatory difficulty. The EMT's prime suspicion must be that the patient *will* develop a tension pneumothorax which will require further actions on the part of the EMT ("burping" the bandage or performing a needle decompression of the chest, etc.)

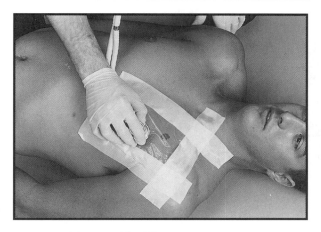

7. Carefully monitor the patient's condition to see if the pneumothorax begins to develop into a tension pneumothorax. If this is suspected, remove the tape and raise a corner of the gauze pad and foil package. If the wound has not clotted shut, removing a portion of the dressing should allow the release of any pressurized air which has been trapped in the thoracic cavity — relieving the tension pneumothorax. If *NO* air is released when the dressing is opened in this manner, but the patient still displays signs of a tension pneumothorax, appropriately trained EMTs may need to perform a needle decompression of the chest.

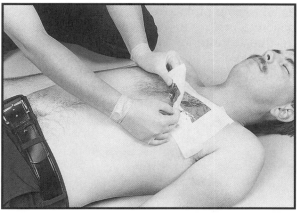

ALS

PERFORMING A NEEDLE THORACOSTOMY

A needle thoracostomy, or needle decompression of the chest, is an advanced life support skill in which a large bore IV needle/catheter (preferably at least 2 inches long) is inserted between the ribs to allow built-up air to escape from the thorax. It is only performed when the patient's ventilatory condition has significantly deteriorated due to the presence of a tension pneumothorax on one or both sides of the chest. The needle is inserted just *above* the selected rib so as to avoid the nerve and blood vessel bundle which exists just below each rib. After determining the presence of a developing tension pneumothorax and establishing its location as either the right or left side of the chest, and after taking appropriate body substance isolation precautions:

1. Locate the second or third intercostal space in the midclavicular line. One way to do this is to feel for the "angle of Louis" — the bump which can be palpated about a quarter of the way down the patient's sternum from his suprasternal notch.

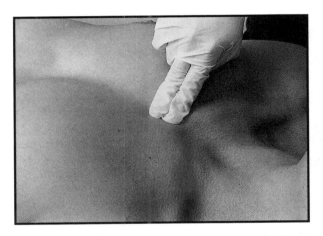

2. Slide your fingers laterally from the angle of Louis and you should feel the second intercostal space. Continue sliding your fingers laterally until they are vertically in line with the midpoint of the patient's clavicle (the "mid-clavicular line"). The point you have just found is the place where you will insert the needle.

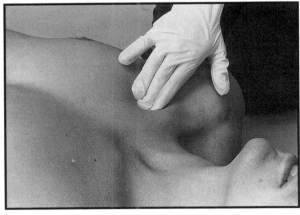

3. In some protocols a lower lateral site is an option to provide an alternative location if needed due to anterior injuries of the chest. This lower lateral site is in the fifth or sixth intercostal space along the mid-axillary line. To locate this, place a finger on the mid-axillary line and palpate the lowest (10th) rib of the rib cage.

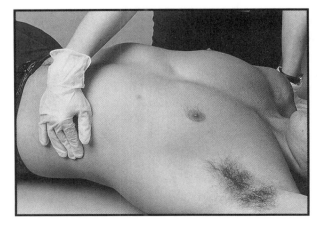

4. Then slide your finger slowly up the ribcage (cephalad), counting the depressions between the ribs as you go. The first depression to be felt will be the 9th intercostal space, the next the 8th, and so on. Keep counting while sliding your finger toward the armpit until you reach the 6th or 5th intercostal space on the mid-axillary line. This will be the needle insertion site. When this site is selected the insertion should be during peak inhalation to assure that the diaphragm is not elevated into the thorax as the needle is entering.

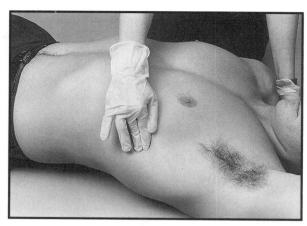

5. Cleanse the site and the surrounding area with alcohol or Betadine antiseptic pads. Use a large bore (14 gauge or larger) IV needle catheter that is preferably at least 2 inches long (the short-length, large bore needle catheters used for trauma fluid resuscitation may be too short to extend through the chest wall to the pleural cavity).

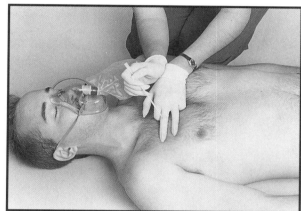

6. At your preference you can hold the needle/catheter directly in your hand, or attach a 10cc syringe to the needle hub for better control. If you use a syringe, pull the plunger halfway up into the barrel before entering the skin. Many EMTs find that it is easier to manipulate the needle if it is first attached to a syringe.

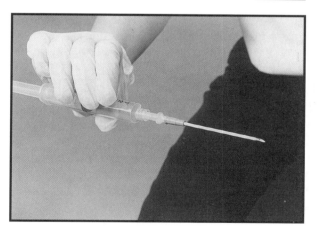

7. If you use a catheter-over-needle device without a syringe, remove the plastic cap from the *needle* hub. This allows air to exit the needle once it passes through the chest wall.

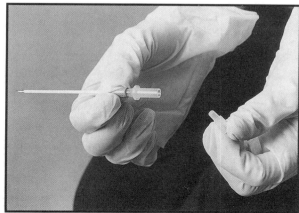

8. Hold the needle perpendicular to the skin. Insert the needle through the intercostal space by riding over top of the rib, never on the bottom of the rib. This is done to avoid the nerve and vascular bundle that exists just below each rib. Push the needle until you feel a "pop" as you enter the pleural space. If there is pressurized air in the cavity (as with a present or developing tension pneumothorax) you should hear a hiss of air exiting through the hub of the needle.

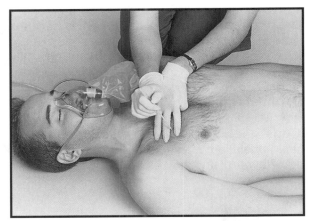

9. When using a needle that is attached to a syringe, if there is a tension pneumothorax present the plunger will be pushed outward in the barrel when the needle enters the pleural space as pressurized air exits the chest. If there is not a tension pneumothorax present the plunger will remain unmoving or on inspiration will be sucked further into the barrel. Once the needle/catheter has been inserted in the chest, detach the syringe.

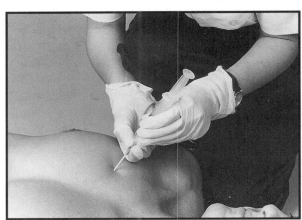

10. Advance the catheter over the needle as if you were starting an IV. Remove the needle, leaving only catheter in place. Depending on the angle of your approach over the rib as you entered the skin, you may need to move the patient's arm or shoulder to prevent the catheter from kinking shut once the needle has been removed. The catheter hub must be fastened to the chest with tape. Be sure that it does not become bent over or kinked shut when you are securing it.

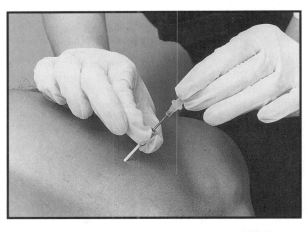

11. The addition of a one-way valve is required so that air is not drawn into the pleural space with each inhalation. The easiest way to make one of these is to attach a commercial device (e.g., Heimlich valve). If one is not available you can use a finger cut from a powder-free latex exam glove and tape it to the hub of the needle with the tip of the glove cut off for air to escape. Be sure the finger is long enough to collapse over the hub of the needle during inhalation.

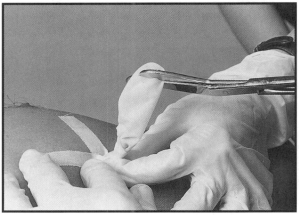

12. Another, simpler method is to attach standard IV tubing to the hub of the catheter and tape it in place. Cut off the drip chamber and spike sections from the other end of the tubing and place it under the surface of the fluid in a bottle of sterile water or saline which is placed below the level of the patient's chest. By placing the end underwater and well below the patient's chest you create a water seal, allowing air to leave the tubing but not to enter it. Whichever is done, make sure the catheter is stable and free-flowing for air movement. If it is kinked closed the tension pneumothorax can easily re-occur.

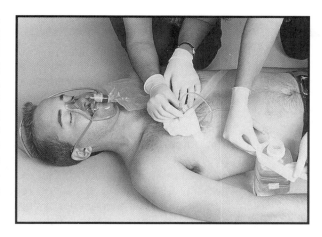

MANAGEMENT OF A FLAIL CHEST

When injury to the rib cage results in two or more adjacent ribs being fractured each in two or more places, or when two or more adjacent ribs and the sternum are fractured, so that a comminuted area without a remaining skeletal connection is formed, the patient is said to have a "flail chest". After such an injury the intercostal muscles will typically spasm and thereby maintain the continuity of the chest wall for a period of time. During that period inspiratory and expiratory chest wall movement will be much as normal and still result in adequate air exchange. Once the intercostal muscles tire (or in some cases immediately post-insult) the continuity between this free section and the remaining chest wall may be lost and it will "flail" and move in an opposite direction to the rest of the ribcage during the chest excursion. This ***paradoxical motion*** of the flail section results in the internal volume of the thorax remaining essentially the same regardless of the degree of movement caused by the chest wall movement. When the chest moves upward and outward to inhale, the flail section collapses inward. Since the shape but not the volume of the thorax is changed, negative pressure is not produced in the lungs and the patient cannot draw an adequate amount of — or in some cases, any — air in. The greater the number of ribs fractured, the greater the potential ventilatory compromise. If a large enough area of the chest has disorganized movement, virtually no air exchange will result even though chest excursion is exaggerated.

Patients found with paradoxical chest movement need immediate positive pressure ventilation to assure a sufficient inspiratory volume. While stabilizing a moving flail segment is important, the most common life-threatening problem for the patient is one of hypoxia resulting from the damage to the pulmonary tissue underlying the injured ribs. This will be covered later in this Section. Once the positive presssure ventilation is underway, firm manual pressure can be applied to the moving flail segment to stabilize it. This support should be sufficiently firm and cover a large enough area to prevent the flail segment from bulging outward as each positive pressure inspiration is provided, or as the uninjured sections of the chest wall move inward with exhalation. The manual pressure provided must be neither so forceful nor so localized that it causes the flail segment to be pushed inward beyond the margins of the intact ribcage and onto the underlying organs.

Stabilization of the flail section, in addition to being necessary for the proper mechanics of ventilation, also minimizes the segment's independent motion and the risk that such movement will cause additional damage to the intercostal nerves or blood vessels or those structures which underlie the injured area.

Once ventilation and mild hand pressure over the flail have been initiated, the EMT should replace the manual stabilization with mechanical support as soon as practical. If a BVM is being used to provide ventilation, supplemental oxygen and a reservoir should be added as well in order to provide a high FiO_2.

For continued support of the flail segment, a folded towel or small pillow should be taped over the flail segment to stabilize it during ventilation. Sufficiently long pieces of tape should be used to provide adequate adhesion but must not completely encircle the chest or extend so far around the circumference of the chest that they inhibit or curtail proper chest rise.

Heavy objects such as sandbags or IV solution bags should not be used to stabilize a flail segment. Their weight can result in so inhibiting the chest movement that an adequate inspiratory volume can no longer be provided. As well, such gross weight localized over the flail segment can push it deeply into the thoracic cavity and cause further injury.

A flail chest can produce lowered blood oxygen levels and increased cellular hypoxia from two different mechanisms: the reduced or absent pulmonary ventilation previously described, and from direct injury to the underlying lung. Due to the cavitation produced by a force sufficient to produce a flail, and the sudden intrusion on the lung that often occurs as the ribs fracture, flail chests are generally associated with significant pulmonary contusions. When an area of the lung is severely contused, oxygen and carbon dioxide can not be exchanged in that area of lung tissue. Blood in the pulmonary circuit passes through this area without any oxygen loading or CO_2 elimination. This oxygen-depleted blood mixes with the oxygenated blood that has passed through healthy sections of the lung, lowering the overall concentration of oxygen in the bloodstream. Even though the EMT has restored ventilation and is providing a proper minute volume, lowered blood oxygen levels will result.

Because of the high probability that the flail has underlying pulmonary contusions associated with it, as soon as practical after ventilation has been initiated and the flail segment stabilized, a reservoir and high flow oxygen should be added if a BVM is being used. By providing ventilation with an FiO_2 of 0.85 – 1.00 the EMT can be sure that, regardless of any mixing of un-oxygenated and re-oxygenated blood, a relatively high blood oxygen level is still maintained and continued cellular hypoxia is avoided.

Even if the patient with a flail chest is found to have no paradoxical movement, it is unlikely that he is providing a sufficient minute volume and oxygenation for himself — therefore the treatment and priorities previously described should be provided by the EMT without alteration.

Once the patient is found to have lowered or absent air exchange and paradoxical movement of a part of the chest wall, or upon palpation two or more adjacent ribs appear to be fractured in two places (or at or with the sternum), you (the EMT) should:

1. Immediately direct another EMT to initiate positive pressure ventilation while you apply mild manual pressure that covers the area of the flail segment and the immediately adjacent rib ends in order to stabilize the segment continuously during ventilation. ***Care must be taken to avoid placing too localized or forceful pressure on the segment.*** If the patient has an altered level of consciousness, airway management must also be provided.

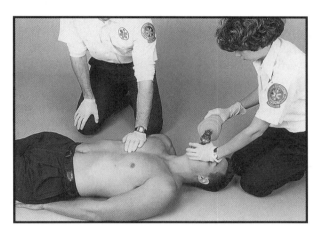

2. Once ventilation and manual stabilization of the flail segment have been initiated, a folded towel or small pillow should be taped over the flail and adjacent ribs to prevent movement during ventilation. When taping the chest wall, tape only between 1/3 and 1/2 of the chest's circumference. Never wrap tape completely around the chest as this will inhibit full chest inflation and impede ventilation. ***Heavy objects such as sand bags or IV solution bags should not be used*** because they can defeat the EMT's provided ventilations and can push the flail segment into the ribcage and cause further damage. Further, the presence of any heavy object on the chest wall will make the process of ventilation more difficult.

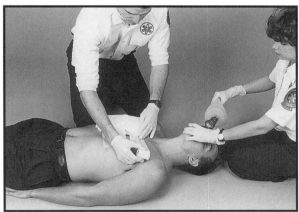

3. Once the segment has been taped, a reservoir and supplemental oxygen should be added if the BVM is being used. Ventilations should be provided with an FiO_2 of 0.85 – 1.00 to maximize blood oxygen concentration. Once other urgent priorities have been met, transport the patient to the nearest trauma center for further assessment and any needed surgical intervention.

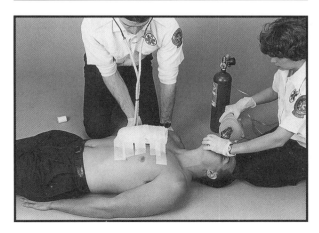

MANUAL RELIEF OF ABDOMINAL DISTENTION FROM GASTRIC INSUFFLATION

Gastric distention can occur when too high a ventilatory pressure, too great an inspiratory volume, or incomplete exhalation occurs during overly energetic positive pressure ventilation from a BVM, Demand Valve, or even mouth-to-mask ventilation. Another cause can be improper alignment of the patient's head and neck while performing ventilation, resulting in some delivered air being directed into the esophagus and stomach instead of into the trachea. Normally, moderate gastric distention will not encumber ventilation and does not need to be relieved.

If the gastric distention is too great it can exert pressure on the diaphragm and impede proper lung inflation even in intubated patients. The EMT should expect and be prepared for the patient to vomit as the distention is manually relieved. If it is suspected that the patient has spinal injuries, every effort must be made to roll him as a unit with due precaution to keep his head and spine in the neutral in-line position throughout.

Whether the patient has spine trauma or not, the procedure requires a minimum of four people: three to roll the patient onto his side and to properly maintain him in this position while purging the stomach, and a fourth person to suction the pharynx. Once ventilation has been stopped the EMT who was providing it can maintain the patient's head in the neutral in-line position. This is necessary even in patients without spine trauma. The EMT at the patient's chest can hold him once he has been rolled onto his side, and the EMT who rolled the hips and legs can compress the abdomen. The fourth EMT should be positioned facing the patient's mouth and nose with a powered suction unit running or a V-VAC held ready. The urgency of purging the stomach to restore adequate ventilation dictates that the procedure neither be omitted nor delayed when the number of people available is less than the optimal number. If only two EMTs are available, one will have to prepare the suction while the other continues to ventilate. When ready, the EMT at the head maintains the cervical alignment and performs the suctioning. The second EMT rolls the torso and supports the patient on his side while purging the stomach. In such cases it is helpful to enlist bystanders to assist with rolling the patient. The need to be able to provide adequate ventilation supersedes the risk of rolling him without enough trained EMTs.

When gastric distention has been identified to be significantly interfering with adequate ventilation the EMT should immediately act to relieve it. With the assistance of several others, he should prepare to roll the patient onto his side and to suction him with a Yankauer or other large bore tip, or with a V-VAC. The EMT who has been ventilating the patient should continue to ventilate with as great a volume as possible without causing further gastric insufflation while the other EMTs take any additionally needed body substance isolation precautions and prepare to roll and suction the patient. In any patient who is being ventilated with a mask, the ventilator and mask will have to be removed from the patient's face before the stomach is decompressed. Attempting to ventilate such patients while they are being rolled onto their side, supported on their side, or returned to a supine position, is impractical at best and usually only results in increasing the actual interruption in effective ventilation. Therefore, except in intubated patients it is recommended that ventilations be interrupted prior to rolling the patient and only reinstituted once he has been returned to a supine position. Everything should be readied before rolling the patient is begun, in order to allow this to be performed in such a way that ventilation is interrupted for no more than thirty seconds. Once the:

- Suction has been prepared and properly placed,
- Any needed body substance isolation precautions have been taken,
- The other EMTs are properly positioned and ready,
- And you are properly positioned at the patient's hips,
  you are ready to initiate the maneuver.

1. Direct the EMT providing ventilation to stop and to support the patient's head and neck. Then direct all of the EMTs to roll the patient onto his side (facing away from the EMTs).

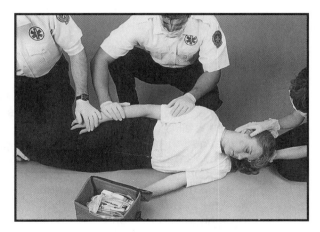

2. If spinal injuries are suspected, the patient will have to be moved and maintained using a suitable logroll or, if immobilized, the patient will have to be rotated onto his side together with the backboard.

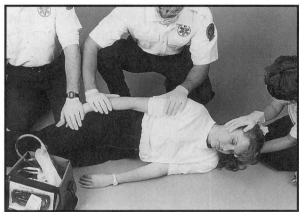

3. With the suction equipment turned on and running at its maximum, gently but firmly apply pressure to the patient's anterior abdomen with the flat of your hand. Prepare for vomitus along with air! Maintain the patient on his side and rapidly suction his mouth and pharynx to make sure that he does not aspirate any gastric contents. Ideally, the patient will have already been intubated before you need to manually relieve the gastric distention.

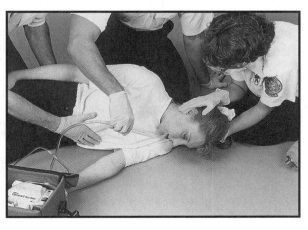

4. Once any gastric contents that are regurgitated into the pharynx have been suctioned, roll the patient back into a supine position and immediately direct the EMT at the head to resume airway management and ventilation. If the gastric distention has been sufficiently reduced, ventilating at an adequate volume should no longer present a problem. If not, or if the problem returns at a later time, ventilate the patient for 30 seconds or more and then repeat the procedure. Further regurgitation following this procedure is common and must be anticipated and the patient immediately suctioned if pulmonary aspiration is to be avoided.

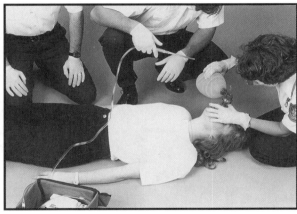

ALS

INSERTION OF A NASOGASTRIC TUBE
(For Relief Of Gastric Distention Or Evacuation Of Gastric Contents)

Although the majority of EMS texts mention or call for the use of nasogastric tubes (NG tubes) for patients with an altered level of consciousness, the prehospital practice of this relatively simple yet very valuable skill is thought to be rare. Certainly, placement of a nasogastric tube should be an early consideration in the management of any seriously injured patient, any intubated patient, any patient for whom ventilations are being or are anticipated to be provided, and any patient who may be expected to vomit or who may benefit from lavage (e.g., poisonings and overdoses). In addition to decompressing the stomach of gases and fluids which have already built up and become pressurized by the time that the NG tube is inserted, placement of a nasogastric tube also provides an ongoing "vent" which can prevent any ensuing accumulation and forestall problems before they develop.

The primary indication for the EMT to insert a nasogastric tube is to relieve gastric distention. As has been discussed earlier in this text, gastric distention can be an unwanted by-product of provided ventilation, and can cause serious compromise of the patient's ventilation or of the EMT's ability to provide ventilations. Gastric insufflation which produces distention exerts pressure on the diaphragm which subsequently limits the expansion of the thoracic cage as well as of the lungs, and can restrict venous return to the heart (limiting cardiac refill). Emergency department and in-hospital use of NG tubes typically involves attaching them to low pressure intermittent suction machines, whereas prehospital powered suction devices usually operate continuously and at higher suction pressures and, if set at lower levels, neither reliably maintain the needed suction nor guard against its undesirable sudden increase. Additionally, EMS vehicle-mounted suction systems are generally linked to the vehicle's engine speed and therefore the suction provided can vary abruptly with sudden speed-ups and slow downs as the vehicle is driven. Unless the ambulance has been outfitted with intermittent low-pressure suction equipment specially designed for this purpose, the prehospital use of an NG tube should be limited to manual aspiration with a syringe and/or allowing the open-ended tube to passively act as a "vent pipe" from the stomach.

Insertion of an NG tube is contraindicated when the nasopharynx is completely obstructed, when the patient has suffered major facial trauma, when the EMT suspects that the patient may have cervical spine injury, or when the patient has a functioning gastrostomy tube already in place. (A gastrostomy tube, inserted through a surgical opening in the abdomen, provides direct access to the stomach from outside the body and — if functioning correctly — should eliminate the need for an NG tube.)

Nasogastric tubes may be inserted in patients who are conscious or unconscious, and in patients who have already been intubated. The equipment needed to perform a nasogastric tube insertion includes an NG tube, a 50ml syringe, water-soluble lubricant, adhesive tape (0.5 or 1.0 inch width), an emesis basin or towel, a stethoscope, and appropriate personal protective equipment for the EMT (gloves, face shield and goggles, gown, etc.) If the patient is conscious, it will be helpful to have a cup or glass of water available with a drinking straw, if possible.

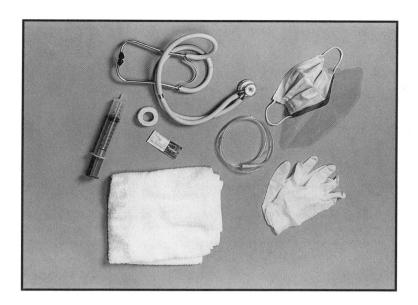

The NG tube should be measured to the patient before beginning the procedure. This will provide an indication of when the distal tip of the NG tube has reached the stomach, and help to avoid inserting the tube too far. While holding the distal end of the NG tube, measure the distance from the patient's earlobe to the bridge of his nose, and additionally from there to a point just below his xiphoid. This length should be marked on the tube with a piece of adhesive tape to serve as a guidepost for how far the tube should be inserted.

The conscious patient should be positioned sitting either fully upright or in a semi-sitting position. The head should be somewhat forward, with the neck slightly flexed, and with the towel draped across the chest. The procedure should be explained to the patient, including why it is important and what to expect. It is advisable to establish a signal — such as raising one finger — that the patient can use to request a pause in the event of excessive gagging or discomfort, however this should not be overemphasized. Most nasogastric tubes are successfully passed with a minimum of patient discomfort — there is no need to prime your patient to expect the worst!

Lubricate the distal 3 – 6 inches of the NG tube liberally and select the most widely patent nostril. With your free hand, support the back of the patient's head and gently move it forward into a slightly flexed position while you insert the tip of the NG tube into the selected nostril. Advance the tube **straight back** *(in an anterior-to-posterior, not cephalad, direction)* into the nostril. If mild resistance is felt, rotating the tube slightly will usually help it to advance. When the tip reaches the posterior nasopharynx the patient is likely to gag slightly. Pause at this point and look into the back of the patient's mouth. You should be able to see the NG tube at the back of the throat. Have the patient swallow repeatedly. If available, have the patient sip water from a cup through a drinking straw. Either of these actions will reduce the sensitivity of the patient's gag reflex and assist him in swallowing the distal tip of the tube past the glottic opening and into the esophagus. Continue to insert the tube into the nose until your pre-measured mark reaches the front edge of the nostril. Sometimes the NG tube will become misdirected and curl up in the patient's oropharynx or pharynx. If this happens, pull back on the tube and again attempt to enter the esophagus. From that point on, inserting the rest of the tube until the taped marker reaches the nostril should be relatively easy.

It is important that the tube not extend too far into the stomach for it can then coil up in the stomach, pass on into the duodenum, or turn and head back up the esophagus.

There may be a slight feeling of resistance as the distal tip of the NG tube passes through the gastroesophageal sphincter muscle at the entrance to the stomach. As the tip enters into the stomach there can be air and gastric contents "shooting" back up the tube if there is a lot of gastric distention. Be careful where you are pointing the *proximal* end of the tube!

When you believe that the distal end of the NG tube is in the stomach, aspirate between 20ml and 35ml of air into the syringe and attach it to the proximal end of the NG tube. While listening over the epigastrium with a stethoscope, have another EMT quickly push the air out of the syringe and into the NG tube. You will hear air entering the stomach if the tube is indeed in the stomach. If air sounds are not heard, advance the tube a little farther and try again. Once air pushed down the NG tube with the syringe has been clearly auscultated over the epigastrium, aspirate the syringe to obtain gastric contents and further confirm proper placement. As mentioned above, if there is a lot of gastric distention you will know it when the tube enters the stomach. If any question of proper placement remains, the NG tube should be withdrawn and, after a brief period, insertion re-attempted. With the distention relieved, detach the syringe from the end of the NG tube. Tape the tube to the patient's nose so that it will not become displaced, however be careful to not cause any pressure against the nasal septum or to obstruct the patient's vision.

Inserting an NG tube in an unconscious patient is complicated by not having the patient's assistance in swallowing the tube past the glottic opening. A common problem is that the tube coils up in the back of the oropharynx. If resistance is encountered soon after the tube has been inserted in the nostril, look into the patient's mouth to see if this is the problem. It may be possible to reach into the mouth with two gloved fingers and manipulate the base of the tongue — directing the tip of the tube along the posterior pharyngeal wall while the other hand continues to advance the tube.

The presence of the endotracheal tube in an intubated patient can also complicate the process of inserting an NG tube, and visualized digital manipulation may again be necessary to direct the NG tube through the glottic opening and into the esophagus. *The EMT is cautioned that the prior placement of an endotracheal tube is no guarantee that the NG tube cannot be placed in the trachea and extend beyond the ET tube's distal cuff.* Even when an endotracheal tube has already been inserted and its proper placement in the trachea confirmed by chest rise and auscultation of the epigastrium and lung fields, the proper placement of the nasogastric tube must still be checked by auscultation of air sounds over the epigastrium when air is injected into the NG tube and ventilation is interrupted, and confirmed by aspiration of gastric fluids into the syringe. As previously mentioned, if proper placement can not be absolutely confirmed the NG tube should be withdrawn and its insertion re-attempted.

As is true with endotracheal tubes, warm nasogastric tubes may become too flexible to push past minor resistance points in the nose, pharynx or esophagus. Should this occur, one possible solution is to chill the tube with ice bags or chemical ice packs to stiffen it and make it easier to pass.

Nasogastric tubes come in different sizes and materials, some with a single opening and others with two lumens. A commonly used tube is the "Salem Sump 16 French" dual lumen tube. The EMT should follow local protocols and preferences for tube selection. After taking appropriate body substance isolation precautions and assembling the needed equipment:

1. Explain to the patient what you are going to do and its importance. Determine the proper length for the NG tube by first placing its distal tip at the patient's nose and measuring from the tip of the nose to the earlobe.

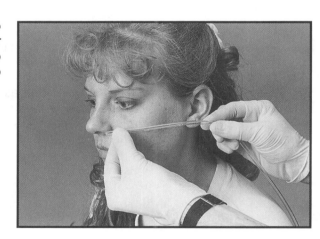

2. Then measure onward from the earlobe to just below his xiphoid. While holding the tube at this measure, place a piece of tape on the tube at that point to mark its maximum insertion length.

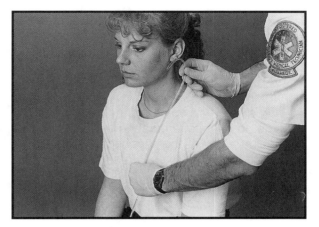

3. Position the patient either sitting fully upright or semi-sitting. Look at the nostrils and select the most widely patent one. Next, drape a towel, if available, across the patient's chest.

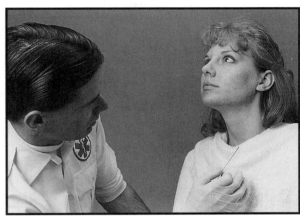

4. Lubricate the distal 3–6 inches of the NG tube with a water soluble material. With one hand support the back of the patient's head and gently lift it forward into a slightly flexed position and insert the tip of the NG tube into the selected nostril.

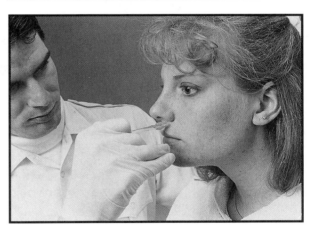

5. Advance the tube *straight back* in an anterior-to-posterior direction — not cephalad. When passing through the posterior part of the nostril and just beyond, some resistance is common. Gently rotating the tube with a back-and-forth motion between your fingertips while advancing the tube is often helpful.

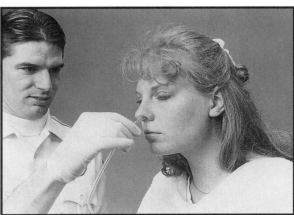

6. The patient will probably gag slightly when the tip of the NG tube reaches the posterior nasopharynx. (You should be able to see the tube in the back of the patient's mouth if you are unsure of its location.) Have the patient swallow repeatedly — or sip water from a glass through a drinking straw — as you continue to advance the NG tube, to help pass the tube through the glottic opening and into the esophagus. If continued resistance is met or if you can see the tube curling up in the patient's mouth, withdraw the tube a short distance and re-attempt to advance it.

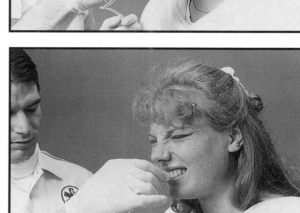

7. There may also be some resistance as the distal end of the tube reaches the sphincter muscle where the esophagus enters the stomach. If there is any gastric distention present, be alert for gas and fluid stomach contents to be rapidly ejected from the *proximal* end of the tube when the distal end enters the stomach. Continue inserting the tube until the tape marker reaches the outer edge of the nostril.

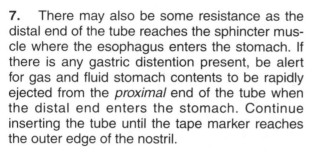

8. Inject between 20ml and 35ml of air from a syringe into the proximal end of the NG tube while an assistant auscultates with a stethoscope over the epigastrium. The sounds of air entering the stomach should be audible through the stethoscope. If they cannot be heard, advance the tube a bit farther and re-check while additional air is injected into the NG tube. Unlike an airway, when the NG tube is properly placed there is direct isolated communication between the stomach and the outside. Therefore, when air is pushed down the NG tube *air sounds should be heard* and are desirable.

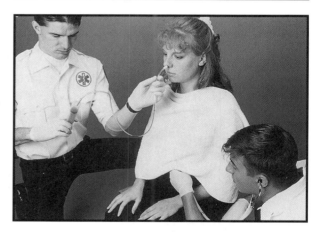

9. Once air sounds are auscultated over the epigastrium when air is injected into the NG tube, confirm the tube's proper placement by drawing back on the plunger of the syringe to create suction in the NG tube. Fluid gastric contents should be drawn into and seen in the barrel of the syringe, further confirming the tube's placement and patency. If its placement can not be confirmed, it will have to be withdrawn and insertion re-attempted after a brief period.

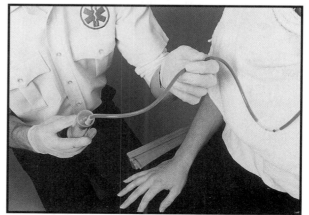

10. Once the tube's placement has been confirmed, remove the syringe from the tube's proximal end and tape the NG tube to the patient's face without putting pressure on the nasal septum or obstructing the patient's vision. In a nonintubated patient it should be secured so that it will not interfere with obtaining a mask seal should it become necessary to provide ventilation. When applying an oxygen mask or ventilating a patient in whom an NG tube has been inserted, care must be taken that the proximal end of the NG tube remains outside of the mask to assure that gastric contents can not be aspirated.

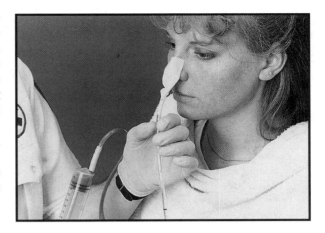

11. Some advanced protocols allow for the emergency insertion of an NG tube for the purpose of purging air from the stomach (to reduce gastric distention), but do not include the evacuation of fluid or solid gastric contents. If evacuation of such stomach contents is allowed, this should be done as soon as the NG tube has been inserted and taped in place. This will help to avoid aspiration of gastric fluids into the lungs if the patient regurgitates. In intubated patients this can be a prudent measure in advance of ET extubation in the event that the patient regains consciousness and can no longer tolerate the ET tube. When the ET tube is removed the patient loses the protection and isolation of his airway that the ET tube was providing.

Similarly, if allowed in cases of poisoning and indicated by the Poison Control Center, activated charcoal and water should be passed down the NG tube in order to collect and dilute the toxin. If this and continued lavage is achieved without unnecessary delay, it will minimize the amount and concentration of the poison which is digested and absorbed into the patient's bloodstream. When the stomach contents are being emptied it is not uncommon for the patient to gag or retch, causing fluid stomach contents to be widely spewed from the mouth of NG tube. To protect against any chance of contamination, proper face protection and a fluid-impervious gown should be added before attempting to evacuate the stomach contents.

Since the portable suction units and those mounted in EMS vehicles are generally unsuitable for gastric suctioning, evacuation of stomach contents should only be done by aspirating with a large syringe unless a low pressure suction unit designed for nasogastric suction is available. The syringe is aspirated while connected to the proximal end or the NG tube, and is then removed for emptying. Alternating between two large syringes (aspirating with one while the other is being emptied) will greatly increase the efficiency of the procedure.

ETI SUMMARY SKILL SHEET

Foreign Body Obstruction: Adult or Child Found Conscious

1. DETERMINE IF the PATIENT is ADEQUATELY MOVING AIR. ASK "ARE YOU CHOKING?," or "Can you speak?" If vocal sounds are not heard, presume that the airway is completely obstructed. IF at any point the PATIENT with a partial obstruction APPEARS TO BE getting WORSE, immediately INTERVENE and attempt TO FORCE THE OBSTRUCTION OUT of the patient's trachea. MOVE BEHIND the patient and PLACE both of YOUR ARMS AROUND the patient's WAIST.

2. FORM A FIST with one hand and place the thumb over your fingers. PLACE the flat side of your FIST AGAINST the patient's ABDOMEN between the navel and the xiphoid.

3. GRASP the outside of YOUR FIST with your other hand. You should be in contact with and BRACE the PATIENT with your own body FROM BEHIND.

4. PULL INWARD AND UPWARD INTO the PATIENT'S ABDOMEN quickly and sharply. COMPRESS the ABDOMINAL CONTENTS TO DISTEND the patient's DIAPHRAGM into his thorax and INCREASE HIS INTRATHORACIC PRESSURE.

5. RELEASE the pressure of YOUR HANDS on the abdomen, but be prepared to support the patient if he "rebounds" forward from the effects of your thrust.

6. REPEAT the THRUSTS continuously UNTIL the FOREIGN BODY is EXPELLED, OR until the PATIENT becomes so weak that he CAN NOT STAND, OR BECOMES UNCONSCIOUS.

If the obstructed adult or child becomes too weak to stand:

7. IF the PATIENT becomes TOO WEAK TO continue STANDing position, you will have to SUPPORT HIM WHILE HELPING HIM TO the GROUND to prevent any injury from occurring during his collapse. INSERT YOUR LEG BETWEEN the PATIENT'S LEGS AND SUPPORT HIM with your arms while he slides DOWN your leg TO the GROUND. DO NOT BECOME so ENTANGED or over-reached that you injure yourself or fall.

8. PLACE the PATIENT in a SUPINE position and REIN-STITUTE abdominal THRUSTS. First STRADDLE his legs so that your hands can easily reach the patient's mid-abdomen. PLACE the heel of one HAND AGAINST his ABDOMEN between the navel and the xiphoid with the fingers pointing cephalad. Place your other hand either on top of the first, or grip the wrist of your first hand with the second.

9. With your ARMS STRAIGHT and your ELBOWS LOCKED, PUSH both cephalad and posteriorly INTO the patient's ABDOMEN.

10. After the compression, RELEASE the pressure of YOUR HANDS until the abdominal wall returns to its original position. CONTINUE abdominal THRUSTS UNTIL the foreign BODY is EXPELLED OR the PATIENT becomes UNCONSCIOUS.

If the obstructed adult or child becomes unconscious:

11. OPEN the patient's MOUTH using a tongue-jaw lift. Insert one or two fingers into the patient's mouth and SWEEP the inside of the mouth if the patient is an adult in an attempt TO EXTRACT the OBSTRUC-TION. IF the patient is a CHILD, perform the same steps but FIRST LOOK into the MOUTH and only insert your fingers if the object can be seen.

12. DIRECT another EMT TO PERFORM a MANUAL AIR-WAY MANEUVER while you ATTEMPT TO VENTI-LATE the PATIENT. IF the first ventilation attempt is UNSUCCESSFUL, REPOSITION the patient's head AND again ATTEMPT TO VENTILATE.

13. IF you are STILL UNSUCCESSFUL, STRADDLE the patient's LEGS (or kneel beside them) and RESUME abdominal THRUSTS. COUNT the number delivered.

14. DELIVER FIVE abdominal THRUSTS then again PER-FORM a TONGUE – JAW LIFT and — if the patient is an adult — a finger SWEEP of the MOUTH in an attempt to remove the obstruction. IF the patient is a CHILD, perform the same steps but FIRST LOOK into the MOUTH and only insert your fingers if the object can be seen.

15. Regardless of whether anything was removed from the mouth, again institute a MANUAL AIRWAY MANEUVER and ATTEMPT TO VENTILATE the patient. IF the ventilation is UNSUCCESSFUL, RE-POSITION the patient's HEAD and ATTEMPT another VENTILATION. IF both attempts are UNSUCCESS-FUL, DELIVER FIVE more abdominal THRUSTS.

16. CONTINUE the CYCLE of five abdominal thrusts, finger sweep (or visualization if a child), and attempted ventilation, UNTIL the obstruction is CLEARED OR other ADVANCED CARE has been INSTITUTED.

17. If spontaneous VENTILATION RESUMES, the EMT should still provide a HIGH FiO_2.

18. IF the airway OBSTRUCTION has been RELIEVED BUT the patient is APNEIC AND PULSELESS, PERFORM CPR.

19. The patient should be TRANSPORTed TO the HOSPI-TAL to be checked for any resulting laryngeal, tracheal, thoracic, or abdominal injury.

20. IF you are UNSUCCESSFUL AFTER performing these cycles of steps for SEVERAL MINUTES, the patient should be RAPIDLY PACKAGED and TRANSPORTed while the steps are continued.

21. ALS PERSONNEL should attempt LARYNGOSCOPY and VISUALIZED REMOVAL with McGill forceps or Kelly clamp. If all attempts to clear the airway have failed after 3 or 4 minutes, CONSIDER a TRANS-TRACHEAL PROCEDURE.

ETI SUMMARY SKILL SHEET
Foreign Body Obstruction Adult or Child Found Unconscious

1. ASSESS RESPONSIVENESS by speaking to the patient and gently shaking him in an attempt to elicit a response.

2. OPEN the MOUTH with a manual airway maneuver (with or without spine protection, as indicated) and LOOK, LISTEN, and FEEL for AIR EXCHANGE.

3. If there is no detectable air exchange, ATTEMPT TO VENTILATE the patient. Do not delay to add supplemental oxygen and a reservoir if you select a BVM — all you want to do at this time is to rapidly initiate ventilation or to identify that there is a problem which defeats your attempt.

4. IF the bag is DIFFICULT TO COMPRESS and there is a lot of AIR LEAKING from AROUND the MASK, REPOSITION the patient's HEAD by tilting it back further. Ensure that the mandible is elevated and that you have a good mask seal.

5. RE-ATTEMPT VENTILATION. IF NO AIR MOVES INto the patient and there is air leakage from around the mask seal, you must ASSUME that there is a foreign body OBSTRUCTION of the airway.

6. Immediately move from the patient's head and STRADDLE his LEGS. PLACE the heel of one HAND ON the midline of the patient's ABDOMEN, between the xiphoid and the umbilicus (but closer to the umbilicus) with the fingers pointing cephalad. Place your other hand on top of the first, and DELIVER 5 abdominal THRUSTS as previously described.

7. Return to the patient's head, PERFORM a TONGUE-JAW LIFT and, if the patient is an adult, insert the index or middle finger of your other hand into one corner of the patient's mouth and SWEEP it deeply across the inside of the MOUTH in an attempt to grasp any foreign objects that may have been dislodged from the trachea into the mouth. If the patient is a child, first look into the mouth and only insert your fingers if an object can be seen.

8. Regardless of whether anything was removed from the mouth, again INSTITUTE a MANUAL AIRWAY MANEUVER and ATTEMPT TO VENTILATE. IF UNSUCCESSFUL, REPOSITION the patient's head and ATTEMPT another VENTILATION. IF still UNSUCCESSFUL, resume the abdominal thrust position and DELIVER 5 more THRUSTS.

9. CONTINUE the CYCLE of five abdominal thrusts, finger sweep (or visualization if a child), and attempted ventilation, UNTIL the obstruction is CLEARED OR other ADVANCED CARE has been instituted.

10. IF spontaneous VENTILATION RESUMES, the EMT should still PROVIDE a HIGH FiO_2.

11. If the airway OBSTRUCTION has been RELIEVED BUT the patient is APNEIC AND PULSELESS, PERFORM CPR.

12. The patient should be TRANSPORTed TO the HOSPITAL to be checked for any resulting laryngeal, tracheal, thoracic, or abdominal injury.

13. IF you are UNSUCCESSFUL AFTER performing these cycles of steps for SEVERAL MINUTES, the patient should be RAPIDLY PACKAGed and TRANSPORTed while the steps are continued.

14. ALS PERSONNEL should attempt laryngoscopy and VISUALIZED REMOVAL with McGill forceps or a Kelly clamp. If all attempts to clear the airway have failed after 3 or 4 minutes, CONSIDER a TRANSTRACHEAL PROCEDURE.

ETI SUMMARY SKILL SHEET
Foreign Body Obstruction: Infant

1. WHEN a complete airway OBSTRUCTION is RECOGNIZED, immediately PICK UP the INFANT and HOLD him FACE DOWN ALONG your FOREARM with his face cupped in the palm of your hand, with his legs straddling your forearm, and with his HEAD held LOWER THAN the rest of his BODY. SUPPORT YOUR ARM on your thigh or on a firm object to prevent it from moving.

2. USE the HEEL OF your other HAND to DELIVER 5 firm BACK BLOWS to the infant between his shoulder blades. PAUSE BETWEEN BLOWS to allow the thorax to "uncompress" and resume its normal shape. Be sure to FIRMLY SUPPORT the INFANT'S BODY with your arm while delivering the back blows.

3. After the 5 back blows, immediately TURN the INFANT over and place him SUPINE on a FIRM FLAT SURFACE or on your supported arm. Place yor free hand on his back, holding his head. Carefully SUPPORT the HEAD AND NECK WHILE TURNING the infant.

4. PLACE the TIPS of your FIRST TWO FINGERS ON his STERNUM one finger-width below an imaginary line drawn from one nipple to the other. Your fingers should be side-by-side and in line with the long axis of the sternum.

5. PUSH directly DOWNWARD with your fingers and COMPRESS the infant's STERNUM approximately 1/3 to 1/2 the depth of the chest (usually about 1/2 to 1 inch). PERFORM 5 of these CHEST THRUSTS.

6. OPEN the infant's MOUTH with a tongue-jaw lift and ATTEMPT TO VISUALIZE the OBSTRUCTION. DO NOT PERFORM a BLIND finger SWEEP UNLESS YOU CAN actually SEE the OBSTRUCTION.

7. IF you DO NOT SEE the obstruction, OPEN the AIRWAY and ATTEMPT TO VENTILATE.

8. IF UNSUCCESSFUL, REPOSITION the head and TRY AGAIN.

9. IF still UNSUCCESSFUL, TURN the INFANT back up on your arm and REPEAT the CYCLE OF 5 BACK BLOWS, 5 CHEST THRUSTS, then OPENING the MOUTH and LOOKING for a foreign body, then RE-ATTEMPTING VENTILATIONS, etc.

10. IF the OBSTRUCTION PERSISTS after a few of these cycles , consider initiating TRANSPORT while you CONTINUE to repeat the CYCLE of back blows, chest thrusts, visualizing, ventilating, etc.

11. If ALS PERSONNEL are present they MAY ATTEMPT a VISUALIZED REMOVAL with Magill forceps — OR if all else fails, a NEEDLE CRICOTHYROIDOTOMY to create an alternate airway.

ALS

ETI SUMMARY SKILL SHEET
Performing A Needle Thoracostomy

1. LOCATE the 2nd or 3rd INTERCOSTAL SPACE in the MIDCLAVICULAR LINE or the 5th or 6th intercostal space in the mid-axillary line.

2. CLEANSE the SITE and the surrounding area with alcohol or Betadine antiseptic pads. USE a LARGE BORE (14 gauge or larger) IV NEEDLE CATHETER that is preferably at least 2 inches long.

3. You can HOLD the NEEDLE/catheter directly in your hand, OR ATTACH a 10cc SYRINGE to the needle hub for better control. If you use a syringe, pull the plunger halfway up into the barrel before entering the skin.

4. If you use a catheter-over-needle device without a syringe, REMOVE the plastic CAP FROM the needle HUB.

5. HOLD the NEEDLE PERPENDICULAR TO the SKIN. INSERT the needle through the intercostal space by riding OVER TOP OF the RIB, never on the bottom of the rib. PUSH the needle UNTIL YOU FEEL a "POP" as you enter the pleural space.

6. When using a needle that is attached to a syringe, if there is a tension pneumothorax present the plunger will be pushed outward in the barrel when the needle enters the pleural space as pressurized air exits the chest. If there is not a tension pneumothorax present the plunger will remain unmoving or on inspiration will be sucked further into the barrel. Once the needle/catheter has been inserted in the chest, DETACH the SYRINGE.

7. ADVANCE the CATHETER over the needle as if you were starting an IV. REMOVE the NEEDLE, leaving only the catheter in place. Depending on the angle of your approach over the rib as you entered the skin, you may need to move the patient's arm or shoulder to prevent the catheter from kinking shut once the needle has been removed. FASTEN the catheter HUB TO the CHEST with tape.

8. ADD a ONE-WAY VALVE so that air is not drawn into the pleural space with each inhalation.

ALS

ETI SUMMARY SKILL SHEET

Insertion of A Nasogastric Tube For Relief of Gastric Distention Or Evacuation of Stomach Contents

1. EXPLAIN to the patient WHAT YOU ARE GOING TO DO and its importance. MEASURE for the proper length of the NG tube by placing its distal tip at the patient's earlobe and then extending it FROM the EARLOBE TO the BRIDGE OF his NOSE.

2. THEN MEASURE onward FROM the bridge of the patient's NOSE TO just BELOW his XIPHOID. While holding the tube at this measure, place a piece of TAPE on the TUBE AT THAT POINT to mark its maximum insertion length.

3. Position the PATENT either SITTING fully UPRIGHT OR SEMI-SITTING. Look at the nostrils and SELECT the most widely PATIENT NOSTRIL. Next, DRAPE a TOWEL, if available, ACROSS the patient's CHEST.

4. LUBRICATE the DISTAL 3–6 inches of the NG TUBE with a water soluble material.

5. With one hand SUPPORT the BACK OF the PATIENT'S HEAD and gently lift it FORWARD into a SLIGHTLY FLEXED position.

6. INSERT the TIP of the NG tube INTO the selected NOSTRIL.

7. ADVANCE the TUBE *straight back* in an ANTERIOR-TO-POSTERIOR direction—not cephalad. GENTLY ROTATE the TUBE with a back-and-forth motion between your fingertips WHILE ADVANCING it to overcome any mild resistance.

8. HAVE the PATIENT SWALLOW repeatedly — or sip water from a glass through a drinking straw — as you continue to advance the NG tube, to help pass the tube through the glottic opening and into the esophagus. IF CONTINUED RESISTANCE is met or if you can see the tube curling up in the patient's mouth, WITHDRAW the tube a short distance AND RE-ATTEMPT to advance it.

9. INSERT the tube UNTIL the tape MARKER reaches the outer edge of the nostril.

10. INJECT between 20ml and 35ml of AIR from a syringe INTO the proximal end of the NG TUBE while an assistant AUSCULTATEs with a stethoscope over the EPIGASTRIUM. IF AIR can NOT be HEARD, ADVANCE the tube a bit FARTHER AND RE-CHECK while additional air is injected into the NG tube.

11. Once air sounds are auscultated over the epigastrium when air is injected into the NG tube, CONFIRM the tube's proper PLACEMENT BY drawing back on the plunger of the syringe and ASPIRATING the NG tube. Fluid gastric contents should be drawn into and seen in the barrel of the syringe, further confirming the tube's placement and patency. If its placement can not be confirmed, it will have to be withdrawn and insertion re-attempted after a brief period.

12. Once the tube's placement has been confirmed, REMOVE the SYRINGE from the tube's proximal end and TAPE the NG TUBE TO the patient's FACE without putting pressure on the nasal septum or obstructing the patient's vision.

13. IF ALLOWED by local protocol, EVACUATE THE STOMACH CONTENTS by aspirating with a large syringe. In cases of poisoning, if indicated and allowed, provide activated charcoal and water and continue gastric lavage and evacuation.

SECTION 7

Supplemental Oxygen Delivery Skills and Patient Oxygenation

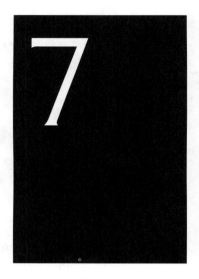

Introduction to Supplemental Oxygen

In normally healthy people, the "room air" we breathe (containing 21% oxygen) provides adequate oxygen to maintain the body's cellular metabolic function and life. When patients have (or have had) a condition which results in inadequate cellular oxygenation, they need to breathe (or be ventilated with, if they cannot provide an adequate minute volume for themselves) air that has an enriched level of oxygen. *The provision of a high percentage of supplemental oxygen to patients with cellular hypoxia is a key priority for the EMT if anerobic metabolism (resulting in irreversible cell death), vital organ death, and ultimately death of the patient are to be avoided.*

Inadequate cellular oxygenation can be caused by a vast number of etiologies affecting any one of the major body systems accutely or chronically. Whether from a primary respiratory problem or when any of the following pathophysiological mechanisms occur, increased supplemental oxygen is needed:

- A respiratory deficit resulting in inadequate pulmonary air exchange and reduced oygen levels in the lungs.

- A systemic circulatory deficit (shock) which, regardless of the adequacy of pulmonary oxygen levels, results in inadequate perfusion (hypoperfusion) of the cells with properly oxygenated blood.

- A deficit in available hemoglobin so there is insufficient oxyhemaglobin bonding and inadequate oxygen transported to the cells, regardless of the adequacy of pulmonary oxygen levels and perfusion.

- A metabolic or other bio-chemical imbalance which deters or interferes with oxygen diffusion across the pulmonary or systemic capillaries, or through the cell wall.

When high percentage supplementary oxygen is administered during the early compensating stages of respiratory distress or shock, it can often be a key contributor to slowing or stopping their progression. In the decompensating patient, the increased oxygen supplied is a key treatment in countering further deterioration until irreversible cell death occurs. In either case, the timely initiation of increased oxygenation represents a key priority treatment in the EMT's intervention.

The percentage of oxygen provided to patients in their inspired air is called the "FiO_2" and is stated as a decimal fraction. The oxygen in normal "room air" is 21% or 21/100 and would be written as: $FiO_2 = 0.21$.

Since the EMT can *NOT* determine the exact amount of increased oxygen that is specifically needed by the patient, any patient with a significant injury or medical emergency associated with respiratory distress and/or shock should be treated with an FiO_2 of 0.85 to 1.00. By providing these patients with such a high FiO_2 the EMT is assured that as much oxygen as *can be used by the body* (in such an acute situation) is provided. This might not be the case, were an FiO_2 of only 0.35 — 0.50 supplied instead. Any surplus oxygen supplied beyond what the body can use, will simply be discarded through the normal exhalation process without causing any undesirable effect. Even in patients with a history of COPD where there is a fear of eliminating the respiratory drive with high levels of oxygenation, oxygen should *NOT* be withheld or lessened if they have acute injuries or other medical conditions commonly associated with cellular hypoxia. Even when their condition is isolated to a severe COPD episode, many believe that enriched levels of oxygen should not be significantly reduced since the EMT cannot determine when this could result in continued hypoxia and cell death, but he can provide ventilation if the patient's respiratory drive is lost. *The EMT will have to follow his local protocol when providing supplemental oxygen for patients with exclusively acute COPD, but should treat patients with a history of COPD who sustain significant trauma or have other acute medical emergencies just as he would any other patient with acute hypoxia or hypoperfusion.*

Supplemental oxygen with a high FiO_2 is delivered to apneic patients or those who can *NOT* provide an adequate minute volume for themselves as a part of provided or assisted ventilations employing one of the various ventilators discussed in Section 5 of this text.

Supplemental oxygen is provided to patients who have adequate spontaneous air exchange by use of a mask or nasal cannula. Use of either must be limited to patients in whom the EMT has confirmed that an adequate minute volume exists and, as a part of their use, the EMT must periodically confirm that the minute volume is maintained. *It must be emphasized that supplemental oxygen by mask or cannula in patients with an inadequate minute volume is dangerous, and progressive cellular hypoxia will continue until proper ventilation is provided or death occurs.*

Supplemental oxygen is supplied using four essential pieces of equipment:

• A tank or piped wall **oxygen source**.

• A **regulator**, with gauges and a flow-meter.

• **Oxygen supply tubing** (also called Low Pressure Gas Delivery Tubing).

• A **delivery device**, either a mask or cannula.

OXYGEN SOURCE

Oxygen is a colorless, odorless gas that is generally stored in tanks. To provide for a significant volume to be stored in the smallest possible space the oxygen in the tank is compressed—resulting in extremely high pressure (about 2,000 psi) within the tank. To safely withstand the high pressure, tanks are of a strong cylindrical shape and are made of heavy gauge steel or, in the case of some portable tanks, a special strong but lighter alloy to reduce their weight. A special valve is screwed into the top of the tank at the factory and remains a permanent sealed part of the tank.

Due to the high pressure within these tanks, extreme care must be used when handling them to assure that they are not dropped, pierced or dented in any way, and to prevent damage to the valve which protrudes from their top. Since oxygen supports combustion it is classified as a flammable gas. Oxygen should never be used near an open flame, embers, or around electrical devices associated with sparking or unshielded non-explosive proof electrical motors. As well, when oxygen is in use there should be a strictly enforced BAN ON SMOKING in the area or room. Similar safety precautions are required when filling or replacing oxygen tanks. To avoid the chance of spontaneous combustion NEVER use or allow grease, oil, other petroleum based products, or fat-based soaps (from hands or greasy tools) to contact any device that will be attached to or used with oxygen. Similarly, NEVER use adhesive tape to cover an oxygen tank outlet, to label a tank, or in any other way with oxygen equipment, as the adhesive contains petroleum oils.

As an additional safety, each tank is required to be hydrostatically tested at the factory to assure that it can withstand pressures well in excess of that normal to its use. The date of that test is stamped onto the cylinder. Most tanks need to be hydrostatically tested every five years. Some newer tanks only require testing every ten years and can be identified by a *star* added after the initial hydrostatic test date on the cylinder. *Filling an oxygen tank that has been injured in any way, or one that is beyond 5 years (or 10 years for those with a "star") from the date at which it was last hydrostatically tested is EXTREMELY DANGEROUS and can result in serious injury or death.*

Oxygen tanks are color coded for the gas that they contain. The United States Pharmacopeia has assigned *light green and white* for all grades of oxygen. Unpainted stainless steel and aluminum cylinders are also used for oxygen. *The EMT must assure that only medical grade oxygen is used for patient care,* as "medical grade" is more carefully cleaned and refined than other commercial types. Medical oxygen cylinders will be labelled "OXYGEN U.S.P."

The compressed gas oxygen tanks commonly used in pre-hospital care come in four sizes. Each size is designated by a letter of the alphabet. The four sizes commonly used are "D" and "E", which are small and portable, and "M" and "H" (sometimes labelled as "K"), which are significantly larger. The larger tanks are commonly used as the on-board oxygen source in the ambulance, and for stationary use in the station for refilling smaller tanks.

The valve at the top of "D" and "E" tanks is designed to fit into the yoke of the type of regulator designed for portable use. The stem at the upper end of the valve is rectangularly shaped, and an "oxygen key" (generally attached to the regulator by a cord or chain) is used to turn the stem and thereby open and close the tank.

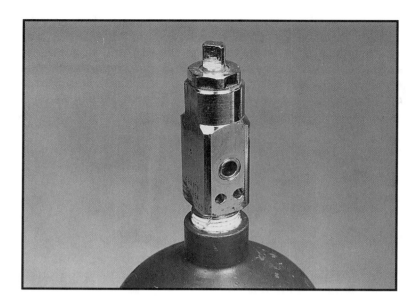

Because portable smaller tanks are changed often, a universal "pin index system" is used for safety to ensure that only a cylinder of the correct gas can be attached to the appropriate regulator. Two specifically located round pins can be seen when you look through the yoke of the oxygen regulator. When a portable oxygen tank is fastened into the yoke these pins align with two matching holes in the tank's valve. The pins on a portable oxygen regulator are differently placed than in regulators for other gases, and will only allow connection of an oxygen tank.

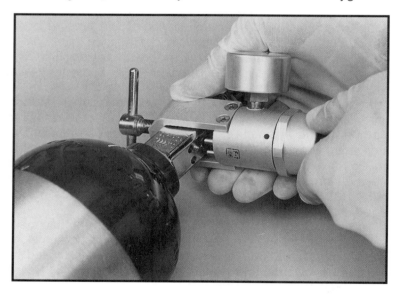

The valve on "M" and "H" or "K" tanks has a round handle (much like an outside water faucet) attached to it to open and close the tank, and has a threaded nipple outlet to allow connection to it.

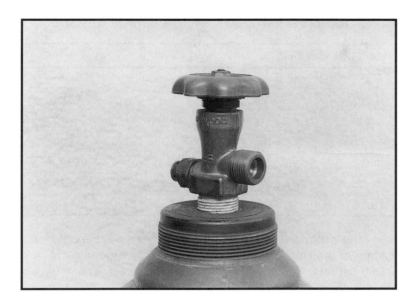

These larger tanks also contain threading on a raised lip at the top of the tank surrounding the valve, so that a rigid steel safety cover can be fastened over the valve to protect it whenever it is being moved.

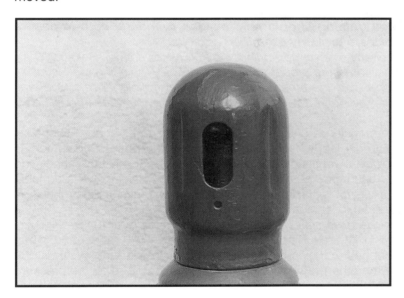

In these larger "M", "H", or "K" tanks there is *NO* pin index safety system such as found in the smaller portable tanks, but the threads on the larger tanks are unique to their respective intended gas. This makes a mistaken connection to most other gases difficult but not completely impossible (as with the pin index system). Therefore, the EMT must take care that only medical oxygen and oxygen regulators are used.

The following chart will serve as a useful guide for the EMT when using the different size tanks.

OXYGEN TANK DATA				
Cylinder Type	**D**	**E**	**M**	**H or K**
Height	17 in.	26 in.	43 in.	51 in.
Diameter	4.5 in.	4.25 in.	7 in.	9.25 in.
Pressure at Which Full	1900 psi	1900 psi	2200 psi	2200 psi
Volume When Full	400 L.	625 L.	3,450 L.	6,900 L.
Approx. Time of Use @ 15L/min	21 min.	37 min.	3 hrs. 28 min.	6 hrs. 48 min.
Cylinder Constant	0.16	0.28	1.56	3.14

The "Pressure At Which Full" indicates the minimum tank pressure when the tank is considered full, but does not indicate the greatest volume or pressure than can safely be accommodated. "D" and "E" tanks are commonly filled to about 2,000 psi and, "M", "H" or "K" tanks to 2,300 psi. These figures are included only to allay any fears of handling tanks with such pressure and not as guidelines for personnel in filling these cylinders.

The skills involved in removing and replacing cylinders for both portable and on-board ambulance oxygen are a normal part of the EMT's function and have been included in this text. The refilling of oxygen tanks from a cascade or other system requires additional training in the handling of gases under pressure and the use of the specific system available, and therefore has not been included in this text. **Only EMTs with specialized additional training should refill oxygen cylinders, both to assure their safety and to ensure that the tanks are properly examined and filled.**

The safe residual pressure for use of any size oxygen cylinder is 200 psi or greater. Below 200 psi there is not enough oxygen in the cylinder to assure proper continuous delivery. Also, if a tank is totally emptied (to zero pressure) condensation inside the tank will require special maintenance to the tank before it can safely be refilled. Therefore, cylinders MUST be replaced before the pressure is below 200 psi.

When returning portable units to the ambulance after a call it is recommended that any tank below 500 psi at a minimum, and preferably 750 psi, be replaced with a full one. Where such equipment is used in conjunction with an oxygen powered ventilator, it is recommended that the tank should be replaced with a completely full tank after each use regardless of the amount remaining in the portable tank. No universally accepted standard exists for replacing the onboard oxygen tanks in the ambulance since this may be a factor of the number of tanks and call frequency.

Onboard systems containing two tanks have several significant advantages over those with only one, even when the single tank is the "H" or "K" size. The second tank serves as a reserve and, when long distance inter-facility transport is needed, doubles the amount carried. In two tank systems, the tanks should be used in relay (one after the other) rather than both simultaneously, so as the pressure approaches 200 psi in the first tank it can be shut down and the second tank opened. This signals the crew that upon return to quarters the first tank needs to be replaced. If the onboard system has only a single tank, it is recommended that it be replaced or refilled after any call where its use has left it below 1,000 psi to ensure it will not fall below 200 psi even if the next call involves high liter-flow usage for the longest possible run time.

The "Cylinder Constant" figure for each tank given in the bottom row of the preceding chart is used to calculate the amount of time remaining to use the tank at any given pressure at the liter flow being supplied. The number of minutes remaining can be calculated by multiplying the psi remaining in the tank (less the 200 psi required as a safe residual pressure) by the constant factor for that size tank, and then dividing that result by the number of **liters per minute (LPM)** at which the flow rate is set.

The formula can be simply stated as:

$$\text{Remaining time in minutes} = \frac{(\text{Gauge psi pressure} - 200\text{ psi residual}) \times \text{Constant factor}}{\text{LPM setting}}$$

For example, if the gauge showed an "E" tank to have 1600 psi pressure and it is being used at a flow rate of 15 LPM:

$$\text{Remaining time in minutes} = \frac{(1600 - 200 \text{ psi}) \times 0.28}{15 \text{ LPM}}$$

$$= \frac{1400 \times 0.28}{15}$$

$$= \frac{392}{15}$$

$$\text{Remaining time in tank} = 26 \text{ minutes}$$

Oxygen tanks should be labelled as "full," "in use," or "empty." *Only tanks that are completely full should be labelled as "full."* Tanks which have been used but still have sufficient pressure to continue their use should be labelled as "in-use" (neither as "full" nor "empty"). Tanks that need refilling before they are again placed in service, regardless of their remaining pressure, need to be labelled as "empty." Remember that tanks labelled as "empty" are truly not "empty," and have a remaining pressure of between 200 psi and 1,000 psi (depending at what minimum pressure tanks are replaced). **All oxygen cylinders, including those which are labelled as "empty," contain gas under high pressure and must be handled with extreme care.** Portable tanks that have been commercially refilled will generally have a plastic strap around the valve which covers the oxygen outlet in order to protect it from dirt. This strap usually contains a spare nylon washer (called an "O" ring) in case the one on the regulator is missing or needs to be replaced.

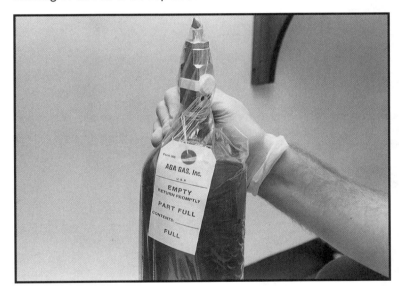

No tank should ever be considered to be full or have adequate pressure just because it is so labelled (or did when last used or checked). The EMT should verify the pressure of all oxygen tanks carried at the start of his shift or on-call duty period to assure that their contents are as labelled and sufficient.

Oxygen cylinders should NEVER be left standing in an upright position unless properly secured. Large tanks should always be held in place by a chain or metal strap bolted around their circumference, and portable tanks should be placed on their side on the floor, or in a case or other secure carrier. When using portable oxygen while moving the patient, the portable tank should be fastened in a container for that purpose on the cot or securely strapped to the stretcher. When strapping a portable tank and regulator to the cot, space is usually available beside or between the patient's lower legs. *All oxygen tanks must be securely fastened at all times in any moving vehicle if injury is to be avoided.*

On-board oxygen systems in most ambulances use "M", "H", or "K" tanks (preferably more than one) secured upright in a special compartment which opens to the outside to facilitate easy tank replacement or refilling.

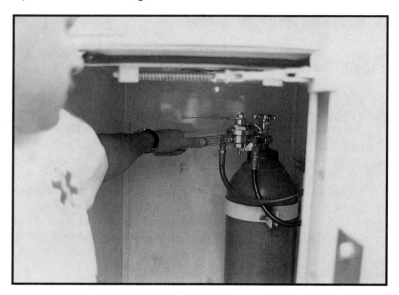

The tank is connected by a flexible high pressure hose to the ambulance's piped system. This piping connects to a pressure reduction regulator and has separate flow regulators (or snap-in connections for such flow regulators) near the head of the patient cot and near the head of the squad bench. A wide variety of configurations exist.

Hospitals have a large central tank from which oxygen at a reduced pressure is piped through the building. A flow meter and gauge is found on the wall at each patient bed. These are either fixed or have a self-sealing snap-in system to allow for their removal.

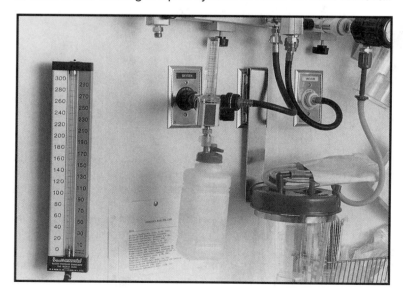

When moving patients from one location to another within the hospital, portable units using "D" or "E" tanks similar to those used in pre-hospital care are used. Often, rather than being in a protective case as is common with pre-hospital use, these are in a small metal cart called a "walker" to allow them to be rolled with the patient's bed.

COPD patients who have oxygen in their home generally have large tanks as well as small portable units that contain oxygen in a compressed liquid form rather than as a gas. *Liquid oxygen systems and their components ARE NOT compatible with the compressed gas equipment (oxygen tanks or regulators) used in pre-hospital and hospital systems, and MUST NOT be used together or interchanged.* Only the masks or nasal cannula remain the same in both systems.

REGULATORS AND FLOW METERS

To maximize the amount of oxygen that can be carried in the smallest space, the oxygen in tanks is compressed and stored at extremely high pressures (200 to 2,200 psi). Therefore, a **regulator** is required to reduce this pressure and control its flow. The regulators used to deliver supplemental oxygen directly to the patient from a standard low pressure oxygen nipple employ a two-stage reduction system. The first stage reduces it to between 50 and 70 psi, and the second stage further reduces it so that the pressure at the universal low pressure supplemental oxygen nipple does not exceed 40 psi. The second stage has a flow meter which includes a liter-flow valve with which the EMT can adjust the volume being delivered. Generally these range from "off" to between 2 and 15 LPM (some newer models may provide up to 25 LPM). The flow-meter has a universal low pressure oxygen nipple ("Christmas tree") at its outlet as shown below.

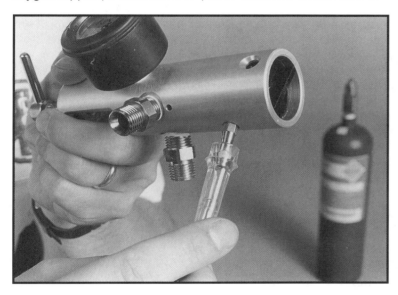

The regulator also includes a pressure gauge which reflects the pressure in the tank (usually in psi) when the tank valve has been opened. Most regulators also include a second gauge which reflects the liter flow being delivered. In portable units these are round aneroid Bourdon type gauges which are rugged and will operate at any angle. It must be noted that this type of gauge is fairly inaccurate, particularly at low flow rates, and will not compensate for back pressure. Should the tubing between the unit and the hose become kinked it may indicate a 15 LPM flow even though only 2 LPM are being delivered to the patient. Instead, some portable units have a constant flow selector valve in which the liter flow is adjusted in stepped preset increments (eg: 2, 4, 6...15 LPM) and no liter flow gauge is usually included.

Regulators for use with "D" and "E" tanks (portable units) have a yoke and pin-indexed system (previously discussed) for attachment to the tank valve. As well as the pin index, the inside of the yoke has a short metal tube surrounded by a nylon washer ("O" ring) that inserts into the outlet hole on the tank valves.

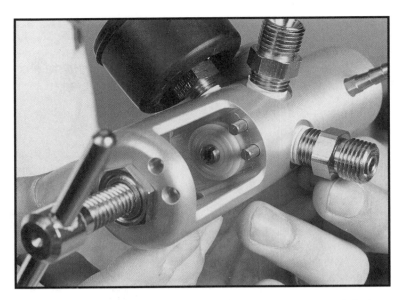

When connecting the tank to the yoke of the regulator it is important to make sure that the two index pins and this metal tube are properly inserted into their respective holes before tightening. A screw clamp with a pointed tip (which fits into a cone-like indentation on the opposite side of the valve from the two pins) is firmly hand tightened to secure the regulator to the tank.

Most regulators which are used with portable units contain one or more DISS threaded outlets that allow for the connection of a high pressure oxygen hose and Demand Valve Resuscitators or Automatic Transport Ventilators directly to the 50 psi outlet of the regulator, rather than to the nipple on the flowmeter. Because this outlet is placed in the system before the flowmeter and liter-flow gauge, a constant 50 psi flow is independently provided from this outlet regardless of the setting of the flowmeter or LPM flow shown on the gauge. *The flowmeter ONLY controls and indicates the flow through the low pressure supplemental oxygen nipple.*

Although rarely used pre-hospital, a two stage regulator (similar to those used in portable units with "D" or "E" tanks) is available for attachment to "M", "H", or "K" tanks to allow for providing supplemental oxygen to patients directly from these large tanks. They are primarily of the same design as the regulators previously described, except that instead of a yoke they contain a screw-on coupling that is compatible with the larger tanks.

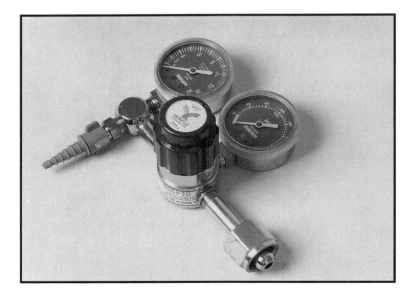

These regulators have a rounded tip which inserts into the opening in the tank outlet to provide a seal when the female coupling which covers the tip is securely tightened onto the male threads on the tank-valve with a wrench. *Only nonferrous metal wrenches should be used since other metals may produce a spark should they strike against another metal object.* These units are primarily used as stand-by equipment to provide oxygen in the hospital should the piped wall system fail, for pre-hospital situations where sustained oxygen use over days or weeks is anticipated, and for home convalescent care.

The on-board oxygen systems in most ambulances have one (or preferably two) "M", "H" or "K" tanks in an outside compartment attached to a single stage regulator which is pre-connected by a flexible hose to the vehicle's oxygen piping. The oxygen is reduced to between 40 and 70 psi (approximately 50 psi), and when the tank valve is opened, is piped to a flowmeter and a series of valves and controls behind a master oxygen control panel generally found near the "attendant" seat at the head of the cot.

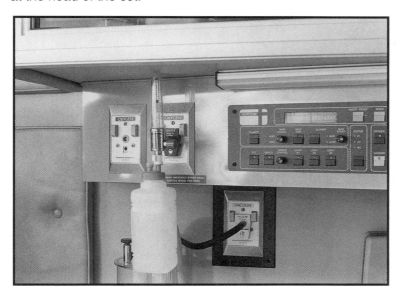

These panels generally contain an oxygen ON and OFF switch with a pilot light which controls an electrically operated valve which, when the tank valve is open, allows for immediate control from this panel of whether or not oxygen flows from the system. In some systems this switch and electrically operated remote valve is replaced by a manual valve. A liter flow control and gauges are also included on the panel. A pressure gauge on the panel, which may be redundant to one at the tank, allows monitoring of the tank pressure from inside the patient compartment at all times when the unit is in use. The liter flow gauge may be the same round Bourdon gauge found on most portable units, or it may be the more accurate pressure-compensated type. These are not used with portable units because they are gravity dependent and must be used in an upright position. This type of flow gauge has an upright calibrated glass tube containing a ball float. The ball rises and falls based upon the amount of gas passing through the tube. It indicates the actual gas flow, so were the oxygen line to become kinked it would reflect the actual reduced flow rather than the intended rate.

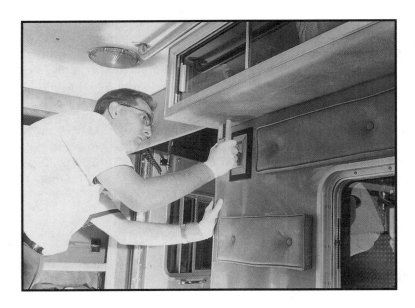

A separate line goes from just beyond the "on/off" valve to other flowmeters near the squad bench and elsewhere to allow for independent use with other patients (only the on/off control is retained at the master panel).

Some of the onboard systems are very sophisticated and include features such as a warning indicator light or audible alarm if the pressure in the system drops below 40 psi or exceeds 70 psi. Some multi-tank systems contain automatic switch-over equipment so that when one tank falls below 500 psi it opens the second into the system, closes the first, and indicates by a warning light that the unit is on its last tank.

Onboard oxygen systems differ. Some have fixed units at each location—others have a two pronged snap-in system with multiple outlets in the patient compartment. In such a system each outlet is self-sealing when a flowmeter is not inserted into it. Two standards for snap-in connections are available, and equipment for one is not compatible with the other.

Since ambulances of different ages and designs are usually in use simultaneously by a service, the onboard oxygen systems in each vehicle may be different. At the start of the EMT's shift or on-call period, he should review the specific operation of the unit he will be using as an essential part of checking the oxygen equipment. *The EMT MUST be fully familiar with the operation of the specific onboard oxygen system in the ambulance he will be responding in, prior to using it with a patient.*

Most regulators, portable or onboard, contain an inlet filter to prevent particulate matter from entering and restricting the flow of oxygen or damaging the mechanism. Such filters need to be periodically checked to be sure that they are free of damage, and cleaned or replaced as necessary. *Disassembly and servicing of regulators, flowmeters, or other sealed oxygen therapy components should ONLY be done by properly qualified authorized service personnel. Tampering with such units by the EMT is extremely dangerous to the individual, others who will ensuingly use the equipment, and patients.*

Unlike piped hospital systems, the portable and onboard oxygen systems common to pre-hospital care are not designed to have pressure in the system at all times. Although they can have pressure in them for sustained periods without harm, they require that after each call (in which the system was charged) the tank be shut and pressure in the line bled-off, so that they are stored without any residual pressure remaining in the system. *Leaving these units with pressure in them for any sustained period between calls is a poor practice inviting inadvertent emptying of tanks if any leak exists in the system, and damage to the regulator, flowmeter and gauges.*

The EMT must be familiar with the oxygen wall units found in the hospital as he will commonly need to use these when transfering a patient to the Emergency Department or patient room.

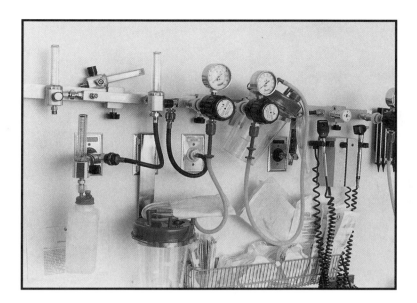

Hospital piped oxygen systems are "charged" — having a constant pressure and flow available at each outlet at all times. Hospital wall units contain a flowmeter with a valve to open the oxygen flow and with which to regulate the LPM delivered. Generally these contain a pressure compensated gauge (floating ball type previously described) and a humidifier. The humidifier generally consists of a clear plastic cannister which is partially filled with sterile water and which has a sealed (gas proof) removable top. A tube connects the cannister top to the standard low pressure oxygen nipple. When the flow valve on the unit is opened, oxygen flows into the water through a supply tube under its surface and "bubbles" through it — being humidified as it rises to the area of the cannister above the water line. The humidified oxygen (but not water) then flows through an oxygen outlet tube (which passes through the top of the cannister) to the universal nipple on the end of the unit.

Currently, such humidifiers are *NOT* generally used with onboard ambulance wall units (as in the past) since road shocks can result in water entering the delivery tubing. Also, if the humidifier requires filling this delays the care of the patient, whereas pre-filled units invite the introduction of bacteria and other organisms. When oxygen is being delivered for less than 90 minutes there is no appreciable benefit to include a humidifier in the ambulance. Therefore, they are not recommended for common pre-hospital use. When run times are prolonged (as with lengthy inter-hospital transfers) humidification should be considered.

UNIVERSAL CONNECTING TUBING

Units used to supply supplemental oxygen to a patient or to a Bag Valve Mask Ventilator or nebulizer, have a *universal low pressure nipple* at their outlet. This male fitting is usually a cone-shaped (5 – 7mm) ridged nipple of approximately 2.5cm to 3.5cm in length which is made of plastic or metal and looks somewhat like an upside-down "Christmas Tree" — from which it derives its nickname. Some variations of this nipple are simply a 1/4 inch metal tube with several ridges or a bulbous flange at their end. To provide for flexibility of movement and use of the delivery device (mask, cannula, BVM or nebulizer) at a practical distance from the flowmeter, these are connected using flexible tubing. For such connections, a disposable single-use *universal oxygen connecting tubing* (commonly just called an "oxygen connecting tube" or oxygen supply tubing) is used. This tubing is of a narrow diameter and will be either clear or light green in color. Only tubing designed for low pressure medical gases should be used for these inter-connections.

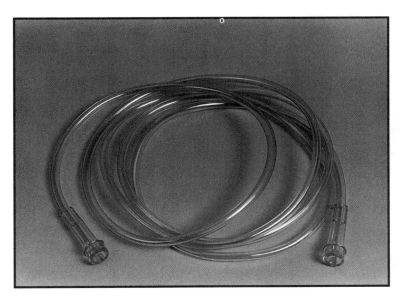

Although shorter lengths are available, this tubing is generally 7 feet (2.1m) long and has a pliable female cone-shaped fitting at each end. These pliable fittings allow for connection to virtually any type of low pressure outlet at one end and to the male 5–7mm (1/4 inch) nipple universally used on oxygen masks, cannulae, BVMs, BVM accumulators, or nebulizers.

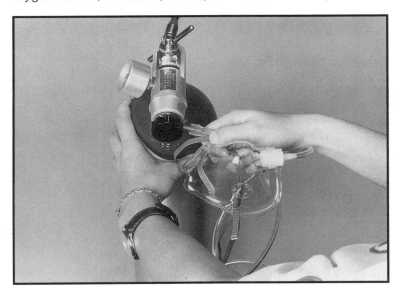

When installing the female connectors onto the flowmeter's outlet nipple or to the 1/4 inch nipple of the delivery device, the flowmeter or mask should be held stationary with one hand while the female connector is slid over the male nipple with a slight back-and-forth rotary motion with the other hand. Care must be taken to assure that the male nipple is sufficiently inserted into the female connector at each end to assure that these connections will not inadvertently separate in normal use.

It should be noted that some masks and nasal cannulae come with 5 to 7 feet of tubing already affixed to the device. These will have the same female connectors as found on the universal connecting tubing, to allow for connection directly to the low pressure delivery nipple on the flowmeter *without* the need for separate connecting tubing.

SUPPLEMENTAL OXYGEN DELIVERY DEVICES

The use of supplemental oxygen equipment to supply a high FiO_2 with provided or assisted ventilations has been fully discussed in the previous section of this text dealing with "Ventilation."

Supplemental oxygen is delivered to patients who have confirmed adequate spontaneous air exchange through either a mask or nasal cannula. Several designs of each are available. The EMT should be familiar with the use and attributes of each one that is commonly found in pre-hospital use. These include:

- Nasal Cannula
- Venturi Masks
- Simple Face Masks (NO Reservoir)
- Partial-Rebreather Reservoir Masks
- Non-Rebreather Reservoir Masks

Contrary to a common misperception, the FiO_2 delivered is most determined by the design of the supplemental oxygen device and NOT by the liter flow per minute (LPM), unless the liter flow is insufficient for the need. For example, the percentage of oxygen delivered with a simple face mask is not significantly increased when the liter flow is increased from 8 LPM to 12 LPM. It would only be affected, causing the oxygen concentration to become lower, if the LPM supplied was **reduced** to below the patient's minute volume.

As long as the liter flow supplied to the device is equal to or greater than the patient's minute volume the degree to which the device's design allows for room air and the patient's exhaled air to mix with the 100% oxygen supplied from the flowmeter is the major factor in determining the maximum FiO_2 the device can deliver. The desired FiO_2 is the key determining factor in deciding which supplementary delivery device to select. The following chart will provide the EMT with a handy overview:

SUPPLEMENTAL OXYGEN DEVICES AND THEIR OXYGEN CONCENTRATIONS			
Delivery Device	**Liter Flow/Min**	**Oxygen Concentration**	
No Supplemental Oxygen	N/A	21%	Normal FiO_2
Nasal Cannula	1–6 LPM	24–30%	Slightly increased FiO_2
Venturi Mask with LOWER Range Adapter Installed	3–6 LPM	24–30% As Set	
Venturi Mask with UPPER Range Adapter Installed	9–15 LPM	35–50%	Moderately Increased FiO_2
Simple Face Mask (No Reservoir)	8–15 LPM	35–60%	
Partial–Rebreather Reservoir Mask	6–15 LPM	60–90%	High FiO_2
Non-Rebreather Reservoir Mask	6–15 LPM	85–100%	

A **nasal cannula** only provides between 3–9% oxygen enrichment beyond normal room air. Because they are only inserted in the nose and do not cover the patient's mouth, the oxygen mixes with a larger volume of unenriched room air that the patient draws in through his mouth. With any significant respiratory distress, patients become predominantly obligate mouth breathers increasing this dilution.

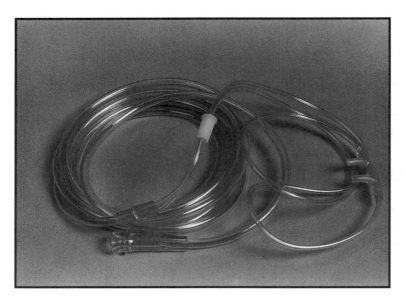

Therefore, a nasal cannula should NOT be used with patients with multi-systems trauma, marked dyspnea, or any acute systemic medical emergency where a high FiO_2 is required.

Simple masks which cover the mouth and nose (but do not include a reservoir bag) can at best only produce an oxygen concentration of up to 50–60%. Without a reservoir the amount of the 100% oxygen provided from the source that actually reaches the patient is limited to the amount the source can deliver into the mask during the 1 to 1–1/2 second period during which the patient inhales. Even at 15 LPM this is less than the normal adult inspiratory volume. Therefore, ambient air must be drawn in through the holes in the side of the mask which, as it mixes with the 100% oxygen, causes a significant dilution in its concentration.

Venturi Masks are simple masks which have either several adaptor rings or "mixing inserts" which determine the amount of ambient air that mixes with the 100% oxygen supply. Depending upon which is selected (and in the case of the rings, to which percentage they are set) between 24–50% oxygen is delivered. These are not commonly used pre-hospital but the EMT may find such a mask is used for home oxygen service or for intra-hospital transfers.

Reservoir Masks have a soft plastic bag which lies below the mask. The oxygen being supplied flows to the reservoir bag and then to the face mask. This reservoir bag fills constantly during the longer period between inspirations. By the time the patient inspires, a sufficient amount of oxygen has accumulated in the reservoir so that no additional outside air is drawn in to dilute the oxygen concentration.

Partial Rebreather Reservoir Masks allow some of the patient's exhaled air to become mixed with the oxygen coming from the reservoir, resulting in lower concentration (between 60–90%, depending on the liter flow and exhaled air ratio). With such masks the EMT can neither control nor ascertain the specific oxygen concentration being delivered, and therefore such masks are rarely used in pre-hospital care.

Non-Rebreather Reservoir Masks have a one-way valve between the reservoir and the mask which prevents any exhaled air from entering the reservoir bag. Additional one-way valves on the sides of the mask open to allow the exhaled air to be purged to the outside. During inspiration these valves keep ambient air out, and the one-way valve between the mask and reservoir opens to allow the patient to draw his total inspiratory volume from the oxygen accumulated in the reservoir.

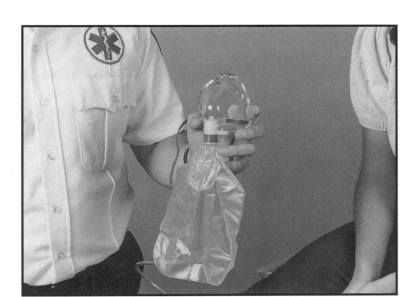

The system of one-way valves which prevents the introduction of exhaled or ambient air with the 100% oxygen supplied to the mask and the inclusion of a reservoir to accumulate sufficient volume between inspirations, results in Non-Rebreather Reservoir Masks delivering a FiO_2 of between 0.85 and 1.00.

Supplemental oxygen with a high FiO_2 is indicated for patients with significant trauma, respiratory distress or an acute systemic medical emergency who have adequate spontaneous air exchange. The EMT should use a Non-Rebreather Reservoir Mask with a high liter flow to ensure that a high FiO_2 is provided. Nasal cannulae, simple masks, venturi masks, and partial rebreather reservoir masks should ONLY be used with patients for whom little or moderate oxygen enrichment is desired, and they should NOT be used in any patient for whom a high FiO_2 is indicated.

Conscious patients, particularly those with respiratory distress, hypoxia or a cardiac condition are often extremely anxious. Such patients may feel "smoothered" and resist having a mask tightly fastened over their nose and mouth. When patients need a high FiO_2, such fears and resistance should *NOT* cause the EMT to use nasal cannula instead of a mask.

Obviously, if the EMT fastens a mask tightly to the patient's head (covering the mouth and nose without an adequate explanation) the patient's fears will be exacerbated. The benefits of the oxygen need to be explained, including that, "in a few minutes the oxygen should make it easier for you to breathe". Additionally, it is helpful to have the patient take as deep a breath as possible as a demonstration. After this demonstration, the EMT should point out that as much air as the patient wanted was available without any restriction caused by the mask.

Experience has shown that it is the tight affixation of the mask with the elastic band, rather than its covering the nose and mouth, which represents the major source of the fear that a mask may generate. Often it is helpful in a cooperative patient with such fears, to have the patient hold the mask firmly over his mouth and nose instead of securing it with the elastic. This leaves control of the mask to the patient, and knowing that he can remove it "if needed" is an effective tool in allaying his fears. Once most patients have seen that the oxygen mask helps rather than restricts their breathing, they will become more calm and the elastic can be fastened without further resistance. Even if the patient who is attempting to cooperate seems to lift the mask off unnecessarily often, he should not be spoken to harshly or threatened with restraint.

When the patient is a small child or is not mentally competent, and is uncooperative or combative repeatedly attempting to remove the mask — his hands will have to be restrained so that the mask can remain fastened and to ensure the EMT's safety.

Significant oxygen enrichment (but not an FiO_2 greater than 0.50) occurs even when the mask — rather than being in contact with the face — is held a few centimeters in front of the nose and mouth. The EMT should lift the mask or move it to one side whenever he asks the patient a question or when the patient wants to talk to the EMT. Similarly, lifting it periodically if the patient appears to become more anxious can be helpful in calming the patient.

The specific use of nasal cannula, 100% non-rebreather reservoir masks, other masks the EMT may encounter in patient transfers, portable and on-board oxygen units (including changing tanks) and hospital wall oxygen units are presented in detailed steps on the following pages. *The description for each of these assumes the EMTs knowledge and understanding of the material presented in this introduction.*

USING NASAL CANNULA

Nasal Cannula are only used in patients requiring low levels of oxygen enrichment. Since they can *only* provide an FiO_2 of between 0.24 and 0.30, they should *NOT BE USED* in patients for whom a high FiO_2 is indicated. Because they deliver the supplemental oxygen to the respiratory system exclusively through the nose, they should *NOT* be applied to patients who cannot breathe through their nose or who are obligate mouth breathers. The method by which these are affixed to the patient's head represents the only significant difference in the two types commonly found in use.

1. The most commonly used style of nasal cannula has a loop which contains at it's mid-point two prongs (the cannula) about a half inch apart with openings at their distal tip. There is a plastic slide over the loop to adjust its size in order to secure it to the patient's head. The loop is generally pre-connected to 5–7 feet of oxygen tubing with a universal low-pressure female oxygen connector at its other end. After confirming that the proper Universal Precautions are in place, the patient has an adequate minute volume, and that a high FiO_2 is **NOT** called for, withdraw the nasal cannula unit from it's packaging.

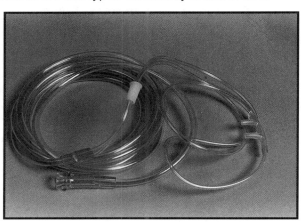

2. Uncoil the tubing and after assuring that it is not kinked, fasten the female connector completely over the low pressure nipple (Christmas tree) on the flowmeter of the oxygen source. Open the tank and adjust the flow valve to the desired LPM flow. Nasal cannula should be used with a flow of between 2–6 LPM ONLY. *Flows greater than 6 LPM should NEVER be used with a nasal cannula since this will NOT increase the FiO_2 and can cause "oxygen burns" to the patient's nostrils.* Check that oxygen properly flows from the cannula's prongs.

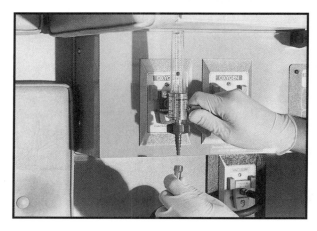

3. After explaining the procedure to the patient, hold the loop in front of the patient's face so that the prongs are oriented on the upper side of the loop. The curverture in the prongs should be oriented so that the tips will face upward and slightly posteriorly once they have been inserted (as shown). Note that the rest of the loop has *NOT* been placed over the patient's head but is held so it remains anterior to the face and neck.

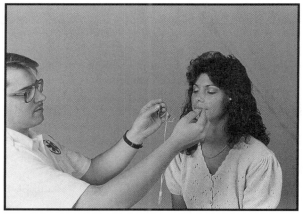

4. While pointing the tips of the prongs directly upward into each nostril, advance them until they are fully inserted. While holding the loop at the nose to keep the prongs inserted, with the other hand carefully pass one side of the loop over and behind the ear on one side of the patient's head. Pull it snug so that there is no slack in the loop between the patient's nose and his ear.

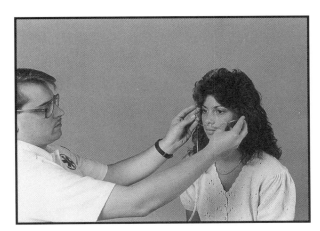

5. While continuing to hold the inserted prongs in place, place the loop at the other side of the cannula snugly over and behind the ear on that side. Once the loop has been placed around each ear, grasp the loop hanging at the neck and, while pulling it gently in a caudad direction, move the plastic slide-fastener up under the patient's chin until the bottom of the loop is held firmly in place as shown. Check that the entire loop is snug enough to keep the cannula inserted but not so tight as to produce any anterior-to-posterior pressure on the trachea or cause any patient discomfort.

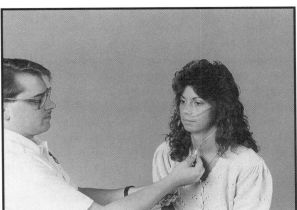

6. The previously described method keeps all of the loop on the anterior and lateral aspects of the head and neck — avoiding any part being under a supine patient's head. In sitting patients, once the cannula have been inserted the loop can alternatively be passed over the head and — with it resting over each ear — be tightened at the posterior lateral aspect of the neck with the posterior part of the loop below the occiput. This method should only be used when necessary, since part of the loop will be under the patient's head or neck if he is placed in a supine position.

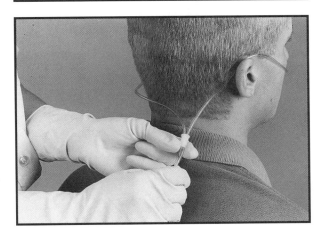

7. In some models there is no loop and the prongs are found at one end of the oxygen delivery tube. In such models the cannula are connected to the main tubing with a flat piece of soft plastic which has an elastic strap connected to the main tubing with a flat piece of soft plastic which has an elastic strap connected to each of its sides. Once the prongs have been inserted into the patient's nostrils, the elastic band is placed over the head so that it rests over each ear and under the occiput. Once the elastic band is in place around the head, it can be tightened (a shown) by simultaneously pulling the strap ends further through the buckles (generally two) found on each side of this elastic "loop."

USING A SIMPLE FACE MASK

Simple face masks without a reservoir have, in the main, been replaced in pre-hospital care by the use of non-rebreather reservoir masks which provide a high FiO$_2$. A simple mask, due to the absence of a reservoir, will only provide an FiO$_2$ of between 0.35−0.60, determined by the relationship between the patient's tidal volume and the liter per minute flow supplied. Simple masks should be used with a LPM flow of between 8 and 15 if any significant oxygen enrichment is desired. Simple face masks should not be used in patients who require a high FiO$_2$.

1. After assuring that the necessary Universal Precautions have been taken and that the patient does not need either provided ventilation or a high FiO$_2$, remove the mask from it's packaging. Next, connect the female connector of the delivery tubing firmly over the low pressure oxygen nipple of the oxygen source. Some brands do not include tubing and require that universal oxygen connecting tubing be attached between the source oxygen nipple and the 1/4 inch male nipple on the mask. Open the tank and adjust the flowmeter to the desired liter per minute flow.

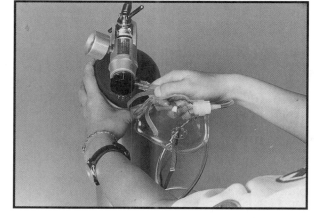

2. After feeling to assure that oxygen is flowing properly from the mask and explaining the procedure to the patient, orient the mask with its narrower nose portion in a cephalad direction and place it over the patient's nose and mouth. Slip the elastic strap over the patient's head, placing it so it is between the ear and the head at each side, and just below the occiput posteriorly. Tighten the elastic as needed.

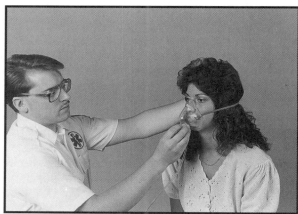

3. If the mask includes a malleable metal strip across the nose portion, squeeze this to a shape which will provide for a better fit without applying any pressure upon the nose. If the maximum FiO$_2$ possible with such a mask is desired, adjust the liter flow until the maximum flow occurs without a vast surplus constantly flowing from the mask's openings and from around its edges. If a high FiO$_2$ becomes needed, the mask must be replaced with a non-rebreather reservoir type.

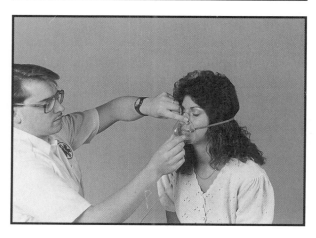

USING A NON-REBREATHER RESERVOIR MASK

Non-rebreather reservoir masks should be used in any patient with adequate spontaneous air exchange who requires a high FiO_2. Presently these masks are the sole oxygen enrichment delivery devices available (except ventilators) which provide an FiO_2 of between $0.85 - 1.00$. Due to their one-way valve systems and the constant filling of the reservoir, these masks provide almost 100% oxygen without dilution with ambient room air or the patient's exhaled gases. Since they appear to be almost identical, care must be taken to ensure that the mask is a non-rebreather rather than a partial-rebreather type. To do this locate the one-way inlet valve between the reservoir bag and mask. If such a valve is not present the mask is a "partial rebreather," *NOT* a "non-rebreather."

1. After assuring that the necessary Universal Precautions have been taken and that the patient has adequate spontaneous air exchange, remove the non-rebreather reservoir mask and pre-connected tubing from it's packaging. After fully uncoiling the reservoir bag and tubing, connect the female connector on the tubing firmly over the universal low pressure nipple (Christmas tree) of the oxygen source flowmeter. Open the tank and set the Liter flow at between 10 and 15 Liters/min.

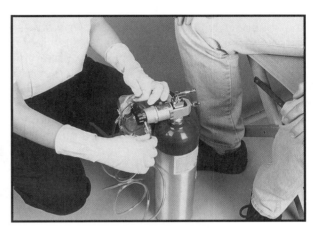

2. Check that the one-way exhaust valves are in place at each side of the mask, and that they appear undamaged. Some brands contain only one such valve. In such models, when a sufficient liter flow is provided almost no ambient air enters through the small sized openings that are provided and, should the patient inspire a greater volume than has accumulated in the reservoir, this provides for any needed additional volume to be drawn in from the ambient air. Place your thumb or a finger over the one-way inlet valve between the mask and the reservoir, to occlude it until the reservoir bag becomes fully inflated. Then, remove your finger.

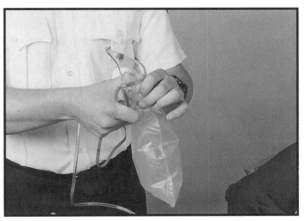

3. After having fully inflated the bag (to eliminate any adhesion of the reservoir's walls that may have resulted from its folded storage), check that oxygen flows properly from the mask and explain what you are about to do to the patient. Next, place the mask over the patient's mouth and nose and slip the elastic strap over the patient's head so it is placed between each ear and the patient's head and just below the occiput. Then, tighten the elastic strap as needed.

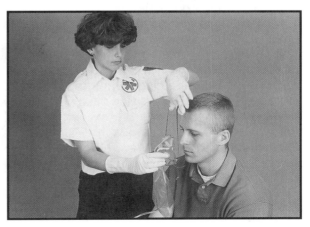

4. If the mask includes a pliable metal strip across the part covering the nose, squeeze it slightly to form the mask so that a better fit is achieved without it pressing on the sides of the nose. Care should be taken to adjust the mask's position and elastic strap so that the entire perimeter of the mask's outer edge seals with the patient's face. This prevents ambient air from being drawn into the mask and lowering the FiO_2 provided.

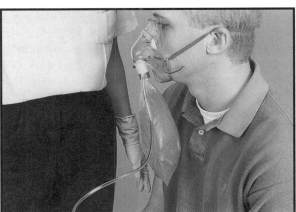

5. If a sufficiently tight fit has been achieved the reservoir will progressively *inflate between inspirations* and will *deflate during inspiration.* Adjust the LPM flow while carefully observing the reservoir bag over several breathing cycles. The correct liter flow setting has been achieved when the reservoir bag remains partially inflated at peak inspiration. The flow is too high when the reservoir bag's capacity is exceeded at any time in the cycle and oxygen flows from the valves on the sides of the mask. With any reservoir mask, this must be 6 LPM or greater to avoid rebreathing the exhaled air from the "dead space" in the mask.

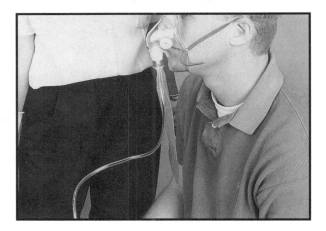

6. *With this type of mask, if the reservoir bag empties and the sides of the bag flatten prior to reaching peak inhalation, a dangerous situation may result. The EMT should immediately increase the oxygen liter flow.* If the reservoir bag has completely emptied prior to peak inhalation, the patient will not be able to obtain a sufficient inspiratory volume since room air cannot enter if the mask and one-way exhaust valves are properly sealed. At best, if air can be drawn in, it will result in a lowered FiO_2.

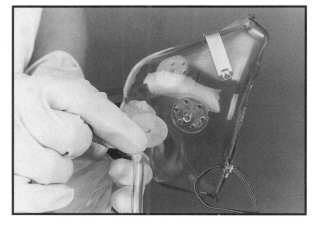

7. *Should a lower FiO_2 be desired, it should NOT be attempted by simply lowering the liter flow below that required to maintain proper inflation of the reservoir bag. This is a dangerous practice which may restrict the patient's ventilation.* Instead, the non-rebreather unit should be modified to allow the introduction of ambient air and/or partial rebreathing. When the valves at the side of the mask are pulled off, ambient air is drawn in and mixes with the oxygen supplied from the reservoir. This lowers the FiO_2 to about 0.70 to 0.80. If the one-way valve between the reservoir bag and the mask is also removed, the device becomes a partial rebreather and the FiO_2 is further reduced to between 0.60 and 0.70.

USING A PARTIAL REBREATHER RESERVOIR MASK

These masks are the same as Non-Rebreather Reservoir Masks except that they do not contain a one-way valve between the reservoir bag and mask, and only one (if either) of the openings at the side of the mask include a one-way exhaust valve.

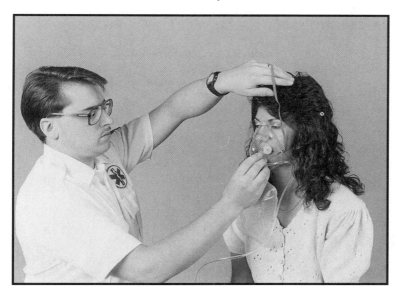

Without a valve between the mask and reservoir which closes upon exhalation some portion of the patient's exhaled air will enter the reservoir bag and reduce the concentration below the 100% supplied from the source. Upon inspiration, the room air which enters through the openings in the side of the mask causes additional dilution and results in an FiO_2 of between 0.60 and 0.90. The actual resulting FiO_2 within this range cannot be measured or controlled by the EMT since it is determined by a multitude of factors including the size of the openings in the mask, the force of the exhalation, the expiratory volume, the inspiratory volume and duration, the oxygen pressure as it arrives at the reservoir, and the liter per minute flow. The EMT can only attempt to adjust the delivered FiO_2 by adjusting the liter flow. In most adult patients an FiO_2 of 0.75 to 0.90 can only be achieved with a partial rebreather at a 12–15 LPM flow. As with any reservoir mask, the liter per minute flow should never be set below 6 LPM in order to avoid the buildup of excess CO_2.

Because a partial rebreather mask is almost never desirable pre-hospital, and since a non-rebreather reservoir mask can be modified to allow partial rebreathing (in the rare case where this may be desirable), partial rebreather reservoir masks are seldom carried or used by EMS Units. Discussion of these masks has been included so that the EMT is familiar with them should he encounter their use in a transfer patient or within the hospital. If the EMT is using such a mask, he should follow the same general directions as have been provided for the use of non-rebreather masks found in the immediately preceding pages.

USING A VENTURI MASK

Venturi Masks are used to deliver a specific selected concentration of oxygen to the patient. Unlike other masks, they are especially designed to allow ambient air to be drawn in. The room air mixes with the 100% oxygen from the source, producing the exact FiO_2 between 0.24 and 0.50 selected. The exact amount of air which mixes with the oxygen is determined by the size opening to the outside that has been selected and the maintenance of a specific LPM flow indicated for that setting. The Venturi mask does not employ a reservoir. Instead, as the oxygen flows past the opening communicating with the outside, produces the "Venturi effect" (from which it's name is derived). This negative pressure draws the correct amount of room air into the mask and creates the desired concentration as it mixes with the 100% oxygen.

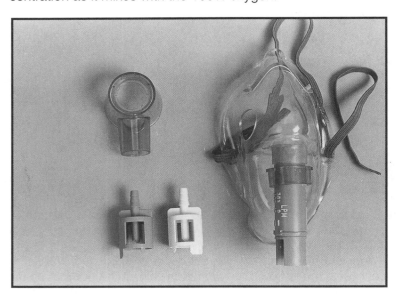

The desired FiO_2 level is determined by which "mixer' is inserted into the mask in some models, or which mixer is inserted and how it is adjusted in others. Some brands have a number of "mixers" with each one providing exclusively one specific FiO_2.

A specific LPM flow should be used with each different "mixer" and is indicated on it. The liter flow must be set to the rate indicated if the selected FiO_2 is to result.

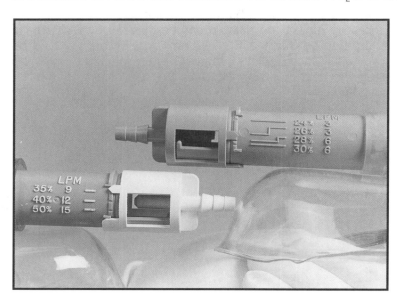

In other models there are only 2 color-coded ring-like "mixers" for insertion into the mask. With this design, the low range ring is used for providing any FiO_2 between 0.24 and 0.30 and the high range ring for any FiO_2 between 0.35 and 0.50. Once the correct ring has been selected and inserted, it is rotated (changing the ambient air opening's size) until the graduated scale on its perimeter is set at the specific oxygen concentration desired. The LPM flow setting required for the specific concentration selected appears on the ring under each possible choice of oxygen concentration.

Use of a Venturi Mask is rarely initiated pre-hospital. Discussion of this type of mask has only been included because the EMT may find such a mask used on a patient he will be transferring from one facility to another, and because he may come into contact with one in the hospital. Should the EMT have a patient with such a mask transferred to his care, he should ascertain and check two points before leaving the hospital:

- Determine the prescribed oxygen concentration and make sure that the mask is properly set and assembled to provide it.
- Check the Liter flow indicated for use with that specific setting on the "mixer insert" and set the flowmeter at this recommended flow level.

As with any mask which only supplies a low or moderate amount of oxygen enrichment, should the patient's condition worsen and a high FiO_2 become indicated the Venturi mask will have to be replaced with a non-rebreather reservoir mask. If the patient's condition worsens, and the EMT is not sure if (for this patient) a high FiO_2 should be maintained, once it has been instituted, the EMT should obtain on-line medical direction for guidance.

USING A PORTABLE OXYGEN UNIT

Portable oxygen units vary slightly from model to model but essentially contain the same overall parts and are used in substantially the same manner. The portable units used in pre-hospital care incorporate "D" or "E" tanks and an oxygen regulator. The connecting yoke, the pressure reducing system, the pressure gauge and the flowmeter are permanently pre-assembled into a single unit which is commonly referred to as the **regulator.** The regulator and portable tank are pre-connected and usually stored ready for immediate carry-in use with nasal cannula, oxygen masks and an oxygen key in a rigid or fabric carrying case. This case allows all of the supplemental oxygen equipment that may be initially needed at the patient's location to be carried in one handy kit, and it protects the included components when they are carried and stored.

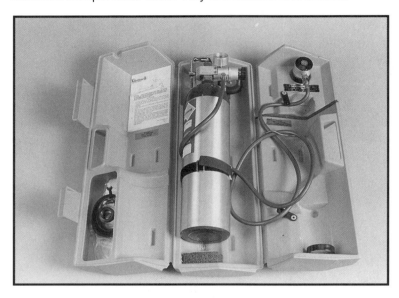

As well as being able to be completely opened for removal of the unit or to change tanks, these cases are usually also generally designed so that just the portion of the case which covers the regulator can be opened and the oxygen unit can be used without having to remove it from the case. Soft fabric cases add less weight than do the stronger rigid ones which are made of wood or plastic. However, fabric cases generally do not provide as much protection for the regulator and tank as a rigid case, and greater care in handling and storing them is required. They are also more vulnerable to absorbing body fluids and other contaminants.

Some services incorporate their tank, regulator, and oxygen supplies into a larger case which also includes all of the airway management and ventilation equipment that may be needed at the patient's side.

Services which use a Demand Valve resuscitator, generally use the same portable oxygen unit to supply both the demand head and a mask or cannula.

When it has been determined in the patient assessment sequence that supplemental oxygen is to be initiated using a portable unit, the following steps should be followed:

1. Place the portable oxygen case flat on the ground near the patient's head and open the top of the case (or remove the unit from the case). Check that no open flame, smoldering embers, persons smoking, etc., are in or near the area in which the oxygen is to be used and confirm that the proper Universal Precautions have been taken.

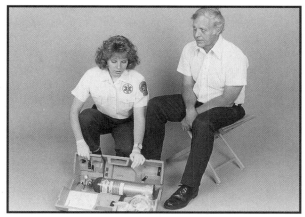

2. Rapidly reconfirm that no additional airway adjunct is required and that adequate spontaneous ventilation exists. Then, based upon the FiO_2 needed, select the mask or nasal cannula to be used and remove it from its packaging. Attach the connector found at its proximal end securely over the low pressure nipple (Christmas tree) of the flowmeter. If the mask selected did not come pre-assembled with tubing, universal connecting tubing should be attached to the flowmeter's nipple and to the nipple on the mask. Check that the hand screw holding the regulator in place to the tank is still as firmly hand tightened as possible.

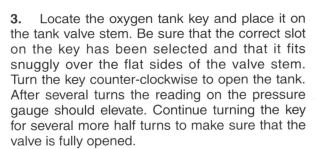

3. Locate the oxygen tank key and place it on the tank valve stem. Be sure that the correct slot on the key has been selected and that it fits snuggly over the flat sides of the valve stem. Turn the key counter-clockwise to open the tank. After several turns the reading on the pressure gauge should elevate. Continue turning the key for several more half turns to make sure that the valve is fully opened.

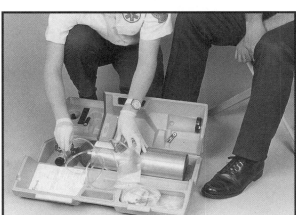

4. Check the pressure gauge to confirm that the tank has a pressure greater than 500 to 750 psi. Next, while observing the flow gauge, adjust the liter flow valve to the desired Liter per minute rate. If it is the pre-set type without a LPM gauge, set it at the desired flow rate marked on the liter flow valve handle.

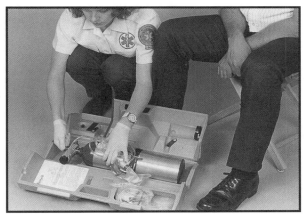

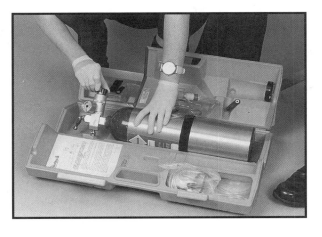

5. By feel, check that oxygen is flowing from the mask or cannula. If a mask with a reservoir is being used, occlude the flow from the reservoir to the mask to fully inflate the bag of the reservoir. Make sure that with such a mask the liter per minute flow selected is no less than 6 LPM, or if a nasal cannula, that it is no greater than 6 LPM. After confirming that oxygen flows properly from the device selected, explain what you are doing to the patient and install the mask or cannula on the patient's face. Then, make any further liter flow adjustment needed.

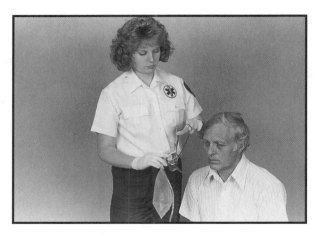

6. After placing the patient on the ambulance cot (or backboard, split-litter, etc.), fully secure the tank and regulator in between or alongside the patient's legs (or if so equipped, in the cot's oxygen carrier). Be sure it is positioned so that you can access the flow valve and tank key, and that the gauge is visible. It is important to the patient's safety that the tank is secured by a strap which fully encircles it, so that the unit can *NOT* move towards the patient's torso.

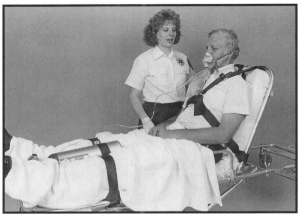

7. Once the patient has been moved and the cot has been installed properly in the patient compartment of the ambulance, turn ON the on-board oxygen system (described in a following skills sequence) and set it to the same desired liter per minute flow. After checking that oxygen properly flows from the low pressure nipple of the on-board flowmeter, disconnect the supply tubing from the portable unit and firmly attach it to the nipple of the on-board system without removing the mask or cannula from the patient. Then, turn off the portable unit's oxygen flow.

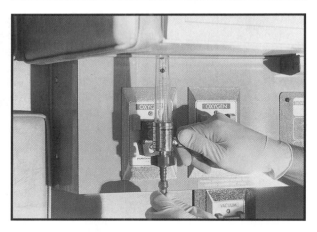

8. When nearing the hospital, reverse the process described in the previous step. Adjust the liter flow of the portable unit back to the correct liter per minute flow and transfer the mask's connecting tubing from the on-board oxygen source back to the portable unit. Then turn off the on-board oxygen. In cases where the run-time is only a few short minutes, the EMT may decide that the transfer from the portable unit to the on-board system and back is unnecessary.

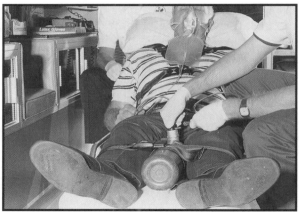

9. Once the cot is next to the Emergency Department bed and you are ready to transfer the patient from the cot onto it, adjust the hospital wall unit's flowmeter to the proper Liter per minute setting and check that oxygen flows from the outlet nipple of the wall unit. Then, transfer the connecting tubing from the portable unit to the nipple on the wall source and turn off the portable unit's flow.

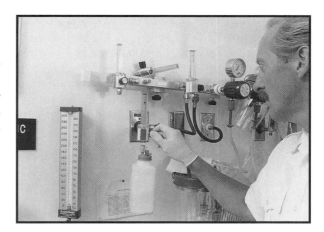

10. After the patient's care has been fully transferred to the hospital staff and the EMTs are preparing their equipment to leave, the portable unit should be put away ready for its next use. First, check the pressure gauge to make sure that the remaining tank pressure is greater than 500 – 750 psi. Then, close the tank by turning the key clockwise until it will turn no further. Note that even with the tank shut off, the gauge continues to read as before, reflecting the pressure left in the system. Open the flow valve to bleed-off this residual pressure. Once the gauge has "pinned out" at "0" pressure, turn the liter flow valve to its off position.

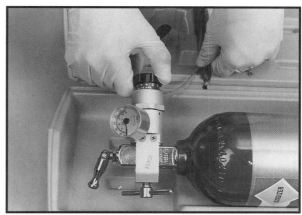

11. Clean the unit by wiping its exposed parts with a suitable antiseptic wipe. ***DO NOT use any wipe containing petroleum oil or soap made from animal fat as this can result in spontaneous ignition and fire or explosion.*** Replace the unit in its case and restock any masks, cannula, or connecting tubing used, obtaining them from the hospital or ambulance back-up stock. Before closing the case make sure that the oxygen tank key is still attached or properly located within the unit.

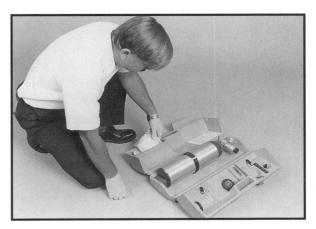

12. If the pressure in the tank was less than 500 psi or whatever minimum level your service allows, the tank should be replaced with a full tank. *If the portable tank needs replacement, this should be done before the ambulance leaves the hospital im case the ambulance comes upon an accident or is dispatched to another call.* Once the EMTs are back in the ambulance the on-board oxygen should also be properly shut off. Changing tanks in the portable unit, use of on-board and hospital wall units, and changing ambulance oxygen tanks are discussed in the following pages of this section.

REPLACING THE OXYGEN TANK IN A PORTABLE UNIT

When the tank pressure in a portable unit approaches 200 psi the tank should be replaced. *Loosening the tank and regulator or any other screw-type connections of any oxygen unit while any residual pressure remaining (except in the closed oxygen tank) is **dangerous** and should **never** be attempted.* Such connections should only be separated once the EMT is sure that the line pressure has been fully relieved and that no flame, embers, spark-producing items or oil are near, if the danger of injury is to be avoided. After confirming that the tank requires replacement:

1. Close the tank by turning the tank valve key clockwise until it will turn no further. These valves should only be closed with the oxygen key. Use of other tools is unnecessary and may cause dangerous damage to the valve. After fully closing the tank, remove the key from the tank's valve stem. Next, open the flow valve to bleed off the residual pressure left in the unit. Once the pressure gauge has "pinned-out" at the "0" psi setting indicating that no pressure remains, the flow valve should again be closed.

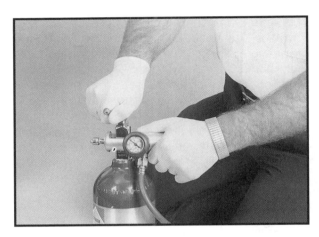

2. After confirming that the tank is closed and that all pressure has been bled-off, hold the tank securely in a lying position and loosen the hand-screw which holds the regulator in place on the valve-stem. Continue turning the handle until the pointed end of the hand screw no longer protrudes into the opening of the yoke.

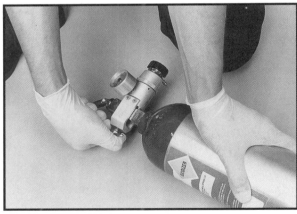

3. Slide the regulator to the side until the tank valve is at the hand screw side of the yoke. Once the valve stem is completely free of the index pins, carefully remove it from the tank valve. Care must be taken not to allow the pins or outlet tube to become reinserted or to make contact with the valve stem when withdrawing the regulator yoke from over the tank valve. After the regulator and tank have been separated, label the tank "empty" and place it flat on the ground, in the spare oxygen cylinder case, or in an "empty" cylinder rack.

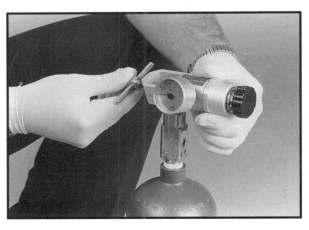

4. Take a "full" tank and confirm that it is labelled as "U.S.P. Oxygen" and "full." Remove the protective band (usually containing a spare "O" ring) which has been placed around the valve stem to protect the outlet from dirt. Carefully look at the "O" ring presently surrounding the regulator's inlet nipple on the inside of the yoke. If it appears flattened or otherwise worn or damaged replace it with a new one. Also check that the two index pins on the inside of the yoke are present and appear undamaged.

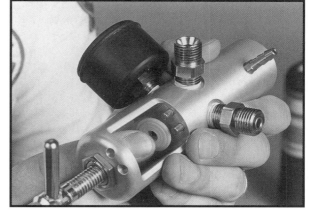

5. Place the oxygen key properly on the full tank's valve stem. Hold the tank so that no part of your body is over (above) the valve stem and that it does not point at any other person. Slowly open the tank valve and, as soon as oxygen is heard to blow from the outlet, rapidly close it. "Cracking" the tank in this way blows any dirt particles from the tank valve's outlet and keeps them from entering the regulator. Next remove the key from the tank's valve stem.

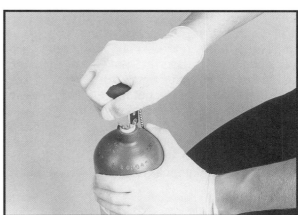

6. Carefully rotate the tank so that the flat side of the tank valve containing the oxygen outlet and pin index holes faces the end of the regulator yoke containing the regulator inlet tube (surrounded by the "O" ring) and the index pins. Once the tank is so oriented, insert the yoke over the tank valve being careful to avoid any contact between the index pins and the valve.

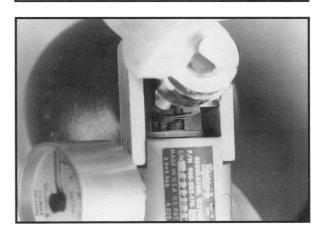

7. Once the yoke has been advanced down the valve so that the pins on the yoke approximate the holes in the tank, carefully adjust the yoke until the index pins and inlet tube align exactly with their respective holes in the tank valve. Once these are aligned properly, move the yoke sideways so that the inlet tube and index pins insert correctly into their respective holes.

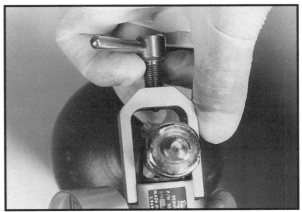

8. Hold the yoke so that it remains firmly pressed against the "O" ring and keep the inlet tube inserted into the outlet hole on the tank valve. Turn the hand-screw of the yoke clockwise until its pointed tip lodges within the cone-shaped indentation found on the side of the valve opposite from the one containing the holes for the index pins and outlet tube. Verify that the outlet tube and hand-screw tip are properly located, and then tighten the hand-screw fully by hand. Since the yoke is usually made of brass or other soft metal, the screw should only be hand-tightened. Excessive force or use of a wrench can result in stripping the yoke's threading and is not necessary to seal the "O" ring.

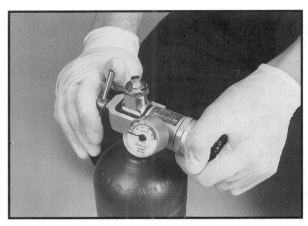

9. Once the regulator and tank have been connected, replace the oxygen key on the valve stem and slowly open the tank valve. If oxygen leaks from the yoke, tighten the hand-screw more firmly. If this does not resolve the problem, the tank will have to be closed, the pressure bled-off, and the tank taken out of the yoke to replace the "O" ring and check the inlet tube for cracks or damage. In most cases, just some additional hand-tightening will stop the leakage.

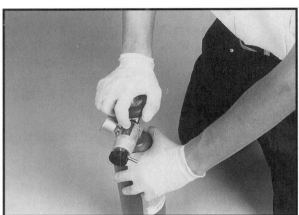

10. Once the tank valve has been opened, check the pressure gauge to assure that the tank is indeed full. The pressure should be between 1900–2200 psi. *NO tank should ever be assumed "full" until it has been checked.* Then open the liter flow valve to between 6–10 LPM and feel that oxygen flows from the low pressure nipple of the flowmeter.

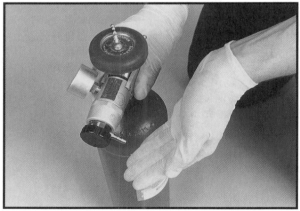

11. If you are changing the tank while the oxygen unit was in use, reattach the connecting tubing from the mask and adjust the liter flow to the desired rate. If the unit is to be stored, shut the tank valve fully and – once all of the pressure has bled off – turn the liter flow valve off. After placing the assembled tank and regulator in its case, check that the proper masks, cannula, and connecting tubes are also packed in the case, before closing it. Lastly, the readied portable oxygen unit in its case should be carefully secured within the vehicle.

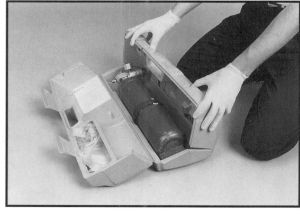

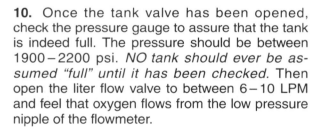

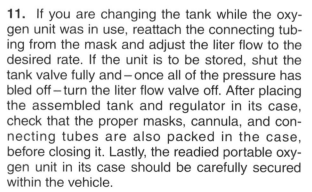

12. If you are using a dual-yoked unit and one tank approaches 200 psi, first make sure that a second tank has been properly inserted tightly in the second yoke. Next, fully close the first tank and immediately open the second one. The pressure gauge should "jump" to a new elevated reading. The gauge now reflects the contents of the "open" second tank *only.* Dual-yoke units contain self-sealing one-way valves for each yoke to allow the replacement of either tank while the unit remains in use on the other one. After 15 seconds or so, the line between the closed first tank and the regulator will be bled-off, and it can carefully be removed. When the hand-screw on this closed first tank is loosened (while the unit is in use on the other tank) a momentary leak will occur. The "hiss" of escaping oxygen will be heard initially as the tank is loosened in the yoke, followed by a "pop" as the one way valve closes to keep any further oxygen from leaving the empty yoke. As needed, replace the empty tank with a full one. In two-yoke units it is recommended that the tanks be used alternately rather than simultaneously. In this method, as each tank empties it is closed before the other tank is opened so that none of the contents of the full tank is diverted into the empty one. If both tanks are open at the same time there is communication between both tanks and oxygen from the full one will flow into the empty one until the pressure in both is equal. With further use, this cross filling will cause them both to approach 200 psi simultaneously, defeating the purpose of a dual-yoked system.

USING AN ON-BOARD, AMBULANCE OXYGEN UNIT

The piped oxygen systems on-board ambulances vary greatly in their exact component design and therefore, the specific steps required to use these parts. The EMT must be experienced in the use of the specific on-board oxygen unit in any ambulance that he will respond in. Since services commonly have different generations and models of ambulances in use at the same time, the EMT should re-familiarize himself with the use of the unit in "his" ambulance at the beginning of his shift or on-call period. The following steps demonstrating the use of one such unit should only act as a general guideline, and needs to be modified for the specific model to be used. Regardless of their differences on-board units universally include:

- One or more large USP oxygen tanks secured in an outside compartment and connected by a flexible hose with a screw-on coupling to the oxygen pipes built into the walls of the patient compartment.

- A regulator to reduce the pressure from the tank. In some units a single stage regulator and pressure gauge are included in this connection. In others, there is only a hose and coupling, and the regulator and pressure gauge are located at the unit's master oxygen control panel.

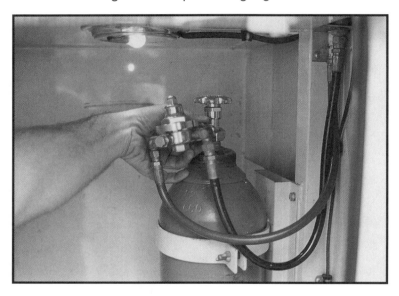

- **Pipes** within the walls of the ambulance between the tank and a master valve and from that valve to each oxygen outlet in the ambulance.

- A **master valve** to open and close the piped system from within the patient compartment of the ambulance.

- A **pressure gauge** with which to monitor the oxygen level remaining in the tank.

- Separate **flowmeters** for each patient oxygen outlet containing a control valve and flow gauge.

- Most newer units have an **oxygen master control panel** (at which many of the controls and gauges are assembled) usually located within easy reach of an EMT in the attendant's seat at the head end of the cot.

Although ambulances commonly carry only one large oxygen tank, on-board units in areas with unusually long run-times preferably contain two. When a two-tank system is used, both tanks are pre-connected. Only one of these should be used at a time, with the second only used as a backup should the first approach empty (200 psi) while on a run. Should this occur the tank in use is closed first, then the full tank opened to avoid cross filling between the full and empty tanks. At the end of the run the full tank is labelled as the "in-use" tank and the empty one is replaced or refilled. In systems which only contain a single tank, it is recommended that it be changed or refilled after any call when it reaches 1,000 psi or less, to assure that it will not run out regardless of the length of use during a run. In some newer models the gauges have been replaced by a computerized display. In some these are constant digital displays, while in others a menu exists and the desired display has to be selected to be brought up on the screen.

Usually, a hatch is built into the wall between the patient and the oxygen tank compartments to allow the EMT to access the tank valve(s) from within the patient compartment of the ambulance while enroute.

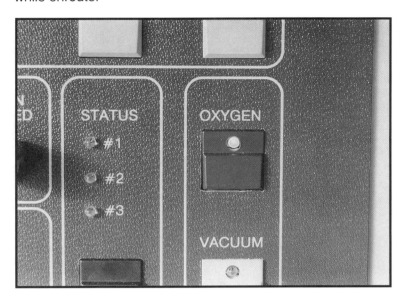

The oxygen from the tanks in the outside compartment is piped first to a master control panel generally found near the attendant seat at the head of the patient cot. This panel will include a master valve with which to open or close the flow of oxygen to the several flowmeters in the system. This valve is generally electrically operated (solenoid or electronic) and is controlled by an "on/off" switch. When the switch is placed in the "on" position the valve opens and an indicator light shows that the system is "on." When the switch is turned "off" the valve closes and oxygen no longer flows to the flowmeters.

The switch which controls the master valve may be near or at some distance from the valve itself. In most ambulances the valve is located near or behind the control panel and therefore considerable piping exists in the walls of the ambulance between the tank and the master valve. In such units, when the ambulance is not in use for any extended period the tank valve should be closed so that there is no chance that a leak can empty the tank. In many recent models, although the switch is at the panel the actual electronic valve it controls is just beyond the tank's valve in the outside compartment. This advantageous design allows for safely using this valve to open and close the system without the need of closing the actual tank valve and without any fear that a potential leak in the wall piping can "empty" the tank. The EMT, based upon which design is incorporated in the ambulance and his service's protocol, will have to determine which method is appropriate when shutting-off the system. Should any doubt exist, closing the tank valve when the unit will not be used between calls is recommended.

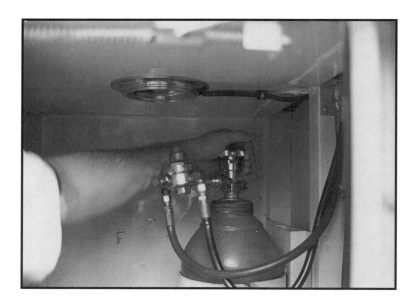

In some units the valve will be a manually operated one, requiring that it be turned to open or close it in the customary manner for gas flow valves.

A flowmeter and flow-valve are also found at (or near) the master control panel to allow for connection of the selected oxygen delivery device and control of the liter per minute flow to the patient on the cot. The panel usually contains a flow gauge and a pressure gauge. In systems where a pressure gauge is part of the regulator in the outside compartment, a second gauge is generally also at the panel to allow for easy monitoring of the oxygen level remaining in the tank from within the patient compartment. Many units contain a warning light and audible alarm which warns the EMT if the system drops below 40 psi or exceeds 70 psi at any time.

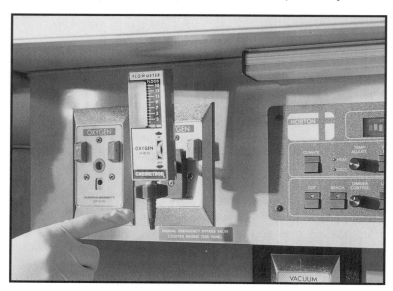

Almost all units have additional piping from the master panel to a second flowmeter placed near the squad bench. This allows the EMT to provide oxygen to a second patient without the need for connecting tubing to lie across the compartment's aisle. Some ambulances have additional flowmeters as well. Each flowmeter consists of a flow gauge plus a flow valve with which to independently control the flow.

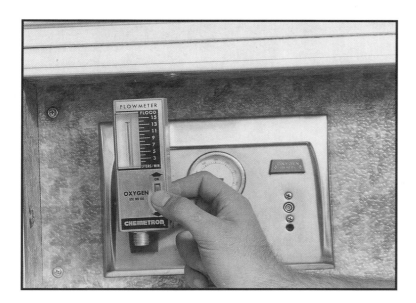

Although each flowmeter can be opened or closed and the flow regulated independently, all of the flowmeters are in-line after the master valve on the panel—requiring that both the tank valve and this master valve be open for oxygen to be available to the flowmeters. In some units there is a sub-switch and indicator light controlling each separate flowmeter location. These are generally found next to the master switch at the main control panel. Some panels also include separate controls for built-in suction units which may be located at some or all of the flowmeter locations.

On-board systems, like portable units, should *NOT* be left with pressure in the lines for any sustained period between calls in order to avoid damage to the regulator, gauges, electronic components or flowmeters. After the tank valve has been closed, the pressure gauge continues to show the same pressure as before. This reflects the residual pressure remaining in the lines rather than the pressure in the tank. Therefore, once the tank valve has been closed the remaining pressure in the line needs to be "bled-off." To achieve this, after closing the tank valve the EMT must open the master valve and open the flowmeter. After a few seconds the oxygen flow will stop and the pressure gauge will read "0." Once this occurs the master valve should be closed and the flowmeter valve should also be set at its "0" or "off" position. In models that have the master valve in the oxygen tank compartment this valve rather than the tank's valve can be closed, and the line pressure bled-off solely by opening the flow valve. Since this advantage is not available in all ambulances, the directions on the following pages assume the need to use the tank valve to close the system, and need to be modified in models with an electrically controlled valve positioned immediately after the tank.

Some units have a snap-in system at each location for a flowmeter. With this type of system the outlets have openings with one-way valves which close when the flowmeter is removed. This allows for oxygen access at several secondary locations in the ambulance without a unit protruding from the wall when not in use. When oxygen is desired at such a location, a flowmeter is attached by inserting the prongs on its back into the keyed opening on the wall. When fully inserted it "snaps" into place and remains locked in until the release button is pressed.

When use of the on-board oxygen is required:

1. Open the tank by turning the handle attached to the valve stem counter-clockwise to provide an oxygen flow to the master control panel.

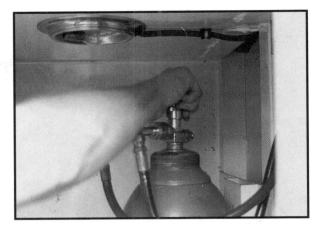

2. To activate the on-board system, open the master valve by placing the master oxygen switch to the "on" position (or with manual valves turning it to its fully opened position). Check that the indicator light shows the system is on, and check the pressure gauge to confirm that the tank is full or contains enough pressure.

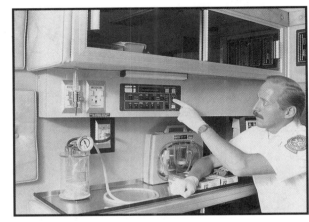

3. Next, open the flow valve near the panel (if each flowmeter has a separate electronic valve and sub-switch also turn "on" the appropriate one) and while looking at the flow gauge, set it to the desired liter flow. Confirm that oxygen flows from the unit by feeling near the open end of the low pressure nipple of the flowmeter.

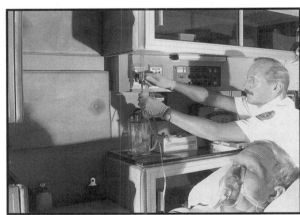

4. Attach the female connector of the supply tubing from the selected delivery device firmly over the "Christmas tree" nipple of the flowmeter. If a reservoir mask is used, adjust the liter flow as needed to maintain a proper volume in the reservoir bag. If the patient was on oxygen from a portable unit, close the valve of the portable tank. Monitor respirations, oxygen flow and tank pressure while enroute and periodically confirm that airway patency and adequate ventilation continue.

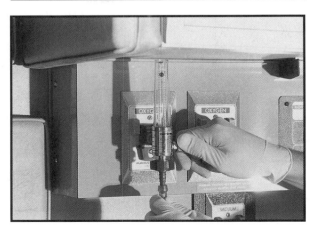

5. If oxygen is needed for a second patient, open the flow valve at the second flowmeter and adjust it to the desired liter flow. After checking that oxygen flows from the "Christmas tree" of this flowmeter, attach the female connector on the mask's tubing firmly over it and adjust the liter flow further as needed.

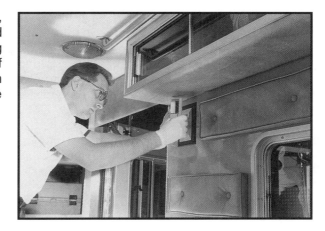

6. When nearing the hospital, open the portable tank secured to the cot and switch the delivery device's tubing from the on-board oxygen flowmeter nipple back to the nipple on the portable unit. Adjust the portable unit's liter flow as needed. If use of oxygen was only initiated in the ambulance, a portable unit will have to be set up and secured on the cot prior to switching over. Next, turn the wall flowmeter off and close the master valve by placing the switch in the "off" position (unless a second patient is still being oxygenated using the system).

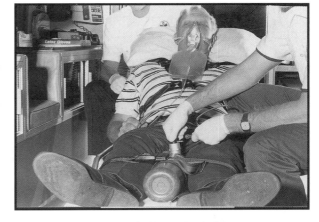

7. After transferring the patient at the hospital and returning to the ambulance, the on-board oxygen system should be shut down. Start by checking the pressure gauge or display to determine how much pressure remains in the tank, and note if the tank will have to be replaced once back at quarters.

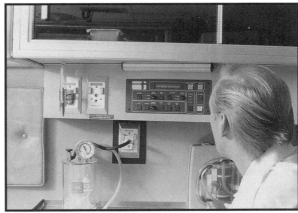

8. Next close the tank valve. The pressure gauge will remain unchanged, reflecting the remaining pressure in the line rather than that in the closed tank. Open the master valve by turning the master switch "on" (be sure that any vehicle battery switches required to power the oxygen unit are "on") and open the valve of the flowmeter. After the oxygen flow has stopped and the pressure gauge drops to an "0" reading, close the flow valve and shut the master valve by placing its switch in the "off" position.

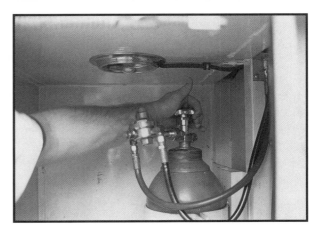

CHANGING TANKS IN ON-BOARD AMBULANCE OXYGEN SYSTEMS

The tanks used for on-board oxygen systems are either "M", "H" or "K" tanks. Because these are extremely heavy and hard to grasp, two EMTs are needed to safely lift and maneuver the tanks when changing them in the ambulance. Whenever these large oxygen tanks are to be lifted or moved any distance, their protective cap should be firmly screwed on over the valve to protect it. If such a tank must be moved any significant distance, it should be secured onto a hand-cart designed for large gas cylinders and only moved by rolling the cart. When it needs to be moved only a short distance it should be leaned slightly from its fully upright position and rotated (continuously or back and forth) on its lower edge to maneuver it into place while a second EMT assures that it does not fall. *Oxygen tanks should NEVER be left standing upright unless firmly secured in place, and should NEVER be moved by rolling them flat on their sides.* When changing the tanks in the ambulance, to avoid having the full tank standing unsecured while the empty one is removed, it is recommended that the empty tank be removed and secured to the wall before the full tank is released and moved to the ambulance.

When oxygen tanks are stored standing against a wall, they should be chained securely in place. Ropes, web strapping, elastic cords, or other forms of "ties" are not sufficiently safe. Tanks mounted in the ambulance should be tightly secured in place with steel straps which surround the tank and are kept closed with either a locking handle or hand bolt.

When large tanks need to be lifted up to or down from the elevated tank compartment of the ambulance—lifting or lowering the tank by encircling it with one's arms invites back injury or injury to the EMT's feet should the tank rapidly slide to the ground, and is extremely dangerous. Therefore, this is not recommended. Instead, when tanks are to be lowered from within the ambulance compartment they should be unstrapped and rotated back and forth until part of the edge of the tank extends beyond the compartment's floor. Then, while one EMT holds the upper tank so that it is leaning slightly back form its fully upright position, a second EMT places his hands under the tank and—lifts the base out—lowering it to the ground by bending his legs. The tank must be held on a slight angle at all times to avoid the possibility that the EMT lifting the bottom will have his fingers crushed under the base of the tank. When lifting the heavier full tank into place, the same general method is used. The tank is placed upright on the ground directly in front of the open door of the compartment. While one EMT securely holds the tank on a slight angle, the second EMT squats and—holding the lower edge of the tank—lifts with his legs until a significant portion of the tank's base has been placed on the compartment floor. Again, care must be taken to avoid the base being lowered onto the compartment floor without it being sufficiently tilted to avoid catching the lifter's fingers between it and the compartment floor.

When the tank for the on-board oxygen system needs to be replaced:

1. Make sure the ambulance is in "Park" and the "Parking Brake" is properly set. Open the oxygen tank compartment door fully and secure it open in some manner. Then turn the tank valve until it is fully closed. (If the system contains two tanks, both the valve on the one to be changed and the second tank that will remain in the compartment must be fully closed.)

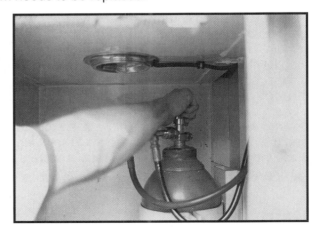

2. Next, make sure to turn on any switches in the driver's compartment that are required to provide electric power at the oxygen panel. Note that even with the tank valve(s) shut, the pressure gauge will continue to indicate the same pressure as before. With the tank valve closed the pressure gauge reflects the line pressure rather than the pressure in the tank. Then, open the master valve by turning the oxygen switch to "on" and open the flow valve on the flowmeter. When the pressure in all of the lines has been bled off the oxygen flow from the nipple of the flowmeter will stop and the pressure gauge will read "0" psi. Next, close the master valve by turning the master switch to "off" and close the flow valve.

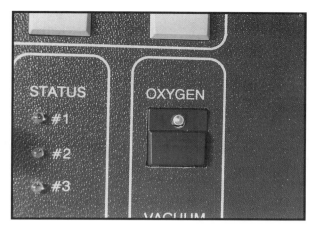

3. Once there is no longer any pressure in the system (except in the closed tanks), it is safe to uncouple the tank. Take a large tank wrench and place it over the female threaded nut which secures the unit's hose stem onto the tank valve, and loosen it. *Only wrenches designed for this purpose should be used. Using other types is dangerous and can result in damage.* Once the nut has been loosened, continue turning it by hand until it is fully unscrewed. Then, separate the hose connection from the tank and screw a protective metal cap firmly over the tank valve.

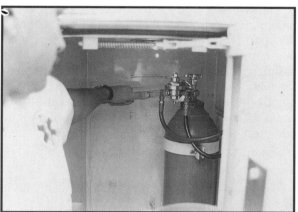

4. Open the handle or bolts that fasten the steel strap around the tank and move the parts of the strapping aside so they will not interfere with removal of the tank. "Walk" the tank carefully towards the compartment door until enough of the tank's base is beyond the door's sill allowing for a good grasp on the base of the tank. Be careful not to walk the tank too far over the edge of the compartment floor.

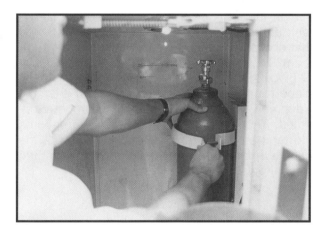

5. While one EMT carefully tilts and stabilizes the top of the tank, the second EMT squats and — with his hands at the base of the tank — lifts it slightly using his leg muscles. He then brings the bottom of the tank entirely out of the compartment and lowers it slowly to the ground. It is essential that the EMT at the upper end of the tank maintains the tilt so that the EMT lowering the base to the ground cannot have his hands trapped between the tank and the floor.

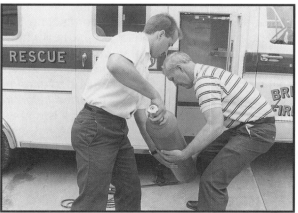

6. With continuous or back and forth rotation, "walk" the tank until it is placed fully upright next to the wall. Secure it with the chain to the wall and, before leaving it, be sure it is clearly labelled "EMPTY." In stations that have separate locations for "full" and "empty" tanks, be sure that it has been properly located in the "empty" section.

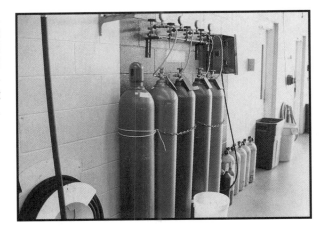

7. Next select the full tank you will place in the ambulance and check that it is labelled "full" and "Oxygen U.S.P." Also, make sure that the protective cap is firmly screwed over the valve. After releasing the chain securing the tank in place to the wall, "walk" it to the open ambulance oxygen compartment. Carefully position it so that it is close to the side of the ambulance and exactly centered on the compartment opening.

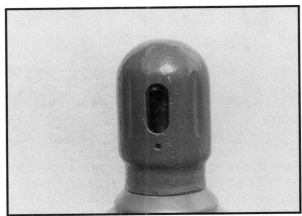

8. In the manner previously described, lift the tank and place it on the compartment's floor so that about half of its base is within the compartment. Then, carefully "walk" it back into its proper place in the compartment. Once the tank is in place remove the protective cap from over the valve end, rotate the tank until it is properly oriented. Then, place the steel band that secures the tank around it, and lock it in place with the handle or bolts provided. Next, rapidly open and close the valve to blow off any dirt.

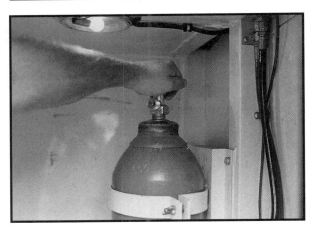

9. Carefully align the stem and female threaded nut at the end of the unit's connecting line with the male threaded outlet on the tank valve. While carefully holding the stem aligned against the tank valve with one hand, turn the nut several times clockwise with the other hand to engage the threaded connection. *Care must be taken to avoid cross-threading.* If any resistance is met as you start tightening, stop. Unscrew the nut, and start again. When the threads are properly engaged the nut can initially be turned easily by hand.

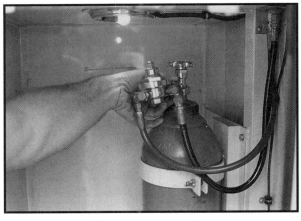

10. After hand tightening the nut as far as possible, use the large tank wrench to complete its tightening. Continue tightening until the wrench can no longer be turned with one hand. Excessive tightening can damage or "jam" the connection. Next, open the tank valve and check the connection for any leak. If a leak is found, tighten the nut in 1/4 turn increments until it is eliminated.

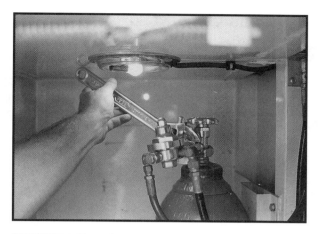

11. With the tank valve open, check the pressure gauge to confirm that the tank is indeed full. In units that have a gauge in the tank compartment and a second one on the master panel, after opening the master valve check that both gauges indicate substantially the same pressure. Next, turn the valve on the flowmeter to about 10–12 LPM and check that oxygen flows from its output nipple.

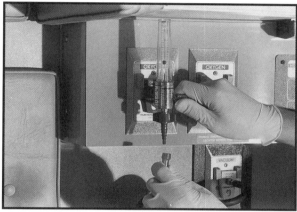

12. After replacing the oxygen tank and confirming that the tank is full and that the on-board oxygen system is operating properly, shut the tank valve, bleed-off the line pressure, and close both the flowmeter and master valves. Next, check the cabinet where the supplemental oxygen supplies are stored in the ambulance and add any masks, nasal cannula, connecting tubing, or spare oxygen keys required to bring each to the proper quantity (indicated in the ambulance inventory list). Lastly, according to your department policy, log the tank change and notify the appropriate individual that there is an empty tank which requires refilling.

USING HOSPITAL OXYGEN WALL UNITS

There is usually an oxygen wall outlet at each bed position within the hospital to provide for delivery of supplemental oxygen. These are connected by a system of pipes to a central oxygen source elsewhere in the building. The system is "charged" at all times, providing a constant pressure and high oxygen flow available at each outlet. Depending upon their design, these outlets have either a screw-on or a snap-in connection for attaching a flowmeter to them. Usually the outlets are self-sealing so that no oxygen flows out of them when the flowmeter is removed for cleaning or service. When connected to the outlet, oxygen is provided to the flowmeter. Adjusting the valve of the flowmeter determines whether the unit is closed or open — and if open, the exact liter flow being delivered. In some systems the flowmeter is permanently attached to each outlet and there is a separate shut-off valve which must be opened prior to adjusting the liter flow.

Whether removable or permanently attached to the outlet, hospital flowmeters contain a gauge and valve with which to identify and control the oxygen flow. Generally these are of the pressure compensated type and will indicate actual liter flow being delivered. If there is a reduced flow (in the event that the oxygen tubing becomes kinked or the end flow becomes obstructed in any manner) this type of gauge will accurately reflect the change.

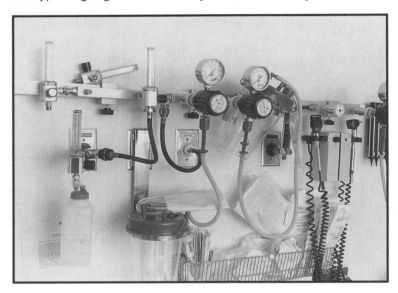

Hospital wall units also commonly include a humidifier. The humidifier contains a clear plastic cannister which hangs on the flowmeter and has a removable "air proof" top. The cannister is partially filled with water and contains a plastic inlet tube through its top which is connected to the flowmeter's outlet nipple by a short piece of tubing. When the flow valve is opened, oxygen flows into the water and is humidified as it "bubbles," rising through the water to the area of the cannister above the water line. Then, it flows through the outlet tube which passes through the sealed top of the cannister to the universal connecting nipple ("Christmas tree") found on the outside of the cannister. Humidifiers may or may not be used with every patient who is given oxygen, depending upon the different policies the EMT may find from one hospital to another. Therefore, the EMT should connect the oxygen mask or cannula initiated in the field to a wall unit without a humidifier unless directed to include a humidifier by a member of the hospital staff. Should any question exist, the EMT should ask the nurse who is assuming responsibility for the patient's care as a routine part of giving the report.

After moving the patient from the ambulance to the bedside the tubing to the mask or nasal cannula being used needs to be transferred from the squad's portable oxygen unit to the hospital wall unit. Whether this should be done before or after moving the patient from the ambulance cot to the hospital bed may be dictated by the physical layout or situation. If not, it is solely a matter of individual preference. In patients who are being furnished with a low FiO_2, experience has shown that the supplemental oxygen can most easily be disconnected during the physical transfer from the ambulance cot to the hospital bed and then re-established once that movement has been accomplished. In patients requiring a higher FiO_2, rather than interrupting it for several minutes the change should be made before or after moving the patient over—whichever will best minimize the time during which it is disconnected. Care must be taken with 100% Non-Rebreather Reservoir Masks, so that room air can enter the mask during this period.

When transferring to a wall unit which does not include a humidifier, the steps followed are similar to those when transferring the oxygen source from a portable unit to the on-board ambulance wall unit. When directed to transfer the oxygen to a hospital unit containing a humidifier the EMT should:

1. Ascertain that the humidifier has not been used for a prior patient and check that it is properly filled with sterile water. If not, fill it with sterile water up to, but not exceeding, the maximum water line marked on the cannister. Then replace the top, making sure that it is properly sealed to exclude the introduction of room air which would lower the FiO_2. If you are not completely familiar with the use of that specific model, ask the nurse who is assuming responsibility for the patient for assistance.

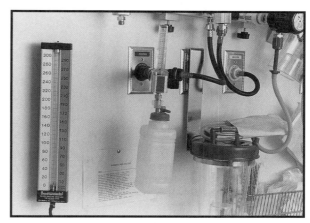

2. Open the flow valve and set the liter flow to the same as that which was being supplied using the portable. (In units that have a separate valve to start or shut off the oxygen flow, open the valve before setting the liter flow.) Check that the oxygen bubbles through the cannister and feel that it flows from the output nipple of the flowmeter. Explain what you are about to do to the patient.

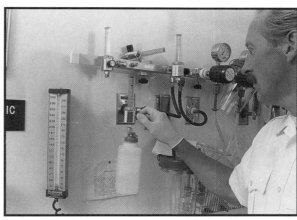

3. Disconnect the proximal end of the mask's tubing from the portable unit and connect it securely over the wall unit's outlet nipple. Be sure to turn off the flow from the portable unit. In the case of a reservoir mask, increase the liter flow until the reservoir bag fills and then re-adjust it to the proper flow. Before leaving the hospital, document the transfer to the wall unit and the liter flow established in your run report, restock any disposable equipment used, clean the portable unit, replace the tank if necessary, and put the portable unit away properly.

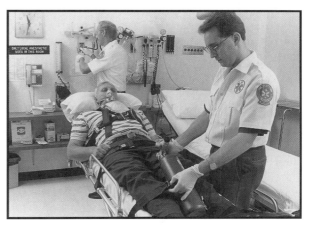

ETI SUMMARY SKILL SHEET
Providing Supplemental Oxygen Enrichment

1. TAKE/CONFIRM proper UNIVERSAL PRECAUTIONS.

2. From the assessment, determine that SUPPLEMEN-TAL OXYGEN is INDICATED and what FiO$_2$ is appropriate.

3. Place the PORTABLE UNIT near the patient's head and OPEN THE CASE for use.

4. CONFIRM that the patient can maintain a PATENT AIR-WAY and ADEQUATE SPONTANEOUS AIR EXCHANGE, and that the area is SAFE FOR USE OF OXYGEN.

5. Place the oxygen key on the tank's valve stem and OPEN THE TANK VALVE.

6. CHECK the TANK PRESSURE to confirm it is suffi-ciently FULL for use.

7. SELECT the appropriate MASK or nasal cannula to deliver the FiO$_2$ desired and ATTACH THE female connector of THIS DEVICE'S TUBING over the outlet nipple of the PORTABLE UNIT'S FLOWMETER.

8. While observing the gauge (if included), TURN the FLOW VALVE TO the DESIRED LPM SETTING.

9. FEEL that the OXYGEN FLOWS from the MASK or CANNULA. If a reservoir mask is being used, occlude the valve between the mask and reservoir to expand the bag fully before attaching it to the patient.

10. IF CONSCIOUS, EXPLAIN TO THE PATIENT what you are going to do.

11. INSTALL THE DELIVERY DEVICE properly ONTO the PATIENT'S FACE.

12. SECURE it to the patient's head with THE LOOP OR ELASTIC BAND provided.

13. ADJUST the liter flow as needed.

14. If available, INITIATE PULSE OXIMETRY.

15. ONCE ON THE COT (or backboard) SECURE THE PORTABLE UNIT properly.

16. MONITOR the PATIENT'S RESPIRATION and signs associated with CELLULAR OXYGENATION.

17. When the patient has been loaded into the ambulance, CHECK that THE AMBULANCE OXYGEN TANK VALVE IS OPEN and OPEN THE ON-BOARD MASTER VALVE by placing the switch in the "on" position.

18. CHECK the AMBULANCE OXYGEN PRESSURE GAUGE to confirm that the tank and on-board system con-tain adequate oxygen.

19. SET the WALL-MOUNTED FLOW VALVE (nearest to the patient's head) at the desired liter flow AND CHECK that OXYGEN FLOWS from its outlet nipple.

20. TRANSFER the mask or cannula's tubing FROM THE outlet nipple of the PORTABLE UNIT TO that of THE WALL UNIT.

21. TURN OFF the PORTABLE unit's oxygen flow.

22. ADJUST THE LITER FLOW of the on-board unit AS NEEDED.

23. WHEN NEARING THE HOSPITAL, turn on the flow from the portable, TRANSFER THE mask or cannu-la's TUBING FROM the ON-BOARD FLOWMETER BACK TO THE PORTABLE UNIT, and turn "off" the on-board oxygen.

24. Once at the patient's bed in the Emergency Department or patient's room, OPEN THE HOSPITAL WALL UUNIT to the desired liter flow and TRANS-FER the female connector on the proximal end of the tubing from the mask or cannula FROM the outlet nipple of the PORTABLE UNIT TO that of THE HOS-PITAL WALL UNIT.

25. SHUT OFF the flow from the PORTABLE UNIT.

26. Before leaving the hospital, CLOSE THE PORTABLE TANK, BLEED OFF THE PRESSURE, CLEAN it, and RESTOCK ANY disposable ITEMS USED. CHANGE the TANK (IF NEEDED), and SECURE THE PORTABLE UNIT so it is ready to be used on the next call.

27. When back at the ambulance, CHECK the PRESSURE OF THE ON-BOARD TANK. Note if it needs replace-ment and, if it does, notify the dispatcher that you need to be out of service until you can return to quarters and replace it.

28. CLOSE and BLEED OFF the ON-BOARD SYSTEM.

29. Once you are back in quarters, REPLACE any MASKS, CANNULA, PORTABLE TANKS, ETC., used from the ambulance stock AND, REPLACE OR REFILL THE ON-BOARD TANKS as needed.

SECTION 8

Quantitative Measurement of Patient Oxygenation and End-Tidal CO$_2$

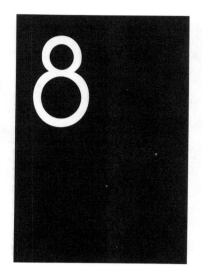

Introduction

Until recently blood oxygen and CO_2 levels were only obtainable by drawing blood and immediately analyzing the blood gases within the hospital. These needed to be rechecked periodically and there was no easy way to continuously monitor the blood gases. In recent years improved technology has added pulse oximetry to provide non-invasive continuous monitoring of blood oxygen levels, and end tidal carbon dioxide (CO_2) detectors make the non-invasive monitoring of exhaled end-tidal CO_2 concentrations possible.

Hospital pulse oximeters and end-tidal CO_2 detectors (capnometers) are generally large and heavy, and require domestic electric current and a stable environment in order to be accurate. Because of their lack of portability and durability and their high cost, these large units are rarely used in pre-hospital care. In the last few years, several lower priced miniaturized pulse oximeters have become available for pre-hospital and in-hospital portable use. As well, inexpensive disposable single-patient—use colorimetric end-tidal CO_2 detectors, and most recently miniaturized electronic infrared CO_2 detectors, have also been introduced.

A number of portable pulse oximeters presently available have proven their durability, reliability, and usefulness in the field. Similarly, the reliability and usefulness of disposable single use colorimetric end-tidal CO_2 (ET CO_2) detectors (Easy Cap®) has been widely documented in intubated patients. However, due to limited experience, further study is necessary to determine the durability and reliability of the several models of miniaturized electronic infrared CO_2 detectors that have recently been introduced.

A pulse oximeter measures the percentage of oxygen saturation of the patient's blood. Because good blood oxygen saturation is *dependent* upon good alveolar oxygenation, oximetry provides the EMT with an indicator of airway patency, plus a quantitative measurement to confirm that both the minute volume (spontaneous or provided) and FiO_2 supplied are resulting in proper blood oxygen levels. In patients with spontaneous ventilation, pulse oximetry provides a quantitative measure indicating whether the increased FiO_2 provided is sufficient, or (when an FiO_2 of $0.85-1.00$ is supplied and a low blood oxygen level persists) an indication of the need to provide an increased minute volume with BVM-assisted ventilations. With apneic patients (or patients for whom ventilation is being assisted), the oximeter serves to quantitatively confirm that the airway management, minute volume, and FiO_2 provided are effective and that proper alveolar oxygenation results. Further, by monitoring the oximeter's continuous measurement the EMT will be warned if the oxygen level suddenly drops, and can evaluate and make whatever adjustments in the airway or provided ventilations are necessary to return the levels to an adequate reading.

The oximeter's measurement of the blood oxygen saturation reflects the airway's patency (including proper placement of an ET tube, if included) and the effectiveness of the ventilation and alveolar oxygenation that results—oximetry does not measure or reflect on cellular oxygenation and metabolism.

Although not usually identified in such specific terms, the maintenance of adequate cellular oxygenation and proper aerobic metabolism is the key objective of emergency care. Almost all of the critical interventions provided by all levels of EMTs either provide the patient with a component necessary to maintain cellular oxygenation or eliminate or reduce items which—without intervention—will result in cellular hypoxia or its increase. Adding the measurement of ET CO_2 (as well as providing an alternate way of confirming airway patency, adequate ventilation, and alveolar oxygenation) provides a quantitative measure which reflects the levels of cellular oxygenation and cellular metabolism that result. A positive finding of adequate end-tidal CO_2, as well as confirming airway patency and proper alveolar oxygenation, also confirms that the circulatory and chemical components required for proper aerobic cellular metabolism are present. Therefore it also indicates that adequate hemoglobin, oxyhemoglobin bonding, circulation and cellular perfusion exist, and that no chemical imbalance which is present can prevent capillary and cell wall gas exchange. If adequate perfusion with properly oxgenated blood (cellular oxygenation) is not present, then high levels of the byproduct of the cellular metabolism (CO_2) will not be transported to the lungs to produce a high concentration of CO_2 in the exhaled air and a high ET CO_2 will not be measured.

Although a high ET CO_2 has proven to be a reliable method for confirming proper placement of an endotracheal tube, the lack of such a finding does not provide a clear indication that the ET tube has been misplaced into the esophagus. Even though the lack of a proper level of ET CO_2 may be due to such misplacement, it can also result from poor perfusion, inadequate hemoglobin, or a chemical disturbance in a patient in whom the ET tube has been properly placed. In cardiac arrest patients or those in whom hemorrhage or other causes of shock result in hypoperfusion, a clinical determination will have to be made as to whether improper tube placement or a circulatory deficit is the cause of poor cellular oxygenation and reduced metabolism resulting in the low ET CO_2 reading. In such cases, the EMT must rely on chest excursion, auscultation over the epigastrium, and auscultation of both midlung fields to evaluate whether the trachea or the esophagus has been intubated.

Pre-hospital intubation is most often performed in patients who are in cardiac arrest or are victims of multi-systems trauma, therefore end-tidal CO_2 measurement will most commonly be used in the field in patients who are hemodynamically **unstable.** The measurement of end-tidal CO_2 should be considered as an important adjunct but should not be used by the EMT to supercede the other prudent assessment skills required to determine whether or not an endotracheal tube has been properly placed. As in most patient assessment, the reliance on any one exclusive indicator without consideration of other signs and symptoms is generally unreliable.

Hopefully, as the capability of these devices is extended, they will eventually result in the development of a single small microprocessor unit which will simultaneously measure blood coloration, pulse waves, and ET CO_2. This could then provide the EMT with a quantitative measure of blood oxygen and ET CO_2 and prompt the determination of whether cellular oxygenation and metabolism are being properly maintained and, if not, whether cellular hypoxia continues due to inadequate pulmonary oxygenation, hypoperfusion, or a lack of adequate hemoglobin.

Even with today's pulse oximetry and ET CO_2 measurement capabilities, the EMT can easily determine the effectiveness of his airway, ventilation and oxygenation efforts on the patient's pulmonary oxygenation. In intubated patients, he can further determine whether or not this results in proper cellular oxygenation and metabolism. These can be important diagnostic adjuncts to his clinical findings, and help the EMT to evaluate the effectiveness of the ventilation and treatments to improve perfusion which are being provided in the field.

Portable pulse oximeters are available from different manufacturers. The exact method for the proper use of each of the various models varies and requires that the EMT be trained in the use of the specific model used by his service. The following discussion is included solely as a general guideline, and the EMT will need to be familiar with, and follow, the specific directions for use recommended by the manufacturer and his local medical authority. Since the current literature surrounding end-tidal CO_2 measurement in the field is limited and predominantly deals with the disposable colorimetric device, the discussion found in the following pages is similarly limited to that unit.

USING A PULSE OXIMETER

The typical pulse oximeters used in the field has a microprocessor contained in a monitor "box" and a sensor which connects to the monitor by a thin wire. Various alphanumeric displays are visible on the monitor. These devices are small, lightweight and battery operated. The sensor is usually clipped to the fingertip in adults and to the toe or distal foot in infants. In patients in advancing shock — rather than using the vasoconstricted and poorly perfusing extremities — more central locations such as the bridge of the nose, forehead or ear lobe are preferred. Areas with bruises, hematomas, burns, stains, nail polish, tatoos, or other conditions producing discoloration must be avoided.

Pulse Oximetry provides non-invasive, continuous "real-time" monitoring of the patient's pulse rate and the percentage of oxygen saturation of the patient's blood (SpO_2). This latter is written, for example, as "$SpO_2 = 99\%$."

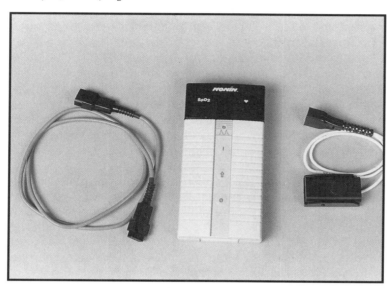

Each of these measurements is continuously visible on the monitor by a lighted digital display. Most units contain an indicator which confirms when a sufficient blood flow exists under the sensor, and a second warning light or other indicator which displays when it is not. Usually, if the unit cannot "read" properly, the problem can be resolved by repositioning the sensor on the finger or relocating it elsewhere. Most units also contain a "low battery" warning light and have an audible alarm which will sound should the oxygen saturation level drop below that to which it has been set.

Measurements are taken by the unit only during each pulse to ensure that the reading is from arterial blood. In order to minimize variability, the microprocessor takes an average of five measurements before displaying the calculated mean SpO_2. This causes a slight delay before the initial reading is displayed. If the average of the last five readings changes, the display changes accordingly. Since most pulse rates have less than one second between pulse waves, it is quite common for the display to fluctuate back and forth between several readings.

The sensor usually contains two infrared light emitting diodes which transmit separate wavelengths of light. After passing through the skin and vascular bed they are "read" by a photo detector on the other side of the sensor and the signal is then relayed through the wire to the microprocessor. By measuring the light absorbed the unit determines from the color of the blood the percentage of oxygen saturation of the hemoglobin remaining in the blood vessels.

Oxygen saturation pressure (SpO$_2$) is a different measurement than the partial pressure of oxygen (PaO$_2$) which is commonly measured by laboratory blood gas analysis. With laboratory blood gas analysis, a drop from a PaO$_2$ of 100 to one of 90mm Hg is not cause for alarm. The oxygen saturation pressure measured by pulse oximetry is evaluated in a scale with a smaller acceptable range and a drop of just a few percent in the reading is significant. At normal levels of oxygenation and perfusion the reading will fluctuate between 96–100%. If the reading is 95% or less, the FiO$_2$ supplied should be increased immediately. If this does not resolve the problem, the patient's minute volume must be reevaluated and assisted ventilation with a high FiO$_2$ considered. If readings are below 90% a loss of airway patency must be considered. If ventilation with a high FiO$_2$ is being provided but the SpO$_2$ is less than 90%, it must be considered to be unsuccessful in achieving proper alveolar oxygenation, and needs to be re-evaluated. It probably requires modification or replacement using another form of provided ventilation. It must be noted that the sensor may be affected by direct sunlight or a nearby strong lamp. resulting in inaccurate (usually lowered) readings. If such a strong ambient light source cannot otherwise be eliminated, the EMT may need to cover the sensor (once installed on the patient) with some opaque material.

Also, the sensor can *NOT* read properly through nail polish. Experience has shown that carrying nail polish remover is useful so that the presence of polish does not exclude using the fingertip. A recent study, however, found that the glue and additional layers of a synthetic material which are added when false nails are worn does *NOT* result in any variation in results or inadequate readings other than from the nail polish which has been added (and which can be removed in the normal manner). In alert patients the fingertip is generally the first choice, since when the clip is attached to other locations some discomfort can be produced.

Pulse oximetry readings have also been shown to be affected by patient movement, hypothermia, the action of vasopressor drugs, peripheral vascular disease, and elevated biliruben levels. As well, oximetry may be significantly inaccurate in patients with abnormal hemoglobin values or if an IV diagnostic dye has been administered in the last 24 hours.

Pulse oximetry is an important diagnostic tool providing the EMT with key additional information about the patient's initial blood oxygenation before and after ventilatory and oxygen enrichment interventions. However, it is not without limits and—as is the case with any monitoring device—it must *NOT* be used to supercede other assessment. **The EMT should treat the patient and not the pulse oximeter's display.** The patient's other key signs and symptoms must be assessed and evaluated so that the oximeter's readings are interpreted within the context of the patient's overall condition.

Cellular oxygenation requires proper pulmonary oxygenation, adequate hemoglobin, a circulatory status capable of maintaining proper cellular perfusion, and an absence of any chemical or metabolic condition which would interfere with the oxygen's on/off loading or diffusion through the capillary and cell walls. Because the oxygen saturation level indicated by the oximeter does *NOT* reflect the level of hemoglobin in the blood or the presence of any chemical or metabolic condition which interferes with oxygen diffusion at the capillary or cellular level, nor the patient's circulatory or metabolic status, no implication or assumptions about cellular oxygenation should be drawn from it. *The percentage of oxygen saturation measured by an oximeter only reflects the supplied pulmonary oxygenation and is NOT an indicator or measure of cellular oxygenation.*

Because the oxygen saturation levels measured by the pulse oximeter reflect pulmonary ventilation and the resulting level of oxygen delivered to the alveoli, it is useful both in the assessment of the patient and as an adjunct for evaluating the effectiveness of the airway management, ventilation, and oxygen enrichment provided by the EMT. The inclusion of pulse oximetry as a local standard of prehospital care is highly recommended.

If possible, it is useful to have a second EMT initiate pulse oximetry when he takes the vital signs in the Initial Systemic Exam. This enlarges the scope of the in-depth respiratory assessment by adding a quantitative measurement of the blood oxygen and indicates whether or not hypoxia is present. It also provides a useful baseline against which the effectiveness and benefit of the EMT's treatment can be compared. Obviously if resources are limited or early initiation of oximetry would otherwise cause delay, it should be deferred until more urgent assessment and care priorities have first been resolved. However, it should not be viewed as simply an ancillary activity with a pre-determined low priority. In patients with marked dyspnea, oximetry may be needed to determine whether a high FiO_2 by mask is sufficient or if assisted ventilation is also required. In patients requiring that ventilation be supported by the EMT, pulse oximetry should soon follow to confirm the effectiveness of the ventilation and oxygenation provided. The EMT will have to determine on a case-by-case basis when in the sequence of his assessment and care the oximetry should be initiated.

When ready to initiate use of the Pulse Oximeter:

1. Place the monitor near the patient where its display can readily be seen. If the patient is being ventilated, place it so that the EMT providing ventilation can easily observe it. Connect the sensor cord to the monitor and clip the sensor over a fingertip properly. In patients in advancing shock, due to the poor peripheral circulation, the bridge of the nose or ear lobe may be preferable to the fingertip, and in infants the toe or distal foot is used.

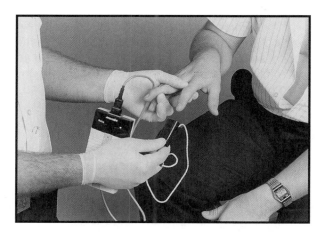

2. After the sensor has been connected to both the monitor and the patient, turn the on/off switch to the "on" position. When the sensor is positioned properly to read the capillary flow, and the flow is sufficient, the "good reading" light or display (depending upon the model) will come on. Check that the "low battery" indicator has *NOT* come on.

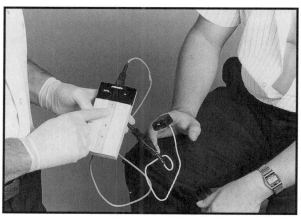

3. If the sensor is not properly located over the vascular bed or if there is an inadequate blood flow underlying it, a "trouble" indicator (rather than the one confirming proper input from the sensor) will display. Reposition the sensor until the display changes and confirms that proper sensing has been established. Should repositioning the sensor on the finger fail to resolve the problem, relocate it to another site.

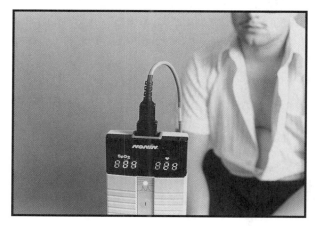

4. Once proper sensing has been confirmed by the oximeter's display, there will be a delay of approximately 3 to 6 seconds before the pulse rate and SpO$_2$ are displayed. To ensure that the readings reflect arterial blood, the sensor only measures the oxygen saturation at each pulse surge (systole). In order to reduce variation in the pulse rate and SpO$_2$ displayed, most models present the average of the last five sensor readings. The initial display is delayed because the microprocessor must receive the result sensed at five consecutive pulse surges before it can calculate these mean averages.

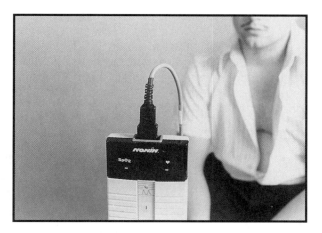

5. After the initial few seconds of delay, the pulse rate and mean SpO$_2$ will each be displayed on the monitor. As long as the sensor remains properly placed, readings will be continuously displayed on the monitor. Even though it reflects a mean average of the last five readings obtained, since the unit measures in small increments, rapid "bouncing" between several adjacent values is common and does *NOT* generally indicate a malfunction. Be sure to properly secure the unit to the cot (or backboard) before moving it, to avoid dropping and damaging the oximeter.

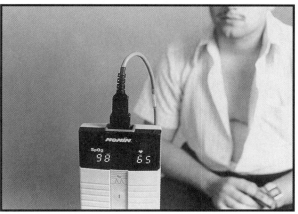

6. Most oximeters are designed to provide either no reading or an unintelligible garbled one if any component fails to operate properly. Although this reduces the chance that an unrecognized malfunction will produce inaccurate results, it does not eliminate the possibility. The oximeter readings should regularly be compared against the values from another unit (which can readily be accomplished after transferring a patient in the Emergency Department). Units should be serviced and checked by factory authorized service technicians in a regularly scheduled maintenance program and at any time after the unit has been dropped, otherwise damaged, or is found to provide inconsistent values.

USING AN END-TIDAL CO$_2$ DETECTOR

A variety of small portable End-Tidal CO$_2$ Detectors (ET CO$_2$) are presently available for pre-hospital use. These are either battery operated electronic devices which employ a sensor attached to the endotracheal tube and a microprocessor, or they are simple colorimetric detectors (such as the Easy Cap®) which are placed between the proximal end of the endotracheal tube and the BVM or other ventilator being used.

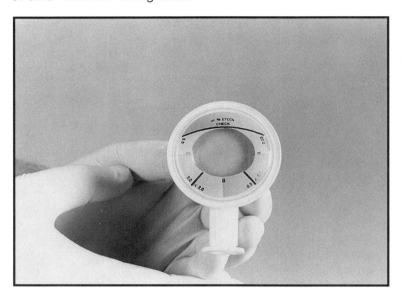

Colorimetric end-tidal CO$_2$ detectors such as the Easy Cap®, are small self-contained units that do not employ batteries or electronics. Instead, the device employs a chemically treated indicator which indicates the approximate end-tidal CO$_2$ produced by it's immediate color changes. The device has two ports, one (the patient end) with a 15mm inside diameter for attaching to the ET tube and the second which has a 15mm outside diameter for attaching to the BVM (or other ventilator). When it is attached in-line between the ET tube and ventilator, the indicator (an oval in the center of the top of the detector) changes color between inspiration and expiration. The ET CO$_2$ level is determined by comparing the color at the peak end of expiration with the color scale printed surrounding the indicator.

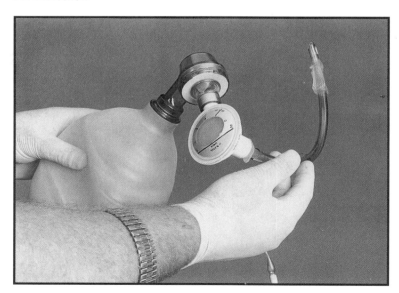

A color "check" to compare the initial color of the indicator when removing it from its airtight package is provided at the top of this scale. *If the purple color of the indicator is not the same, or is darker, than that of the "check", the unit should not be used.* The color scale on the Easy Cap is divided into 3 parts labeled "A", "B" and "C". This is from vivid purple at the lowest end of the "A" portion of the scale (representing an absent or low percentage of 0.03% ET CO_2) through a brownish and tan color on the "B" portion, to bright yellow at the highest end of the "C" part of the scale (representing a high percentage of 5.0% ET CO_2). Although each alphabetically separated area contains several color variations, the device is not accurate enough to make a more exact distinction of the CO_2 level other than to approximate that it lies somewhere within the entire range represented by that section of the scale. A reading in the "A" section represents an absent or minimal ET CO_2 level of less than 0.5% (less than 4mm Hg). Any color match in the "B" section indicates a low end-tidal CO_2 level of between 0.5% and 1.9% (4mm to 14.9mm Hg). Only a color match in the "C" area, which ranges from 2–5% (15–38mm Hg) indicates a desirably high ET CO_2 reading.

A reading in the "C" range is a useful adjunct to the other customary clinical indicators in confirming proper endotracheal tube placement, since airway patency is required for sufficient ventilation and the cellular oxygenation and metabolism needed to produce a good ET CO_2 level.

Readings in the "B" range are equivocal. Such readings most commonly indicate proper ET tube placement but also reflect the lowered cellular metabolism which results from poor perfusion. However, they can result from some continued problems with the airway or delivered ventilations. A compromise in the condition of the ET tube or with the provided ventilation should be ruled out by clinical confirmation of good pulmonary ventilation before the EMT is willing to accept that the lowered "B" level readings are the result of poor perfusion.

It must be noted that a false positive yellow reading in the "C" range, or a tan reading in the "B" range, may occur when the endotracheal tube is first misplaced into the esophagus. If gastric distension has resulted from insufflation prior to intubation, or if a sizable amount of a carbonated beverage has recently been consumed, CO_2 levels as high as 4.5% can be introduced into the detector when the ET tube is initially placed into the esophagus. Although with such misplacement the CO_2 concentration will be diluted (thereby eliminating the positive reading) when ensuing provided ventilations with a high FiO_2 enter the stomach, this may not always be the case when ventilating with room air.

Readings in the "A" range in patients who have signs of adequate perfusion must conservatively be assumed to indicate misplacement or other compromise of the ET tube. In such cases the tube should be removed and the patient re-intubated. In patients with poor perfusion (such as with CPR or profound hemorrhagic shock) and a reading in the "A" range, it is unclear whether the absent or minimal CO_2 readings are resulting from improper placement or other compromise of the ET tube, or from the patient's reduced metabolism stemming from inadequate perfusion. In such cases clinical signs, chest excursion, auscultation over the epigastrium and auscultation over the midlung fields must be used to determine if the ET tube is properly placed or if it needs to be withdrawn and re-inserted.

In summary, readings in the "C" range confirm proper placement of an ET tube, readings in the "B" or "A" ranges require clinical evaluation of tube placement and delivered ventilation to determine whether they are caused by misplacement, airway compromise, or poor perfusion or other conditions which reduce cellular metabolism.

It should be noted that either pulse oximetry or end-tidal CO_2 measurement can be used as an adjunct to confirm that a patent airway and adequate ventilation exist. Pulse oximetry, by measuring the oxygen saturation level in the blood, reflects the alveolar oxygenation resulting from ventilation. It does not, however, equate to or confirm that adequate *cellular* oxygenation results.

ET CO_2 does reflect cellular oxygenation since adequate oxygenation of the cells is needed for proper metabolism and the elimination of excess CO_2 from the lungs. An ET CO_2 reading in the "C" range provides the EMT with confirmation, beyond that provided by blood oxygen saturation levels, that the oxygen provided to the lungs is being properly transported to the cells and is being exchanged for CO_2 from them.

Although generally used as an indicator in confirming proper ET tube placement, the ET CO_2 can be a useful indicator of the other key components required for proper cellular metabolism in patients in whom proper ventilation and oxygenation of the lungs has been otherwise verified. In cases of cardiac arrest without hemorrhage, ET CO_2 readings in either the "C" or "B" range (a "C" or even "B" reading may not be obtainable with CPR in all cases) confirm that chest compressions are effectively producing levels of circulation, and that cellular perfusion and oxygenation are occurring at the higher end of the range possible with CPR. When a reading in the "C" or "B" range has been sustained for some period in an intubated patient during CPR, a sudden shift to the "A" range (or from "C" to "B") should warn the EMT that either effective ventilation or effective chest compressions have been lost. In such cases when ventilation is found to be properly performed, the ET CO_2 readings generally reflect blood flow and can be a useful guide in establishing which alterations in chest compressions best produce improved perfusion and cause a return to earlier or better readings. In one study of pre-hospital use of colorimetric ET CO_2 , all cardiac arrest patients who survived to hospital admission had an ET CO_2 *value* in the "C" range. This suggests that, after further study, the device may have value in predicting outcome in cardiac arrest patients.

In patients without cardiac arrest, significant circulatory deficits may be masked by the physiologic reserves common in younger, healthy people, or in cases where conditions such as hidden bleeding (such as GI bleeding), developing anemia, or reduced cardiac efficiency develop slowly over an extended period of time. In such cases the reduced hemoglobin or perfusion levels may *NOT* be readily evidenced by a clear clinical picture of progressing shock, a history or signs of bleeding, or any overt signs of reduced cardiac function. In such cases the ambulance is often summoned due to general weakness, "dizziness", or the "unexplained" collapse of the patient. Once such patients have been intubated and proper ventilation confirmed, a "B" range ET CO_2 reading may be a key indicator of reduced blood flow and poor perfusion or a significant reduction in available hemoglobin. In such cases the EMT will have to use other clinical findings to determine if hypoperfusion is the problem and which pre-hospital interventions are immediately indicated.

Whether due to hypoperfusion, inadequate hemoglobin, or a chemical imbalance interfering with cellular metabolism, continued ET CO_2 readings in the "B" range (or worse, in the "A" range) in a properly intubated and ventilated patient warns the EMT that cellular hypoxia and reduced cellular metabolism have not been resolved, and that rapid initiation of transport to an appropriate facility is key if the patient is to have a chance of survival.

The perception of colors is affected by the type and color of the light in which the colors are viewed. The color chart printed on the Easy Cap detector is color matched for use in fluorescent lighting which is the common standard in emergency departments. When the device is used in incandescent lighting (flashlights, ambulance compartment lights, most home lighting other than kitchens, etc.) or direct sunlight, an "Incandescent Color Chart" which is furnished in the package should be attached over the color scale printed on the device (as shown below) and should be used as the color guide instead.

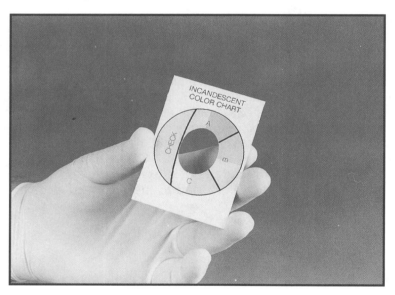

The Easy-Cap readings should only be considered to indicate the ET CO$_2$ level:

- *If the initial check confirmed that the proper chemical state of the indicator has been maintained, and the detector appears undamaged.*

- *At peak end-tidal expiration*

- *After 6 full ventilations have been provided with the device properly in place between the BVM and endotracheal tube.* Interpreting results before 6 initial breaths have been supplied through the detector can result in initial false negative or false positive readings.

- *Only during the first two hours of use.* Use of the device should not exceed 2 hours from the time it was initially opened and ambient air was allowed to come in contact with the indicator. With the passage of time the color change on inspiration may not be as obvious or detectable as at first, however there should not be a deterioration of the end-tidal color during the two hour time limit.

- *IF the patient's body weight is 15 kg or more.* The Easy Cap should not be used with patients having a body weight of less than 15kg.

Several other WARNINGS must be noted by the EMT when using an EASY CAP®:

- If gastric distension has occurred prior to intubation, a false positive reading as high as 4.5% may occur initially if the ET tube is misplaced into the esophagus.

- Similar or higher readings can also be obtained if the ET tube is misplaced in the esophagus following any significant intake of carbonated beverages (such as beer or soda pop) shortly prior to intubation.

- The device will not detect hypercarbia (excessive CO$_2$) or intubation of a main stem bronchus.

- Because the device depends upon all of the expired gases to pass through it for an accurate reading of peak ET CO$_2$, an inaccurately low reading may result if the distal cuff of the ET tube is inadequately inflated and a proper seal is not maintained.

- The device should *NOT* be used in conjunction with significantly humidified air or with a nebulizer. Excessive humidity affects accuracy. Contamination of the Easy Cap detector with gastric contents, mucous, edema, or intratracheal epinepherine can result in patchy unreactive areas on the indicator. If this occurs the detector should be replaced.

- Contamination of the Easy Cap with particulate matter (i.e., vomitus, activated charcoal, etc.) may increase airway resistance and affect patient ventilation.

- The presence of the Easy Cap on the ET tube causes an increase in airway "dead space" and in the strength needed to draw air through it. Therefore, when an Easy Cap is used on an intubated patient who is breathing spontaneously, the respiratory effort required should be evaluated prior to use. This must also be evaluated in cases where spontaneous ventilation returns and the ET tube is to remain inserted.

- The Easy Cap has been designed for use with an endotracheal tube. It will not accurately reflect the ET CO$_2$ with airways that do not provide for all of the expired gases to be exclusively and directly discharged through it. The Easy Cap cannot provide accurate readings when used with airways which produce any significant additional dead space enlargement, or which allow for communication with gastric gases or ambient air. Therefore, the detector should not be used to indicate airway patency when using manual airway maneuvers, simple airway adjuncts, esophageal opturator airways, or dual lumen airways that have been placed in the esophagus.

Even though a dual lumen airway which has been placed in the trachea is in essence an endotracheal tube, there is presently not sufficient experience or scientific evidence to establish that the detector is a reliable and useful adjunct to confirm that the distal end of the dual lumen airway tube is in the trachea and that the correct port for ventilation has been selected. Therefore, use of the Easy Cap is presently only recommended with a standard ET tube.

For several years the Easy-Cap disposable Colormetric End Tidal CO_2 detector was the only such device available in the market. Because it is to date the most prevalently used, it was selected for the preceding discussion of color values and the values and the following demonstration. Recently, the Resuscitation ACE and an ET tube with an analagous colormetric $ETCO_2$ detector built into it have been introduced. The following demonstration and general discussion will be useful regardless of which is used, however if one other than the Easy-Cap is used the values and some steps must be modified.

When preparing to intubate and after checking and assembling the laryngoscope and ET tube, if an Easy-Cap is to be used (after assuring that the patient weighs 15 kg. or more:

1. Open the airtight foil package and remove the Easy-Cap and incandescent light adaptor. Examine the detector to make sure that it has not been cracked or otherwise damaged. *DO NOT loosen or remove the end caps at this time.* Next, check the color of the indicator against the "check" color provided on the printed scale (fluorescent light) or the Incandescent Color Chart (incandescent light or sunlight). If the purple color of the indicator is *NOT* the same as the check color (or darker) or if the unit appears damaged, replace it.

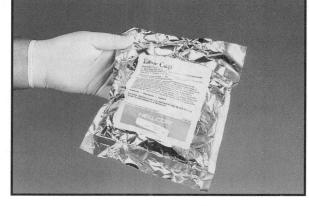

2. With the detector (and incandescent light adaptor) readily at hand, intubate the patient, inflate the cuff of the ET tube, and direct the EMT providing ventilation to discard the mask and reinstitute ventilation. While the ET tube is held firmly in place, confirm that the tube is in the trachea by observing chest rise and auscultation over the epigastrium and each midlung field. Once proper placement has been confirmed, secure the tube with tape or a commercial ET tube holder.

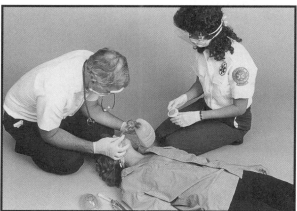

3. After successful tube placement has been clinically confirmed, you are ready to install the Easy-Cap. Remove the end caps from both ports of the detector and note the time. Have the EMT providing ventilation stop, and disconnect the BVM from the ET tube. Rapidly attach the de-tector by placing the larger plastic tube at the bottom of the detector over the adaptor at the ET tube's proximal end. Then direct the second EMT to connect the BVM to the smaller tube at the side of the detector, and to reinstitute ventilation.

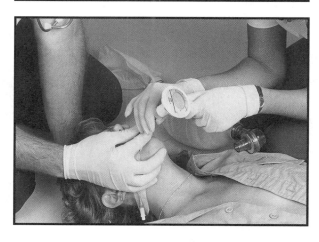

4. To avoid possibly causing a distraction or delay in first gaining positive control of the airway, the detector has not been added until successful intubation and proper bilateral pulmonary ventilation have first been confirmed. Once experienced in the detector's application, the EMT may want to have the EMT providing ventilation attach the detector to the BVM when he discards the mask, so that it is installed when the BVM is initially connected to the ET tube. This avoids the need to interrupt ventilation a second time. *With either method, tube placement and a good bilateral pulmonary ventilation must be clinically confirmed prior to evaluating the ET CO₂.*

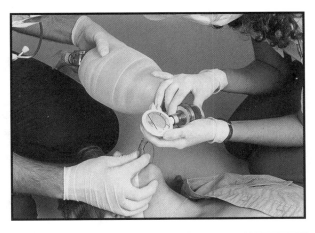

5. If you are in fluorescent lighting, place the Incandescent Color Chart in your pocket for use at a later time in the ambulance. If you are in incandescent light, sunlight, or are using a flashlight, place the Incandescent Color Chart over the top of the detector and secure it by placing its tab ends under the flange at the side of the detector as shown.

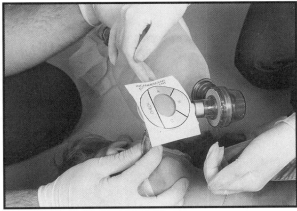

6. After 6 breaths or more have been delivered with the Easy Cap in place, verify that the color of the indicator fluctuates properly and carefully compare the indicator's color with the color scale during the peak end expiration of several breaths. Determine whether the ET CO₂ is in the "C", "B", or "A" range. If in the "C" range, the ET CO₂ is between 2–5% (15–38mm Hg), and the tube is properly placed. A "C" reading indicates that airway patency, ventilation, cellular perfusion, and cellular oxygenation are all occurring. *Interpretation before 6 breaths with the Easy Cap installed can yield false results.*

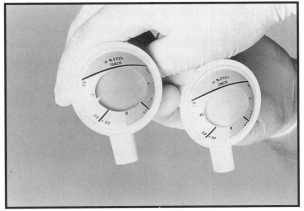

Values in the "B" range (ET CO₂ of 0.5–1.9%), generally indicate proper placement of the ET tube and simply reflect lowered cellular oxygenation (and metabolism) resulting from poor perfusion or reduced levels of available hemoglobin. They can, however, also result from some compromise in the ET tube, intubation of a main stem bronchus, lack of a proper distal cuff seal, or inadequate provided ventilation. "B" range values can even result at first when the ET tube has been misplaced into the esophagus, due to the gastric CO₂ levels from air insufflation or from the intake of carbonated beverages prior to intubation.

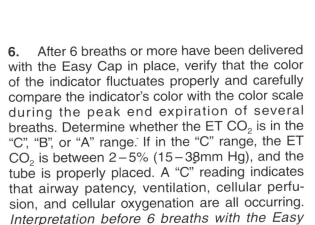

7. When a reading in the "B" (rather than "C") range is obtained, rapidly check the ET tube's pilot bulb for proper inflation and listen for expired gases leaking around the cuff. If any leaks are heard, inflate the cuff further until a seal is achieved. Then repeat the steps in clinically confirming that the tube is properly placed. If a BVM is being used, also evaluate the bag's compliance. Only after proper tube placement and pulmonary ventilation are confirmed by the chest rise, the absence of breath sounds over the epigastrium, and good bilateral breath sounds, can the EMT assume that the "B" reading results from poor perfusion or some other circulatory compromise.

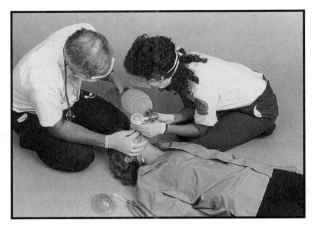

8. In a patient with signs of *adequate perfusion*, if the initial reading after intubation is in the "A" range (ET CO_2 of 0.03–0.5%), the EMT must assume that the ET tube has been misplaced. In such cases it must be removed and the patient re-intubated. If the patient is in cardiac arrest or has other signs indicating severely compromised perfusion, since a reading in the "A" range may result from either misplacement of the ET tube or inadequate perfusion, the EMT must re-evaluate the pulmonary ventilation and determine from the clinical findings whether or not the tube is properly placed.

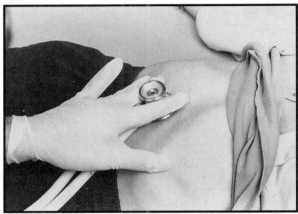

9. In a patient to whom CPR is being furnished, if a "B" or "A" range reading persists once proper tube placement and good pulmonary ventilation have been re-confirmed clinically, chest compressions should be adjusted to see if better perfusion and an increased ET CO_2 can be achieved. Compressions should be similarly adjusted if a "C" reading suddenly drops to a "B", or if a "C" or "B" reading deteriorates to an "A".

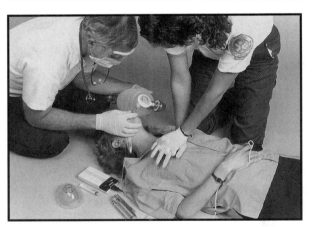

10. After use of the Easy Cap has been completed, the detector should be properly disposed in a bio-hazard waste container. If use of the device is transferred to hospital personnel, the EMT should make sure that they are familiar with it, and should indicate the time elapsed since the onset of its use so that it is not continued (without replacement) beyond the 2 hour maximum limit.

SECTION
Cardiopulmonary Resuscitation Skills

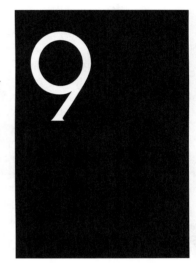
9

Introduction

Cardiopulmonary Resuscitation—known as "CPR"—involves as its name implies a two-pronged effort to resuscitate a patient whose heart has stopped and who is not breathing. Artificial ventilations are delivered to replace the absent breathing, and chest compressions are performed to cause blood to circulate through the lungs and throughout the body.

Classically, the lay management of "Foreign Body Airway Obstruction" is taught as a part of CPR. In most EMT texts it is included as one of the skills of "Airway Management." Such sequencing would seem to imply that the EMT's discovery of the obstruction occurs during airway manipulation and *before* ventilation is attempted. In reality an airway obstruction is the primary presenting problem only in cases of conscious witnessed obstruction. The EMT is much more likely to identify a foreign body obstruction only through his inability to ventilate an unconscious apneic patient—that is, *after* beginning/attempting ventilation. We have, therefore, placed the discussion of foreign body airway obstruction in the Section dealing with Special Problems of Ventilation rather than in this Section.

The material presented here also does not go into great detail on the issues and techniques of opening the airway, maintaining a patent airway, using airway adjuncts, or ventilation and oxygenation —as these have all been presented in earlier Sections of this text. When appropriate, they are included here by name without the earlier detail of how they are best performed.

The cardiopulmonary resuscitation (CPR) format presented here follows the Guidelines for CPR and the Emergency Cardiac Care recommendations of the American Heart Association as published by the Journal of the American Medical Association (JAMA). CPR is different from many of the other subjects in this text because of its dependence upon the national protocols put forth by the American Heart Association. Rather than directing the reader to local protocols or local medical direction, the references here are exclusively to the published guidelines of the American Heart Association.

This Section also includes situational CPR procedures for EMTs, such as moving a patient while performing CPR. Unless otherwise stated, we presume that at least two EMTs are involved and that they will employ appropriate adjuncts for airway management, ventilation, etc.

CPR is best performed by two operators working in concert to provide ventilations and deliver chest compressions. There are, however, times when you as an EMT will be alone with an unresponsive and pulseless patient. This can occur when there are multiple patients and your partner is occupied elsewhere, or when the logistics of the scene are such that you have to act alone for a short period while your partner obtains and prepares resuscitation equipment, calls for assistance, etc. You may have to initially provide CPR alone, or you may begin two-operator CPR and then revert to the one-operator mode while your partner gets the cot or other equipment.

And even the busiest EMT is sometimes off-duty; you may encounter a heart attack victim or other critical patient and have to function as a "lay rescuer" without your usual EMS equipment and adjuncts until an on-duty crew can respond.

CPR must be performed on a patient who is supine and laying on a hard flat surface. Although artificial ventilations can be delivered to a patient who is in a sitting position or who is found on a soft bed or couch, chest compressions cannot. The effects of gravity on blood flow, combined with the poor efficiency of chest compressions in circulating blood to the cells of the body under the best of circumstances, mandates that chest compressions only be performed with the patient supine. Similarly, the mechanics of trying to compress the patient's thorax to decrease its size and increase the intrathoracic pressure—thereby forcing blood out of the heart—requires that the patient be positioned on a hard surface to maximize the effects of the EMT's compressions against the patient's sternum. If the patient is on a yielding surface, much of the energy delivered with each compression will go to compressing the surface rather than the thorax. When a patient in full cardiopulmonary arrest is found in a posture or location in which CPR cannot be adequately performed, it is pointless to attempt CPR before quickly moving the patient to a position and place where CPR can be effectively administered.

CPR is delivered to patients who do not have a palpable carotid pulse and when the EMT has no reason to believe that CPR should *NOT* be performed. In recent years there has been growing acceptance that CPR should not automatically be performed on everyone found to be pulseless. Examples of when CPR should *NOT* be begun include the presence of obvious clinical signs of death, cases where attempts would place the EMT at significant physical risk, or cases where there is clear documentation to believe that CPR is not wanted or in the patient's best interest. "Obvious clinical signs of death" have classically included decapitation, the presence of dependent lividity and/or rigor mortis, and actual decomposition of the body. The American Heart Association notes that CPR is not indicated for traumatic arrests in cases of extended response or transport times after a patent airway has been obtained. Significant programs have also been initiated to allow patients with their physicians to establish "advance directives" regarding their desire to have resuscitative measures performed or withheld in the event of death. From one state to another, "living wills" or physician "Do Not Attempt Resuscitation" orders have different legal value and interpretations. Their validity is also questionable if an original written copy cannot be furnished immediately to the EMTs, or when resuscitation is requested by a family member, or when the immediate cause of death varies from terminal diseases which the patient has been suffering. Documents known as "living wills" are usually written by the patient to his or her physician, outlining the scope of care which the patient desires should they become unable to articulate it themselves. These are frequently not binding on prehospital providers. Written physician orders, commonly known as "DNAR" (Do Not Attempt Resuscitation_ or "No-CPR" orders, are binding upon the EMT but usually *apply only to the provision of CPR*—other care such as administering oxygen, stopping bleeding, splinting fractures, etc., is not prohibited by the existence of a DNAR order. EMTs must be careful that their actions are in accordance with their local state laws regarding adherence to such directives.

CPR procedures for adults and children are very similar, varying principally only because of the differences in body size. The American Heart Association, for CPR purposes, identifies a "child" as anyone with a body size consistent with a person between the ages of one year to eight years of age. "Adults" are individuals with body sizes greater than that of an eight-year-old, regardless of the patient's true chronological age. Thus, a large seven-year-old might be treated as an adult while a frail nine-year-old would be considered to be a child. CPR is a vigorous (some might say violent) activity, and it is certainly not inappropriate to differentiate treatment methods and forces by the size (and resilience) of the patient's body. In the majority of this Section we present the Adult techniques in detail, and then identify the alternatives that should be used when the patient qualifies as a Child.

The hallmark procedure of performing "CPR" is the delivery of closed chest cardiac compressions. Adding chest compressions to "rescue breathing" or "artificial ventilation" converts the resuscitation to "full CPR." While the exact technique for delivering compressions varies according to the size of the patient, the intent is the same: to decrease the size of the thoracic cage in order to *increase* the intrathoracic pressure and thus cause blood to be "pumped" from the heart to the lungs and other parts of the body. Compressions are delivered over the sternum and are directed straight downward toward the spinal column.

Although it was long thought that such compressions caused blood to circulate by directly squeezing the heart between the sternum and the vertebrae, mounting evidence shows that changes in intrathoracic pressure are at least equally responsible for the artificial circulation that is produced. Techniques not yet widely endorsed but which are currently being studied with some enthusiasm include "pneumatic vest CPR," "interposed abdominal compression CPR," and "active compression-decompression CPR." As more data is obtained it may be that CPR in the future will be performed in a markedly different fashion than we employ today.

While they can be life-saving, performing chest compressions can also produce serious damage to the patient. At a minimum, damage to the cartilage between the sternum and the ribs can be expected, as well as fractures of the ribs and possibly the sternum. If the lower end of the sternum is depressed too far, damage can also occur to the liver and other underlying structures. Finally, if the rescuer's hands are improperly located or move out of the correct location, the compression force can cause injury and damage.

The proper hand position on an adult or child patient's chest is centered on the lower half of the sternum. The long axis of the heel of the compressor's hand should be aligned with the long axis of the patient's sternum. For an adult patient, the compressor's other hand should be placed directly on top of his first hand. The only part of the compressor's hands that should touch the patient is the heel of the bottom hand—fingers can be interlaced with those of the other hand, or both sets of fingers can be extended, but they should not be allowed to touch the patient's chest. This will focus the force on the sternum and help to prevent avoidable chest wall trauma.

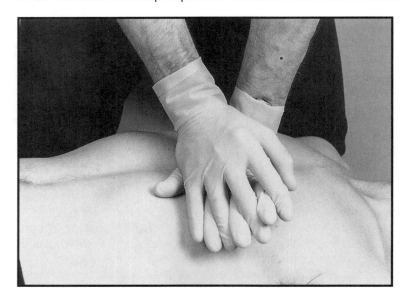

Some rescuers may find it helpful to establish the bottom hand in the correct location and to then grasp that wrist with their other hand rather than pushing down directly on the bottom hand.

For smaller children in whom less force is needed, compressions can be delivered with only one hand on the chest. For infants, it is recommended that only the tips of two fingers be used to depress the sternum. While the correct location on adults and children is the lower sternum, a slightly different placement technique is recommended for infants. With the chest bared, imagine a line drawn between the infant's nipples and position your fingertips approximately one finger's width below that line and centered on the sternum. This should locate the fingertips on the lower third of the infant's sternum.

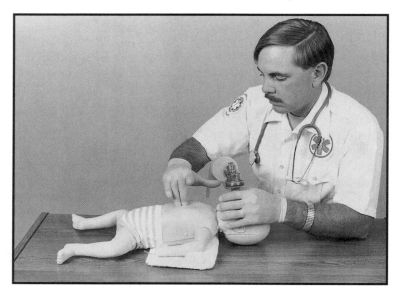

As a starting point, the sternum of an adult patient should be depressed approximately one and one-half to two inches; for a child, approximately one to one and one-half inches; and for an infant, approximately one-half to one inch. The amount of force needed to be effective must be adjusted based upon the patient's clinical response in terms of palpable pulses, skin color, and pupillary dilation.

For adults and children the chest compressions should be smooth and rhythmic, delivered straight down from the rescuer's shoulders with his elbows locked. It is desirable for the rescuer to use the weight of his own body to push down on the sternum. The chest should be compressed and then allowed to rise again to its normal position. The rescuer should not allow his hands to leave the patient's chest even though the "touch" on the chest wall should be so very light that no pressure is exerted between compressions. The most effective technique is for the downward part of each compression to represent fifty percent of the maneuver, and for compressions to be delivered at a rate of eighty to one hundred times per minute.

With infants, the torso must be firmly supported by the rescuer's arm or—preferably—a tabletop or other stationary object. When holding the infant in your arms, it is helpful to use your thigh or torso as a brace for added support. While delivering chest compressions, it is also important to keep the infant's head properly aligned with the torso if possible. This may make it possible to interpose the ventilation between each set of five compressions without having to pause to reposition the head each time a ventilation is to be delivered. Usually the hand supporting the head can maintain the minimal head tilt necessary to keep the airway open without the hand which is doing compressions needing to move from the chest to perform a chin lift. If the hand which is doing compressions must move back and forth to assist with the airway, the rate of delivered chest compressions will fall.

TWO RESCUER CPR, ADULT PATIENT

"Two-rescuer" or "two operator" is the version of CPR most likely to be done by EMTs, allowing for those occasions when due to limited personnel one EMT may have to perform single-operator CPR while the second EMT obtains and assembles equipment, brings the stretcher, calls for assistance, etc. By utilizing additional resuscitation equipment such as airways, ventilators, oxygen, or intubation, the task of ventilating and oxygenating the patient can be greatly improved. The initial steps of two-rescuer CPR are always the same, but can be upgraded and improved as equipment and additional personnel become available.

Your initial step when approaching a patient is to first assess the scene for potential hazards to your own safety. If there are none, after taking all necessary Body Substance Isolation precautions you should:

1. Assess the patient for unresponsiveness by shouting and by physically stimulating him such as by tapping his shoulder.

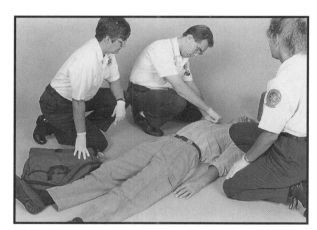

2. If the patient remains unresponsive, open his airway using a head tilt/chin lift or jaw thrust maneuver, or a cervical spine-controlled airway maneuver if trauma is suspected. While maintaining the open airway maneuver, bend over the patient's face with your cheek directly above his nose and mouth while you look toward his chest. Listen and feel for any air movement from his mouth and nose, and watch for chest movement that is coordinated with the sound or feel of air movement. When you are outdoors a breeze can mimic the feel of an exhaled breath; timing it to chest rise eliminates mistaken impressions.

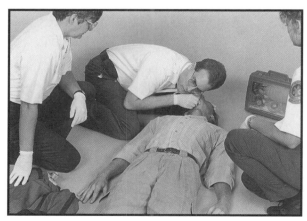

3. If there are adequate spontaneous ventilations, place the patient in the recovery position on his side with his head turned so that secretions can drain away from his airway. If the spontaneous ventilations are *NOT* adequate, provide assisted ventilations. If there are no spontaneous ventilations, insert an oral airway and deliver two slow, full ventilations with a bag-valve-mask or demand valve. Your partner should be simultaneously palpating for a carotid pulse.

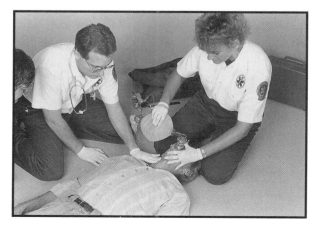

4. If no pulse is found, the second EMT should bare the patient's chest and locate the landmarks for correct hand position as the first EMT continues to ventilate the patient. Whenever possible the two EMTs should work from different sides of the patient. To locate the correct hand position, bare the patient's chest and find the xiphoid process. Place your ring finger over it. Place your middle and index fingers over the lower end of the sternum.

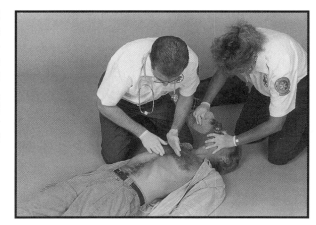

5. Place the heel of your other hand directly over the midline of the sternum, so that it is touching the index finger of the landmark.

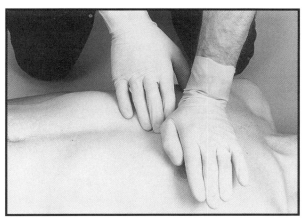

6. Now, remove the landmark hand and place it directly on top of the hand over the sternum so that your wrists touch. Only the heel of your bottom hand should be touching the victim. Interlace your fingers and pull up on them, or extend the fingers of both hands, to avoid any fingers touching the chest.

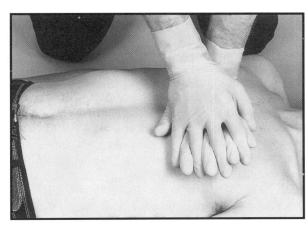

7. Your shoulders and arms should be directly over the victim's sternum with your arms straight and your elbows locked. Use the weight of your body to drive straight down on the sternum so that you compress the chest between one and a half and two inches. Do not rock on your knees or push with the muscles of the arms. The chest should be compressed for less than a second. Be sure you are close enough to the victim so that your compressions are delivered by pushing straight down.

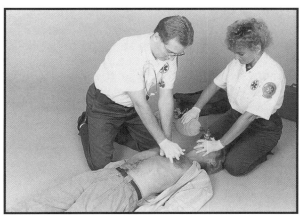

8. Allow the chest to rise again to its normal position but don't take your hands off the chest. Avoid bouncing off! Compress and release the chest at a rate of eighty to one hundred times per minute. Eighty compressions per minute is the minimum rate, one hundred per minute is desirable. Count out loud "One-and-two-and-three-and-four-and-five."

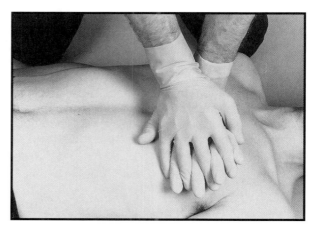

9. When you have finished delivering five compressions, pause to allow the EMT at the head to deliver one slow, full ventilation. *DO NOT* remove your hands from the patient's chest! The breath should take one and one-half to two seconds to blow in (inspire). As soon as the ventilation has been delivered, perform another set of five compressions.

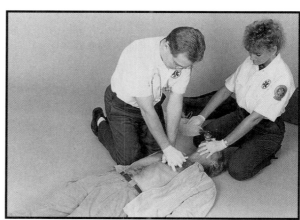

10. While the EMT at the chest delivers chest compressions, the EMT at the head is responsible for monitoring the patient's condition and response to the CPR being provided. He should regularly palpate the carotid pulse during compressions to monitor the adequacy of the chest compressions. Proper depth and rate of compression should produce a palpable carotid pulse.

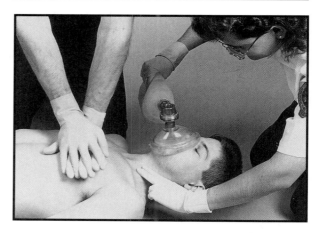

11. Continue compressions and ventilations at the ratio of five compressions to one ventilation for about one minute, then stop and re-check for the presence of a spontaneous carotid pulse. If absent, resume CPR and re-check periodically for the return of a spontaneous pulse. Once CPR is begun, you don't stop except to periodically check for a pulse.

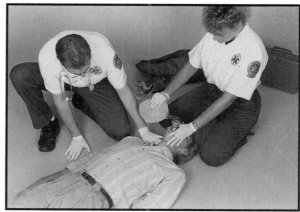

12. While compressions are being delivered, the EMT at the head can begin to upgrade the level of equipment being used by attaching oxygen supply tubing to the BVM, connecting it to an oxygen source, and attaching an oxygen accumulator ("reservoir").

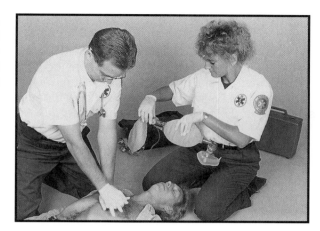

13. If advanced personnel are available to intubate the patient, it should be done once the patient has been well oxygenated. The EMT performing the intubation should assemble the needed equipment and prepare to intubate while the EMT at the head continues to ventilate the patient.

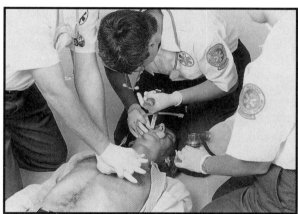

14. Once the tube has been placed, ventilations should be resumed and proper tube placement assessed.

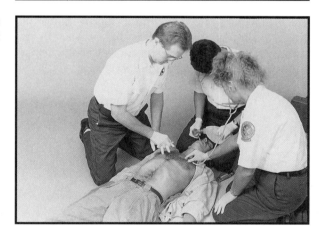

15. If at any time a spontaneous pulse is found, compressions should be discontinued and a check made to determine whether or not spontaneous ventilations have also been restored. If not, ventilations should be continued at a rate of 10 to 12 times per minute. Regardless of whether the full arrest continues or if spontaneous circulation and/or ventilation returns, preparations should be made to transport the patient as soon as possible.

TWO-RESCUER CPR, CHILD PATIENT (1 To 8 Years)

The recommended steps for Child CPR are virtually identical to those for adult victims, with only slight modifications that take into account the child's smaller body size and immature musculoskeletal development. The three major differences are that ventilations are performed at a faster rate and quicker—twenty times per minute and with each delivered breath taking a maximum of only one and a half seconds to blow in; that chest compressions are delivered with only one hand; and finally, a ratio of five compressions to one ventilation is maintained *for both single and two-rescuer performances.* Compression depth on a child should be only one to one and one-half inches, and are delivered with the heel of only one hand.

Your initial step when approaching a patient is to first assess the scene for potential hazards to your own safety. If there are none, after taking all necessary Body Substance Isolation precautions you should:

1. Assess the child for unresponsiveness by shouting and by physically stimulating him such as by tapping his shoulder.

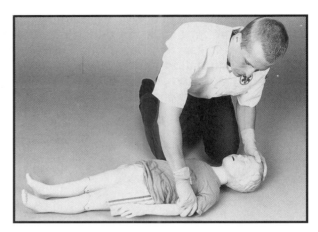

2. If the child remains unresponsive, open his airway using a head tilt/chin lift or jaw thrust maneuver, or a cervical spine-controlled airway maneuver if trauma is suspected.

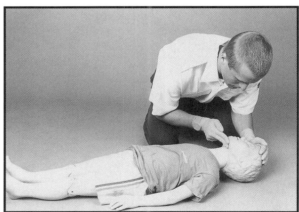

3. While maintaining the open airway maneuver, bend over the child's face with your cheek directly above his nose and mouth while you look toward his chest. Listen and feel for any air movement from his mouth and nose, and watch for chest movement that is coordinated with the sound or feel of air movement. When you are outdoors a breeze can mimic the feel of an exhaled breath; timing it to chest rise eliminates mistaken impressions.

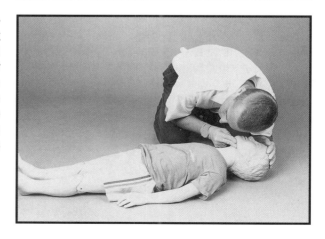

4. If there are spontaneous ventilations, place the child in the recovery position on his side with his head turned so that secretions can drain away from his airway. If the spontaneous ventilations are inadequate, provide assisted ventilations. If there are no spontaneous ventilations, insert an oral airway and deliver two slow, full ventilations with a bag-valve-mask or demand valve. Your partner should be simultaneously palpating for a carotid pulse.

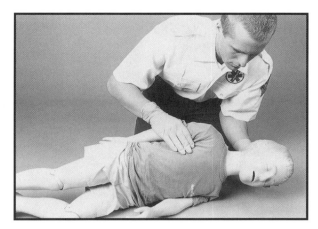

5. If no pulse is found, the second EMT should bare the child's chest and locate the landmarks for correct hand position as the first EMT continues to ventilate the patient. Whenever possible the two EMTs should face each other from opposite sides of the patient. To locate the correct hand position, find the patient's xiphoid process and place the ring finger of your caudad hand over it, then place your middle and index fingers over the lower end of the sternum.

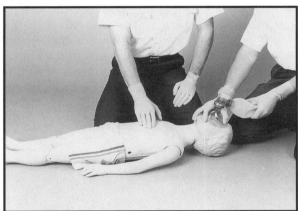

6. Place the heel of your cephalad hand directly over the midline of the sternum, so that it is touching the index finger of the caudad hand.

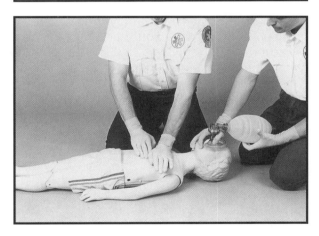

7. Only the heel of your cephalad hand should be touching the victim, and due to the child's smaller size you should not have to use both hands to perform adequate compressions.

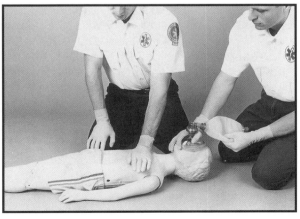

8. Your shoulders and arms should be directly over the victim's sternum with your arms straight and your elbow locked.

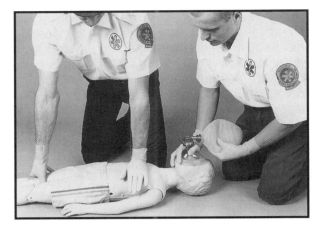

9. Use the weight of your body to drive straight down on the sternum so that you compress the chest between one to one and one-half inches. Do not rock on your knees or push with the muscles of the arm. The chest should be compressed for less than a second. Be sure you are close enough to the victim so that your compressions are delivered by pushing straight down.

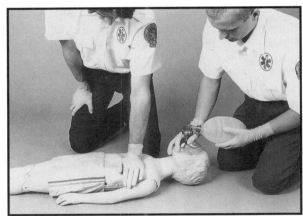

10. Allow the chest to rise again to its normal position but don't take your hand off the chest. Avoid bouncing off! Compress and release the chest at a rate of one hundred times per minute. Count out loud "One-and-two-and-three-and-four-and-five."

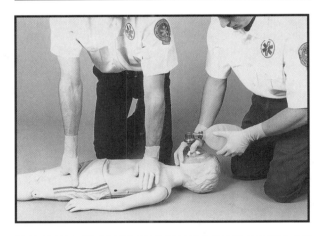

11. When you have finished delivering five compressions, pause to allow the EMT at the head to deliver one slow, full ventilation. *DO NOT* remove your hand from the child's chest! The breath should take one to one and one-half seconds to blow in (inspire). As soon as the breath has been blown in, deliver another set of five compressions.

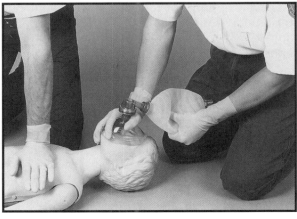

12. While the EMT at the chest delivers chest compressions, the EMT at the head monitors the child's condition and response to the CPR being provided. He should regularly palpate the carotid pulse during compressions to monitor the adequacy of the chest compressions. Proper depth and rate of compression should produce a palpable carotid pulse.

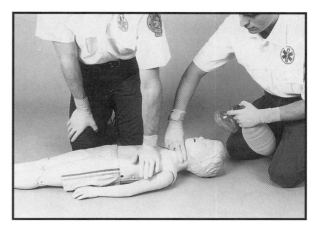

13. Continue compressions and ventilations at the ratio of five compressions to one ventilation for about one minute, then stop and re-check for the presence of a spontaneous carotid pulse. If absent, resume CPR and re-check periodically for the return of a spontaneous pulse. Once CPR is begun, don't stop except to periodically check for a pulse.

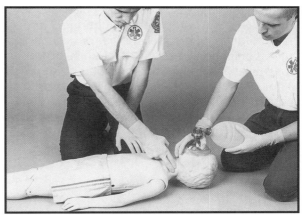

14. While compressions are being delivered, the EMT at the head can begin to upgrade the level of equipment being used by attaching oxygen supply tubing to the BVM, connecting it to an oxygen source, and attaching an oxygen accumulator ("reservoir").

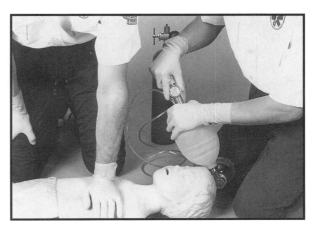

15. If advanced personnel are available to intubate the child, it should be done once he has been well oxygenated. The EMT performing the intubation should assemble the needed equipment and prepare to intubate while the EMT at the head continues to ventilate the child.

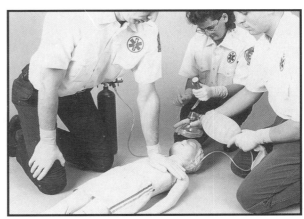

16. Once the tube has been placed, ventilations should be resumed and proper tube placement assessed.

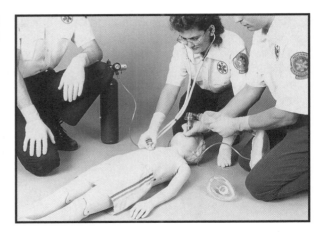

17. If at any time a spontaneous pulse is found, compressions should be discontinued and a check made to determine whether or not spontaneous ventilations have also been restored. If not, ventilations should be continued at a rate of 10 to 12 times per minute. Regardless of whether the full arrest continues or if spontaneous circulation and/or ventilation returns, preparations should be made to transport the patient as soon as possible.

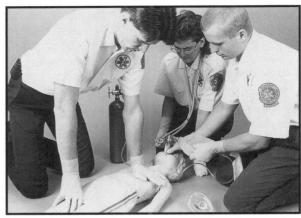

SINGLE RESCUER CPR, ADULT PATIENT

Your initial step when approaching a patient is to first access the scene for potential hazards to your own safety. If there are none, after taking all necessary Body Substance Isolation precautions you should:

1. Assess the patient's level of responsiveness by speaking loudly and tapping or shaking his shoulder.

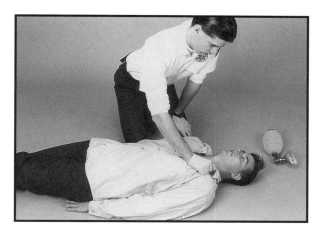

2. Establish an open airway by performing a head tilt/chin lift or jaw thrust maneuver, and position yourself to look for chest rise and listen for air movement from the mouth or nose. Perform a cervical spine-controlled airway maneuver if trauma is suspected.

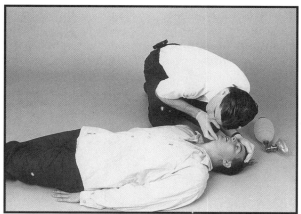

3. If there are spontaneous ventilations, place the patient in the recovery position on his side with his head turned so that secretions can drain away from his airway. If the spontaneous ventilations are inadequate, provide assisted ventilations. If there are no spontaneous ventilations, insert an oral airway and deliver two slow, full ventilations with a bag-valve-mask or demand valve.

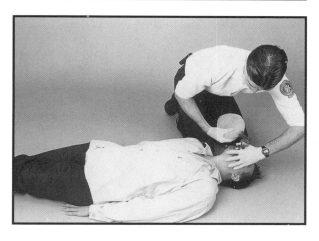

4. Deliver each ventilation over one and one-half to two seconds, with approximately three seconds allowed between breaths for the patient to exhale. Seeing the patient's chest rise coincident with your provided inhalation is the best indicator that your ventilation has entered the patient's lungs.

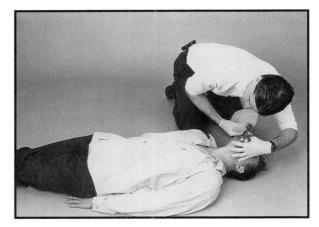

5. With the index and middle finger of one hand, attempt to palpate the patient's carotid artery for the presence of a pulse. Palpate the carotid area for five to ten seconds to insure that a pulse cannot be found. If a pulse is located, continue to ventilate the patient at a rate of ten to twelve times a minute.

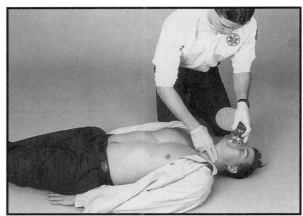

6. If no pulse is located, move down to the patient's chest and remove any clothing that is covering the anterior chest wall. Locate the patient's xiphoid process with the ring finger of your caudad hand, and place your middle and index fingers down next to it on the very end of the sternum.

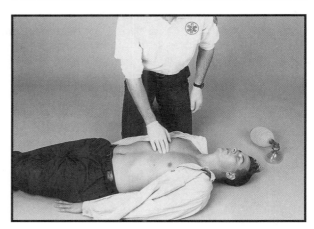

7. Then place the heel of your other hand next to your index finger on the lower half of the sternum and place your caudad hand on top of it with the fingers extended or interlaced or by grasping the wrist of the hand on the chest. Your shoulders should be positioned directly over the top of the patient's chest with your arms extended and elbows locked.

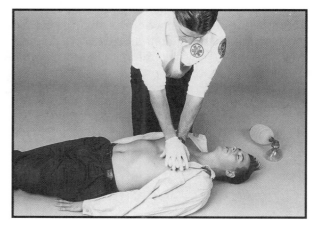

8. Compressions should be done rhythmically by bending at the waist and pushing down on the chest one and one-half to two inches in depth at a rate of 80 to 100 compressions per minute. Ideally, the downward compression should represent one-half of the entire stroke — fifty percent down and fifty percent up. Hand placement and contact on the chest wall should be continuous — removing your hand between compressions can cause you to lose your landmark position on the chest.

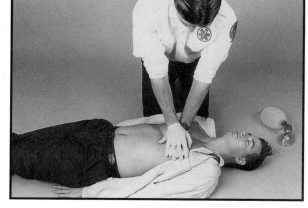

9. After completing fifteen compressions, move quickly to the patient's head and re-open the airway with a chin lift-head tilt. Provide two slow full ventilations again using a ventilator or barrier device. Each breath should take 1.5 to 2 seconds to blow in, and three seconds should be allowed for exhalation after the first breath.

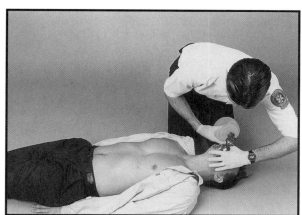

10. After the second ventilation, move back to the chest and re-establish proper hand placement on the lower half of the sternum. Perform fifteen more compressions at a rate of 80 to 100 per minute.

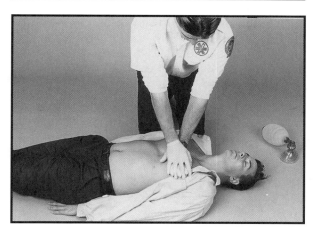

11. After the fifteenth compression, return to the patient's head and again provide two slow full breaths. This cycle of two ventilations and fifteen chest compressions should be done four times — that is, four complete cycles of 2 breaths followed by 15 compressions — and then you should palpate over the carotid artery for 5 to 10 seconds to assess for the return of a spontaneous pulse. If no pulse is found, ventilate the patient twice and continue to perform chest compressions and ventilations.

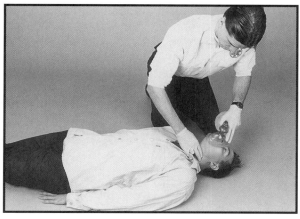

SINGLE RESCUER CPR, CHILD PATIENT (1 To 8 Years)

The recommended steps for Child CPR are virtually identical to those for adult victims, with only slight modifications that take into account the child's smaller body size and immature musculoskeletal development. The three major differences are that ventilations are performed at a faster rate and quicker—twenty times per minute and with each delivered breath taking a maximum of only one and a half seconds to blow in; that chest compressions are delivered with only one hand; and finally, a ratio of five compressions to one ventilation is maintained *for both single and two-rescuer performances.* Compression depth on a child should be only one to one and one-half inches, and are delivered with the heel of only one hand.

Your initial step when approaching a patient is to first assess the scene for potential hazards to your own safety. If there are none, after taking all necessary Body Substance Isolation precautions you should:

1. Assess the child's level of responsiveness by speaking loudly and tapping or shaking his shoulder.

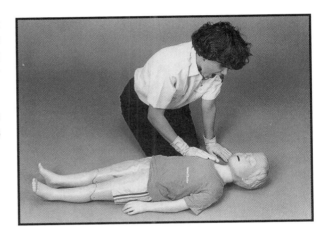

2. Establish an open airway by performing a head tilt/chin lift or jaw thrust maneuver, and position yourself to look for chest rise and listen for air movement from the mouth or nose. If trauma is suspected, perform a jaw thrust or chin lift without tilting the head.

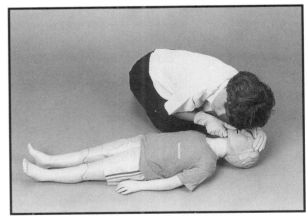

3. If there are spontaneous ventilations, place the child in the recovery position on his side with his head turned so that secretions can drain away from his airway. If the spontaneous ventilations are inadequate, provide assisted ventilations. If there are no spontaneous ventilations, insert an oral airway and deliver two slow, full ventilations with a bag-valve-mask or barrier device.

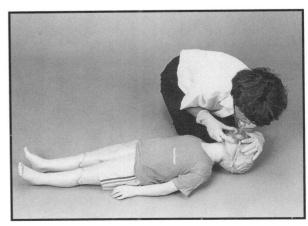

4. Deliver each ventilation over one to one and one-half seconds, with approximately three seconds allowed between breaths for the patient to exhale. Seeing the child's chest rise coincident with the delivered ventilation is the best indicator that your provided inhalation has entered the patient's lungs.

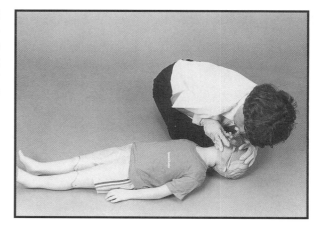

5. Palpate the child's carotid artery for the presence of a pulse. Palpate the carotid area for five to ten seconds to insure that a pulse cannot be found. If a pulse is located, continue to ventilate the patient at a rate of twenty times a minute. If the child is particularly small and the neck is difficult to palpate, you should consider assessing the brachial pulse in the upper arm.

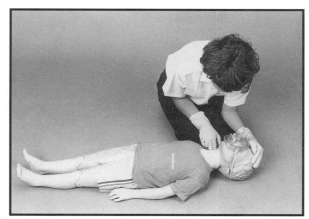

6. If no pulse is located, move down to the patient's chest and remove any clothing that is covering the anterior chest wall. Locate the child's xiphoid process with the middle finger of your caudad hand, and place your index finger down next to it on the very end of the sternum.

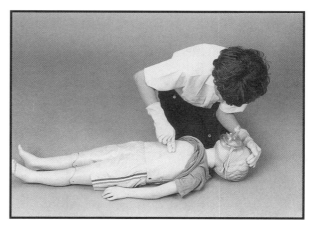

7. Lift your caudad hand and place the heel of that hand next to the point over the lower third of the sternum where your index finger had been. Use your cephalad hand to hold the mask in place and to maintain the head tilt. Your shoulders should be positioned directly over the top of the child's chest with your arm extended and elbow locked.

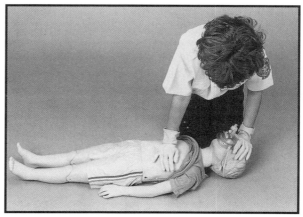

8. Compressions should be done rhythmically by bending at the waist and pushing down on the chest one to one and one-half inches in depth at a rate of 100 compressions per minute. Ideally, the downward compression should represent one-half of the entire stroke—fifty percent down and fifty percent up. Hand placement and contact on the chest wall should be continuous—removing your hand between compressions can cause you to lose your landmark position on the chest.

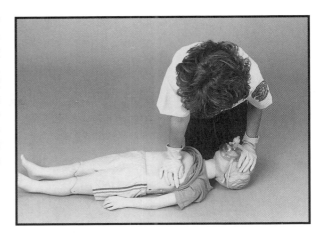

9. After completing five compressions, move quickly to the patient's head and re-open the airway with a head tilt-chin lift or head tilt-jaw thrust. Re-establish the mask seal over the child's mouth and nose. Provide one slow full ventilation again using a bag-valve-mask or barrier device. Take 1 to 1.5 seconds to blow in.

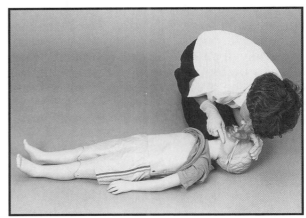

10. After ventilating the child, move back to the chest and re-establish proper hand placement on the lower half of the sternum. Perform five more compressions at a rate of 100 per minute.

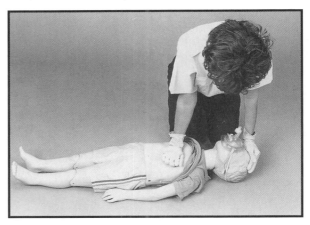

11. After the fifth compression, return to the patient's head and again provide one slow full breath. This cycle of one ventilation and five chest compressions should be done twenty times—that is, twenty complete cycles of one breath followed by 5 compressions—and then you should palpate over the carotid artery for 5 to 10 seconds to assess for the return of a spontaneous pulse. If no pulse is found, ventilate again and continue to perform cycles of chest compressions and ventilations.

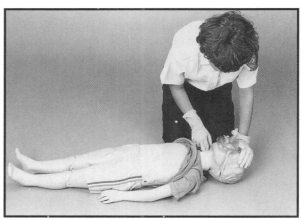

INFANT CPR (Birth To 1 Year)

Cardiopulmonary arrest in infants (less than 1 year of age) is predominantly caused by respiratory problems. Rarely do infants and children suffer acute myocardial infarctions as the prime cause of their cardiac arrest. Unlike with an arrested adult patient (whose problem is most likely to be cardiac in origin and who will benefit most from Advanced Life Support defibrillation and medication), the arrested infant most often needs *ventilatory* resuscitation that should be begun immediately. While the JAMA guidelines direct rescuers to activate the EMS system before beginning CPR on adult patients, the priority with infants is to open the airway and begin ventilations — and if necessary, chest compressions — *before* activating the EMS system.

Unlike with an adult, ventilations and CPR on an infant are best performed by a single rescuer due to the small body size — at least until moving the patient is no longer a concern or endotracheal intubation can be performed. The following demonstration, therefore, includes mouth-to-mask (or barrier) ventilation. For a more detailed discussion of infant airway management and ventilation, the reader should refer to Sections 4 and 5. After taking all appropriate Body Substance Isolation precautions:

1. First establish unresponsiveness by gently but firmly tapping the infant's shoulder or chest and speaking loudly.

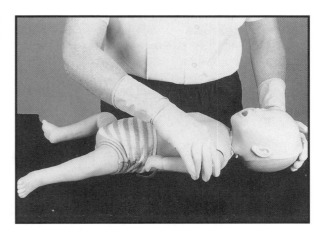

2. If they are unresponsive, open the airway with a head tilt/chin lift maneuver. Use a jaw thrust without head tilt if spinal trauma is suspected.

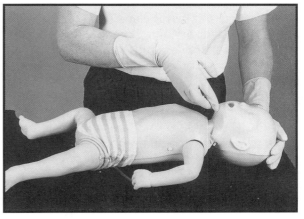

3. Once the airway has been opened, carefully look, listen and feel for signs of air exchange.

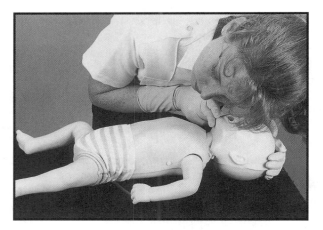

4. If the infant is not breathing, quickly apply a mask with one-way valve or other barrier device over the patient's mouth and nose and deliver two small slow breaths over one to one and one-half seconds. Allow the infant to exhale completely after the first breath. Watch for chest rise with each ventilation as confirmation that the breaths are reaching the lungs.

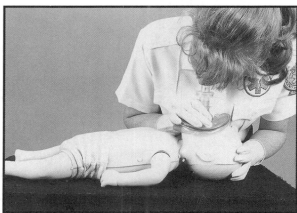

5. After the two initial breaths, check for the presence of a pulse. As infants have very short chubby necks, it is easier and more reliable to palpate for the brachial artery in the upper arm. If a pulse is found, maintain the open airway and continue to ventilate the infant at a rate of 20 times per minute while periodically verifying the continued presence of a pulse.

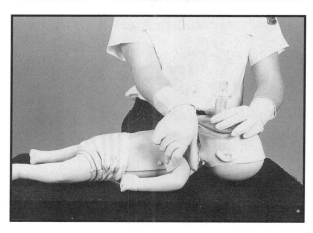

6. If no pulse is found, immediately bare the infant's chest and either place him on a hard flat surface or support him across your forearm. Individual preferences and comfort vary greatly in this regard. Some EMTs prefer to have the infant on a hard surface in front of them, while others are most effective holding the infant in their arms or on their lap. The guiding principle is that the EMT must be able to effectively compress the infant's sternum against firm counterpressure, and to deliver ventilations in a coordinated manner.

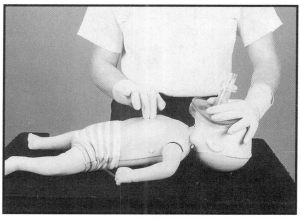

7. Chest compressions for an infant are delivered with the tips of the EMT's index and middle fingers. The compressions are delivered over the sternum, approximately one finger's width below an imaginary line drawn between the infant's nipples. This should locate the fingertips on the lower half of the infant's sternum. Compression depth should be one-half to one inch, and delivered at a rate of at least 100 per minute.

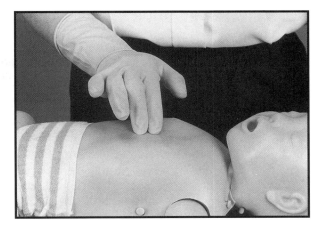

8. The ratio of compressions to ventilations for both infants and children is five to one, with a pause after each fifth compression to allow a slow breath to be delivered over 1 to 1.5 seconds and allowing for good chest rise. Keeping one hand on the patient's forehead will help to maintain a patent airway during compressions and allow for complete exhalation when the next compression is delivered. This will also help to keep the airway ready for the next ventilation.

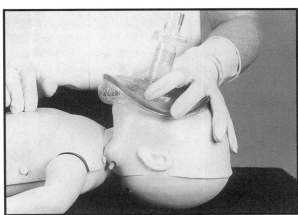

9. As with an adult patient, periodically stop CPR to assess for the return of spontaneous circulation. If the pulse remains absent, continue CPR. If the pulse returns, evaluate the patient's ventilation. If the patient is not breathing or if the breathing is inadequate, continue to provide ventilations. If the patient is breathing adequately, supply oxygen with a high FiO_2 and continue to monitor the patient's breathing and circulation. In any case, initiate transport without delay.

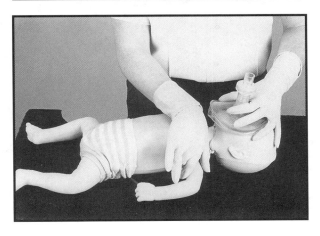

NEONATAL MODIFICATION

While technically fitting into the "birth-to-one-year" definition of an "infant," the American Heart Association recognizes the need for some modifications in CPR techniques when resuscitating a brand-new "newborn," or **neonate.** A key concern is to keep the baby as warm as possible even during resuscitation to promote the recovery from acidosis and to support the neonate's extremely unstable thermoregulatory mechanism.

Positive pressure ventilation is indicated when the neonate is apneic or displays only gasping ventilations, when the heart rate is less than 100, or if central cyanosis persists despite the administration of 100% oxygen. The AHA recommends ventilating the neonate at a rate of 40 to 60 times per minute, with careful observation of chest wall movement to assess adequate inflation.

Chest compressions are indicated whenever the neonatal heart rate is less than 60 beats per minute, or is between 60 and 80 beats per minutes *but is not increasing despite adequate ventilation with a high FiO$_2$.* The AHA's preferred technique for delivering chest compressions to a neonate is for the rescuer to place both of his thumbs on the middle third of the infant's sternum, with the rest of his fingers encircling the chest and supporting the back. The thumbs should be placed on the chest just below an imaginary line drawn between the nipples. Compressions are delivered in a smooth rhythmic "half squeeze — half relax" movement that compresses the sternum between one-half and three-quarters of an inch. For very small newborns the EMT may have to lay one thumb on top of the other to avoid putting pressure on the ribs rather than the sternum.

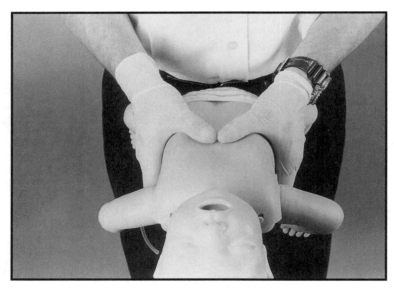

If the EMT's hands are too small to encircle the neonate's chest and provide both compression and back support, chest compressions should be delivered with two fingers on the sternum just as previously described for older infants. The American Heart Association recommends that chest compressions and positive pressure ventilations be delivered in a 3:1 ratio — that is, 3 compressions followed by a pause to deliver one effective ventilation. The recommended rate of compressions is 120 per minute, which should yield about 90 compressions and 30 ventilations per minute when actually delivered. As with infants and older children, however, the EMT must remember that adequate ventilation is of prime importance in resuscitating newborns, and deliberate effective breaths must take precedence over rapid chest compressions.

RE-LOCATING TO A SUITABLE PLACE PRIOR TO INITIATING CPR

In many cases, the location where you find the patient is not optimal for performing CPR. The patient may be in a bathroom or other confined area, or on an unsuitable surface such as a soft bed or couch. When this occurs you must quickly assess the patient and, upon determining the need for CPR, move them to an area which allows you room to provide effective resuscitation.

When called to a scene where a patient is in a confined area, first assess the scene to assure that there are no hazards. Not all unconscious patients in bathrooms have had a primary cardiac arrest!

With the scene safe, assess the patient by establishing unresponsiveness, open the airway and check for breathing. If spontaneous ventilations are not present and the environment is such that you cannot effectively provide sustained ventilation where you are, carefully drag the patient to a nearby larger area that is immediately available. Once there, quickly re-assess for breathlessness and if found, provide two slow full breaths while observing for chest rise. When the breaths have been delivered, palpate for a carotid pulse and, if none is found, begin chest compressions and full CPR.

CPR WHILE MOVING TO THE AMBULANCE AND DURING TRANSPORT

At some point during a cardiac arrest you will need to move the patient from the location where you found him to your ambulance. This takes some forethought to evaluate where you are and what obstacles are between you and the ambulance — such as sharply angled corners, narrow hallways, stairs, or steep terrain. When stairs are encountered it is usually best to perform CPR until you reach the stairs and then to interrupt CPR on a coordinated signal, move the patient quickly but safely to the next level or landing, and resume CPR at that location for a few minutes before again interrupting CPR to move to the next level, and so on. Although there can be a terrific urge to rush when moving a patient while performing CPR, a slower, more controlled move is actually more productive in terms of effective CPR. Ventilations and chest compressions must be maintained except in the most adverse circumstances. While moving the patient on the ambulance cot, the person performing compressions must be able either to walk alongside the cot and maintain the proper hand-arm-shoulder alignment to deliver effective compressions, or must straddle the patient on the cot. With most ambulance cots, "riding the rails" of the cot's undercarriage by standing on the tubing which extends between the wheel mounts is not advised as this tends to bend the tubing and impair the ability to lock the stretcher into the cot mounts in the ambulance.

Your safety and that of the patient are paramount. Be sure to have enough manpower to lift and transport the patient so that no one is injured.

With CPR in progress and all of the available adjuncts in place (such as endotracheal intubation, cardiac monitoring, etc., according to the certification level of the responders present):

1. Continue CPR while one EMT prepares a backboard and straps.

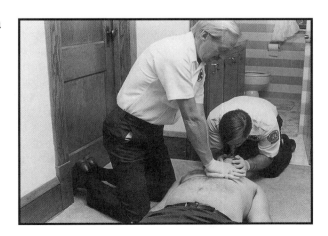

2. Using a standard logroll method, quickly stop CPR, roll the patient onto his side, and slide the longboard underneath the patient.

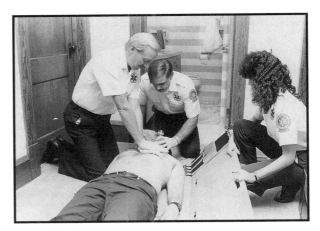

3. Immediately resume CPR while the patient is being strapped to the board. The oxygen cylinder can be placed between the patient's legs with the leg straps going over the tank and legs. Be sure to leave the tank gauges visible.

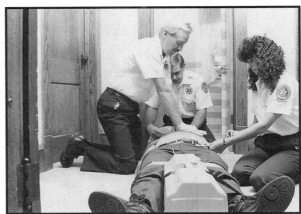

4. With an EMT on each end of the board, carefully lift the patient and board. Continue ventilations, however chest compressions cannot be effectively done if the board is not supported from underneath by the wheeled ambulance stretcher or the floor. When a stretcher can be used, the EMT performing chest compressions may be able to walk alongside the stretcher or may climb onto the bed of the stretcher to straddle the patient and perform compressions. In any event, the posture is awkward, the effectiveness of the compressions is minimal, and there is risk of injury to the EMT.

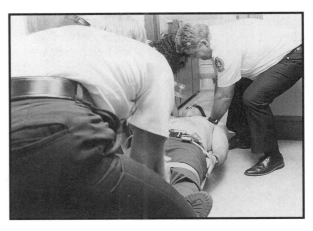

5. If it is not feasible to bring the wheeled stretcher directly to the patient, you will have to perform CPR and move the patient in stages. Perform 1 or 2 cycles of ventilations and compressions while the patient is in a stable position, then interrupt compressions to move the patient a short distance before resuming. The interruptions should not be for more than 30 seconds at a time, with good CPR performed between moves. Effective ventilations should be able to be continuously provided while the patient is being moved in most cases.

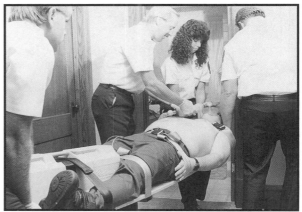

6. If the patient and backboard are being moved on a wheeled stretcher and chest compressions are being performed from the side, moving through narrow doorways or tight passages can be accomplished with teamwork and good communication. Once the EMT doing compressions has reached one side of the narrow area the compressions should be interrupted while the patient and stretcher are moved through the doorway.

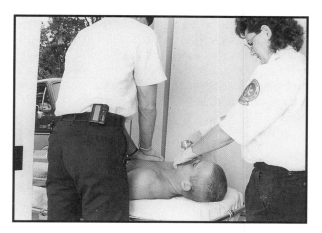

7. As soon as the patient is accessible on the far side of the doorway or passage, compressions should be resumed as quickly as possible. Once they have been reliably re-instituted, the patient and stretcher should again be moved toward the ambulance.

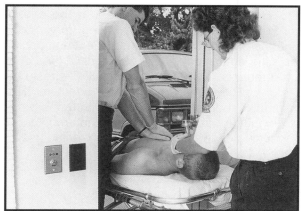

8. If stairs are encountered, several cycles of CPR should be performed with the patient in a stable position. *BOTH* compressions and ventilations should then be interrupted while the patient is moved as quickly as safely possible to the next landing or level where CPR can be resumed. As soon as the patient is again in a location where CPR can be performed, effective ventilations and chest compressions should be re-instituted before the patient is again moved.

9. Once the patient can be placed on the wheeled cot, CPR can be continuously provided while the patient is moved to the ambulance. If the EMT providing chest compressions is walking alongside the cot, experience has shown that it is often easier to do effective compressions if the cot elevation is set at about bed level. The most common failure at this point is to move the cot too quickly — making it difficult if not impossible for the EMT at the chest to provide effective compressions, and even interfering with the delivery of adequate ventilations.

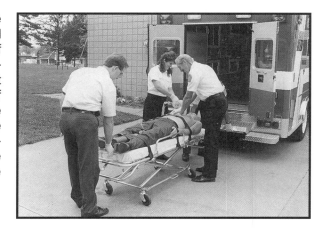

10. There are several options for performing CPR while transporting the patient in the ambulance, including leaving the cot behind and placing the patient and backboard on the floor of the ambulance so that the compressor can kneel beside the patient.

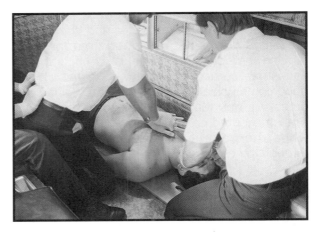

11. Other options leave the cot in the ambulance, with the compressor working from alongside the patient, straddling the patient and cot, or kneeling on the cot over the patient. If the cot is to be returned to the ambulance, CPR should be performed until the ambulance is reached. The cot should then be raised or lowered to the proper height for it to be inserted into the ambulance, depending on the model of stretcher being used.

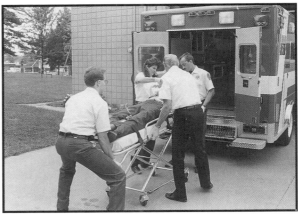

12. With good communication among all of the EMTs, both compressions and ventilations should be halted and the stretcher lifted into the ambulance. If there are extra EMTs available, one or more can be waiting inside the ambulance to receive the patient and resume CPR.

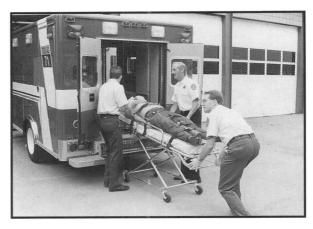

13. If there is only a basic complement of EMTs, those who are to perform ventilations and compressions should follow the stretcher into the ambulance as quickly as possible and re-institute CPR. Once CPR has been re-instituted inside the ambulance, switch from the portable oxygen tank to the on-board system to conserve the portable's capacity.

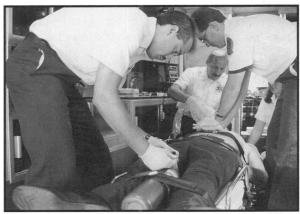

14. Upon arrival at the hospital, the process of loading the patient is reversed. The oxygen line can be re-attached to the portable oxygen cylinder as everyone prepares to unload the patient.

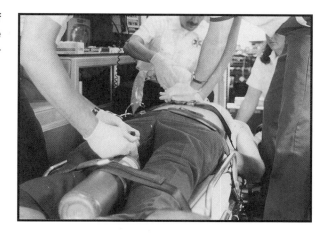

15. With CPR still in progress, one EMT steps out of the ambulance and releases the cot — remaining at the foot of the cot. A second EMT stands at the right side of the rear door of the ambulance, ready to lock the undercarriage as the cot is pulled out of the ambulance.

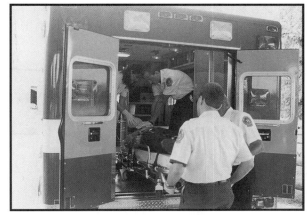

16. As the cot moves halfway out of the ambulance the EMT doing compressions stops CPR and steps to the ground while the EMT providing ventilations remains in the unit still bagging the patient.

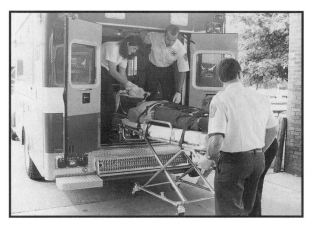

17. As the cot is pulled from the ambulance ventilations stop as that EMT steps out. The cot is lowered to bed level, then CPR ventilations and compressions resume. The patient is then moved into the hospital while the EMTs continue CPR.

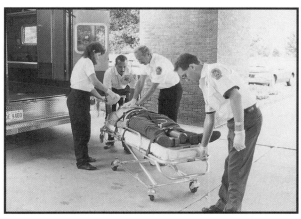

18. Next to the Emergency Department bed the cot rails are lowered and EMTs and hospital staff position themselves to transfer the backboard and patient to the ED bed.

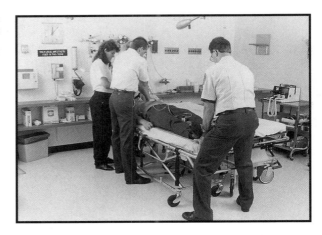

19. The board and patient are moved from the cot to the bed, and CPR is resumed with the patient on the ER bed.

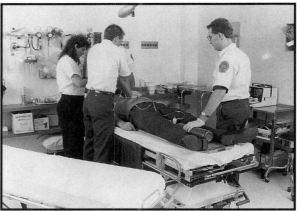

Once the patient is on the ER bed the EMTs should continue ventilations and chest compressions until relieved by the hospital staff. Due to the height of most ER beds, the use of a small stool to elevate the EMT providing compressions is recommended.

Patient movement during CPR takes a lot of communication between the various team members. The least amount of time possible should be taken when CPR is stopped. The faster CPR can be resumed, the better the patient's chances will be. Coordination in moving equipment with the patient, such as IVs, monitors oxygen tanks, etc., is essential for the best transfer of a patient. If the patient is intubated, care must be taken to minimize the chance of endotracheal tube displacement during the movement of the patient. Tube placement should always be re-assessed each time the patient is moved.

ETI SUMMARY SKILL SHEET
Two Rescuer CPR, Adult Or Child Patient

Note: As explained earlier in this Section, the procedures for performing CPR on adult and child (1–8 years of age) patients are remarkably similar. We have, therefore, combined them in this Summary Skill Sheet—identifying only the three areas of significant difference: the length of inspirations, the number of hands used for chest compressions, and the recommended compression depth.

1. ASSESS the patient FOR UNRESPONSIVENESS.

2. IF the patient remains UNRESPONSIVE, OPEN his AIRWAY using a head tilt/chin lift or jaw thrust maneuver, or a cervical spine-controlled airway maneuver if trauma is suspected.

3. While maintaining the open airway maneuver, BEND OVER the PATIENT'S FACE with your cheek directly above his nose and mouth while you LOOK toward his chest. LISTEN AND FEEL FOR any AIR MOVEMENT from his mouth and nose, and watch for chest movement that is coordinated with the sound or feel of air movement.

4. IF the patient is BREATHING, PLACE the PATIENT IN the RECOVERY POSITION on his side with his head turned so that secretions can drain away from his airway.
IF the patient is NOT BREATHING, INSERT an oral AIRWAY AND DELIVER TWO slow, full VENTILATIONS with a bag-valve-mask or demand valve. Your partner should be simultaneously palpating for a carotid pulse.
ADULT: Each inspiration should take 1.5 to 2 seconds.
CHILD: Each inspiration should take 1 to 1.5 seconds.

5. IF NO PULSE is found, the second EMT should BARE the PATIENT'S CHEST AND LOCATE the CORRECT HAND POSITION FOR CHEST COMPRESSIONS as the first EMT continues to ventilate the patient. The correct hand position is found by identifying the xiphoid process and placing your ring finger over it. Place your middle and index fingers over the lower end of the sternum.

6. PLACE the HEEL OF your OTHER HAND directly OVER the MIDLINE OF the STERNUM, so that it is touching the index finger of the landmark.

7. **ADULT:** REMOVE the LANDMARK HAND AND PLACE IT directly ON TOP OF the HAND OVER the STERNUM so that your wrists touch.
CHILD: REMOVE THE LANDMARK HAND. ONLY the heel of YOUR CEPHALAD HAND SHOULD be touching the victim, and due to the child's smaller size you should not have to use both hands to perform adequate compressions.

8. Your SHOULDERS AND ARMS SHOULD BE DIRECTLY OVER the victim's STERNUM with your ARMS STRAIGHT and your ELBOWS LOCKED.

9. **ADULT:** Use the weight of your body to DRIVE STRAIGHT DOWN ON THE STERNUM so that you COMPRESS the CHEST 1.5 to 2 INCHES.
CHILD: Use the weight of your body to DRIVE STRAIGHT DOWN ON THE STERNUM so that you COMPRESS the CHEST 1 to 1.5 INCHES.
BOTH: DO NOT ROCK on your knees or push with the muscles of the arms. The chest should be compressed for less than a second. Be sure you are close enough to the victim so that your compressions are delivered by pushing straight down.

10. ALLOW the CHEST TO RISE again to its normal position but DON'T TAKE your HANDS OFF the CHEST. Avoid boucing off! COMPRESS AND RELEASE the chest AT A RATE OF 80 TO 100 times per minute. Eighty compressions per minute is the minimum rate, one hundred per minute is desirable. Count out loud "One-and-two-and-three-and-four-and-five."

11. AFTER DELIVERING 5 COMPRESSIONS, pause to allow the EMT at the head to DELIVER ONE slow, full VENTILATION. Do not remove your hand(s) from the patient's chest! The breath should take 1.5 to 2 seconds to blow in. As soon as the ventilation has been delivered, PERFORM ANOTHER SET OF FIVE COMPRESSIONS.

12. While the EMT at the chest delivers chest compressions, the EMT at the head is responsible for MONITORing the PATIENT'S CONDITION AND RESPONSE TO the CPR being provided. He should regularly PALPATE the CAROTID PULSE during compressions.

13. CONTINUE compressions and ventilations at the RATIO OF FIVE COMPRESSIONS TO ONE VENTILATION FOR about ONE MINUTE, THEN stop and RE-CHECK FOR a SPONTANEOUS carotid PULSE. If absent, resume CPR and re-check periodically for the return of a spontaneous pulse.

14. While compressions are being delivered, the EMT at the head can BEGIN TO UPGRADE the LEVEL OF EQUIPMENT being used BY ATTACHING OXYGEN supply tubing to the BVM, connecting it to an oxygen source, and attaching an oxygen reservoir.

15. If ADVANCED PERSONNEL are available the patient SHOULD be INTUBATED once the patient has been well oxygenated. The EMT performing the intubation should assemble the needed equipment and prepare to intubate while the EMT at the head continues to ventilate the patient.

16. Once the tube has been placed, ventilations should be resumed and proper tube placement assessed.

17. IF at any time a spontaneous PULSE IS FOUND, DISCONTINUE COMPRESSIONS. EVALUATE VENTILATIONS AND CONTINUE VENTILATIONS at a RATE OF 10 to 12 times per minute IF ABSENT OR INADEQUATE. PREPARE TO TRANSPORT the patient as soon as possible.

ETI SUMMARY SKILL SHEET
Single Rescuer CPR, Adult Or Child

Note: As explained earlier in this Section, the procedures for performing CPR on adult and child (1–8 years of age) patients are remarkably similar. We have, therefore, combined them in this Summary Skill Sheet—identifying only the four areas of significant difference: length of delivered inspirations, number of hands used for chest compressions, the recommended compression depth, and the ratio of compressions and ventilations delivered in a "cycle."

1. ASSESS the patient FOR UNRESPONSIVENESS.

2. IF the patient remains UNRESPONSIVE, OPEN his AIRWAY using a head tilt/chin lift or jaw thrust maneuver, or a cervical spine-controlled airway maneuver if trauma is suspected.

3. While maintaining the open airway maneuver, BEND OVER the PATIENT'S FACE with your cheek directly above his nose and mouth while you look toward his chest. LISTEN AND FEEL FOR any AIR MOVEMENT from his mouth and nose, and LOOK FOR CHEST MOVEMENT that is coordinated with the sound or feel of air movement.

4. IF the patient is BREATHING, PLACE the PATIENT IN the RECOVERY POSITION on his side with his head turned so that secretions can drain away from his airway.
IF the patient is NOT BREATHING, INSERT an oral AIRWAY AND DELIVER TWO slow, full VENTILATIONS with a bag-valve-mask or demand valve.
ADULT: Each breath should be 1.5 to 2.0 seconds of inspiration and approximately 3 seconds exhalation.
CHILD: Each breath should be 1 to 1.5 seconds of inspiration and approximately 3 seconds exhalation.

5. After delivering the two breaths, PALPATE FOR A CAROTID PULSE. (IF the child is particularly small and it is difficult to locate the carotid pulse, the brachial pulse is recommended.)

6. IF NO PULSE is found, BARE the PATIENT'S CHEST AND LOCATE the CORRECT HAND POSITION FOR CHEST COMPRESSIONS. The correct hand position is found by identifying the xiphoid process and placing the ring finger of your caudad hand over it. Place your middle and index fingers over the lower end of the sternum.

7. **ADULT:** PLACE the HEEL OF your OTHER HAND directly OVER the MIDLINE OF the STERNUM, so that it is touching the index finger of the landmark. REMOVE the LANDMARK HAND AND PLACE IT directly ON TOP OF the HAND OVER the STERNUM so that your wrists touch with the fingers extended or interlaced or by grasping the wrist of the hand on the chest.
CHILD: LIFT your CAUDAD HAND AND PLACE the HEEL of that hand NEXT TO the point WHERE YOUR INDEX FINGER WAS over the lower third of the sternum. Due to the child's smaller size you should be able to PERFORM adequate COMPRESSIONS WITH ONLY ONE HAND. Use your cephalad hand to hold the mask in place and to maintain the head tilt.

8. COMPRESSions should be done rhythmically BY BENDING AT the WAIST and pushing down on the chest AT a RATE OF 80 to 100 COMPRESSIONS PER MINUTE. DELIVER 5 COMPRESSIONS.
ADULT: Compression depth is 1.5 to 2 inches. DELIVER FIFTEEN COMPRESSIONS.
CHILD: Compression depth is 1 to 1.5 inches. DELIVER FIVE COMPRESSIONS.

9. After completing the compressions, move quickly to the patient's head and RE-OPEN the AIRWAY with a chin lift/head tilt.

10. VENTILATE the patient using a ventilator or barrier device.
ADULT: DELIVER TWO BREATHS. Each breath should take 1.5 to 2 seconds to blow in. Pause for approximately 3 seconds after the first breath to allow full exhalation.
CHILD: DELIVER ONE BREATH. The breath should take 1 to 1.5 seconds to blow in.

11. After delivering the ventilation, immediately move back to the chest and RE-ESTABLISH PROPER HAND POSITION on the lower half of the sternum.
ADULT: Physically re-locate the correct hand position and PERFORM FIFTEEN more COMPRESSIONS at a rate of 80 to 100 per minute.
CHILD: Keeping your cephalad hand on the child's forehead to maintain head tilt, visually re-locate the correct hand position for your caudad hand. PERFORM FIVE MORE COMPRESSIONS at a rate of 80 to 100 per minute.

12. After the fifteenth (Child: fifth) compression, return to the patient's head and again PROVIDE two (Child: one) SLOW FULL BREATHS. REPEAT this CYCLE of ventilations and chest compressions FOR approximately ONE MINUTE.

13. Then interrupt the cycle to PALPATE over the CAROTID ARTERY for 5 to 10 seconds to assess for the return of a spontaneous pulse. If a pulse is found, EVALUATE VENTILATIONS and determine if provided ventilations are still necessary. If no pulse is found, ventilate the patient twice (Child: once) and continue to perform chest compressions and ventilations.

ETI SUMMARY SKILL SHEET
Infant CPR (Birth To 1 Year)

1. First ESTABLISH UNRESPONSIVENESS by gently but firmly tapping the infant's shoulder or chest and speaking loudly.

2. If unresponsive, OPEN the AIRWAY with a head tilt/chin lift maneuver. Use a jaw thrust without head tilt if spinal trauma is suspected.

3. Once the airway has been opened, carefully LOOK, LISTEN AND FEEL FOR signs of AIR EXCHANGE.

4. IF the infant is NOT BREATHING, quickly APPLY a MASK with one-way valve OR other BARRIER device over the patient's mouth and nose and DELIVER TWO small slow BREATHS over one to one and one-half seconds. Allow the infant to exhale completely after the first breath. WATCH FOR CHEST RISE with each ventilation to confirm that the breaths are reaching the lungs.

5. After the two initial breaths, CHECK FOR the presence of a PULSE. Palpate the brachial artery in the upper arm. IF a PULSE is FOUND, maintain the open airway and CONTINUE TO VENTILATE the infant at a rate of 20 times per minute while periodically verifying the continued presence of a pulse.

6. IF NO PULSE is found, immediately BARE the infant's CHEST and either PLACE him ON a HARD FLAT SURFACE or across your forearm.

7. Chest COMPRESSions for an infant are delivered WITH the TIPS OF the EMT's index and middle FINGERS. The compressions are delivered OVER the sternum, approximately one finger's width below an imaginary line drawn between the infant's nipples. This should locate the fingertips on the LOWER HALF OF THE infant's STERNUM. Compression depth should be one-half to one inch, and delivered at a rate of at least 100 per minute.

8. DELIVER FIVE COMPRESSIONS, THEN pause to provide ONE BREATH over a 1 to 1.5 second interval. Keep one hand on the patient's forehead to maintain a patent airway during compressions and allow for complete exhalation when the next compression is delivered. This will also help to keep the airway ready for the next ventilation.

9. As with an adult patient, PERIODICALLY STOP CPR TO ASSESS FOR the RETURN OF SPONTANEOUS CIRCULATION. IF ABSENT, continue CPR. IF A PULSE IS FOUND, evaluate breathing and provide airway management and ventilation as indicated. IF SPONTANEOUS CIRCULATION AND BREATHING ARE BOTH RESTORED, provide a high FiO_2 and continue to check each periodically.

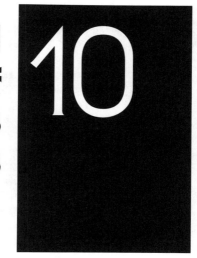

SECTION

Use of Cardiac Monitors and Defibrillators

10

Introduction

The use of a cardiac monitor and defibrillator are essential tools for providing advanced cardiac life support. The cardiac monitor furnishes the advanced EMT, together with the results of the history and physical examination, the identity of the specific cardiac rhythm or dysrhythmia that is present. From his clinical findings and this information the EMT can determine the specific treatment sequence (ACLS protocol) that is appropriate for that patient. The monitor depicts the heart's electrical activity as a continuous dynamic rhythm on an oscilloscope. With most equipment this image can also be recorded onto a roll of paper whenever desired in order to provide a more permanent record. The paper moves past the printer stylus at a specific rate, assuring that the printed image reproduces the original time intervals accurately. The paper typically contains printed markers on it to facilitate interpreting the time intervals. Printed "strips" make possible a more detailed measurement and interpretation of the cardiac rhythm than can be done with the moving image on the screen, and allow comparisons to be made between different time intervals.

Cardiac monitors were initially developed in Germany and the "K" in "EKG" comes from their original German name—**"electrokardiograf."** The name has since been Anglicized to **electrocardiograph,** and it is typically abbreviated as either **"EKG"** or **"ECG"** (not to be confused with the term electroencephalograph which refers to tracings of the brain's electrical activity and is abbreviated as "EEG").

Although most cardiac monitors have a defibrillator associated with them, the units most commonly used in pre-hospital care feature a defibrillator that can be separated from the monitor and has its own power source. The defibrillator is used to deliver controlled electrical shocks to the heart in an attempt to stop certain extreme life-threatening dysrhythmias. When this therapy is successful the heart actually stops for a few seconds and then resumes beating—this time with a functional life-sustaining rhythm which provides effective circulation. In addition to defibrillation, cardiac medications and other therapy are commonly also needed in such cases to maintain a life-sustaining rhythm.

Most defibrillators are electronically connected to the monitor in such a way that electrical impulses can be sensed through the defibrillator paddles and reproduced on the monitor screen. This allows the EMT to obtain a *quick-look* or "snapshot" view of the heart's electrical activity before taking time for the more conventional and long-term electrode and cable attachments. The electrical interface between the defibrillator and monitor also provides for **synchronized cardioversion** when the electrical shocks must be delivered only at certain times in the heart's electrical cycle.

A few cardiac monitors commonly used for pre-hospital care also allow the EMT to set alarm limits for the patient's heart rate. This feature is very common in units designed for in-hospital use. When the rate detected by the monitor becomes faster or slower than the high or low limits established by the EMT, an audible alarm sounds and the strip recorder starts creating a printed record of the rhythm at that time. Some pre-hospital models which include the latest technology will also sound an audible alarm and print a strip each time that the patient's underlying cardiac rhythm changes.

One feature that is almost exclusively found only in pre-hospital units is a recording capability that permits later playback of each event from when the machine was turned on including the voices and sounds heard in the vicinity of the monitor when it was being used, the exact times of each event, and each EKG pattern that the unit sensed. It can indicate when and at what level defibrillatory shocks were delivered. The EKG can be printed through the strip chart recorder and/or displayed on the monitor screen, and in some units the reviewer can select whether to see them in their entirety or only for short periods before and after any rhythm change or shock delivered. The ability to replay the sequence of EKG rhythms and delivered shocks is invaluable for retrospective quality assurance review as well as for recalling the actual sequence and times of events on a call to assist in completing the necessary written documentation.

Additionally, some monitor/defibrillator units include the capability of providing **transcutaneous pacing.** This allows the external non-invasive delivery of electrical stimuli to produce cardiac contractions in patients whose cardiac dysrhythmia has not responded to drug therapy. The ability to provide transcutaneous pacing to such patients outside the hospital has been shown to produce significantly higher survival rates than when this capability is delayed until the patient reaches the hospital.

Cardiac monitors and defibrillators which are designed for pre-hospital use (or for portable use within a hospital) are extremely durable in order to withstand the impact of being carried and used in the various situations which EMTs commonly encounter. These units are typically lighter and smaller than stationary models, and are generally powered by externally available and easily exchanged rechargeable batteries. Depending upon the manufacturer's design, pre-hospital models may require one or two such batteries — one to power the monitor and a second for the defibrillator. For most EMS services, three batteries are needed to provide around-the-clock power for each battery actually used to power the unit: one installed in the unit, one carried as a back-up on the ambulance, and a third left in the charger. The batteries must be rotated after each use and on a periodic basis to ensure that they are fully charged and ready whenever the unit is needed.

Until recently, pre-hospital cardiac monitoring and defibrillation was limited to advanced EMTs who had been trained in EKG recognition and the Advanced Cardiac Life Support (ACLS) course or an equivalent. In 1978 a program was piloted in King County, Washington, in which specially trained basic and intermediate EMTs were allowed to use a new "EMT-D" protocol. Under this program the EMT-Ds were able to defibrillate patients in whom they detected ventricular fibrillation. During the first year of the pilot study, twenty percent of the patients who were found to be in ventricular fibrillation and who were treated by EMT-Ds and early defibrillation survived to be discharged alive from the hospital. This compared very favorably to the less than four percent survival rate that had been historically reported and that was found in parallel control groups. Based upon the success reported in this study, early defibrillation by basic and intermediate EMTs became widespread in many areas of the country and is now an accepted practice nationwide.

As the benefit of early defibrillation became better understood, a new generation of cardiac monitor/defibrillators emerged. Today a large number of automatic and semi-automatic monitor/defibrillators are in service with EMT-D personnel. These machines identify ventricular fibrillation and ventricular tachycardia without the need for the EMT to do so. They then alert the EMT that a defibrillatory shock is therapeutically indicated, and — depending upon the unit — issue an audible warning and deliver the shock automatically *or* signal the operator to do so manually. Some models of automated monitor/defibrillators display the patient's cardiac rhythm while others only indicate by electronic voice or other signal when the patient is in a "shockable" rhythm.

The essential difference between fully automatic and semi-automatic units is that when a shockable rhythm is detected by a fully automatic monitor/defibrillator, it issues an audible warning and then proceeds to deliver the defibrillatory shock without any confirmation or action by the EMT (except if he needs to intervene and *stop* the process). A semi-automatic unit makes the audible warning but pauses until the EMT consciously confirms the decision to defibrillate and pushes the appropriate button to activate the delivery of *each shock.*

There are many different makes and models of monitor/defibrillator units available today, each with their own capabilities and special function. They all possess, to some degree, the basic two needs of any such unit: monitoring of cardiac electrical activity and delivery of electrical energy to the cardiac muscle. Regardless of which type of unit (manual, semi-automatic, or fully automatic) or which brand is used, the EMT must be familiar with the operation of that specific model and must be fluent in the protocol for its use as permitted at his level of certification.

Cardiac monitoring and defibrillation deal with the heart's electrical activity. The cardiac muscle is a unique muscle in that it can contract or depolarize completely on its own without stimulation from the brain or central nervous system. The contraction of the cardiac muscle is caused by the movement of electrically charged chemicals within the cardiac cells. This movement produces electrical current. When all of the cardiac cells are stimulated to contract (depolarize) there is a large electrical current created. Using electrodes placed on a patient's chest, this current can be detected by a cardiac monitor and displayed as a dynamic "live EKG" on an oscilloscope. This allows the EMT to "see" and assess the patient's cardiac electrical activity as it occurs. Most monitoring units also have the capability of printing a static visual image of the EKG onto a moving strip of time-gridded paper for more detailed analysis and later review. This chapter will *NOT* deal with cardiac rhythm interpretation but just with the sequential manipulative skills required when using the monitoring and defibrillation equipment.

As noted earlier, many monitor/defibrillators allow the EMT to obtain an EKG reading by placing the defibrillator paddles on the patient's chest. Although such a "quick-look" may be helpful when assessing pulseless or critical patients, it is not as accurate nor as functional for ongoing monitoring as the use of adhesive electrodes which are attached to the patient's chest.

The electrodes that are used to sense the heart's electrical activity and carry it to the monitor are generally round and about 2 inches in diameter. On the side that contacts the patient's skin there is an adhesive surface to keep the electrode in place on the patient, as well as a gelled sensing surface that must be in firm contact with the skin in order for accurate readings to be made. On the outer side of the electrode there is a male electrical snap connector which mates with the female connector on the wire lead coming from the monitor.

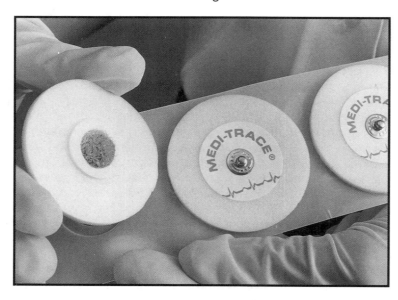

When the patient is diaphoretic or has a particularly hairy chest it may be very difficult to get the electrodes to adhere properly to the skin. Wiping the skin with alcohol or betadine swabs may help, and shaving portions of the chest may be necessary on occasion. If the image on the monitor becomes bizarre or inconsistent or disappears completely, the EMT must remember to check the wire connections to each electrode and also the electrode attachments to the skin.

Some monitoring electrodes are designed to replace the defibrillator paddles, allowing EKG signals to be conveyed to the monitor and the defibrillation current to the patient. These electrodes are typically three to four times larger than conventional "monitor-only" electrodes, and only two are used—placed in the same locations as when the paddles are being used to defibrillate. Combination electrodes are common with automatic and semi-automatic machines, and relatively inexpensive conversion kits are available for most models of manual monitor/defibrillators. Many EMTs find this type of

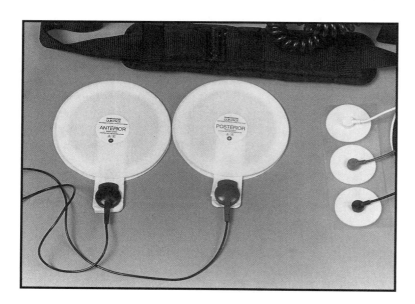

electrode very convenient to use when managing a full arrest patient, as they do not have to repeatedly manipulate the paddles and stretch themselves over the patient to deliver shocks. The cost of these electrodes is considerably higher than the cost of conventional "monitor only" electrodes, and they can only be used with machines that are specially designed to use them or that have been adapted for their use.

When using the paddles to defibrillate or cardiovert a lethal cardiac arrhythmia, the defibrillator delivers several thousand volts and a small amount of amperage to the cardiac muscle in a very short period of time. The energy level is counted in **watt/seconds**, and is calculated as voltage multiplied by amperage producing watts delivered over time (in seconds). Another common term for watt/seconds is **joules**. The defibrillator is capable of delivering between 50 and 360 watt/seconds (joules) with each shock. The energy delivered is intended to cause a strong electrical charge to pass momentarily through the major portion of the cardiac muscle and cause complete myocardial depolarization. By defibrillating the heart muscle and causing all of the myocardial muscle cells to contract at once, it is hoped that a single pacemaker cell in the sino-atrial node will begin firing before any ventricular pacemaker cells initiate a dysfunctional rhythm.

Defibrillation and cardioversion are virtually identical, with one major difference. With defibrillation, the EMT delivers the electrical shock to the heart at a random point in the cardiac cycle whenever the red discharge buttons are pushed. With cardioversion, once the discharge buttons are pushed the defibrillator waits until a precise moment in the heart's electrical cycle to deliver the shock. Generally, rhythms that are still producing a pulse but that need to be slowed (or "converted") are the targets of synchronized cardioversion. By synchronizing the cardioversion to the time when the heart is in the absolute refractory period, the potential for causing ventricular fibrillation is limited. When the synchronization button is pushed the monitor synchronizes with the "R" wave of the patient's cardiac rhythm. When the discharge buttons are pushed the defibrillator discharges the energy on the down slope of the next "R" wave that it detects — which is the absolute refractory period of the heart. It is important that the monitor be properly calibrated so that the patient's "R" waves are clearly discernible by the monitor. If the gain is turned too low the "R" wave can be hidden in the rest of the EKG tracing and the synchronizer will be unable to identify it and cardiovert the heart.

INTRODUCTION TO USING A MANUAL MONITOR DEFIBRILLATOR

For the purposes of this Section, the authors have selected the Physio-Control LIFEPAK 5 manual monitor-defibrillator to illustrate the information and skills being presented. While this does not represent an endorsement of this manufacturer nor this product per se, it is an acknowledgment that this particular model is the most widely used among pre-hospital EMS services at this time. As noted earlier, this text does not include a review of EKG interpretation; nonetheless, that is prerequisite knowledge for using the *manual* equipment and techniques demonstrated in this Section.

Monitor Unit Controls And Features

The dominant feature on the front of the monitor unit is a 36mm x 60mm *oscilloscope screen*. It takes approximately three seconds for an EKG image to travel from one edge of the screen to the other. To the left of the monitor screen is the *paper recorder*. The recorder, when activated, prints what is on the screen 2.4 seconds later, and uses moving heat-sensitive paper and a thermal stylus to produce the EKG tracings.

The controls on the monitor unit are located on the top of the case, and are either pushed or turned to operate. The *On/Off switch* is incorporated into the *EKG lead select button*. When this green switch is turned fully clockwise the monitor is turned off; the operator rotates it counter-clockwise to select—in turn—first the "paddles" position and then Lead I, Lead II, and Lead III. As the switch is moved from the "off" position it not only selects the desired monitoring lead but also powers up the monitor and screen.

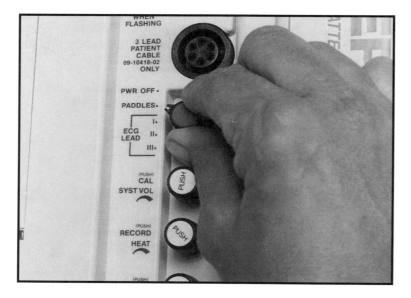

In the "paddles" mode, the two paddles from the defibrillator are used to sense the electrical activity in the patient's heart. Physio Control calls this the "Quick Look"—a registered name that has become a generic term used with all monitor/defibrillators with the ability to monitor through the paddles. In addition to "quick look" monitoring, defibrillation or synchronized cardioversion can be performed with the "On/Off/Lead Select" switch in the "paddles" setting. Although monitoring through the paddles can be effectively done, it is not foolproof. If the patient is in a moving ambulance, or if the EMT is unable to hold the paddles securely on the patient's chest, the external motion of the paddles may cause a distortion or misrepresentation of the cardiac electrical pattern displayed on the monitor screen. For this reason most protocols allow "quick look" monitoring only when the patient is unmoving and in a fixed location rather than during ambulance transport.

The more conventional and definitive way to obtain a reading of the cardiac electrical activity is with adhesive chest electrodes or "leads." With the adhesive electrodes placed on the patient and with the leads that make up the cable from the monitor connected to the electrodes, turning the "On/Off/Lead Select" switch to the desired Lead setting (I, II, or III) will cause that view of the heart's electrical activity to be displayed on the monitor screen.

When using the cabled leads to view the patient's cardiac rhythm, snap a monitoring electrode onto each of the three leads. Remove the backing on each electrode before you place it on the patient's chest.

Proper electrode placement is essential for correct viewing and interpretation of the cardiac rhythm. The white negative lead should be placed on the patient's right upper chest wall, below the clavicle and close to the shoulder joint. The black or green ground lead should be positioned in the corresponding place on the patient's left chest wall. The red positive lead is placed on the patient's left chest wall. The red positive lead is placed on the patient's left chest wall. The red positive lead is placed on the patient's left side, usually just above the belt line on the abdomen at the anterior axillary or mid-clavicular lines. While this positioning is beneficial for monitoring the heart, it also keeps the monitoring electrodes away from where the paddles will need to be placed if defibrillation is needed. The *polarity* of each of these electrodes determines which view or *Lead* is viewed on the monitor — the description just given (white = negative, black = ground, red = positive) refer to the respective polarities only when the LIFEPAK 5 Lead Select switch is set to Lead II. If the white and black electrodes are reversed and the switch is still set for Lead II, the rhythm shown on the monitor screen will be Lead III — and changing the switch to Lead I will cause Lead II to be displayed. In other words, it is very important for the EMT to know the polarities of the electrodes in at least the three basic Leads and also to be careful in positioning the electrodes and selecting the Lead to be viewed.

Once the electrodes are placed on the chest, select the monitoring Lead you want to view. Most monitors are capable of internally changing the polarity of the three leads so that different electrical "views" of the heart can be seen without having to physically move the electrodes on the patient's chest.

For *Lead I*, the right chest electrode would be negative and the upper left chest electrode positive, with the lower left chest electrode being the ground.

Selecting *Lead II* would cause the right electrode to remain negative, the lower left chest electrode to become positive, and the upper left chest electrode the ground.

For *Lead III*, the upper left chest electrode would be negative, the lower chest electrode positive, and the right chest wall electrode ground.

Another common monitoring Lead is the *Modified Chest Lead I, or "MCL I."* By placing the negative electrode on the upper left chest, the positive electrode on the lower right chest wall and the ground on the upper right chest you can view the electrical activity of the heart from yet another vantage point. On a LIFEPAK 5 the "lead select" switch must be in the Lead II position and the electrodes arranged as described above in order to view MCL I.

The lead most commonly selected for prehospital use is Lead II. Rather than turning the green "On/Off/Lead Select" knob click-by-click from "Off" to "Paddles," then "Lead I," and then to "Lead II," it is simpler to rotate the knob counter-clockwise as far as it will go (Lead III), *and then to rotate it back clockwise one click to the Lead II position.* This technique can be particularly helpful in poorly lit settings.

The *paddles* are important to the monitoring process only in the absence of the chest electrodes and when the Lead Select switch is in the "Paddles" position. Once the electrodes are in place the EMT should select one of the Lead positions and monitor the patient through the electrodes. If defibrillation or cardioversion is needed, there is no need to switch back to paddle mode. Defibrillation or cardioversion can be done with the "On/Off/Lead Select" switch in a "Lead" position.

Above the Lead select button is the *patient cable jack* for the three lead electrode cable. This cable has been referred to already, and includes the wires ("leads") which go to the chest electrodes. Most prehospital cardiac monitors, including the LIFEPAK 5, use a three wire cable. Most hospital monitors use four wires, or more. The essential wires are color-coded the same in all monitors: white, red, and black and/or green. A mnemonic that may prove helpful is "White to right, smoke over fire" — which translates as *white wire to right shoulder, black (smoke) wire to left shoulder, above red (fire) wire at left anterior lower chest.* If the monitor has a fourth wire, or if you encounter one at the hospital when transferring the patient, it should attach at the right anterior lower chest — across the torso from the red wire.

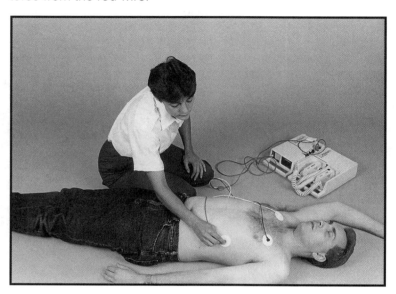

Above the patient cable jack is a one volt *EKG output jack.* This jack is used to connect the monitor to a modulator so that the patient's EKG can be transmitted as telemetry by radio or telephone to a hospital. The receiving monitor must have a compatible "demodulator" with which to unscramble the signal.

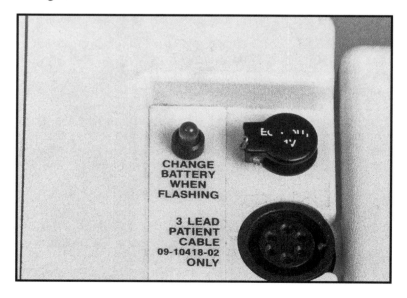

Next to the EKG modulator jack is the *low battery indicator light.* When flashing, this indicates that the battery powering the monitor is low on stored energy and needs to be replaced.

Immediately below the lead select button is the *CAL/SYST VOLUME* button. This is a dual function button which adjusts the volume of the "systolic beeper" and is also used when calibrating the monitor display. Turning this button controls the volume of a beeping noise which can be made to sound whenever the monitor senses an "R" wave in the patient's EKG. This allows the EMT to "hear" the rate and rhythm of the EKG without looking at the monitor screen, however it can become irritating and distracting on long and otherwise uneventful transports. In emergencies, however, when there are only a few people to watch everything that is going on, it can be an important help in keeping track of the patient's continuing cardiac activity. Turning the knob clockwise increases the volume, turning it counterclockwise decreases the sound to fully off.

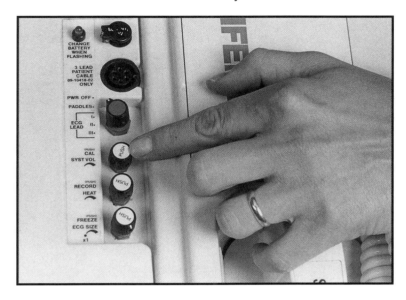

The same button is used to calibrate the EKG wave form being displayed by the monitor and printed on the strip recorder. When the button is depressed it sends a one millivolt (1mv) electrical pulse to the monitor. The interpretation of EKGs printed on a LIFEPAK 5 are standardized in that every 10mm deflection is expected to represent a 1mv electrical current. Ten millimeters is printed as a deflection of two "big boxes" on the graph paper. By pushing the button while the recording paper is running, the EMT commands the monitor to display its response to a 1mv current.

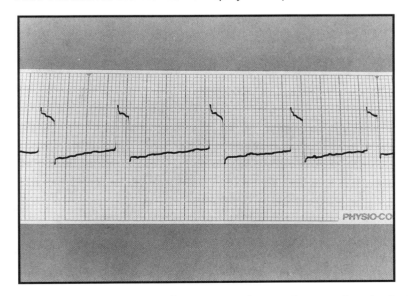

Using the *FREEZE/ECG SIZE button,* the monitor can then be "calibrated" or tuned so that it prints just a 10mm deflection when the 1mv current is present. The calibration button should be pushed, the calibration adjusted, and then the calibration button pushed again to confirm the correctly calibrated setting whenever a printed EKG record is being made. If a 10mm calibration mark can be seen on an EKG strip, the person interpreting the rhythm is assured that the size of the image is accurate to the strength of the electrical activity in the patient's heart and that the "synchronized" mode will work properly for cardioversion.

The *FREEZE/ECG SIZE button* is the bottom one. To adjust the calibrated height of the wave form, turn it clockwise or counter-clockwise. By calibrating the size of the EKG, you will consistently be seeing the same EKG deflections on all patients. Having the EKG size too high will depict large bizarre EKG complexes on the screen and recording paper when the pattern may actually look very normal when correctly calibrated. Having the EKG gain too low will cause the EKG to be very small and flat looking. When the size adjustment is too low, any rhythm (including ventricular fibrillation) can look like asystole.

Between the "calibration" button and the "EKG Size" button is the *RECORD/HEAT button.* This turns the paper strip recorder on and off and controls the recording of a *static* EKG record on a moving strip of paper. It also allows the EMT to adjust the temperature of the stylus which actually marks the paper. Pushing the button starts the recorder paper. There is a 2.4 second delay between when an electrical impulse appears on the monitor screen and when it is recorded on the EKG paper. Turning the button clockwise increases the temperature of the stylus tip, turning it counter-clockwise reduces the heat level. The temperature of the stylus should be adjusted to obtain the most legible printout on the recording paper.

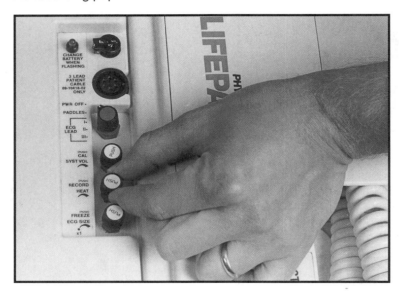

As noted earlier, the bottom button adjusts the EKG size and is used when calibrating the monitor and recorder. By turning the button the EKG shown on the screen can be made larger or smaller. Once you have properly calibrated the EKG size, there should be minimal further adjustments needed.

This button is also used to *freeze* the EKG rhythm on the screen. When you push the button down and hold it, the image on the monitor screen stops moving but remains visible. This allows you to carefully view a group of EKG complexes should you notice something abnormal. If the recorder is turned on it will continue to print the "live" EKG rhythm (with the 2.4 second delay) while the depressed freeze button is holding the original image on the monitor screen. When the button is released the image that was "frozen" on the screen will be immediately printed on the recording paper. Once the frozen complexes have been printed, the recorder will again return to its normal 2.4 second delay.

If you are watching the monitor screen with the paper recorder turned off, and see something of interest on the screen, you should first reach for the "freeze" button and hold the image on the screen. Then, with your other hand, turn on the paper recorder so that it is printing the "live" EKG rhythm and release the "freeze" button to print the "frozen" rhythm or complex. In this way you can preserve the complex or abnormality that caught your attention and allow you time to study it more carefully without it disappearing off the monitor screen. Simply turning on the paper recorder may not start the recording rapidly enough to capture the image, as the printer takes a few seconds to warm up and begin printing legible patterns.

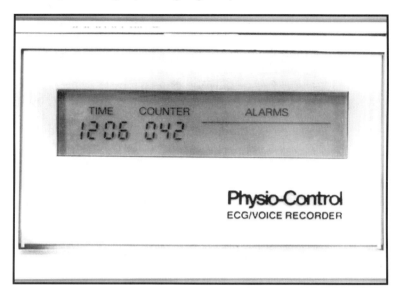

EKG/Voice Recorder

There is an optional EKG/voice recorder available for the LIFEPAK 5 which records both the EMTs' voices as well as the patient's EKG. When the tape is replayed in an appropriate machine, it will recreate the patient's EKG and let the reviewer hear the EMT's actual simultaneous conversation. This device is excellent for quality assurance review and run critiques.

To install the unit, press the lock release button between the monitor and defibrillator units and slide them apart. Slide the recorder unit into the slots in the side of the monitor and defibrillator until they all lock into place.

Insert a cassette tape into the recorder. The controls are similar to those found on any cassette tape recorder. When the monitor is turned on, if a tape is not present in the recorder a warning tone will be heard and appropriate message will appear on the LCD display on the recorder.

Defibrillator Unit Controls and Features

The most commonly used parts on the defibrillator side of the LIFEPAK 5 are the two paddles. The paddles are labelled "Sternum" and "Apex" to remind the user of their preferred placement locations, however they will still effectively defibrillate the heart if they are placed in reverse position. "Apex" refers to the apex of the heart; just below and to the side of the left nipple. "Sternum" refers to the position just to the right of the upper sternum. The "Sternum" paddle should be placed on the right side of the patient's chest, lateral to the upper sternum and below the right clavicle. The "Apex" paddle should be placed on the lower left side of the patient's chest, below and lateral to the apex of the heart. The cardiac monitor is configured electronically to display the patient's EKG pattern in the conventional "R up" style when the electrical current coming to it is consistent with the "Sternum" paddle being in the "Sternum" position and the "Apex" paddle being in the "Apex" position. If the position of the paddles is reversed the monitor will still depict the EKG activity being sensed, but the image on the monitor screen will be inverted—that is, the "R" wave will point downward rather than up (provided that when conventionally monitored the patient's "R" wave would have pointed upward!)

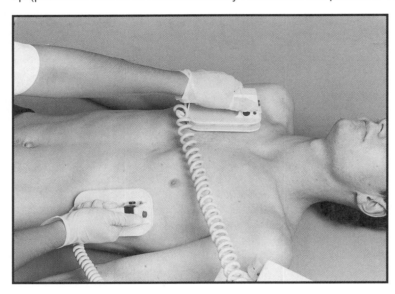

Each paddle consists of a handle, the electrode plate that is placed on the patient, and a number of buttons and switches which allow the operator to perform various operations while holding the paddles and without turning back to the main unit itself. The "Sternum" paddle contains the *On/Off power button* for activating the paddles, and also one of the two red "discharge" buttons.

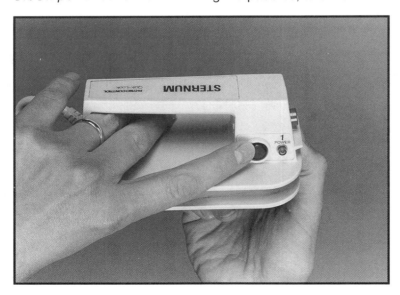

A *discharge button* is located on the front of each paddle. To avoid accidentally discharging the defibrillator's electrical charge, *both of the discharge buttons must be pressed simultaneously for the defibrillatory shock to be delivered.*

The Apex paddle contains the "Energy Joules" dial switch, the "Charge" button, and the second discharge button. The round *Energy dial switch* found on the medial side of the handle is labelled for a variety of electrical power settings, including 20, 50, 100, 200, 300, and 400 "joules." The desired power setting is selected by rotating the dial until the arrow on the dial points to the desired energy level.

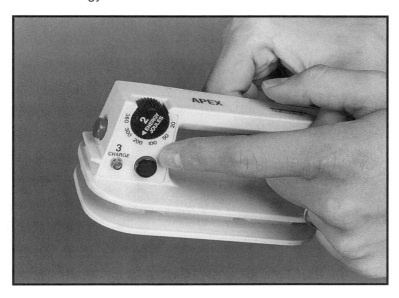

To *charge the defibrillator paddles*, first turn the lead select to either paddles or to a specific lead (I, II, III). Push the power button on the sternum paddle so that the green light is lit.

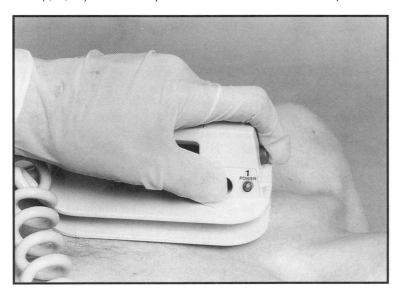

Next, select the energy level desired by rotating the energy level dial on the Apex paddle and then push the *Charge button* located next to it. The amber light will flash and a tone will increase in pitch until the energy level is reached. Once the tone stops and the amber light remains on, the paddles are charged to the selected energy level. If the amber light begins to blink again soon after the charge level is reached, the defibrillator battery level is probably too low to provide effective counter shocks. Turn off the defibrillator power, change batteries, and then power up and charge the paddles again.

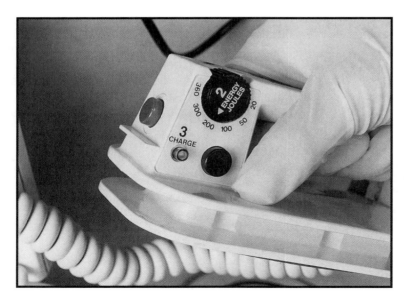

If you wait too long (about a minute) between charging the paddles and delivering a shock, the defibrillator will automatically "dump" the charge. If you see the amber light begin to blink after you have had the paddles charged for several seconds, this is a warning that the charge is about to be "dumped." If you are not immediately ready to deliver a shock, dump the charge and then charge the paddles again.

"Dumping" the energy load in the paddles can be accomplished in any one of three ways: change the energy setting by rotating the dial to a new position, place the paddles back into the holders on top of the defibrillator case, or turn off the defibrillator function by pushing the "Power" button on the Sternum paddle to "off" (the green light turns off). Turning the "energy joules" selection dial disables or dumps everything except the power to the paddles. Pushing the "Power" button or replacing the paddles in the holding case dumps the power load and also turns the paddles completely off — as noted by the green power light turning off.

When defibrillating a patient, a *conductive medium* must be used to reduce the resistance to the flow of current from the paddles to the skin. One option is to apply a conductive gel to the electrode surfaces of the paddles, which are then rubbed on the patient's chest to assure that the gel is applied evenly to the skin where the paddles will be placed. An earlier practice of smearing the paddles together to spread the gel too often results in uneven contact with the skin. If gel is used, the EMT must also periodically check the paddle surfaces between shocks to make sure that enough gel remains on the electrode plates. The chest usually needs to be wiped off to prevent warmed gel from extending so far over the chest that the gel from each paddle site runs together — or to keep it out from under the hands of the EMT doing CPR compressions. While part of the attention to making sure the gel is properly spread relates to delivering effective shocks and protecting the patient's skin, proper care will also protect the surface of the paddles from becoming pitted and scarred. Whenever they are not being applied to the patient's chest, the paddles should be returned to their holders on the LIFEPAK main unit to keep them from being damaged or from accumulating dirt on the electrode surface.

Special adhesive defibrillator pads are commercially available which make it unnecessary to apply anything to the paddles themselves. These are much larger than the monitoring electrodes and much neater than using gel. They also provide the EMT with a visual reminder of where the paddles are to be applied on the chest. An alternative to the commercial "defib pads" is to soak standard 4" x 4" gauze dressings in normal saline and, after squeezing the excess fluid from them, apply them on the chest in the locations where the paddles will be applied. These have the advantage of being inexpensive and readily available, but they can also be time-consuming to prepare and apply (and if too much saline is applied it will run all over the chest).

When a defibrillatory shock is delivered and the saline or conductive gel has spread from the paddle location to other areas of the chest, the electrical current tends to follow the path of least resistance — namely through the conductive material rather than the chest wall. *If the saline or gel from both paddle locations comes too close or merge together, an electrical arc will travel across the outside of the patient's chest rather than internally through the axis of the heart. This does the patient no good, and can be dangerous for the EMT and others nearby.* When special defibrillation pads are not used, care must be taken to wipe the paddle locations and chest area regularly so that neither conductive gel nor saline spread too far and interfere with the delivery of an effective defibrillatory shock. ***Do not use any type of alcohol soaked pads as the passage of electricity through them can cause them to ignite.***

Although an electrical shock delivered to a cardiac patient can be life-saving, it can also be *very harmful* if delivered to someone whose heart is functioning normally — namely the EMT and other rescuers crowded around the patient. As the paddles are applied to the patient's chest, but before any fingers are placed near the red "defibrillate" buttons on the paddles, *the EMT operating the defibrillator must visually and verbally "clear" all personnel.* This entails making sure that no one, including the operator, is touching the patient. A loud statement such as "CLEAR" or "ONE I'm clear, TWO you're clear, THREE we're all clear" while deliberately scanning the patient's body from head to toe allows for everyone to safely move away from the patient before the shock is delivered.

To insure the effective delivery of the electrical current, the electrode plates on each paddle must be applied to the patient's chest with enough force to provide complete contact between the plates and the skin. Incomplete contact can result in increased resistance to the flow of current and diminish the effectiveness of the defibrillatory shock. *The EMT manning the paddles must push them forcefully downward onto the patient's chest or defibrillation pads to obtain maximum contact.*

It is also somewhat natural for the person operating the paddles to lean in toward the patient in preparation for delivering the shock, in part to assure that firm equal pressure is being exerted on the paddles. This has the disadvantage, however, of bringing the EMT's body closer to the patient at the time that the shock is delivered. Again, exercise care and be sure that you (and everyone else except the patient) are clear!

On the front edge of the defibrillator unit is the red *synchronized cardioversion button.* To activate the synchronizer the paddles must first be turned on, and then the synchronizer button must be pushed. When the synchronizer is active the button will illuminate.

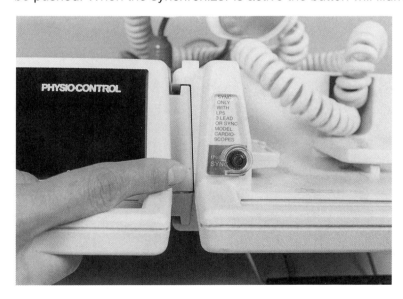

When using the synchronizer, you may have to increase the size of the EKG image on the monitor screen so that the monitor can "read" the peak of the "R" wave of the QRS complex. If the monitor is reading the "R" wave the synchronizer light will flash and a small dot will appear above each "R" wave on the monitor screen. If the synchronizer light is illuminated but not flashing and if dots are not visible above the "R" waves, adjust the "EKG size" button until these are noted. The synchronizer will not discharge if the monitor cannot detect the "R" wave of the QRS complex.

Once the synchronizer light is flashing and the highlighted dots are visible on the monitor screen, the paddles should be charged to the desired setting and placed on the chest. Defibrillation pads, saline pads, or conductive gel should be used just as when performing unsynchronized defibrillation. Although the defibrillator will not fire exactly when both red defibrillation buttons on the paddles are pushed, it *will* fire as soon as both buttons are held in *AND* it reads an "R" wave on the monitor — therefore before placing the paddles on the patient's chest you should be certain that everyone is clear of the patient and that all necessary precautions have been taken from patient and rescuer safety.

The synchronizer function on the LIFEPAK 5 is a "one time" thing — the synchronizer automatically turns off after a synchronized shock is delivered and also if any changes are made to the unit's various settings between when the synchronizer is activated and when the shock is delivered — such as a change in energy level. It is recommended that, when preparing to deliver a synchronized shock, the synchronizer button be one of the *LAST* things activated before delivering the shock. This will help to assure that the synchronizer is still activated when the shock is desired.

Changing Recording Paper

The paper used in the strip chart printer comes in fifty foot rolls. During continuous recording of a monitored rhythm, a full roll of paper will last about ten minutes. The usual practice is to print strips only on an intermittent basis — such as when a change is noted in the patient's rhythm or when a medication is being administered — and therefore a single roll of paper can typically be used for several patients without running out. *A red line* will appear on the top edge of the paper during the last three feet of the roll, warning the EMT that the roll is almost exhausted and needs to be replaced.

To replace a roll of EKG paper, open the paper holder by pulling on the black metal grasp at the bottom of the holder. The paper roll and cardboard center can then be lifted off of the spindle.

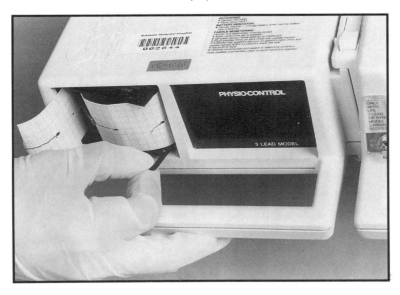

Take a new roll and slide it back onto the spindle, making sure the three second markers are toward the top edge of the paper.

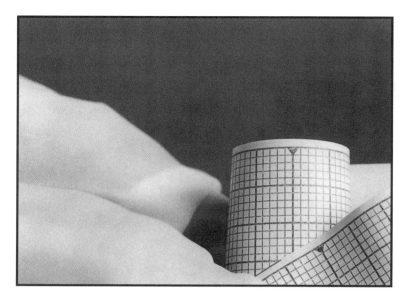

Pull out a few inches of the paper from the roll and then push the paper holder back into the recorder. If necessary, trim the end of the paper to make sure that the vertical edge is cleanly cut. Turn on the monitor and then push the appropriate button to turn on the paper recorder. Feed the end of the paper under the rubber power rollers until it is caught by the rollers and feeds freely through the printer assembly, emerging from the far left side of the paper recording area on the monitor case. The width and clarity of the recorded image will vary as determined by the heat of the stylus. To do this, adjust the previously discussed "Heat" button on the monitor's control panel.

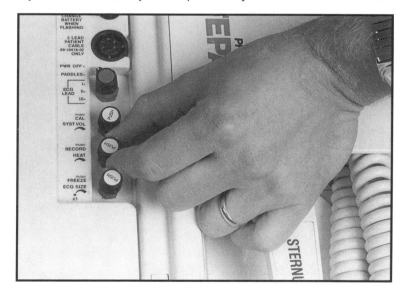

Separating The Units

The LIFEPAK 5 is unique in that its monitor and defibrillator sections can be separated and still perform their respective basic functions. Separating the monitor from the defibrillator does, however, disable both the "quick look" function of the defibrillator and the ability to perform synchronized cardioversion. *The two units must be connected together for either of these two functions to be performed.*

To separate the two units, push the lock release tab which is found between the two units near the front of the machine. While holding the lock release tab down, pull the monitor unit forward while holding the defibrillator half still until the monitor portion has been completely separated from the defibrillator half.

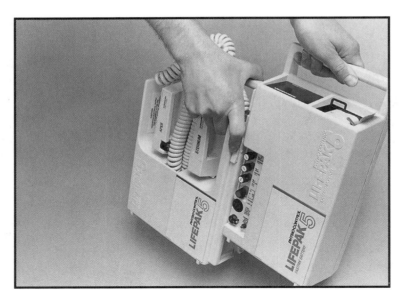

With the units separated, notice the small copper strips on the side of each unit where they slide together in the track. These are the electrical connectors which allow the two halves to work together, and it is important that they be kept clean. The strips should be inspected periodically. A standard pencil eraser makes a good "cleaner" for removing any build-up on the copper surfaces. Any eraser material left on the connectors after cleaning should be brushed off.

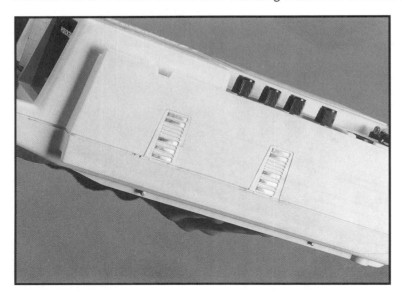

To reconnect the two units simply slide the monitor half back into the track on the side of the defibrillator half until the lock release clicks.

When picking up or carrying a LIFEPAK 5 that does not have an external carrying case and strap, it is best to grasp the handle of the defibrillator side (or both handles) in case the lock release is broken or not secure. Because the monitor slides into the attachment from forward of the defibrillator and is stopped from sliding beyond it, this prevents the two units from accidentally sliding apart and the monitor being dropped and damaged.

Changing And Charging Batteries

The LIFEPAK 5 uses two rechargeable nickel-cadmium ("NiCad") batteries to power the monitor and defibrillator. Although the batteries are interchangeable, they serve only the half of the unit into which they are inserted — the battery on the monitor side does not supply power for the defibrillator, and vice-versa. A specific checklist should be used to charge and rotate the batteries to maximize their stored charge and effective life. Label each battery with its date of manufacture and date placed in service, and maintain a record for each battery. With periodic testing and reconditioning, a typical battery can be expected to perform dependably for at least two years. Performing a re-conditioning or "exercise" procedure every three months will help to maintain the batteries at maximum effectiveness. The exercise procedure consists of fully discharging and then recharging the batteries three times in a row, and then checking the battery's capacity. Physio Control has a specific battery conditioning device that automatically conditions and recharges LIFEPAK batteries, and then displays the battery's actual power capacity. Typically, batteries should be able to store at least 70 per cent of their rated capacity after the exercise procedure. If not, the battery should be retired from service. Well maintained batteries should be able to power the monitor side of a LIFEPAK 5 for 1.7 hours of continuous EKG monitoring. For defibrillation, a fully charged battery should be capable of delivering more than thirty 360-joule discharges in a normal temperature environment. For best results, follow the recommendations of the specific battery manufacturer for optimum care and treatment of rechargeable batteries.

On a LIFEPAK 5 monitor/defibrillator, the batteries are secured in their respective slots by means of two thin metal pins and a tension clip. The "pins" are actually the electrical connectors through which current is drawn from the battery into the monitor or defibrillator, and can easily be bent or broken if they are mishandled. The pins point upward from inside the recessed battery slots in the top of the LIFEPAK case, and can be damaged by carelessly inserting a battery into the recess without visually lining up the pins with the matching holes in the battery.

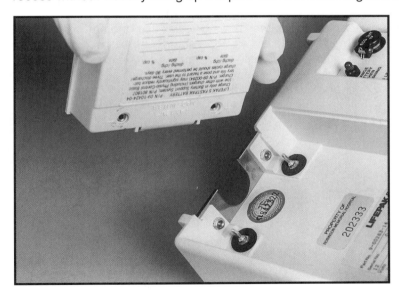

The tension clip is found on the posterior edge of the battery, and must be pushed in with the EMT's finger to latch the battery in place. To remove a battery, again push in on the clip and lift first the posterior portion and then the entire battery out of the recess.

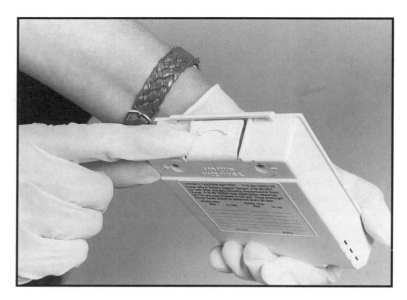

The preceding discussion is specific to the LIFEPAK 5 model produced closest to the time of this book's publication. Due to its wide proliferation in the field, it is beneficial for all advanced EMTs to be introduced to and familiar with the use of this model as a part of their training. The LIFEPAK 5 was selected because in a large number of cases this will be the equipment that the EMT will need to be able to use. Although the location and use of each control and function on the unit are specific to this model, this introduction can also be useful in a wider context.

Since all monitor/defibrillators have analogous functions and controls, the preceding discussion will be useful as an introduction and general overview of the use of any such units. By viewing each specific reference to the LIFEPAK 5 as solely an example, the EMTs who will use another unit can use this introduction as a generic framework of knowledge to aid in understanding the specific operating instructions when learning the use of different units. Regardless of similarities, however, the EMT must be fluent in the set-up and use of the specific model he will be using, and should be required to demonstrate his level of competence in every aspect of its use on a mannikin before he can safely employ it with patients in the field.

ALS **USING THE LIFEPAK 5 MONITOR/DEFIBRILLATOR**

As noted in the Introduction to this Section, most monitor/defibrillator units allow the EMT to assess the patient's electrical cardiac activity both through the paddles and also with the more conventional adhesive electrodes. When first encountering a patient whose heart is to be monitored, the EMT must choose between these two methods. The choice is typically based upon the patient's overall presentation and appearance; that is, a patient who is responsive and obviously has a pulse is most likely to be monitored with adhesive electrodes, whereas an unresponsive patient in whom pulselessness is a possibility should more appropriately be first evaluated with the paddles.

After determining that the scene is safe and that all indicated body substance isolation precautions have been taken, assess the patient's responsiveness and determine that the airway is open, whether or not the patient is breathing, and whether or not there is a palpable pulse. If the patient is pulseless begin CPR and bring the monitor-defibrillator to the patient's side.

1. To use the paddles to take a "quick look" at the patient's cardiac status, first turn the "lead select" switch to paddle mode. This also turns the monitor on. Position the monitor so that you can easily observe both the patient and the monitor screen, and so that the paddles can easily reach the patient's chest.

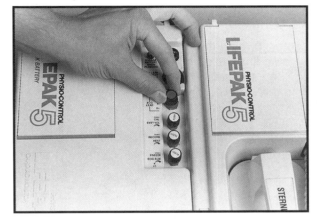

2. Bare the patient's chest and place the sternum paddle over the patient's right anterior chest wall—above the nipple line and below the clavicle, to the right of the sternum.

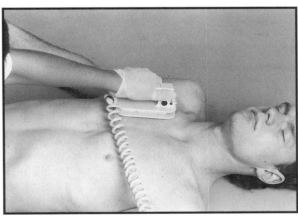

3. Place the apex paddle over the lower left anterior chest wall below the left nipple line at the anterior axillary line of the thoracic cavity. Apply firm pressure to both paddles so that the metal paddle plates are in full contact with the patient's skin. Conductive gel or defibrillator pads are not needed to do a limited "quick look."

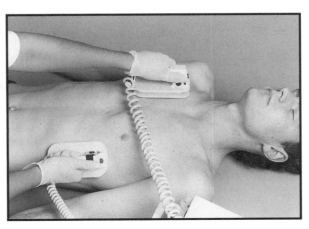

4. With the paddles in place, look at the monitor to assess the rhythm. Keep the paddles and the paddle cables as motionless as possible to help eliminate any movement artifact on the monitor screen. If the monitor screen shows asystole, verify that the "Lead select" switch is in "paddle" mode — if it is set for a cabled Lead and you are using the paddles, you will obtain a false image (possibly appearing to be asystole) on the monitor screen!

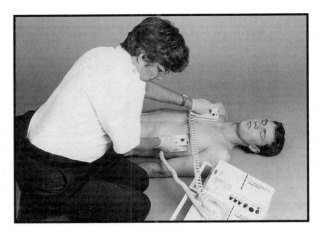

Similarly, if the paddles are removed from the chest wall the rhythm will disappear from the screen and all that will be visible will be the iso-electric line which can be confused for asystole or fine ventricular fibrillation. Do not confuse this with the patient's rhythm!

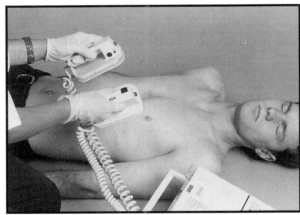

5. A final consideration if asystole appears on the monitor is whether this is true asystole or if it could be fine ventricular fibrillation which is indistinguishable on the small monitor screen for the axis of the heart being sensed between the paddles. As there is a major difference in therapy between asystole and fibrillation, it is important to rapidly and accurately determine which it is. To view a different axis of the heart, move *ONE* of the paddles — for example, switch the apex paddle to the left upper chest wall or the sternum paddle to the lower right side. Moving both paddles might result in simply reversing the original axis and not provide a second view of the heart to confirm asystole.

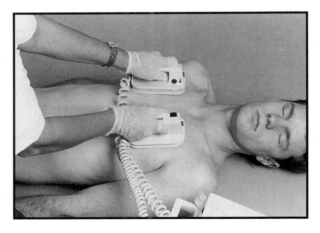

If the rhythm on the monitor is determined to be one that is best treated by defibrillation or synchronized cardioversion, provide that intervention. Those techniques will be addressed in a later part of this Section. If the rhythm is asystole or pulseless electrical activity, institute CPR and provide appropriate ACLS therapy. One element in that evolution will be to change from monitoring through the paddles to applying adhesive electrodes to the patient's chest and monitoring through the cabled leads. This would involve the same steps as if the patient had been initially found to be responsive and have a pulse, and the option of monitoring through the paddles had not been selected.

6. Return both paddles to their holders on the main unit. Connect an adhesive electrode to each of the three cable leads. Attach the white lead to the patient's upper right chest, just below the clavicle and lateral of the nipple line. If the patient is extremely diaphoretic, wipe the skin dry before applying the electrode. You may wipe the skin with an alcohol swab if it is particularly oily or wet. It may be necessary to shave the electrode placement spots on especially hairy patients.

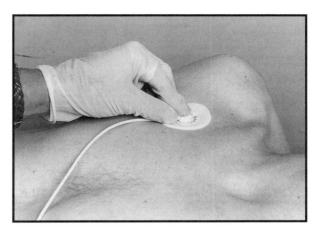

7. Attach the red lead to the patient's lower right side, just below the lowest margin of the ribs on the anterior axillary line. Unless the patient is wearing a one-piece garment this can usually be placed without completely opening all of their clothes by simply pulling out the shirt or blouse at the beltline.

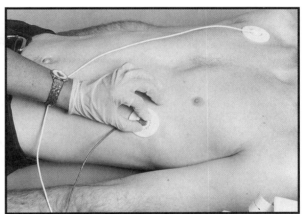

8. Attach the remaining black (or green) lead to the patient's anterior left chest just below the clavicle and lateral of the nipple line. This should be comparable to the location of the white lead on the right side of the chest. If you are using a four-wire cable, attach the remaining lead on the patient's lower right side, just across from the red lead.

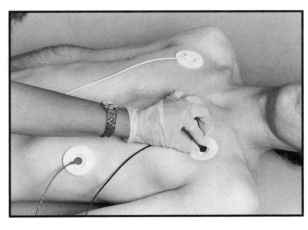

9. Switch the "Lead Select" control on the monitor from "Paddles" to "Lead II" and evaluate the rhythm display. If the image seems distorted or bizarre, yet the patient is responsive, the problem is probably with the cable and lead connections rather than with the patient. If, when you have secured the leads, you initially see asystole, *IMMEDIATELY* confirm that you have indeed changed the Lead Select control from the "Paddles" position and are *NOT* monitoring the isoelectric line from them rather than the patient.

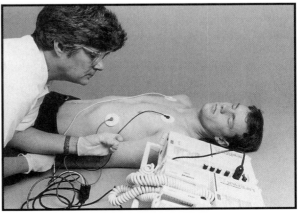

10. If at any other time while monitoring through the cable the machine displays asystole, you can view the heart's activity through a second Lead by simply changing the setting on the "Lead Select" switch from Lead II to either Lead I or Lead III. Be careful not to switch to "Paddles" unless you actually have them on the patient's chest!

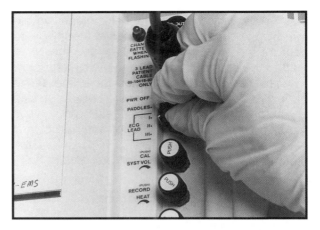

11. Whichever monitoring technique you use, either by the quick look method with the paddles or the chest electrodes, you can create a printed record of the cardiac rhythm by simply pressing the "record" button on the monitor. Allow at least ten seconds of recording time, and somewhere on the paper strip you should mark the time and the patient's last name so that it can be used for review and documentation purposes later.

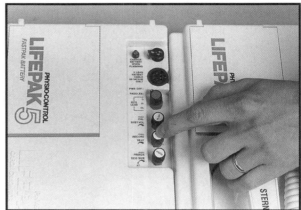

Using The Defibrillator

12. To defibrillate a patient, first remove the paddles from their holder and apply conductive gel to the electrode plates. Alternately, place defibrillation pads or saline-soaked gauze pads on the patient's chest where the paddles will be placed.

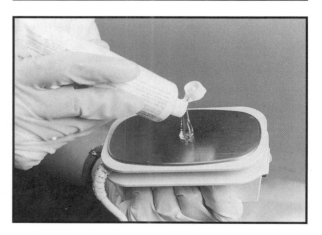

13. Place the "sternum" paddle on the patient's right anterior chest wall, just to the right of the patient's upper sternum and below the clavicle. The paddle should not cover the EKG monitoring electrode if one is in place, and the EMT should avoid placing the paddle over the site of an implanted pacemaker if one is detected.

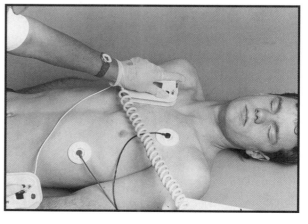

14. Place the "Apex" paddle to the left of the patient's left nipple with the center of the paddle plate in the mid-axillary line.

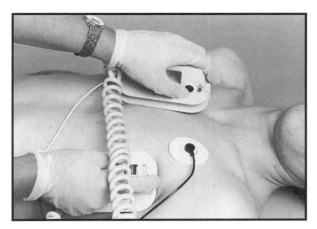

15. Push the defibrillator "power on" button on the side of the "Sternum" paddle. When the defibrillator function is enabled the green light next to the button will illuminate.

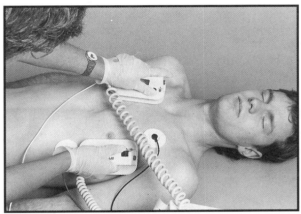

16. Select the energy level (joules setting) on the apex paddle by dialing the appropriate number, typically 200 joules for the first unsynchronized shock in adults and 2 joules per kilogram in children.

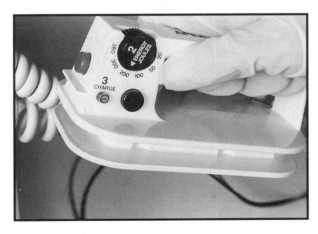

17. Press the charge button located below the energy select dial. You should hear an increasing tone and see the amber light flashing. When the tone stops and the amber light stays lit, the paddles are charged to the selected level.

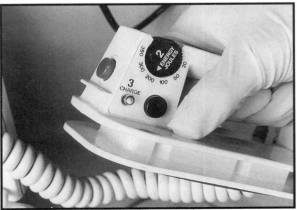

18. Visually and verbally "clear" all personnel from the area around the patient — making sure that no one (including yourself) is touching the patient. A loud statement such as "CLEAR" or "ONE I'm clear, TWO you're clear, THREE we're all clear" should be used. Be sure to allow enough time for everyone to move back from the patient. Press firmly against the patient's skin with the paddles to assure good electrical contact.

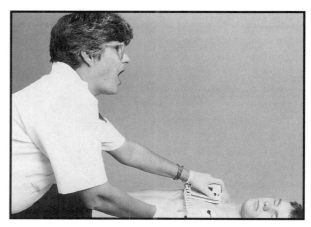

19. After both viewing the monitor to verify the rhythm one more time and scanning to ensure that all are clear, press the red buttons at the front of each paddle simultaneously to deliver the charge.

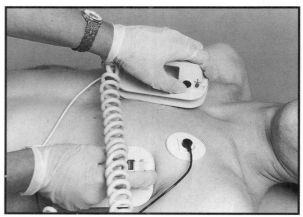

20. After the shock has been delivered, and while you still maintain paddle placement, select the desired energy level for the next shock in the event that one must be delivered (usually between 200 and 300 joules for a second shock in adults and 4 joules per kilogram for second and subsequent shocks in children). Press the charge button to begin the process of re-charging the defibrillator.

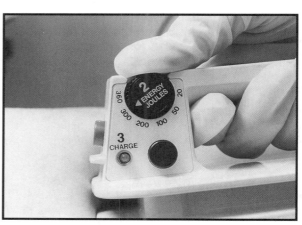

21. While the defibrillator is charging, reassess the rhythm for any changes or for the continued presence of ventricular fibrillation. Depending upon your protocol, you may wish to have another EMT check for a carotid pulse while the charging process continues.

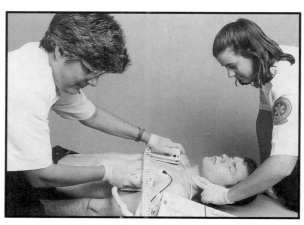

22. As soon as the whining charging sound ends and the amber light stops flashing, repeat the "clear" warning and scan to assure that all personnel are clear and discharge the paddles again. Be sure to maintain firm pressure on the paddles against the patient's skin.

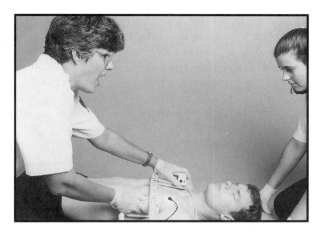

23. After the shock has been delivered, and while you still maintain paddle placement, select the desired energy level for the next shock in the event that one must be delivered (usually 360 joules in adults for the third shock and 4 joules per kilogram for children). Press the charge button to begin the process of re-charging the defibrillator.

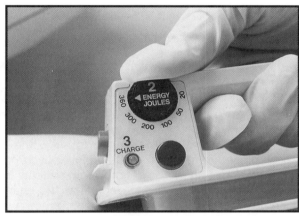

24. While the defibrillator is charging, reassess the rhythm for any changes or for the continued presence of ventricular fibrillation. Depending upon your protocol, you may wish to have another EMT check for a carotid pulse while the charging process continues.

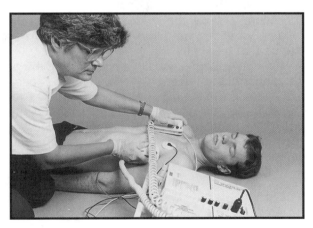

25. As soon as the whining charging sound ends and the amber light stops flashing, repeat the "clear" warning and visual scan and discharge the paddles again.

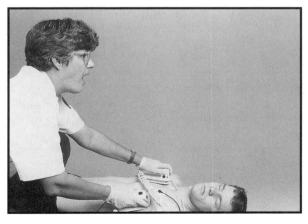

26. After delivering the third shock, re-assess the monitored rhythm and palpate for a carotid pulse. If the patient remains pulseless, re-institute CPR and follow the ACLS algorithm for the rhythm being displayed on the monitor. Subsequent use of the defibrillator will not substantially change from this point on, with shocks delivered at the last energy setting used and interspersed with medications per the ACLS protocols.

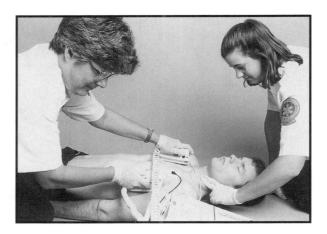

ALS

Synchronized Cardioversion

The electrical shocks for synchronized cardioversion are performed in the same manner as for unsynchronized defibrillation, however the synchronizer button must be turned on and the monitor display must have sufficient gain to allow the defibrillator to read the presence of an "R" wave. Synchronized cardioversion is employed with patients in supraventricular tachycardia, atrial fibrillation, and atrial flutter, and at times with patients in ventricular tachycardia with a pulse. Unlike defibrillation, in which the goal is to depolarize the entire myocardium at one time in hopes that an effective pacemaker site will emerge that can produce a viable cardiac rhythm, synchronized cardioversion is performed to convert an undesirable rhythm without increasing the possibility of producing ventricular fibrillation. V-fib can be induced in a patient if the defibrillatory shock is delivered during the relative refractory period (the "R-on-T" phenomenon)—synchronized shocks are specifically timed to avoid that period.

Cardioversion is usually easier to do if the patient is on chest leads. Conductive gel or defibrillation pads must be used. If the patient is conscious, consideration should be given to sedating the patient to lessen the pain and memory of the event.

To perform synchronized cardioversion, first monitor the patient with the cabled leads or with the quick look paddles and verify the rhythm you need to cardiovert. Apply a conductive medium on the chest or paddles, or apply defibrillation pads, and place the paddles on the patient's chest just like for defibrillation. Then:

a. Press the power button on the sternum paddle and select the desired energy setting by rotating the selector on the apex paddle.

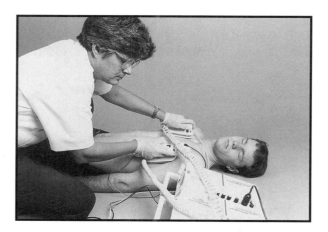

b. Push the synchronizer button until the red button lights up. The light should be flashing, indicating that the monitor has identified the "R" wave of the QRS complex.

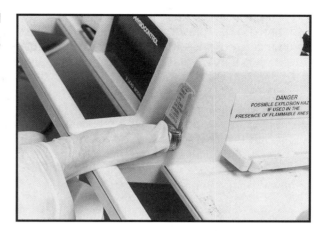

c. If the light is not flashing but is lit, turn up the EKG size button until the light begins to flash. Without the synchronizer button flashing, the paddles will not discharge. An added precaution with many defibrillators is that any readjustment of the energy selector after the synchronizer is pushed will turn off the synchronizer. Make activation of the synchronizer button the last step prior to cardioversion so that you do not accidentally turn it off by adjusting the energy setting after you engage the synchronizer.

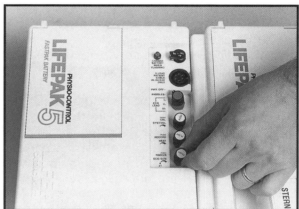

d. Visually and verbally "clear" the area around the patient just as you would with unsynchronized defibrillation. Once everyone is away from the patient, press the discharge button at the front of each paddle *AND HOLD THEM "PUSHED."*

Once you push the discharge button, there may be a slight delay before the defibrillator fires — the defibrillator must wait for the monitor to select a QRS complex to fire on. Once the energy is delivered, verify the rhythm and determine if another cardioversion shock is needed. If so, repeat the same steps using the next energy level per your protocol.

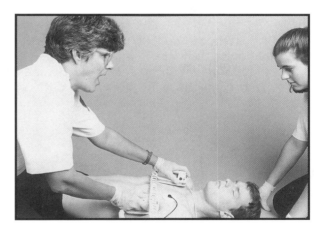

e. With many defibrillators, once you have discharged the paddles in a synchronized cardioversion the synchronizer automatically turns off. If you need to cardiovert again, you must push the synchronizer button each time. Failure to do this will deliver the shock to the patient as soon as the discharge buttons are pushed (unsynchronized defibrillation). This may cause the energy to enter the heart during the relative refractory period of the cardiac cycle and put the patient into ventricular fibrillation. Again, you must turn the synchronizer on each time you repeat the cardioversion.

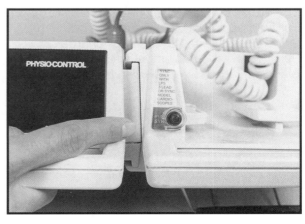

27. Regardless of whether the unit was used to only monitor the patient or if either defibrillation or synchronized cardioversion was performed, it is recommended for most EMS services that the unit remain turned on — that is, with the rechargeable batteries activated — until the ambulance is returned to service at the station and the batteries can be exchanged for fresh ones. When the battery is turned on but only used briefly and then turned off — and then exchanged for a new battery and placed in the charger, it is susceptible to developing a false "memory" of exactly what its capacity is. By allowing the battery to run for a considerable period of time it gets "exercised," and the subsequent charging period restores it to its full capacity. The EMT will have to use some discretion in this regard — busy services may not have the opportunity to return to a station and exchange batteries after each call; if you are already using the back-up set of batteries on the ambulance, it may be more prudent to turn the unit off and conserve whatever power is left in case yet another call is received before you can return to the station.

Putting The Equipment Away

After every use the monitor/defibrillator should be checked and re-stocked as a routine part of putting it back in service and making it available for immediate use on the next call.

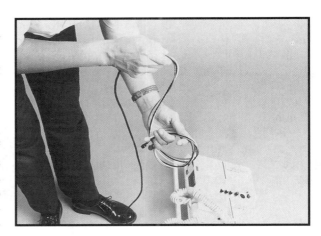

28. The equipment should be visually inspected for cleanliness and damage. Check the cables and cords for cracks or frays in the insulation. If the defibrillator was used, examine the paddles to be sure they are clean, dry, and free of cracks and pitting. Reset the energy select switch to 200 joules. Replace all used monitoring electrodes and defibrillator pads. Restock the conductive gel if any was used.

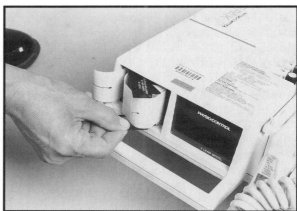

29. Check that the strip paper advances smoothly and that there is adequate paper for the strip chart recorder. Also verify that a spare roll of paper is carried in the storage pouch.

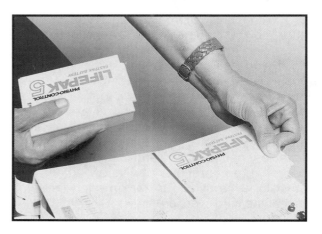

30. Replace any batteries that were used. Follow proper battery maintenance and recharge any used batteries to assure full charge capacity. Finally, store the equipment in its proper location, ready for immediate use when next needed.

![ALS]

EMERGENCY CARDIAC PACING

Transcutaneous pacing, which may also be called "external" pacing, is a "non-invasive" procedure in which the heart is stimulated with externally applied electrodes that deliver an electrical impulse through the skin. External pacing requires use of a special pacemaker unit or a monitor/defibrillator which includes this capability. EMS services which provide this skill typically use portable monitor/defibrillators which also pace. In most cases, transcutaneous pacing is performed with a pair of large "hands off" monitoring/defibrillation electrodes that are applied to the anterior and posterior chest walls. Unlike unsynchronized defibrillation, the amount of electrical current is minor and there is no danger to providers when pacing is being performed. CPR can even be continued during pacing with the compressor's hands touching the non-conductive upper surface of the electrode pads.

Transcutaneous pacing is primarily indicated for the treatment of significant bradycardias that have *NOT* responded to (are "refractory" to) drug therapy. Patients who are hypothermic and bradycardic are poor candidates for transcutaneous pacing, as the pacing process may induce ventricular fibrillation. Also, patients who have been asystolic for more than twenty minutes are rarely resuscitated despite the application of pacing. Bradycardia in children is typically from hypoxia or hypoventilation and will respond best to treatments focused directly at those problems; however, bradycardia in children stemming from congenital cardiac defects or following open heart surgery may be responsive to pacing.

Transcutaneous pacers are adjustable according to the desired cardiac rate — usually between 30 and 180 beats per minute (bpm) — and the level of electrical stimulating current — usually adjustable from 0 to 200 milliamperes (mA).

Transcutaneous pacing is not without potential complications. There are reported instances in which underlying treatable ventricular fibrillation has gone unnoticed during pacing, and operators have also failed to detect that the pacing process is not working — that the pacemaker is not "capturing." While it is regarded as theoretically possible that delivering an electrical stimulus across the heart may induce fibrillation or other dysrhythmias, the prevalent belief is that the machines presently in use do not deliver enough current to induce fibrillation.

Another complication with earlier machines and techniques was significant pain experienced by the patient. Again, more modern machines appear to operate well without producing more than "mild" discomfort, although some patients still report intolerable pain. Following the manufacturer's recommendations and using modern-day defibrillation pads can markedly reduce this potential or that of producing burns on the patient's skin. In the past, tissue damage — and even third degree burns in children — have been reported, and the EMT should frequently inspect the patient's skin and be prepared to adjust the location of the electrodes if problems are detected.

Because an electrical impulse is generated from the external pacing device, the patient may experience skeletal muscle contraction or pectoral muscle twitching. This should be expected and may be described by the patient as tingling, twitching or a "tap" or "thud" sensation. The patient's comfort level may be tolerable or intolerable. In cases where patients complain of an intolerable sensation from the pacemaker, it may be necessary to administer an analgesic or sedative medication to reduce the discomfort.

The preferred placement for the pacing electrodes is the "Anterior-Posterior" position. The electrodes are color-coded and identified as positive or negative. The negative pacing electrode (usually black) is labelled ANTERIOR and is placed on the left *anterior* chest to the left of the sternum and centered as closely as possible over the apex of the heart. The posterior electrode (usually red) is labelled POSTERIOR and is placed on the left *posterior* chest lateral to the thoracic spine and directly aligned with the anterior electrode.

An alternative method of electrode placement is the Anterior-Anterior position. This can be used when the conventional Anterior-Posterior position is contraindicated. The position of the pacing electrodes in this fashion may interfere with the placement of the defibrillator paddles and may cause pectoral muscle stimulation.

In Anterior-Anterior positioning, the negative electrode is placed on the left chest, over the 4th intercostal space at the mid-axillary line. The positive electrode is placed on the anterior right chest below the midclavicular hollow just to the right of the sternum.

The patient must be monitored at all times when transcutaneous pacing is initiated. It is essential to confirm that capture is occurring and that functional beats are being produced. To evaluate capture of the pacer, the patient must be assessed for both electrical capture and mechanical outcome. Mechanical (or ventricular) capture is determined by improvement in cardiac output as evidenced by a palpable pulse, improved level of consciousness, increase in blood pressure and improvement in skin color and temperature. Electrical capture is evidenced on the monitor by a wide QRS and tall broad T-wave and a visible "pacer spike" preceding each QRS.

To perform transcutaneous pacing, first identify the need for the use of the non-invasive external pacer. The patient should display significant symptomatic bradycardia which is unresponsive to Atropine and/or Isuprel, or be asystolic. Connect the patient to the cardiac monitor to obtain an initial rhythm strip. Follow usual ACLS treatment and resuscitation guidelines, including maintaining a patent airway, assuring adequate ventilation, and assisting with circulation as needed. If the patient is conscious and alert enough to understand, explain the procedure and the possible discomfort from the device. Then:

1. Apply the adhesive pacing electrodes to clean, dry skin in the left anterior—left posterior position (or if this is not practical, in the left anterior—right anterior position), and attach the pacing cables to the electrodes. If the cables and electrodes are color-coded, make sure that you have connected them correctly.

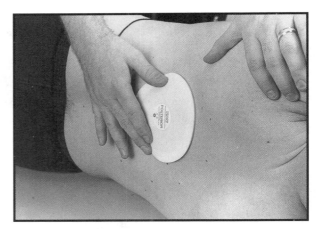

2. Turn on the pacemaker function and observe the EKG monitor screen to verify that the pacer is properly sensing the QRS complexes. A bright dot should appear superimposed on the "R" wave on the screen when there is proper sensing. Adjust the EKG gain/sensitivity control if needed. You can use the QRS volume button to assure that the device is sensing an "R" wave with each QRS complex visible on the monitor screen. If the patient is asystolic, this step should be omitted. Turning on the pacer does not mean that current is being sent to the patient—it is the initiation of the *sensing* portion of the overall pacing operation.

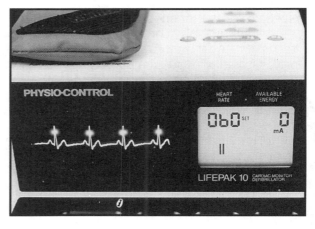

3. Set the initial pacing rate at 80 BPM or whatever level is called for in your local protocols.

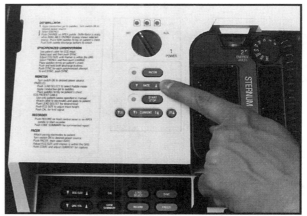

4. Set the electrical current at the minimum setting. Activate the pacemaker by pushing the appropriate control button on the machine. A sharp pacing "spike" should appear on the monitor screen at the beats-per-minute rate previously set. Most pacing machines also have a flashing light or another indication that the pacer is firing. Activating the pacer begins the second step in pacing — delivering the pacing current to the heart. The next step is to gradually increase the amount of current until the level is reached at which the heart responds.

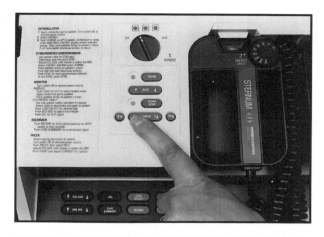

5. Adjust the electrical current upward, constantly observing the patient for signs of improvement. Mechanical/ventricular capture can be identified by signs of improving cardiac output. The return of a palpable carotid pulse is the obvious goal, with an increase in blood pressure, improvement in level of consciousness, skin color and temperature also very desirable. Remember, due to the low current levels, it is SAFE to touch the patient during pacing to palpate pulses, assess the condition of the skin, or even to perform CPR.

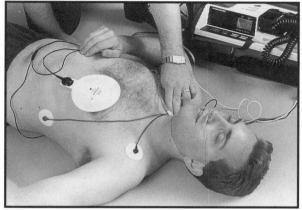

6. Verify electrical capture by the appearance on the monitor of the pacer spike and a wide QRS followed by a tall "T" wave. Continuously observe the monitor for continued pacing and capture.

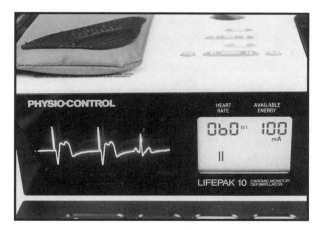

7. During pacing, continuously monitor the patient's condition to confirm that proper cardiac output continues. Consider the use of an analgesic and/or sedative if the patient describes the pain as intolerable.

8. Document the date and time that pacing was initiated, and save both baseline and pacing strips. Note the level of electrical current required for capture, the pacing rate and mode, the patient's response, and any medications used.

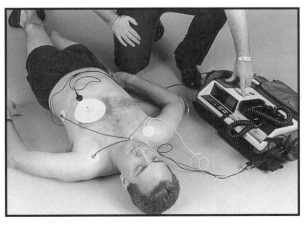

AN INTRODUCTION TO AUTOMATIC AND SEMI-AUTOMATIC DEFIBRILLATION (EMT-D)

Automated electrical defibrillation (AED) is typically performed by EMTs and other medical providers who have not been trained or equipped to provide manual defibrillation in accordance with the conventional ACLS treatment protocols. The development of simplified dysrhythmia recognition programs in King County, Washington, in the late 1970's which allowed basic EMT's to perform defibrillation when they identified ventricular fibrillation is undoubtedly one of the high points of modern EMS care. While the King County program utilized manual defibrillators, as did subsequent programs in Iowa and many other locations, the present-day emphasis is on automated machines which perform most — if not all — of the rhythm analysis and recognition of "shockable" rhythms.

The capabilities and features of the monitor/defibrillators available today for use in "EMT-Defibrillation" programs vary widely. Some are very simple "black boxes" — an on/off switch and an electronic voice that announces when a shock is being delivered or when the EMT should check the patient's pulse or consider performing CPR. Others can function at the same very basic level but have highly sophisticated software options which allow ACLS providers to use them as fully manual machines with pacing capabilities and the full range of synchronized and unsynchronized electrical monitoring and therapy. The generic definitions which apply to all of these devices are:

- **(Fully) Automatic Defibrillator** — A monitor/defibrillator which automatically determines the underlying rhythm. The decision to countershock is made by the monitor/defibrillator, and it will be delivered unless the EMT acts to STOP a shock if he believes that it is not needed.

- **Semi-Automatic Defibrillator** — A monitor/defibrillator which automatically determines the underlying rhythm. The machine indicates when a countershock should be delivered, however the EMT must consciously act to deliver the shock.

- **Manual Defibrillator** — Any monitor/defibrillator which requires monitoring and analysis of the EKG by the EMT to determine the underlying rhythm. If the rhythm requires defibrillation, that determination and the delivery of the countershock are made by the operator.

The practice of leaving to automated machines the issues of recognizing EKG rhythms and setting electrical current levels is admittedly scary to providers who are accustomed to manual equipment and practices, yet AEDs have proven themselves to be effective and reliable in the two critical areas of function: they can reliably identify ventricular fibrillation and they can deliver therapeutic electrical countershocks as fast or faster than human providers. For defibrillatory therapy to be effective, it must be provided as early and as quickly as possible. By eliminating the need for extensive rhythm recognition training and competency maintenance, large numbers of first responders equipped with AED machines can bring front-line emergency cardiac care to thousands of patients who would otherwise have to wait for arrival at the hospital to benefit from this type of care.

Although using an AED is much simpler than using a manual monitor/defibrillator, it is not without its rules and procedures. Before an AED can be employed, the EMS responder must first assess the patient's condition and establish that he is indeed unresponsive and pulseless. CPR should be provided while the AED is obtained and being readied for use. Each EMS system establishes standard practices, or "protocols," for the EMS personnel who are operating the AEDs. These protocols are designed to allow prompt defibrillation of patients who have confirmed circulatory arrest due to ventricular fibrillation or pulseless ventricular tachycardia, while insuring that inappropriate or unwanted usage is avoided. Protocols vary from service to service and are customized according to the type of equipment utilized. The protocols typically spell out who can use the machine and when, how to operate it, how to document each usage, and the frequency of use or supervised practice that is required. Most AED machines have a cassette recording or some type of computerized memory module or chip that can replay the patient's EKG, provide information as to energy levels and shocks delivered, and in some cases even the voices of the responders during the resuscitation.

The most common protocol for AED defibrillation is to deliver up to three sets of three shocks each before beginning transport. The first shock is delivered at 200 joules, followed immediately by having the AED re-analyze the rhythm but *NOT* by having the EMT check for a palpable carotid pulse. Pulse checks are *NOT* performed after the first two shocks in each set of three due to the potential for delay and operator errors, unless the "no shock needed" message is displayed. The AED's "analysis" phase must be performed without anyone touching the patient. Following a defibrillatory shock, the heart enters a brief period of "stunned" asystole — that is, the electrical current briefly stops all muscular activity. Immediately following those few seconds of inactivity, the heart resumes muscular activity: either a rhythmic functional beat of some type, or continued asystole, or a non-functional a-rhythmic fibrillation. In either of the first two cases, the AED will signal "no shock needed/check patient" and will *NOT* begin the sequence for delivering another shock. The EMT should assess for a palpable carotid pulse and act accordingly: if a pulse is palpated, assess breathing and support ventilation and oxygenation; if a pulse is not detected, perform CPR for one minute before having the AED again analyze the patient's cardiac activity.

Only if the AED detects fibrillation will it prepare to deliver a second shock of 200–300 joules. Following the second shock the AED is again allowed to analyze the patient's cardiac activity, and if fibrillation is detected it will deliver or call for a third shock at no more than 360 joules. After the third shock the machine is not again put in "Analyze" mode, but the patient *is* checked for a palpable carotid pulse. If no pulse is felt, CPR is performed for one minute and then the patient's cardiac activity is re-analyzed by the AED.

A second set of three shocks, usually all delivered at 360 joules or the last highest setting, are then delivered with AED analysis again after the first two shocks. A pulse is again palpated after the third shock *(but NOT the first two)*. If the patient remains pulseless, perform CPR for another minute and then repeat the sequence of analyzing and defibrillating for three more shocks.

If the patient remains pulseless and unresponsive after nine shocks (some protocols call for only two sets of three shocks), the decision should be made to initiate transport to the nearest qualified ACLS facility.

The AED must never be allowed to "analyze" the patient's cardiac activity while being moved — whether on an ambulance stretcher or while the vehicle is being driven. "Road noise" artifact has been proven to confuse AED's into interpreting this muscle movement as fibrillation and incorrectly calling for or delivering a shock. While some protocols allow the AED to be left "on" during transport and simply not operated in the "analyze" mode, a much safer procedure is to simply turn the entire unit off during transport.

Local protocols differ as to whether or not an AED-level service should stop during transport to allow the AED to re-analyze the patient's cardiac activity, however the prevailing opinion appears to be that if the patient has not responded to the two or three sets of three shocks, he probably will not revive without the addition of ACLS-level treatment. Many protocols require or strongly suggest that when an AED service is transporting a patient who did not respond to the initial sets of three shocks, an "intercept" be made with a paramedic-level service whenever this will hasten the delivery of ACLS treatment. A patient who has not responded to defibrillation is either beyond help or needs the ventilation and medication treatments available through ACLS-level care, and the sooner that therapy can be made available the better the patient's chances are. The decision as to whether or not to interrupt transport to allow the AED to re-analyze the patient's cardiac activity is usually left to on-line medical direction on a case-by-case basis.

On rare occasions the EMT is justified in either interrupting the defibrillation process (of a fully automatic AED) or not heeding the "shock indicated" instruction (of a semi-automatic AED). Generally speaking, current models of AED are well-designed and very reliable — but the EMT must not blindly follow the machine's directions in every case.

The first reason to interfere with the delivery of a shock results from an error on the part of the EMT — the machine has been allowed to "analyze" a patient whose body is being moved or transported, or who has not been confirmed as being pulseless. When the AED announces the decision to deliver a shock, the EMT in charge must inactivate the AED before a shock can be delivered.

Hypothermic patients (core temperatures below 85°F) are not known to respond well to defibrillation — and the electrical charge may even be harmful to frozen cells. The American Heart Association's guideline for such patients is to deliver up to three shocks if called for by the AED, but then to halt AED intervention if the patient does not respond at that point and continue with only CPR and rewarming attempts until an advanced treatment facility can be reached.

Major trauma patients who suffer cardiac arrest as a result of their injuries are also not candidates for defibrillation. Their best chances for survival hinge on an early and "all around" approach that includes spinal immobilization, airway management and ventilation and oxygenation, chest compressions, hemorrhage control, *and then* defibrillation if ventricular fibrillation is present.

The EMT in charge of a fully automatic AED is also responsible for making sure that everyone near the patient is indeed "clear" when the machine announces that it will deliver a shock. If everyone cannot be cleared, the EMT must turn off the unit or otherwise interrupt the delivery of the shock. When using a semi-automatic machine, the EMT in charge must make a verbal announcement and visually scan the patient's body to verify that everyone is clear before activating the machine to deliver the shock. The procedure, described earlier, is exactly the same as would be done with a manual defibrillator.

The procedures described in this Introduction and in the following sub-sections on using fully automatic and semi-automatic AEDs presume that the operator is an "EMT-D" — that is, *NOT* someone trained in full rhythm recognition and the ACLS algorithms of the American Heart Association. Certainly, AEDs can be used effectively by EMT-Paramedics and other ACLS providers, and many semi-automatic machines include at least the capability of displaying the patient's cardiac rhythm if they can not be converted to fully manual use as well.

ALS

USING THE AUTOMATIC DEFIBRILLATOR (EMT-D)

Assess the patient and confirm that he is unresponsive and does not have a palpable carotid pulse. Also confirm, in accordance with your local protocols, that the patient is a candidate for resuscitation. In some areas, "advance directives" may dictate that a patient is not to be revived. If the patient is pulseless, begin CPR while the AED is being brought to the patient's side. Take all appropriate body substance isolation precautions.

1. Place the device close to the patient's left ear. The principal operator should work from the left side of the patient. Better access to the defibrillator controls and placement of the defibrillator pads on the chest is achieved with the AED and the operator in these positions. Confirm that adequate ventilation and chest compressions are being performed.

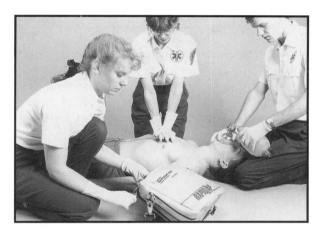

2. Turn the power ON and make sure the tape recorder or memory module is functioning. If the machine has a voice recorder, identify yourself and your EMS unit and briefly describe the clinical situation. Report each step as it is being performed. Verbally report as the shocks are delivered, even though the machine will log these also. Provide a continuous explanation of the actions taking place, decision to transport, problems, etc. that occur during the course of the resuscitation.

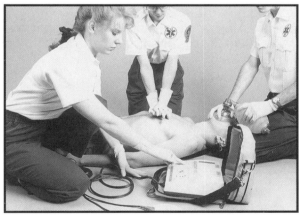

3. Attach the adhesive defibrillation pads to the patient's chest. The white or sternum pad goes just to the right of the sternum with its top edge touching the bottom of the clavicle.

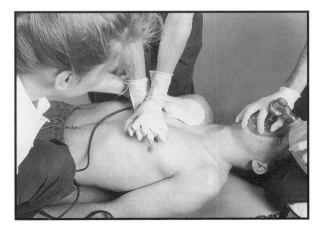

4. The red or Apex pad is positioned at the lower left chest, at the anterior axillary line but above the distal margin of the ribs.

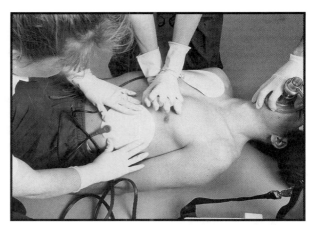

5. Direct that CPR be stopped and verify that everyone is physically clear of the patient. Although there is no danger of being shocked at this time, it is essential to the proper operation of the rhythm recognition system that the patient be as still as possible and that he not be touched by anyone during this time. If the patient is being transported in the ambulance, the vehicle should pull to the side of the road and be completely stopped during this step.

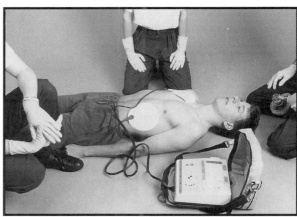

6. While the machine is assessing the patient's rhythm, it is important that none touch the patient. Assessment should take less than 30 seconds.

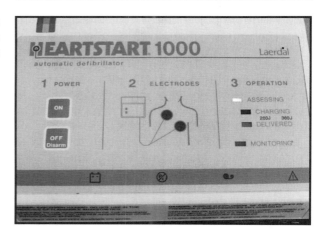

7. If a fully automatic AED detects a "shockable" rhythm according to its software protocols, it will indicate that a shock is needed by announcing a warning to "stand back" and remain clear of the patient. Some machines will also announce the rhythm, such as "V-Fib, stand back, stand back!," while it is charging the defibrillator.

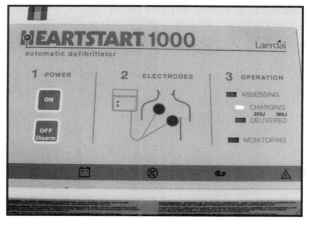

8. After several warnings, a fully automated machine will deliver the first shock. Follow the voice or displayed instructions of the AED exactly to prevent any hazards to the operator or patient.

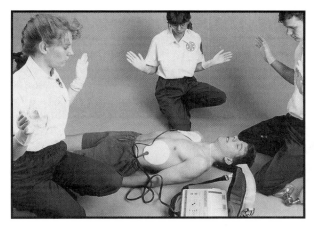

9. If for any reason it is not safe for the AED to deliver a shock, turn off the AED to interrupt the process of delivering a shock until it is safe to do so.

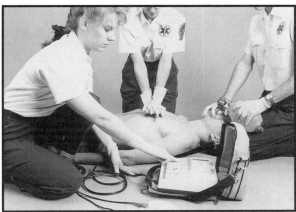

10. After a shock has been delivered, the machine will revert to its analyzing mode. If a treatable (shockable) rhythm is still detected, the device will again announce a warning, charge the defibrillator to the energy level established in the software protocol, and deliver the next shock. It is most important that none touch the patient during this time. *DO NOT* check for a palpable carotid pulse at this time.

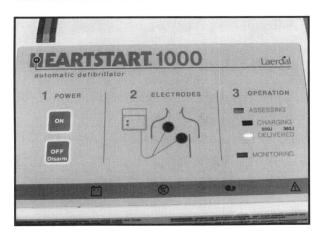

11. If the AED signals "check patient" or "no shock indicated," THEN check for a palpable carotid pulse. If the patient is pulseless, resume CPR according to AHA standards for cardiac arrest resuscitation. Follow your local protocols for how often you should return to the AED for additional rhythm analysis and possible defibrillation, and when you should initiate transport.

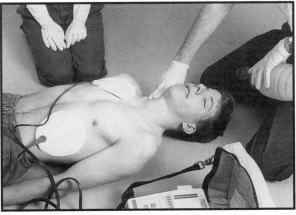

ALS

USING THE SEMI-AUTOMATIC DEFIBRILLATOR (EMT-D)

Assess the patient and confirm the absence of a carotid pulse. Also confirm, in accordance with your local protocols, that the patient is a candidate for resuscitation. In some areas, "advance directives" may dictate that a patient is not to be revived. If the patient is pulseless, begin CPR while the SAED is being brought to the patient's side. Take all appropriate body substance isolation precautions.

1. Place the device close to the patient's left ear. Turn the power ON and make sure the tape recorder or memory module is functioning. If the machine has a voice recorder, identify yourself and your EMS unit and briefly describe the clinical situation. Report each step as it is being performed. Verbally report as the shocks are delivered, even though the machine will log these also. Provide a continuous explanation of the actions taking place, decision to transport, problems, etc. that occur during the course of the resuscitation.

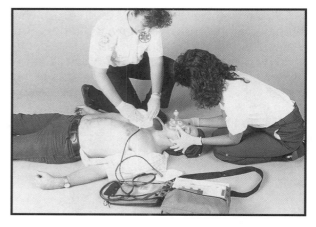

2. Attach the adhesive defibrillation pads with their cables to the patient's chest. If the cables are color-coded, be sure to attach them correctly. The white or sternum pad goes just to the right of the sternum with its top edge touching the bottom of the clavicle.

3. The red or Apex pad is positioned at the lower left chest, at the anterior axillary line but above the distal margin of the ribs.

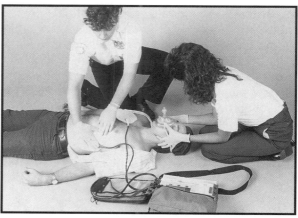

4. Direct that CPR be stopped and verify that everyone is physically clear of the patient. Although there is no danger of being shocked at this time, it is essential to the proper operation of the rhythm recognition system that the patient be as still as possible and that he not be touched by anyone during this time. If the patient is being transported in the ambulance, the vehicle should pull to the side of the road and be completely stopped during this step. Once this has been done press the "Analyze" control switch on the SAED.

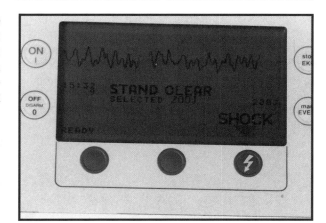

5. While the machine is assessing the patient's rhythm, it is important that no one touch the patient. Assessment should take less than 20 seconds. If a semi-automatic AED detects a "shockable" rhythm according to its software protocols, it will call for the EMT to deliver the shock by pushing the "shock" or "defibrillate" button.

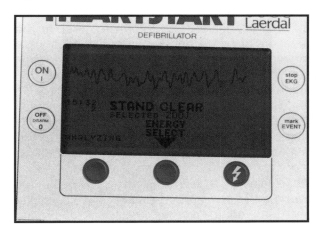

6. Follow your local protocols for energy level settings when a shock is to be delivered. Assure that everyone is clear of the patient by using the same warning announcement recommended for manual defibrillation — "One, I'm clear; Two, you're clear; Three, we're all clear."

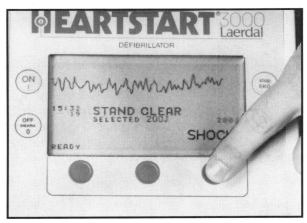

7. As soon as possible after the SAED calls for a shock and everyone is clear, push the "shock" button to defibrillate the patient. The only reasons to interrupt the process would be if someone could not get clear or if you realized that the patient was being transported and that the SAED should never have been put in "analyze" mode.

8. As soon as the first shock is delivered, push the "analyze" button and keep everyone clear of the patient. *DO NOT* check for a palpable carotid pulse at this time.

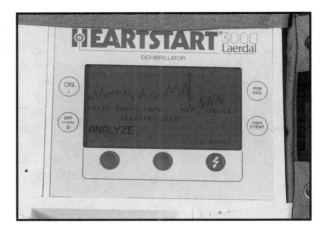

9. If the SAED signals "check patient" or "no shock indicated," *THEN* check for a palpable carotid pulse. If the patient is pulseless, resume CPR according to AHA standards for cardiac arrest resuscitation. Follow your local protocols for how often you should return to the SAED for additional rhythm analysis and possible defibrillation, and when you should initiate transport.

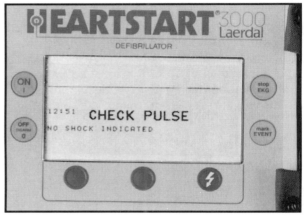

10. If the SAED signals that a shock is indicated first assure that everyone is clear of the patient and out of danger. If your protocol calls for an increase in energy level for the second shock, adjust the machine accordingly. Then push the button to deliver the shock. Following the delivery of the second shock, again immediately push the "analyze" button and keep everyone clear of the patient. *DO NOT* assess for a palpable carotid pulse unless the SAED advises "no shock indicated." If the SAED announces that a third shock is indicated, again assure that everyone is clear of the patient and make any necessary energy level adjustments.

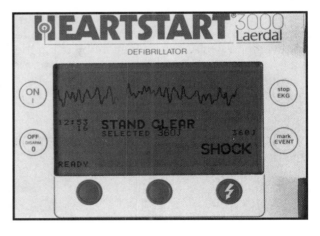

11. Following delivery of the third shock, *DO NOT* push the "analyze" button but *DO* assess the patient for a palpable carotid pulse. If the patient is pulseless, perform CPR for one minute and then begin the second set of three shocks before again pausing to perform one minute of CPR. Use the energy level setting last used — do not reset the SAED to its initial setting. If your protocol includes a third set of shocks before transporting, and the patient remains pulseless after the second set of three shocks has been delivered and followed by a minute of CPR, deliver the third set and then initiate transport to the nearest ACLS facility.

ALS

ETI SUMMARY SKILL SHEET
Manual Cardiac Monitoring And Defibrillation

1. Determine that the SCENE IS SAFE and TAKE all indicated BODY SUBSTANCE ISOLATION PRECAUTIONS.

2. ASSESS the patient's RESPONSIVENESS and AIRWAY, and whether or not the patient is BREATHING and has a palpable PULSE.

3. IF the patient is UNRESPONSIVE AND PULSELESS,BEGIN CPR and BRING the MONITOR-DEFIBRILLATOR TO the PATIENT'S side.

4. TURN the "lead select" SWITCH TO PADDLES mode. Position the monitor properly.

5. BARE the patient's CHEST. PLACE the STERNUM PADDLE OVER the patient's UPPER RIGHT ANTERIOR CHEST WALL and place the APEX PADDLE OVER the LOWER LEFT ANTERIOR CHEST WALL. APPLY firm PRESSURE to both paddles.

6. LOOK AT the MONITOR to ASSESS the RHYTHM while keeping the paddles and cables as motionless as possible.

7. IF the monitor screen shows ASYSTOLE, VERIFY that the "Lead select" SWITCH IS IN "PADDLES" mode. VERIFY ASYSTOLE BY VIEWING a DIFFERENT AXIS of the heart. MOVE ONE PADDLE to a different location on the chest and verify if asystole still appears or if fine ventricular fibrillation can be detected.

8. If the rhythm is not one that should be defibrillated or cardioverted, RETURN both PADDLES TO their HOLDERS and prepare to monitor through the CABLED LEADS. This provides a better quality of image for the monitor and is less subject to interference when the ambulance is moving.

9. CONNECT an adhesive ELECTRODE TO each of the three cable LEADS and, if the patient is extremely diaphoretic, wipe the skin dry before applying the electrodes.

10. Attach the WHITE LEAD TO the patient's UPPER RIGHT CHEST, attach the RED LEAD to the patient's LOWER LEFT SIDE, and the remaining BLACK (or green) LEAD TO the patient's UPPER LEFT CHEST.

11. CHANGE the "LEAD Select" CONTROL on the monitor from "Paddles" TO "LEAD II" and EVALUATE the rhythm DISPLAY. If the image seems distorted but the patient is responsive, inspect the cable and lead connections. If you initially see asystole, immediately confirm that you have changed the Lead Select control from the "Paddles" position.

12. TO VIEW the heart's activity through A SECOND LEAD simply CHANGE the SETTING on the "Lead Select" switch from Lead II to either Lead I or Lead III. Be careful not to switch to "Paddles" unless you actually have them on the patient's chest.

13. TO create a PRINTed RECORD of the cardiac rhythm, simply DEPRESS the "RECORD" BUTTON on the monitor. Allow at least ten seconds of recording time, and write the time and the patient's last name on the paper.

14. TO DEFIBRILLATE a patient, remove the paddles from their holder and APPLY conductive GEL TO the electrode plates on the PADDLES OR PLACE DEFIBRILLATION pads OR SALINE-soaked gauze PADS ON the patient's CHEST where the paddles will be placed.

15. PLACE the "STERNUM" PADDLE ON the patient's RIGHT ANTERIOR CHEST wall and PLACE the "APEX" PADDLE to the LEFT OF the patient's LEFT NIPPLE.

16. Push the "power on" button on the side of the "Sternum" paddle to TURN ON the DEFIBRILLATOR. When the defibrillator function is enabled the green light next to the button will illuminate.

17. SELECT the ENERGY LEVEL — typically 200 joules for the first unsynchronized shock in adults and 2 joules per kilogram in children.

18. Press the "Charge" button on the Apex paddle to CHARGE THE DEFIBRILLATOR. You should hear an increasing tone and see the amber light flashing. When the tone stops and the amber light stays lit, indicating that the unit is charged, verbally instruct ALL PERSONNEL to "CLEAR" the area around the patient.

19. VIEW the MONITOR to verify the rhythm AND visually SCAN to ensure that all are clear.

20. PRESS FIRMLY against the patient's skin WITH the PADDLES to assure good electrical contact, and THEN PRESS the RED BUTTONS at the front of each paddle simultaneously TO deliver the SHOCK.

21. After the shock has been delivered, and while you still MAINTAIN PADDLE PLACEMENT, SELECT the desired ENERGY LEVEL for the next shock in the event that one must be delivered (usually between 200 and 300 joules for a second shock in adults and 4 joules per kilogram for second and subsequent shocks in children). PRESS the CHARGE BUTTON to begin the process of re-charging the defibrillator.

22. REASSESS the RHYTHM for any changes. Depending upon your protocol, you may wish to CHECK FOR a carotid PULSE WHILE the CHARGING process continues.

23. If a "shockable" rhythm remains, REPEAT the "CLEAR" WARNING AND SCAN to assure that all personnel are clear and DISCHARGE the PADDLES AGAIN. Be sure to maintain firm pressure on the paddles against the patient's skin.

24. MAINTAIN PADDLE PLACEMENT fand SELECT the desired ENERGY LEVEL for the next shock (usually 360 joules in adults for the third shock and 4 joules per kilogram for children). PRESS the CHARGE BUTTON to begin the process of re-charging the defibrillator.

25. REASSESS the RHYTHM for any changes and CHECK for a carotid PULSE while charging.

26. If a "shockable" rhythm remains, REPEAT the "CLEAR" WARNING AND visual SCAN, and DISCHARGE the PADDLES again.

27. RE-ASSESS the RHYTHM and PALPATE for a carotid PULSE.

28. IF the patient remains PULSELESS, RE-INSTITUTE CPR. CONTINUE TO FOLLOW the appropriate ACLS algorithm for the rhythm being displayed.

29. If the patient's condition requires treatment by synchronized cardioversion, first be sure that MONITORing is being done THROUGH the CABLE LEADS and that defibrillation electrode pads or CONDUCTIVE PADS are in place OR that the skin is protected with conductive GEL where the paddles will be placed. If the patient is conscious, CONSIDER the use of SEDATION to lessen the pain and memory of the event.

   a. Press the power button on the sternum paddle to TURN THE DEFIBRILLATOR ON and SELECT the desired ENERGY SETTING on the apex paddle.

   b. Push the "charge" button on the Apex paddle to charge the unit, and wait until the light and sound verify that charging has been completed.

   c. PUSH the SYNCHRONIZER BUTTON until the red button lights up. The light should be flashing, indicating that the monitor has identified the "R" wave of the QRS complex.

   d. ADJUST the EKG SIZE button if necessary until the light begins to flash. Without the synchronizer button flashing, the paddles will not discharge.

   e. Visually and verbally "CLEAR" THE AREA around the patient just as you would with unsynchronized defibrillation. Once everyone is away from the patient, PRESS the DISCHARGE BUTTONS at the front of each paddle AND HOLD THEM "PUSHED."

   f. Once the shock is delivered, ASSESS the RHYTHM and determine if another cardioversion shock is needed. If so, repeat the same steps using the next energy level per your protocol.

30. After use of the monitor/defibrillator on the patient has been completed, ALLOW THE BATTERY(ies) TO RUN for a considerable period of time to get "exercised." VISUALLY INSPECT the equipment FOR CLEANLINESS AND DAMAGE. CHECK the CABLES AND CORDS for cracks or frays in the insulation and STORE THEM APPROPRIATELY as suggested by the manufacturer.

31. If the defibrillator was used, EXAMINE the PADDLES to be sure they are clean and dry and free of cracks and pitting. RESET the ENERGY select SWITCH TO 200 joules.

32. REPLACE all used MONITORING ELECTRODES AND DEFIBRILLATOR PADS. RESTOCK the conductive GEL if any was used.

33. CHECK that the STRIP RECORDER works properly and VERIFY that there is ADEQUATE PAPER for the strip chart recorder. Also VERIFY that a SPARE ROLL of paper is carried in the storage pouch.

34. REPLACE any USED BATTERIES.

35. Finally, STORE the equipment IN its PROPER LOCATION, READY FOR IMMEDIATE USE when next needed.

ALS

ETI SUMMARY SKILL SHEET
EMT-D Use of a Manual Monitor/Defibrillator

1. CONFIRM that PATIENT is UNRESPONSIVE AND PULSELESS.

2. BEGIN CPR while the monitor/defibrillator is being brought to the patient's side. TAKE all appropriate body substance ISOLATION PRECAUTIONS.

3. PLACE the MONITOR/DEFIBRILLATOR CLOSE TO the patient's LEFT EAR FOR better access to the controls and chest.

4. CONFIRM that ADEQUATE CPR is BEING PERFORMED.

5. TURN the MONITOR ON and ACTIVATE the RECORDER. If it includes voice recording, IDENTIFY YOURSELF and BRIEFLY DESCRIBE the clinical SITUATION AND EACH STEP as it is performed.

6. REMOVE THE PADDLES FROM THEIR HOLDER and PLACE them in the proper positions ON the patient's CHEST. Maintain firm even pressure with the paddles against the patient's skin.

7. STOP CPR and VERIFY that EVERYONE is CLEAR of the patient.

8. LOOK AT monitor SCREEN and ASSESS the RHYTHM.

9. IF the RHYTHM is NOT one that is "SHOCKABLE" and the patient remains pulseless, RESUME CPR FOR ONE MINUTE and then re-analyze the rhythm. If a "shockable" rhythm is not identified after three intervals of CPR, continue CPR and prepare the patient for transport.

10. IF you detect a "SHOCKABLE" RHYTHM, press the green button on the Sternum paddle to TURN ON THE DEFIBRILLATOR.

11. APPLY CONDUCTIVE GEL OR PADS TO the patient's CHEST where the paddles will be placed.

12. ADJUST the ENERGY LEVEL to 200 JOULES with the control on the Apex paddle. (For children, set the level to 2 joules/kg).

13. CHARGE THE DEFIBRILLATOR by pushing the amber "Charge" button on the Apex paddle. When the whine stops and the amber light remains constantly lit, the selected charge level has been reached. PLACE the PADDLES ON the patient's CHEST and apply firm pressure against the chest wall.

14. Direct all personnel to CLEAR THE AREA around the patient and visually make sure that no one is touching the patient.

15. PUSH BOTH RED discharge BUTTONS on the paddles to deliver the shock. KEEP the PADDLES ON the CHEST AFTER the SHOCK is delivered.

16. Immediately CHANGE THE ENERGY LEVEL TO the NEXT SETTING, usually between 200 and 300 joules for adults and 4 joules/kg for children, and PUSH THE CHARGE BUTTON.

17. LOOK AT the monitor SCREEN and ASSESS the RHYTHM.

18. IF a SHOCKABLE RHYTHM is IDENTIFIED, CLEAR THE AREA around the patient and DELIVER the SECOND SHOCK.

19. KEEP the PADDLES ON the CHEST AFTER the SHOCK is delivered.

20. Immediately CHANGE THE ENERGY LEVEL TO the NEXT SETTING, usually 360 joules for adults and 4 joules/kg for children, and PUSH THE CHARGE BUTTON.

21. LOOK AT the monitor SCREEN and ASSESS the RHYTHM.

22. IF a SHOCKABLE RHYTHM is IDENTIFIED, CLEAR THE AREA around the patient and DELIVER the THIRD SHOCK.

23. ASSESS the patient's carotid PULSE and IF ABSENT, RESUME CPR for one minute.

24. AFTER ONE MINUTE of CPR, PLACE the PADDLES ON the patient's CHEST AND RE-ANALYZE the RHYTHM.

25. IF the rhythm is SHOCKABLE, REPEAT the SEQUENCE OF DELIVERING THREE SHOCKS as before, but with the ENERGY LEVEL for each shock SET AT 360 JOULES.

26. IF the patient is STILL PULSELESS AFTER the SECOND SET OF THREE SHOCKS, again PERFORM ONE MINUTE OF CPR.

27. AFTER ONE MINUTE of CPR, PLACE the PADDLES ON the patient's CHEST AND RE-ANALYZE the RHYTHM.

28. IF the rhythm is SHOCKABLE, REPEAT the SEQUENCE OF DELIVERING THREE SHOCKS as before, with the ENERGY LEVEL SET AT 360 JOULES.

29. IF the patient is STILL PULSELESS AFTER the THIRD SET OF THREE SHOCKS, RESUME CPR and PREPARE FOR TRANSPORT. RETURN THE PADDLES TO their HOLDER to avoid damaging the electrode surface.

30. FOLLOW your LOCAL PROTOCOL ABOUT IF AND WHEN TO RE-ANALYZE DURING TRANSPORT.

ALS

ETI SUMMARY SKILL SHEET
EMT-D Use of an Automated Defibrillator (AED) — Automatic or Semi-Automatic

1. CONFIRM that PATIENT is UNRESPONSIVE AND PULSELESS and not in a moving vehicle.

2. BEGIN CPR while the monitor/defibrillator is being brought to the patient's side. TAKE all appropriate body substance ISOLATION PRECAUTIONS.

3. PLACE the MONITOR/DEFIBRILLATOR CLOSE TO the patient's LEFT EAR FOR better access to the controls and chest.

4. CONFIRM that ADEQUATE CPR is BEING PERFORMED.

5. TURN the MONITOR ON and ACTIVATE the RECORDER. IDENTIFY YOURSELF and BRIEFLY DESCRIBE the clinical SITUATION AND EACH STEP as it is performed.

6. ATTACH the ADHESIVE DEFIBRILLATION PADS TO the patient's CHEST. ATTACH the defibrillator CABLES TO the adhesive PADS.

7. STOP CPR AND CLEAR EVERYONE from around the patient.

8. If there is one, PRESS the "ANALYZE" control SWITCH.

9. FOLLOW the AED's voice or displayed INSTRUCTIONS exactly TO PREVENT any HAZARDS to the operator or patient. ASSURE that EVERYONE is CLEAR of the patient WHEN the AED is ANALYZING.

10. IF at any time in the following sequence the "NO SHOCK INDICATED" message is given, ASSESS the patient for a palpable carotid PULSE and IF it is ABSENT PERFORM CPR for one minute, THEN HAVE the AED RE-ANALYZE the patient's RHYTHM. IF the AED SIGNALS "NO SHOCK INDICATED" AND the PATIENT REMAINS PULSELESS, RESUME CPR and follow your protocol for how often you should return to the AED for additional rhythm analysis and possible defibrillation, AND when you should initiate TRANSPORT.

11. IF the "SHOCK INDICATED" message is given, VERIFY that EVERYONE IS CLEAR of the patient and that it is safe for the shock to be delivered. If it is not, turn off the AED or otherwise interrupt the process of delivering a shock until it is safe to do so. IF USING a SEMI-AUTOMATIC AED, PUSH the "SHOCK" BUTTON WHEN you have verified IT IS SAFE to do so.

12. AFTER the first SHOCK is DELIVERED, PUSH the "ANALYZE" BUTTON on a semi-automatic machine and KEEP EVERYONE CLEAR of the patient. DO NOT CHECK for a palpable carotid PULSE at this time.

13. IF the AED SIGNALS that a SECOND SHOCK is INDICATED, first ASSURE that EVERYONE IS CLEAR of the patient and out of danger.

14. IF your PROTOCOL CALLS FOR an INCREASE IN ENERGY level for the second shock, ADJUST the MACHINE ACCORDINGLY if this is not incorporated in its software.

15. WHEN USING a FULLY AUTOMATIC AED, INTERRUPT the machine IF it is NOT SAFE FOR the SHOCK to be delivered. WHEN USING a SEMI-AUTOMATIC AED and it is charged and everyone is clear, PUSH the shock BUTTON TO deliver the SHOCK.

16. AFTER the SECOND SHOCK, again IMMEDIATELY PUSH the "ANALYZE" BUTTON on a semi-automatic machine and KEEP EVERYONE CLEAR of the patient. DO NOT CHECK for a palpable carotid PULSE unless the AED advises "no shock indicated."

17. IF the AED CALLS FOR a THIRD shock, again ASSURE that EVERYONE is CLEAR of the patient and MAKE any necessary ENERGY LEVEL ADJUSTMENTS.

18. WHEN USING a FULLY AUTOMATIC AED, INTERRUPT the machine IF it is NOT SAFE for the SHOCK to be delivered. WHEN USING a SEMI-AUTOMATIC AED and it is charged and everyone is clear, PUSH the shock BUTTON TO deliver the SHOCK.

19. AFTER the THIRD SHOCK, DO NOT push the "ANALYZE" button but DO CHECK the patient for a palpable carotid PULSE.

20. IF the patient is PULSELESS, PERFORM CPR FOR ONE MINUTE and THEN BEGIN the SECOND SET OF THREE SHOCKS before again pausing to perform one minute of CPR. Use the energy level setting last used — do not reset the AED to its initial setting. If your protocol includes a third set of shocks before transporting, and the patient remains pulseless after the second set of three shocks has been delivered and followed by a minute of CPR, deliver the third set and then initiate transport to the nearest ACLS facility.

SECTION

Hemorrhage Control and Shock Management Skills

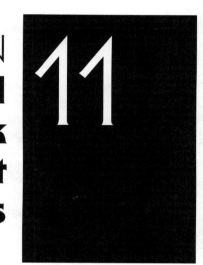

Introduction

Shock and hemorrhage control should be considered together since a patient with any significant blood loss will be in shock. Although commonly associated with blood loss, shock can also result from other pathological mechanisms even when no hemorrhage has occurred.

HEMORRHAGE CONTROL

Bleeding from a lacerated blood vessel is primarily caused by the greater pressure inside the vessel than outside of it. Significant bleeding will continue until the intravascular pressure is approximately equal to or less than the extravascular pressure. This can occur without intervention when the systolic blood pressure becomes so low that at each pulse surge the intravascular pressure is approximately equal to or less than that exerted against the outside of the vessel by the muscles, organs or other tissue surrounding it. The difference in pressure can also be reduced or eliminated—regardless of changes in the blood pressure—by treatments which increase the extravascular pressure. The application of *direct pressure* over a wound increases the pressure outside of the injured blood vessels to a higher level than that inside them, and in almost all cases will stop the bleeding. Although some of the external pressure is dissipated as tissue between the skin and the vessel reshapes and moves, most of it is reflected against the underlying vessels. This, together with the "static" pressure brought by the bones, organs, and other tissue underlying the vessels, results in increased pressure against the vessels. When the pressure reflected against a severed vessel is significantly greater than that of the fluid pumped through it, the vessel will be squeezed shut—obstructing further distal blood flow and controlling the bleeding. Even if the vessel is not completely shut, its size will be significantly reduced. The flow of blood through a vessel is reduced by four times the reduction in its size, therefore even if some flow continues it will be significantly less.

A second effort of increasing the pressure surrounding a breached vessel is that it produces a form of "back pressure" against the blood exiting from the vessel. This promotes tamponading and further reduces the flow of blood from the opening. Thirdly, when the vascular wall is squeezed it reduces the tissue tension which has been keeping the breach open, thereby reducing the size of the opening and the loss of blood through it. Because of these three simultaneous effects, direct pressure is effective in controlling most external bleeding. When these same factors are applied using the Pneumatic Anti-Shock Garment, most internal bleeding located under the garment can also be controlled. Direct pressure should be used to control bleeding from open fractures as with any other wound. It should not be bypassed because fractured bone ends are protruding from the wound, but care must be taken to assure that any sharp bone ends do not pierce the EMT's glove or skin.

When applying direct pressure, sterile gauze dressings should be placed directly over the wound and the area immediately adjacent to it and firmly held in place by the EMT's gloved hand. The layers of gauze provide a framework which promotes clotting and, once in place, should generally not be removed. If they become saturated, several additional layers should be added instead.

Large gaping wounds, except when in the cranium, may require packing with sterile gauze dressings as well as the application of direct pressure over them to control the various sources of bleeding commonly associated with such large wounds. After significant bleeding has been successfully stopped with direct manual pressure over the gauze dressing and wound, the EMT's gloved hand should be replaced by a pressure bandage over the dressing. Care must be taken to assure that this bandage is neither so loose that bleeding resumes nor so tight that it becomes a tourniquet. Once applied a pressure bandage should be checked frequently to ensure that progressive swelling or edema do not cause it to impair or occlude the distal circulation.

When bleeding is from an extremity, as well as applying direct pressure the EMT should elevate the limb (above the heart) to help reduce the blood flow in the extremity. Even though this is of significant benefit in supine patients, it is particularly important in seated patients. In seated patients the force of gravity increases the flow of blood (and therefore the bleeding in inferiorly-positioned extremities), whereas if the limb is elevated the blood must circulate *against* the force of gravity. This produces some reduction in the distal circulation and bleeding. Maintaining as much elevation of the wound as is practical should be a consideration once a pressure dressing has been applied and the patient is being packaged.

In most cases where movement of a blood vessel (or its location) prevents direct external pressure from being effectively referred against it, significant bleeding can continue despite the application of direct pressure. In such cases, while maintaining direct pressure, the EMT must further reduce the flow of blood by adding pressure at a *second* more proximal location on the injured blood vessel or the vessels supplying it. *Pressure points* have been identified at numerous locations throughout the body where vessels lie near a bone and where there is a minimum of tissue between them and the skin. Firm pressure applied over the vessel at a pressure point will reduce the vessel's size — significantly limiting or occluding the flow of blood through it. Generally, the pressure squeezing the vessel against the bone is best applied using the fingertips in order to limit the area pressed and to concentrate the pressure directly over the vessel and underlying bone. When applying pressure over the femoral artery use of the heel of the hand is generally required instead due to its location and the muscles overlying it.

In the rare case when simultaneous use of direct pressure, elevation, and pressure on a proximal pressure point fail to control significant extremity bleeding, a tourniquet is used. Application of a tourniquet generally stops the flow of all blood in the limb distal to its placement and may jeopardize the ultimate survival of the limb. ***A tourniquet is only used when otherwise uncontrollable significant bleeding threatens the patient's life.***

A tourniquet can be made from a 3–4 inch wide cravat bandage, a blood pressure cuff, or a wide buckled strap especially designed for such use. In the rare case that a tourniquet is needed on a call, EMS services generally use a BP cuff for this purpose. The tourniquet is placed on the limb 1 to 2 inches proximal to the bleeding site at a location where the tourniquet is not over or immediately adjacent to a joint. When a bleeding site on the lower leg or lower arm is within approximately 2 or 3 inches of the knee or elbow, or at either of these joints, the tourniquet should be placed 2 or 3 inches proximal to the joint on the thigh or upper arm, respectively. Once the tourniquet has been properly placed it is tightened (inflated if a BP cuff) until just beyond the point when the bleeding is stopped. It is then secured so that it will not loosen. When the tourniquet is tightened it increases the pressure on the blood vessels underlying it, progressively occluding blood vessels inward from the surface of the skin to the vessels deep within the extremity. When the bleeding stops the arterial blood supply to the wound has been occluded and effective circulation (or often, all circulation) distal to the tourniquet has been stopped. *Once a tourniquet has been applied and tightened it is not released until at the hospital.* The length of time that a tourniquet remains in place is a key factor. The exact time that the tourniquet was applied should be recorded on the patient's skin in an easily visible location (usually the forehead) as well as on the tourniquet and on the run report.

A tourniquet should not be covered by bandages or otherwise masked from view unless absolutely necessary to the overall care of the patient. Since hemorrhage is identified and managed early in the initial assessment, fractures and other injuries may exist which have not yet been identified. The EMT's assessment prior to initiating transport should be limited to locating life-threatening injuries only, and he should *NOT* delay transport to perform a head-to-toe musculoskeletal exam. Instead, once all urgent ABC needs have been met the patient should be rapidly immobilized to a longboard. In this way all of the body is supported and immobilized, thereby protecting any fractures from harm without the unnecessary delay of identifying and splinting each individual fracture. Further detailed assessment and any fluid replacement should only be initiated once enroute. It is important that the EMT clearly identify in his radio report, his written report, and the verbal report he gives at the hospital that a tourniquet is in place, its specific location, and the time it was applied.

Whenever a tourniquet has been applied there is a possibility of permanent blood vessel and nerve damage and the chance that circulation in the limb cannot be restored. It must be emphasized that the need for a tourniquet is extremely rare. However, hemorrhage that can not be otherwise controlled presents an immediate threat to the patient's life and a tourniquet should *NOT* be avoided. In such cases the patient's survival must be placed above any possible loss of limb. When needed, the EMT should not hesitate to apply a blood pressure cuff as a tourniquet, since these distribute the pressure over a broad enough area to cause little or no permanent nerve, blood vessel, or tissue damage.

Capillary or minor venous bleeding will generally resolve itself prior to the EMT's arrival. If some small amount continues to issue from a wound, it can be stopped by placing gauze dressings over the site and securing them with a suitable bandage.

SHOCK AND ITS MANAGEMENT

Shock is most commonly defined as inadequate perfusion of the cells of the body with properly oxygenated blood. Although this limited definition is accurate to advanced stages of shock, it does not accurately describe the early phase of shock in which the body's defense mechanisms maintain adequate cellular perfusion.

Shock occurs when a localized injury or condition produces a body-wide circulatory deficit. If unchecked, shock is progressive and the circulatory deficit continues to advance at an increasing rate. When the deficit outstrips the body's compensatory mechanisms, the blood pressure falls below the minimum pressure needed to circulate blood components to surround the cells (hypotension), and inadequate cellular perfusion (hypoperfusion) results. When hypoperfusion is present, regardless of the adequacy of pulmonary oxygenation and blood oxygen levels, sufficient oxygen is not delivered to the cells and cellular hypoxia results. When an inadequate supply of oxygen is delivered to the cells, the cells switch from normal aerobic metabolism to anaerobic metabolism. The increased production of acids as a by-product of anaerobic metabolism makes the blood increasingly acidic and toxic (metabolic acidosis), prompting cell death. As cells begin to die in the vital organs, the organs' ability to function is reduced. The interactive effect of failing organs on each other (sometimes described as "hypoperfusion syndrome") further accelerates the patient's deterioration until such a level of toxicity and cell death has been reached that the shock is irreversible and profound vital organ death occurs — soon followed by the death of the patient. *Shock can be most accurately defined as a progressive systemic circulatory deficit which, when it becomes profound, will result in hypoperfusion, cellular hypoxia and anaerobic metabolism. If unchecked it will progress to cellular death and ultimately to the death of the vital organs and subsequently of the patient.*

The EMT's recognition and prompt intervention to counter shock are key to the patient's survival. After airway patency and adequate pulmonary ventilation, treatment that eliminates or limits the initial insult's further contribution to circulatory compromise becomes the EMT's top priority. As well as survival in the field, the EMT's recognition and treatment of shock can determine the patient's ultimate outcome. If shock progresses until vital organ hypoperfusion occurs, and then continues without cellular perfusion and oxygenation being restored in a relatively short time, even though the patient may survive to the hospital he will die days or weeks later from the irreversible damage which occurred in the first hours after the incident. How long shock can progress before it becomes so profound that the patient's defense mechanisms can no longer maintain adequate vital organ perfusion (decompensated shock) depends upon the patient's age, health and the nature and severity of its cause. Even though the body's defense mechanisms direct most of the available blood to the brain and other vial organs once hypotension commences (so that their perfusion is maintained the longest), trauma studies show that if hypoperfusion continues beyond the "Golden Hour" there is a marked reduction in the possibility of the patient's survival. Further, published studies show that survival rates drop geometrically for each few minutes that this time is extended.

Shock commences when there is a reduction in cardiac output. This may be due to reduced venous return or to a cardiac or central nervous system problem which reduces the heart's pumping ability. When this occurs the patient enters the early **compensated phase** of shock. In compensated shock the body's sympathetic defense mechanisms increase the heart rate and the volume pumped with each beat and cause the peripheral blood vessels to constrict. This restores the heart's output and directs the available blood to the vital organs. As a result, the patient becomes tachycardic and the skin becomes pale, cool, and moist. Throughout the compensatory phase of shock, these defense mechanisms maintain the blood pressure within the normal range. Since adequate cerebral perfusion is maintained, there is no significant change in level of consciousness. As shock advances the heart rate increases further and the skin becomes paler, cooler, and more moist. When the shock has become so profound that the defense mechanisms can no longer overcome the deficits, the patient enters the decompensated phase. At this point the blood pressure drops and, if it continues to decline, produces progressively lower levels of consciousness. As shock progresses, if the systolic blood pressure drops below 90mm Hg in a male adult, under 80mm Hg in a female, or under 70mm Hg in a child, and is accompanied by the other presenting signs and symptoms of shock, the patient should be considered to be in profound shock. Such blood pressure levels indicate that shock has progressed beyond the early compensated phase and that the patient has deteriorated into the decompensated phase. It is a *late* — rather than early — sign of shock. In otherwise healthy adult patients with hemorrhage, a loss of 30–40% of the blood's volume from the vascular system is required before the blood pressure will drop.

The preceding overview of the pathophysiology of shock has been included to provide a suitable context for the skills in this section. A more detailed discussion of the mechanisms of shock and its specific signs and symptoms will be found in the *Patient Assessment* section of this book and in the discussion of shock found in your primary textbook.

When shock progresses into the decompensated phase it results in impairment and collapse of all of the body's vital systems — requiring intervention for many of them. The EMT's treatment in the field, however, is of a more limited scope and will have to primarily focus on the cardiovascular and respiratory systems and, if needed, on protecting the musculoskeletal system from additional harm.

The presence and degree of shock should be identified early in the assessment. The general clinical presenting picture is found in the *Global Survey* of the patient, prior to identifying its causes or exact etiology. Once any airway or ventilation deficits, cardiac arrest or external hemorrhage have been ruled-out or managed, the EMT should provide the general support treatment for shock regardless of its exact cause. The patient should be placed in a supine position with his body horizontal and his legs elevated approximately 10 to 12 inches.

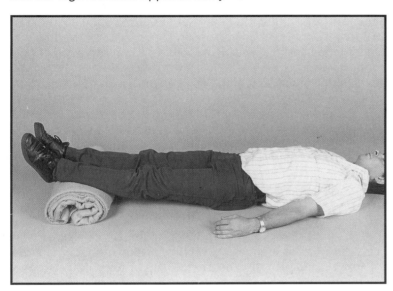

This *modified Trendelenburg position* places the head at the same level as the heart and with the legs higher than it. Since blood is a fluid, pumping it at the same level (height) is easier than pumping it to a higher level or height. Therefore, placing the patient's head and vital organs at essentially the same height as the heart maximizes venous return and reduces the cardiac effort required. Elevating the legs also directs the available circulating blood to the vital organs rather to the lower extremities. The classical position described by Trendelenburg places the patient in a fully supine position with the foot end of the bed elevated at least ten to twelve inches above the head end. This is *NOT* recommended as it causes the weight of the abdominal organs to press onto the diaphragm and promotes increased respiratory effort and distress. The previously described modified Trendelenburg position, with the head and torso horizontal and only the legs elevated, provides the same circulatory benefits without the possibility of increased respiratory impairment.

Since the circulation of blood to the cells is reduced as shock progresses, it is desirable to provide as much oxygen to the blood as possible to maximize the oxygen delivered to the cells when perfusion is compromised. Therefore, oxygen enrichment with an FiO_2 of between 0.85 and 1.00 should be provided to any patient in shock to help compensate for the circulatory deficit. By providing the highest possible percentage the EMT eliminates the need to evaluate how much the patient needs, and any excess is simply exhaled without any negative side effects.

When the body gets too hot or too cold, its thermoregulatory mechanisms cause the peripheral blood vessels to dilate (overriding any other stimulus causing them to constrict). Because the thermoregulatory controls can reverse the peripheral vasoconstriction generated by the sympathetic defense mechanisms, the treatment for shock must include preserving normal body temperature. As well as covering the patient to avoid evaporation and heat loss by radiation and convection, the EMT must insulate the patient from the cold ground to avoid heat loss through conduction. Patients in shock will lose heat even at room temperature, and require covering to retain body heat. Although assessment of the patient requires removing clothing to perform parts of the examination, heat loss must remain a concern and the area exposed and the length of the exposure should be limited in any environment where the ambient temperature is lower than normal body temperature. Heat is not added except in special circumstances, as too high a body temperature will also result in vasodilation. If the environment is exceptionally cold or wet, such as outside in rain or in cold winter climates, the initial care should include moving the patient rapidly into the ambulance's heated patient compartment once the most immediate ABC's have been managed and before further assessment and care are provided. ***Prolonging the shock patient's exposure to the elements in freezing temperatures, even for several minutes, can result in a significantly increased circulatory compromise, hypothermia, and certain death.*** In extremely hot environments the excessive temperature (and lying in the sun) can also result in vasodilation. To avoid this, in excessively hot situations the patient should (once the most immediate ABC needs have been met) be moved to cooler location or into the air conditioned ambulance.

Elevated blood CO_2 levels can similarly override the sympathetic vasoconstriction, resulting in vasodilation and increased levels of shock. The EMT must be sure that adequate ventilation exists so that hypoxia and CO_2 build-up are avoided. If spontaneous ventilation is marginal, or there is any question of its adequacy, the EMT should provide assisted ventilation both as a consideration of providing adequate pulmonary oxygenation and of avoiding retained CO_2. With any patient in shock who requires assisted ventilation, the ventilations should include a high FiO_2 and particular attention must be paid to allowing ample time for full exhalation of CO_2.

Once any immediate ABC needs and the general treatment for shock have been provided, the EMT should continue his assessment to determine if the shock is a result of previous external bleeding, "hidden" internal bleeding, a cardiac problem, an allergic reaction or another cause requiring additional specific intervention. When a patient is initially found to be unresponsive and pulseless, or when the history of the episode includes chest pain or an overt suggestion of a cardiac or serious medical problem in the absence of trauma, cardiac monitoring and ACLS procedures should be initiated early on if appropriately certified personnel are present. This is appropriately included in the circulatory ("C") part of the initial A,B,C's, prior to any further and more detailed assessment. In cases of trauma without cardiac arrest, EKG monitoring can provide key information on cardiac performance, however extensive and ACLS procedures other than airway and ventilation management are usually deferred until the possibility of any internal bleeding has been identified or ruled out.

Intracranial bleeding is evidenced by neurological changes that include an alteration in level of consciousness and often motor and sensory deficits in one side of the body. Increases in intracranial pressure are followed by unconsciousness, rising blood pressure, lowering pulse rate, pathological respiratory patterns and pathological posturing. Adults cannot lose enough blood into the closed cranium to produce hypovolemic shock. Generally, if shock is present in a patient with a significant head injury, the shock is either produced by hemorrhage in another location or it is an immediately pre-terminal event. Therefore, if shock is present in conjunction with head trauma the EMT should presume that it may be caused by another injury — and should actively search for that injury.

Although early intrathoracic bleeding may not be specifically identifiable in the field, as bleeding into either side of the thorax exceeds about 250ml it will impinge on the lung and produce evident respiratory distress. As bleeding progresses the respiratory distress increases and breath sounds become reduced or absent on the injured side.

Intra-abdominal bleeding is often more difficult to detect. Although free blood irritates the abdominal cavity's lining and results in a distended, rigid abdomen and pain, this does not always occur. In young otherwise healthy trauma victims with unexplained levels of shock, intra-abdominal bleeding must be assumed. In any patient with a pelvic fracture, intra-abdominal bleeding must also be assumed since it is frequently associated with such fractures. Significant bleeding can also occur with closed fractures of the femur. The pathological *third-space* that is produced when the bone ends override each other allows for between 1200 and 1500 ml of blood loss without any open wound. Bilateral fractures (often seen in head-on motorcycle collisions when the rider's thighs become trapped under the handlebars as he is ejected upwards) can result in lethal blood loss if not promptly identified and treated.

Present studies are unclear and there is is vast debate about whether or not there is any benefit or increased survival from the use of the Pneumatic Anti-Shock Garment (PASG) in the general treatment of shock. However, there is irrefutable scientific evidence and unaltered medical consensus that, by promoting tamponade, the garment successfully controls most bleeding in body areas underlying it—whether external or internal. Although the garment may or may not continue to be included as a treatment for shock from other causes, the garment does provide the EMT with a unique and often life-saving prehospital device to control intra-abdominal and lower extremity third-space bleeding.

An important part of the assessment and treatment of shock is identifying those patients that have intra-abdominal hemorrhage or internal bleeding in other areas covered by the garment, as well as those who do not. In those who do, the Pneumatic Anti-Shock Garment should be used to limit further bleeding (unless otherwise contraindicated) as a key element in treating shock. In those that do not have such bleeding, whether or not the garment provides a benefit remains a matter of individual physician interpretation and the EMT must follow local protocols. Considerations, use and contraindications for the PASG will be discussed in greater detail later in this section.

When the hemorrhage and shock result from a closed overriding femur fracture, similar tamponading and control of internal bleeding can be obtained by the use of a traction splint in place of the PASG. In such cases the traction reduces the overriding bone ends, lessening the size of the pathological third-space and limiting the additional blood loss into it.

Fluid resuscitation is an important consideration when treating shock. In patients who have shock from hemorrhage or other hypovolemic causes, rapid fluid replacement is important in restoring their blood pressure and cellular perfusion to an acceptable level. In such cases the EMT must rapidly begin to temporarily restore the lost volume in the field by initiating two or more IV's of Normal Saline or Lactated Ringer's in larger peripheral veins, using large bore IV cannulas and maxidrip tubing or blood delivery sets. To most rapidly supply replacement fluid, these IV's are run at a "wide open" rate. Starting IV's and the modifications necessary in infants and children, the elderly, and the various considerations and complications attendant to this skill, are discussed in detail in a later Section of this book. Due to the transitory nature of crystalloid fluids in the vascular system, three times the amount of blood volume lost must be infused to restore the vascular volume. While it is unrealistic to expect IV's alone to fully restore the lost volume, it is important to the patient's long term survival that the fluid replacement process begin as quickly as possible.

When shock has been caused by a significant fluid loss, the effectiveness of field treatment in stabilizing the patient is heavily determined by the *nature* of the hypovolemia. If it results from fluid loss without bleeding (such as dehydration or a lack of fluid intake), the prehospital of IV fluid replacement can begin to restore the fluid volume and return the blood pressure to a normal level. When fluid loss has occurred *without any bleeding* and adequate hemoglobin remains in the system, infusing sufficient crystalloid IV fluid to return the blood pressure to an acceptable level and restore adequate perfusion reinstitutes adequate cellular oxygenation. In neurological shock the vascular tone is lost, resulting in widespread vasdilation. Because the drop in blood pressure results from the significant enlargement of the vascular container and the loss of an effective ratio between the fluid volume and the size of the vascular system, rather than from any actual fluid loss, this condition is called **relative hypovolemia**. When shock has been caused by relative hypovolemia, an adequate blood pressure and cellular perfusion can be temporarily restored by crystalloid fluid infusion and a return to a favorable ratio between the vascular size and the available fluid. Since no blood loss occurred, adequate hemoglobin remains and—once a sufficient fluid volume is supplied to re-establish adequate perfusion—cellular oxygenation will be restored.

In cases of hemorrhagic shock, whether or not (and to what degree) the temporary improvement in the blood pressure and perfusion results in cellular oxygenation will be determined by the amount of hemoglobin that has been lost from the vascular system. If the remaining hemoglobin level is not adequate, cellular hypoxia and cell death will continue. Since oxygen is only transported to the cells by bonding with hemoglobin and can *NOT* be transported freely in fluid, regardless of the adequacy of pulmonary ventilation with a high FiO_2 and the restoration of adequate blood pressure and perfusion, without adequate hemoglobin the oxygen will not be transported from the alveoli to the cells.

Patients who have had any significant bleeding rapidly need to have blood replacement if adequate cellular oxygenation is to be assured. In such patients the only warranted delay in initiating transport to the nearest hospital should be for the management of other urgent ABC needs, rapid packaging to avoid further injury, or entrapment or safety considerations. Blood replacement is a key treatment for hypovolemic shock in cases where hemorrhage has been the cause, and no additional delay should occur in the field to initiate IV's. Instead, infusions for fluid replacement should usually only be started once enroute to the hospital. Only when there are sufficient resources in the field, or when transport must be delayed by the patient's entrapment or other causes, is it recommended that IVs for fluid replacement be started in the field. In such cases this will initiate fluid replacement earlier but will add "zero time" to the patient's stay in the field.

As well as the urgent need for blood replacement in some patients, all significant hemorrhage can not be controlled (or even identified) in the field. The possibility of continued hemorrhage must remain a concern. Though the EMT can identify and control significant extremity bleeding, and with the use of the Pneumatic Anti-Shock Garment (PASG) can control suspected intra-abdominal bleeding, he can *NOT* control intracranial or intra-thoracic bleeding. Laboratory and radiological studies are required before the presence of such hidden internal bleeding can be completely ruled out. Even though the EMT can provide support treatments to help counter the resulting shock and offset any respiratory impact, definitive surgical intervention is generally required before intra-thoracic or intracranial hemorrhage can be stopped. *In cases where the bleeding which is causing the shock cannot be controlled without surgery, identifying such patients and rapidly initiating transport to an appropriate facility to minimize the delay to the operating room becomes an essential pre-hospital treatment.*

Although hemorrhagic shock is most commonly the result of trauma it is important that the EMT does not discount it as a possibility in patients who present without openly apparent injuries or a clear history of events which suggest that previous trauma may have occurred. Significant internal bleeding and rapidly progressing hemorrhagic shock can result spontaneously from medical conditions such as a dissecting aneurism, an ectopic pregnancy, a miscarriage or abortion, a spontaneous pneumo-hemothorax, or from sustained unrecognized gastro-intestinal (GI) bleeding. Although rarely producing shock, intracranial bleeding can also occur without trauma from a cerebrovascular accident (CVA). When trauma is not apparent the EMT may also be misled because the patient purposely denies such an event (for social or legal reasons), or because the injury occurred days, weeks, or even months prior to the call and the patient does not relate it to this event. Chronic sub-dural bleeding, for example, may result from a seemingly unimpressive blow to the head and may not present any obvious signs for days or even weeks afterward.

With cardiogenic shock, the circulatory deficit causing the hypoperfusion results from impaired or absent cardiac pumping—rather than from bleeding or other fluid loss. The treatment, once any needed airway management, ventilation, or CPR has been initiated, focuses on restoring a functional cardiac rhythm and rate and eliminating the factors contributing to the dysrhythmia or other cardiac dysfunction. Although survival is greatly increased by providing a high FiO_2 and airway management, ventilation, CPR or early defibrillation as needed, ultimately the survival of patients in cardiogenic shock depends on the rapid initiation of full Advanced Cardiac Life Support (ACLS) treatment.

When ACLS personnel are present, the initial care of patients in cardiogenic shock should be focused upon providing adequate pulmonary ventilation, oxygenation, and treatment to restore a proper cardiac rhythm and rate. Only once this has been achieved should any further treatment to restore the blood pressure (such as vasopressors) and other support treatment for shock be initiated. In most cases, since the reduced cardiac output resulted from a dysfunctional cardiac rhythm, if a proper rate and rhythm is restored then an acceptable blood pressure will result and adequate perfusion and cellular oxygenation will follow. Unlike hypovolemic shock, the early initiation of IVs to allow access for needed medications (beyond those that can be provided down the ET tube) is an early field priority. Except when fluiFd loss precipitates or contributes to the cardiac problem, the infusion of a substantial amount of fluid will usually be deleterious rather than beneficial to the patient (resulting in fluid overload, increased cardiac stress and pulmonary edema), and IV fluid input should be limited to that required to keep the IV open (TKO or KVO) and to properly transport the medications being administered. Regardless of his apparent lack of severity or even with a positive outcome after ACLS field resuscitation, a patient in any cardiogenic episode must be considered to remain highly unstable until more definitive evaluation and treatment have been provided at the hospital. Therefore, even though ACLS capability is present, any unnecessary delay in the field increases patient risk and should be avoided.

When a patient has signs of cardiogenic shock (or any possible cardiac episode) and ACLS capability is *NOT* available, the EMT's treatment must focus on five priorities essential to patient survival:

- Providing a high FiO_2 and any BLS interventions needed (airway management, ventilation, or CPR).
- Early defibrillation (if indicated and available).
- Aiding the patient in taking any medication prescribed for the problem he is presenting with (if indicated and available).
- Positioning the patient properly and keeping him from standing, walking, unnecessary anxiety, etc. — anything that would contribute to cardiac stress.
- Initiating transport to the hospital or to an earlier intercept with an ACLS EMS unit without additional delay.

Once it has been established that a cardiac episode is or may be involved, the EMT should limit his immediate concerns in the field only to the above items and to any other key ABC needs which require immediate intervention prior to transport. When ACLS capability is *NOT* available in the field, the EMT must be careful not to waste time with any assessment that does not address immediate life-threatening needs or which will not cause a change in the interventions he can provide for life-threatening conditions. Except for any needed ABC interventions, providing a high FiO_2, and early defibrillation (if indicated and available), the key element in determining survival in such situations is the amount of time taken until the patient is in a facility or EMS unit with full ACLS capability. In such cases, further assessment checking, vital signs or starting IV's to establish a KVO "lifeline" should only be done once enroute. Even when a patient with chest pain or other signs or history suggesting a cardiac episode appears stable, a rapid sudden change to a dysfunctional rhythm or the commencement of potentially deadly side effects (such as pulmonary edema) is common. If this occurs prior to arrival at a place where ACLS can be provided, death may result — whereas with such a capability it often can be prevented or treated successfully.

Successfully countering cardiogenic shock is dependent upon accurately identifying the specific problem involved, and the administration of the appropriate medications and other treatments in a timely fashion. *For EMTs limited to BLS (even with EMT-D and IV capability), the two essential factors in promoting survival are to immediately meet any ABC and early defibrillation needs, and to initiate transport to an ACLS capability without any needless delay.*

Respiratory shock is caused by either hypoventilation or by being in an environment which does not contain sufficient oxygen to sustain life. Hypoventilation and pulmonary hypoxia have been discussed in detail in the preceding sections on *Ventilation and Oxygenation Skills*. When the pulmonary hypoxia is sustained and the resulting cellular hypoxia leads to a progressive circulatory collapse, the patient is said to have *respiratory shock*. The immediate treatment for respiratory shock is to manage the airway, to ventilate the patient with a high FiO_2, and to resolve any problem which would inhibit proper alveolar ventilation and oxygenation. Once proper alveolar ventilation and oxygenation have been restored, the cardiac and circulatory deficits caused by the hypoxia are addressed. In small children the prime cause of cardiac arrest are respiratory exhaustion developing to respiratory arrest and apnea. Often, with respiratory shock in all ages, once proper ventilation is provided the cardiac arrest resolves. If it does not, it is treated the same as cardiogenic shock requiring the timely availability of full ACLS resources or immediate transport to a facility which can provide ACLS treatment.

Anaphylactic shock is a severe systemic allergic reaction to foreign substances (allergens) such as a drug, vaccine, insect venom, certain foods, or chemicals which have been injected, ingested, or absorbed into the body. Anaphylactic reactions are marked by the development of signs and symptoms of a progressing systemic reaction, generally including increasing respiratory distress and advancing shock. In some cases the systemic impact will be slow: localized redness and edema may radiate to adjacent areas, followed by hives (a splotchy white or red rash) appearing on other parts of the body, then increased difficulty breathing, wheezing, and worsening shock. In some cases, however, the patient will rapidly develop marked respiratory distress, marked diaphoresis, decompensated shock, dysrhythmia, and even respiratory or cardiac arrest within seconds or minutes. Generally, the quicker the systemic reaction occurs, the more severe the shock is likely to be. As with cardiogenic shock, in severe cases the patient's outcome depends upon meeting any basic ABC needs *and* the rapid initiation of the proper drug therapy. The immediate administration of epinephrine has proven to be effective in countering anaphalaxis in the field. This should be followed by the administration of benadryl or another antihistamine in the field or at the hospital.

When Epinepherine-trained EMTs are present and a patient develops the signs and symptoms of a systemic anaphylactic reaction, the EMTs should immediately administer epinepherine to counter the developing anaphylactic shock (giving the initial dose, a repeat dose as needed, and any antihistamine or other medication included in their local protocols). When a patient who has a diagnosed history of anaphylactic reaction is exposed it is recommended that the initial dose of epinephrine be given without waiting for the signs of anaphylaxis unless otherwise dictated by local protocols. A repeat dose or another medication should be given according to local protocol or, if the EMT is uncertain, with on-line medical direction. Many patients confuse a previous episode of nausea, a mild rash, or another unpleasant but benign side reaction from exposure to a substance as being an allergic reaction. The administration of epinephrine before any signs of anaphylaxis are present should be limited to patients for whom epinephrine has been prescribed, or when the history of their "reaction(s)" clearly describes anaphylactic shock.

Many patients who have a history of anaphylactic reactions carry kits prescribed for them which contain pre-measured self-injecting epinephrine devices (EPi Pens), or pre-loaded dose-controlled syringes (anakits, etc.) so that they or a companion can administer the medication if they are exposed to the substance. When EMTs who are *NOT* trained and certified to carry epinephrine but have been trained in the use of such kits have been called to a scene where such a kit has been prescribed and is available, after assuring that the kit has been prescribed for the patient and not another family member they should assist the patient or relative in its use unless such practice is prohibited by State or local regulations.

When a patient develops signs of anaphylaxis, or when a patient with a known history of anaphylactic shock from a substance is exposed to it, and the EMTs responding are not trained and certified in the administration of epinephrine (or no kit is available for the patient's self-use), a critical time-line emergency exists. Even though the EMTs can provide airway management, ventilation with a high FiO_2 and general supportive treatment for shock, if the reaction is severe the resulting airway edema may make continued ventilation impossible. The hypoxia and progressing shock may therefore lead to cardiac dysrhythmias and cardiac arrest. In such cases, once the primary problem has been identified as an anaphylactic reaction, transport to a hospital where more definitive airway management, epinephrine, and an ACLS capability are available becomes the key priority in patient survival. When the hospital is far away, intercepting with a unit that has epinephrine capability or stopping at a closer physician's office or urgent care center (once you have confirmed that it is staffed by personnel capable of administering epinephrine) should be considered. Many BLS squads have pre-existing protocols for such intercepts established by their medical director with a nearby advanced squad or non-hospital physician facility. Although death from anaphylactic shock is a rare event, when BLS units have long run times to a hospital the additional simple training and certification for administration of IM epinephrine that is being allowed in more and more states is highly recommended, since countering anaphylactic shock is dependent upon its timely administration.

The onset of septic or metabolic shock is generally slow and associated with a history of a substantial illness. Definitive treatment is generally of a complex bio-chemical nature requiring a wide range of laboratory tests to determine the exact nature and treatment for the problem. Pre-hospital treatment is limited to meeting any ABC needs, general treatment for shock, steps to reduce a dangerously high fever (if present), and initiating transport to the hospital without delay. Even when the patient has proper air exchange and a high FiO_2, either septic or metabolic shock can chemically interfere with the transfer of oxygen from the blood to the cells and cause cellular hypoxia. Although the onset is rarely rapid the EMT must assume that the condition has been progressing for some time and that it has now reached a critical level if the changes in the patient have precipitated summoning of an ambulance.

SUMMARY

The management and treatment of shock varies, based upon the underlying pathophysiological mechanism which is impacting the circulation and causing the shock. Therefore pre-hospital treatment for shock surrounds four key considerations:

- Provide any ABC needs.
- Provide the general support treatment for shock (position, retain body heat, high FiO_2).
- When possible, address and reduce any further circulatory deficit at its source (hemorrhage, cardiac, anaphylaxis, etc.).
- Initial transport to the hospital without delay.

Although the EMT may not always be able to identify the exact location of the problem, or in some cases the specific cause of the shock, in most cases he can identify the nature of the cause. Whether it is respiratory, hemorrhagic, hypovolemic (without blood loss), neurologic, cardiogenic, anaphylactic or either septic or metabolic shock is determined by reviewing the situation and history of the episode, the patient's past history, and the findings of the Initial Systemic Exam.

When advanced level EMTs are present, making the distinction is key to including specific treatment which can address the cause in conjunction with the general treatment for shock. In cases of hypovolemia, cardiac failure, respiratory failure, and anaphylaxis, for example, countering shock depends upon recognition and treating of the cause as a primary priority. Without this distinction and differentiated treatment in the field, a successful outcome is less likely.

Even for basic EMTs, distinguishing the etiology of the shock is key and will often result in different treatment and priorities. For example, when a patient has cardiogenic shock or intrathoracic hemorrhage, rapidly initiating transport is essential. However, when a patient has intra-abdominal hemorrhage the timely application of the PASG prior to transport may be essential in avoiding irreversible shock and death.

At any level of training, determine the need for essential field intervention on a case-by-case basis and recognizing patients with urgent needs that cannot be met in the field, are key components in providing intelligent and meaningful pre-hospital care.

Even when the immediate pre-hospital care for patients in shock successfully restores perfusion (by restoring adequate volume, pressure, and cardiac pumping) and a high level of oxygen in the blood (by ensuring a patent airway, adequate ventilation and a high FiO_2), a variety of complex biochemical, cardiological and blood chemistry considerations and treatments — including blood replacement and surgical intervention in some cases — are required before shock can be definitively resolved. Although the patient may appear to be improved because his blood pressure has been restored and ventilation with a high FiO_2 is being provided, perfusion and cellular oxygenation *may or may not* be restored or maintainable in the filed. **Any patient in shock must continue to be considered unstable and in critical condition until definitive assessment and treatment are provided at the hospital, regardless of the initial presenting level of shock or seeming improvement in the field.**

CONTROLLING EXTERNAL BLEEDING WITH DIRECT PRESSURE (And Elevation)

Direct pressure remains the most effective method for control of external bleeding. Pressure is applied by using the fingers held together or the heel of the hand over the wound site and the area immediately adjacent to it, so that the pressure is referred to the underlying injured vessel and to those vessels which supply the bleeding site. Gauze dressings are placed over the wound to promote clotting and the patient is usually placed supine. If bleeding is from the scalp or from a limb the site is elevated to obtain the additional advantage of gravity in reducing blood flow to the wound.

1. Assure that the proper body substance isolation precautions indicated by the extent of the bleeding have been taken, and rapidly examine the wound to ascertain its size and nature. Look for and remove any sharp, loose fragments of glass, bone or other foreign substance which, if pressed upon, could result in additional damage to the patient or to the EMT. This should not be confused with cleaning and debridement of the would which is inappropriate in the field. If an impaled object is found it should *NOT* be removed. Rather, it should be held in place to stabilize it from any movement or deeper insertion while the direct pressure is carefully applied around it.

2. Cover the bleeding site with several gauze dressings so that their edges extend slightly beyond the outer perimeter of the wound. If there are sharp bone ends protruding from the wound additional dressings may be needed to protect against piercing the EMT's glove *and* hand. In any case, care must be taken to avoid using so many dressings that they interfere with the application of pressure to the underlying vessels.

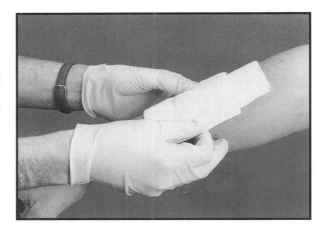

3. While firmly holding the limb with one hand so that it cannot move when pressure is applied, apply firm (substantial) pressure directly over the gauze covering the wound with the flat of the fingers, heel, or palm of the other hand. To be most effective pressure on a wound should be directed so that the injured vessels lie between the point where the external pressure is applied and an underlying bone.

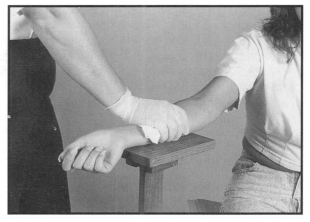

4. When the circumference of the limb is small enough, the direct pressure can be applied using only a single hand keeping the other hand available. This can be achieved by partially encircling the limb with the hand so that the flattened finger ends lie over the bleeding site and the heel of the hand lies on the opposite side of the limb (or vise-versa), and squeezing firmly.

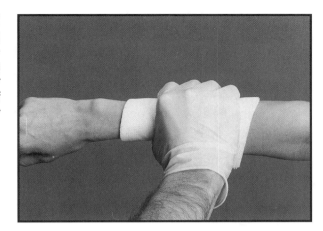

5. Gravity promotes distal blood flow when a limb is extended downwards, is neutralized when the patient is supine and the limbs are at the same level as the heart, and reduces distal flow when a limb is elevated above the heart. Therefore, when the bleeding site is on a limb it should be elevated once direct pressure is applied, thereby raising the bleeding site above the heart. When packaging the patient, maintaining the wound even slightly higher than the heart will be of benefit in preventing the reinstitution of bleeding.

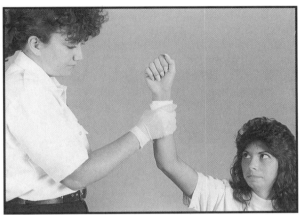

6. Even when bleeding control from an open fracture is needed, direct pressure remains the initial method of choice. With extremity fractures the limb needs to be supported from beyond the distal and proximal joints to prevent unnecessary movement and damage when the direct pressure is applied. In such cases, early elevation may need to be limited. If a bone end is protruding from the open fracture, additional dressings need to be applied to protect the EMT's glove and hand from being pierced.

7. Direct pressure is also the initial method of choice for controlling hemorrhage at locations other than the extremities. When direct pressure is applied to a larger or flatter body area than the limbs, it is often easier to obtain the force required by using the palm and heel of the hand rather than just the ends of the fingers. Pressing with the EMT's elbow locked and using some of his body weight is easier than pushing with only the arm muscles when the arm is bent.

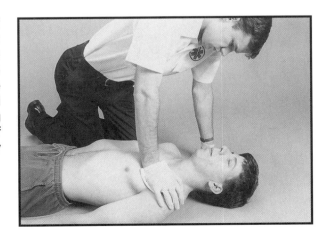

8. Once manual direct pressure has stopped or minimized the bleeding, it can be replaced — freeing the EMT for other priorities. Although less pressure results, generally enough force can be maintained by applying a snug pressure bandage over the dressing. It is important that this bandage be tight enough to provide continued adequate pressure but not so tight (initially or if swelling occurs) as to become a venous constrictor or tourniquet.

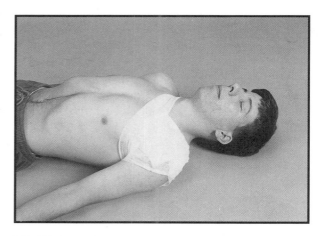

9. An inflatable splint or (when pressure is required at a site that would lie under the garment) the pneumatic anti-shock trousers can be used as "pressure" bandages. Due to the wider physiologic effect of the PASG on the underlying and distal circulation, they should not be used for solely controlling external bleeding when a smaller pressure bandage would suffice.

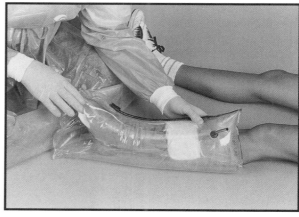

CONTROLLING EXTERNAL BLEEDING USING A PRESSURE POINT

Although direct pressure and elevation are effective in controlling most external bleeding, this is not always the case. When the mobility of the underlying vessels (or the organs and tissues surrounding them) results in the dissipation of the external force being applied, significant bleeding will continue. When this is the case the blood supply proximal to the injury must be occluded or reduced to control the hemorrhage. Many arteries, at some point along their length, lie near the body's surface. Locations where this occurs so that the amount of tissue between the surface, the artery, and the underlying bone is not great, have been identified as **pressure points**. When the firm pressure is applied over an artery at a pressure point, the artery becomes squeezed against the bone and becomes occluded or greatly reduced in size. This stops or significantly reduces the distal blood flow through the vessel and any distal vessels that it supplies. With most pressure points pressure is applied using on the first two or three fingertips to limit the area pressed and to maximize the force against the artery and the underlying bone. Where an artery, such as the femoral, lies deeper and the pressure must include keeping the vessel from escaping while angling it towards a nearby bone, pressure will have to be applied over a larger area than is possible with only a few fingertips. At these pressure points all of the fingers held together (or the heel of the hand) will have to be applied if the artery is to be successfully squeezed against the bone.

Although the list of possible pressure points is too extensive for the EMT to remember, he should be able to locate the axillary, brachial, radial, femoral and popliteal. It will also be useful to be able to locate the sub-maxillary, ulnar, and pedal pressure points. One of these can be effective in controlling almost any extremity, scalp or mandibular bleeding when direct pressure and elevation fail to do so. In order to limit the area of compromised circulation to only that required to control the bleeding, the proximal pressure point nearest to the bleeding site should be selected. Only if the nearest proximal pressure point cannot be located, or fails to control the bleeding, should a more proximal one be sought.

Although pressure points are employed when direct pressure and elevation have failed to control the bleeding, they should not be abandoned when use of the pressure point is initiated. Experience has shown that the combination of all three simultaneously is the most effective method to stop previously uncontrollable external bleeding. Sometimes this requires the availability of a second EMT. *Initiation of a proximal pressure point exclusively, rather than in combination with continued direct pressure and elevation, should only occur when dictated by needs at the scene and should not be elected by choice.*

To use pressure on an artery proximal to a bleeding site to promote control of bleeding:

1. While direct pressure and elevation are maintained, remove any clothing from the area immediately proximal to the bleeding site. Carefully identify the *nearest* proximal *pressure point* to the bleeding site and, by palpating with your gloved fingertips, identify the specific artery to be occluded. In most cases, the pulse can be easily felt when the fingertips are lightly pressed directly over the vessel at a pressure point.

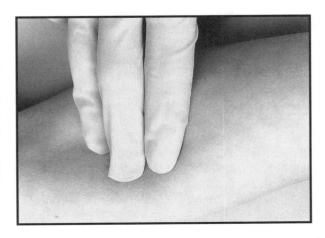

2. Once the underlying artery has been located at the nearest proximal pressure point, support the limb with your hand and firmly press the artery against the underlying bone with several fingertips. Maintain the pressure without interruption. When the vessel supplying the wound site is successfully occluded or substantially reduced in size by the pressure applied at the proximal pressure point, the bleeding should stop or be significantly reduced. Sometimes slight alterations in the fingertip location or in the direction of the pressure are needed before this is accomplished.

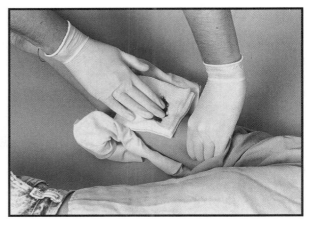

3. When the femoral pressure point must be used to control distal bleeding in a leg, pressure will generally need to be applied using the fingers of one hand held together or the heel of the hand. When bleeding results from an override fracture of the femur, a traction splint or the PASG should be considered to reduce bleeding into the third-space.

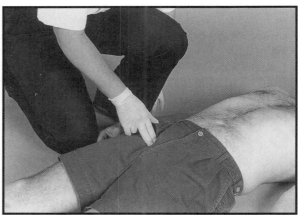

4. Once use of the pressure point has successfully reduced the bleeding, it should (if possible) be maintained for at least five to eight minutes before its attempted release in order to promote clotting at the bleeding site. While it is being maintained, additional dressings and a firm pressure bandage should be applied over the wound so that the continued direct pressure they provide is in place before release of the pressure point. Once the pressure point is released, some bleeding may recur. The EMT must evaluate its extent and take the appropriate action.

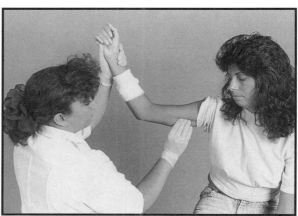

5. If significant bleeding resumes when the pressure point is released, pressure will have to be reinstituted. In such cases the EMT must decide whether to maintain pressure on the pressure point for a longer period before again attempting to release it, or only until it can be replaced by a tourniquet. The decision should be based on the patient's other injuries, overall condition, and whether this would cause additional delay in meeting other priorities or initiating transport. If significant bleeding recurs after the second application and release of the pressure point, the use of a tourniquet (or the PASG, if the bleeding site would underlie the garment) is indicated.

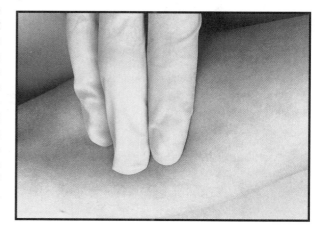

CONTROLLING EXTERNAL BLEEDING USING A TOURNIQUET

A tourniquet is a wide band applied around a limb which, when tightened, occludes the arteries and other blood vessels under it, stopping distal blood flow and therefore any continued significant bleeding from an injury distal to its placement. Since it occludes all of the distal blood supply, the application of a tourniquet can place the limb in jeopardy and should only be used after direct pressure and pressure on a proximal pressure point have failed to control significant external bleeding. In rare situations, when there are several sites with severe hemorrhage, multiple urgent life-threatening conditions needing immediate intervention, or more than one critical patient needing simultaneous care, or even when a single patient with profuse extremity bleeding needs to be moved to another location without significant delay, the EMT may have to consider the use of a tourniquet.

Once a tourniquet has been applied and tightened it should NOT be loosened or removed until the patient is at the hospital and its release is ordered by a physician. As well as the risk that bleeding will be reinstituted, loosening a tourniquet allows acids and other toxic byproducts which have been produced by the cellular hypoxia in the area affected by the tourniquet to be released into the blood stream. The reintroduction into the systemic circulation of the blood that was isolated by the tourniquet can result in a sudden drastic chemical imbalance which unfavorably affects patient outcome.

When a tourniquet is indicated it should be placed around the extremity with its distal edge about two inches proximal of the bleeding site. This keeps it a safe distance from the wound's edge while still limiting the distal area in which circulation will be occluded. A tourniquet will not be effective if it lies over a joint, therefore when the wound is immediately distal to a joint the tourniquet should be placed two inches proximal to the joint so that it lies over a long bone where it can occlude the artery when it is tightened.

A number of commercial tourniquets are available and a suitable tourniquet can be made from a variety of materials. Commercially available tourniquets have a strap and buckle which, when fastened allow it to be tightened without becoming loose unless the buckle is purposely released. In addition, these tourniquets have a pad under the buckle to keep it from damaging the tissues under it. Although commonly included in first aid kits, strap tourniquets are generally too narrow (less than two or three inches) and are not recommended for use by the EMT. The rubber strips or tubing used when starting an IV or drawing blood are commonly erroneously called "tourniquets", but are only *venous constrictors.* These are limited to stopping only venous blood flow and, if mistakenly used as a tourniquet, will usually increase the bleeding. Since material with any elasticity will not produce sufficient pressure to occlude arterial blood flow, its use for a tourniquet should not be attempted. A sphygmomanometer with its wide inflatable cuff, rubber bulb pump, and one-way valve (allowing air to be inflated into the cuff but not escape when the screw valve has been closed) provides the EMT with the easiest to use and best tourniquet, and is usually immediately at hand when needed. The proper use of a sphygmomanometer as a tourniquet is described in the sequence on the next pages and is followed by the steps for making a tourniquet from a wide cravat bandage and tongue blades (or other stick-like object). These two methods are preferred and recommended as the EMT's first and second choices, respectively. Due to the danger of producing permanent underlying tissue damage, use of other objects is only recommended when off duty and in the remote case that material to fold into a suitably wide cravat is not available.

When other conditions, such as intra-abdominal bleeding, a fractured pelvis, or overriding femur fractures indicating the use of the PASG are also present with severe lower extremity external bleeding, a tourniquet is redundant to the use of the PASG. In such cases, several dressings should be placed over the bleeding site and the PASG applied and inflated instead. *A tourniquet should never be left in place under the inflated PASG* as this can result in damage to the patient's limb or damage the garment, possibly resulting in a loss of the circumferential pressure. The need for the PASG should be evaluated and ruled out before a tourniquet is placed on the legs, or the EMT may have no choice but to release and remove it when applying the garment.

When use of a tourniquet is indicated:

1. In your own mind, rapidly confirm that the failure of other methods to control external bleeding, or the situation, dictates the application of a tourniquet. Select a BP cuff of sufficient size to fully surround the limb proximal to the bleeding site. Be sure that the gauge and pump are firmly attached to the cuff. Although the gauge will not be used, it must be in place for most cuffs to hold air. Also prepare 2 or 3 one inch adhesive tape strips and, if available, a medium sized Kelly clamp.

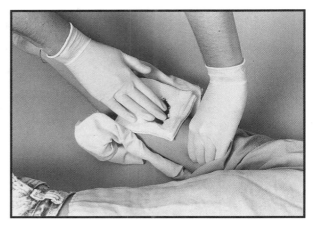

2. Place the distal edge of the cuff about 2 inches proximal to the wound's edge — or if the wound is immediately distal to or at a joint, two inches proximal to the joint — and fasten the velcro snugly around the arm. Carefully rub over the velcro'd areas to obtain the maximum fastening possible. Be sure that there is sufficient velcro contact so that it will not precipitously release.

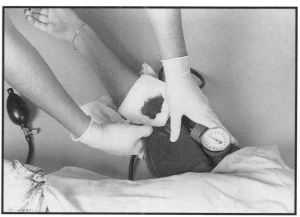

3. Rotate the cuff until its inflatable bladder lies over the artery. Most cuffs are marked to identify this area. Close the valve and inflate the cuff. Keep inflating the cuff (bleeding may initially increase) until the bleeding is reduced to an insignificant amount or is stopped. Note the reading on the BP cuff's gauge.

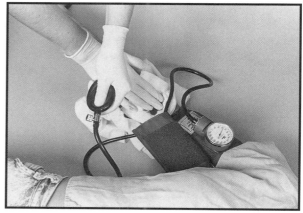

4. Add slightly more air to the cuff to act as a reserve against any pressure changes in the cuff or an increase in the patient's blood pressure. Once you are sure that the cuff is effectively tourniqueting the limb, carefully place 2 or 3 strips of adhesive tape across the end and part way around the inflated cuff to protect from accidental release.

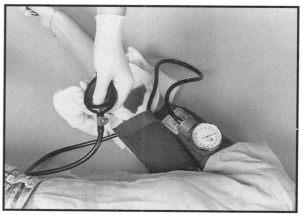

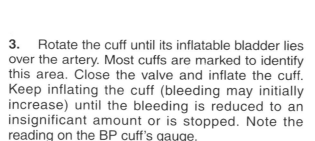

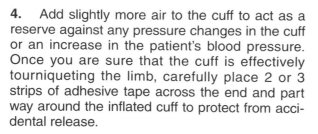

5. It is not uncommon for the air release valve of a BP cuff to leak slightly even when it has been firmly tightened. To avoid this, kink the hose between the valve and cuff by folding it back on itself, and tape it or clamp it with a Kelly clamp. This will have to be released before the cuff can be deflated at the hospital, or in the rare event that additional air is required to maintain the cuff pressure in transit.

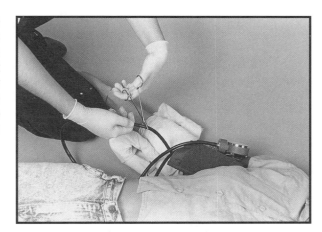

6. Mark the time that the tourniquet was applied on a piece of tape (or directly) on the patient's forehead. The letters "TK" should be included, and the tape should be clearly visible on the forehead. On your run report record the time the tourniquet was applied and its specific location. Rapidly examine the wound(s) and cover it with dressings and a pressure bandage. Initiate transport to the hospital as soon as other urgent priorities allow. The BP cuff tourniquet and any distal bleeding sites should not be hidden from view and, along with the patient's vital signs, need to be continuously monitored by the EMT to detect any significant bleeding that resumes or any drop in cuff pressure. If the pressure noted on the gauge suddenly drops drastically, lost air must be replaced to maintain the tourniquet.

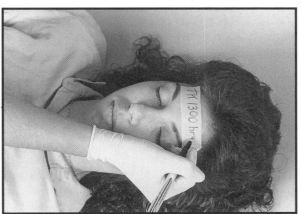

7. The time that the tourniquet was applied and its specific location on the patient should be included in the EMT's radio report and should be highlighted in a separate highly visible place on the written run report. As well, the EMT should include this information in his verbal report when transferring the patient at the hospital, and should visually identify the location of the tourniquet to the nurse or physician assuming responsibility for the patient.

USING A WIDE CRAVAT AS A TOURNIQUET

When a sphygmomanometer is not available, or when the available cuffs are too small to assure good closure around the limb, a wide cravat bandage can easily be used to make a tourniquet. The EMT will need a cravat bandage, 3 or 4 tongue blades (or another approximately 6 inch long strong stick-like object), and 1 to 2 inch adhesive tape. Individual ball point pens are too flexible and fragile for safe use and should be avoided. Although there are accounts of individuals who have successfully applied a tourniquet to themselves, it can be most rapidly and safely applied when two EMTs are available for the task.

When use of a tourniquet is indicated:

1. Make sure that the bandage is neatly folded into a cravat between three and four inches wide. Prepare the tongue blades by rapidly taping them (stacked one on top of another) together and prepare 4 additional strips of tape approximately 12 inches long. When this has been completed, hold the cravat almost perpendicular to the limb so that its distal edge is approximately 1 to 2 inches proximal of the bleeding wound's edge.

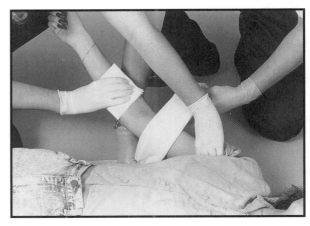

2. Without attempting to pull it very tight, snugly wrap each end in the opposite direction all of the way around the limb. Repeat, taking full turns around the limb with both ends approximately overlapping each previous layer (without widening the covered area beyond 4 to 5 inches) until 10 to 12 inches of each end remains. Tie the ends together (using a normal half-knot) so that the finished knot ends up over the cravat — not over bare skin — and approximately over the artery. Sometimes, in order to properly locate the knot over the artery, the tied bandage may have to be slightly rotated. It should be applied and tied snugly but loose enough that this is still possible.

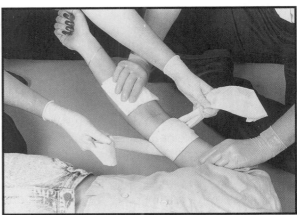

3. Next take the taped tongue blades (or other stick-like object) and center it over the knot. While holding it in place, have the second EMT tie the cravat ends tightly over its midpoint with a square knot so that an approximately equal length of the stick is on each side of the knot. Although knots other than a square knot can be used, it is important that a knot be used that will neither loosen nor "walk" when pressure is applied.

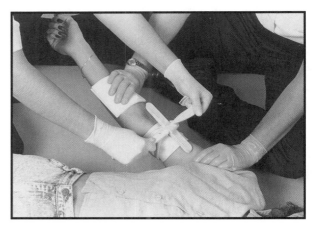

4. To tighten the tourniquet, turn the stick in either a clockwise or counterclockwise direction. Care must be taken when the tension on the stick increases (as the cravat becomes progressively tighter) not to lose control of the stick and allow it to unwind when the hand-hold changes are made. Continue to turn the stick, tightening the cravat until the bleeding is minimized or stopped.

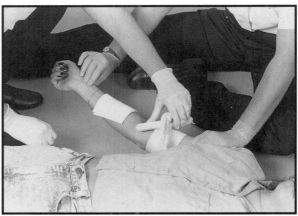

5. Once the bleeding has been controlled, turn the stick an additional 1/4 to 1/2 turn until it is aligned with the long axis of the limb. While one EMT carefully holds the stick to keep it from unwinding, the second EMT places the center of one of the prepared strips of the tape under one end of the stick so that its outer edge is between a half and three quarters of an inch from the end of the stick. Next, wind each end of the tape tightly around the stick several times to secure it to the stick's end.

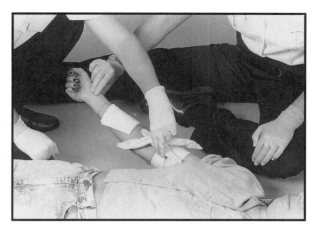

6. Then fasten one end of the tape carefully around one side of the limb and the other end around the other side of the limb. The tape ends should overlap each other on the underside of the limb to assure they are sufficiently secured to avoid coming off. Some EMTs may prefer to tie the tape ends together at the underside of the limb as an extra margin of safety. Now, with another strip of tape, secure the other end of stick in the same manner.

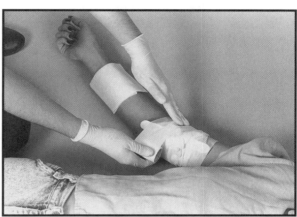

7. For an extra margin of safety to keep the stick from unwinding, place an additional strip of tape around one side of the limb, over the end of the stick, and back around the opposite side of the limb at each end of the stick. With four separate long pieces of tape securing the stick to the limb, it is a highly unlikely event that the tourniquet will accidentally become loose. Next follow the steps previously outlined for patients who have had a tourniquet applied.

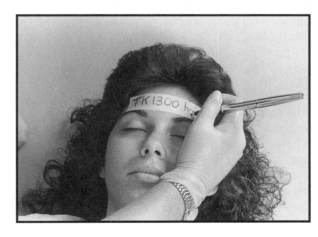

USING THE PNEUMATIC ANTI-SHOCK GARMENT (PASG)

The use of the Pneumatic Anti-Shock Garment (PASG) for the general treatment of profound hypovolemic shock has become the subject of a vast medical debate. At the core of the discussion is the question of whether or not the temporary restoration of the patient's blood pressure which commonly results from use of the garment actually produces or contributes to increased survival.

As well, the question has been raised of whether or not this may even accelerate hemorrhage and thus adversely affect survival in patients who have bleeding (such as intra-thoracic) which can only be controlled by surgical intervention. A variety of recent studies have resulted in widely differing interpretations from physician to physician, and a lack of consensus often from the same literature. Some observers conclude that the garment provides little or no benefit in the treatment of shock (Bickell, Mattox, et al). Others maintain that the data clearly shows an increase in survival in hypovolemic patients with a blood pressure lower than 50mm Hg (Cayten et al, MacKersie et al, and the data from Bickell et al). Still others maintain that the garment is of benefit except in patients with open (some include closed) intrathoracic bleeding. The issues, which include questions of the validity of the controls and of the conclusions presented in recent studies, are so complex as to be outside the scope of the research interpretation of most observers and cannot be resolved by the individual EMT. Whether the garment should remain as an adjunct in the treatment of hypovolemic shock, and for which patients it is indicated and for which it is contraindication, remains a question of individual interpretation which must be made in the absence of irrefutable scientific evidence or a clear consensus among most physicians.Until further study results in such a consensus, use of the garment in treating hypovolemic shock will have to be determined by the best opinion of the local medical authority — and the EMT must follow the local protocols.

The benefit of using the garment in patients with shock resulting from relative hypovolemia (such as neurogenic shock) also remains a question. Recent PASG studies have failed to isolate this etiology for independent evaluation. The pathophysiology involved (shock resulting from enlargement of the vascular container due to a loss of ability to maintain vascular constriction rather than blood or other fluid loss) suggest that the PASG would be of benefit. When the application of external pressure reduces the capacity of the underlying vessels in patients who have no loss of hemoglobin or other blood components, it should restore the blood pressure to an acceptable level and result in the return of adequate cellular perfusion and oxygenation. Although such benefit is suggested by the physiological effect the garment produces, its true benefit in such cases is also presently without clear scientific proof and such use for the garment remains a matter that must be determined by the local medical authority.

Although the PASG's benefit and use in countering shock remains a question of debate, irrefutable scientific evidence that the PASG is an effective tool for controlling internal and external hemorrhage underlying the garment remains unaltered. In such patients, regardless of whether or not the garment otherwise promotes survival, its use to control further blood loss represents a key element in countering the advancement of shock. The control of bleeding is beyond question a key intervention in the treatment of hemorrhagic shock. Other debate surrounding the garment's benefit should not be misinterpreted resulting in the discounting of the garment's unique pre-hospital usefulness in controlling intra-abdominal and third-space lower extremity bleeding, or its usefulness as an option in controlling copious or multi-site external bleeding underlying it. As well, since significant intra-abdominal bleeding must be assumed with any pelvic fracture, the PASG is the clear treatment of choice for such injuries. When used with pelvic fractures the inflated PASG promotes tamponading of the internal bleeding and provides support and immobilization for the fracture(s). At a minimum, regardless of the interpretation of whether or not the garment is of other benefit, the PASG should still be viewed as an essential adjunct for the control of internal and external bleeding from areas underlying it.

The Pneumatic Anti-Shock Garment includes two essential components:
- A three-chambered garment (with a supply hose for each chamber)
- A pump (with a 3 branched hose)

In most current models, the hose from each of the three chambers (abdominal and each leg) is attached to one of the branches of the air supply hose coming from the pump. The abdominal section hose is usually longer than those for each leg. The hose coming from each garment chamber contains a stop-cock. This allows for directing air exclusively into one or more chambers at a time while the other(s) are closed, and provides a way when the stopcocks are closed to make sure that air does not escape from the chambers should a hose become disconnected.

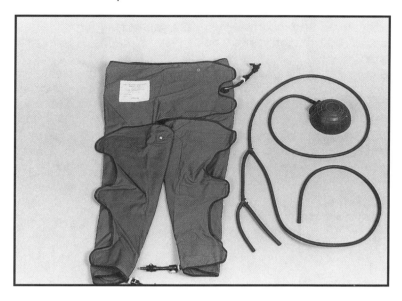

Some units contain gauges, others do not. When gauges are included there may be a single gauge in the supply hose before it branches into 3 sections, or there may be 3 gauges—one for each chamber.

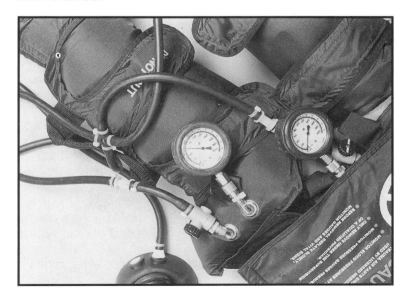

In some earlier models all three gauges were located in the removable top of the PASG's storage box. ***PASG gauges solely indicate the pressure in the garment and DO NOT measure or reflect in any way the patient's blood pressure or condition.*** Gauges are not necessary when applying or inflating the garment, but are useful in assuring that the garment pressure is maintained without air being lost from leakage. PASG hoses are sometimes color-coded as a guide to identifying each chamber's hose and to which chamber air is being pumped. The ends of the branches of the pump hose have either a male or female plastic connector and the end of each hose from the garment has the other. When the male connector is fully inserted into the female a tight airproof pressure fit is achieved. Experience has shown that a slight twist when these are being inserted will produce a tighter more secure connection.

The exact design of the trouser-like garment is slightly different from one model to the other. The garment has three major sections: a left leg, a right leg, and an abdominal section. Each section separates at one side so that it can be opened and folded out of the way when being applied to the patient. The garment can be easiest applied by drawing it under the patient's legs and buttocks while each is slightly lifted. The garment can also be applied by logrolling the patient onto the garment or by lifting the patient onto the garment. Sliding *the patient* onto the garment (rather than drawing the garment under the patient) usually results in its becoming misplaced and unraveled and is not recommended.

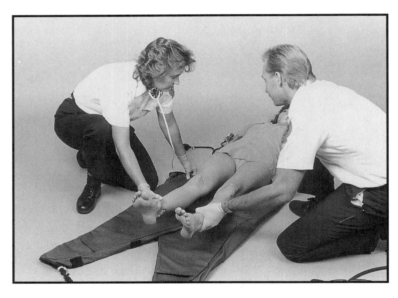

In patients with a pelvic fracture, applying the garment and fully inflating it prior to moving the patient onto a longboard is important since this immobilizes and protects the pelvis. Once the patient is properly positioned on the folded garment each section is unfolded and wrapped snugly around each leg and the abdomen. The sections are then secured by large velcro tabs. Once the patient is fully installed in the garment and all of the velcro tabs have been fastened, the hoses are connected.

Most brands of PASG have two sizes of trouser-like garment available: "adult" and "child". The "child" size should be considered a "small adult" since it is often the correct size for teenagers or smaller adults as well as for some children. Some brands allow for adjustments in the size of each garment. If the EMT is using such a model, he should adjust its size according to the specific directions provided by the manufacturer. The PASG should only be used on patients who approximate the size of the garment. Any alteration in the garment or modification of its use in order to accommodate patients of a size different than that for which it was intended is dangerous and should not be attempted.

The lack of even smaller sized garments is intentional — due to respiratory and other physiologic differences the use of a PASG for small children and infants is contraindicated.

The small foot pump is self-filling, and is repeatedly depressed and released to inflate the garment. The first pump or two does not provide pressure against the patient but simply fills the dead space voids between the garment and the patient. Once all of the voids are filled, each depression of the footpump increases the circumferential pressure against the patient by the chamber or chambers into which the air is being directed. The garment is fully inflated when the pressure in it is between 100mm and 104mm Hg. When a chamber is about half inflated the velcro will start to "crackle". On gauged models, when the compartment is full the gauge will reach its maximum reading, and on models without gauges a maximum pressure limit valve will open and any excess air volume will be purged through it. This indicates to the EMT that the maximum inflation has been reached. Most garments presently sold, even if gauged, contain a high pressure relief valve as a safety device to protect the patient and garment from over-inflation.

The garment should only be inflated using the pump and hosing designed for that model, as the connectors from other brands or models may not be compatible. ***Inflation using a larger pump, portable air compressor (such as used for inflating tires), compressed air or oxygen tanks or any device not specifically supplied by the manufacturer for use with the garment can be extremely dangerous to the patient and responders, and should NEVER be attempted.*** The practice of rapidly eliminating the voids between the garment and patient by initially blowing into the tubes for each section as has been suggested in several "street sense" articles, is also a dangerous procedure that can cause an unnecessary life-threat to the EMT. Placing the tube in your mouth can result in contact with infectious body substances which contaminated the inlet hoses when the garment was placed under the patient, or which — regardless of cleaning — have remained from a prior use. As well, the moist dark interior of the bladder is an ideal breeding ground for disease organisms that can easily spread to anyone whose mouth contacts the air tubes.

There is *NO* universal agreement on the best sequence for inflating the garment. Whether all three chambers should be simultaneously inflated, or if the leg sections should be inflated first and then the abdominal section, remains a matter of preference. *However, to avoid entrapment of blood in the legs the pressure in the abdominal section should never exceed that in the leg sections.* Due to the high frequency of asymptomatic undetected intra-abdominal bleeding, the inflation of only the leg sections, without the abdominal section, is *NOT* recommended (unless use of the abdominal section is contraindicated) since if intra-abdominal bleeding exists this would increase rather than control it. How much circumferential pressure is needed to control external bleeding, internal third-space bleeding in the thigh, or intra-abdominal bleeding is also not known. Although wide experience with the garment has shown that many patients have their blood pressure restored when the garment is inflated to only half of its capacity, and the blood pressure could only be so restored if the underlying vessels had been compressed (although it is unlikely that any external bleeding continues), one cannot be sure at what garment pressure level that some significant internal bleeding does not remain. Until further study, when the PASG is used to control underlying bleeding the most conservative and therefore recommended approach is to inflate the garment to its maximum pressure. If the garment is being used to counter hypotension, the garment should be inflated to the level where the blood pressure is restored. Additional inflation is not necessary unless the restored blood pressure cannot be maintained.

The steps for using the Pneumatic Anti-Shock Garment which are found on the following pages should serve solely as a guideline and the EMT should follow his local protocols. If he is unclear as to whether the existing general protocol for inflation reflects the practice desired when the garment is used to control underlying bleeding, the EMT should consult with his Medical Director.

There *is* clear universal agreement that use of the PASG is contraindicated in patients with pulmonary edema (generally from congestive heart failure or other primary cardiac deficiency). Based upon the interpretation of recent studies, some protocols also contraindicate their use with an open (some may include open and closed) intrathoracic hemorrhage. Rather than relying on previous knowledge or instruction, the EMT must be familiar with, and follow his *current* local protocols in this regard.

Regardless of whether the protocol limits the contraindications solely to patients with pulmonary edema or if they include intrathoracic bleeding, bilateral auscultation of the lungs is required to rule out the presence of either of these conditions and therefore must be performed prior to initiating use of the garment. The area that will be covered by the garment (anteriorly, posteriorly, laterally and medially) should be bared and rapidly evaluated before the garment is applied. This allows the EMT to locate any impaled objects and also to check for any underlying injuries that will be covered and hidden from view until the garment is deflated at the hospital.

Use of the abdominal section of the PASG is generally considered to be relatively contraindicated in any patient with an impaled object in the abdomen, a pregnancy beyond the second tri-mester, or an evisceration. If any of these are present the leg sections of the garment will have to be used exclusively. Labeling these as "relative contraindications" means that using the abdominal compartment with them presents a particular danger to the patient. Removing an impaled object without x-rays may result in additional injury or increased hemorrhage. The circumferential pressure of the PASG may cause injury to a fetus or its blood supply. Pressure on the eviscerated bowel may interfere with the flow of blood to non-eviscerated but distal sections of bowel and produce necrosis of otherwise healthy and uninjured tissue. However, there may also be a significant life-threatening danger if uncontrolled intra-abdominal bleeding continues. Use of the abdominal section with these conditions is deemed a "relative contraindication" since the physician may decide in certain individual cases that the danger from progressing shock and continued abdominal bleeding outstrips the danger that may be inherent in also using the garment's abdominal section with that patient. This complex decision must be made on a case-by-case basis and is solely a physician's prerogative. Should the EMT be faced with a patient in whom the use of the PASG's abdominal section has been withheld due to one of these three conditions, and who has continued uncontrolled abdominal hemorrhage and deterioration, he should seek on-line medical direction to allow the medical control physician to make the determination.

Once applied and inflated, the garment should only be deflated and removed at the hospital by a physician's order (generally after fluid replacement has occurred and blood replacement and surgical intervention are available). *Precipitous, sudden, or rapid deflation of the garment is dangerous and can result in irreversible deterioration of the patient.* With one exception, deflating any or all of the garment is not a pre-hospital prerogative or skill and is therefore not included in most protocols or this text. In rare cases where the diaphragm has been traumatically herniated, inflation of the abdominal section can push a piece of bowel or other abdominal contents into the thoracic cavity. This can result in immediate extreme respiratory embarrassment. If, as the EMT is inflating the abdominal section, an increasing respiratory problem occurs with a clear causal relationship between progressive inflation and the increasing respiratory difficulty, the EMT must stop any further inflation of the abdominal section and proceed to deflate it exclusively *(NOT deflating the leg sections)*. Because it is not uncommon for some patients to complain that inflation of the abdominal section has made it more difficult to breathe, the EMT must carefully differentiate between this perception and true respiratory embarrassment.

Extreme care must be taken when applying the garment to ensure that the upper edge of the abdominal compartment is distal to the lower edge of the rib cage and does not cover a part of it. The EMT must palpate the lower margin of the lateral rib cage (at the mid-axillary line) to make sure that the fastened garment lies several inches distal to the 10th rib and will be unable to encircle any of the lower rib cage when it is inflated. When properly placed, except in cases with diaphragmatic herniation, inflation of the garment should not cause any significant respiratory distress.

No section of the PASG should be fastened or inflated over an impaled object even if the protruding length is small enough to allow it. Upon inflation, the object can be driven deeper or otherwise moved — increasing the injury to the patient — and possibly piercing the garment — resulting in loss of the circumferential pressure. Also, no leg section of the garment should be fastened or inflated over an appliance (such as a knee brace, cast, or traction splint). these can create a space between the garment and the patient's leg which defeats the application of full circumferential pressure. In addition to encouraging internal third-space bleeding, with an open wound this can also provide a new space for hidden external bleeding. Also, when the section is inflated the appliance can be uncontrollably pressed into a part of the limb and produce additional injury. In such cases either the appliance must first be removed, or the garment will have to be used by only applying and inflating its other sections.

If the EMT anticipates the possible need for the garment should the patient's condition deteriorate at a later time, the garment can be opened and placed under the patient when he is moved onto the longboard or packaged—but not immediately inflated. The garment should not be wrapped or fastened around any part of the patient until immediately prior to its inflation, as the opaque and fluid impervious fabric could allow significant external bleeding to remain undetected.

After use, the garment and its accessories should be carefully cleaned and disinfected to assure that proper body substance isolation is maintained between patients and for the EMTs next using the garment. Only detergents (or soaps), disinfecting solutions and cleaning methods specified by the manufacturer should be used when cleaning the parts of the PASG. The soiled components need to be isolated and properly handled in keeping with the precautions required for any item which has contacted blood or other body substances. The pump and all hoses including connectors and stopcocks need to be cleaned and then wiped with an antiseptic solution.

With some models, the inflatable bladders and gauges can be removed from each section to allow machine washing of the fabric shell of the garment. Once removed, the bladders should be wiped with an antiseptic solution and the fabric portion flushed with cold water to remove any excess blood or other body substances before this part is placed in a washing machine. Even if machine washable, the fabric portion should *NOT* be placed in a heated drier to be otherwise machine dried unless specifically recommended by the manufacturer.

Garments that do not have removable bladders should be laid open on a flat surface, and after copious flushing with cold water should be scrubbed clean with a hot water solution (unless prohibited) containing a suitable detergent and antiseptic. After washing, the garment should be fully air dried and the velcro closures cleaned with a brush specifically designed for that purpose.

When the Pneumatic Anti-Shock Garment is to be used:

1. Ascertain that the indicated Universal Precautions have been taken and that any higher ABC priorities have been initiated. Direct another EMT to bring the PASG and a backboard from the ambulance. Examine and auscultate the chest to make sure that there is no pulmonary edema (or if included in your protocol, an open or closed hemothorax) contraindicating the use of the garment.

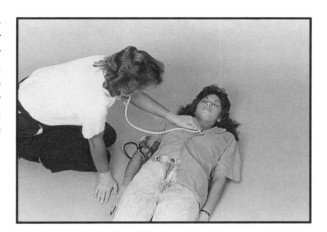

2. Remove or cut away clothing that will be covered by the garment if not removed. If not previously assessed, observe the abdomen for any apparent injuries and palpate the abdomen, pelvis and posteriorly the retroperitoneal area and lower spine in the usual manner. Although generally not done at this point in the assessment sequence when the PASG is *NOT* indicated, carefully look at and palpate each leg to identify and note any injuries because application of the garment will preclude their future examination.

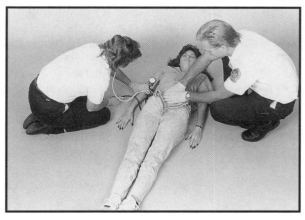

3. Place the garment and pump on the ground next to the patient. Prepare the garment by opening the top (anterior) part of each section and laying the open flaps on the ground (or folding or rolling them) so that the patient will only be placed upon the bottom (posterior) part of the garment and not on the parts that will be wrapped over each area.

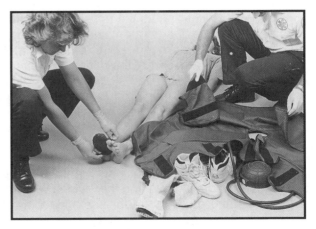

4. To slide the garment under a supine patient, place the prepared garment on the ground with the upper edge of the abdominal section just beyond the patient's feet and the opened leg sections extended straight out from them. Next, one EMT should kneel at each side of the patient's legs at about the level of the knee and facing the patient's midline.

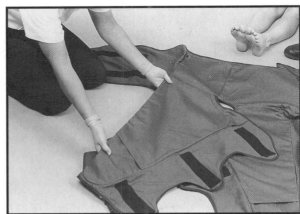

5. With the arm nearest to the patient's foot, each EMT grasps the ankle nearest him and lifts the leg an inch or so off the ground. Then with his other hand he reaches under him arm and takes hold of the garment's waist (proximal edge) as shown.

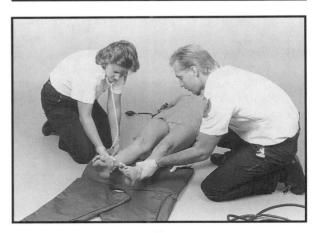

6. Both EMTs then draw the garment under the patient until the waist is at the patient's buttock and cannot go further. While keeping the leg elevated with one hand, each EMT releases his other hand from the garment's waist and places it at a more distal location on the leg section and continues to pull it proximally until the distal edge of the leg section is under the patient's ankle. Once the leg sections have been fully drawn under the patient's legs, the EMTs can lower the patient's legs onto the garment.

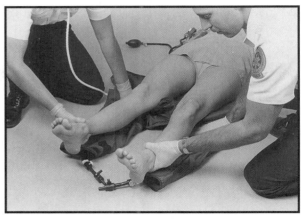

7.   Next, both EMTs move to a position beside the patient's waist. While slightly elevating the buttock, (without actually lifting the patient off the ground), each EMTs grasps the garment's waist and continues to draw it under the patient until it is completely under the buttocks.

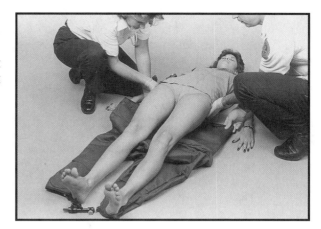

8.   Once the garment is fully under the patient's buttocks they can be released. Palpate the lower edge of the rib cage (10th rib) at the mid-axillary line with one hand and continue drawing the garment under the patient. The proximal edge of the garment should be no closer than one or two inches distal to the lower edge of the rib cage to ensure that the garment does not cover any of the top 10 ribs when it is inflated.

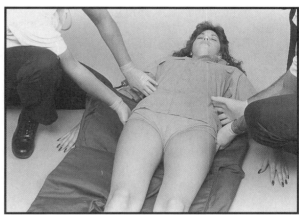

9.   Rather than drawing the garment under the patient as shown in the preceding steps, placing the patient onto the opened garment may be more desirable in some situations. This can be done using a logroll. Place the opened garment at the correct level alongside the patient. Logroll the patient away from the garment and slide the garment in behind the patient while he is being held up on his side. Bunch some of it up so that after the patient has been rolled back onto the garment, it can be easily pulled out from under him.

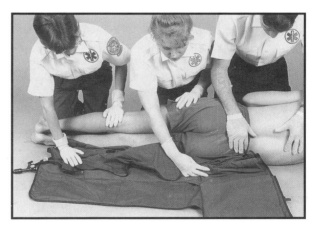

10.   Once the garment has been repositioned, roll the patient back onto it. Slide him as needed to center him on the garment and pull the bunched-up fabric out from under him. Palpate the distal edge of the rib cage and slide the patient or the garment as needed to assure that its proximal edge is correctly placed below the rib cage. In cases of suspected spine trauma, the prepared garment can be placed on a long-board so that the patient only needs to be logrolled once.

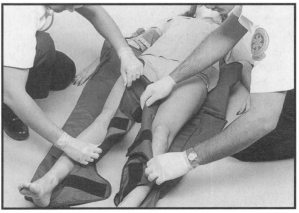

11. Alternately the patient can be placed on the garment by the use of any appropriate body lift (with or without spinal immobilization as indicated) or by use of a scoop stretcher. When a scoop stretcher is used, once the patient and scoop have been lowered onto the opened garment the scoop will have to be separated and carefully removed. Regardless of method, once the patient has been lifted onto the garment he must be properly centered and the garment positioned so that it is below the rib cage.

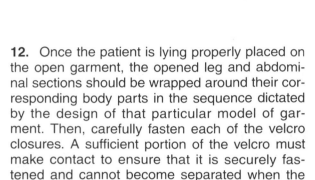
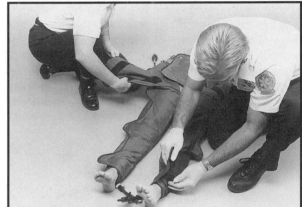

12. Once the patient is lying properly placed on the open garment, the opened leg and abdominal sections should be wrapped around their corresponding body parts in the sequence dictated by the design of that particular model of garment. Then, carefully fasten each of the velcro closures. A sufficient portion of the velcro must make contact to ensure that it is securely fastened and cannot become separated when the garment is inflated.

13. The adult garment is purposely of such a girth that it can accommodate large patients. Therefore, with most normally sized patients the garment will appear overly large and loose fitting when the top parts of each section are properly overlapped to maximize the velcro's contact. The sections should *NOT* be made more snug as this will result in less of the velcro making contact. The voids between the garment and the patient will be filled when air is initially pumped into each section. Once the garment is fastened, run your hand over each velcro fastener to assure that its entire length makes firm contact.

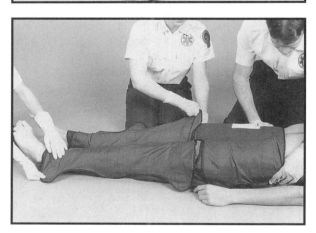

14. The proper placement of the garment caudad of the rib cage can cause the lower edges of the leg sections to extend too far. If the leg sections extend beyond the distal margin of the ankles, undesirable (plantar) extension of the feet will occur when the garment is inflated. To shorten each leg section, fold any excess that extends distal of the ankle inward under the leg section. Do not fold it *outward* and back over the leg as, even if taped, it will unfold as the garment becomes inflated.

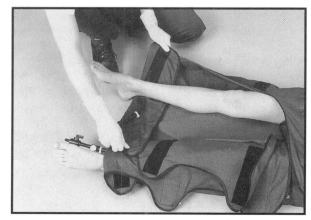

15. After each section has been fastened, look at the hose coming from the pump. Select one of the three hose ends, and if so marked, match and attach it to the same colored hose from a section of the garment. The connectors at the end of each of the hoses form a firm pressure fit when one is fully inserted into the other. Turning the connector a quarter of half turn once it has been inserted will ensure that a good connection is achieved.

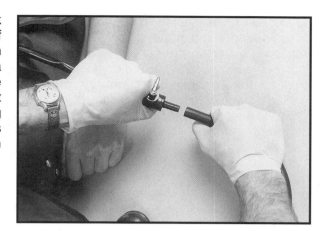

16. Repeat this procedure, connecting the remaining branches of the supply hose to the hoses from each of the other sections. In units that are not color coded one of the three branches of the supply tubing is often longer. This one should be connected to the abdominal section to provide for the distance between the leg and abdominal sections. Place the pump on the ground near the patient.

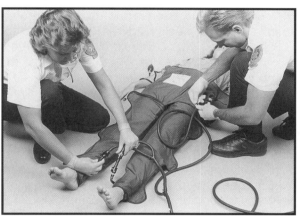

The recommended sequence for inflating the garment's sections varies from place to place. Some users prefer to inflate all three sections simultaneously, while some inflate both leg sections together, and then immediately inflate the abdominal section. Others inflate all three sections simultaneously if any intra-abdominal bleeding is suspected (or if there is profound shock), and use the two-step approach when it is not. The specific sequence selected is a matter of personal preference. With any method, the guidelines listed below should be considerations:

- Inflating one leg at a time provides *NO* advantage and simply produces unnecessary delay.
- To avoid the unnecessary risk of failing to control unidentified intra-abdominal bleeding, inflating only the leg sections should *NOT* be elected except in cases with a specific relative contraindication against use of the abdominal section.
- The inflation sequence should *NOT* at any time result in greater pressure in the abdominal section than has already been established in the leg sections.
- When used to control bleeding underlying the garment, it should be inflated to its maximum pressure even if the blood pressure is restored at a lower pressure in the garment.

17. If you have elected to inflate the leg sections first, open the stopcock for each of the leg sections by turning the handle (or indicator) so that it is in-line with its hose, and close the stopcock for the abdominal section by turning the handle (or indicator) perpendicular to its hose. With the stopcocks in these positions air from the pump can flow to each of the leg sections and, since they are now commonly connected, the pressure will rise equally in both. In single gauge units the gauge reads the pressure common to each open section; in units with three gauges, the gauges for the open sections should reflect approximately the same pressure.

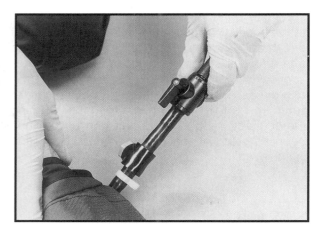

18. Depress and release the pump alternately to inflate the leg sections. Pressure is not exerted against the patient (therefore, in gauged models the gauge will return to zero each time the pump is released) until the open sections have been sufficiently inflated to fill the voids between the garment and the patient. Once these are filled the pressure within the sections being inflated will rise with each successive depression of the pump and increasing circumferential pressure will be applied. When the pressure in a section reaches about one half of its capacity the velcro will normally start to "crackle". Continue inflating until the gauge(s) indicate that the section(s) is at maximum pressure, or excess air purges from the high pressure relief valve.

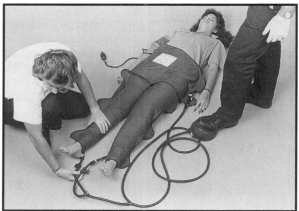

19. Once the leg sections have been fully inflated, stop pumping and close the stopcock for each leg section. Then open the stopcock for the abdominal section. It is imperative that the leg sections be closed before the abdominal section is opened or air will flow from the leg sections into the abdominal section and cause a sudden vast drop in the leg section's pressure. Next, continue pumping until the gauge or high pressure relief valve indicates that the abdominal section has reached its maximum desired pressure.

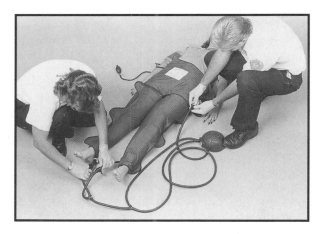

20. Alternatively, if simultaneous inflation of all three chambers is elected, all three stopcocks are opened (in-line with the hose) and air is pumped into the garment as previously described until the gauges(s) or high pressure relief valves (or a single common one) indicate that each section has been inflated to its maximum capacity. In this mode all sections are common to each other, causing the pressure to equalize between them and they should all reach their capacity at almost the same instant.

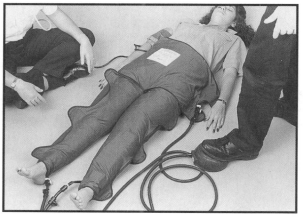

21. Once the inflation of all three section of the garment has been completed, the patient's blood pressure and other vital signs should be rechecked. As well as obtaining the respiratory rate, the patient's air exchange should be carefully observed and breath sounds should be auscultated bilaterally. The patient should be monitored and vital signs and breath sounds rechecked periodically. *In gauged models, the gauge is solely an indicator of the garment's condition and does NOT reflect the patient's condition.*

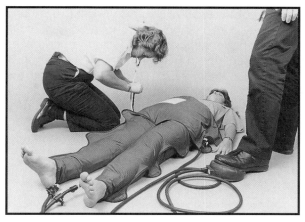

22. Once the PASG has been properly inflated and other urgent priorities have been met, the patient should be packaged and transported to the hospital should be initiated without delay. *Whenever the patient is to be moved, all three stopcocks should be closed to protect against sudden precipitous deflation of a section if the hose becomes separated.* In units where the gauge is on the pump side of the stopcocks, they must be re-opened to monitor the garment pressure. Models with gauges on the garment side of the stopcocks will do this whether the stopcock is open or closed, and in these or ungauged models all of the stopcocks should be kept closed to isolate any leaks.

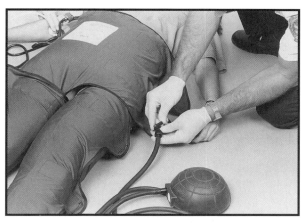

23. Once enroute to the hospital, if appropriately certified personnel are available, two large bore IV's should be established and fluid replacement initiated.

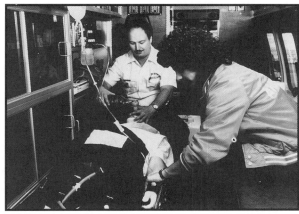

24. When periodically rechecking the patient's vital signs, the inflated pressure in each section of the garment should also be checked. This can be done by pressing each section with your hand to ensure that it remains as rigidly inflated as before, or in models so equipped by monitoring the gauges. Patient movement, passing gas, voiding, or vehicular movement will cause the pressure to alter slightly from time to time.

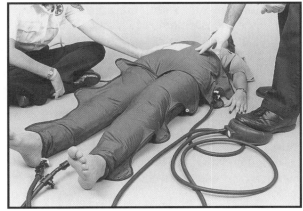

25. If continued lowering of pressure in one section occurs, it should be re-inflated periodically to maintain sufficient pressure. In such cases the stopcock for that section should be left open to facilitate the periodic addition of air and the stopcocks for the other two sections should be kept closed to isolate them from the leaking section. Fortunately, the garments are extremely durable and such leaks are extremely rare.

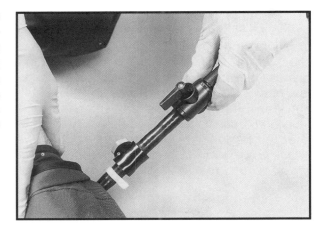

26. Substantial changes in ambient temperature or in altitude (or cabin pressure in aircraft) can also result in the significant lowering of the garment's pressure. Should any significant drop occur, the EMT should add air to restore the garment to full inflation *before* the drop in garment pressure can result in any adverse affect on the patient. However, care must also be taken *NOT* to become so preoccupied with the garment and with slight meaningless pressure changes that the EMT becomes distracted from the patient.

27. The PASG should be left inflated on the patient until volume replacement has been initiated and blood and surgical intervention are available. This requires that the garment and pump/hose unit be left at the hospital (in case reinflation is later needed) and that another PASG be placed in the ambulance before it is back in service. When removing the garment the pressure is lowered in small increments (usually about 10mm Hg) to avoid a rapid physiologic change caused by the sudden release of the external pressure. The patient's stability and vital signs are checked after each release of air. The abdominal section is deflated first, followed by each leg section.

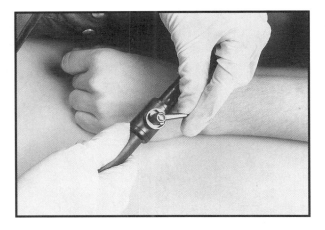

28. Clean the garment, pump and all hoses and, once the garment is fully dry, reassemble it so that each section is properly folded to avoid fouling when put away or next removed. After checking that all of the components are present, the garment should be folded and placed in the unit's protective carrying case. Care must be taken to assure that the parts do not become kinked or otherwise damaged when stored, and that no part of the garment or hose becomes crimped between the edges of the lid and bottom when a rigid case is used.

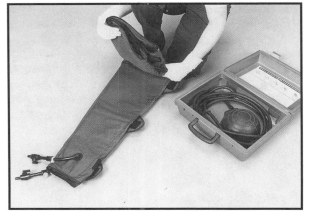

If the garment is being used to counter hypotension from internal or external bleeding *from a location that does NOT underly the garment,* from other fluid loss, or from relative hypovolemia (where no blood or other fluid loss has actually occurred) — the three sections of the garment only need to be inflated until there is sufficient pressure in the garment to restore the patient's systolic blood pressure to 100mm Hg or greater. When this is the sole purpose for the use of the garment, limiting the pressure in the garment to that needed to restore the blood pressure is the preferred conservative approach. No benefit is gained from additional inflation, and the possibility of physiologic complications which could occur from additional external pressure by the garment are avoided.

Since blood pressure cannot be continuously monitored in the field but only periodically checked, the question of when to interrupt inflation of the garment in order to check if the blood pressure has been restored must be addressed. Were this to be done too frequently it would result in unnecessary delay in achieving the desired effect of the garment and also in initiating transport. Several studies have shown that hypotension is rarely resolved with low pressure in the garment and that in a large number of patients this occurs by the time the garment is about one-half of its pressure capacity. Therefore, it is recommended that the garment be inflated until the velcro's crackling or the pressure gauge(s) indicates that about half of the garment's pressure capacity has been reached. The patient's blood pressure and other key signs should then be checked. If the blood pressure has been restored, no further inflation is needed at that time. If it has not been restored, the garment should again be inflated until the maximum pressure is achieved in each section, and then the blood pressure and other key patient indicators should be re-checked.

If the EMT prefers to inflate first the leg sections and then the abdominal section, the leg sections should be simultaneously inflated to half their capacity and then the abdominal section to the same pressure *before checking the patient's blood pressure.* If this does not restore the patient's blood pressure this sequence should be repeated to the maximum pressure of the leg sections, and then similarly the abdominal section, before the patient's blood pressure is again checked.

Inflation of the leg sections to half their maximum pressure and then, if the patient's blood pressure is not restored, to the maximum garment pressure — followed by inflation of the abdominal section only if the maximum pressure in the leg sections alone fails to restore the blood pressure — *is NOT recommended* unless use of the abdominal section is contraindicated. Two dangerous effects can result from this method:

- The blood pressure is rarely restored without including pressure on the abdominal vasculature, in which case the increased number of steps involved causes unnecessary delay until the garment is effective.

- If the blood pressure is restored using solely the leg sections and there is a missed intra-abdominal bleed, it will be increased rather than controlled. By the time this is identified from the patient's continued deterioration, sufficient additional blood loss may have occurred so that the hypotension and shock become irreversible.

When the garment is used to counter marked hypotension in the absence of any identified hemorrhage underlying the garment, whether all three sections are inflated simultaneously or whether the leg sections are inflated to a given pressure first, followed immediately by inflation of the abdominal section to the same level, or even if the garment's sections are initially inflated to their maximum capacity — is a matter of individual preference. However, regardless of which is elected, the abdominal section should always be inflated (unless its use is specifically contraindicated) to the same pressure as the leg sections before checking the patient's blood pressure and determining whether or not additional inflation of the garment is needed.

To be conservative in cases with either a surgical abdomen, a history of GI bleeding, females with abdominal pain and a history of missed period(s), or trauma patients with unexplained levels of shock (without cardiac symptoms or other conditions sufficient to explain the level of shock seen), intra-abdominal bleeding must be suspected and use of the garment with all three chambers inflated to maximum pressure (unless contraindicated) is recommended.

The preceding discussion of the use of the anti-shock trousers has been necessarily complicated due to the need to include a complete discussion of all of the choices that may be possible in the vastly different protocols found from one place to another. The decisions that must be made under any one area's protocols for use of the garment are extremely more limited and, once familiar with the local protocol and garment, the EMT will find the device quite easy to use.

COUNTERING SHOCK

The identification of shock and its severity, and its general treatment and any additional management related to its cause, have been discussed in the preceding Introduction to this section and in the section on Patient Assessment. The discussion on this and the next few pages organizes that information into a more specific sequence of steps to be followed. The ability to apply a sequence to meet the various differing needs that a patient in shock may have is in itself a key skill in countering shock and in reducing its immediate or long range effect on morbidity and mortality.

1. Take/confirm the appropriate body substance isolation precautions and, from the initial size-up, determine the mechanism of injury or event and chief complaints that precipitated summoning EMS. If indicated, direct immediate manual immobilization of the spine. From the Global Survey determine the patient's gross level of consciousness and whether or not spontaneous ventilation is present. If the patient has a lowered LOC, manage the airway. If apneic, provide ventilation. If unresponsive, apneic and pulseless— initiate CPR and, if indicated, immediate defibrillation. By observing, and palpating while checking for a pulse, note if and what level of shock appears to be present.

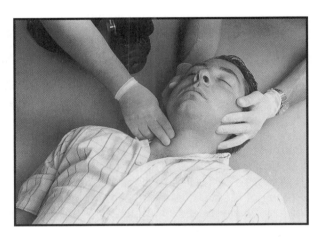

2. Scan the patient from head-to-foot for any signs of external bleeding or clothing that could mask it. Remove any such clothing, and control any significant external bleeding that is identified. Once any immediate ABC needs have been met, if there is a presenting clinical picture of shock (regardless of level or whether or not it includes blood loss) aggressive management for shock should be initiated.

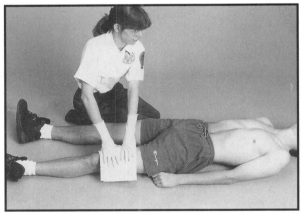

3. If the patient is not already lying down, place him in a supine position and elevate his legs so that his feet are between 10 and 12 inches above the level of his heart unless this is contraindicated by obvious injuries of the legs or other concerns. If an unstable spine is suspected the patient will have to be moved to a supine position while spinal immobilization is maintained. The foot end of the longboard should be elevated once he is immobilized. If the patient has labored breathing or if he is bleeding from the head, he will have to be positioned in a semi-sitting position with his legs elevated.

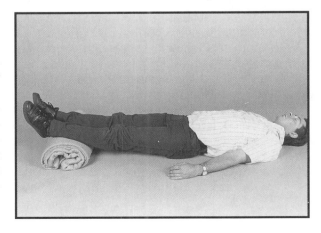

4. Retain body heat by covering the patient. If he is on the cold ground a blanket or backboard must be placed under him as well to prevent heat loss by conduction. If he is wet from immersion or rain his clothing should be removed and he should be surrounded above and below with blankets. If the patient is outside and the temperature is extremely cold, consider placing him on a backboard and moving to the heated ambulance before examining further. *DO NOT* add heat or otherwise allow the patient to become overheated as this — like heat loss — can contribute to increasing shock.

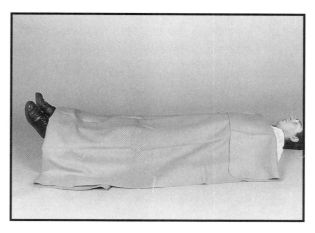

5. Provide the patient with an FiO_2 of 0.85–1.00 as soon as practical and evaluate his respiratory rate and depth. As other priorities allow, auscultate the chest to confirm whether or not an adequate minute volume exists. If the air exchange is adequate, provide oxygen enrichment with a non-rebreather reservoir mask and a high liter flow of oxygen. If the patient's minute volume is *NOT* adequate provide assisted ventilation using a BVM with an accumulator and a 12 LPM or greater flow of oxygen connected to it. If the patient is being ventilated this should include a high FiO_2 and consideration of initiating more definitive airway management.

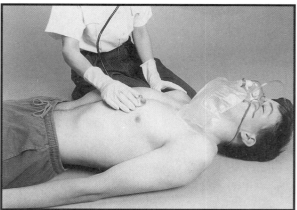

6. Determine the general underlying cause of the shock. From your size-up and ongoing in-depth Initial Systemic Exam (including the history of this episode and the patient's pertinent past history), form an impression of the general pathophysiological nature of the shock. Determine if it appears to be hemorrhagic, hypovolemic other than bleeding, cardiogenic, anaphylactic, neurologic, septic or metabolic, *or* if none of these are identifiable and it is undeterminable. In adult non-trauma patients any chest pain with a clinical picture of shock must be assumed to be cardiogenic.

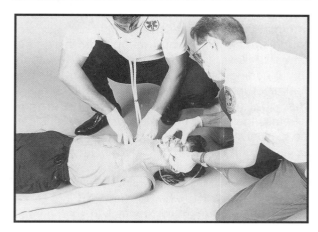

7. If the shock is cardiogenic or anaphylactic, care for the specific problem becomes the key priority for advanced personnel. If cardiogenic, initiate cardiac monitoring and treatment as recommended in the ACLS Guidelines. If anaphylactic, provide an intramuscular injection of epinephrine (and if included, benadryl or another antihistamine) according to your local protocols. With either of these etiologies, if properly trained/certified EMTs are *NOT* available, transport to the nearest appropriate facility (or intercept point with an ALS squad) should be initiated without delay.

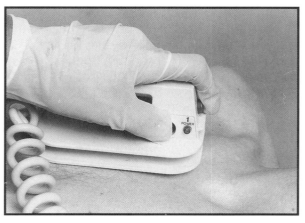

8. If the shock is *NOT* cardiac or anaphylactic in origin, continue the in-depth systemic examination to locate any signs of possible internal bleeding. From your examination identify or rule out intracranial, intra-thoracic, intra-abdominal or significant urogenital bleeding, dehydration, a closed overriding femur fracture or pelvic instability. From the history, identify or rule out any GI bleeding, any other blood or fluid loss previously not indicated to you, anemia, and in females either confirmed pregnancy or abdominal pain with missed menstrual periods.

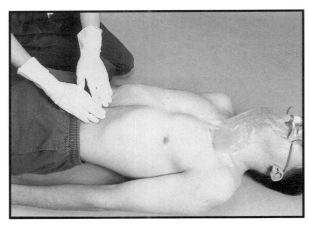

9. If either intra-abdominal bleeding, an unstable pelvis, bilateral overriding closed femur fractures (or a simple overriding femur fracture for which use of a traction splint is contraindicated) are found, or if there is a high suspicion of intra-abdominal bleeding with unexplained levels of shock, use of the pneumatic anti-shock garment should be considered to promote tamponade and control of the bleeding. If substantial external bleeding in areas underlying the garment is found, use of the PASG for their continued control should also be considered. If there is solely an isolated femur shaft fracture, a traction splint rather than the PASG can be applied to control any internal third-space bleeding.

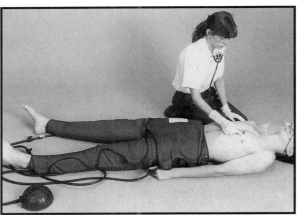

10. Whether the PASG should be used to improve the blood pressure in patients with profound shock and hypotension from bleeding, other fluid loss, or relative hypovolemia — without any bleeding site underlying the garment — is a matter of individual medical judgment. Similarly the local medical authority must determine whether the use of the garment is contraindicated exclusively in patients with pulmonary edema or if the contraindications also include patients with open or both open and closed intrathoracic bleeding. The EMT must follow his local protocols in determining whether the PASG is to be included in the treatment of shock in such cases.

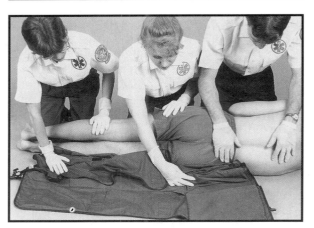

11. In patients with septic or metabolic shock, or when the cause of the shock cannot be identified, field intervention will have to be limited to meeting any A,B,C needs found, providing general supportive treatment for shock (position, retain body heat, high FiO_2), and rapidly packaging the patient appropriately.

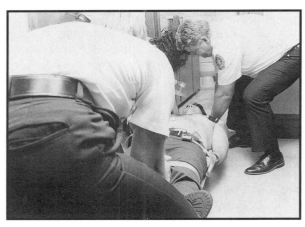

12. After completing the Initial Systemic Examination, meeting any urgent priorities of care, and rapidly packaging the patient, initiate transport to the nearest appropriate hospital without delay. Patients in shock, regardless of whether field care produced an apparent improvement or not, *urgently* need more definitive evaluation and care. All patients with any sustained shock (shock which did not resolve between insult and the EMT's arrival) are to be considered unstable. The pre-hospital care in some cases can lessen the degree of instability, but it cannot eliminate it.

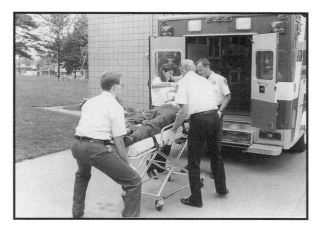

13. The initiation of IV fluid replacement is an important treatment for patients with hypovolemic shock (or relative hypovolemia). Although IV's may be required in the field to provide immediate medication access, *initiating IVs for fluid replacement in unstable patients — except in special circumstances — should be deferred until once enroute to the hospital.* Opening and connecting the bag and tubing, filling the drip chamber and tubing, and selecting and preparing the catheter and insertion site — the most time consuming part of starting any IV — can be done in the moving ambulance. In this way the transport time is only extended by the 30 to 90 seconds that the ambulance may have to be stopped to allow for cannulation once the IV has been readied.

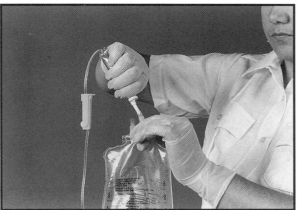

14. In adults and selectively some pediatric patients with shock and no other need of an IV, the initiation of an IV "lifeline" run at a KVO (TKO) rate to establish IV access, in the event it is needed later when initiating an IV may be more difficult, is highly recommended. This should only be considered once enroute, since actually causing a delay in the field simply to avoid the chance that one might occur in transit is contradictory and lacks reason.

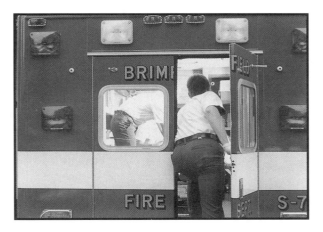

15. Once enroute to the hospital and while any vital needs being supplied are continued, any urgent key items that were deferred earlier should be performed. Once those indicated (such as initiating IVs, EKG monitoring, initiating pulse oximetry, etc) have been addressed, one EMT should complete the assessment by — as indicated from the earlier assessment — doing a detailed head-to-toe examination, a more in-depth examination pertitent to the patient's complaints/conditions, or by obtaining a more detailed history.

16. The patient should be continuously monitored while enroute and the vital signs should be rechecked periodically. It is important that the EMT compare his findings with earlier ones to determine if there is any deterioration in the patient and to measure the effectiveness of the interventions that have been provided. The need for increasing or otherwise modifying the present interventions and the potential need for any additional ones should be constantly evaluated.

ETI SUMMARY SKILL SHEET

Control of Bleeding

1. TAKE/Confirm UNIVERSAL body substance isolation PRECAUTIONS.

2. From your initial size-up DETERMINE THE MECHANISM OF INJURY and, if indicated, DIRECT a second EMT to initiate manual SPINAL IMMOBILIZATION.

After assessing the gross LOC and patient appearance and ruling out or providing any immediate airway, ventilation or CPR needs:

3. SCAN the patient's body FROM HEAD-TO-FOOT for any signs of significant EXTERNAL BLEEDING.

4. REMOVE any fluid impervious or other CLOTHING THAT COULD MASK underlying BLEEDING, AND EVALUATE any DARK SPOTS ON DARK FABRICS to ascertain if they are blood or not.

If a wound with significant bleeding is found:

5. PLACE several DRESSINGS OVER THE WOUND (unless this would cause undue delay).

6. APPLY DIRECT PRESSURE over the dressing and wound.

7. POSITION THE PATIENT appropriately and, IF EXTREMITY BLEEDING, ELEVATE the limb.

8. IF BLEEDING IS CONTROLLED, ADD A PRESSURE BANDAGE securely over the dressings and bleeding site, INITIATE the basic TREATMENT FOR SHOCK, and CONTINUE the patient ASSESSMENT.

9. IF SIGNIFICANT BLEEDING CONTINUES, while maintaining direct pressure and elevation (if possible) identify and APPLY PRESSURE over the artery AT the nearest PROXIMAL PRESSURE POINT.

10. IF BLEEDING IS CONTROLLED, after a short time FOLLOW the procedures indicated in STEP 7.

11. IF SIGNIFICANT BLEEDING CONTINUES OR RESUMES when the pressure on the proximal pressure point is released, APPLY A TOURNIQUET at a point 1 to 2 inches proximal to the bleeding site (or any joint adjacent to the wound which would interfere with the tourniquet's tightening.

12. TIGHTEN (or inflate) THE TOURNIQUET until the bleeding stops AND SECURE IT. RECORD the TIME applied, and MARK "TK" and the time ON THE PATIENT'S FOREHEAD (or tape placed on the patient's forehead).

IF THE BLEEDING SITE(S) WOULD UNDERLIE THE PASG, the EMT will have to ELECT WHETHER TO USE THE PASG OR A TOURNIQUET. If the PASG is elected, Step 10 should be: Install the patient in the garment and fasten it; and Step 11: Inflate it to maximum pressure in all three sections.

13. ONCE BLEEDING has been CONTROLLED, CONTINUE the initial SYSTEMIC EXAMINATION and as soon as possible CHECK the patient's VITAL SIGNS.

14. IF SIGNS OF INTRA-ABDOMINAL BLEEDING OR PELVIC INSTABILITY (fracture) are found, APPLY AND INFLATE THE PASG. If there is a FEMUR shaft fracture apply either a TRACTION SPLINT OR USE the PASG.

15. PROVIDE the general TREATMENT FOR SHOCK INCLUDING initiation of oxygen enrichment with a HIGH FiO_2.

16. IF NOT previously APPLIED to control underlying bleeding, CONSIDER USE OF PASG TO COUNTER MARKED HYPOTENSION. IF INDICATED and included IN YOUR PROTOCOL, APPLY AND INFLATE the garment.

17. Once all urgent immediate needs have been met, PACKAGE the patient (support and immobilize any fractures and limbs not yet examined) AND INITIATE TRANSPORT without further delay.

18. Once enroute, if indicated and available, INITIATE IVs AND FLUID REPLACEMENT.

19. Continue the patient assessment by doing a DETAILED HEAD-TO-FOOT EXAM and any other additional steps previously deferred. Dress and BANDAGE any OTHER WOUNDS found.

20. MONITOR the patient AND PERIODICALLY RECHECK VITAL SIGNS AND any previously controlled BLEEDING SITES.

ETI SUMMARY SKILL SHEET

Shock Management

1. TAKE/CONFIRM proper UNIVERSAL body substance isolation PRECAUTIONS.

2. From your initial size-up DETERMINE MECHANISM OF INJURY OR EVENTS CAUSING SUMMONING OF EMS and direct INITIATION OF MANUAL SPINAL IMMOBILIZATION if indicated. Note any obvious injuries/deformities and the position in which the patient presents.

3. From your Global Survey, EVALUATE GROSS LOC and confirm the presence of each of the A,B,Cs. Also, ESTIMATE the apparent SHOCK LEVEL.

4. IF UNRESPONSIVE or patient has a lowered level of consciousness, MANAGE THE AIRWAY and CHECK FOR the presence of spontaneous BREATHING.

5. IF APNEIC, PROVIDE VENTILATION immediately AND after two breaths CHECK for a palpable CAROTID PULSE.

6. IF also PULSELESS, PROVIDE full CPR.

7. Once the presence of a patent airway, breathing and circulation have been confirmed (or provided), SCAN FROM HEAD-TO-FOOT to identify or rule out any external bleeding (remove any obstructive clothing) AND CONTROL ANY SIGNIFICANT EXTERNAL BLEEDING.

8. PLACE the patient IN the MODIFIED TRENDELEN-BURG POSITION (or other appropriate position indicated by his conditions).

9. RETAIN BODY HEAT by covering the patient and, if applicable, insulating him from the cold ground.

10. Further EVALUATE the patient's RESPIRATION. IF the minute volume is ADEQUATE, INITIATE supplemental oxygen with A HIGH FiO_2. IF the minute volume is INADEQUATE, DIRECT PROVISION OF ASSISTED VENTILATION with a high FiO_2.

11. From the history of your findings, DETERMINE IF the underlying pathophysiological CAUSE OF THE SHOCK IS CARDIOGENIC, ANAPHYLACTIC, OR OTHER. IF CARDIOGENIC, INITIATE ACLS and IF ANAPHYLACTIC, GIVE EPINEPHERINE and any other medications in your protocol — OR — if advanced personnel are not present, RAPIDLY INITI-ATE TRANSPORT to a facility that can provide it.

12. IF the shock is NOT cardiogenic or anaphylactic, CONTINUE your initial systemic EXAM to IDENTIFY OR RULE OUT ANY INTERNAL BLEEDING (in medical and trauma patients), AND OBTAIN VITAL SIGNS.

13. IF signs and symptoms of INTRA-ABDOMINAL BLEEDING OR A PELVIC FRACTURE are present, APPLY and inflate the PASG to control underlying bleeding. IF FEMUR FRACTURE(S) without intra-abdominal bleeding are found, APPLY either A TRACTION SPLINT OR PASG.

14. IF no signs of bleeding that would underlie the garment are found, CONSIDER USE OF PASG to restore the blood pressure IN PATIENTS WITH MARKED HYPOTENSION. FOLLOW YOUR local PROTOCOL in determining such use.

15. RAPIDLY PACKAGE the patient as indicated AND INITIATE TRANSPORT to the nearest appropriate facility without delay.

16. ONCE ENROUTE, IF the patient is HYPOVOLEMIC from bleeding or other fluid loss, OR has marked RELATIVE HYPOVOLEMIA, INITIATE 2 LARGE BORE IVs and FLUID REPLACEMENT (if properly trained/certified EMTs are present).

17. Regardless of the shock's cause or degree, IF NO IV has been initiated for medication access or fluid replacement, INITIATE A KVO (TKO) IV "LIfeline".

18. Continuously MONITOR the patient AND PERIODI-CALLY RE-CHECK VITAL SIGNS to evaluate for any changes and the effectiveness of the interventions. MODIFY OR ADD any additional available INTER-VENTIONS INDICATED.

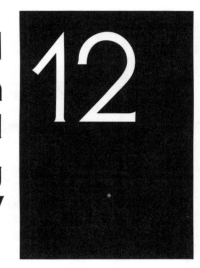

Introduction

Medications can be given to patients through a variety of specific methods, and come in a number of forms to accommodate their recommended method of administration and the desired rate of absorption into the body. The methods for administration are classified into two major categories based upon the pathway they employ to introduce the drug into the body. Substances which are taken by mouth and swallowed, so they enter the digestive (alimentary) tract and are absorbed by the intestines through the normal process of ingestion, are said to be *enterally absorbed*. Substances which are introduced into the body *NOT* through ingestion and absorption in the intestines are said to be *parenterally absorbed*. Medications prepared in a form for injection, IV use, or other non-ingested methods of introduction into the body are described as **parenteral**. Some medications are available in two different forms — one for oral use and ingestion and one, generally as an injectable, for parenteral administration.

Medications designed for oral administration will include language on their label or in their directions indicating that they are for oral use, and may even have the word "oral" preceding their name. *No medication should ever be given orally unless it is specifically designated for oral use either on its label or in the directions included with it. The ABSENCE of a warning stating that it is "NOT for oral use," should never be misconstrued to imply that oral administration is a safe option.*

Medications given by mouth and then absorbed in the digestive system are said to be administered *Per Ora* (by mouth) or simply *PO*. The term *per ora (PO)* does not include medications, which although passing through the mouth, are absorbed by a means other than through the digestive tract. Medications that are held under the tongue and absorbed into the blood stream through the mucosa (such as nitroglycerine tablets or oral glucose gel) are ordered and indicated as *sublingual (SL)*. Sprays introduced into the mouth or nose and absorbed through the pulmonary system are ordered and indicated as *"nebulized" or "nebulizer."* If a medication is administered as droplets for absorption through the pulmonary system and is delivered through an endotracheal tube, it is indicated as *"by ET tube" or "by transtracheal administration" (TT)*.

Oxygen and other gases, although inhaled through the mouth (and nose) are not considered to be an oral medication and are not designated as PO. Unlike other medications, oxygen and other gases are *NOT* prescribed to include a specific dose. Instead they are ordered by route of delivery and either the rate of flow or concentration desired. Because the use and administration of oxygen is such a large unique topic and so closely relates to other respiratory considerations and skills, it is detailed in a separate prior Section. Therefore, although oxygen is a prescribed drug, it is not included further in this Section.

The labels on medications intended only for parenteral administration, or when a drug which can be given by either route is in a form limited to parenteral administration, usually include the term "parenteral" in their name or wording elsewhere on the label warning that it is "For Parenteral Use." Some drugs which are only administered parenterally may *NOT* include such a designation on their label. It can only be found on the package or in the manufacturer's directions.

The EMT should note two exceptions from what appears apparent. One type of *parenteral medication* is taken by mouth, and one type of *enteral medication* should *NOT* be taken by mouth. Sublingual medications, absorbed through the mucous membranes of the mouth rather than the intestines, are *parenteral* even though taken by mouth. Anal suppositories or medications sprayed into the rectum, although not passing along the digestive tract and being ingested (in the common sense of the term), are absorbed through the intestine. Therefore, these are *enteral* medications even though they are not for oral use.

Some medications can only be safely applied externally, and if ingested or parenterally administered internally will be harmful or even toxic. These substances will generally include the word "topical" in their name or bear a warning that they are "For EXTERNAL Use Only." However, the absence of either of these warnings on a substance should *NEVER* be assumed to imply that internal administration is safe. *Only a medication specified for internal use can be safely administered by mouth or other internal parenteral route.*

Medications must only be given by the specific method for which the available form is designed, and only by the method and exact dose prescribed by the physician.

COMMON FORMS OF MEDICATION AND THEIR ADMINISTRATION

Medications come in a wide variety of forms. Although in some cases this is dictated by the unique properties of the substance, generally it is determined by the method by which the medication is to be administered. Medications are rarely limited to only their therapeutic active ingredients. Usually pills are compounded with binding or *coating agents* and in some cases may include buffers to expedite their absorption. Coatings prevent the breakdown of the pill from beginning when it comes in contact with the saliva in the mouth, thereby reducing or preventing an associated unpleasant taste. Some pills, which contain substances that may be injurious to the upper digestive tract, have an *enteric coating* designed to delay their breakdown and absorption until they have passed beyond the stomach and are in the intestines.

Medications that are in a liquid form are generally dissolved and diluted in an *aqueous solution* (a solution made primarily of water or a water-like fluid). Aqueous solutions can be given as a liquid or in most cases can be nebulized into a mist of fine droplets and administered as a spray. When a liquid form of a medication is required and the therapeutic agent is not water soluble, it is often mixed with a different type of solution. In many of these the therapeutic agent does not dissolve in the solution but instead remains as particles suspended in the fluid. These are called *suspensions* and, in order to assure that the therapeutic particles are properly mixed throughout the solution, must be vigorously shaken prior to each use. Since the specific gravity of the therapeutic particles and the fluid in which they are suspended are usually different, when the suspension is allowed to stand for any period of time they will separate. The indicated dosage (and milligrams delivered per milliliter) are based upon the assumption that the therapeutic agent is equally distributed throughout the fluid carrier. If these are separated, even though the correct fluid measure is administered, it will either be significantly below the dose therapeutically needed and ordered or it will be a significant overdose.

Oral Liquid Medications

With the possible exception of oral glucose gels, medications should only be given by mouth to alert, capable patients.

Many oral medications are supplied in a liquid form as this is easy to take or because it is of benefit to their therapeutic purpose. Because infants and small children can not take pills, most oral pediatric medications are supplied in liquid form. Many of these are dissolved or suspended in a sugar solution. The terms "Syrup of…" or "Elixir" preceding the name indicates this and should be viewed as a warning in patients who must limit their sugar intake. Elixirs also contain alcohol. Although in almost all oral liquid medications the therapeutic agent is "mixed" (either dissolved or suspended) in a fluid carrying agent, the term "Mix" in the medication's name has a different meaning. When the term "Mix" appears after the name of the medication, it indicates that a second (or more) therapeutic agent has been added to the primary one. Therefore, if one is prescribed it can *NOT* be substituted for by the other. For example, although both contain Maalox, Maalox and Maalox Mix are *different medications.*

Liquid oral medications are generally administered to adults and larger children by cup or spoon. With small children and infants it is easier and more certain to administer them into the mouth using a graduated rubber bulb syringe (similar to a large eye dropper) or a needleless syringe. In the home, a graduated test tube-like container whose open end is spoon shaped is also commonly used for small children.

Oral Nebulized Solutions

Some liquid medications which are introduced orally are used to provide a localized effect in the respiratory system and a systemic benefit by absorption through the lungs. Generally these medications are in a solution which can easily be converted into a fine spray by the use of a nebulizer. Nebulizers contain a nozzle-like orifice at which the liquid is mixed with air, oxygen, or an inert gas under pressure which acts as a propellent to form it into a fine spray or mist. A mouthpiece extending from the nebulizer is placed in the mouth and held sealed by the lips. When the unit is activated and the patient inhales, the medication spray delivered into the mouth is distributed by the inspiratory pressure into the bronchi, bronchioles, and alveoli

The most common nebulizer has a medication cup or container in which the EMT places the prescribed medication solution, and that is attached by a connecting hose to the portable or onboard oxygen flowmeter for use.

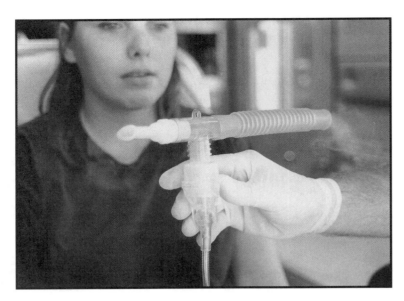

The oxygen pressure serves to nebulize the solution and to propel it deeply into the lungs. This provides the patient with respiratory distress with both the benefit of the medication's therapeutic effect and a high percentage oxygen enrichment. With this type of nebulizer the type of medication, concentration, and dose supplied are variable, and must be prepared by the EMT who is administering the medication.

The second type of nebulizer often found in emergency use is the *metered dose* type. These come from the manufacturer containing the specified medication and, although they contain sufficient medication for multiple doses, each dose is preset and unalterable. Metered dose inhalers are small and lightweight (allowing the patient to easily carry one in a pocket or purse) and do not require an oxygen source.

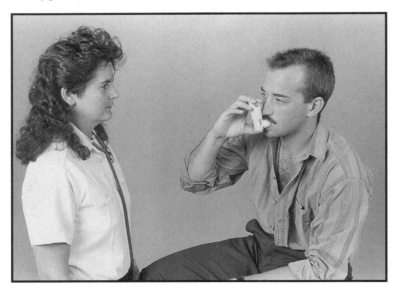

Metered dose nebulizers include a small metal cylinder containing a pressurized inert gas which serves both to nebulize the liquid medication and propel the spray deep into the lungs. When the cylinder is placed into the plastic medication container and pressed, the preset metered dose is delivered from the unit's outlet port. Another identical limited preset dose is delivered each time the cylinder is pushed, until the unit is empty. Although EMT experience with metered dose nebulizers has generally been limited in the past, because of their speed and ease of use and reliability in exact dose delivery, they are becoming more frequently carried on advanced squads.

Several other types of nebulizers are common for administering topical sprays benefit to the nose and throat. These devices and medications are primarily for home use, and are not within the scope of emergency care.

Pills And Other Oral Medications

The term "pill" is a generic label for any small solid form of medication taken by mouth. There are several different forms of pills in which medications are commonly made available. Most of the medications that are made into pills are first produced as a powder. When the powder—by itself or with a binding agent—is compressed, it is formed into a single solid pill called a *tablet*. Tablets generally are round, oval, or oblong in shape and can be of any color. Some tablets are then coated in order to either provide additional solidness, prevent their breakdown from exposure to ambient air and moisture, or to retard their digestion and absorption. Tablets that are coated so their active ingredients are only released when they have passed into the intestine are said to have an *enteric coating* and are often identified by the word "enteric" preceding the medication's name.

Instead of being pressed into a tablet, the powdered medication may alternatively be placed into a small open pre-formed cylindrical gelatinous capsule which is then sealed with the second half of the same material and shape. Medications available in this form are described as *capsules*. When the capsule is taken into the mouth and swallowed, the gelatinous cover dissolves as it passes along the alimentary canal and, after being digested, the therapeutic agents are absorbed into the bloodstream in the intestines.

Some capsules contain very small round bead-like coated tablets. Individual beads are covered with coatings which require different amounts of time to be digested and release the medication each contains. This causes the automatic periodic controlled release and absorption of the medication over an extended period of time. In this way a sustained therapeutic level of the drug can be maintained over long hours (8 to 12) without the need to take it again during the workday or through the night.

Tablets which are designed for sublingual absorption (such as nitroglycerine) are generally small and formed with ingredients that are almost instantly dissolved by saliva—allowing the therapeutic agents to be rapidly absorbed into the bloodstream through the highly vascular mucous membranes of the mouth and underside of the tongue.

The gels used in the various brands of "Instant Glucose" have analogous characteristics to expedite their absorption. When they are squeezed into the pouches of the cheeks and under the tongue the saliva and body temperature cause them to dissolve allowing for their rapid sub-buccal absorption (through the mucous membranes of the "pouches" of the cheeks), or liquification and swallowing for absorption through the digestive system. To further expedite the availability of sugar to the brain, these gels contain monosaccharides (simple sugars) instead of the more complex sugars which would require greater time for the body to process.

Although it is generally not within the intended scope of this Section to discuss any particular medication, the skill of administering sub-buccal glucose gels can not be separated from a discussion of the indication and contraindication for their use. A study published several years ago found that when these glucose gels were placed sub-buccally in healthy volunteers who held them *without swallowing* (as would an unconscious patient), they did not produce any significant increase in the subject's blood sugar levels. Because of the lack of benefit to unconscious patients that this implied, and the general medical fears of the possible adverse affects of inadvertent aspiration of any substance, many textbooks and protocols were changed to only recommend the use of such gels in patients who were alert enough to swallow, and contraindicating their use for those who had a lowered level of consciousness or were unconscious.

Because of the controlled nature of the study, it did not address two key issues. It neither explored the amount of the gel which may flow into the digestive system and be effectively absorbed enterally in an unconscious patient, nor did it explore if some aspiration of the gel is deleterious and indeed produces a danger.

There is no question that it is safer and of more rapid and of greater benefit to hypoglycemic patients to administer $D_{50}W$ or other sugar concentration by an IV route. However, in cases where ALS is not available, the withholding of oral glucose in patients who have developed such a degree of insulin shock that their level of consciousness is lowered beyond the point where they can swallow, also produces a substantial danger. Providing simple sugar to hypoglycemic patients who have already progressed to unconsciousness is of particular urgency, since without increased blood sugar levels brain cell death can commence in six to ten minutes.

There is vast anecdotal evidence of hypoglycemic patients with marked lowered levels of consciousness who responded sufficiently to an initial sub-buccally inserted dose of a glucose gel that they could swallow ensuing amounts. Also, at the time of publication of this text, the authors could not find significant published scientific evidence to prove that some inadvertent aspiration is produced, or that if it occurs it may adversely effect outcome. Until additional scientific study is available, the Medical Director of a service where ALS is *NOT* available (or IV glucose is not available within a few minutes) must decide whether, in hypoglycemic patients who have progressed to stupor or unconsciousness, such gels are effective and if the known danger of delay in rapidly restoring the blood sugar levels is greater or less than the potential dangers associated with possible aspiration. As with any medication, the EMT must strictly follow his protocols.

Medications For Injection

To allow for their introduction, transport and absorption, medications for injection must be in liquid form. Because of their invasive administration they are sterile, and must be handled in such a way that their sterility is maintained. Injectables are generally supplied in one of four formats:

- Vials
- Ampules
- Pre-loaded syringes
- Pre-loaded cartridges

Vials and ampules require that the desired dose be *drawn up* from them into a syringe prior to administration. This is obviously *NOT* necessary with pre-loaded syringes or cartridges.

Vials are small bottles which are capped with a thin rubber stopper to maintain their seal. The rubber stopper is designed to allow for a needle mounted on a syringe to easily be inserted through it, to facilitate drawing up the liquid contained in the vial.

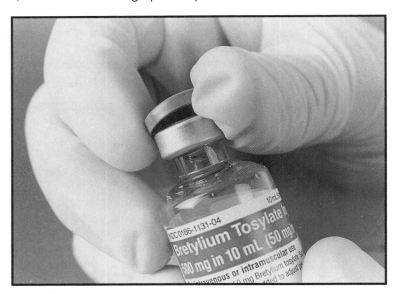

To protect the stopper prior to use, vials have a metal or plastic tear off cover. If such a cover or other outer seal is not found intact, the medication should be considered contaminated and, rather than being administered, should be discarded.

Most vials contain more than the single dose commonly prescribed, however, some may only contain a single measured dose while others may contain sufficient to provide for multiple doses. Once the outer seal has been broken and the initial and any repeated doses required for an individual patient have been used, the vial is discarded.

In order to maintain the proper stability of some medications for injection (e.g. Glucagon), they are only supplied in vials in powder form. This requires the EMT to add *sterile water for injection* (a purer distillate than other forms of sterile water) into the vial using a needle and syringe, and to vigorously shake the vial until *NO* undissolved residue of the powder remains. Once the medication is fully dissolved and in a liquid form, it can be withdrawn, the needle changed and drug administered in the same manner as customary.

Ampules are continuous glass containers which surround the fluid medication completely without any opening.

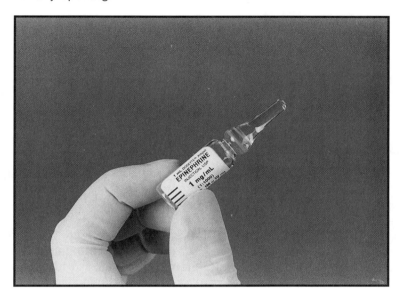

To access their contents, a portion of their top must be carefully "snapped off" to produce an opening. The vial must be covered with gauze pads and great care must be exercised when doing this in order to ensure that the EMT does not cut himself or his gloves, and that the contents are not contaminated by any pieces of glass. As an additional safety a *filter needle* is recommended when drawing up the medication, however, these are rarely available in the field. As an alternative, the use of a narrow gauge needle is recommended and, once the medication has been drawn up, the needle should be changed prior to administering the medication. As an additional caution the glass portion that was snapped off should be immediately discarded into a "sharps" container. Once the medication has been administered and the EMT has rechecked the vial's label, it should be similarly discarded. Should the EMT cut himself when opening any ampule, the ampule should be discarded and another used to avoid any potential chance of communicating blood to the patient.

Prefilled syringes generally contain the maximum single dose of the medication commonly prescribed for a large adult, or a sufficient amount for several or more doses. A suitable needle for the recommended administration route is usually attached to the syringe or separately included within the package. When the anticipated use of a medication is exclusively for adding the contents to an IV bag or line, the chance of an accidental needlestick is eliminated in some brands by the provision of a special needleless adaptor to replace the customary needle for such insertion.

Prefilled cartridges are relatively small in circumference, between one and two inch long sealed glass or plastic cylinders that generally have a permanently attached and covered needle at one end. The other end of the cylinder is sealed by a rubber stopper inserted into it, which in almost all brands (such as the Tubex) has a small screw protruding from its upper surface. The cartridge comes or must be inserted in a special cartridge syringe designed to be used with it. Some cartridge syringes are made of metal to provide for multiple uses and proper sterilization between uses from one patient to another. The most prevalent type are made of plastic and are disposed after a single use. This allows the used syringe and cartridge to be discarded after use and minimizes the chance for a needlestick when removing the cartridge from the syringe, as is required with those designed for multiple use.

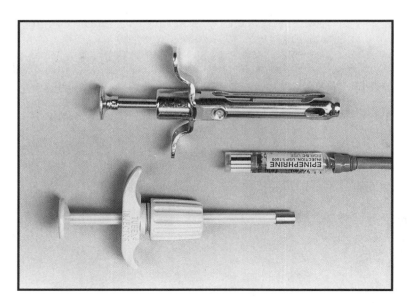

To use a multiple use cartridge syringe, the syringe is opened, the cartridge is inserted into it, the syringe is snapped shut and its plunger is extended down until its end enters the cylinder of the cartridge and is screwed onto the stopper. Once the rubber cap over the needle has been carefully removed, the syringe is used in the same manner as any other.

After the injection has been given, the label on the cartridge is checked one last time, then the syringe's barrel is unscrewed from the cartridge stopper and, after the syringe has been opened, the cartridge and its needle can be dropped directly into a suitable sharps container. Handling the cartridge any further invites a needlestick injury and is a clear violation of current infection control regulations.

Orders for medication by injection (by needle) are specified by the route of the injection desired, written after the medication's name and dose.

Routes For Injection

A medication can be injected just under the skin's outer dermal layers into the immediate fatty tissue, deeper into a muscle, or directly into a vein. When it is given just below the dermal layers it is designated as *subcutaneous* or by the abbreviations, "SQ" or "Sub-Q." When it is given into a muscle it is designated as *intramuscular*, or by the abbreviation "IM." When injected directly into a vein, the administration is *intravenous,* and designated by the abbreviation "IV." IV medications can be injected from a syringe whose needle is inserted directly into a vein or into the line of a previously established IV. IV access for injection of medication into a vein can also be established and maintained by the introduction of a heparin or saline lock into the vein. Either of these, when attached to a needle inserted into a vein, automatically dispense minute amounts of the drug contained sufficient to produce an anti-coagulant dose through the needle. This keeps the vein open and available without the continuous infusion of any (significant) fluid volume.

Whether a medication is injected subcutaneously, intramuscularly or into a vein determines the time that is required for its absorption into the blood stream and its availability throughout the body. Medications which are injected subcutaneously are absorbed slower than those injected intramuscularly, and both of these routes require transport to and absorption through the walls of the vascular system. This requires significantly greater time for absorption into the blood stream than medications administered directly through a vein. In cases of advanced shock, the resulting circulatory deficit and reduced perfusion and metabolism may delay or even prevent medications given by mouth or injected other than directly IV from being absorbed in a timely manner. Therefore, in patients with any form of circulatory deficit, the IV route should generally be used. (However only IV drugs should be administered IV.)

Particularly in patients with profound shock and reduced circulation and hypoperfusion, medication provided into central veins (such as the subclavian) will circulate to the vital organs, where their effect is the most urgently needed, more rapidly and surely than if introduced through peripheral and more distal veins. However, due to the difficulty and secondary dangers associated with central vein cannulation, prehospital IVs are only recommended to be started in peripheral veins. Similarly, intracardiac or arterial injection is not used prehospital.

Administration Of Medications Through An IV Line

Except for rare cases when a medication is supplied from a syringe attached to a needle which has been inserted into the vein exclusively to provide a single injection, IV medications are most usually administered through the establishment of an *IV line*. This provides a continuous uninterrupted flow of fluid through the needle or cannula placed in the vein, both during and between the administration of a medication. This prevents the formation of a clot or collapse of the vein, resulting in losing the patency of the IV line (providing the potential medication access) and necessitating the establishment of another line.

When the IV is solely being run to keep the line open, the drip rate is kept at the very minimum (about 8 to 12 drops per minute with a minidrip set) to prolong the duration of the bag's use, and to minimize the possibly deleterious introduction of significant extra fluid into a usually normovolemic patient (one without fluid loss). When an IV is to be established and run in this way it is ordered to be run at a keep vein open or to keep open rate and is designated by either the abbreviation "KVO" or "TKO," respectively. *Whenever the rapid or repeated need for IV medication is anticipated (and properly certified personnel and an order is available), an IV line should be established to provide easy and fast venous access without the need for multiple IV insertions and repeated delays.*

An IV line is established by the use of three essential connected components: a bag containing sterile IV fluid, an IV administration set which contains a drip chamber, a drip rate regulator and shut off, and about 5 feet of tubing, and a needle or needle-and-catheter which is used to cannulate the vein (enter through its wall and provide a firm hollow tube into it, through which the fluid runs). IV Administration Sets are also commonly called "drip sets" or "IV Sets" and are often referred to simply as "the set."

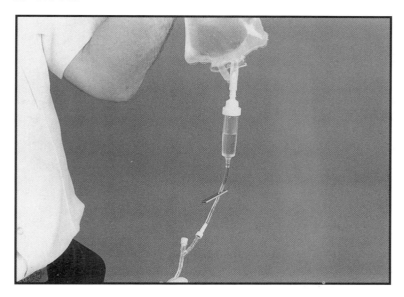

As each drop falls from the IV bag into the drip chamber of the IV set, an equal amount is delivered through the needle or cannula into the vein. The size of each drop is pre-determined by the specific design of the unit, and is constant from one drop to the other. It remains unchanged in size when the rate (number of drops per minute) is adjusted or if a pressure infuser is added. The specific size of the drops produced by a given IV administration set determines the number of drops required to deliver one milliliter (ml) of fluid with it. The number of drops that is needed to produce one milliliter by a set is called the **gtt** of the set. IV Sets with large drops and 10 gtt are commonly called *maxidrip*

sets and those which produce small drops and have a 60 gtt are commonly called *mini-drip sets*. A more detailed discussion of the three components used for IV lines, and the different types that can be selected, will be included in later pages of this section.

An IV line is also established when the transfusion of blood (or blood components such as packed cells) or fluid replacement is required or anticipated. Crystalloid fluids, either Lactated Ringer's (LR) or Normal Saline (NS) solution, are the most prevalently used for fluid replacement in the field. D$_5$W (pronounced Dee-five-double-you) is so transitory and rapidly lost from the vascular system that it is *NOT* generally considered for fluid replacement, but is primarily used for IVs established to keep a vein open for the administration of medications or as the IV solution into which other medications for IV drip administration are mixed.

When both fluid replacement and medication access are anticipated, Normal Saline or Lactated Ringers are preferred for the primary line as these provide fluid replacement and in almost all cases can also be used to deliver IV medications. When administering a medication through an IV line the solution which is selected for the primary IV must be carefully considered. D$_5$W is five percent dextrose in water, Normal Saline is 0.9% sodium chloride in water, Half-Normal Saline is 0.45% sodium chloride in water, and Lactated Ringers contains sugar, sodium chloride and other electrolytes (and if noted, a buffer) in water. Therefore medications that are known to precipitate or crystallize or have another adverse reaction if added to a salt should only be administered through an IV line of D$_5$W and *never LR, NS or 1/2 NS IV solutions*. Similarly medications which have the same possible reaction with a sugar should only be administered through an IV of NS or 1/2 NS and *never through one of D$_5$W or Lactated Ringers.*

When a medication (other than the primary IV fluid) is to be administered through an IV line, it can be given as a single bolus at one time or as an IV drip with a continuous controlled slow administration over a sustained period of time. When it is to be administered as a *bolus*, the medication is injected into the IV line by inserting the needle of the syringe through the rubber cover of a special "Y" port provided in the tubing for this purpose or through a rubber injection site near the end connected to the needle or cannula. In IV systems designed to avoid an accidental needle stick during this process, one or more ports for the insertion of a needleless syringe are supplied instead. When a medication bolus is introduced by pushing it into the IV line with a syringe, it is said to be given by *IV push* and is either designated by that term, the abbreviation "IVP," or the term *IV bolus.*

When administering a medication from the syringe into an IV line, the rate at which the plunger is pushed (and the medication delivered into the line) should generally be moderate, similar to that used when administering any injection.

Some medications *require* a significantly faster or slower push. For example, for Adenosine to be able to achieve its desired therapeutic effect, the entire administered dose must enter the vein simultaneously. This requires the most rapid push possible when introducing it into the IV line, followed immediately by the rapid push of 20 ml or more of NS, using a second syringe which was previously inserted into the line. Adenosine requires such a rapid push and flush from the line into the vein that, even if the drip rate is opened to its maximum rate as is customary for flushing other drugs from the line, the delivered rate is too slow.

Conversely, because of the fear of "blowing a vein" when administering D$_{50}$W which, if the vein blows and it is delivered to the tissues outside of the vein, can result in serious damage, it should only be administered by relatively slow push.

When a faster or slower push than normal is ordered or described in the administration directions, it is customarily described as *Fast IV push or Fast IVP, or conversely as, Slow IV push or Slow IVP*. Immediately after the medication has been injected into the line, the line should be run at a fast or wide open rate for one or two minutes to flush the bolus as a single concentrated fluid column into the vein without delay. The drip rate should then be returned to its previous KVO or other selected rate.

When an IV medication is to be delivered by drip over a sustained period, a primary IV line is first established using D$_5$W, NS or LR run at a KVO or other desired rate. Then the medication is mixed into a second bag of IV solution to an appropriate concentration (or comes pre-mixed) and, using a minidrip set to maximize control is connected to a needle (or needleless connector) which is inserted into the previously established primary IV's drip set line. Once the piggyback line has been installed, its drip rate is adjusted to deliver the desired dose, and the primary line is shut off. Medications by IV drip should always be administered using a second bag and IV administration set inserted into a primary IV line's administration set, so if at any time the medication must be stopped the primary IV line can be reopened to maintain the IV's patency despite having the piggybacked medication line shut off. Even if no other IV need is anticipated, it is an unsafe practice to establish an IV drip with a medication added to the bag of a sole primary IV line. The piggyback method should always be used to supply medication by IV drip unless a totally separate committed non-medication IV line is established and successfully running prior to initiating the administration of the drip medication. If the medication were to be mixed into the bag of the only primary line and the patient had a hypersensitive reaction to the medication being supplied, the medication drip IV would have to be closed in order not to further fuel the reaction and, until another line was established in the crashing patient, no IV access would exist through which to bolus the drugs urgently needed to counter the reaction. By use of the piggyback method, should such a reaction occur the piggyback medication line can instantly be shut off and the primary line reopened to keep the line patent and provide immediate access for boluses of any urgently needed countering drugs.

Since the establishing of an IV line becomes more difficult as shock advances and the veins become less full and distended secondary to the progressive hypotension, many protocols recommend early establishment of a KVO line in all patients with advancing shock or other systemic deterioration in order to establish immediate IV access for medications or fluid replacement if they should be urgently needed at a later time. This follows a basic tenet of emergency care: preplan and always prepare for the worst. An IV line established solely in anticipation of its future potential need is often termed "a lifeline." The practice of establishing an IV "lifeline" of NS with a large bore needle and run at a KVO rate is highly recommended in any patient where the potential need for IV medications or fluid replacement is anticipated. Such an IV can readily be used for either purpose, should it be needed.

In the event that an IV line has *NOT* yet been established in an intubated patient, four emergency IV drugs can be administered through the endotracheal tube.

Administration Of Some IV Medications Through An Endotracheal Tube

Particularly in arrested patients, it is common that an endotracheal tube has been inserted and placed prior to the establishment of an IV line. In such cases, four medications can be administered through the endotracheal tube until IV access can be obtained. The acronym **LEAN** is useful in remembering these. It stands for:

L—Lidocaine

E—Epinephrine

A—Atropine

N—Naloxone (Narcan)

Based upon studies and the recommendations of the American Heart Association (1992 JAMA) for endotracheal administration of these drugs, they should be further diluted in 10 ml of Normal Saline or injectable distilled sterile water and, using a syringe attached to a catheter which is inserted into the ET tube, should be sprayed quickly down the tube. Immediately, the BVM should be reattached to the endotracheal tube and several quick ventilations should be provided to aerosolize the medication and hasten its absorption. If CPR is being provided, chest compressions should be withheld during the brief period that is required to insert the medication through the tube and provide the several ventilations described for furthering its absorption. The chest compressions should then be resumed to circulate the medication.

When drugs are administered by the endotracheal route, they should be instilled as deeply as possible into the tracheobronchial tree. The loss of medication delivered caused by adhesion of the solution to the walls of the tube can be significantly reduced by the use of an ET tube which contains a medication administration port and a catheter which extends to its distal tip. If an ET tube without such a built in medication catheter along its length has been placed, an adaptor which adds this feature to the ET tube should be used. Carrying such adaptors is recommended for any ALS squad which carries these medications.

Several studies have shown that the use of a catheter through the length of the ET tube only increases the amount of the administered dose that is delivered, but does not eliminate some remaining therapeutic loss. Due to the loss between the dose administered and that actually delivered beyond the tube, and the slower absorption rate provided by endotracheal rather than IV administration, the AHA JAMA Guidelines recommend that 2 to 2.5 times the recommended IV dose of lidocaine, epinephrine or atropine should be diluted in 10 ml of NS or sterile water and administered down the ET tube (except in neonates). Although not specifically addressing the dosage for Narcan, they noted that the doses of other resuscitation drugs should probably also be increased from the intravenous dose when administered endotracheally. Unless this is resolved in his protocols, the EMT should ask the service Medical Director for the specific dose of Narcan that he wishes used, when this needs to be administered endotracheally. Even when the dose of one of these drugs is so increased for endotracheal administration, only the normal IV dose is considered as that therapeutically delivered and in determinations of the total accumulated dose that has been delivered.

The Intraosseous administration and infusion of drugs is an excellent alternative when IV access is not readily available, particularly in pediatric patients.

Administration Of Drugs By Intraosseous Infusion (IO)

The administration of IV drugs or fluid replacement by intraosseous infusion—particularly in but not limited to pediatric patients is an increasingly growing prehospital skill. Establishing an Intraosseous line requires special equipment, knowledge, and skills and should only be attempted by EMTs who have been trained and certified in the skill and whose protocols include this method. Red blood cells are produced in the marrow of the central shafts of longbones (the diaphysis), and large veins connect the medullary (marrow) cavity with the rest of the systemic circulatory system. To administer drugs through this route requires a special IO needle which includes a steel catheter attached to a handle (which is removable in some models), and which contains a trocar. A trocar is a rigid steel (or other hard metal) shaft that is inserted into the length of a hollow needle or tube to strengthen it during insertion, and is then removed to allow access through it. Most trocars have a sharp point or bevel at one end which, when it extends beyond the end of the hollow needle or tube, aids in facilitating its insertion. Once the metal catheter containing the trocar has been inserted through the overlying tissue and hard outer layers of the tubular bone shaft into the medullary canal and marrow, the trocar is removed and the catheter's position should be secured. Then, an IV line is connected to it, preferably using an IV extension set and the usual methods. The medication, in the same dose and form as would be used intravenously, can then be administered through the placed IO catheter, either by pushing a bolus into the tubing of the IV set, or by mixing it into a second bag of IV fluid and hanging it as a piggyback drip. Medications provided by this route are designated as **IO Push** or if mixed into the IV solution bag and run in over a sustained period, as **By IO Drip**. The same "flushing" after a bolus has been injected into the line, and separate piggyback cautions and set up, should be followed for IO lines as are followed for IV lines.

In recent years, contrary to earlier belief, the ability to provide fluid at the required volume and rate for fluid replacement via the intraosseous route has been proven to serve as a singular effective alternative if the customary IV route is not available.

Rectal Medication Administration

In some cases such as Valium in small children, rectal rather than IV administration may be preferred. To administer an appropriate medication solution by rectum, the desired dose is drawn into a syringe and, after removing the needle and inserting the tip of the syringe through the anus, is sprayed into the rectum.

Some medications are compounded with a semi-soft low heat soluble carrier, such as a soap or cocoa butter, and are formed into cone shaped suppositories designed for use as a rectal suppository. When the suppository is inserted into the rectum the body temperature causes the carrier to dissolve, and similar to medications sprayed into the rectum the active therapeutic ingredient is enterally absorbed through the lower intestine. Similar suppositories designed for insertion into the vagina or urethra are also available and used to administer some medications, however through those locations the therapeutic ingredients are parentally (rather than enterally) absorbed. Except for the administration of Valium by rectum in small children, these forms of medication are not common to emergency care, and have only been included for general background knowledge.

Administration Of Topical Medications

Few topical medications are used in emergency prehospital care. Generally the EMT's use of these is limited to iodine or other antiseptic solutions (which are discussed in another Section with wound care), bactericide ointments such as Bacitracin, and opthalamic ointments.

When applying an ointment such as Bacitracin to a small cut, it should not be placed on the skin directly from the tube. To prevent the tube and ointment from contact which could needlessly contaminate either, the ointment should be squeezed out onto a sterile gauze pad first and then applied to the cut with this pad. Should the EMT be asked to assist in covering burn areas with an ointment such as Silvadene from a tube that is commonly used for multiple patients, the previously described method should be followed without breach in order to prevent possible contamination of the reusable tube or its contents. If the ointment is provided in a large tub-like jar, one tongue blade should be used to disperse a large amount onto a sterile pad without contacting the pad and another tongue blade used to apply the ointment to the skin and spread it. The one which is introduced repeatedly into the container should not touch the pad, previously touched ointment remaining on it, or the patient, and the one used to transfer and spread the ointment over the patient's skin areas should not come in contact with the container or its contents.

Opthalamic ointments generally come in a tube which has a small nozzle-like tip. Open the tube (and in some cases pierce the seal found at its tip) and hold it about 3/4 to an inch above the eyes near one of its corners. Positioning the patient so he is supine or sitting with his head rotated back and he is facing almost directly upwards. Open the tube and if necessary pierce any seal found at its tip. Hold the tube between your thumb and several fingers and rest the side of your hand on the patient's upper cheek to steady it. While holding the eye open by spreading the skin over both the superior and inferior orbital ridges with the other hand, move the tube's tip until it is about 3/4 of an inch from the eye's surface and squeeze a small amount out of the tube—moving so as it falls a narrow strip of ointment is formed across the center of the exposed surface of the eye. Finally, remove the tube and allow the patient to close his eye. Have him rotate his eyes while closed through the entire range of their normal movement to spread the ointment fully across the surface of the eye and eyelids.

Other Forms Of Medications And Medication Administration

Although they are not a part of prehospital emergency care, no introduction to medication administration would be complete without at least some mention of several other methods commonly used to externally or internally administer medications used in daily care. Ointments to treat various topical conditions common in the ear or vagina are supplied in containers with applicators or tips particular to their insertion. These should be used following the manufacturer's directions or those supplied by the physician prescribing them.

Many fluids are prescribed for application to the ears, nose, or eyes. Generally these are used in one of two forms, as prescribed. Some are used to irrigate the area and should be used exactly as specified. Generally if a solution is for irrigation of the eyes it is furnished with an eye cup to facilitate this procedure. Most commonly liquid medications are applied to these areas by inserting them carefully as drops using a rubber bulb syringe (dropper) included in the cap for this purpose. Some nasal sprays are furnished in either a soft squeeze bottle with a nebulizer tip or a pump top bottle to nebulize them and allow them to be sprayed into the nostrils as a fine mist.

Special ampules for the direct administration of iodine solutions or such medications as "Sting Kill" to a small localized area of the skin are also available. The ampules designed for this purpose are made of a thin capsule-shaped sealed glass which is, except for one end, entirely encased in a protective flexible shield made of plastic or cardboard. The end which is not so encased has a cotton-wool like tubular plug inserted into it which slightly protrudes beyond the end of the shield. When the ampule is squeezed and the glass broken, the shield encasing it protects the hand from the glass fragments and contains them. The solution from the ampule saturates the cotton pad at the unit's end and is used to apply and spread the medication on the skin.

The ammonia inhalants carried by most squads are analogous to these ampules, and are activated in the identical manner *except that the cotton tip should never be placed in contact with the skin or mucous membranes of the nose.*

Some liquid medications are designed to be placed in the cups of electrical nebulizers, vaporizers, or room humidifiers which deliver them as a cool spray or steam into the ambient air. When the ambient air is inhaled the medication in the droplets of mist produced is inhaled into the mouth and nose and absorbed.

AUTHORIZATION TO ADMINISTER A MEDICATION

Although many medications are available as "over-the-counter" drugs and do not require a physician's prescription, *an EMT may not administer ANY medication to a patient—or even assist him in taking any—without an order prescribing it by a licensed physician.* The physician's order prescribing his administration may be in one of four different forms. It can be:

- *A direct verbal order, by radio or telephone, from the EMS physician providing on-line Medical Direction for a specific patient and call.* In most EMS systems, the validity of such orders is limited to EMTs properly certified to administer the medication, administration within the dosage and other parameters defined in the squad's protocols, and orders directly given by a designated on-line EMS physician.

- *A "Standing Order" in the EMTs protocols.* The protocols of many advanced squads include a number of separate standing medication orders by which the physician who serves as the service's Medical Director prescribes the specific medication, method, and dose to be administered to *ANY PATIENT* who is found to meet certain specified criteria and conditions indicated for its use, and does not have any contraindications for administration by the EMT. Some of the standing orders specify one drug (or one followed by a second) routinely in all cases with the proper indication. Others, outline a more complex and branching progression of medications including repeated doses and differing drugs to be administered in a sequence determined by a continued assessment of the patient, and the effect of those previously given.

- *A direct order from a properly identified physician present at the scene.* Such orders must be in keeping with the EMT's protocols and countersigned by the physician. When a properly identified physician is present and (under local regulations) has assumed the responsibility for the patient's care, and orders doses, methods of administration, or a sequence of medication different than those specifically directed in your protocols—explain this limitation to him. Should he persist in his non-conforming order, obtain on-line Medical Direction to confirm or deny the order before following it.

- *A prescription previously ordered by a physician treating the patient and filled by a pharmacy.* Reasonable confirmation of such a prescription is witnessed for the EMT by the pharmacy label on the container. This must include the name of the specific patient for whom it was prescribed, the name of the medication, the dose to be administered, the frequency and/or special occurrence with which it should be taken, the pharmacy's prescription number, the date filled, and the name of the physician who ordered it.

Due to the possibility that the medications in the container have been replaced with another, and the possible uncertainty of when these were last taken, how many were taken, and if they should be continued or not in light of the conditions and events in this episode—EMTs should *NOT generally* administer or assist or permit the patient to take any previously prescribed medication available in the home.

Cases in which a BLS unit which does not carry epinephrine, nitroglycerine, or nebulized bronchial dilators is summoned to a patient for whom one has been prescribed and it is available in the home—may represent an exception to the general rule. In such cases once the patient has been clearly identified as the one for whom the medication was prescribed and his condition is confirmed to match that for which its use was ordered after contacting his on-line Medical Control for concurrence the EMT may be directed to assist the patient in taking the medication.

Even in cases when the patient's medication is the same as that ordered in the protocols and carried by an advanced squad, since its viability is unknown and the form carried by advanced units may be faster acting (and is within the EMT's training and experience), the EMT should only administer the medication from the ambulance stock and in accordance with his protocols. Because of the chance for an excess resulting from cumulating doses in such cases, the EMT must carefully ascertain when and how much the patient has taken prior to the arrival of the ambulance. Should there be any uncertainty in this regard, or in the dose that the EMT should additionally administer, the EMT should obtain on-line Medical Direction to resolve the question before providing any further medication.

Viability Of A Medication

Any medication must be extensively tested before it is permitted to be generally distributed and used. Before a drug is licensed by the Federal Government, the U.S. Food and Drug Administration reviews vast controlled test information and assures that the medication is both effective in producing its claimed therapeutic effect, and is safe when used as directed. As part of this process the common side effects of the drug and the percentage of patients who had an adverse hypersensitivity and the nature of their reactions is noted. These are required to be included as *warnings* in the directions which are packaged with the substance. It is also required that this testing include establishing the viable *shelf life* of the substance.

All medications have a limited viable time frame during which their potency and safety can be ensured. This period is called the *shelf life* of the drug. After that period the drug may be ineffective or, worse, may be unstable and dangerous to use. When the shelf life is *less than one year*, the label must include a warning which clearly displays the specific expiration date. These notices are generally written as, "Do NOT Use After (the expiration date)" or may be in the affirmative as, "Use Before (the expiration date)." When dispensing these medications and repackaging them, a pharmacist is required to clearly include any specific expiration date warning provided on the original manufacturer's package on the label he provides on the individual patient container.

Federal law also requires that all medications be labeled with a lot identification number, and the date on which they were manufactured. When a pharmacist repackages and dispenses a medication, he is required to include the date on which he dispensed the medication and, if the remaining shelf life is *less than one year,* the appropriate expiration date.

Any medication which does NOT contain a specific expiration date to the contrary on its label, should be considered to automatically have an expiration date one year from its noted date of manufacture or the date on the pharmacist's label indicating when it was dispensed.

*If a medication is in a manufacturer's original container and does NOT legibly include the date of manufacture or is in a pharmacy container that does NOT legibly include the date on which it was dispensed, it must be considered to have expired, and should **NOT BE USED.***

The EMT administering a medication or assisting the patient in taking one that was previously prescribed is responsible to, among others, check the date and ascertain that it has NOT expired.

Some medications require constant refrigeration to maintain their viability and safe use. Such medications are labeled with a warning that specifies that they must be refrigerated at all times. If there is any significant lapse in their refrigeration, these must be considered spoiled and dangerous. Once these have been allowed to warm, they should NOT be returned to the refrigerator. Instead they should be "wasted" by discarding them into a suitable drain. Some medications require refrigeration once they have been opened or mixed. These will be labeled accordingly and should their refrigeration lapse once it has been initiated, should similarly be discarded.

Medications which do not require (and which are not labeled as needing) refrigeration, must nevertheless be assumed to need some climate control to maintain their viability and safe use. If any medication is frozen or exposed to an extremely low temperature (generally below 50 degrees Fahrenheit) or exposed to unusually high temperatures (generally over 100 degrees Fahrenheit), or it or its container are exposed to direct sunlight for any sustained period it should be considered unusable, and should be suitably discarded.

Even if none of these forces act upon a medication, if it appears to have changed in color, clarity, or form from that which is normal, or appears to include any foreign matter, it should *NO LONGER* be considered usable and should be suitably discarded. *As well as the other checks required prior to administering any medication, the EMT must assess the appearance of the medication and confirm that no visible change or foreign matter has developed or become introduced.*

When medications have NOT been re-packaged by a pharmacist and remain in the manufacturer's original packaging, the container should be sealed. Should the seal be broken, removed, or otherwise tampered with, the medication should NOT be used. IV fluid bags are usually packaged in a second sealed transparent or translucent bag. Only by using IV fluids that are so sealed can one be reasonably sure that no other substance has been injected into the IV fluid, or that it has not otherwise been altered or contaminated. In the case of injectables or any medication that must be drawn up or mixed, the EMT should only use those that he has so prepared or were prepared on this call by another properly certified EMT within his direct sight. *NO other unlabelled syringe containing a medication or other form of unlabelled medication should ever be administered, in spite of the representations offered by others regardless of their known or apparent reliability.*

By definition, any medication introduced internally is a relatively highly concentrated foreign substance (compared to the absorption of normally ingested substances) which, in order to achieve its desired therapeutic effect, produces significant physiological alteration. Due to their potency and therapeutic effect the physiological alteration produced by some medications is profound while others, being of a less potent concentration or having a less devastating physiological impact, only commonly produce minor changes. Due to the potential impact of any physiological alteration regardless of its degree, and the potential secondary systemic effects it can produce — NO internal medication should ever be considered benign. All medications *must be considered potent and administered only with the greatest of care.* Some are simply *more* potent and devastating than others.

Regardless of the potency and common effect associated with a particular medication, some segment of the population will be hypersensitive to it. In such patients, it can cause a variety of atypical side effects. These can range from producing mild discomfort (itching, nausea, etc.) to vast systemic deterioration and the interruption of key vital functions.

Prior to administering any medication, the EMT is responsible to check for any known history of allergies and any previous reactions. If the patient is unconscious, or has an otherwise altered level of consciousness so that he can not provide a reliable pertinent past history, you should check for any medical alerting jewelry or — in the presence of a witness — the wallet or pocketbook for a card warning of any previously identified allergies. Sometimes the potential allergy to a medication must be deduced from other known allergies. For example, most patients who are allergic to shrimp are actually allergic to the high concentration of iodine they commonly contain. Therefore, iodine-based (or containing) medications should not be used if an individual has a history of allergic reactions after eating shrimp.

In order to have an allergic reaction, generally the patient must have been exposed to the substance at a previous time. Because medications are compounded of a variety of chemical substances, many of which are common to a wide variety of other medications or foods (and because in rare cases such reactions can occur without any prior contact with the substance), the fact that a drug is being introduced to the patient for the first time does not rule out the chance of anaphylaxis. Even when a medication associated with an extremely low incidence of patient hypersensitivity is administered to a patient who has *NO* known allergies and has repeatedly taken it in the past without ill-effect, an anaphylactic reaction can result. *Whenever administering any medication, the EMT must be prepared for an anaphylactic reaction or other unusual adverse side effects.*

Proper Identification And Selection Of A Medication

The individual administering a drug is responsible to assure that the medication given is the exact one specified in the prescription, and can NOT be any other regardless of similarities. Identifying and confirming that you have the correct medication must *NEVER* be a casual process nor abridged regardless of urgency. The responsibility can *NOT* be assigned or transferred to any other individual — but in all cases remains with the individual administering the drugs.

The vials, ampules, pre-loaded syringes, or cartridges in which an injectable or IV medication is supplied, are *identical* in appearance to those of countless other drugs. Conversely the container in which the same drug is supplied by different manufacturers may vary substantially. The appearance of almost all injectable or IV solutions is that of clear water, or in some cases clear salad or cooking oil. Even when a solution has a seemingly unique appearance, some other totally different medication will have the same.

Even though pharmaceutical companies attempt to provide unique colors and shapes to assist in differentiating between pills, there is always a large number that are identical or have a similar appearance. The only safe way to identify the correctness of a medication is by detailed, careful attention to its label.

Each medication may go by one of four different names. It will have an official *USP name* which is assigned to it by the Federal government, a *generic name* which is used regardless of the manufacturer, a *trade name* which is the unique consumer identification used by a single manufacturer to identify and differentiate its brand from others, and a technical *chemical name* which reflects its chemical composition. Generally each of the four names used for a single drug is different from the other three, however in some cases the official name and the generic name will be the same.

Fortunately for the daily identification of a drug for administration, the EMT must only be familiar with its generic and different possible trade names. For example, when identifying one anti-arrhythmic drug commonly used in advanced prehospital care, the EMT must know its:

Generic Name — Xylocaine Hydrochloride

Trade Names — Lidocaine Hydrochloride

Procaine Hydrochloride

Novocain Hydrochloride

Xylocaine Hydrochloride

With some medications, common chemical designations or abbreviations may be used in the name, and the EMT must be familiar with those he administers. For example *hydrochloride* is chemically often identified by the chemical abbreviation HCl. Therefore, using the previous example, *Xylocaine Hydrochloride* may be labeled as *Xylocaine HCl*. It is important to note that the absence of, or a difference in, a single letter in a chemical abbreviation, or an even slight difference in the sequence of the letters, may make the drug described to be a vastly different substance.

Normal Saline serves as another example. It may be identified in the physician's order simply as NS and, on the IV bag, it may be identified only as *0.9% Sodium Chloride* with or without the inclusion of the term, *Normal Saline* or its common abbreviation, *NS*.

The EMT must be sufficiently knowledgeable of any drug he commonly administers to be able to make the necessary translation and to be alerted when there appears to be some discrepancy. Due to the possible dire consequences from a medication error, if any uncertainty exists it should not be resolved by any assumption or logical deduction by the EMT. What appears logical may *NOT* in truth be the fact. *Any question surrounding the identification or administration of a medication in the field should be resolved by the physician providing on-line Medical Direction, before the drug is administered by the EMT.*

The letters USP following the name is not indicative of any chemical variation in the drug, but simply certifies that it has been formulated exactly to the description and standard in the United States Pharmacopeia or National Formulary, which is officially established and maintained by the U.S. Food and Drug Administration.

As has been discussed earlier, the same medication may be commonly available in a variety of grades of purity or different formulations (containing different solvents, carrying, binding, or flavoring agents). *When identifying the medication for a particular ordered administration, the EMT must be sure that as well as being the correct substance, the medication selected is in a formulation designated for the route by which he will administer it.* This should be identified and confirmed by the inclusion of designations on the label such as: *Oral, For oral use, PO, Injection, For Injection, Intravenous, For Intravenous Infusion, IV, etc.*

DETERMINING THE AMOUNT AND CONFIRMING THE DOSE TO BE ADMINISTERED

The amount of the therapeutic agent of a drug that is provided, the actual dose delivered, is most commonly measured in *milligrams (mg)*. There are 1,000 milligrams (milli = a thousandth) in a gram, so larger doses may be measured and described in *grams (G)*. When a dose is required which is a fractional part of a milligram, it may be measured and described in *micrograms (μg)*. There are 1000 micrograms in a milligram (or 1,000,000 micrograms in a gram). Micrograms are properly abbreviated as μg, however, when using a typewriter that does not contain the unique metric symbol for micro (μ), it may be alternatively abbreviated as, *mcg*.

Although rare, some medications are still commonly prescribed and measured in *grains(gr)* from the old Apothecary System used before the metric system became the accepted standard. There are 60mg in 1 grain, or inversely viewed, a milligram is 1/60th of a grain. To aid in avoiding possible confusion between the abbreviations used for grams and grains, gram is always abbreviated as a capital **G** and grains is abbreviated using only lower case letters as **gr** — or is fully spelled out.

With some PO medications whose concentration is either defined as a constant by the drug's name or included in the order, the dosage may be ordered and measured in *ounces (oz.), tablespoons (tbsp.) or teaspoons (tsp.)*. Orders to administer one or more teaspoons or tablespoons, should be considered to define the exact quantity to be delivered but not interpreted literally to limit the exact method by which the medication is to be delivered into the mouth. These do not preclude the use of a syringe or dropper, should this be a better delivery method such as when administering the dose to a small child. Ounces, tablespoons, and teaspoons are remnants from the old Apothecary system and translate into metric measure as:

One Ounce   = 30 milliliters

One Tablespoon = 15 milliliters

One Teaspoon   = 5 milliliters

Except for a few PO medications, these are no longer a common standard measure used to quantify fluids for drug administration.

Liquids are measured and calculated for drug administration in the common metric fluid measures. The volume of a liquid drug is measured and stated in **milliliters** (ml). A milliliter of any fluid measures **one cubic centimeter** (an amount which if formed into a square, would be 1 centimeter (an amount which if formed into a square, would be 1 centimeter wide by 1 centimeter high by 1 centimeter deep). Usually, when describing a fluid, since the shape is transitory, cubic centimeter is expressed as a **cc** and not with its other possible abbreviation **cm³** — although the EMT may see this form occasionally. Since one milliliter equals one cubic centimeter (1ml=1cc), these can be used interchangeably. There are 1,000 milliliters in a Liter (L) and when describing large amounts, such as the fluids in IV bags, they may be described using the latter. Although a milliliter can be divided into 1,000 microliters (μL), this small measure is not used in prescribing or administering drugs.

The number of milligrams of a drug that are delivered in one milliliter will vary depending upon the concentration of the drug in the solvent or suspension. For example, epinephrine is commonly used prehospital in both 1:1,000 and 1:10,000 concentrations. One ml of the 1:1,000 concentration delivers 10 times the dose that is delivered in one ml of the 1:10,000 solution. Similarly, when a drug is added into an IV bag for drip administration, the dose delivered in each ml will vary depending on the amount of the drug that was added to the bag — called the *mixing dose* — and the size (amount of fluid that it contains) of the bag. If 200 mg are added to a 500 ml bag the amount of the drug delivered in 1 ml will be twice that which would be delivered if instead it was added to a 1,000 ml (IL) bag. However, if 200 mg of a drug are added to a ml bag or if 400 mg is added to a 1,000 ml bag, the per ml dose will be the same. To avoid any confusion in the amount of the drug desired, fluid medications are ordered and administered in the milligrams to be delivered rather than in milliliters or another fluid measure (except some PO, constant mixtures). To avoid the chance for confusion caused by possible different concentrations, liquid medications which are for injection or IV administration are labeled with the number of milligrams that are delivered in one milliliter. When mixing or diluting a drug further, the EMT should always include the resulting mg/ml on the medications label as a clear indication of the concentration that results.

The amount of a drug added to the IV bag must never exceed the maximum allowed dosage. When using an IV medication that comes in pre-mixed bags, should the total milligrams supplied exceed the maximum recommended dose for an individual patient, the surplus should be calculated and an appropriate number of milliliters be run out and wasted before the piggyback is hung and installed into the primary line. When mixing a drug into an IV bag the ratio between the dose (mg of the drug to be placed into the IV fluid) and the size of the bag (ml of IV solution in the bag) should be selected so that the desired dose per minute is delivered when the 60 gtt drip set used for this purpose, is adjusted to a 30 gtt/minute (0.5 ml/min) rate of flow. This allows for the maximum possible range of dose/min adjustment to either increase or decrease the delivered per minute dose if needed.

The amount of a medication (with most drugs) that is the appropriate dose for an individual patient is determined by the size of his body. Body size is measured for this purpose by the patient's weight, stated in *kilograms (kg)*, and is described as a number of *milligrams per kilogram (mg/kg)*. If the patient's weight is only known in pounds, it will have to be translated into its metric equivalent in kilograms. There are 2.2 pounds in one kilogram. Therefore, to translate a patient's weight in pounds into kilograms, the number of pounds is divided by 2.2. To avoid a dangerous major error that would result if the calculation was done in the wrong direction or a decimal point misplaced, the EMT should remember that *the number of kilograms is approximately one half of the number of pounds,* and should check that any more accurate calculation done in translating these produces an answer which is near this estimate.

One cannot intermix measures from different systems of measurement (metric and the former British Standard or others) in the same calculation. *All components must be in metric measures (the metric scale) when calculating drug doses, or an invalid answer and the WRONG dose will result from the calculation.*

In the case of many drugs, the therapeutic effect to be delivered is not materially affected by the possible difference in size from one adult to another, and a single adult dosage is used regardless of weight. Due to the vast differences in size from neonate or infant to full adult body size, doses for pediatric patients are ordered and administered based upon the individual patient's kilogram weight, and must be considered to be weight sensitive.

Studies done by Breselow and several other pediatricians in recent years conclude that a child's height (length from the top of the head to the bottoms of the feet) in centimeters (cm) may be a more valid measure of size for the determination of proper drug doses and normal vital sign expectations. Although an increasing number of squads use the *Resuscitation Tape* developed by Breselow to rapidly measure a child's length and indicate the proper dose for common emergency drugs, *kilogram weight still remains the prevailing criteria in determining size and individual dosage of pediatric drugs.*

When administering a drug by IV drip, the therapeutic dose delivered is determined by both the amount of the drug in each milliliter (the concentration) and the rate at which the drip is run. Orders for IV drips contain both and are customarily written as either a given number of milligrams per minute (mg/min) or as a number of milligrams per kilogram per minute (mg/kg/min).

Sometimes only the entire dose and duration of administration are provided with the name of the drug (eg: Administer 720 mgs over 60 minutes). In such cases once the size of the IV bag into which the drug is to/has been added is known, the mg/ml must be determined, and then the per minute rate (gtt/minute) required to deliver all of the medication in the 60 minutes prescribed must be calculated.

In the case of some drugs administered by IV drip (such as Dopamine) the dose necessary to produce the desired therapeutic effect in an individual patient can neither be exactly known nor calculated. For such drugs, only the safe range of administration for an individual is known, and the exact amount needed within this range must be determined clinically. In such cases the drip is initially provided at the low end of the range and is slowly increased by small increments, until the desired therapeutic change is seen to occur and be sustained. This is described as *titrating* the dose to the desired effect and is ordered by indicating the name of the medication and range (from the lowest to the highest number) of mcgs, mgs, or Gs that may be administered, followed by "titrate to BP between 90 and 100 mmHg Systolic." Other drugs are titrated to different specific desired therapeutic effects, whether restoring an adequate BP, the pulse rate, or providing pain relief, as examples.

The dose of some drugs, such as Valium, is also primarily titrated to the desired effect when they are administered by IV Push. Rather than an increased rate of infusion such as when titrating a drug by drip, when titrating a drug by IV Push one slowly continues to push an increasing amount of the drug (enlarging the loading dose amount cumulatively delivered) until the desired effect is achieved or the maximum allowable dose is reached. This is ordered and described as, "Given Valium up to 10 mgs by IVP—titrate to desired effect."

Most IV push drugs that require determining the specific dose and therapeutic level needed for an individual patient by increasing the delivered dose until the desired effect can be clinically observed, are NOT titrated in this way. Instead, an exact initial dose is administered first, shortly followed by one or more specific repeated doses of the same or different quantity until the desired therapeutic result occurs and is clinically seen, or the maximum recommended dose is reached. For example, to suppress ventricular ectopy (PVCs or other undesirable irregular heart beats) lidocaine is generally given with an initial IVP dose of 1.5 mg/kg and if the ectopy is *NOT* resolved, repeated doses of 0.75 mg/kg are administered IV Push as/if needed every 3–5 minutes until the ectopy is resolved or the total accumulated dose administered has reached 3 mg/kg. A group of abbreviations are customarily used to shorten the writing of such orders and EMTs who administer drugs must be familiar with them:

Repeat   — r

Every   — $\bar{q}$ or q

As needed   — prn (from the Latin *pro re nata*)

Not to exceed — "to" or "up to"

Repeat (a specific number) of times — rX (the number such as rX2, etc.)

The previous example of lidocaine would commonly be ordered or written as:

"Give 1.5 mg/kg lidocaine IVP r 0.75 mg/kg

q 3–5 min prn, to 3 mg/kg."

The letters "q" and "prn" are also used in giving verbal orders, however, for clarity "repeat every" or "repeat" are stated fully.

Maintaining The Desired Effect Of A Drug

Once an adequate dose of a drug is administered and absorbed to provide a proper therapeutic level, it is metabolized by the body. This causes the therapeutic level to become progressively lowered and the degree of benefit to decay with time. Finally, the therapeutic agent and other elements included are reduced to waste products, and eliminated from the body.

From a simpler perspective, the therapeutic agents, in producing the desired benefit, are progressively used up by the body and, once the level remaining in the body is below the necessary therapeutic level, the benefit is no longer provided. The duration that drugs remain at a sufficient therapeutic level in the body to provide the desired benefit is different from one drug to the other, and is also varied by the patient's metabolism. It can also be extended by coatings (in the case of pills) or ingredients included with the therapeutic agent which slow the rate of absorption, enlarging the time period in which the necessary therapeutic level is maintained. Regardless of these variations, *the duration during which any drug is effective is always limited*—whether as with adenosine for only a very short 6 second period, or as with many enteric oral cold medications for an extended 10 to 12 hour period.

The duration during which a drug remains at a sufficient therapeutic level to provide its desired benefit is called the drug's *half-life*. If the benefit must be provided beyond the half-life of the drug, the therapeutic level must be maintained by administering a repeat dose or by another means.

Regardless of whether the necessary therapeutic level of a drug is initially achieved by the administration of a single dose or the accumulation of several closely repeated boluses until the desired effect is observed, the initial quantity of the drug needed to obtain the necessary therapeutic level in the patient is called the *loading dose*. As the level of the drug in the body declines during its half-life, any additional amounts administered to restore and maintain a sufficient therapeutic level are called *maintenance doses*.

Except for most oral medications, the repeated dose is commonly administered within the half-life of the drug and at a lower dose than initially provided. In this way, as the therapeutic level decays and becomes reduced (but before it is so low as to no longer be of benefit), an additional, generally smaller, *maintenance dose* is added to keep it at an adequate level at all times in order to maintain "the desired effect" without interruption.

In the case of some drugs (generally those initially administered by IV Push) once the initial therapeutic dose has been administered, or reached as evidenced by the initiation of the desired effect, the therapeutic level is maintained by the infusion of a continuous dose per minute, administered by IV drip. In some cases the IV drip maintenance dose is the same regardless of the initial dose used, while in others such as IV lidocaine (where the initial dose is accumulated using repeated boluses until the necessary benefit is achieved), it is generally varied based upon which cumulative amount was needed to produce the desired therapeutic effect.

After the initial dose of some drugs such as epinephrine, the therapeutic level can be maintained *either* by repeated IV push boluses or by the institution of an IV drip. Generally the method selected and ordered is based upon the purpose for which the drug is being administered. When the epinephrine is being administered to stimulate the heart and accelerate its rate, repeated boluses are elected so maintenance, discontinuance, or reinstitution can be easily effected as rhythm and rate changes occur. If it is being used primarily as an adjunct to improving alveolar ventilation, the continuous maintenance of the therapeutic level provided by IV drip administration is often preferred.

In some cases, drugs such as lidocaine whose therapeutic levels are customarily maintained by an IV drip, may instead be maintained by periodic repeated boluses when run times are relatively short (and if allowed in the EMT's protocols), in order to avoid additional time and confusion prior to arrival at the hospital.

With drugs such as dopamine which are administered exclusively by the titration of an IV drip to the desired effect, there is no distinction made between the loading and maintenance dose. However, the desired effect must be maintained and monitored. Should the effect become lost or too great, the rate of infusion must be adjusted (or re-titrated) to restore the desired level of effect.

The amount and interval between which a drug is repeated to provide a maintenance dose (or the mg/min selected for maintenance by IV drip) is selected to approximate the amount of the drug that is progressively metabolized during the drug's half-life. Maintenance doses are selected so they will only restore the amount of the drug in the body to that of the therapeutic level in the loading dose, and do not increase the circulating level beyond it.

Maximum recommended doses in published drug guidelines or maximum doses detailed in a protocol apply to the loading dose and, unless specifically to the contrary, do *NOT* refer to or include the maintenance doses. For example, the recommended dose of lidocaine is an initial bolus of 1.5 mg/kg IVP with repeated doses of 0.75 mg/kg every 3 to 5 minutes as needed to produce the desired effect, *not to exceed a total cumulative dose of 3 mg/kg*. If the cumulative dose of 3 mg/kg was necessary and succeeded in suppressing the ectopy, an IV drip to deliver 4 mg/min is recommended additionally. Since the IV drip maintains rather than increases the therapeutic level, it is not considered to be included in the 3 mg/kg recommended maximum dose. The maintenance dose is limited to the amount and intervals ordered but not to any specified total amount.

In the rare case where a guideline or order wishes to include both the loading and maintenance doses in its recommended maximum dose restriction, this is indicated by language such as, "not to exceed 1000 mg in any 6 hour period," etc.

DOSES FOR IV FLUID NOT CONTAINING OTHER DRUGS

When running IVs which do NOT contain any drug other than that of the basic fluid selected (D_5W, NS, 0.5NS, LR) the administration dosage surrounds considerations of the volume of fluid infused rather than milligrams delivered. Orders for base IV fluids are usually limited to the type of fluid, overall quantity and rate of infusion.

An example of such an order is, "Administer an IV of 1L. of NS to run at 4 ml/min." To calculate the number of drops at which the IV should be run, you simply multiply the ml/min ordered, times the number of drops in one milliliter (gtt/ml) of the specific IV Administration set to be used.

For the above order if using a 10 gtt/ml administration set the following calculation would be used:

Required Drops/min = (ml/min ordered) X (drops/ml of drip set used)

gtt/min = (ml/min) (gtt/ml)

= (4 ml/min) (10 gtt/ml)

= 4 X 10

To administer the 1L. of NS at the 4 ml/min rate ordered, the drip should be adjusted to a rate of 40 drops per minute and the IV run until the entire bag has been infused.

In most orders for fluid replacement in the field, the overall quantity to be infused is also usually specified. In such orders the maintenance of the infusion at the rate specified from the time of institution of the IV line in the field until arrival at the Emergency Department (or the maximum fluid replacement volume specified in the protocols is reached), is implicit except in small children, the elderly, or patients with congestive heart failure (CHF). An example of such an order would be, "Initiate 2 IVs of NS, run at a wide open rate." The terms *wide open* or *full rate* are interchangeably used to indicate that the IVs should be run at the maximum rate possible for the vein. They also include implicitly a direction to select a large vein, use a large bore catheter (the largest possible for the vein selected but generally not smaller than 18g.), and use a maxidrip (10 gtt) infusion set.

When providing fluid replacement particularly in children, the elderly, or patients with CHF, but not limited to these groups, *homeostasis* (fluid balance) is a concern. If too much fluid is delivered it can result in fluid overload and such problems as pulmonary edema. *When IV fluid replacement is being provided, the lungs must be auscultated repeatedly every 3 to 5 minutes and, should signs of pulmonary edema or any other significant adverse effect appear, the infusion rate should be reduced to KVO until further instructions are obtained from on-line Medical Direction.* To avoid fluid overload in small children, IV fluid replacement is generally administered in rapid 250 ml (or 20 ml/kg) amounts at a time, between which the child's status should be carefully checked before this is repeated. As well, most protocols limit the total crystalloid volume replacement in small children as *not to exceed 50 – 60 ml/kg.*

The EMT should note that in hypovolemic patients, the paramount prehospital problem is in restoring and maintaining a sufficient circulatory volume to produce adequate perfusion, and only rarely one of developing fluid overload. Except in small children, the elderly, or others with CHF, due to the limited duration and transitory nature of the crystalloid fluids generally used to provide fluid replacement prehospital, it is difficult to provide excessive fluid to patients with a significant fluid loss.

Orders to run IV fluids at a wide open or other rapid rate include an *implicit order* to:
- Monitor the patient and IV continuously.
- Periodically recheck the vital signs and IV site.
- Periodically auscultate the lungs. Reduce the rate to KVO if pulmonary edema or other untofore signs appear.
- Obtain on-line medical direction immediately if any problems occur.

Although rare, an order for IV fluid, rather than specifying ml/min rate, may only order the total fluid volume to be delivered and the overall time over which this is to be done. For example, "Start an IV of 1L of NS and run it over 2 hours."

Since one can not include *liters* or *hours* in a calculation before going further, the EMT should rewrite the order so as to convert these to milliliters and minutes. There are 1000 ml in a liter and, since there are 60 minutes in an hour (to convert hours into minutes, multiply the number of hours by 60), the restated order would read, "Run 1,000 ml of NS over 120 min."

The Formula used to calculate the number of drops/min at which the IV should run is:

$$\text{Required drops per minute} = \frac{(\text{TOTAL ml VOLUME ORDERED}) \times (\text{Drops per ml of Set})}{(\text{Ordered time in minutes})}$$

$$\text{Desired gtt/min} = \frac{(\text{ml of IV fluid}) \times (\text{gtt/ml})}{(\text{Number of minutes})}$$

If using a maxidrip as is customary for fluid replacement, the set produces (or requires) 10 drops per ml (10 gtt/ml).

Therefore:

$$\text{Desired gtt/min} = \frac{(1{,}000 \text{ ml}) \times (10 \text{ gtt/ml})}{(120 \text{ min})}$$

$$x = \frac{(1000)\,(10)}{(120)}$$

The numerator and denominator can both be reduced by dividing each by ten without altering the fraction's value. This can rapidly be done by eliminating the (10) in the numerator and, in the denominator, moving the implied decimal point after the 120.00 one space to the left (or more simply by removing the last zero, changing it from 120 to 12.)

$$x = \frac{(1000)\ (10)}{(120)}$$

$$x = \frac{1,000}{12}$$

$$x = 12\overline{)1000.00}$$

$$x = 83.3$$

Therefore, if the IV is run using a 10 gtt/ml set at 83 drops per minute, the Liter of NS will be administered over two hours as was ordered.

If given a similar order including hours and for which a minidrip (60 gtt/ml) set is to be used, those who are familiar with the reduction of fractions by the cancellation of equal factors in both the numerator and denominator, can save a great deal of math by a slight alteration from the preceding.

For example, if given the order to "Run 100 ml of NS over 2 hours," it is expressed as:

$$\text{Desired gtt/min} = \frac{(100\ ml)\ X\ (60\ gtt/ml)}{2\ (60\ min)}$$

$$x = \frac{(100)\ (60)}{2\ (60)}$$

$$x = \frac{(100)}{(2)}$$

$$x = 50$$

$$\text{Desired rate} = 50\ gtt/min$$

Sometimes an order such as this is given as an ordered number of milliliters to be run per hour (*NOT* to be confused with ml/min). Whenever an order for IV fluid is for a stated number of ml/hour *and* a 60 gtt/ml set is used, the number of drops per minute at which the IV should be run equals the number of mls/hour ordered, and no calculation is required.

FORMULAS AND CALCULATIONS FOR PARENTERAL LIQUID DRUG ADMINISTRATION

Since the ordered dose for drugs to be administered by injection, IV Push, or IV drip is given in milligrams (or micrograms, or Grams, or milliequivalents) and the drugs for this purpose are supplied in a liquid form, one or more calculations is necessary to determine the milliliters of the drug fluid that must be administered in order to deliver the number of milligrams (or other specified measure) ordered.

When setting up the formulas and calculations necessary six definitions or terms are commonly used, and the EMT must be familiar with each:

The **Desired Dose** (DD) is the number of milligrams, micrograms or grams (grains, milliequivalents, etc.) that is prescribed and ordered to be administered. IF ordered for IV drip administration it will be stated as milligrams (or similar weight measure) per minute. Other terms used instead of desired dose may be, *Ordered Dose* or *Dose Ordered*.

The **Concentration on Hand** (COH) is the total number of milligrams (or other weight measure) of the drug that is supplied in the vial, ampule, pre-loaded syringe, or IV bag. This can also be designed as *Total mg On Hand* or *Total mg Supplied*.

Warning: "Concentration," when not further qualified, generally refers to the number of milligrams supplied in one milliliter of the drug solution (mg/ml) or the ratio of the number of parts of the drug to the number of parts of the solvent (1:1,000 etc.). However, when qualified as "Concentration On Hand," it is limited to describing the total number of milligrams supplied.

The **Volume On Hand** (VOH) is the total amount of fluid supplied in the vial, ampule, pre-loaded syringe, or IV bag in which the drug is dissolved, *stated in milliliters*. It can also be designated as *Total ml ON Hand or Total ml Supplied.*

The **Volume to be Administered** is the number of milliliters (ml) that is calculated to be needed administered in order to provide the ordered milligram dose. It may also be designated as *Number of ml to Administer or ml To Administer.*

The **gtt** or **drops per milliliter** (gtt/ml) is the number of drops that, in a given IV Administration Set (drip set), equal one milliliter. The drops per milliliter of a set is indicated on its package as its gtt/ml or simply as its gtt.

In almost all cases a 60 gtt (minidrip) set is used for medication delivery as this provides more finite adjustment than those producing larger drops.

The **IV Rate** is the number of drops per minute (gtt/min) at which the IV drip is run. In the case of calculations, *it is the number of drops per minute needed to provide the ordered dose* with the administration set being used. Because the volume being infused at a given drip rate varies with the IV administration set being used, *the rate of infusion* is generally stated as the ml/min being delivered and not as a drip rate.

Two analogous rules must always be followed when setting up and doing any drug calculation:

- *Units of measure from different systems of measurement (Metric, Apothecary, etc.), must NEVER be used in the same formula or calculation.* Should an element which needs to be included in a calculation be in a system other than the metric standard, it must separately be converted into its metric equivalent before it is included in any of the following formulas and calculations.

- *Terms describing different collective standard values for one area of metric measurement* (eg: Liters and milliliters for fluid volume, or micrograms, milligrams, and grams for drug weight/ therapeutic quantity) *can NEVER be used in the same formula or calculation.* All fluid amounts must be in milliliters or converted into them, and any patient weight into kilograms. All drug quantities must be converted to *one* — either micrograms, milligrams, or grams — whichever is the smallest unit stated in the order — or in the case of a few drugs, milliequivalents.

These rules often require that a measure from another system be converted into its metric equivalent, or that one unit of metric measurement is converted into another (eg: Liters to milliliters or Grams to milligrams, etc.). To assist the reader in making such conversions, a Table of common measures and their equivalents, has been included in the Summary Skill Sheets found at the end of this Section.

Drug calculations are introduced in most textbooks in a diverse series of complex classical formulas. Because each of these combines a variety of elements and steps in a single formula and calculation, both their recall and the math that commonly results is often unnecessarily difficult. The same problems can be solved using a short sequence of simpler and logically self-evident formulas which promote much simpler math. Regardless of the different drug problems that must be formulated and calculated when giving drugs by injection, IV Push, or IV piggyback drip, they can be solved by using a single generic sequence of steps.

Note: to avoid redundancy, in the following steps milligrams have been used to indicate the drug's weight/amount. When the order is specified in micrograms or milliequivalents, these are used instead. When doing prehospital drug calculations the sequence recommended is:

Step 1 — Do any conversions needed.
　　　　If applicable, change any fluid measures to milliliters.
　　　　If applicable, change any drug weight/strength to either milligrams or micrograms *whichever is the smallest unit of measure appearing anywhere in the order.*
　　　　If applicable, convert patient's weight from pounds to kilograms.

Step 2 — Determine the number of milligrams (or µgs, etc.) ordered.
　　　　If the number of milligrams to be administered is given as a specific number in the order, note it.
　　　　If the order is dependent upon the patient's weight (mg/kg or mg/kg/min), calculate the number of milligrams (or mg/min) this represents *for this patient*.

Step 3 — Determine the number of milligrams per milliliter (mg/ml) in the specific concentration of the drug supplied.

If the mg/ml is specified on the label, note it.

If not specified, calculate it from the total milligrams and total milliliters supplied and indicated on the container label.

Step 4 — Calculate the number of milliliters (or ml/min) **to be administered to provide the milligrams ordered.**

Step 5 — If an IV drip, determine the gtt/ml of the administration set to be used, and calculate the drip rate (gtt/min) at which it is to be run — to provide the mg/min dose ordered.

Except for the last step, *the steps and calculations* are the same whether the drug is to be administered by injection, IV Push, or a pre-mixed drug for IV drip.

Because the components included in any formula are each reduced to an unqualified numerical value (a simple number) before the mathematical functions (multiplication, division, etc.) are performed, they must be based upon a single common unit of measure for each area of measurement (fluid volume, weight/amount of the drug, patient weight, etc.) included.

If any components needed in a drug calculation are indicated by a measure not in the metric scale (such as grains) these must be converted into their equivalent value in a metric measure. Prehospital orders for parenteral drugs which require calculation to fluid amounts to be administered are stated in metric measure and therefore a calculated conversion in the field is not needed when administering these drugs.

Orders for parenteral drugs do commonly contain references to a given area of measurement (volume, drug/weight amount, etc.) in 2 different metric units of measurement (L and ml, or G and mg, or mg and mcg). If any fluid volume is given in liters it must be converted to milliliters. The prefix *milli* means a thousandth so 1L = 1,000 milliliters. Therefore, liters can be converted to mls by multiplying the number of liters by a thousand.

Number of milliliters = (number of Liters) X (1,000)

The advantage of the metric system is that such conversions can be done without the need of calculation simply by moving the decimal point. Although not generally written, the decimal point is immediately to the right of any whole number. Therefore 4 liters is really 4.000 liters. To multiply any number by a thousand the decimal point is simply moved three spaces to the right,

therefore: 4 liters = 4.000 liters = 4,000 milliliters.

The reader should note that to move the decimal point three spaces to the right of any whole number (one without a decimal point in it), one simply adds three zeros (000) behind it. If the number is a decimal fraction such as 1.5 L, the decimal point will actually need to be moved three spaces to the right.

1.5 L = 1.500 L = 1,500 ml

Since 1 Gram = 1,000 milligrams the same mathematics and method is used to convert from Grams to milligrams:

Number of milligrams = (Number of Grams) X (1,000)

Similarly, since 1 milligram = 1,000 micrograms, the same method is used to convert milligrams to micrograms:

Number of micrograms = (Number of milligrams) X (1,000).

Next, if the number of milligrams ordered is variable dependent upon the patient's weight (a kilogram reference is included in the order), the patient's weight must be converted into kilograms and the number of milligrams (or mg/min) ordered for a patient of this weight calculated. This is necessary to determine a specific number of milligrams as the dose ordered in the additional calculations that are required.

When translating a problem into a mathematical formula, it is often a good idea to write out the relationships using words or familiar abbreviations before writing a more precise formula. When working an equation a lower case "x" is generally used to signify the unknown entity and an upper case "X" to signify "times" or the multiplication function.

If a dose of 4 mg/kg is ordered for a 150 pound patient, one starts by translating the patient's weight from pounds to kilograms. Since there are 2.2 lbs/kg, this can be done exactly using the following formula:

$$\text{Kilogram Weight} = \frac{\text{(Weight in Pounds)}}{2.2}$$

$$x = \frac{150}{2.2}$$

To eliminate a decimal point in the denominator the decimal point is moved one space to the right in both the numerator and the denominator. This is the same as multiplying each by 10 and does *NOT* change the value of the fraction.

$$x = \frac{1500}{22}$$

$$x = 22\overline{)1500.0}$$

$$x = 68.1$$

Patient's Metric Weight = 68 kg

Alternatively, this can be rapidly calculated by dividing the weight in pounds by two, and then subtracting 10% of that number from itself to provide the equivalent weight in kilograms. Since the patient's weight is 150 pounds, when divided by two this becomes 75. To divide it by 10 (in order to find 10% of the number) move the decimal point one place to the left, giving you 7.5. When is is subtracted from the 75, it leaves 67.5 — or a metric weight of 68 kg.

Once the patient's weight has been converted to kilograms the number of milligrams needed is calculated by multiplying the patient's kilogram weight by the number of mg/kg ordered.

Ordered dose = (Patient's kg. weight) X (milligrams per kilogram ordered)

= (kg wt) (mg/kg ordered)

Since the patient's weight is 68 kg and 4 mg/kg were ordered:

mg ordered = (68 kg) (4 mg/kg)

$$x = (68)\ (4)$$

$$x = 68$$
$$X4$$
$$x = 272 \text{ mg.}$$

The dose ordered = 272 mg.

Once any necessary conversions have been done and the mg ordered dose has been determined from the order (and if applicable, calculated from the patient's weight, the next step is to determine the number of milligrams of the drug provided in one milliliter (mg/ml) in the concentration supplied. For the next few steps the following will serve as a good demonstration.

You are ordered to administer 10 mgs of a drug which is provided in a vial containing 4 ml of fluid and a total of 20 mgs of the drug. If, as with many drugs, the mgs/ml is included in the label, it would read "5 mg/ml".

If the number of milligrams in each milliliter (mg/ml) is not indicated on the label, it can be calculated from the total number of milligrams and total number of milliliters supplied (which must be indicated on all drug labels, using the following method:

$$\text{Number of Milligrams in One ml} = \frac{\text{Concentration on Hand}}{\text{Volume on Hand}}$$

or:

$$\text{Number of Milligrams in one ml} = \frac{\text{Total Number of Milligrams Supplied}}{\text{Total Number of Milliliters Supplied}}$$

$$\text{mg/ml} = \frac{\text{Total mg}}{\text{Total ml}}$$

or:

$$1 \text{ ml} = x \text{ mg} = \frac{\text{Total mg}}{\text{Total mg}}$$

$$x \text{ mg} = \frac{20 \text{ mg}}{4 \text{ ml}}$$

$$x = \frac{20}{4}$$

$$x = 5$$

Therefore, 1 ml = 5 mg

Or, the drug concentration = 5 mg/ml.

Once the mg/ml concentration is known, the number of ml needed to provide the desired dose can be easily calculated by using the following simple formula:

$$\text{Volume to be administered} = \frac{\text{Desired Dose in mg}}{\text{Number of mgs in One ml}}$$

or:

$$\text{Number of ml to administer} = \frac{\text{mg in ordered dose}}{\text{mg/ml supplied}}$$

$$\text{ml to administer} = \frac{\text{mg ordered}}{\text{mg/ml supplied}}$$

$$\text{ml to administer} = \frac{10 \text{ mg}}{5 \text{ mg}}$$

$$x = \frac{10}{5}$$

$$x = 2$$

Volume to be administered = 2 ml

To deliver the desired dose of 10 mg to the patient, 2 ml of the fluid in the vial should be drawn up and administered.

When an order is for IV drip administration, the dose is stated as a number of milligrams per minute (mg/min) or as a number of milligrams per kilogram per minute (mg/kg/min). Except that the milligram dose ordered is specified as per minute (mg/min), and therefore the calculated number of milliliters to administer is per minute (ml/min), the calculations necessary to determine the number of milliliters required are exactly the same as the previous ones demonstrated.

If the order had been for 10 mgs/min to be administered by IV drip, and the pre-mixed IV bag contains 500 mg of the drug in 100 ml of IV solution by using the previously demonstrated methods you would have calculated that the concentration in the IV bag is 5 mg/ml (or this would be indicated on the IV label) and, that to deliver the ordered mg/min dose, the infusion must be run at a rate of 2 ml/minute. An additional step is necessary to translate this into a usable drip rate (gtt/min).

To determine the number of drops per minute at which the IV should be run, ascertain the number of drops that provide one ml (gtt/ml) for the particular IV administration set that will be used, and multiply this times the calculated ml/min required (to provide the ordered mg/min). In this case a minidrip set (60 gtt/ml) will be used.

Drops per minute required = (ml/min desired) X (drops per ml of the administration set)

gtt/min = (ml/min) X (gtt of set used)

gtt/min = (2 ml) X (60 gtt)

$$x = (2)(60)$$

$$x = 120$$

Drops per minute required = 120

If the IV is run at 120 drops per minute this will deliver 2 ml/minute and the 10 mg/minute ordered. Though the method is shown as a mini-formula for the sake of completeness, this does not need to be learned. The EMT must only remember that once the number of ml/min has been calculated, it is converted to the drip rate needed (gtt/min) by simply multiplying it by the gtt of the IV administration set used.

When, instead of using a premixed IV solution, the EMT must first mix the drug into a prescribed solution the order will be in two separable parts. For example, "Place 800 mg in 100 ml of D_5W *and* run an IV drip at 8 mg/min."

The first part prescribes the mixture and concentration to be made up by the EMT, and the second the amount to be administered by IV drip. The drug is supplied in a vial with 100 mg/ml. The preceding described formulas and steps will need to be applied twice. Once to determine the number of mls of the supply of the drug that must be drawn up and inserted into the IV bag to add the 800 mg ordered added, and a second time (as with a pre-mixed IV bag of the drug) to determine the ml/min required to provide the mg/min ordered. Lastly, from the gtt of the administration set, this must be translated into the number of drops per minute at which the IV should be run to provide the ml/min infusion rate necessary.

In order to avoid confusion and error between the initial concentration in which the drug is supplied and the vastly different concentration of it once it has been diluted further by mixing it into the IV bag solution, the part of the order and all calculations needed to place and mix the drug into the IV bag should be completed first. Then, separately as with any pre-mixed IV drip, the EMT should determine the mg/ml in the mixed IV bag and the drip rate that the IV must be run at to deliver the mg/min ordered. *Whenever a drug is to be mixed into an IV solution and administered by drip, the two parts of the order and all calculations and steps required for each, should always be kept completely separated as if they were being performed by two different individuals.*

In order to provide simple demonstrations, the examples used were selected so that the calculations always resulted in whole milliliters. Often, however, the calculation of the number of milliliters needed to provide the ordered mg dose results in a fraction.

When a drug calculation provides an answer which is a fraction, the fraction should be reduced to the lowest possible denominator and then translated into its decimal equivalent (or form). Because most syringes used in the field are only marked in milliliter and 2/10ths (0.2) of a milliliter graduations, the calculation does not have to be extended beyond hundredths (eg: 3.28) of a milliliter. This allows it to be rounded off to the nearest tenth of a milliliter (eg: 3.3 ml), which can be determined on the scale provided on most syringes.

The proper handling of answers to drug calculations which are fractions is demonstrated in the following example. If, when the calculation is done, the answer results in:

$$\text{Milliliters to be Administered} = \frac{620}{60}$$

$$x = \frac{620}{60}$$

To reduce a fraction to its lowest common denominator, both the numerator (number above the line) and the denominator (number below the line) can be divided by an equal amount without affecting the fraction's value. In this case they can both be divided by 10 by simply moving the decimal point one place to the left (or more simply just eliminating the 0 in each units column).

$$x = \frac{620}{60} = \frac{62}{6}$$

The fraction can be further reduced by dividing both the numerator and denominator by 2.

$$x = \frac{62}{6} = \frac{31}{3}$$

Once the fraction has been reduced to its lowest possible denominator, it can be translated into the necessary decimal equivalent by dividing the numerator of the fraction by the denominator.

$$x = \frac{31}{3} = 3\overline{)31.00}$$

$$x = 10.33+$$

To round the answer off to the nearest tenth, if the number in the hundredths column is five or greater the answer is raised to the next tenth, and if it is below five it is not. In this case it is less than five so the answer is rounded off to be:

Volume to be Administered = 10.3 ml.

If you have been confused by any of this process, it is recommended that you ask an instructor for help in reviewing the mathematics necessary for doing such calculations.

Whichever system or formulas are used in calculating the amount to administer to provide the dose ordered, the EMT must solve the same two essential problems regardless of the parenteral fluid drug ordered or the method by which it is to be administered.

These can be summarized as:

- *Translate the order into a form which can be used in the calculations required.* All quantities must be translated into compatible units of measure and, if the dose ordered is in a form generic to any patient (mg/kg or mg/kg/min), to translate this into an exact specific mg dose *for this patient.*

- *To calculate the fluid volume required to be administered in order to provide the mg dose ordered* (For injection or IV Push or mixing into an IV solution, the number of mls or, if an IV drip, the gtt/min rate at which the IV should be run).

There are a number of other classical formulas and methods used to calculate the volume to be administered.

The method shown on the preceding pages is recommended over others used because it employs only the same two *simple formulas* to calculate the necessary volume to be delivered, whether the drug order is for injection, IV Push, or IV drip administration. Two essential components make this system universal to any of the parenteral routes ordered in the field, as well as simple and reliable. First, *the concentration of the drug is always separately identified* (either from the supply's label or by calculation) and then becomes the key factor in calculating the required volume to be administered. Second, the number of milliliters (or ml/min) is always calculated and identified, whether for an injection or IVP, or for IV drip administration.

Because IV administration sets are not graduated or indicated in ml/min, it is self-apparent that an additional step is required for an IV drip, and the EMT can not inadvertently forget to do this. Since to convert a desired ml/min infusion rate to the required drip rate (gtt/min) one simply multiplies it by the gtt of the IV administration set, no unique formulas need to be remembered for this additional task or to replace those in the previous calculations.

Solely to provide a comprehensive reference, the alternative formulas that are often used have been included below, since no discussion of drug calculations would be complete without them. The reader should note that regardless of the formulas selected, any translations in the order that are required must always be made before any further calculations are set up and made.

Three classical formulas that can alternatively be used are:

I. Volume to be Administered $= \dfrac{\text{(Volume on Hand)} \times \text{(Desired Dose)}}{\text{(Concentration on Hand)}}$

ml to be Administered $= \dfrac{\text{(Total ml supplied)} \times \text{(mg Ordered)}}{\text{(Total mg supplied)}}$

II. Drops per Minute To Infuse $= \dfrac{\text{(Volume on Hand)} \times \text{(Desired Dose)}}{\text{(Concentration on Hand)}} \times$ Drops per ml of set

gtt/min $= \dfrac{\text{(Total ml in bag)} \times \text{(mg/min ordered)}}{\text{(Total mg in bag)}} \times \text{(gtt/ml of set)}$

gtt/min $= \dfrac{\text{(Total ml)} \times \text{(mg/min ordered} \times \text{(gtt/ml)}}{\text{(Total mg)}}$

or, if the mg/ml in the IV gag is given:

III. Drops per Minute to Infuse $= \dfrac{\text{(Ordered Dose)} \times \text{(Drops/ml of Set)}}{\text{(mg/ml concentration in IV Solution)}}$

gtt/min $= \dfrac{\text{(Ordered mg/min)} \times \text{(gtt/ml of set)}}{\text{(mg/ml in IV Solution)}}$

Calculating The Dose When Administering Pills

Pills, regardless of their specific form, are supplied in a predetermined unalterable milligram strength (dose) per pill. Orders to administer pills include the milligram/pill strength desired and the number of pills to be administered, therefore no calculation is generally necessary in administering them. In two rare cases limited calculation may be necessitated. If the order is in milligrams and the medication is supplied in a different scale such as grains, the EMT may have to use a table and simple calculation to make the conversion. In another rare case, the dose ordered may (for example) be for 650 milligrams, and the tablets supplied contain 325 milligrams each, therefore the number of pills to be given must be calculated.

Unless a pill is scored for the purpose of breaking it in half to supply one-half of the per pill dose when ordered, pills should never otherwise be broken into parts, since the percentage of the pill's milligram dose which will be delivered can *NOT* accurately be determined.

As with any drug, if more than one pill is taken within the drug's half-life, the total milligrams cumulatively taken must be added together to assure that it is *NOT* beyond the maximum recommended dosage.

Minimizing Potential Medication Problems

There is no such thing as a benign drug or medication—just some which are more potent and some less potent. To achieve its therapeutic effect any drug must cause a significant unnaturally introduced chemical and physiological alteration in the body. Any induced alteration in the body's chemistry can touch off a wide range of unpredictable events and side effects.

Any side effect which proves harmful to a patient is called an *untoward effect*. Untoward effects can result from:

Hypersensitivity — A reaction to a substance which normally is more profound than seen in the general population, such as an allergic reaction to a drug.

Idiosyncrasy — An individual reaction to a drug which is unusually different from that or those that are common for the drug.

Side Effects — Effects in addition to the primary therapeutic effect of a drug. **Common side effects** are those which are known to be associated with the drug in a prevalent percentage of the population. **Adverse** or **untoward side effects** are those which are harmful to the patient.

Potentiation — The enhancement of a drug's effect by another drug or substance which may inadvertently cause the effect of the drug to be too great and dangerous.

Synergism — The combined action of two (or more) drugs, or a substance with a drug which causes the effects of either to be stronger than if administered separately (eg: barbiturates and alcohol).

Accumulation — Even when a drug is administered in the correct prescribed dosage, if the body can not temporarily metabolize and discard a drug within its half-life, a greater than safe therapeutic level may be accumulated.

Although not an untoward effect, if a drug is rendered ineffective or otherwise fails to provide the therapeutic benefit for which it was ordered, the lapse can be harmful to the patient. If a patient does not therapeutically respond to a drug or dose he is said to be **refractory** to it. Patients may be refractory to a drug as a result of:

Tolerance — When a patient has taken the same drug or one of similar components for a long time he may develop a tolerance to it so that it no longer produces the desired therapeutic effect from a normal (or even greater) dose.

Antagonism — Chemical antagonism signifies the opposition between two or more medications. If the patient is administered or has taken a drug which is an **antagonist** to the drug of the desired therapeutic effect, its opposing action may prevent the desired therapeutic benefit.

Hypoperfusion — If the patient has such a reduced circulation to produce hypoperfusion and/or cellular hypoxia, circulation through the body, cellular absorption and metabolism may not occur sufficiently to produce the necessary therapeutic level being achieved in the blood stream or the therapeutic agent being delivered throughout the body.

Idiosyncratic Ineffectiveness—Without any predictable reason, a drug may simply fail to provide its commonly proven therapeutic effect in an individual patient.

Although the unscheduled occurrence of any of these undesirable physiological reactions or reactions which render a drug ineffectual can *NOT* be predicted and prevented in all cases, the possibility can be greatly reduced with knowledge. *The EMT should only administer drugs with which he is familiar and has demonstrated sufficient understanding and knowledge.* Even if a drug is ordered by a physician in a specific dose for a specific patient, it can *NOT* be safely administered unless the EMT has the necessary pre-requisite knowledge of the particular drug ordered. The EMT must know the following about each drug that is carried by the squad and is included in his protocols:

Necessary Knowledge About Each Drug

- The Generic and common Trade Names.
- Indication for use.
- Its classification (type) and general expected actions.
- All contraindications (relative or absolute).
- Any restrictions, warnings, and precautions for its use.
- How Available and Supplied.
- Proper appearance.
- Common side effects.
- Normal dose(s) and administration requirements.
- Maximum recommended dose (singular and accumulative).
- Any other drugs with which it may have an adverse or reduced effect, or may cause to similarly alter.
- Any drugs which can be used to *counter* its effects or reactions caused by it, and their specific doses and method of administration.
- Any special "shelf" or administration requirements.
- The conditions, methods, doses and restrictions specifically prescribed for its prehospital administration by protocol (whether administered per direct or standing order).

As well as this general knowledge about the drug to be administered, the EMT must know the following information about the specific supply of the drug that he will use to administer it.

Information Needed About the Specific Provided Vial, Ampule, Pre-loaded Syringe, or IV Bag Mix

- Drug Name.
- Expiration Date.
- Method of administration INDICATED or specifically WARNED AGAINST for *this supply.*
- Any other warnings, precautions, or requirements specific to *this supply.*
- Expected appearance and form of both *the usual* and *this supply.*
- Total milligrams included (concentration or dose on hand).
- Total milliliters included (fluid volume on hand).
- Milligrams supplied in one milliliter (mg/ml in the dilution supplied).
- If an IV bag, the gtt/ml of the specific administration set used must be known.
- If the drug is solely the basic IV fluid (D_5W, NS, 1/2NS, or LR WITHOUT any other drug added) knowing the total milligrams or mg/ml of the electrolytes and other base ingredients is unnecessary.
- If mixing a drug into an IV drip, as well as the preceding information necessary about the provided supply of the drug, the total number of milligrams, milliliters, and the mg/ml of the drug in the mixed IV bag must also be known.

The EMT must also have some key information about the patient's pertinent past history, events immediately preceding this episode (and call), and the patient's condition, before a drug can be administered safely. On a call, these are routinely obtained from the Initial Systemic Examination and S-A-M-P-L-E history which are generally completed prior to the administration of a drug. Even when the patient is unable to provide the pertinent history, the previous history required (or salient parts of it) can be elicited from a relative or others at the scene, or from medical alerting jewelry, medical identification cards, or prescription drugs carried by the patient. In cases of full arrest or other emergencies requiring immediate intervention in a patient who can not communicate and is unaccompanied, the EMT may only be able to obtain *some of the information desired* from spectators and his assessment, before he must initiate the administration of emergency drugs. *Initiating the drug administration prior to completing the Initial Systemic Examination and History in such cases presents less of a potential danger than the known danger to survival caused if the administration of emergency drugs is delayed.* When this is not the case, the following information should be obtained *prior* to administering any drug:

Key Patient Information Needed Prior to Administration of A Drug

- Patient's approximate age.
- Patient's approximate weight.
- Any previous or known allergies.
- Any history of an allergic reaction including what occurred and when.
- Any previous history of heart, sugar (Diabetic), or seizure problems, including which and when.
- Pertinent other past medical history.
- Any medications prescribed (including those for prn use only.)
- Any prescription or non-prescription medications taken in the last 24 hours, including when and how much.
- Events preceding this episode and what predicated summoning the ambulance.
- A clinical estimate of the patient's overall general condition/health.
- The patient's vital signs.
- Signs and symptoms supporting a specific clinical impression (provisional diagnosis) for which the drug is *indicated.*
- Identification of any other conditions or injuries present.
- A reasonable rule-out for each condition which would *contraindicate* the administration of the drug or drugs selected (absence of contraindications).
- The confirmed absence of drugs or other substances in the presence of which the selected drug is contraindicated or not advised.
- Although not prior to administration, a repeated set of vital signs and evaluation of the therapeutic effect of any drug must be obtained after it has been given and sufficient time has occurred to let it be absorbed and circulated.

Even though the EMT must have the nearly forty separate pieces of key information detailed in the three preceding lists before administering a given drug to a specific patient, the task is not as difficult or insurmountable as this would imply. All of the general information which pertains to the drug is learned and added to the EMT's knowledge in his initial and ongoing advanced education. This, together with the development of the key patient information as an automatic by-product of the initial examination and history done routinely in all patients, leaves only a reasonable limited number of items which must be uniquely determined or checked prior to the administration of the drug.

AVOIDING DANGEROUS MEDICATION ERRORS

Any error in the administration of a drug may have disastrous, even fatal, results. Although the chance of an error can not be totally eliminated, it can be greatly reduced by teaching and assiduously following practices which are useful in reducing errors or, should one occur when preparing a dose, will provide a warning prior to its administration to the patient.

As one would expect, the two most common medications errors are the administration of the wrong medication or the administration of an incorrect dose of the correct medication. Errors in standing orders can be minimized by constant review of the orders and dosages prescribed in the protocols, and periodic tests to confirm that each advanced EMT is fluent in his recall and ability to interpolate them.

When following an order prescribed for a particular patient by a physician providing on-line medical direction, the EMT should write the complete order down as it is being given to him over the radio or phone, and should immediately read it back to confirm that he has correctly recorded it before the communication is ended. In the field a similar two party check can be provided by one advanced EMT "announcing" his intent (or giving a verbal order to a second advanced EMT) and having its appropriateness confirmed by a repeated order from the second.

Errors in the drug selected for administration can be minimized by following two practices. Only use the drug name as displayed directly on the vial, ampule, pre-loaded syringe, or IV bag—never the one on the exterior packaging. The second key in assuring a drug's correct selection is the use of the 3-Read system. If the EMT routinely uses this system, it becomes second nature and does not require specific thought. With the 3-Read system, the name and concentration of the drug are read three times: once when the drug is selected and prepared for administration, a second time just prior to its administration, and a third time immediately after its administration when this event is being documented. Although the third check does not prevent the error, it provides a final check against the written order and immediate timely identification of an error should one have occurred.

Experience has shown that dosage errors in most cases are caused by either:

a. Using the wrong formulas to convert or calculate the desired dose

b. Making a math error

c. Misplacing a decimal point (or number of zeros used)

Writing out of the formula in full plain English, only abbreviating "mg," "ml," "kg," "gtt/min," etc., in the same manner as they have initially been displayed on the proceeding pages, causes a "thinking" evaluation of whether the formula makes sense or not, as written.

When doing this it is essential that two pieces of information are initially correctly identified. From the order it is key to determine whether the order is for a number of *mg*, or a number of *mg/kg*, or a number of *mg/min*, or a number of *mg/kg/min*. This should always be noted and recorded first, as an incorrect choice will affect the dose calculation to a vast magnitude. Secondly the mg/ml supplied, should always be identified. When calculating an IV drip dose, the gtt/ml of the administration set is also a key piece of information that should be noted initially. Although it appears to be a pedestrian habit, many formulation errors can be avoided by identifying and writing these components down separately before establishing the formulas and doing the calculations needed.

For example, prior to calculating the dose the EMT would write:

Desired Dose = 2 mg

Supply = 5 mg/ml

This not only aids in correctly setting up the formula(s) to be calculated but also provides the necessary information to *estimate* the correct answer. The key method for avoiding errors—whether in setting up the formula or in doing the necessary math—is to estimate the answer prior to proceeding further. In the above example one first notes that the desired dose is *less* than the number of mg in one ml, therefore, the answer must be *less* than one ml. Going on to get a more specific estimate, one notes that the desired dose is less than a half (2x2=4) and more than a third (2x3=6) of the number of the milligrams (5) in one milliliter of the supply provided. Therefore one concludes that the correct answer should be a number between 1/3 and 1/2 of one milliliter or, in decimal terms, between 0.33 and 0.50 ml. When the formula is established and calculated, should the EMT's calculated answer be 2.5, or 40, or 0.04 ml, he will immediately know, because any of these is outside of the estimated correct range, that it is incorrect. (As a point of information for the reader, in the first case the formula was incorrectly inverted so the wrong items were divided one into the other, and in the last two the decimal point was incorrectly placed.)

When the order is for a given number of mg/kg, the EMT should first estimate the number of total milligrams this represents. This can be easily done by simply halving the weight in pounds.

For an order to provide 2 mg/kg to the patient and a supply of 50 mg/ml the EMT would initially write:

Desired Dose = 3 mg/kg

Pt's Weight = 150 pounds

Supply = 50 mg/ml

Next he would estimate the weight in kilograms to be 75 kg, and then to determine the total dose he would multiply it by the 3 mg/kg ordered. This shows him that the total milligrams delivered should be about 225 mg (actually slightly less, since there are 2.2 kg/lb, rather than 2). Then, since there are 50 mg in one ml and less than 225 mg are desired, the dose in ml should be slightly less than about 4.5 ml (because 50 goes into 225 about 4-1/2 times). The actual calculation yields an answer of 4.09 (or 4 ml) to be given. Had the EMT arrived at any answer that did not approximate an amount less than his estimate of 4.5 ml or which was equal or greater than this estimate, he would know that it had to be incorrect.

When estimating an order for a number of *mg/min* or *mg/kg/min*, the EMT should always first estimate the number of ml/min that this represents using the previously described concepts. Once the ml/min dose has been estimated, multiplying it by the gtt/ml of the IV administration set to be used (60, 10, etc. gtt/ml) will produce an estimate of the number of drops per minute (gtt/min) that the IV should be run at in order to provide the mg/min ordered.

As well as providing the EMT with a good numerical guide against which to compare his actual calculated answer and warn him when an error of any substantial proportion has occurred, writing down the significant components and doing such an estimate also provides the EMT with an understanding of the problem or problems (and any conversions necessary) that must be solved. This is often useful in determining the steps and formulas that should be used when actually doing the exact calculation.

The simple estimate should warn the EMT regardless of whether an error occurs from using an inappropriate or incorrectly stated formula, entering an incorrect measure or equivalent, a math error, or a combination of these. *The value of such notations and estimating as a routine practice prior to doing any drug calculation, regardless of how simple it may appear, can not be emphasized enough.*

Even when the drug, its concentration and quantity administered to the patient is correct, the therapeutic amount delivered can be far greater or far less than desired if the dose (or part of it) becomes inadvertently diverted from the intended route of administration. If a Sub-Q or IM dose is accidentally administered into an artery or vein a dangerously high level of the drug or an adverse reaction may be precipitated. If the dose of a drug for IV administration is instead infiltrated into the muscles surrounding the vein, its therapeutic action may be lost or so delayed as to be ineffectual and, such as with $D_{50}W$, severe local damage may result. To guard against such inadvertent delivery by a route other than that desired, the EMT must check that this is *NOT* occurring when administering the drug.

Whenever a drug is being delivered by injection, the correct placement of the needletip is confirmed after it has been inserted and correctly located, by careful observation and aspiration of the syringe prior to the administration of the drug. If a significant amount of blood enters the syringe at any time *prior to aspiration of the syringe*, an artery or arteriole has been entered (or lacerated and accessed), and if the drug was delivered it could result in dangerous intra-arterial administration. If a significant amount of blood flows into the syringe, hold the plunger of the syringe from being pushed further out of the barrel by the arterial pressure, but do *NOT* push on it or in any way chance injection of any amount of the drug.

Immediately remove the needle and syringe from the patient and apply direct pressure firmly over the site to control the bleeding that results. Once the direct pressure has been initiated, discard the syringe and needle in a sharps container without delay. After the bleeding has been controlled, another syringe with the proper dose should be prepared and the administration re-attempted at another site.

When giving a Sub-Q, IM or IV injection, only sites that are *NOT* near an artery are generally selected. Therefore, chance arterial sticks are relatively infrequent. After the needle has been inserted through the skin and properly located visually, check the syringe to confirm that *NO* blood has or is entering it. (When cannulating a vein, a small amount of blood—which generally appears as a thin floating strand much different from that coming from an artery—may seep into the syringe). Then, aspirate the syringe by retracting the plunger slightly in the barrel and observe if this causes blood to enter it.

If the needletip is properly placed for a Sub-Q or IM injection, *NO* blood will enter the syringe upon aspiration and the dose can be safely injected. Should any blood enter, the needle and syringe should be withdrawn and the injection and administration re-attempted at another site.

When giving an IV injection the opposite result when aspirating the syringe is desired. If the distal tip of the needle has been successfully inserted into the vein, one or two milliliters of blood should be easily drawn into the syringe when it is aspirated. If this occurs easily, the dose can be injected.

If, upon aspiration, blood does not enter the syringe or a sufficient quantity can not be drawn easily without resistance, the tip of the needle is *NOT* properly located in the vein. Attempt to reposition it first, but if this still does not allow for the easy aspiration of blood, the needle and syringe should be removed and another site selected for cannulation. If the same limb is to be used, a more proximal site than that originally attempted should be selected.

Once the proper placement of the needle in the vein has been confirmed by aspiration, the EMT must ensure that the fluid being injected is being delivered into the vein, rather than infiltrating into the surrounding tissues. The drug should be pushed at only a moderate rate and the site carefully observed throughout the administration of the drug. Should a hematoma or lump appear as the drug is being injected, infiltration must be assumed and, instead of proceeding further, the syringe and needle should be removed. Then, cannulation and administration at another site should be attempted.

When providing a drug by piggyback drip or IV push through an established IV line, infiltration rather than intravenous delivery must also be guarded against. Before pushing the dose into the IV line or connecting the drug piggyback into it, the patency of the primary IV line should be checked. Look at the cannulation site for any signs of infiltration and gently palpate the area for any present fluid "lump". If the line is only running at a KVO rate, the rate should be slowly increased to a higher rate for a few seconds to confirm its viability and any lack of infiltration. The timely delivery of the desired dose must also be assured after any IV bolus is inserted, by properly flushing it into the vein with the primary IV solution or, to avoid interference after introducing the piggyback into the line and adjusting its flow rate, by shutting off the flow of the primary IV fluid before the connecting "Y".

The EMT administering the drug or series of doses and drugs is responsible to record (or direct another EMT to record) the drug, dose, and time immediately following each administration, and ultimately for the proper necessary documentation on the run report. When a number of urgent simultaneous interventions are needed in emergency situations such as a complex dysrhythmia or full arrest, it is usually impractical to document each event and drug's administration on the run report in a full and proper manner as it occurs. In such cases a chronological *work sheet* using suitable abbreviations must be used. The use of a single cumulative work sheet instead of loose separate notes is essential if confusion is to be avoided. *The time, drug, dose and route of each drug (and the time and other key interventions, and if applicable their level) must be recorded by an EMT immediately as done, regardless of other priorities.* This is an essential safeguard against giving an extra repeated dose (or missing one), or giving greater than the maximum recommended cumulative dose of a drug in the field, because the EMT forgets where he is in the progression of his protocol or when the patient changes from one rhythm to another. It provides a similar safeguard when transferring the responsibility for such a patient upon arrival at the hospital. As the run report in such situations is generally completed by the EMT only after the transfer, a copy of this work sheet will provide a total itemized overview of the times and drugs administered in the field which is essential immediate information required for the safe continuation of urgent interventions and emergency drug administration in the Emergency Department.

Although the entries on such a work sheet must be legible and clearly understandable by others, the use of abbreviations and lack of inclusion of non-essential information (that can easily be reconstructed later when completing the formal documentation on the run report), makes it possible to maintain a complete up-to-the-minute record without delaying the provision of care, even when resources in the field are less than preferred. Recording on such a work sheet can be limited to simple entries such as:

"0815 — Epi 1 mg IVP

0816 — Shock 360

0818 — Lido 100 mg IVP

0819 — Shock 360"

    etc.

The following list of items to be checked when administering a drug will serve as a useful summary.

Summary of Checks When Administering A Drug

When selecting the supply:

1. Check the drug name on the lavel (and compare with order).
2. Check the expiration date.
3. Check the fluid for clarity, absence of foreign matter, and confirm it appears as usual/expected.
4. Check form supplied is for route prescribed.
5. Check concentration.

When calculating the necessary ml or gtt/min dose:

6. Re-read entire order and confirm or "echo" it.
7. Check mgs ordered.
8. Check if order is for mgs, mg/kg, mg/min, or mg/kg/min.
9. Check mg/ml supplied.
10. If an IV drip, check gtt/ml of administration set.
11. Check ml or ml/min and gtt/min dose calculated to be required, against earlier estimate and order.

When preparing the drug:

12. If for injection, check the amount in the syringe (drawn up or pre-loaded) is the exact amount to be administered (no more and no less).
13. If an IV drip, check gtt/ml of set is correct and same as used in calculations. Check that the piggyback runs properly and that the drip chamber and line are appropriately filled with fluid. Check that no air remains in the line and that the drug has *NOT* precipitated.

When about to administer the drug:

14. Recheck name and concentration of drug supplied.
15. If an IV push or IV drip, check patency of primary IV line and that it is *NOT* infiltrating. Also check that the drug to be administered is compatible with the primary IV fluid.
16. Review, or as needed recheck, the patient's condition and vital signs.
17. Check for the absence of conditions which would contraindicate the use of the drug.
18. Check for any history of allergic reactions or medications taken in past 12 hours which would contraindicate the drug or dose, or cause a change in either.
19. *If for injection,* check needle and proposed site for any irregularities.
    If for IV drip, check that the piggyback is shut off and has been properly connected into the primary IV line.

When administering the drug:

20. *If by injection,* check the proper placement of the distal end of the inserted needle by aspirating the syringe.
    If an IV injection, check that no infiltration occurs as the drug is being injected.
    If by IV push, check that the line above the access port is pinched off while inserting the drug into the line and that the drug is properly "flushed" into the vein immediately afterwards.
    If by IV drip, check that the piggyback drip is adjusted at the desired rate and that the primary IV is shut off.

After administering the drug:

21. Recheck the drug and concentration used as a supply, for the third time.
22. Check that you have recorded the drug, amount, route administered, and time given on the work sheet.
23. Once the drug has been absorbed and circulated, check appropriate signs and symptoms for the initiation/successful therapeutic effect desired.
24. Check for any adverse side effect.
25. Monitor the patient's condition and periodically recheck quality of ventilation and vital signs.

Once at the Emergency Department:

26. Check that ALL drugs used are accounted for, and each drug and dose administered is documented in proper and complete form on your run report.
27. Check that all needles, syringes, glass containers, etc. are properly discarded and are replaced at the hospital or when back in quarters.

Although when provided as a single list, the numerous checks seem almost unmanageable, they soon become second nature and are done by habit in the field.

Regardless of how knowledgeable or experienced the advanced EMT is with the drugs carried on the ambulance, the wide range of problems encountered in the prehospital emergency setting periodically present a unique problem. Should the EMT at any time have a question or doubt about the indication, drug to use or use next, dose, a possible precaution or contraindication in a specific patient—the key check against a potential error is to immediately obtain on-line medical consultation and direction. *The only stupid drug administration question is one that, rather than being asked, is either NOT asked or is answered by a guess.*

Even when the most careful administration practices and checks are followed, a drug error can occur. Should this happen the potentially disastrous—even fatal—results can generally be mitigated by an immediate counteraction. Determining the appropriate immediate therapy needed following a drug error is a highly complex physiological and chemical problem beyond the training and knowledge of even the most knowledgeable EMT, and requires the immediate judgment of a physician. If any drug error occurs or is suspected at any time, the EMT *MUST* immediately report this to his on-line Medical Control and seek directions.

Whenever possible this should be done by phone or other discrete means of communication, but if no other choice than the open radio is available it must be used since the extent of the danger may increase as each few minutes passes. For obvious reasons, the communication should be limited to the essential facts and words such as "error", "drug mistake", "wrong drug", "excessive dose", etc., and defensive or apologetic statements, should be avoided.

After obtaining the physician on-line, identify the unit, give a brief account of the patient's conditions and *present* status and then, detail the drug administration that represents the error or potential error that was made without editorializing. An example of such a detailed error is:

"We have administered four boluses of lidocaine IVP for a total of three point seven five milligrams per kilogram, I repeat 4 boluses for a total of three point seven five milligrams per kilogram, and the patient has gone from a normal sinus rhythm at 74 with ectopy to a bradycardia at 40 without ectopy. His BP has dropped to 70 over 44. We are transporting to your location and should arrive in about five minutes. Are there any special orders at this time."

The emergency physician who is knowledgeable in the emergency drug protocols will be alerted by the emphasis provided by the call itself and the strange repeated portion of the message indicating the excessive dose. The patient's reported deterioration followed by the odd request for *"special"* orders, serves as an additional emphasis that all is not as it should be. Without any unnecessary delay or additional potential overheard exposure, the physician will know that an extra dose was administered and the accumulated dose is 0.75 mg/kg in excess of the maximum recommended. Since the occurrence and dosage was unique, his orders may likely be different from anything in the EMT's protocols and must, after confirmation is obtained by repeating them back, be followed exactly.

Once at the emergency department, and in private, the specific details of the error must be verbally retold directly to the physician without delay. The run report should only include the facts that occurred, without judgments or any other indications or commentary except that, "After administering the last bolus of Lidocaine, we contacted Medical Control immediately".

All of the information surrounding the error and salient information about the patient's condition and the call situation should be summarized in a separate chronological written incident report (which is referenced to the run report number, time, and date, without specific identification of the patient). This should be done as soon as practical while each of the EMTs involved can easily recall and reconstruct the events accurately.

Once the patient responsibility has been transferred to the hospital staff and the EMT is no longer needed to assist, he should contact his supervisor (or watch officer) and report the events. Then, as soon as practical, he should furnish the supervisor (and any others required by local regulation) with a copy of the completed incident report.

Although the seriousness of any drug error can not be sufficiently emphasized, only a few who routinely administer emergency drugs can honestly say that they have never made one over the years. Although such an error may be excusable, the increased danger to the patient that may result from delay in contacting Medical Control or attempted "masking" of the error, is *NOT*. Regardless of any fears surrounding his job security, advanced status, or financial security, anything but the immediate reporting to Medical Control, as outlined, and again upon arrival to the physician in the emergency department, is unethical, a callous and unprofessional lack of regard for the patient's well-being and, in many cases, criminal. It violates the very essence of medical ethics and, if violated, any possible future trust.

If the error is made by another EMT on the call, loyalty to a partner or friend does not mitigate or excuse any EMT present from requiring such *immediate* notification to Medical Control. Anyone who is a party to the purposeful delay or omission of such reporting shares equally in the unethical and dangerous behavior this represents and in its consequences. A good EMT and truly good friend will protect both the patient and the EMT making the error and about to compound it, by making it clear that any action other than immediate communication and disclosure to Medical Control is *NOT* a possibility and can *NOT* even be entertained for further discussion.

Since the EMT administers all drugs as an extension of the responsible physician's license, *the service should notify its Medical Director of any drug error which has occurred in a timely manner.* Since it is a medical issue and a question of ongoing medical trust, the ultimate disposition of the event must be determined or approved by the service Medical Director, and should not be handled solely as an administrative prerogative.

Individual Drug Administration and IV Skills

The individual skills needed to administer drugs and initiate and maintain intravenous infusions (IVs) in the field, are detailed in the following pages of this Section. The guidelines, formulas, calculations, and necessary checks outline in this Introduction should be employed with any of these. In order to avoid needless redundancy and keep the reader's focus on the new information presented, they have not been included in the following demonstrations of each individual skill. As in the rest of this book, the reader's knowledge of the material covered in the Introduction to each Section is assumed and must be integrated and considered to be an inseparable part of each of the skills presented individually.

ALS

GIVING ORAL MEDICATIONS (Liquids, Pills, Or Gels)

In terms of equipment needed and technique of administration, the simplest and most uncomplicated way to administer medication to a patient is "per os" (po) — through the mouth. This is not to say that this route is without its considerations, nor that medicine delivered by mouth cannot cause serious complications if given inappropriately or in the wrong dose. Some drugs with potentially very serious effects are administered by the "po" route.

Oral medications in the liquid form can be given by a dose cup, spoon, or squirted into the mouth with a syringe. A dose cup or spoon is typical for older children and adults, while a syringe may be most effective for infants and small children.

ALS

Administering A "po" Liquid Medication

1. To administer a liquid medication by mouth, first check and confirm that you have selected the correct medication in the prescribed concentration, and that the expiration date has not been reached. Carefully read the label to also verify that this formulation of the drug is intended for oral administration. Check to see if the dose to be administered is dependent upon the patient's weight or other variable factors. After completing these checks and those described in the Introduction, assess the patient to be sure that they are conscious and sufficiently alert to tolerate the oral administration of the medicine, and that they are not allergic to this family of drugs.

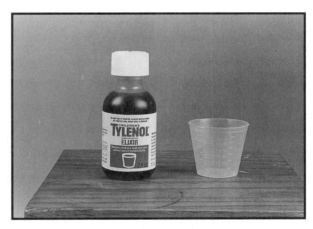

2. Carefully recheck if the order is for milliliters, ounces, tablespoons, or teaspoons. Then, transfer the prescribed amount of liquid from its container to the medication cup or spoon. If this is for a small child, you may also elect to draw it up into a syringe.

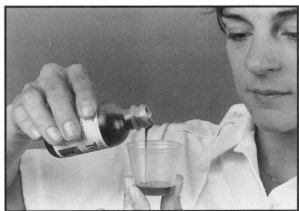

3. Instruct the patient to drink the liquid, or in the case of a small child tell him what you are going to do. Observe the patient while he drinks the liquid to make sure that all of it is swallowed. Discard the cup or syringe in a suitable container, and observe the patient for any adverse reactions to the medication. Document the time of administration, route, medication, quantity, concentration, the patient's reaction (if any or none) and the initials of the EMT who administered it.

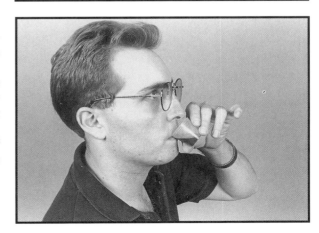

ALS Administering A Pill

While unusual, the EMT may be called upon to administer medication to a patient in the form of a tablet or capsule. As with liquid medication, the patient must be sufficiently alert and capable of swallowing the medicine. A dose cup is often used to present the pill to the patient. The EMT must carefully read the label to verify that he has the correct medication in the prescribed mg strength of tablet or capsule ordered, and that the expiration date has not been reached. At times, some calculation may be required to determine how many pills are to be given if the order is for a certain number of milligrams and the pills come in a smaller size, however tablets and capsules should never be broken to reach a smaller size. If the order is for 100mg of a drug and the only pills available are in 200mg size, advise the physician that you are unable to administer the desired dose. Breaking the pill in half will not reliably produce half of the packaged dose unless the tablet is specifically scored for this purpose.

1. To administer an oral medication in pill form, first inspect the outer container for the identity of the drug, pill size, concentration, and expiration date. Carefully open the container and inspect the pill or capsule to assure that it is intact and appears unspoiled.

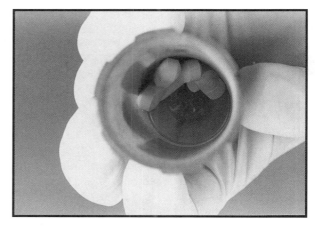

2. After completing the checks indicated in the Introduction, transfer the pill to a medication cup and allow the patient to put the pill in his own mouth. Have a cup of water available to assist the patient in swallowing.

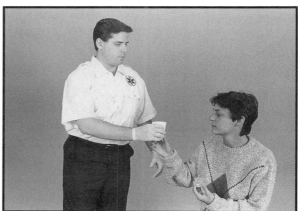

⊙ALS Administering A Sublingual Tablet

Certain medications are administered "sublingually" — that is, under the tongue. The most common of these in the prehospital arena is nitroglycerine, which in recent years is also being administered by a metered-dose spray or externally with a gel-like topical absorbent paste. Nitroglycerine tablets are extremely soluble and crumble easily. As it is not dependent upon the patient's ability to swallow, it may be given to a patient with a lowered level of consciousness and a reduced gag reflex.

1. As with any medication, inspect the container for the identity of the drug, concentration supplied, size of the tablet, and expiration date, as well as the other checks indicated in the Introduction. Nitroglycerine commonly comes in 0.3 or 0.4 mg doses per tablet.

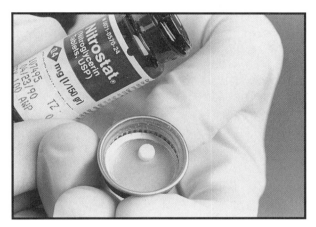

2. With a gloved hand, take one tablet from the container and place it under the patient's tongue. Some alert and oriented patients may prefer to place the tablet themselves. If you are using the metered-dose spray, have the patient elevate his tongue toward the roof of his mouth while you spray one dose into his mouth to the underside of his tongue. Document the administration and its effects in the customary manner.

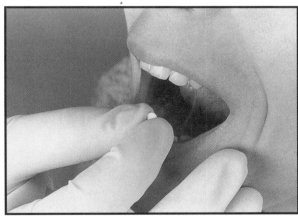

Administering Oral Glucose

Concentrated glucose is supplied in gel form for the emergency administration of sugar to patients who are hypoglycemic (low blood sugar concentration). Frequently known as "oral glucose" or "instant glucose", the gel is packaged in a metallic or plastic tube resembling those used for toothpaste. The oral administration of glucose in this form is generally employed when IV access is unavailable, and is frequently permitted for EMT-Basics when ALS personnel are not present. As noted in the Introduction to this Section, there is some controversy as to the necessary level of consciousness on the part of the patient for the appropriate use of this route. The EMT must be familiar with his local protocols and know whether or not the administration of concentrated oral glucose is limited to conscious and alert patients with a gag reflex, as is done in some areas, or whether it can be given to patients whose level of consciousness has lowered due to their suspected hypoglycemia.

1. To administer oral glucose to a patient who is conscious, inspect the outside of the tube to verify the contents and concentration, and to assure that the expiration date has not been reached. You will need a tongueblade, appropriate personal protective equipment, and the tube of glucose.

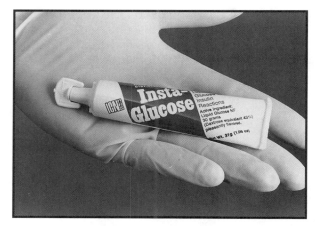

2. There are two methods of administering oral glucose to a conscious patient. The first involves inserting the tongueblade into the patient's mouth between his teeth and cheek. Use the tongueblade to create a pocket between the cheek and the teeth, then insert the tip of the tube of oral glucose into the space between the tongueblade and teeth and squeeze the tube to administer the concentrated glucose.

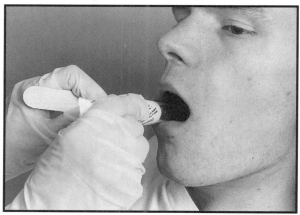

3. The second method is to liberally apply glucose to the tongueblade while it is still outside the patient's mouth, and then introduce it into the mouth against the cheek. This requires the patient to make a sort of chewing motion to move the glucose from the tongueblade into his mouth.

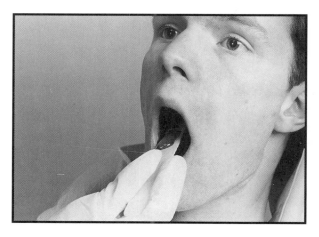

4. When the patient is unconscious or has a markedly lowered level of consciousness, and if your protocol allows oral glucose to be administered to such patients, position the patient on his side if possible or at least turn his head to the side to reduce the possibility of aspiration of the glucose.

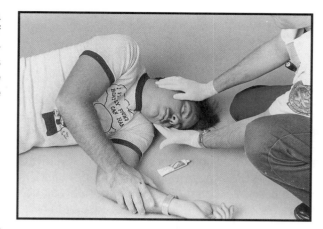

5. Slowly squeeze the tube to instill the glucose into the patient's open mouth alongside the cheek. Do not try to squirt it deeply into the back of the patient's mouth.

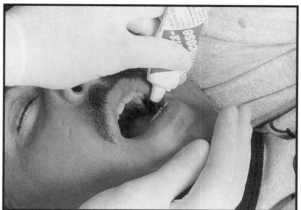

6. Maintain the patient in a lateral position and continue to monitor his condition. In particular, carefully assess the patient's level of consciousness and airway status for any changes. It may be necessary to administer more glucose, but do not allow too much to accumulate in the patient's mouth at any one time.
7. Document the administration and its effects in the customary manner.
8. Repeat the dose prn at the intervals prescribed, up to the maximum needed or allowed by protocol.

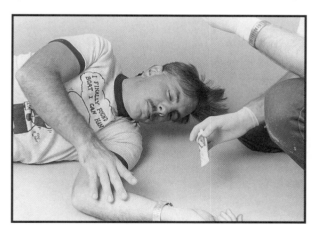

Although given through the mouth, medications which are given by aerosol mist using a nebulizer are not considered po drugs and are discussed separately in the next pages.

ALS

USING A METERED-DOSE INHALER

Metered-dose inhalers (MDI) or nebulizers are prefilled dispensers with an attached propellent gas cannister that deliver a single measured dose of aerosolized medication each time the cannister is triggered. Patients who are prone to episodes of acute ventilatory distress, such as those with severe asthma or emphysema, often have one or more MDIs prescribed for them. Typically, the patient will have already self-administered one or more doses by the time the EMT arrives, and not infrequently the ambulance was summoned because this self-treatment did not provide sufficient relief. The EMT must remember that not all MDI medications are the same—some are designed to dilate bronchial passages, some act to break up mucus deposits in the bronchi and bronchioles, and some are primarily "moisteners"—also helping to improve the flow of air to and from the lungs.

1. As with any medication, carefully read the label to verify its identity, concentration, and expiration date. Establish the dose to be administered, and remove the cap that covers the discharge opening.

2. Some MDIs are designed with an integral tube or mouthpiece, while others have a separate tube that must be attached over the discharge opening. In some the propellent cartridge is packaged connected in place, while in others it must be inserted into the dispenser unit. Prepare the inhaler appropriately, depending upon which type you have, and insert the outlet tube into the patient's mouth.

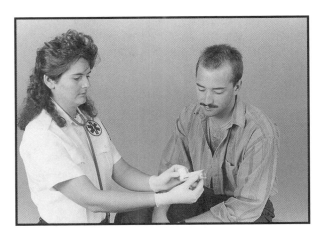

3. Instruct the patient to take a slow deep breath as the medicine is being administered. Either you or the patient can administer the spray by squeezing the top and bottom of the unit together. One squeeze will administer one dose, and holding the ends squeezed together for a prolonged period will not increase the dose delivered per squeeze.

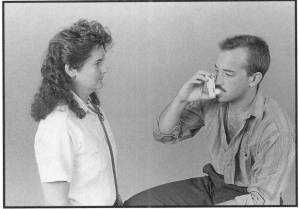

4. Continue to monitor the patient's condition, and re-assess breath sounds and ventilatory adequacy as well as vital signs. Administer additional doses if needed and prescribed.

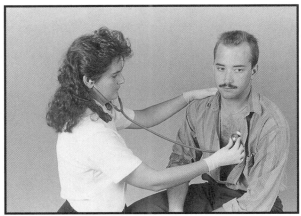

ALS

GIVING AEROSOL MEDICATIONS BY OXYGEN POWERED NEBULIZER MIST

Mist aerosols or nebulizers are used to dilate the bronchi and break up secretions in the bronchial tubes during times of acute ventilatory distress, such as asthma attacks. With these, the patient benefits from immediate local delivery to the tracheobronchial tree and the systemic absorption of the drug, as well as from the supplemental oxygen delivered simultaneously. Prior to administering an aerosol treatment, assess the patient's history and degree of distress as well as identifying any medications that have been prescribed for him — and which, if any, he has already taken. The assessment should include thorough auscultation to evaluate the breath sounds.

1. When an aerosol treatment is indicated, assemble the necessary equipment. You will need a nebulizer unit, oxygen connecting tubing, an oxygen source, and the medication to be administered. Review the order and inspect the medication package to verify its identity, concentration, expiration date, and amount to be administered.

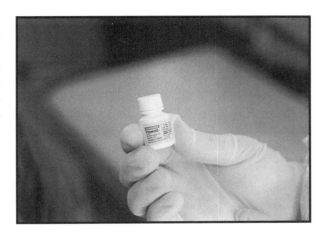

2. Unscrew the lid on the nebulizer to expose the medication cup.

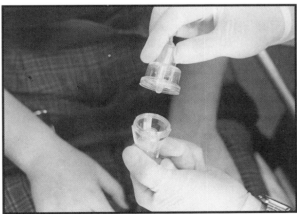

3. Add the medication to the cup and reattach the lid.

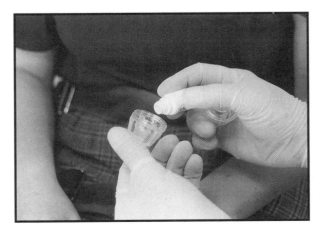

4. Attach the mouthpiece and any extension tube to the nebulizer. Connect the oxygen connecting hose to the appropriate connector on the nebulizer cup.

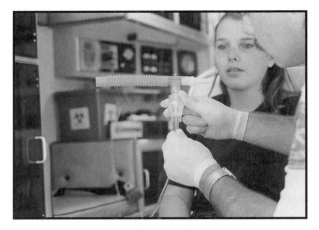

5. Attach the other end of the oxygen tubing to an oxygen source, and adjust the flow of oxygen to about 6 liters per minute. With the oxygen running, you should be able to see a mist coming out of the nebulizer's mouthpiece.

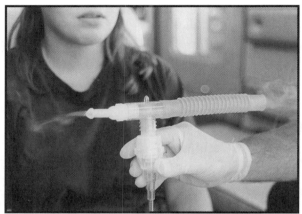

6. Instruct the patient to hold the nebulizer mouthpiece firmly in his mouth, and to breathe as deeply as he can through his mouth in order to inhale the mist. He should continue to use the nebulizer until the full amount of liquid has been used up.

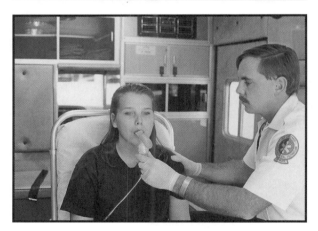

7. Monitor the patient throughout the treatment, and re-assess vital signs and ventilatory adequacy when the treatment is completed. Re-auscultate for breath sounds and compare your findings to those obtained before the treatment.

8. As needed, and if a prn repeat dose is included in your orders or protocol, repeat this process.

9. After the administration of the nebulized drug has been completed, provide supplementary oxygen if and as needed.

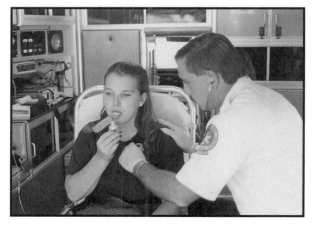

ALS

PREPARING AND USING A SYRINGE

A syringe is one of the most used items when administering medication to a patient. Because it is a tool for measurement, an understanding of how to use and read a syringe is important. Syringes are graduated and marked to measure fluid volume in milliliters (ml) or cubic centimeters (cc). Since 1ml = 1cc, these are interchangeable. Common sizes of syringes, determined by the amount of fluid that they will hold, range from 1cc to 60cc. A syringe is used to either administer fluid volume or to aspirate fluids or air.

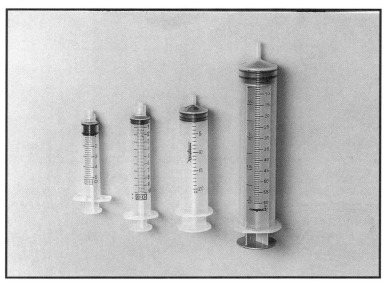

1. A syringe has basically two parts. The barrel of a syringe has markings along the side which measure the volume or amount of fluid contained in the barrel. A 10cc syringe can hold a maximum of 10cc, and between the full ml markings there are additional marks (generally in 0.2 ml graduations) which allow the fluid to be measured in tenths of a ml, such as 9.6ml. One ml syringes can measure fluid volumes to 1/100th of an ml, such as 0.25ml. At one end of the barrel is the tip which connects to the needle.

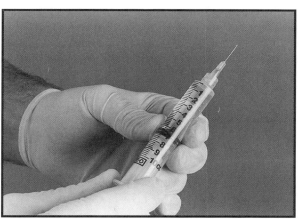

2. The plunger slides inside of the barrel, either pushing fluid or pulling it into the barrel by suction. With new syringes the plunger seal is sometimes stuck to the inside of the barrel. Pull back on the plunger to loosen the seal as you prepare the syringe for use.

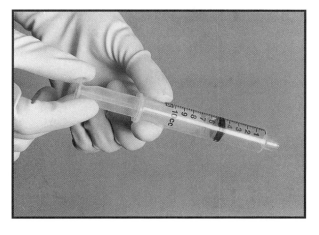

3. To read the correct fluid volume within a syringe, look at where the inside plunger seal line is in relation to the milliliter markings on the barrel of the syringe. The plunger seal line shown in this picture is at the 2.2 ml mark. When a syringe is only graduated in 0.2ml divisions between the whole ml marks, and an odd number such as 2.3 ml is needed, center the plunger seal line between the 2.2 and 2.4 marks.

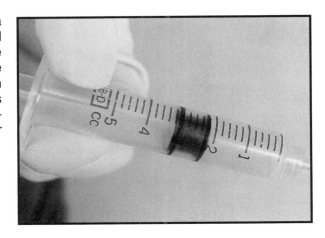

ALS Drawing Up Medication From A Vial Into A Syringe

At times the EMT will administer medication that is supplied in a "vial"—a multi-dose rubber-topped glass or plastic container from which the medication can be removed with a syringe and needle. The liquid medication withdrawn from the vial is then administered to the patient by injection, IV push, or by adding a specific amount of it to the contents of an IV bag to achieve a particular concentration which is then "dripped" into the patient over a specified period of time. Although the multi-dose vial permits medication to be removed more than once, such vials are never used for more than one patient.

1. To draw up medication from a vial, first carefully inspect the vial to insure that it contains the correct drug in the proper concentration. Inspect for color, integrity of the vial, and the absence of foreign matter in the fluid.

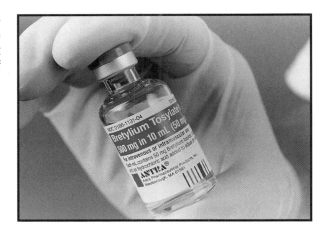

2. Remove the protective cap from the top of the vial and wipe off the rubber stopper with an alcohol prep swab or other antiseptic.

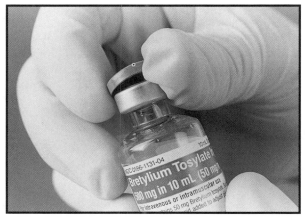

3. You should have already done the mathematical calculations to determine the number of milliliters of medication to withdraw from the vial. Attach a standard hypodermic needle to the syringe and aspirate air into the syringe equal to the amount of fluid that you will extract from the vial. If you intend to withdraw all of the fluid at one time, only aspirate about half that much air into the syringe, as overfilling the vial with air can cause the rubber stopper to dislodge.

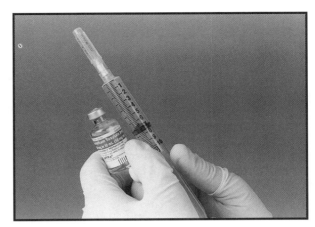

4. Hold the vial upside down with one hand and, holding the syringe and plunger in the other, insert the needle through the stopper so that its tip can just be seen inside the vial. Be careful not to insert the needle so forcefully that it contacts the side or bottom of the vial once it has been inserted.

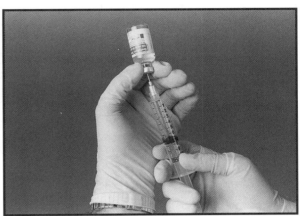

5. Depress the plunger on the syringe and inject the air into the vial. This will pressurize the container and make it easier to aspirate the medication from the vial.

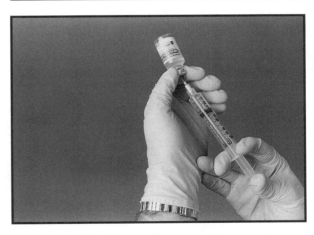

6. Once the plunger has been fully depressed and the vial has been pressurized, simply release the plunger. The increased pressure within the vial will cause some of the medication to enter the needle and syringe. You may need to pull back gently on the plunger to obtain the full amount of medication that you wish to withdraw. When you have obtained the desired amount, withdraw slightly more of the fluid to compensate for what will be lost in the rest of the preparation process.

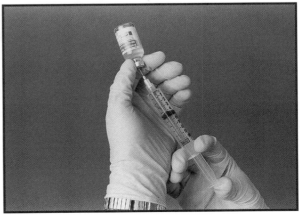

7. With the full amount desired plus a bit extra drawn into the syringe, withdraw the needle from the rubber stopper. Hold the syringe with the needle pointing directly upright and, while tapping the barrel with your other hand to cause any air that has been drawn up with the medication to rise to the top, push the plunger in until only the desired amount of medication remains in the syringe barrel. This will cause the excess to be squirted into the air—aim carefully away from yourself or others!

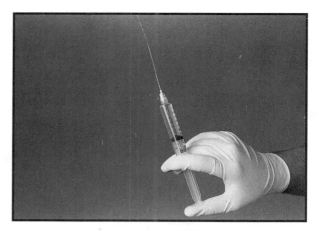

8. Administer the medication from the syringe into the patient, IV tubing, or IV bag appropriately, then discard the syringe and needle into a sharps container.

NEVER attempt to recap the needle prior to discarding it after it has been used. If there is absolutely no possibility that any remaining medication in the vial will be used for this patient, discard the vial in a biohazard container. If a repeat dose may be given to this patient with the remaining medication, save it in an appropriate location until it is needed.

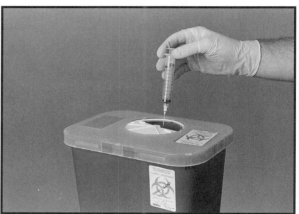

ALS Drawing Up Medication Into A Syringe From An Ampule

Ampules are small glass containers designed for single-dose medication administration. Commonly used prehospital drugs which may be packaged in ampules include Bretylium, Atropine, and Epinephrine. Because they are made entirely of glass, the elongated top or "neck" of an ampule must be cut or snapped off in order to access the medication inside. The neck of an ampule is scored to assist in opening it, however this remains a dangerous part of the procedure as the glass edges are sharp and the EMT can be wounded while attempting to open an ampule. Further, small glass shards that may be created when the top is removed can fall into the ampule and contaminate the medication. For this reason, some EMS systems require that only filter needles or syringes or IV tubing with in-line filters be used when medication from an ampule is being administered.

1. To draw up medication from an ampule, first verify the name of the drug, expiration date, concentration of medication, and color and clarity of the fluid.

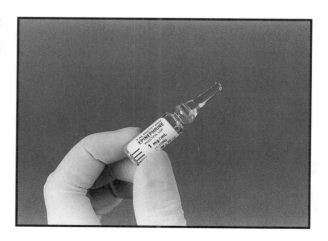

2. Before opening an ampule, you must first insure that all of the liquid is in the base of the ampule. Look closely at the head end or tip of the ampule to see if there is fluid there. Especially with 1cc ampules, there will be some medication trapped in the elongated tip of the ampule. Any trapped fluid must be moved to the larger body of the ampule before you can open it.

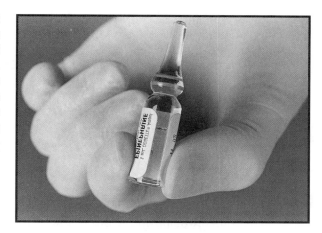

3. One way to do this is to hold the ampule upright and "flick" the body of the ampule with your finger. Tilting the ampule slightly as you flick it sometimes helps to move the fluid from the tip to the body of the ampule.

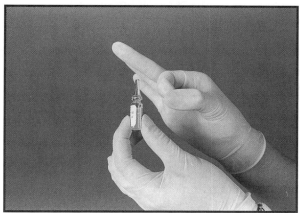

4. Another way to move the liquid to the body of the ampule is to hold the ampule firmly in one hand between your fingers and to shake the medication out of the head by flicking your wrist — similar to shaking down a thermometer. Once all of the liquid medication is in the base of the ampule, you can proceed to open the tip of the ampule.

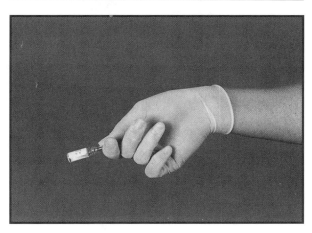

5. Breaking off the tip of the ampule presents the risk of lacerating the EMTs fingers. There are simple plastic caps designed to help with this process, or you can use an alcohol prep swab's foil wrapper or some 2x2 gauze pads to protect yourself. Whichever you use, grasp the tip of the ampule with it while you hold the base of the ampule with your other hand. Never attempt to snap off the head of the ampule with only your bare or gloved hand. Ampules have been known to break unevenly and to slice fingers.

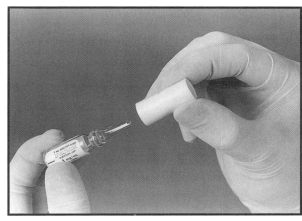

6. Holding the ampule out in front of you at arms length, point it away from your body and pull back on the tip to break off the head. *By pulling the tip toward you, any glass particles that might be created will fly away from you.*

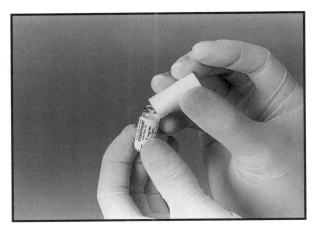

7. Carefully inspect the ampule to insure that it was cleanly broken along the score mark on its neck. If there are any pieces of the head still attached, discard the ampule into a sharps container and repeat the preceding steps with a new ampule. If the break was clean, inspect the ampule for any signs of glass fragments that may have fallen into the ampule. If any are detected, discard the ampule and start again. Using a needle and syringe, there are two ways to draw the medication from the ampule. The first way is to simply insert the needle into the upright ampule and aspirate the contents. You may need to tilt the ampule slightly to get the needlepoint into the bottom angles of the ampule if you need to withdraw all of the fluid.

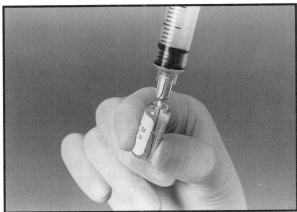

8. The second method involves turning the ampule upside down. Because of the design of the ampule's neck, the fluid in the body of the ampule will remain there even with the ampule inverted. This method is useful when you have a short needle that, when inserted into the ampule, cannot reach the base.

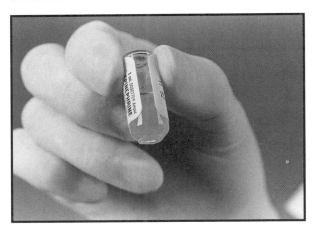

9. With the ampule upside down, carefully insert the needle into the opening. By angling the needle slightly (*NOT* the ampule) you will draw less air into the syringe as you aspirate the fluid from the ampule. Maintain contact between the hand holding the ampule and the one holding the syringe to lessen the chance of accidentally withdrawing the needle from the ampule before all of the fluid is withdrawn. As the medication enters the syringe, you must carefully pull the end of the needletip down toward the open rim of the ampule so that you are always aspirating liquid and not air from beyond the top of the fluid in the ampule.

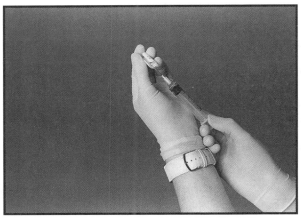

10. Frequently you will have aspirated some air into the syringe despite your best efforts. Accordingly, draw more liquid into the syringe than you need to administer. Then, with the medication in the syringe, hold the syringe with the needle pointing upwards and tap the syringe while you push in on the plunger to expel the unwanted air and the excess medication. After again checking the name of the drug, discard the empty ampule into a sharps container. Remove the needle from the syringe and place it into a sharps container also.

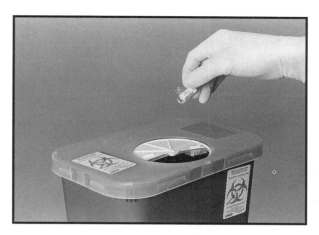

11. Attach a new unused needle to the syringe. After double-checking the medication order, dosage and concentration, and taking all appropriate body substance isolation precautions, administer the medication as prescribed. When you are done with the needle and syringe, place them in a sharps container also.

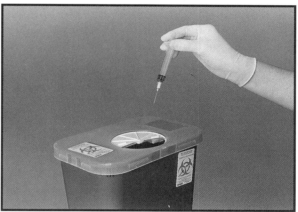

ALS Preparing Injectable Medications Supplied In Powdered Form (Glucagon, Etc.)

Some medications are supplied in powder form but must be dissolved into a liquid solution before being drawn up into a syringe and administered to the patient. While such medications are fairly rare among the list of common prehospital medications, the process is worth reviewing. The conversion from powder to liquid is made by adding sterile water to the powder. In some cases the powdered medication and the sterile water are pre-packaged in a special dual-vial system. When a rubber stopper between them is pushed, it allows the water and powder to mix. When the two are combined, the EMT has only to shake the vial well to promote complete mixing and, once the powder is completely dissolved and no residue remains, draw the needed medication from the vial as previously described. When the powder is supplied in only a standard vial, these steps must be followed:

1. When using a medication to which you must add fluid before drawing it up and administering it to the patient, first carefully inspect the vial to verify the medication's name, expiration date, concentration, and integrity of the vial. Also determine the amount of sterile water that you need to add to the vial.

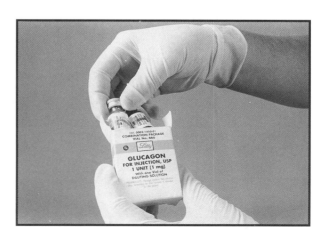

2. Remove the protective cap from the top of the vial and cleanse the rubber top with an alcohol prep swab.

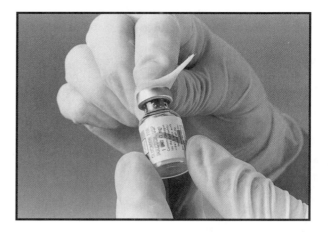

3. Appropriately prepare the container of injectable sterile water from which you will draw the amount necessary to add to the powdered medication. This may be a multi-dose vial, single-dose ampule, or IV bag. Expose and cleanse the top of a vial, remove the head of an ampule, and cleanse the needle port on an IV bag—whichever is appropriate.

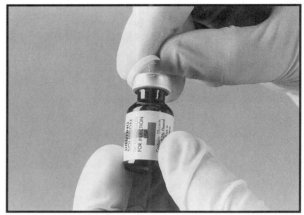

4. Draw up the needed amount of sterile water into a syringe as demonstrated in the preceding description on working with vials of medication.

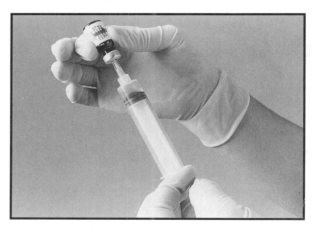

5. Insert the needle through the rubber top of the vial which contains the powdered medication, and inject the sterile water into the vial. Withdraw the needle when all of the sterile water has been added to the vial.

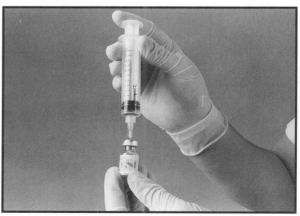

6. Shake the vial vigorously and thoroughly to mix the sterile water and powdered medication into complete solution (so no powder or solid residue remains unmixed).

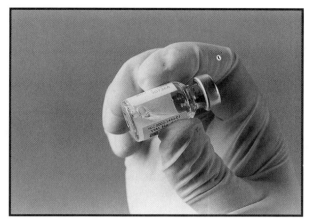

7. Aspirate the same volume of air into the syringe as the volume of mixed medication that you plan to withdraw, then re-insert the needle through the rubber top on the vial and inject the air into the mixed vial. Aspirate the desired amount of medication into the syringe, plus a little more for waste when you aspirate the air out of the syringe before administering it to the patient.

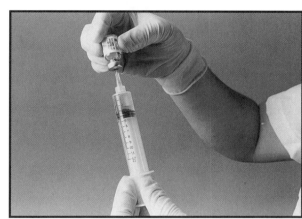

8. With the desired amount of medication aspirated into the syringe, remove the needle from the vial. Because of the possibility of having burred or even bent the needlepoint during the above steps, replace the needle on the syringe with a new one. This also allows for a shorter or smaller needle to be selected for the actual administration to the patient. With the new needle attached and while holding the syringe upright, flick any air bubbles to the needle end of the syringe and push the plunger until the rubber stopper on the end of the plunger is exactly aligned with the volume that you wish to deliver. This will cause both air and unwanted medication to be ejected from the syringe.

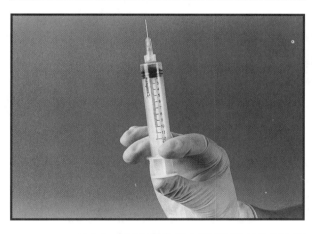

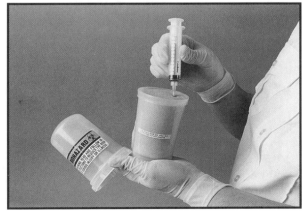

9. Administer the medication via the appropriate route. When done, discard the syringe and both needles into a sharps container as well as the vials which contained the original powder and liquid.

ALS

USING PRELOADED SYRINGES

"Preloaded" or "prefilled" syringes are glass or plastic syringes filled with medication which allow relatively quick and easy administration of a drug. Most of these need just minimal assembly prior to use, usually involving screwing the plunger and barrel together. Some prefilled syringes intended exclusively for IV piggyback use have some type of unusual needle or syringe design that alerts the user to its particular purpose. This special tip makes it difficult to routinely inject the contents of the syringe directly into an IV administration line and on into the patient. Although this feature is well-intended, it is by no means foolproof.

1. As with all medications, you should inspect the package containing the drug to insure that you have obtained the proper medication in the desired concentration, that the expiration date has not been reached, and that the designed route of administration for this version of the drug matches the route of administration you intend to use. Then open the package and inspect the label on the prefilled syringe itself to verify that it matches the information on the outer package. Finally, check the contents of the syringe for color, clarity, and the absence of any particles.

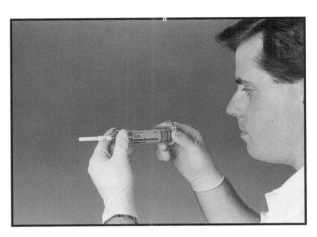

2. Some prefilled syringes come with the plunger separated from the barrel. These require simply screwing the plunger into the back of the syringe barrel to ready it for use. Note that the syringe has a needle already attached. Most often this type of prefilled syringe is intended for direct patient administration — however always read the information on the label before administering the medication. Other prefilled syringes, which are intended solely for IV piggyback administration, will have a cup around the needle to prevent the EMT from easily inserting the needle into a medication port on an IV tubing line. This same cup does not hinder your ability to inject the syringe's contents into the medication port on the bottom of an IV bag.

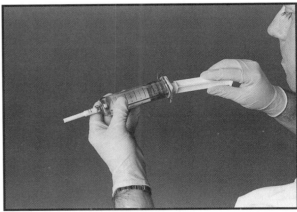

3. Some prefilled syringes are packaged with the medication in a special cartridge that is separate from the syringe barrel and needle. When using this type of prefill, the EMT must first remove the protective caps from the container and the barrel.

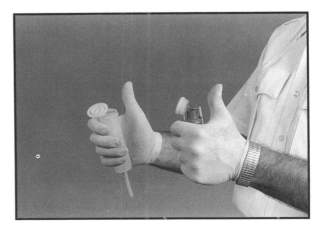

4. Inside the barrel is a special channel that includes a needle which is designed to puncture the medication cartridge when it is screwed into the barrel. With the cartridge threaded onto this needle, the other end of the cartridge becomes the "plunger," and when pushed into the barrel of the syringe the medication is ejected through the needle.

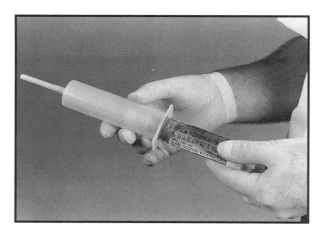

5. With the unit now fully assembled, purge any air and excess medication from the medication cartridge/barrel by pointing the syringe upward and pushing on the plunger. With the syringe assembled and any air purged, administer the medication in the appropriate manner for the route selected. When you are done, immediately discard the syringe in a sharps container for safe disposal.

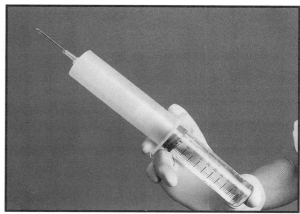

ALS

USING PRE-LOADED CARTRIDGES (Tubex®)

Injectable medications are sometimes supplied in pre-loaded cartridges, unaccompanied by a syringe barrel and plunger. Most "Schedule II" drugs—ones that have a high potential for misuse and are addictive, such as morphine sulfate—are supplied this way. Other medications, however, may also be supplied in such cartridges. Popularly known as "Tubex" cartridges for the overwhelmingly prevalent manufacturer, these glass cartridges must be inserted into a holder which serves as a barrel and provides the plunger. With the current emphasis on avoiding needlestick injuries, the original reusable metal Tubex holders have been replaced by plastic holders that can be discarded with the cartridge and holder still attached, or which allow the cartridge and its needle to be released from the holder/plunger without any risk of a needlestick injury.

1. Plastic Tubex holders, whether reusable or disposable, look considerably different than their metal predecessors. They consist of a screw-on clamp that holds the distal end of the cartridge, a curved plate to support the fingertips, and the plunger. Unlike the older metal version, the disposable/reusable models do not have a barrel section—the cartridge extends unsupported from the clamp.

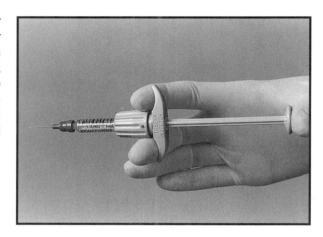

2. With the plunger fully retracted, the distal end of the cartridge is inserted into the opened clamp. The collar of the screw-clamp is rotated counter-clockwise to secure the cartridge in place.

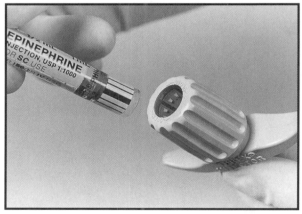

3. After attaching the cartridge to the clamp, rotate the plunger to screw its female tip onto the screw extending from the rubber stopper at the back end of the cartridge. The EMT must be careful to not loosen the screw-on collar while attaching the plunger. The disposable/reusable Tubex injector is now ready for use.

4. Administer the medication in the prescribed amount and by the appropriate route, and then dispose of both the cartridge and the holder by simply dropping them in a suitable sharps container.

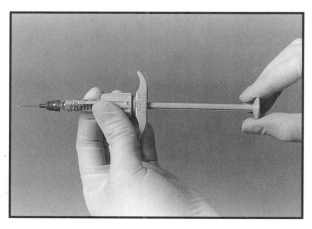

ALS

GIVING A SUBCUTANEOUS INJECTION

Subcutaneous injections are used to place medication under the skin (the fatty cutaneous layer) from where it can be absorbed into the bloodstream at the capillary level. This route of administration delivers the medication much slower than when the medication is injected intravenously. The most common prehospital medication administered by the subcutaneous route ("SQ" or "subQ") is epinephrine in its 1 : 1,000 concentration—typically in cases of anaphylaxis. With most subcutaneous injections, the maximum amount of medication delivered is 0.5 milliliters in volume at any one site. For this reason, a 1cc tuberculin syringe with a 5/8 inch needle attached is most commonly used. With this type of syringe, the EMT can give very ac-curate doses to the hundredth of a milliliter.

1. Subcutaneous injections can be given almost anywhere on the body, as long as the skin can be "pinched up" between the EMT's fingers. The most common site is the posterior lateral aspect of the upper arm. You will need a TB syringe and needle, alcohol prep swabs, personal protective equipment, and the medication. First draw up the appropriate amount of medication.

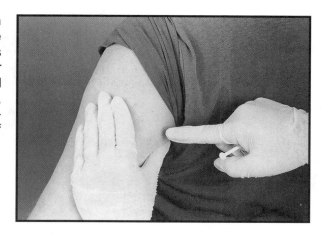

2. After taking appropriate body substance isolation precautions, cleanse the selected injection site on the patient's upper arm with an alcohol swab, moving in a circle from the inside out. Re-check the amount of medication drawn up to reduce the possibility of an error. Pinch up the subcutaneous tissue in the selected area with your index finger and thumb—making sure that you do not touch the area of the selected injection site after it has been cleansed.

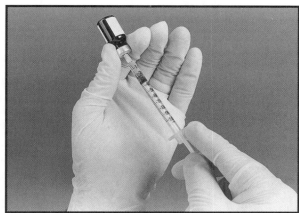

3. Hold the syringe between the thumb and index finger of your other hand as if you were holding a dart. Tell the patient what you are going to do, and that he will feel a small poke or pinch when the needle enters the skin.

4. With the needle held bevel-up and at a 45 degree angle to the patient's skin, insert the needle tip into the patient's arm so that the tip remains in the subcutaneous space under the top layer of skin.

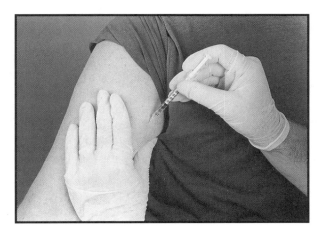

5. Gently release the pinched-up skin while holding the syringe so the needle remains inserted properly in position. Use your free hand to pull back on the plunger slightly to check for a blood return. If there is any blood aspirated into the syringe, this indicates that the needle is in a blood vessel and that if the medication is delivered, it will *NOT* be subcutaneously. In such a case, withdraw the needle and begin again by discarding the syringe in a sharps container and drawing up a new dose with a new syringe.

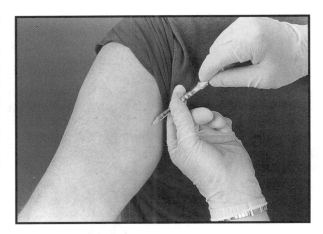

6. If there was not a blood return when the plunger was retracted, slowly depress the plunger and administer the medication. You will usually be able to see a bump or weal develop under the skin where the fluid accumulates in the subcutaneous space.

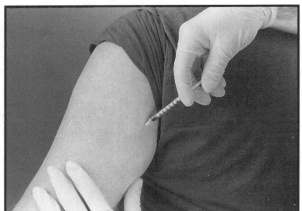

7. Using another alcohol prep swab, gently rub the injection site as you withdraw the needle from the patient's skin to help disperse the medication into the tissues.

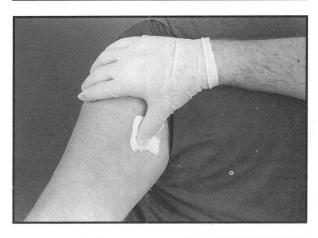

8. Immediately place the syringe and needle into a suitable sharps container, then place a bandaid over the injection site. This helps to reduce the possibility of infection, and also serves to trap the medication in the subcutaneous layer. Document the time of administration, medication and dose, size of syringe and gauge and length of needle, and the location of the injection site. Assess your patient for any adverse reaction to the medication, and document its presence or absence.

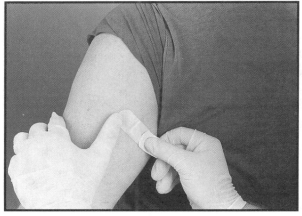

ALS

GIVING AN INTRAMUSCULAR INJECTION

Intramuscular (IM) injections are used to deliver certain medications deep into the patient's muscle fiber. The rate of absorption for these injections is between the slower SQ and the very rapid IV. The most commonly used sites for IM injections are the posterior deltoid muscle in the upper arm, the gluteus medius muscle of the buttock, and the vastus lateralis muscle of the lateral thigh. Of these, the upper arm and thigh are most commonly selected for prehospital administration because the patient is usually transported in a supine or semi-Fowler's position in the ambulance. In the following steps, the posterior deltoid muscle will be used as the example.

1. Since IM injections are intended to place the medication deep into muscle tissue, 1 and 1.5 inch needles are used. Some judgement is needed to determine the appropriate length so that the needle selected is not so long that it might touch the bone which underlies the muscle. Generally, the maximum liquid volume delivered intramuscularly is 5ml, however local protocols may vary this. Some medications which are rarely given by prehospital personnel, such as penicillin, are frequently given in a larger number of milliliters.

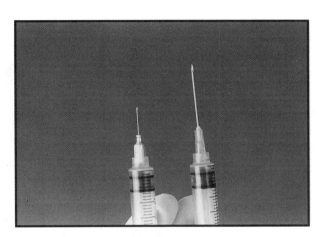

2. Just as with any medication, check and recheck to be sure that you have the correct medication, that its expiration date has not been reached, and that the fluid is of the correct color and clarity. Verify that you have drawn up the correct amount of medication for the prescribed order, based on the concentration on hand. To administer an IM medication, you will need a 5-10cc syringe and appropriate needle, alcohol prep swabs, the medication, and suitable personal protective equipment.

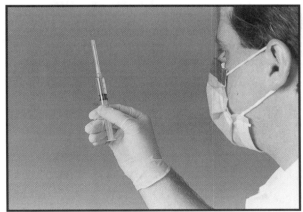

3. If the posterior deltoid muscle is used, first identify the landmarks of the upper arm in order to correctly locate the site. This helps to avoid injecting the nerves and blood vessels which are also found in the arm. Find the top bony portion of the shoulder where the clavicle and scapula meet (the acromioclavicular joint). Measure three to four finger-widths down the arm from the AC joint.

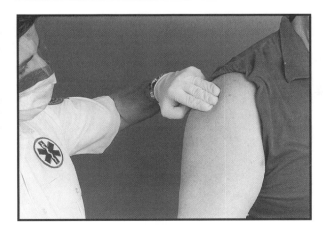

4. Next, slide one to two finger-widths posteriorly on the arm. This is the injection site.

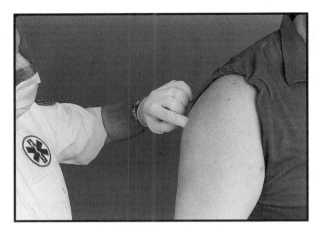

5. After confirming that the appropriate body substance isolation procedures have been taken, cleanse the injection site with an alcohol swab, moving circularly from the inside out.

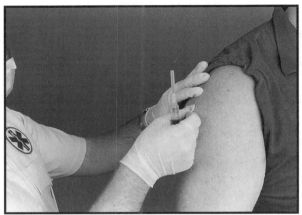

6. Hold the syringe as you would a dart between your thumb and index finger.

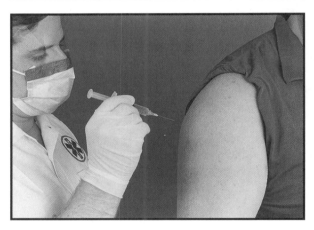

7. Either pinch up the skin and muscle with your free hand, or spread the skin tight between two fingers. Alternately, pull the skin downward to stabilize the skin over the site. Hold the syringe with the needletip just one-half to one inch away from the injection site. You do not need to "wind up" to enter the skin!

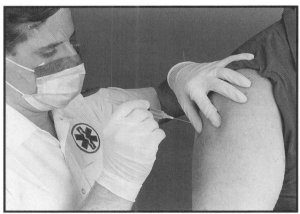

8. Tell the patient what you are going to do, and that he will feel a poke or pinch when the needle enters his arm. Quickly but not forcefully, insert the needle into the arm at a 90 degree angle. Push it in until the hub of the needle is against the skin.

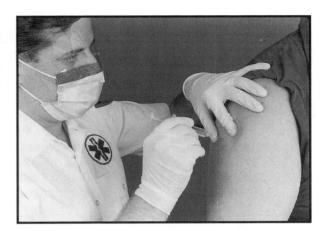

9. Release the skin with your one hand while continuing to hold the syringe with the other. Try to rest the hand holding the syringe on the patient's arm to help stabilize the needle. In this way, if the patient flinches or moves, the needle will remain in place and at the same depth.

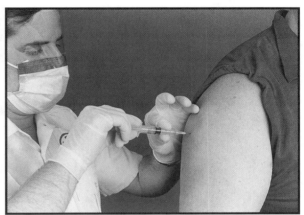

10. With your free hand, grasp the plunger and draw it slightly to assess for any blood return. If blood is aspirated in this way, you have inadvertently entered a blood vessel and the medication will not be delivered by the intended IM route. Withdraw the syringe and needle and discard them in a sharps container, then begin again using a new supply and syringe. If there is no blood return when the plunger is retracted, slowly depress the plunger and administer the medication.

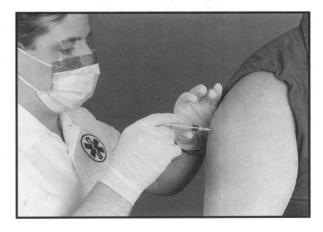

11. Once all of the medication has been administered, quickly withdraw the syringe and needle and cover the injection site with an alcohol swab or gauze pad. Rub the area gently to help minimize the pain and to promote dispersion of the drug within the muscle.

12. Discard the syringe and needle in an appropriate sharps container, and place a bandaid over the injection site. Document the time of administration, medication and dose, size of syringe and gauge and length of needle, and the location of the injection site. Assess your patient for any adverse reaction to the medication, and document its presence or absence.

ALS

USING AN ANAKIT OR AN EPI-PEN

Physicians often prescribe a prefilled set-dose self-injection device for patients who are extremely susceptible to anaphylactic reactions. There are two principal types of devices available: the AnaKit and the Epi-Pen. The AnaKit contains a special syringe prefilled with Epinephrine in a 1 : 1,000 concentration and intended for subcutaneous injection. The syringe is designed to hold two individual doses of epinephrine—one delivered by simply depressing the plunger as with any injection, the other obtainable after the first dose has been administered by rotating the plunger 180 degrees and again depressing the plunger. The AnaKit is packaged in a red plastic box that includes the syringe as well as alcohol swabs and frequently some oral Benadryl tablets.

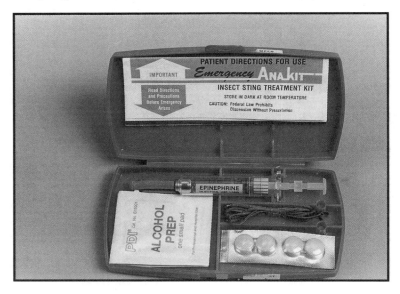

To use an AnaKit, the patient or a family member or the EMT must be abe to open the box, remove the syringe, and administer the injection into a muscle much like any IM injection.

Although an Epi-Pen is similar in purpose to an AnaKit, its design and mode of operation are significantly different. The Epi-Pen resembles a large felt-tip marker pen. The outer shell houses a recessed intramuscular needle, a pre-measured dose of Epinephrine 1 : 1,000, and a spring-loaded device that propels the needle and medication into the patient.

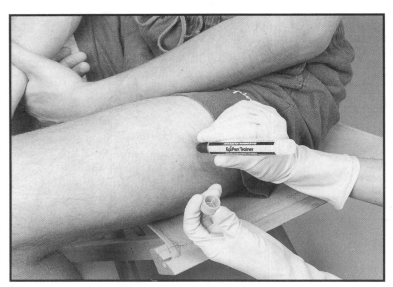

When the needle end of the Epi-Pen is pushed against a large muscle, such as the vastus lateralis of the thigh or the deltoid muscle, the resistance encountered is registered by the spring-loaded mechanism. When the resistance exceeds a preset limit, the mechanism activates and drives the needle from the barrel and into the muscle. This also disperses the Epinephrine stored within the device through the needle and into the muscle. The Epi-Pen is much easier to operate than the manipulation required in using an AnaKit, and also avoids much of the reluctance or apprehension caused by the sight of the syringe and needle. It can be used through clothing if necessary, although if time permits a more conventional approach should be used.

To use an Epi-Pen, remove the gray safety cap from the back end of the device and place the black tip firmly against the outer thigh. With a smooth motion, push in hard until the needle enters the skin *AND THEN HOLD THE EPI-PEN IN PLACE FOR TEN MORE SECONDS* to allow the epinephrine to be injected through the needle and into the muscle. Continue to monitor the patient for signs of improvement or the need for additional treatment. Take and record vital signs on a regular basis, and provide prompt transport to a hospital.

ALS

DRAWING BLOOD SAMPLES — INTRODUCTION

Phlebotomy (drawing blood from a vein) is the procedure used to acquire blood samples from a patient for analysis. A great deal of information can be gained about the patient through the various laboratory tests that can be performed on a sample of blood, including evaluating the hemoglobin and hematocrit levels, determining clotting time, blood sugar levels, the presence of medications or poisons, cardiac enzyme evaluation, and many more. Most prehospital blood samples are used to determine what the "baseline" conditions are before prehospital and Emergency Department treatment (drugs or fluid replacement) causes the blood values to change. The most common example of this is blood glucose (sugar) levels in suspected hypoglycemic (low blood sugar) patients prior to administering Dextrose 50% Water.

There are several different ways to obtain blood samples, however the "best" way is usually the one which involves the fewest skin punctures or needle sticks for the patient. When an IV is to be initiated, all of the needed blood can be obtained through one needle stick when the catheter is inserted into the vein, and then the catheter is used as a route for administering IV fluids and/or medications. When an IV is not indicated, or if the quality of the patient's veins is poor and drawing blood could jeopardize the patency of the IV or cause undesirable delay in cases where emergency drug administration is rapidly needed, the vein will need to be separately cannulated for the purpose of obtaining drug samples.

There are several different sizes and types of tubes used to collect and hold the blood samples. The rubber caps on the tubes are differently colored, and are frequently called "red tops," "purple tops," "gray tops," or "jungle tops" depending upon their colors and patterns. Some of these tubes have small amounts of liquid or other agents inside the tube to prevent coagulation or to assist in preserving the blood in a way necessary to a particular type of test. Other tubes need to be placed in ice after the blood is added (light blue top). The tubes most commonly used for prehospital samples are red tops, green or "jungle" tops, and gray tops. When obtaining a blood sample, it is desirable to fill each tube completely so that an adequate amount will be available for the laboratory.

When the tubes are manufactured, a vacuum is introduced into the tube which aids in sucking blood into the tube when the sample is drawn. The most common brand for blood collection tubes is the *Vacutainer®*. For these a special holder is generally used. The holder is analogous to the barrel of a large syringe and contains a threaded tip. When a Vacutainer needle is inserted through the tip and screwed into place, one of its sharp ends extends from the holder much like any hollow needle from a syringe. This needle is used to cannulate the vein. The other end of the hollow needle protrudes into the holder and also has a sharpened end. Once the needle has been properly located in a vein and a collecting tube is inserted into the holder, the tube is pushed down into the holder and the sharp end within the holder pierces and enters the tube through the rubber stopper.

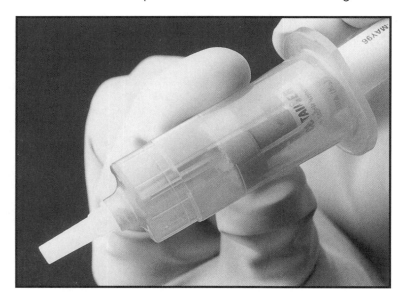

Blood collection tubes have expiration dates printed on their labels, and the EMT needs to check this information before using a tube to collect a blood sample. Once the blood has been collected, you should immediately write the patient's name, the date, the time, "drawn by" and your name, and any other information that will be helpful—such as "prior to $D_{50}W$" or "after Narcan"—on each tube's label. If you are caring for more than one patient, be sure not to mix up the tubes once the samples have been drawn. *Tubes containing samples from different patients should never be handled at the same time.*

The classic method of drawing a blood sample is to do so directly with a needle, Vacutainer holder, and blood collection tubes. This method is most often used in laboratories and clinics when an IV line is not contemplated and the primary interest is in simply obtaining the blood sample. As with any procedure, preparation of the equipment prior to puncturing the skin is necessary. This technique requires a venous tourniquet, an alcohol prep swab, a few 2x2 gauze pads, a bandaid, the indicated blood collection tubes, a Vacutainer holder and a Vacutainer needle.

Inasmuch as the procedure of drawing a blood sample does involve venipuncture and the removal of blood from the patient's body, appropriate body substance isolation procedures should be employed even though this process is usually performed without any direct contact with the blood or other body substances by the EMT. In recent years the original style of vacutainer holder has been replaced with a single-use disposable one that permits the contaminated needle to be retracted into the barrel of the holder, thus removing the danger of a needlestick injury after the needle has been withdrawn from the patient and before it is placed in a sharps container. Whichever holder is available to the EMT, it should only be used for a single venous cannulation. Once it has been used and withdrawn, it should be disposed of in a sharps container *WITHOUT* any attempt to remove the needle from the holder. Removal of the needle or any re-use of the holder produces unnecessary risk of an accidental needlestick injury and contamination to the EMT, or from one patient to another, and is no longer an acceptable practice.

ALS

Drawing Blood With A Vacutainer®

1. Twist the protective cap off of the shorter end of the Vacutainer needle. This will reveal a rubber sleeve covering this end of the needle, which is threaded at its base.

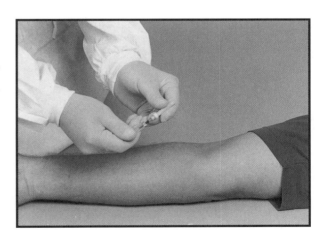

2. Insert the rubber covered end of the Vacutainer needle into the small hole at the bottom of the holder. Screw the needle tightly into the holder.

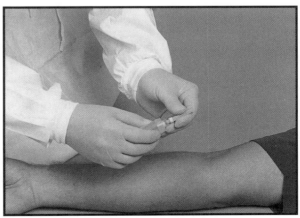

3. Select an appropriate vein on the back of the hand or on the arm. The most commonly used is in the antecubital fossa, although any large vein can be used. Apply a venous tourniquet proximal to the selected site just as you would when starting an IV. Cleanse the site with an alcohol or Betadine prep swab, circling from the inside outward.

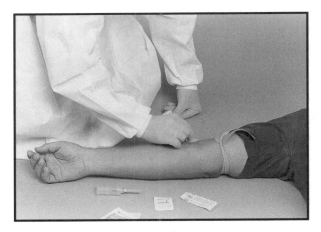

4. Remove the protective cap from the exposed end of the Vacutainer needle. Talk to your patient and let him know what you are going to do and what to expect. Explain that he will feel the needle pinch as it enters the skin, and that it is important that he *NOT* move his arm as you further position it and change the tubes to obtain the necessary blood samples.

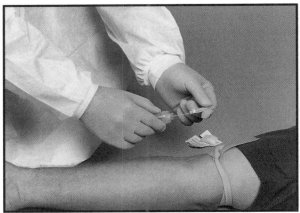

5. Select the first blood collection tube and slide it into the Vacutainer holder—but *DO NOT* push down on the tube or allow the rubber top to be punctured by the needle inside the holder. Puncturing the top now will release the vacuum inside the tube and make it unusable for drawing blood.

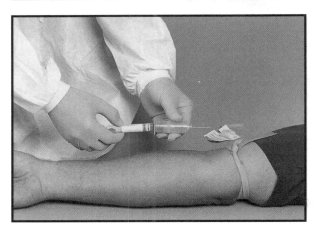

6. While holding the Vacutainer at about a 45 degree angle and with the bevel on the needle facing upward, quickly but gently enter the skin and the vein as you would when giving an intravenous injection or starting an IV, using both hands to hold and guide the Vacutainer and the patient's arm. Remember that you want to place the tip of the needle into the lumen of the vein, so be careful to not insert the needle too deeply, causing it to pass through both walls of the vein.

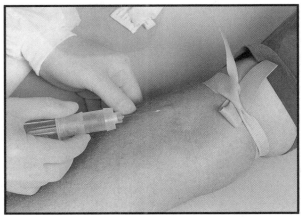

7. As soon as you feel that the needle is in the vein, lower the Vacutainer and thread the needle one or two millimeters further into the vein. Continue to hold the Vacutainer chamber securely with one hand and use your other hand to push the collection tube down onto the needle inside the chamber. Blood should immediately begin to fill the collection tube. If blood does not begin to flow immediately, re-assess the position of the needle in the vein and either advance or retract it slightly until you do get a good blood flow.

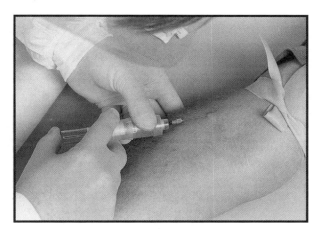

8. When the first collection tube is filled, remove it by pulling back on the tube while holding the barrel of the holder from moving to keep the needletip in place in the vein. If additional tubes are to be filled, insert each one in turn and push them onto the needle in the holder to collect the needed blood. Be careful while removing and adding tubes that you do not change the position of the needle in the vein. When you have filled all of the required tubes, release the tourniquet from the patient's arm and remove the last tube from the holder.

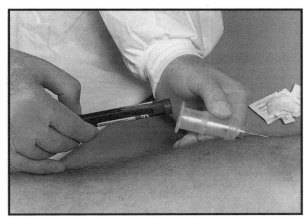

9. Place a folded 2x2 gauze pad over the puncture site and gently remove the Vacutainer needle from the vein. Apply direct pressure through the gauze pad to the puncture site. If the patient is cooperative, they can be recruited to hold the pad in place.

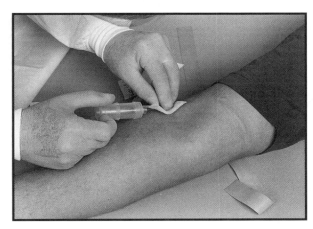

10. Discard the Vacutainer with its needle into an appropriate sharps container. Label all of the tubes with the date and time, the patient's name, "drawn by" and your name, and any pertinent information such as "before $D_{50}W$," etc. Replace the gauze pad over the puncture site with a bandaid.

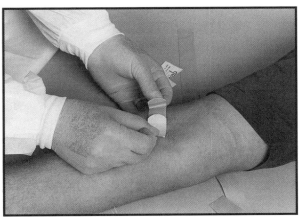

ALS **Drawing Blood Using A Syringe**

   At times it may be preferable to obtain the blood sample with a needle and syringe, and then transfer the blood sample from the syringe to the blood collection tubes. The process is very similar to that described above using a Vacutainer holder, and requires the same supplies except that a hypodermic needle and 20cc syringe are used instead of a Vacutainer holder and needle.

1. To obtain a blood sample by syringe, take all appropriate body substance isolation precautions and assemble the materials needed. Cannulate the vein with the hypodermic needle attached to the syringe with the plunger fully depressed into the barrel of the syringe.

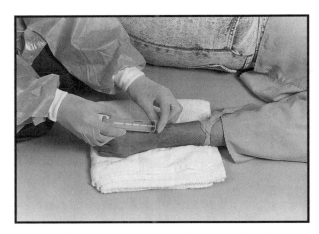

2. Slowly but steadily pull back on the plunger and draw blood into the barrel of the syringe. The walls of the vein may be drawn to the tip of the needle if you aspirate too vigorously, or the red cells can become "bruised" — making the sample unusable for some tests if the syringe is aspirated too rapidly.

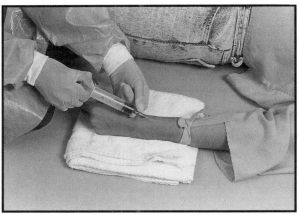

3. When the syringe is full, cover the puncture site with a folded 2x2 gauze pad and carefully withdraw the needle. While the patient or a second EMT applies direct pressure over the puncture site, insert the needle straight down into the top of a blood collection tube. The vacuum in the tube will pull the blood from the syringe into the tube. If more than one tube is to be filled, control the plunger so that too much blood is not drawn into the earlier tubes and none remains for the last. At least 1/2 inch of blood is desirable in each tube if only a limited amount was able to be drawn.

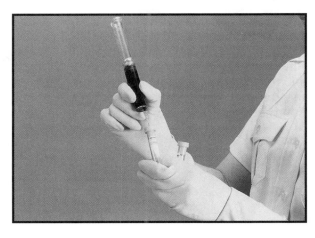

4. Once the tube is full of blood, carefully withdraw the needle from the tube. If you have more tubes to fill, repeat this procedure with each collection tube until you are done or have run out of blood.

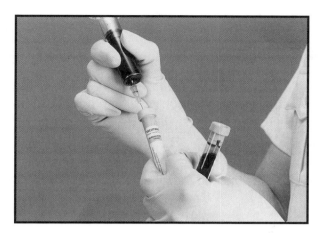

5. Discard the syringe and needle into an appropriate sharps container, and label the collection tubes with the date and time, the name of the patient, your name, and any other key information such as "prior to $D_{50}W$."

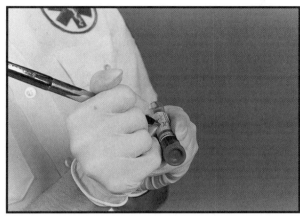

ALS

DRAWING BLOOD WHILE ESTABLISHING AN IV

Drawing a blood sample through an IV catheter during the process of initiating an IV is the simplest and most commonly used prehospital method of obtaining a blood sample. After advancing the IV catheter into the vein and applying pressure with your finger over the vein at the location of the tip of the catheter, attach a 20cc syringe to the catheter hub instead of connecting the IV tubing. You can also use a Vacutainer holder with a multi-sample IV Luer-lock adapter fitted to it. When blood is to be drawn while establishing an IV, it is done immediately after the vein has been cannulated and the needle is removed from the catheter, but before the administration set is connected to the catheter.

1. Whether you use a syringe or a Vacutainer, be especially careful to not disturb the IV catheter's placement while connecting the syringe or Vacutainer to it. Leave the tourniquet in place while obtaining the blood samples.

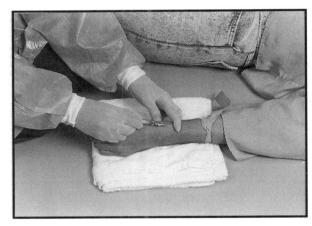

2. If you are using a Vacutainer, slide the collection tube into the holder and push the tube down on the needle to begin collecting blood. If you are using a syringe, retract the plunger very slowly to aspirate blood into the barrel. Again, be careful to not dislodge the catheter. It may be necessary to rotate and carefully slide the catheter outwards a bit or forward further into the vein in the event that a vein wall or valve occludes the tip of the catheter as you aspirate.

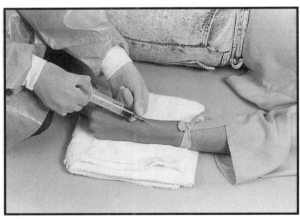

3. Once the syringe is completely full or you have collected enough blood using the Vacutainer, release the tourniquet from the patient's arm. Occlude the vein at the catheter's tip by pressing down with your middle or ring finger over the area just proximal to where the end of the catheter lies under the skin. Grasp the IV catheter hub with the thumb and index finger of the same hand and carefully disconnect the syringe or Vacutainer from the IV catheter hub without dislodging the catheter.

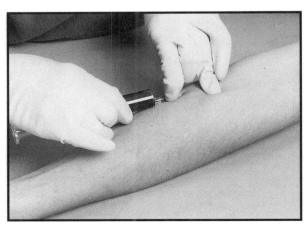

4. At this point two tasks need to be accomplished simultaneously, requiring two EMTs. First, the IV tubing must be connected to the IV hub and, once the desired drip rate has been adjusted with the flow control clamp on the IV tubing, the catheter and tubing taped into place. Second, the collected blood must be managed.

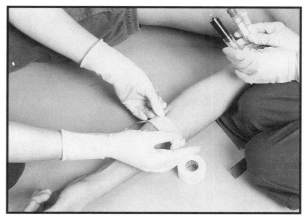

5. If you collected blood in Vacutainer tubes, now is the time to safely dispose of the Vacutainer holder in a sharps container and to label the tubes with the time and date, patient's name, "drawn by" and your name, and any pertinent additional information. Depending upon your local protocols or the preference of the hospital to which you are transporting the patient, "package" the filled blood collection tubes appropriately and secure and label the package.

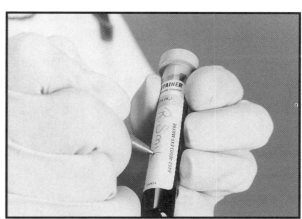

6. If you collected the blood in a syringe, it must now be transferred to Vacutainer tubes. This is perhaps the most hazardous part of the operation as it poses the possibility of incurring a needlestick injury and bloodborne pathogen exposure. First attach an 18 gauge hypodermic needle to the syringe, then insert the needle through the rubber top of the first blood collection tube and fill it with blood from the syringe. Continue until you run out of blood or tubes. Properly dispose of the contaminated needle and syringe in a sharps container, and label the collection tubes as described above.

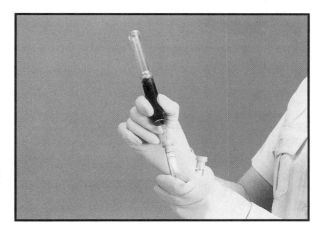

DOING A FINGER/HEEL STICK
(Obtaining Blood Droplets For Dextrostix or Glucometer Evaluation)

A finger or heel "stick" is used to obtain a small sample of blood for quick blood analysis — usually to measure a patient's blood glucose level. The equipment needed includes an alcohol prep, a bandaid, a lancet for piercing the skin, and a gauze pad. In addition, you will need whatever blood analyzing device your service uses. This can range from Dextrostix® paper strips to One Touch® automated glucometers. The lancet used for this test is commonly a very short needle housed in a plastic holder to facilitate grasping it properly. The needletip is covered by a twist-off protective top. When this top is removed, about one eighth of the needle tip is exposed and the plastic holder acts as a depth stop to prevent the lancet from being inserted too deeply. The following demonstration portrays the use of the Dextrostix system, however the general sequence of events is similar regardless of the equipment being used. Explain the procedure to the patient and:

1. Choose an appropriate site for the stick. The fleshy finger tip of an adult and child over two, or the heel of an infant are the most commonly selected. Check that the expiration date on the Dextrostix has not been passed, and that the individual stick appears as it should. Cleanse the area with an alcohol prep swab, circling from the inside outward, and allow the area to dry.

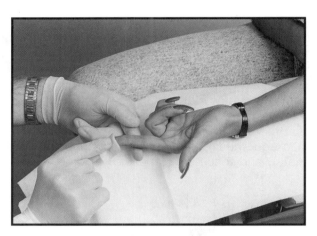

2. After confirming that the appropriate body substance isolation precautions have been taken, remove the protective cap from the tip of the lancet and hold it directly over the selected site.

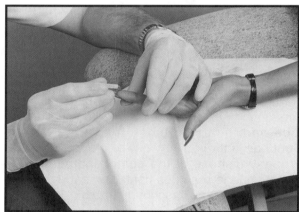

3. Lower the tip of the lancet until it is just touching the skin's surface and, in a quick firm stab-like movement, puncture the skin with the lancet so that blood flows from the site. Wipe off the initial show of blood with the gauze pad.

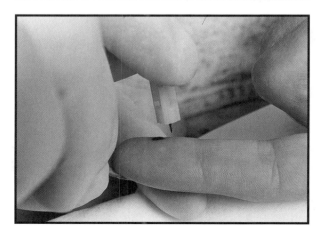

4. Squeeze the site to encourage further bleeding, and draw the treated end of a Dextrostix through the new blood. Clean the site with an alcohol swab and apply a gauze pad or bandaid over the site.

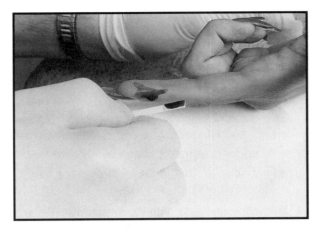

5. After wiping the blood onto the treated end of the Dextrostix, wait the manufacturer's prescribed time before reading the results. This is usually one minute. It is important that this wait be accurate, so use your watch to keep track of the time.

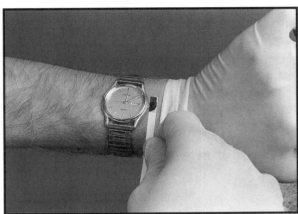

6. After waiting the designated period of time, "read" the results. With a Dextrostix this involves matching the color of the strip that was exposed to the blood, to the color chart on the package.

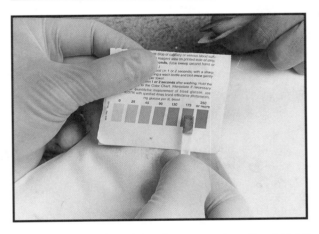

7. When using a glucometer or similar automated device to obtain a blood sugar value, the "stick" and elimination of the first one or two drops of blood are done in the identical manner. The specific method for then obtaining the sample and its evaluation with the device will vary depending upon the design and brand being used. The EMT must be familiar with the specific directions and use of the particular model carried on his ambulance, and should follow the manufacturer's directions exactly. Automated devices usually provide a numeric result that corresponds to the patient's blood glucose level. Depending upon the results of this test, follow your local protocols for the further management of the patient.

INTRAVENOUS THERAPY—INTRODUCTION

Intravenous (IV) therapy is an invasive procedure which is used to obtain venous access to the circulatory system for one or more of the following reasons:

- To administer fluids for volume replacement, using crystalloid solutions (Normal Saline, Lactated Ringer's, or D_5W) or colloids (whole blood, packed red cells, Dextran, etc.)
- To administer medications by either a bolus or "drip."
- Finally, as a "just in case" lifeline for medication access or fluid volume replacement when the patient's condition is presently stable but deterioration is anticipated.

In the prehospital setting, peripheral IVs are most commonly used for both pediatric and adult patients. Peripheral cannulation includes veins in the fingers, hands, forearm, upper arm, lower legs and feet. In the adult patient, the external jugular vein can also be considered a peripheral vein. Infant scalp veins are also used as peripheral IV sites when other locations fail to provide venous access. Intraosseous ("in the bone") routes are also considered to be peripheral. The alternative to peripheral routes are "central" routes. Central veins are typically used only in the hospital and primarily when internal hemodynamic monitoring is being performed.

When selecting a peripheral IV site, try to avoid using an extremity that contains a possible fracture, is burned, shows signs of infection, has fresh tatoos, venous cutdowns, or any dialysis shunts. Also avoid extremities that are paralyzed (including stroke patients with unilateral paralysis), upper extremities on the same side as a mastectomy, and extremities which display signs of multiple venpuncture (such as with IV drug abusers.)

Equipment

Prior to starting an IV, selection of the proper equipment is necessary.

IV Needle/Catheters: There are three common types of IV needles used in pre-hospital care: Catheter-Over-Needle (most common), Butterfly, and Intraosseous. Typical Catheter-Over-Needle sizes range from 24 gauge (smallest) to 14 gauge (largest). Butterfly needles are sized in odd numbers and range from 27 gauge (smallest) to 19 gauge (largest).

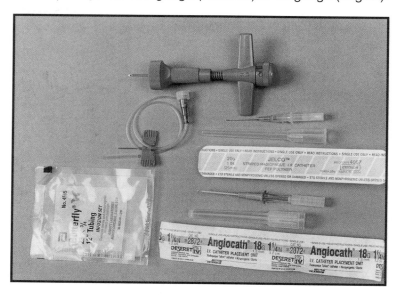

IV Administration Sets: Common types of IV tubing include "Macro drip" tubing (10, 15 or 20 gtts/ml flow rates) for large volume infusion and "micro drip" tubing (60 gtts/ml flow) for smaller infusion volumes and medication administration.

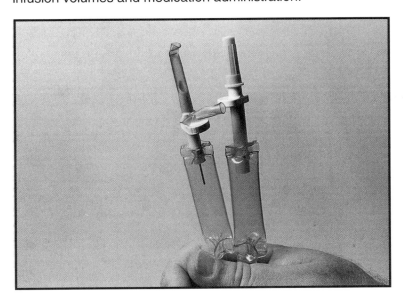

Specialty IV tubing: IV "blood tubing" has a particularly large internal diameter plus a special blood filter. It can be used in place of macro drip tubing. If blood tubing is used with the prehospital IV, blood can then be "hung" in place of a crystalloid solution with a minimum of tubing change-over once the patient is at the hospital. "Volutrol chamber" IV tubing is commonly used when specific amounts of fluid are to be administered. They are common for infant and pediatric infusions.

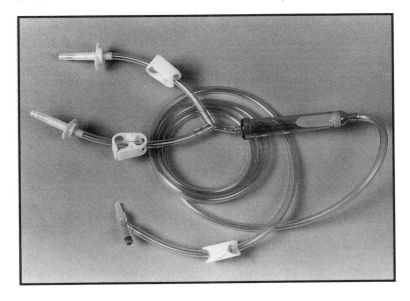

Other equipment items needed to initiate and maintain an IV infusion include tape, bandaids, gauze pads, armboard, Opsite® dressing, alcohol or betadine swabs, anti-bacterial ointment, the fluid or IV medication solution to be administered, and protective gloves.

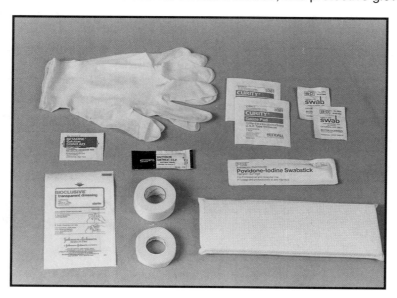

IV Fluid: IV fluids generally come in 50, 250, 500, and 1000mL volume bags. Fluids commonly used in prehospital care include 5% Dextrose in Water (D$_5$W), Lactated Ringer's (LR), Normal Saline (NS) which is 0.9% Sodium Chloride, 5% Dextrose and Lactated Ringer's (D$_5$LR), 5% Dextrose and Sodium Chloride (D$_5$NS), and Half-Normal Saline (0.45% Sodium Chloride). Each type of fluid has a particular special application, although Normal Saline and Lactated Ringer's are frequently recommended for volume replacement purposes and D$_5$W is more often identified for medication administration. Local preferences vary widely in such choices, and in recent years many areas have moved to using Normal Saline almost exclusively.

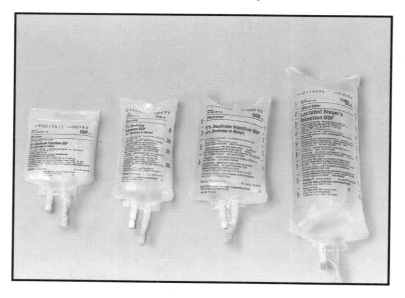

Venous Tourniquets: Different types of rubber venous tourniquets can be used, including flat Penrose drain tubing and round rubber tubing. Commercially manufactured venous tourniquets are also available which use rubber and Velcro®. A blood pressure cuff inflated to between 20 and 30 mmHg can also be used as a tourniquet. A venous constrictor or tourniquet should not be confused with the type of tourniquet used to obstruct all distal circulation to control external bleeding. A venous constrictor should only be tightened to the point where it obstructs the underlying venous flow without preventing continued distal arterial circulation.

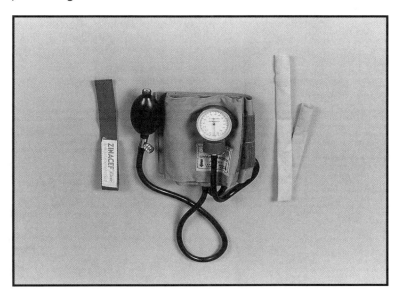

An IV is established in three separately identifiable major parts:
• Preparing and "hanging" the IV
• Obtaining IV access
• Connecting the IV catheter and tubing, and regulating the flow rate.

When there are ample resources the IV can be prepared and hung by one EMT while a second completes the assessment and prepares to obtain venous access. Cannulation of a vein should not be attempted before the IV bag and administration tubing are ready to be connected to the catheter so that the patency of the venipuncture will not be lost due to the lack of IV fluid promptly flowing through it. The demonstration of establishing an IV line in the following pages is shown in a continuous sequence as if it was performed by an individual EMT. It has been separated by headings into the three parts identified above. When two EMTs are available, then one should follow the steps in preparing the IV and the second should start at the sub-heading for gaining IV access. In such cases, the EMT who actually inserts the needle and catheter remains responsible for checking the work of the first EMT—verifying that the correct solution and administration set has been used—and for documenting the IV start.

ALS

ESTABLISHING A PERIPHERAL IV LINE
Preparation Of The Equipment — Hanging The IV

1. Based upon the patient's condition (and your standing orders) or the physician's specific order, select the appropriate IV solution, size of IV bag, and administration set. Also gather an IV "start kit" (or the equivalent loose components: antiseptic swabs, gauze pads, venous tourniquet, bio-occlusive venipuncture site bandage, antibiotic gel, etc.) and several needle/catheters of the general size desired. The exact size needle/catheter that is eventually used will not be determined until the particular vein to be cannulated has been identified. Examine the covering of the IV bag for leakage or other damage. Some moisture from condensation may be present in this outer protective bag, however this is normal and should not be of any concern.

2. To open the outer bag, tear the bag at the pre-cut slit at either end. If using scissors, be careful to not cut or puncture the inner IV bag itself. Once removed from the protective outer bag, the inner IV bag should be examined to re-check the name of the fluid, to assure that the expiration date is still valid, and that the fluid is clear and free of any particulate matter.

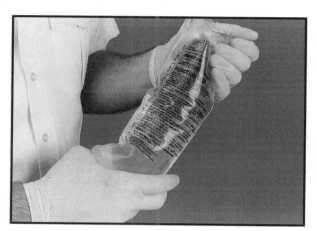

3. Check that the drip rating of the IV tubing set is the size desired, and remove the tubing from its package. Uncoil the tubing, making sure it is completely untangled. Both ends should have protective caps in place or plastic covers to maintain sterility. Both of these end caps must remain sterile at all times, even after the protective caps have been removed.

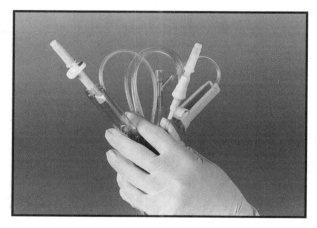

4. To "spike" the IV bag, first remove the covering on the IV tubing at the top of the drip chamber. This will expose a beveled spike.

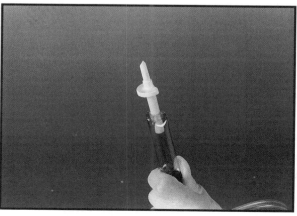

5. The IV bag will have two tail ports at the bottom of the bag, one with a rubber stopper for the infusion of medications, the other with a plastic tab similar to the IV tubing. This is where the IV tubing plugs into the IV bag. (The bag shown here is being held bottom-end-up to show the tail ports.)

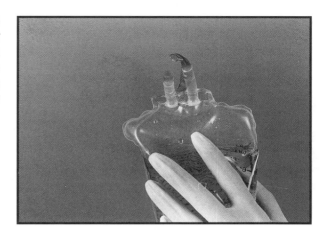

6. While holding the IV bag upside down, remove the plastic covering from the port by pulling the plastic tab. The port has not yet been punctured, so holding the bag upright will not cause it to leak. Remember that this port must also remain sterile.

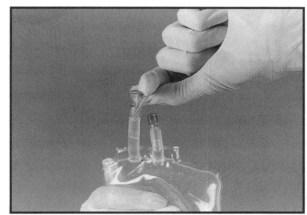

7. With the IV bag upside down, take the IV tubing spike and insert it into the port by pushing and twisting the spike until it punctures the seal at the port.

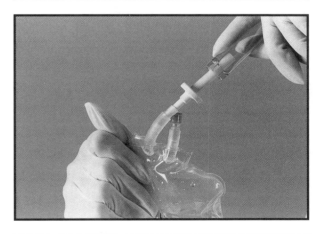

8. Slide the flow adjustment clamp up the tubing toward the drip chamber so that it can easily be found and tighten it just enough to keep it in place.

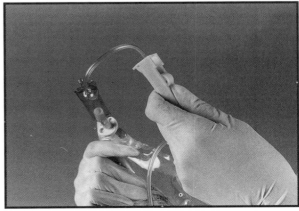

9. Turn the IV bag upright. Fluid should begin to flow into the drip chamber. Squeeze the drip chamber once or twice to fill the chamber half-full. Failure to do this now will add excess air bubbles into the IV line.

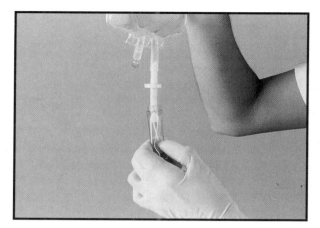

10. If too much fluid enters the chamber, just turn the IV bag and drip chamber upside down and squeeze a little fluid back into the bag until the chamber is about half-full.

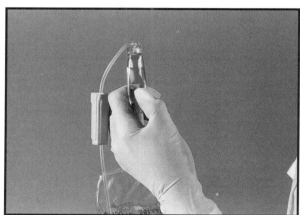

11. Place the other end of the tubing into a container such as a wastebasket or the IV cover bag to collect any excess fluid draining from the IV tubing. You can remove the end cap to increase the flow of the fluid but this is not necessary in most makes. If you do, remember the tubing end must remain sterile.

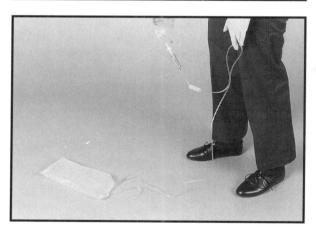

12. Allow the IV tubing to completely fill with fluid, removing any large air bubbles, and then clamp the line shut. Small air bubbles can usually be seen clinging to the sides of the tubing. These are not of concern. (Your patient might want to hear you tell them this information because they usually are looking at them as well.) Recap the end if you had removed it.

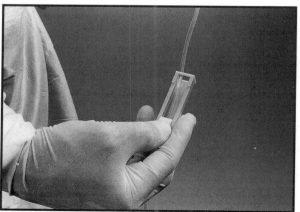

13. Hang your IV bag on an IV pole or IV hanger or have someone hold the bag for you. Locate the end of the IV tubing and place it near where you will be starting the IV. Locate your "sharps" container and position it within easy reach on the side of the patient on which you are going to start the IV.

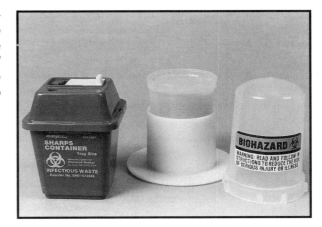

14. Prepare the other equipment. Tear three or four pieces of tape into 1/4 inch strips about six to eight inches in length. Open the alcohol or Betadine prep, bandaid, gauze pads and antibacterial ointment or Opsite® package so they will be ready to use.

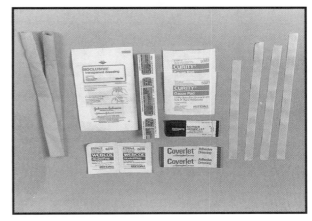

Obtaining IV Access — Peripheral Intravenous Cannulation In An Extremity

Once you have assembled the IV bag and tubing, and all of the other equipment has been assembled and prepared, you are ready to select a vein and insert a needle/catheter into it. Examine the extremity you have selected, making sure that there are no contraindicated conditions present in it. You may want to apply a tourniquet to each upper extremity, one at a time, to determine which extremity has the best veins. Keep in mind that you may not always be able to see a vein, so you have to practice feeling for veins with the tips of your fingers. Experience and practice will make you familiar with the location of veins commonly used for cannulation.

It is also important to attempt IVs in the more distal locations on an extremity and work your way proximally if a cannulation is unsuccessful. By starting too proximal, such as always beginning in the antecubital fossa, the hand and forearm veins will become invalid for use if you were to miss the first attempt. Any fluid administered distal to a "blown" IV site will leak into the surrounding tissue through the hole in the proximal vessel. If this is the only vein suitable for cannulation, you have no choice and must start at the proximal portion of the extremity.

When selecting a vein, make sure that you choose one that is fairly straight. This will make "threading" the catheter into the vein easier. Also, look for an area where two veins come together to form a larger vein (anastomosis). Many feel that by starting the IV at the "Y" of the two veins, cannulations can be more successful. When using a hand vein, visualize where the entry site will be and where the tip of the catheter will end up in relation to the location of the wrist joint. Starting the IV too close to the joint, or using a long catheter, will cause the catheter to cross the wrist joint. If the patient bends his wrist the catheter may become kinked and an arm board will have to be used to keep the wrist and catheter straight. Once the vein and site have been identified, palpate a short distance along the vein proximal to the site to assure that no valves lay where the catheter will be threaded into the vein.

When you have confirmed that everything is ready and have chosen the general location in which you plan to start the IV:

15. Take/confirm the proper body substance isolation precautions. Bare the selected extremity to make sure that the patient's clothing will not accidentally cover the tourniquet once it is applied. At a point about 4 to 8 inches proximal of the anticipated site (or beyond the proximal joint if necessary), wrap the tourniquet around the back of the extremity and stretch both ends outward and upward towards the front of the extremity. Slight counterpressure of the extremity against the EMT's arm or body may be necessary if the patient cannot hold his own arm down against the EMT's upward pull.

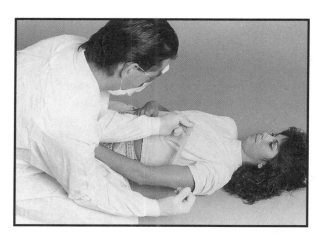

16. Bring the ends toward each other and, while they are still pulled outward away from the arm, loop one end around the other — like tying a shoelace.

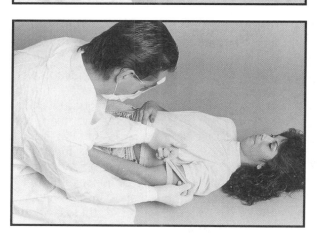

17. Instead of allowing the entire end to wrap under the crossover point, tuck only the middle portion of one end under it using the index finger and leaving a tail extend. At the same time, allow the tourniquet to relax against the extremity so that the crossover loop will hold its tightness against the skin.

18. After a few seconds for the distal veins to become distended, identify a suitable vein and specific site to cannulate. Palpate the vein at the proposed site and for a short distance proximal to it to locate any valves that may be present. Don't hurry — make a careful selection. Often a few additional seconds to identify a site you "like" can save minutes later.

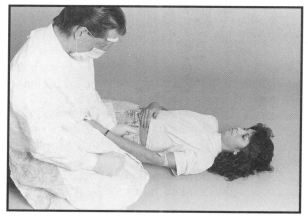

19. With an alcohol or Betadine prep, cleanse the IV site, starting from the center of the area and moving outward in a circular motion. This procedure may have to be done more than once to insure that the site is clean. Allow the alcohol to dry.

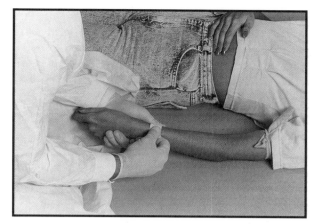

20. Based upon the IV's purpose and the size of the chosen vein, select an appropriate gauge needle/catheter. Remove the IV needle and catheter from its package and take the protective cap off the end of the needle — making sure that the catheter remains sterile. Depending on the type of catheter, there may be a small white cap at the other end of the needle beyond the "flash-back" chamber. Do not remove this cap.

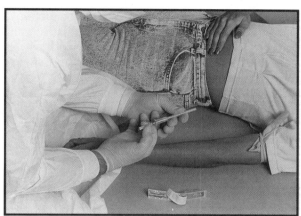

21. Inspect the point of the metal IV needle and the tip of the plastic catheter for any defects such as burred edges. Note that the catheter is about 1/8 of an inch shorter than the metal needle. Also note the bevel of the needle point. Some IV catheters have a tendency to stick at the connection of the catheter hub and flashback chamber. Twisting the catheter hub now while holding onto the flashback chamber will break this connection and prevent sticking when the needle and catheter are inside the patient's vein.

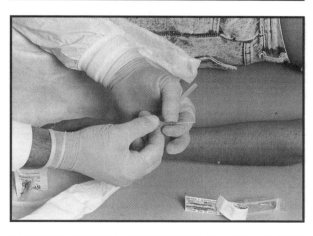

22. NEVER slide the end of the catheter over the point of the needle to break this seal. This can cause a small plastic splinter to be scraped off the inside of the catheter as it slides back onto the needle. The photograph on the right is obvious — small fragments which can wind up in your patient's bloodstream may not be as obvious.

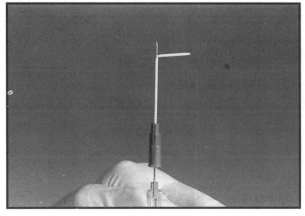

23. Grasp the patient's extremity near the area where the IV is to be started using your non-dominant hand. Using your thumb, stretch the skin near the vein by pulling downward. This will help anchor the vein and prevent it from rolling away from the IV needle.

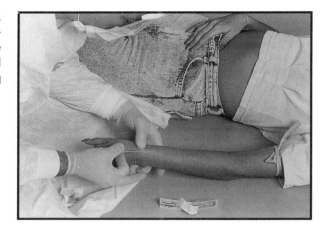

24. If a hand vein is used, grasp the patient's hand as shown and use your thumb to stretch the skin while slightly bending the patient's wrist. Do not place your thumb directly on the vein to be cannulated or the blood flow will be occluded and the veins will flatten.

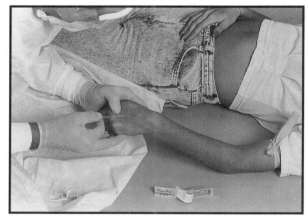

25. Determine where the bevel of the IV needle is. Turn the needle/catheter until the bevel is "up" in relation to the patient's skin. This will allow the sharp point of the needle to enter the skin first. Hold the end of the IV needle with your thumb and index/middle fingers—similar to how you would hold a pool stick. This allows you to see what you are doing and enables you to see the flashback chamber.

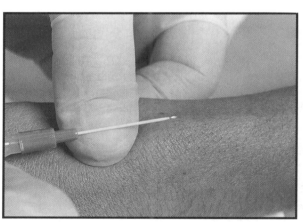

26. Approach the skin with the bevel of the IV needle up and the needle held at about a 35 to 45 degree angle to the skin. Tell the patient that they will feel a small poke or pinch as the needle enters the skin. Continue to talk to your patient and reassure him as you continue the procedure. Entry into the skin and vein can be done in either of two ways. The first is to enter the skin directly above the vein so that the needle goes through the skin and right into the vessel. (The other will be discussed later.)

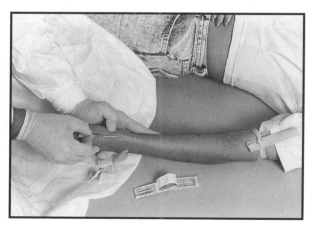

27. While applying traction to the vein, and with the needle's point directly over the vein, quickly but carefully enter the skin with the needle and continue until the needletip is on the wall of the vein itself.

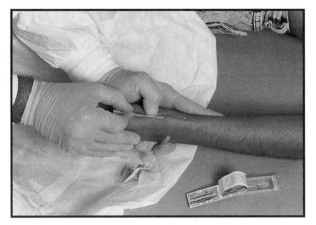

28. So as not to go through the back of the vessel as you enter the vein, lower the angle of the IV needle towards the skin (so that the needle is on less of an angle to the extremity) and slowly advance the needle through the vein's wall and into the lumen. Normally you will feel a slight "pop" or "give" as the needle passes through the wall of the vein. Care must be taken not to enter too fast or too deeply, as the needle can go through the back side of the vein.

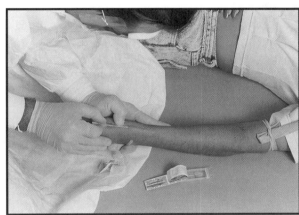

29. If the needle entered the vein, you should notice blood filling up the clear flashback chamber. If not, continue advancing the needle slightly along the vein until you do see a blood return in the chamber. As a general rule of thumb, if you need to continue advancing the needle in an attempt to enter the vein, no more than half of the catheter should be under the skin. If you enter the vein with less than half the catheter showing outside the skin, only a small portion of the catheter will be able to enter the vein itself.

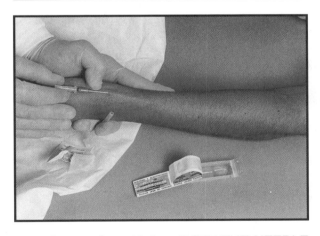

30. If you are unable to locate the vein after advancing the needle, *withdraw BOTH THE NEEDLE AND THE CATHETER slightly*—making sure that you do not pull the needle entirely out of the skin—and re-attempt to advance it into the vein. If the needle is pulled entirely out of the skin, get a new needle/catheter and re-attempt the IV. Again, in such cases *ALWAYS* pull back on the IV needle and catheter as a unit.

31. Once you have entered the vein and have blood in the flashback chamber, with the needle in line with the vein advance the needle another 1/8 to 1/4 inch further into it. You want the catheter to be inside the lumen of the vein, and since the catheter is shorter than the needle you must move the distal tip a bit further inside the vein to make sure that the catheter is properly placed. Be sure to advance the needle along the path of the vein so as not to poke through the opposite side of the vein.

32. When you are sure the tip of the catheter is well within the vein, slowly advance the *catheter* along the needle, threading it into the vein until the hub meets the skin. Simultaneously, withdraw the needle stylet backward toward the catheter hub but *DO NOT* pull the needle all of the way out yet.

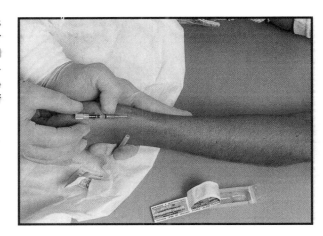

33. If you wish to draw blood from the IV for later laboratory analysis using a Vacutainer® or a syringe, have this equipment ready for use and leave the tourniquet in place. If you are going to immediately attach the IV tubing, release the tourniquet now. To release the tourniquet, simply pull on the tail piece to undo the half knot.

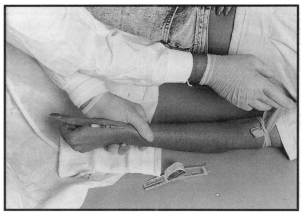

34. Palpate to find the end of the catheter under the skin, or approximate where the end is located. Apply direct pressure on the vein just proximal to the tip of the catheter to block blood from coming out of the catheter when the needle is removed from inside it.

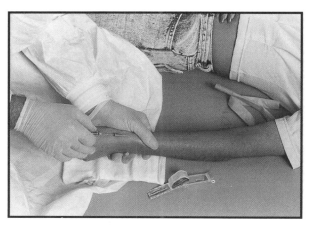

35. Withdraw the needle/stylet all the way out of the catheter and immediately drop it into the sharps container.

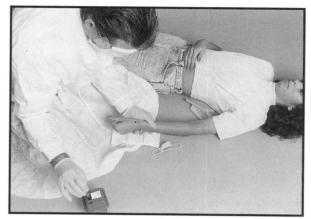

36. With your free hand, remove the protective cap from the end of the IV tubing. Without removing the pressure from over the vein, slide the end of the tubing into the hub of the IV catheter and gently push the tubing and hub together—making sure not to push the catheter further in or pull it out of the vein. Release the pressure from the vein above the catheter tip and use that hand to stabilize the catheter hub while you attach the tubing more securely.

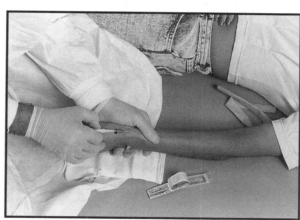

37. While continuing to hold the IV catheter hub, find the IV tubing flow clamp and open it. Slowly increase the rate to allow fluid to flow into the vein at a fast rate. You can set the desired drip rate after you have secured the IV.

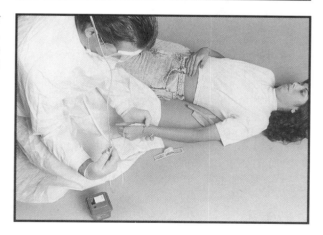

38. If the IV fluid does not begin to flow, check to make sure that you have released the tourniquet. If the tourniquet has been released, carefully pull the catheter back between 1/8 and 1/4 inch in case the tip is laying against a valve or against the wall of the vein. Pull back just enough to allow fluid to begin flowing without withdrawing a substantial amount of the catheter from the vein.

39. The alternate approach to cannulating a vein is to approach it from the side. Using the same approach as previously described with a 35–45 degree angle and bevel-up position, enter the skin with the needle poised alongside rather than directly above the vein. Once you have entered the skin, rotate the needle one quarter turn so that the bevel is away from the vein wall under the skin.

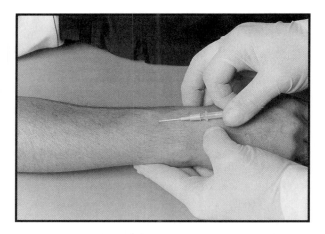

40. Once the tip of the needle is under the skin, move it sideways and enter the vein from the side. You may have to angle the catheter hub slightly away from the vein to allow the needle point to enter the wall of the vessel rather than running alongside it. Once you have entered the vein and obtained a good flashback, align the angle of the catheter to match the direction of the vein, advance the catheter and remove the needle, then connect the IV tubing and start the flow of IV solution as described earlier.

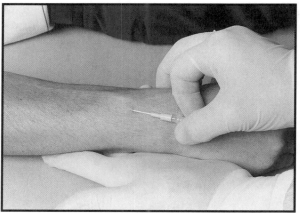

Either approach is an acceptable way to start an IV. Practice will assist you in learning which approach works best for you. The "on top" entry approach is frequently preferred for veins that move easily under the skin no matter how well you attempt to anchor them down. The disadvantage to this approach is the tendency to enter the vein too quickly and too deeply—going through the other side of the vein and "blowing" the IV. The side approach avoids this complication. The most painful part of an IV for the patient is the needle entering the skin. With the side approach you can quickly enter the skin without worrying about going too deep or blowing the vein. The disadvantage of the side approach is that, if you cannot secure the vein, you may push the vein away with the needle tip as you advance and never puncture the blood vessel.

41. With the IV fluid running and before covering the site with a bandaid or tape, inspect the venipuncture site for infiltration of fluid to insure that no fluid is leaking out of the vessel into the surrounding tissue. Clean up any blood that has dripped out of the catheter hub with a gauze pad or alcohol prep.

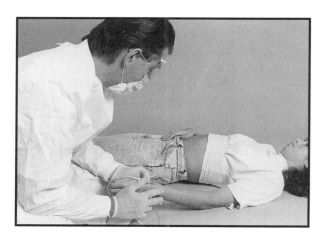

42. The signs and symptoms of infiltration include complaints of pain or burning at the site and swelling around the site. When an IV infiltrates, the IV drip rates usually slows and then stops. To check the patency of the IV, do a retrograde flow check by lowering the IV bag below the IV site. Blood should enter the IV catheter and tubing if the IV is patent. If not, or if any other sign or symptom of infiltration is present, immediately stop the IV, withdraw the catheter and apply digital pressure over the site with a sterile gauze pad. Restart the IV at another site.

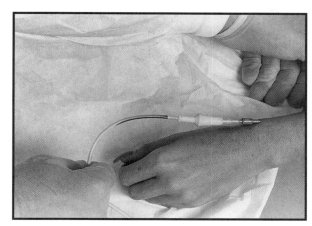

43. Once you are sure the IV is patent, secure the IV with tape or a manufactured IV closure such as an Opsite®. If an Opsite® is used, open the package and remove the clear covering — making sure the sticky sides do not touch each other. Carefully cover the IV site with the Opsite® keeping the site near the middle of the covering, and the press along the surface of the Opsite® — except over the catheter — to secure all of its sides.

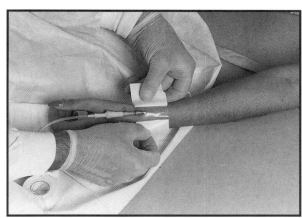

44. If tape is to be used, a bandaid over the IV entry site will insure that no tape touches the puncture area. Depending upon local protocol, an antibiotic gel may be added under the bandaid for further protection from infection.

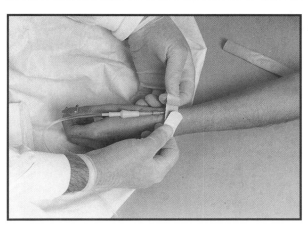

45. Take one strip of the 1/4 inch tape you have previously prepared, and slide it up under the IV tubing and catheter hub with the sticky side up. This can be tricky wearing gloves.

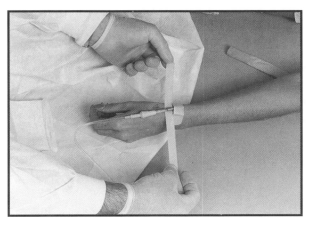

46. Being careful to not dislodge the catheter, cross each end over the catheter hub to the opposite side and encircle the hub snugly. Then secure each tail to the patient's skin, forming a chevron to anchor the catheter. When securing the tape tails to the skin, care must be taken to not pull them so tight that the catheter hub is pulled flat against the skin, or that it is otherwise moved from its naturally slightly angled position, as this can kink the catheter.

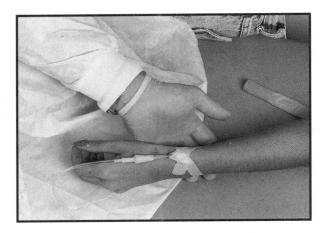

47. Take another piece of tape and repeat this process, or lay it directly over the hub of the IV line and secure it to the skin. Do not conceal all of the hub or the hub/tubing connection. This allows others to see what size catheter has been used by the color of the hub, and also allows for a leaky connection to be quickly spotted.

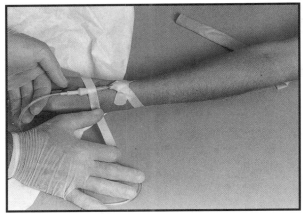

48. Make a loop with the IV tubing and secure this to the extremity at a point 8 to 10 inches proximal to the last tape strip you applied. This slack in the line helps insure that if the IV bag is pulled away from the patient the tubing will be pulled tight but the IV catheter will not be pulled out. Whether you have used a bandaid or an Opsite® to cover the entry site, the same general taping method should be used to secure the IV tubing to the patient's arm.

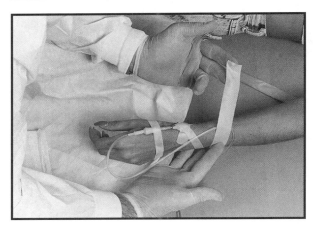

49. If the IV is "positional," where the fluid will only flow if the extremity is in a specific position, an armboard may be needed. This is common if the IV is in or near a joint. Carefully wrap or tape the armboard to the extremity making sure that the wrap or tape is not so tight as to impede venous blood flow or inhibit the distal circulation.

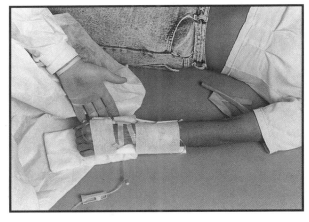

50. Once the IV is secured, check that it is still properly flowing and there are no signs of infiltration. Then adjust the flow of the IV to the specific drip rate desired. When the IV is solely an IV solution, running it at a fast rate while taping provides a clear demonstration of its patency and the absence of any infiltration. In the rare case that the IV solution in a primary IV line contains a drug, it should only be run at the prescribed rate and therefore must be adjusted immediately after the catheter hub has been secured and before completing the taping of the line to the extremity.

Adjusting The IV Infusion Rate

Before an IV has been started, the rate of infusion must be determined. "KVO" ("Keep Vein Open") or "TKO" ("To Keep Open"), are common terms used to describe a minimal flow of fluid into a vein to prevent the venous blood in the IV catheter from clotting. "To Keep Open" flow rates are usually around eight to fifteen drops per minute (8–15 gtts/min) as counted in the drip chamber. By contrast, "wide open" means just that—there is no restriction of fluid flow from the IV bag to the patient.

Even when an IV is set to run "wide open," fluid movement from the IV bag into the vein is determined by seven factors:

1. The size of the vein. The amount of blood flowing through a vein is relative to its size, and venous blood flow past the tip of the catheter creates a venturi effect that pulls IV fluid into the blood vessel.

2. The size and length of the catheter. A large-bore short-length catheter creates less resistance to fluid flow, so the fluid flows faster.

3. The size of the drops produced by the drip chamber (gtt/ml) ("mini-drip" versus a "macro-drip").

4. The diameter and length of the tubing in the administration set. The longer the tubing the slower the flow.

5. Gravity, in relation to the height of the IV bag above the patient. The higher the bag, the greater the affect of gravity and the faster the flow.

6. External pressure applied to the IV bag, such as a pressure infuser or blood pressure cuff, or simply squeezing the bag with your hands.

7. The adjustment of the IV tubing flow clamp.

If you want to administer a lot of fluid to a patient, you should use a large-bore short-length catheter (14 or 16 gauge, 1" or 1 1/4" long), large diameter short-length "maxi-drip" tubing set with a low gtt/ml number (10, 15, etc.), a pressure infuser to squeeze the fluid out of the IV bag, and an IV pole that will hold the bag high above the patient.

Except when running TKO or "wide open," the order for IV infusion will be for a specific number of milliliters per minute (ml/min), or for a given amount of IV solution to be run over a given period of time. To determine the drip rate (gtt/min) at which the specific administration set used must be set in order to provide the fluid volume per minute ordered, one or more calculations are necessary. These have been fully discussed and demonstrated in the Introduction to this Section. To determine the drip rate at which the IV should be run, the reader should refer to that earlier information.

Once the number of drops per minute (gtt/min) that is needed to provide the ordered rate of infusion has been calculated, the infusion rate should be set in the following manner.

In the hospital, most IV lines are run through an electronic fluid infuser which, when the line into it is fully opened, automatically maintains the exact flow rate to which it is set. In the field, however, the infusion flow rate is regulated with the flow rate clamp which surrounds the IV tubing at one point along its length. Two different clamps are provided on the IV tubing of most administration sets. One is a piece of flat plastic with a narrowing notch through its center that is used to simply open or stop the flow of fluid through the line. When it is fully pushed onto the line it squeezes the sides of the tubing together and clamps off the flow past that point. The second clamp (which is generally box-like in shape) contains an adjustment knob which, when it is turned, squeezes progressively onto the tube to reduce the diameter of its lumen and therefore regulates the amount of fluid which can pass through it.

The amount of fluid which enters the vein is equal to the amount which drops into the drip chamber, therefore the drops per minute that enter the chamber are used as the index by which the flow rate clamp is set. To set the drip rate of the IV, hold the flow rate clamp in your hand so that a thumb or finger is placed upon the turnable part which adjusts the flow rate. Hold the clamp with the hand of the arm on which you *DO NOT* wear your watch. Hold your other hand up so that your watch is clearly visible next to the drip chamber. you can also remove your watch and hold it up next to the chamber.

Using the second hand on the watch, you are now ready to count the number of drops per minute that are set as you vary the adjustment of the flow rate clamp. To provide a timeframe that is more practical than counting for a whole minute, divide the desired gtt/min by four and count the number of drops that occur for a 15 second period. For example, if a rate of 100 drops per minute is desired, the flow rate should be adjusted so that 25 drops fall into the drip chamber during a 15 second period.

Initially, open the clamp all the way and then slowly close it in progressive increments until the correct number of drops (one-fourth the desired gtt/min) is counted in a fifteen second period. Once it has been properly set, count the drip rate for an additional 15 second period (or, preferably, for a full minute) to confirm that the desired gtt/min rate has indeed been set.

Once you have adjusted the IV flow clamp to deliver the ordered amount of fluid, it is your responsibility to continuously recheck that the IV is flowing properly. There are a variety of reasons why an IV flow may become compromised, including positional IV catheters, movement of the catheterized extremity by the patient, pinched or squashed tubing by the patient's movement or by being accidentally laid upon by the patient. There is nothing more frustrating than to have an IV line become closed off by a clot because the tubing became kinked and the flow was insufficient to keep the line open. By the same token, the pulmonary edema patient does not need a runaway IV line that adds another 500ml of fluid to his already overloaded circulatory system. Monitor the IV closely!

When supplying fluid to a patient over an extended period of time, *time taping* the IV bag is a further useful adjunct to ensuring that the flow is maintained at the correct drip rate.

Time Taping an IV Bag

To produce a *time tape* on an IV bag, a piece of 1/2 inch fabric adhesive tape is secured down the side of the IV bag next to the ml markings printed on the front of the bag. Care must be taken when affixing the tape to not cover the ml graduations, the name of the IV solution, the expiration date, or any medication label that you have added.

Write the ordered rate at the top of the tape (e.g.: 250 ml/hr). Note that when the IV is initially hung the fluid is at the "0" ml mar on the bag. Customarily, IV bags are marked by the manufacturer from 0ml when first hung and full, to the total amount of fluid they contain (e.g.: 1,000 ml) at their bottom, so that the graduations marked on the bag indicate the amount of fluid that has been given and *NOT the amount remaining*. Always check that the particular bag being used is marked in this manner.

Write the time that the IV was started next to the 0 ml mark (e.g.: 0900 hours). Then determine or calculate from the ml/min ordered how many mls of IV solution should be run out each hour and half hour (or if a shorter time is desired, each 15 minutes) when the IV is run at the correct rate from the time it was started. At each appropriate ml marker, place a line across the tape and write the time at which it should be reached (e.g.: 0915, 0930, 0945, 1000, etc.)

From this guide, the maintenance of the desired rate can be confirmed at a glance at any time by comparing the present time with the times and amounts marked on the tape. There are a variety of different ways in which a time tape can be graduated and marked, however regardless of which is used the general principle remains the same. With any time tape, the number of mls of fluid that should have been infused at a series of determined times (if the IV continues to flow at the desired rate) is calculated and marked with a line and the time at which the fluid should be at that ml level on the tape.

If an IV bag has been time-taped and the ordered/desired rate is later changed, the tape should immediately be removed from the IV bag to avoid possible confusion as it no longer displays the correct information.

ALS

CHANGING THE SOLUTION BAG OF AN ESTABLISHED IV LINE

At times, either because the bag that was previously hung is almost empty or because a different solution is ordered/desired, you will need to change the IV bag on an established IV line while it is running. By periodically checking an established IV you can anticipate the need to change the bag before it completely empties and the patency of the line is lost.

1. When you notice that the IV bag is about 3/4 empty, select another bag of the same solution and size as that initially ordered and hung. If your orders include a limit on the amount of fluid to be given, and it will be reached at the end of the presently hung bag, or if you are not sure how to proceed, obtain on-line medical direction now so that enough time exists to handle the situation before the fluid is totally expended and the IV's patency is jeopardized. Open the replacement IV solution package and remove the IV bag. As previously described, check the name of the solution, the expiration date, and the clarity of the contents.

2. When the IV bag is almost empty, shut off the flow clamp to prevent air entry into the IV tubing. Without delay, remove the IV bag from the IV pole or hanger on which it is elevated, and turn the empty IV bag upside down so that when you pull out the tubing spike the fluid remaining in the bag will not run out. Next, pull the spike out of the empty IV bag port. Be sure to keep the spike from touching anything in order to maintain its sterility.

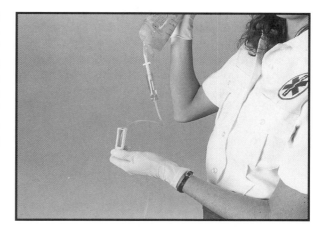

3. Pick up the new IV bag and remove the tail port cover. Spike the new bag using a twisting motion until the port has been punctured. You may need to add a little fluid to the drip chamber by squeezing and releasing it until it is half full of fluid.

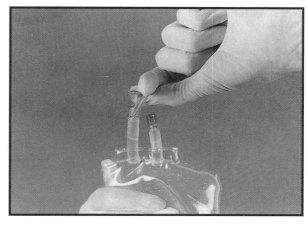

4. Place the replacement bag that is now connected to the IV line on an IV pole or hanger. Once the bag is hung, open the IV line shut-off clamp and re-adjust the flow clamp as needed to obtain the desired drip rate. After a few minutes, recount the drops per minute against your watch to confirm that the desired rate is being continued.

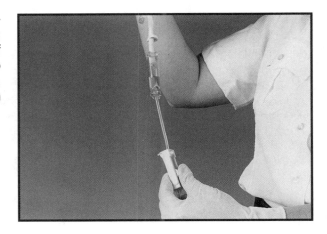

Removing Air From The IV Tubing

The introduction of a significant amount of air into the IV tubing can generally be avoided by monitoring the amount of solution remaining in the bag and replacing it in a timely manner as described above. Occasionally, you may not notice that the bag is empty until the drip chamber is empty and air has entered a significant portion of the upper end of the tubing. Should this occur, immediately shut off the line with the flow clamp or the slide clamp, and without delay replace the empty bag with a full one as just described. After the new bag has been spiked and the IV re-hung, a column of air will generally remain in the tubing. This must be removed before the flow of fluid into the patient is resumed. This can be easily achieved without the need to change the administration set. To purge air from the IV tubing in such cases:

1. Check that the tubing is clamped shut, and gather the necessary supplies. You will need an alcohol swab, a standard IM needle and optionally a syringe. Locate the injection port on the IV line that is below the level of the air in the line and clean this port with the alcohol swab.

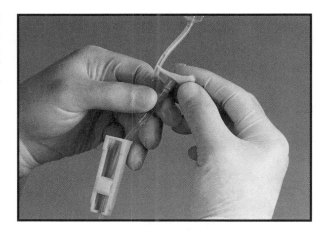

2. Insert the needle into the port. Prior to insertion you can attach a syringe to the needle to provide a better hold on the needle while it is inserted through the cap of the insertion port, but it is not necessary to this procedure.

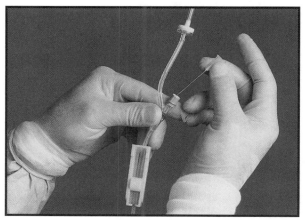

3. With the needle in the port, fold over the IV tubing to completely pinch it off below the port with the needle in it (between the port and the patient).

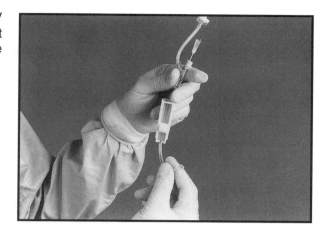

4. Fill the drip chamber half full of IV fluid by squeezing and releasing the drip chamber. By filling the chamber first you prevent small air bubbles from entering the tubing as it fills.

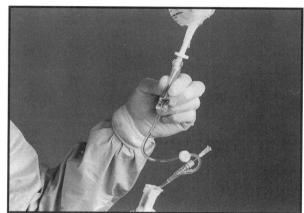

5. With the IV tubing pinched off between the injection port and the patient, and the open needle in the IV tubing, open the shut-off or flow clamp until a flow of fluid is demonstrated by fluid dripping into the drip chamber. As the IV fluid enters the tubing from the drip chamber, the air will be forced out of the tubing through the needle inserted in the injection port. If you have a syringe attached to the needle you can aspirate the air out of the line faster by drawing back on the plunger.

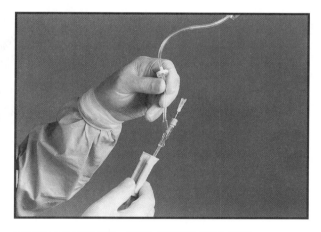

6. Once the air is completely evacuated from the IV tubing, remove the needle from the port, release the IV tubing, and then re-adjust the IV drip to the desired rate. Be sure to immediately discard the needle into a sharps container. Should the column of air extend beyond the level of all the injection ports, the needle will have to be inserted carefully through the wall of the tubing at a level where it will enter the fluid remaining in the line. Once the air has been purged and the needle removed, a piece of tape should be wrapped around the tubing where it was pierced to prevent any leakage. Note: the injection port on the catheter hub cannot be used to purge air from the tubing, as there is no tubing to pinch shut beyond that point.

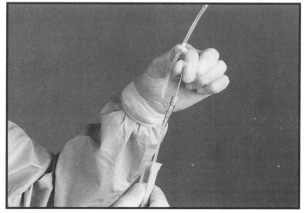

ALS

GIVING A MEDICATION BOLUS THROUGH AN ESTABLISHED IV LINE

Intravenous bolus medications are commonly given by "IV push" through an established IV line. Depending upon the medication, some are given rapidly (as fast as you can push the plunger on the syringe, such as adenosine or epinephrine), while others are given more slowly either due to the effects of the drug or its thick viscous consistency (such as $D_{50}W$). Knowing how fast a particular medication should be administered is an important part of the knowledge necessary to its correct administration.

To administer an IV medication bolus, first identify the drug to be used, the desired concentration, and the dose to be administered, and confirm that there are no contraindications to using this drug with this patient. Then check that the supply is correct and that the expiration date has not been reached. Draw up the desired amount of medication in a syringe using the calculations and methods described earlier in this Section. Although the following example will involve using a syringe with a needle, many IV administration sets now include "needle-less" access ports for IV bolus and piggy-back administrations that use Luer-lock connections rather than needles. Regardless, the key steps are essentially the same whichever type of access is being used.

1. With the IV line established and running, and with the correct medication and quantity drawn up, cleanse the IV tubing's medication access port that is closest to the actual IV infusion site with an alcohol prep swab.

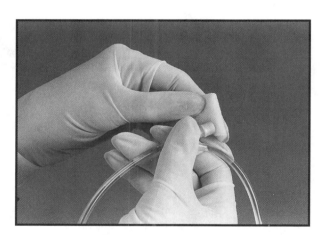

2. With the port cleansed, carefully insert the needle of the syringe containing the prescribed dose of the medication into the rubber cap covering the access port.

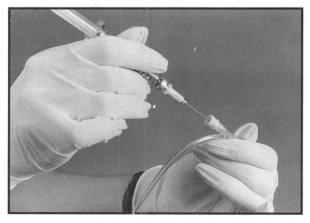

3.   Next, bend back the IV tubing *above* the access port to pinch it closed and stop the flow of IV fluid. This prevents the medication bolus from travelling in the wrong direction when it is injected into the line and possibly entering the IV bag.

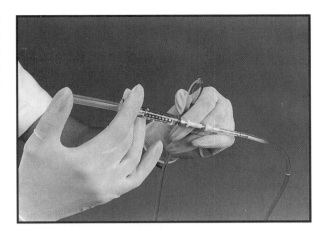

4.   While continuing to hold the IV line pinched shut, push the plunger on the syringe and inject the medication through the access port and into the IV line. Even though you are injecting it into the IV line and not the patient directly, administer the medication at the rate suggested for that drug.

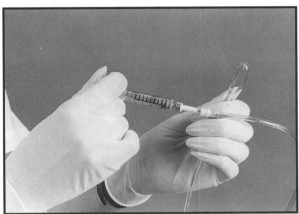

5.   As soon as all of the medication has passed from the syringe, release the IV tubing and allow the fluid to flow again. Open the IV flow clamp so that fluid is running at a "wide open" rate for at least 50ml, to thoroughly flush the added medication into the patient.

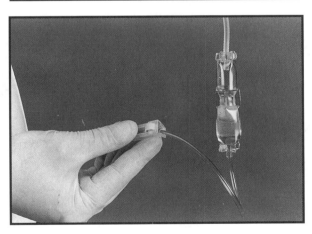

6.   Holding the barrel of the syringe, withdraw it to remove the needle from the rubber stopper in the medication access port, and discard the syringe and needle in an appropriate sharps container. Monitor the patient for signs of improvement or adverse reaction. Adjust the IV flow clamp to the previous drip rate, and document the drug given, concentration, dose, route, time, etc.

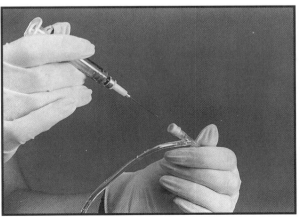

ALS

GIVING A MEDICATION BY IV PIGGYBACK DRIP

Piggyback drug infusions are used to administer medication to a patient over a longer period of time and frequently at a lower concentration than is done with an IV bolus. Many times a drug bolus is given to quickly *load* the desired therapeutic level of the drug into the bloodstream. Then, a piggyback drip mixture of the same drug is used to *maintain the therapeutic level*, and can be increased or decreased as needed by changing the drip rate.

A piggyback drug is just that—a separate IV bag containing NS, D₅W, or sterile water into which the medication has been dissolved. This second bag is then "piggybacked" onto an existing IV line. Medication should never be added to the primary IV bag, for if there is a sudden need to stop the drug your only option is to discontinue your entire IV access route.

1. To hang an IV piggyback medication drip, a primary IV line must already be established and running. The amount of the drug to be added to the secondary piggyback bag should be known or calculated. Confirm that it is the ordered IV solution and quantity, and inspect the IV bag and its contents for color, clarity, and expiration date.

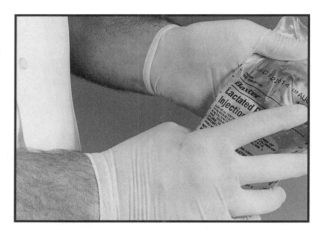

2. If the IV piggyback drug comes premixed in an IV bag, calculate the mg/ml and the gtt/min that will need to be run to provide the ordered mg/min as described in the Introduction. If the piggyback drug has to be mixed, check the drug supplied for name, concentration, expiration date and proper appearance. Draw up the appropriate amount of drug to be added to the piggyback bag. Double check that you have the right drug and correct amount in the syringe.

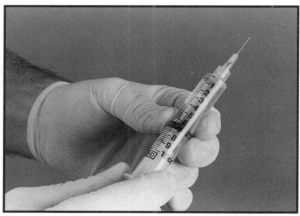

3. Cleanse the medication port on the piggyback IV bag with an alcohol prep swab, then carefully insert the needle of the syringe into the medication port—making sure that you do not accidentally poke through the IV bag and into your hand. Depress the plunger on the syringe to inject the drug into the piggyback IV bag.

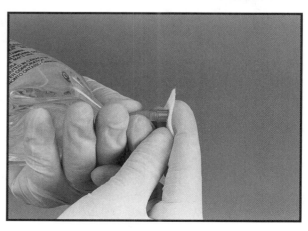

4. When all of the drug has been injected into the secondary bag, withdraw the needle and syringe and discard them immediately in a sharps container. Thoroughly mix the drug and IV fluid in the bag by manipulating it to assure a uniform dispersion of the drug throughout the IV solution.

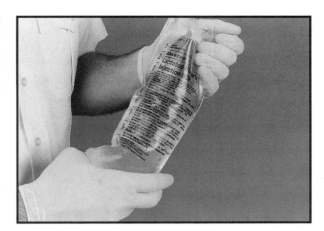

5. Spike the secondary IV bag with an appropriate IV tubing set. Most piggyback drugs are administered through a mini-drip (60 gtt/ml) set. Fill the drip chamber and flush the IV line to purge any air bubbles.

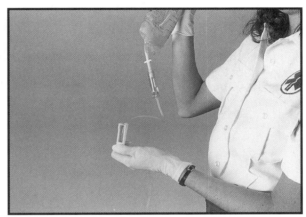

6. Depending upon the type of primary and secondary IV tubing you are using, you may have to attach a needle to the piggyback line so that it can be connected to the primary line. Alternately, the sets you are using may employ needleless connectors. When a needle is required a 21-gauge hypodermic needle is usually used, and should be connected to the hub of the IV line at this time.

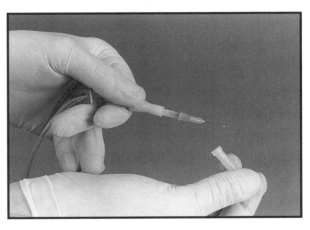

7. With the secondary bag and IV tubing ready, select a medication access port on the primary IV tubing and cleanse it with an alcohol prep swab. Insert the needle of the secondary IV line into the access port on the primary line, and tape the primary and secondary lines together for stability. If you are using a needleless set, fasten the connectors together to secure them.

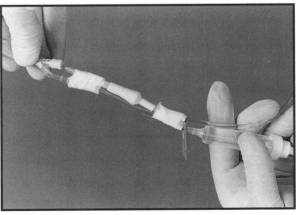

8. Open the flow control clamp on the piggy-back IV tubing and observe the flow in the drip chamber to assure that the line is patent. Adjust the piggyback's flow control clamp to the gtt/min rate required.

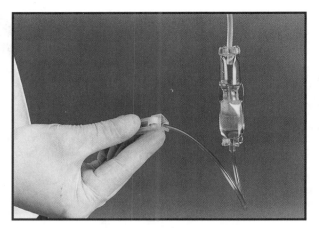

9. With the piggyback line running, close the flow control clamp on the primary IV line. This insures that the only fluid passing on to the patient is that coming from the piggyback medication bag. Once the primary line has been shut off, recheck the gtt/min rate of the piggyback line and adjust it as needed.

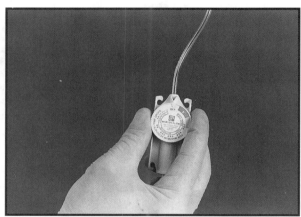

10. Prepare a medication label and attach it to the piggyback bag. The label should indicate what drug is being given, the amount being administered, the concentration in the bag, the patient's name, the date and time that the piggyback was started, and your name or initials. Continue to monitor the patient, and document all of the above information in your run report as well as the patient's subsequent reaction to the medication.

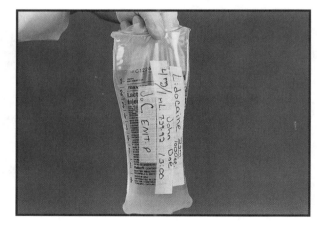

STARTING AN IV USING A BUTTERFLY NEEDLE (Infant Scalp Vein Cannulation)

Butterfly needles are used to establish intravenous access in very small veins, such as in elderly and infant patients. Butterfly needles are made of hollow steel. They do *NOT* have a plastic catheter which is threaded into and remains in the vein when the needle is removed—in the case of a butterfly needle, the steel needle remains in place. Because of this, the vein used must be straight for about an inch proximal of the venipuncture site. Butterfly needles are only 1/2 or 3/8 inches long. Although they can be inserted in any vein, the most common pre-hospital usage for a butterfly needle is in an infant scalp vein, as demonstrated here with an infant head mannikin.

1. Butterfly needles are rigid hollow steel needles which, once placed in a vein, remain there until the IV is discontinued. The name "butterfly" comes from the two plastic "wings" or side flaps which are bonded to the hub of the needle and onto which the EMT holds when inserting the needle. These are also used to stabilize the needle in place once the vein has been cannulated. Butterfly needles also feature an attached flexible extension tube to which the regular IV tubing can be connected without directly contacting or moving the butterfly needle.

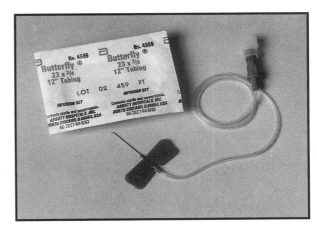

2. Prior to applying the tourniquet, all of the needed equipment and supplies must be assembled and prepared. If a volume regulation chamber is being used it should be prepared and filled, and all of the standard IV accessories should be available as well as a 3cc syringe.

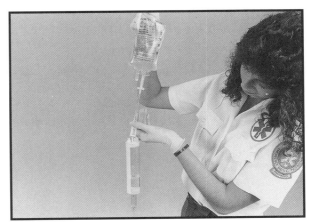

3. Scalp veins are usually the easiest to find on small infants and neonates. Hand and foot veins can be difficult at best to locate because of all the "baby fat" on infant extremities. To promote distention of the scalp veins and make them easier to cannulate, place a large rubber band around the infant's head. As soon as the equipment is prepared the rubber band can be placed around the infant's scalp. The band needs to be tight enough to impede venous blood flow without being so tight that the skin is injured. With the rubber band in place, select the vein to be used and clean the site with a Betadine or alcohol prep swab.

4. Select the appropriate size butterfly needle, open the package and remove it. Connect the butterfly's flexible extension tubing to the IV tubing and charge the tubing with IV fluid to purge all of the air. Lay the IV bag at the same level as the child's head to avoid any fluid flow due to gravity. (Alternately, fill a 3cc syringe with fluid taken from the IV bag. Empty the syringe into the butterfly's tubing and needle so that they will be full of fluid.) Grasp the butterfly needle by the two wings and remove the plastic cover from the needle.

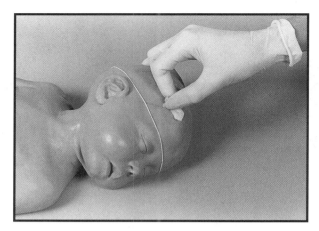

5. When cannulating a scalp vein the needle should be held with its tip pointing in a caudad direction directly over the vein. Enter the vein with the bevel up and the needle held at a 15 degree angle.

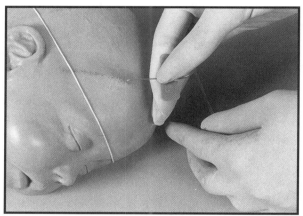

6. Once you are in the vein, lower the hub of the needle and insert it slightly further into the vein. Then, lower the IV bag (or gently aspirate with the syringe) to see if you get a blood return into the butterfly's extension tubing. Be sure that you hold onto the IV needle securely until you have it taped down. Carefully check that the IV is patent and that there is no infiltration around the IV site.

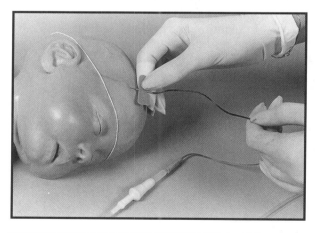

7. With the IV in place, gently pull out on a piece of the rubber band and then cut off the rubber band with a pair of scissors.

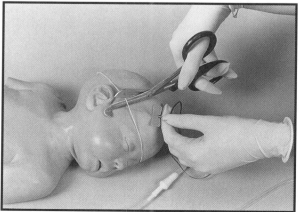

8. Open the flow clamp on the IV tubing or Volutrol chamber, whichever is being used, and reassess the patency of the IV.

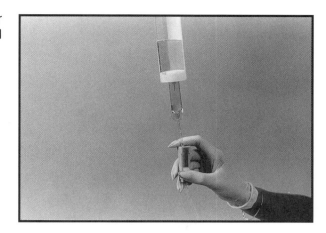

9. Tape the butterfly and tubing to the infant's scalp, making sure to not tape over the venipuncture site itself. Once the needle and tubing have been secured, adjust the drip flow clamp to the desired rate.

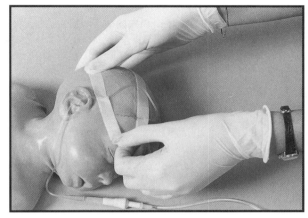

ALS

CANNULATION OF AN EXTERNAL JUGULAR VEIN

The external jugular vein of the neck is often forgotten by EMS personnel as a "peripheral" IV site. Because it is such a large vein, it can be easily cannulated when other peripheral veins have collapsed. Although it can be accessible when the head is in a neutral in-line position, the vein is most easily cannulated when the patient's head is turned to the side. In the trauma patient, in-line cervical spine control must be maintained and a cervical collar is usually placed on the patient—making the external jugular more difficult to access. For this reason, the external jugular is utilized most often in the non-trauma patient such as the patient in cardiopulmonary arrest where cervical spine control is not a concern.

1. The external jugular veins are located on each side of the neck. They start between the earlobe and the angle of the mandible, travelling downward toward the mid-clavicular line before passing beneath the clavicle and out of sight as they enter the subclavian vein.

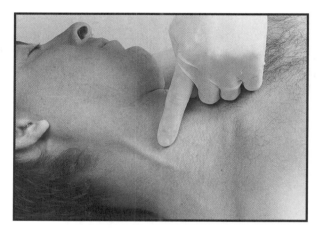

2. Prior to starting an external jugular IV, you must prepare all of the necessary equipment just as with any other IV. There is no special equipment needed to start an external jugular IV—the usual IV fluid, tubing, tape, antiseptic swab, sharps container and IV catheters are used. Over-the-needle catheters between 14 and 18 gauge in size are most often used.

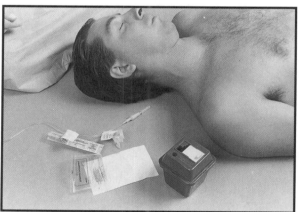

3. Carefully clean the area of the puncture site with an alcohol or Betadine prep swab. Note that the patient's head is turned away from the vein being used so as to provide the best angle from which to approach the vein.

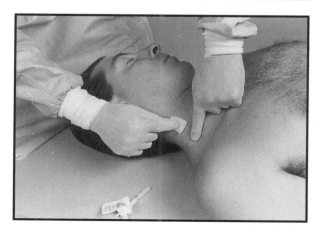

4. Because a tourniquet is obviously not to be used, promote venous distention by occluding the vein near the clavicle with one hand. Hold the IV needle in the other hand with the bevel of the needle facing up and the tip facing caudally. Enter the skin and vein directly from the top, with the needle catheter held at a 35–45 degree angle. Depending upon the size of the patient's neck, your hand which is holding the catheter will usually have to slide across the side of the patient's face and jaw as you advance into the vein.

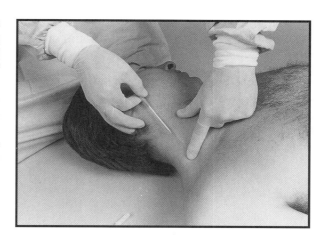

5. Once you have obtained a flashback and are sure you have entered the vein, advance the needle and catheter slightly to insure that the catheter is placed inside the lumen of the vein. Lower the angle of insertion of the catheter until it is more parallel to the vein. At this point you can release your finger that has been occluding the vein.

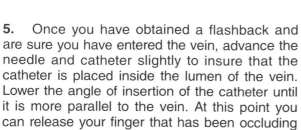

6. Advance the catheter into the vein up to the catheter hub by sliding the catheter off the needle. Place your finger on the vein just caudad of the area where the catheter tip lies under the skin, and press down to occlude the vein beyond the point of the catheter tip. Because the external jugular vein is so large, any blood flow past the tip of the catheter before the IV tubing is connected will draw air into the vein and can create an air embolism.

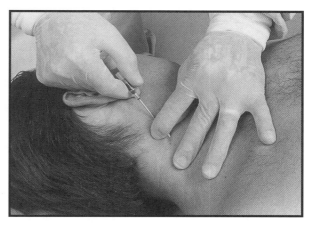

7. Once the catheter is occluded, the needle can be removed and placed into the sharps container. The IV tubing should then be connected to the IV catheter hub and digital pressure over the vein released.

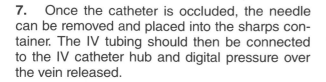

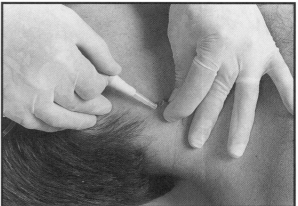

8. While holding onto the IV tubing, release the flow clamp. Before taping the catheter and tubing into place, carefully inspect the puncture site for any signs of infiltration.

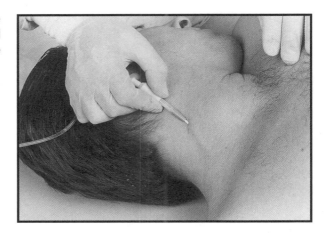

9. Now carefully secure the catheter in place using tape or an Opsite-type dressing. Securely tape the tubing to the patient's neck and face so that the IV cannot be accidentally pulled out. Once the IV has been taped, adjust the drip flow to the desired rate and re-evaluate the patient.

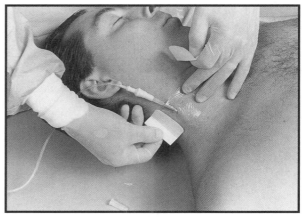

ALS

USING AN IV VOLUME REGULATION CHAMBER (Volutrol®, etc.)

In some patients the need for rapid fluid volume replacement must be balanced by the possibility of causing fluid overload and/or pulmonary edema due to their age or overall medical condition. In such cases it becomes very important to not only rapidly infuse the fluid but to also precisely measure and control the amount of fluid being administered. A fluid volume regulation chamber can hold up to 250ml of IV solution, which can be administered at the desired rate and then the patient reevaluated as to the need for additional fluid or other therapy. A fluid volume regulation chamber is an IV administration set which contains an additional flow valve and a graduated cylinder in the IV line before the drip chamber. This allows the EMT to run the desired quantity of fluid into the chamber, and then to close the line between the IV bag and the chamber. In this way, only the pre-measured amount of fluid that has been run into the chamber can be infused into the patient.

1. Select the appropriate type of fluid to be administered, and "spike" the IV bag using the volume control chamber in the same way that you would for a regular IV administration set.

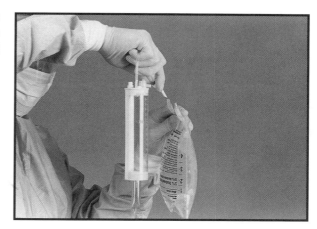

2. Once the bag and drip set are connected and hung, close the flow clamp *at the bottom* of the volume control chamber.

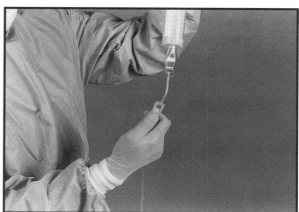

3. Open the flow clamp *above the chamber* which regulates the flow from the IV bag into the volume chamber. Fill the chamber with the appropriate desired ml volume of the IV solution. Then close the clamp to stop any further flow of fluid from the IV bag at this time.

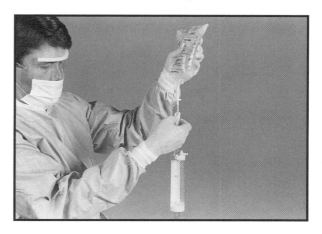

4. Open the flow clamp at the bottom of the chamber and fill the drip chamber and tubing with fluid in the customary manner.

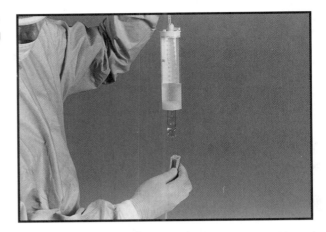

5. Once the drip chamber and tubing are properly filled, cannulate the vein, connect the IV tubing, tape the IV and, using the flow regulation clamp below the volume chamber, set the drip at the desired rate. Carefully monitor the amount of fluid remaining in the chamber at all times.

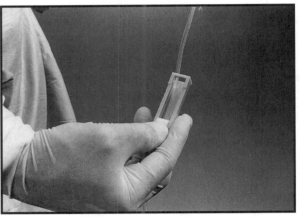

6. When the volume regulation chamber is almost empty, re-assess the patient's condition and lung fields to determine whether to repeat the infusion of a pre-measured fluid volume or whether the IV should only be continued at a TKO rate. If a pre-measured volume is to be used, repeat the procedure outlined above to refill the chamber with the desired amount of fluid. IF the flow is to be maintained at a TKO rate, open the flow clamp above the chamber so that IV fluid from the bag can flow through the chamber and to the drip rate regulation clamp below the chamber.

ALS

USING AN IV PRESSURE INFUSER

IV pressure infusers are used to force fluid out of the IV bag to infuse fluid volume into a patient's circulatory system more rapidly than would be possible using only gravity and the customary drip method. Commercial IV pressure infusers are designed to cover a one Liter or smaller IV bag. A commercial infuser is shown below, but a blood pressure cuff wrapped around an IV bag will work just as well. When using a BP cuff, you have to continuously inflate the cuff as the bag of fluid empties so that the cuff maintains its pressure upon and does not slip off the IV bag. An extra pair of hands squeezing the IV bag will also work well as a pressure infuser.

1. A commercial IV pressure infuser consists of a nylon bag with an inflatable bladder sewn into it. The bladder is inflated with a rubber bulb pump similar to that on a blood pressure cuff. There is a thumb-screw as well to maintain the pressure in the bladder. Most commercial IV pressure infusers are equipped with a high pressure release valve to prevent overinflation of the bladder.

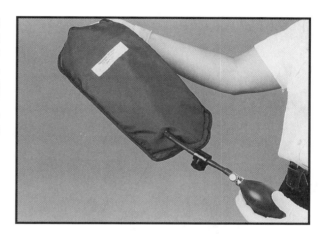

2. When using the commercial IV pressure infuser, slide the IV bag into the cover until it is completely inside the infuser. With the IV started and running wide open into the vein, begin inflating the bladder with the bulb pump until the drip chamber fills up and you get a good stream of fluid running through the tubing. Monitor the IV site to insure that the vein is handling the volume of fluid being forced through it. When an infuser is being used the IV bag does not have to be hung or carried above the patient, since the flow is not dependent upon gravity as long as the inflation pressure in the pressure infuser is maintained.

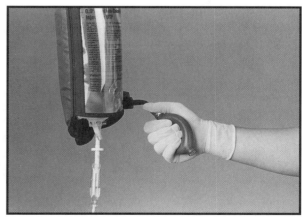

ALS

DISCONTINUING AN IV

Established primary IV lines are rarely discontinued in the pre-hospital setting. If the maximum fluid volume ordered is infused prior to arrival at the hospital, the IV is generally continued at a KVO rate to maintain the IV access. In some cases, however, the EMT will be ordered to D/C a line in the field or when assisting in the ER. Should an established IV become occluded or infiltrate, the same general steps are followed except that the IV bag and administration set are connected to the hub of another cannula inserted at a different site, instead of being discarded. To D/C an IV:

1. Begin by shutting the flow clamp on the IV tubing.

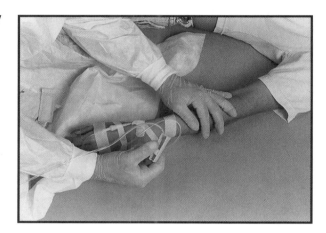

2. Next, assemble the necessary equipment. A sterile 2x2 gauze pad, bandaid, and antibacterial ointment will be needed.

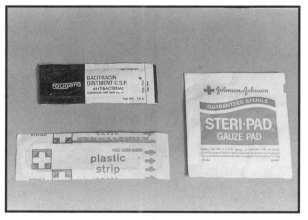

3. Next gently remove the tape from the IV tubing. Pull on the tape in a downward direction if it is stuck to the patient's hair or skin. Be sure to hold the hub of the catheter when doing this to ensure that it is *NOT* prematurely pulled from the vein.

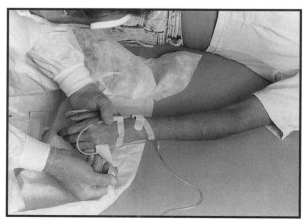

MEDICATION AND IV SKILLS **615**

4. Carefully undo the tape or Opsite dressing that covers the venipuncture site.

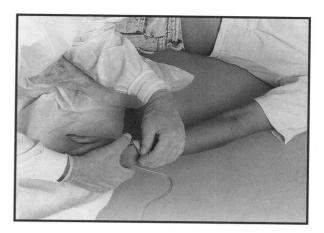

5. Gently grasp the IV catheter hub with one gloved hand and lightly lay a folded sterile 2x2 gauze pad over the venipuncture site. Withdraw the IV catheter straight back out of the vein and then apply mild digital pressure over the site with the gauze pad.

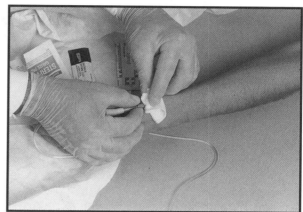

6. Inspect the IV site for any signs of infection. If there is any redness or swelling, note this on your run report and include it in your verbal report when you transfer care of the patient at the hospital. Also inspect the end of the IV catheter for missing pieces or signs of damage. If the tip is damaged, contact medical control immediately.

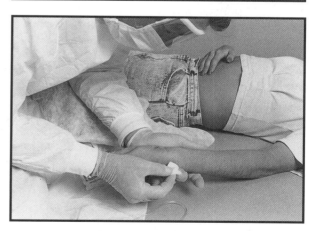

7. Once the site has been inspected, place a dab of anti-bacterial ointment on the bandaid pad and use it to cover the former IV puncture site. Properly dispose of the IV catheter, tubing and remaining IV fluid.

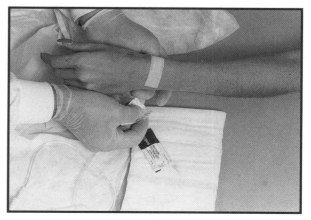

ALS

ADMINISTERING A MEDICATION THROUGH AN ET TUBE

Certain emergency medications can be administered through a properly placed endotracheal tube when IV access has not yet been obtained. This is most often performed in the setting of cardiopulmonary arrest. The cardiac medications that can be administered in this manner are lidocaine, epinephrine and atropine. A fourth prehospital medication that can also be given by this route is narcan (naloxone). Together, these four drugs can be recalled by the mnemonic "LEAN."

Originally, drugs given through an endotracheal tube had to be administered by syringe between ventilations. That is, ventilation had to be stopped, the bag-valve-mask or demand valve had to be removed from the end of the ET tube, the medication injected into the ET tube, and then the ventilation device re-attached and ventilations resumed. While effective, this requires an interuption in ventilations and also causes the medication to be added at quite some distance from the actual tracheal tissues.

More recently, two new devices have improved the way in which medications can be administered through an ET tube without interrupting the ventilations. One is a specially modified endotracheal tube which incorporates a medication access port at the proximal end of the tube, resembling the traditional one-way valve used for filling the tube's distal cuff. This port connects to a catheter which is built into the wall of the ET tube and extends to the tube's distal tip. Using this device, fluid medications injected into the medication port are transmitted directly to the patient end of the ET tube and, as they emerge from the special medication tube, are immediately nebulized and carried on to the trachea and bronchi.

The second device involves a collar which fits over the top of any endotracheal tube, and has an attached catheter which is fed down the inside of the ET tube. With the collar in place between the top of the ET tube and the BVM or demand valve, ventilations can proceed while medications are administered through a medication access port and down the catheter. With both of these devices, ventilations can be continued uninterrupted while the drugs are supplied to the patient. With any method of providing these medications down an ET tube, a significant amount of the drug adheres to the ET tube or catheter walls and is either not delivered to the patient or is so slowly delivered with subsequent ventilations as to not be a part of the initial loading dose. To compensate for this, when these drugs are administered transtracheally, many protocols recommend that 2 to 2.5 times the normal IV dose be administered and it be diluted with an additional 10ml of NS or sterile water to facilitate its transport into the tracheobronchial tree.

The reader is cautioned that this practice is highly dependent upon the particular drug being used, as some could involve considerable and dangerous fluid volumes if the recommendation is followed blindly. A more detailed discussion is found in the discussion of medication doses in this Section's Introduction. To administer a drug through an ET tube:

1. With CPR in progress and the patient being ventilated with a bag-valve-mask attached to the endotracheal tube, select the appropriate medication to be given. Perform the checks described in the Introduction to verify its identity, concentration, etc. Draw up the medication as ordered for administration down an endotracheal tube (generally double the normal intravenous dose), and add 10ml of sterile water or normal saline to the syringe.

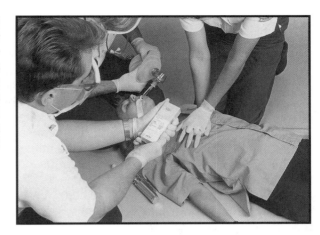

2. If the medication must be injected directly into the proximal end of the ET tube, direct the EMT who is operating the BVM to hyperventilate the patient for approximately 30 seconds with CPR still being applied.

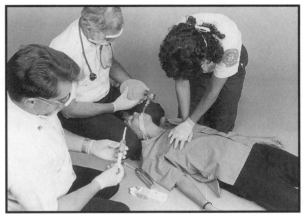

3. Stop CPR and remove the BVM from the ET tube. Insert the needle into the end of the tube and squirt the contents of the syringe into the tube quickly. As soon as the syringe is empty, direct the ventilator to re-attach the BVM and re-institute ventilations and to again hyperventilate the patient for approximately 30 seconds. *DO NOT* resume chest compressions immediately, however, as the increased thoracic pressure will cause the medication to blow back up the tube.

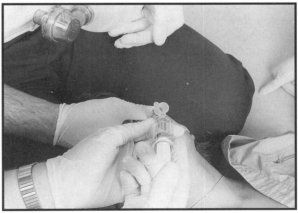

4. If an endotracheal tube with a medication port has been placed, or if the special "collar-catheter" device is available, insert the needle into the medication port and inject the medication by this route. Ventilations should be paused while the injection is made, and then hyperventilation should be instituted for about 30 seconds after the administration to help speed the distribution of the drug.

5. Resume chest compressions following the brief period of hyperventilation. Discard the syringe and needle in an appropriate sharps container, and document the medication administration and its effects in the customary manner.

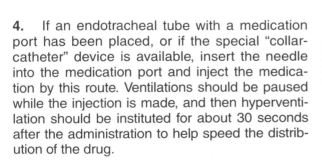

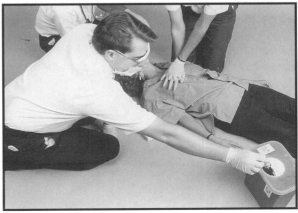

ALS

ESTABLISHING AN INTRAOSSEOUS INFUSION ("IO" Line)

Intraosseous ("in the bone") infusion is another method of obtaining access to a patient's circulatory system. The inner core of certain bones can be accessed with the use of a special intraosseous needle to which standard IV tubing can be attached. Fluid volume replacement, medications, and blood can be administered through an intraosseous infusion. Large longbones such as the tibia, humerus and femur can be used, as well as the medial malleolus (ankle bone).

Intraosseous infusions are most often used with pediatric patients when conventional peripheral IV access has not been successful, and in a growing number of EMS systems it is the preferred route to use in unconscious seriously ill children. Although the "IO" technique can also be used on adults, it is usually a much lower priority choice due to the ease of access with other IV methods. In pediatric patients the proximal tibia is the preferred site due to its availability and ease of access, and because of its shape and prominent landmarks. Most IO protocols require that the patient be unconscious before an IO insertion is attempted. To establish an IO line:

1. An IO needle is somewhat of an awkward-looking device. The needle or trocar slides down the middle of the actual steel catheter which remains in the bone. There is usually a hand or palm plate at the top of the trocar to make penetration of the bone easier. Aside from the IO needle, you will also need an alcohol prep pad, 20cc syringe filled with IV fluid, and IV extension tubing.

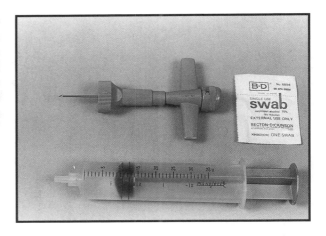

2. With the IV bag spiked and all equipment ready, find an appropriate landmark. When selecting the tibia, slide your finger caudally from the patella onto the tibia. You will feel a bump just below the kneecap, called the tibial tuberosity.

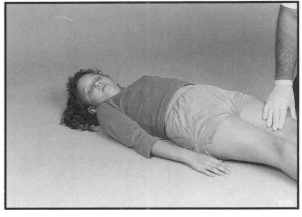

3. Using this as a landmark, measure two to three finger's-width below the tuberosity.

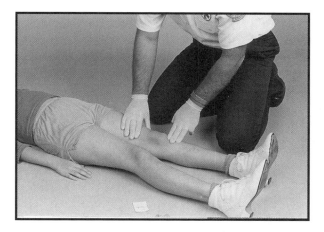

4. Slide your fingers to the medial (inside) plane of the tibia. The surface of the bone here is flat and easy to puncture with the IO needle.

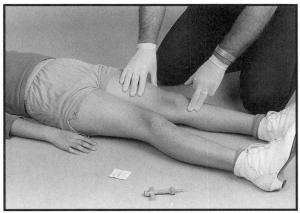

5. Because the face of the bone here is flat, there is less danger of sliding off the bone while introducing the IO needle.

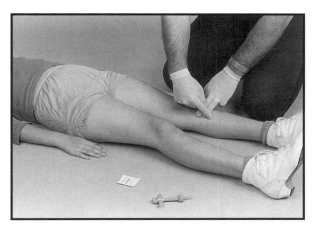

6. Cleanse the site with an alcohol or Betadine prep swab, beginning at the intended puncture site and circling outward.

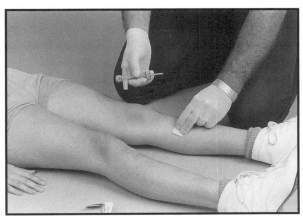

7. Hold the IO needle in one hand with the palm plate against the palm or heel of your hand.

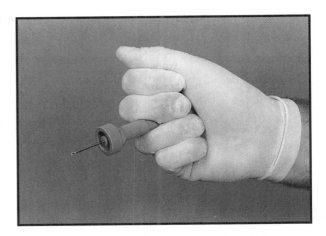

8. Stabilize the patient's lower leg by placing your free hand under the leg but not directly under the intended insertion site. A complication of this procedure is pushing too hard on the needle and having it pass completely through the bone.

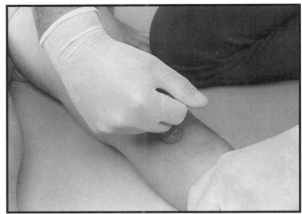

9. Place the tip of the needle over the IO site. Direct the needle at about a 90 degree angle to the surface of the tibia.

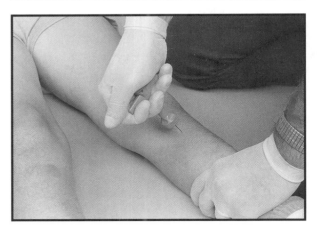

10. Push downward and, using a twisting back-and-forth motion, advance the needle into the bone. Once you enter the bone's core you will feel a "pop." As soon as this happens, stop pushing on the needle.

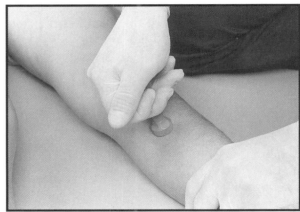

11. Remove the trocar from the catheter by unscrewing and sliding the trocar out. The IO catheter should stand up unsupported if it has been properly placed in the bone.

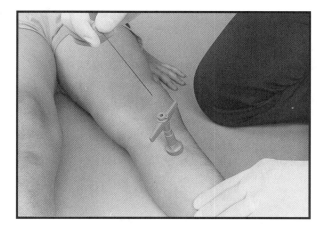

12. Attach the syringe to the extension tubing and prime the tubing with Normal Saline, then attach the extension tubing to the IO catheter and inject the fluid into the bone. Watch around the injection site for any signs of infiltration.

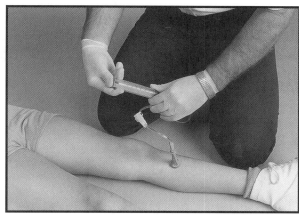

13. If there is any sign of fluid leakage or swelling at the injection site, remove the IO needle from the bone and apply firm but gentle pressure over the site. Do not attempt to re-cannulate at that same site, but select a suitable site on the other leg and attempt the same procedure again using a new needle.

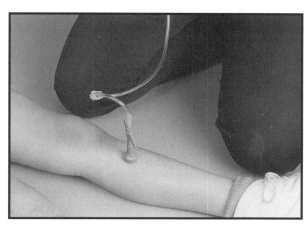

14. If no signs of infiltration appear after flushing the line and checking for patency, draw back slightly on the plunger of the syringe. You may be able to aspirate a cloudy fluid into the syringe from the marrow cavity. While this confirms proper placement of the IO needle in the bone, being *UNABLE* to aspirate marrow does not mean that the IO is incorrectly placed. A "dry tap" is not uncommon with an IO insertion. After checking for aspiration, remove the syringe and attach the IV tubing to the extension set tubing. Adjust the drip rate to the desired flow.

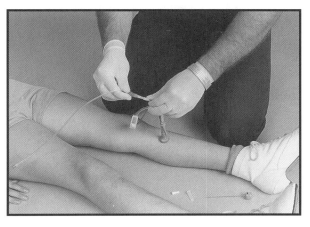

ALS

ETI SUMMARY SKILL SHEET
Establishing A Peripheral IV (Primary Line)

1. OBTAIN ORDER or refer to "Standing Orders".

2. CONFIRM FINDINGS and history PROVIDE INDICA-TION for establishing an IV line. CONFIRM THAT NO MORE URGENT PRIORITIES, REQUIRING the IV START BE DELAYED to a later time, are present. If for rapid fluid replacement, confirm that no relative contraindications to such rate are present. (If yes, establish the line, at a KVO rate and obtain on-line Medication Direction).

3. From its indicated purpose, DETERMINE AND SELECT THE FLUID AND QUANTITY, ADMINISTRATION SET, AND SEVERAL NEEDLES OR over-the-needle CATHETERS OF AN APPROPRIATE SIZE. (Note the following steps assume the use of an over-the-needle-catheter and, should a butterfly needle be used instead, must be modified accordingly).

4. OBTAIN AND OPEN AN IV START KIT AND PREPARE 3 or 4, 6 inch STRIPS OF NARROW TAPE. (If a pre-packed kit containing antiseptic wipes, antiseptic ointment, adhesive tape, a venous constrictor and a plastic film or fabric adhesive site cover is not routinely used and available, obtain and prepare the separate components that will be needed.)

5. Remove IV bag from outer package and CHECK THE NAME AND QUANTITY OF THE IV SOLUTION is that ordered.

6. CHECK THE solution's EXPIRATION DATE.

7. CHECK THE CLARITY of the IV solution and that the bag does not contain any foreign matter or leaks.

8. CHECK THE **gtt** OF THE ADMINISTRATION SET is that desired/ordered. REMOVE THE SET FROM ITS PACKAGE and confirm that the line is clamped shut.

9. Remove the protective seal at the IV bag's outlet port and, INSERT THE hard plastic TUBE FROM THE DRIP CHAMBER INTO THE IV BAG outlet port, so both components are properly assembled.

10. HANG THE IV BAG (or otherwise have it elevated) AND, after removing the protective cover from the needle end of the IV tubing, RUN THE IV SOLUTION INTO THE DRIP CHAMBER AND IV TUBING until each is properly filled.

11. SHUT OFF THE LINE AND PROTECT THE NEEDLE END OF THE TUBING FROM CONTAMINATION, by recovering it or "handing" it in a suitable manner.

12. TAKE/CONFIRM all necessary BODY SUBSTANCE ISOLATION PRECAUTIONS.

13. DETERMINE the desired potential LOCATION FOR THE IV AND, APPLY A venous CONSTRICTOR snugly around the arm PROXIMAL TO IT. If blood is to be drawn when establishing the IV, assemble the necessary vacutainer holder tubes, etc., and place them easily within reach.

14. After waiting for the veins to engorge, IDENTIFY A SUITABLE VEIN AND PALPATE THE SPECIFIC SITE selected in order to ensure that a valve does not lie under or just proximal to it.

15. Once the specific vein and site have been selected, CLEANSE THE AREA WITH AN ANTISEPTIC WIPE, AND SELECT A (over-the-needle) CATHETER OF THE APPROPRIATE SIZE for the vein.

16. After peeling back the package cover and removing the over-the-needle catheter, GRASP THE NEEDLE AND CATHETER HUB AND REMOVE THE PLASTIC PRO-TECTOR from over their tips. CHECK BOTH for any irregularities AND LOOSEN THE CATHETER (without pulling it more than one millimeter or beyond the end of the needle).

17. While anchoring the vein with one finger pressed over it proximal and one distal to the exact site selected, LOCATE THE TIP OF THE NEEDLE OVER (or aside) THE VEIN AND while holding it at about a 45 degree angle) ADVANCE IT through the skin UNTIL IT IS FELT TO "POP" THROUGH THE VEIN WALL.

18. LOWER THE NEEDLE'S HUB, AND ADVANCE THE NEEDLE ALONG THE inside of the VEIN FOR ABOUT 1/4 OF AN INCH AND STOP.

19. WHILE STILL FIRMLY GRASPING THE NEEDLE HUB with one hand, GRASP THE HUB OF THE CATHETER WITH THE OTHER HAND AND slowly carefully THREAD IT INTO THE VEIN.

20. SECURELY HOLD THE CATHETER FROM MOVING between the thumb and first finger of one hand, OCCLUDE THE VEIN by pressing on it with another finger of the same hand. THEN CAREFULLY WITH-DRAW THE NEEDLE FULLY with the other hand AND DISCARD IT PROPERLY in a sharps container.

21. CONNECT THE HUB OF THE IV LINE INTO THE HUB OF THE CATHETER. Make sure these are sufficiently tightly secured together. (If drawing blood before initiating the IV, the vacutainer holder should be connected and the necessary tubes filled, before the hub of the IV line is connected replacing it in the catheter's hub).

22. WHILE STILL HOLDING the hub of THE CATHETER with one hand, RELEASE THE VENOUS CONSTRIC-TOR AND OPEN THE IV LINE with the other hand.

23. Regardless of rate desired, SLOWLY INCREASE THE FLOW RATE OF THE IV SOLUTION (to at least 1/2 of the gtt rate of the administration set) AND CHECK THAT THE IV IS PATENT (runs freely and without infiltrating).

24. SECURE THE HUB OF THE NEEDLE properly IN PLACE WITH one or more TAPE strips AND, with some slack provided along its length (or a loop), ALSO SECURE THE LINE TO A SECOND POINT on the arm and PROXIMAL TO THE CANNULATION SITE with additional prepared strips of tape.

25. ADJUST THE FLOW RATE (gtt/min) of the IV TO THAT DESIRED.

26. RECHECK THE SOLUTION AND INFUSION RATE ARE THOSE ORDERED, AND THAT THE IV LINE CONTINUES TO BE PATENT AND WITHOUT signs of INFILTRATION after it has been taped in place.

27. RECORD ALL PERTINENT INFORMATION surrounding the IV start. This should include the time, IV solution, rate, needle or catheter type and size, location (e.g.: left antecubital space, back of left hand, etc.), and initials of the EMT who established the line.

28. Since a significant period of time has elapsed, RECHECK THE QUALITY OF VENTILATION AND VITAL SIGNS.

29. MONITOR THE PATIENT'S CONDITION AND THAT THE IV REMAINS PATENT AND AT A PROPER RATE. PERIODICALLY RECHECK THE patient's VITAL SIGNS.

30. IF THE IV BAG BECOMES NEAR EMPTY at any point, PREPARE ANOTHER of the same solution and quantity as the previous one ordered. CHANGE THE LINE OVER TO THE REPLACEMENT BAG before the first is fully run out and the drip chamber and line empty, AND RUN IT AT THE RATE INITIALLY PRESCRIBED. IF the ORDER LIMITS the total FLUID to be INFUSED, WHEN this is REACHED, REDUCE the RATE TO KVO, and OBTAIN on-line MEDICAL DIRECTION.

ALS

ETI SUMMARY SKILL SHEET
Administration of A Drug By Injection, IV Push, or Pre-Mixed IV Piggyback Drip

1. OBTAIN ORDER or "echo" the standing order.

2. CONFIRM FINDINGS and history PROVIDE INDICATION for use of the drug AND DO NOT INCLUDE ANY allergies, adverse drugs, or other CONTRAINDICATIONS excluding its use.

3. SELECT the supply of the prescribed DRUG, AND GATHER all OTHER NEEDED ITEMS (needles, syringes, administration sets, etc.)

4. CHECK NAME of drug on actual container.

5. CHECK supply is in APPROPRIATE FORM AND, if applicable, CONCENTRATION for the desired route of administration.

6. CHECK EXPIRATION DATE of the drug supplied.

7. CHECK APPEARANCE for clarity, absence of foreign matter, and conformity with customary expectation.

8. NOTE TOTAL MILLIGRAMS supplied (Concentration On-hand).

9. NOTE TOTAL MILLILITERS supplied (Volume On-hand).

10. NOTE (or calculate) the MILLIGRAMS PER MILLILITER (mg/ml) of the supply.

11. CHECK IF the DESIRED DOSE (DD) is in **mg, mg/kg, mg/min,** or **mg/kg/min.**

12. If applicable, DETERMINE the PATIENT'S approximate WEIGHT AND CONVERT IT from pounds TO KILOGRAMS (kg).

13. DETERMINE the TOTAL **mg** or **mg/min** ORDERED ADMINISTERED for this patient (Specified for him exactly, or calculated from the mg/kg ordered and his kg weight).

14. ESTIMATE, from the **mg/ml** SUPPLIED and the total **mg** (or **mg/min**) ordered, the number of **ml** (OR **ml/min**) REQUIRED delivered TO PROVIDE the DESIRED DOSE.

15. Based upon the mg/ml supplied, set up the necessary formulas and CALCULATE THE EXACT **ml** (or **ml/min**) REQUIRED TO PROVIDE THE DESIRED DOSE.

16. CHECK THE CALCULATED ANSWER AGAINST THE EARLIER deduced ESTIMATE or estimated possible range.

17. *If drug is supplied in a vial or ampule,* DRAW UP THE EXACT AMOUNT TO BE ADMINISTERED.

    If using a pre-loaded syringe or cartridge for injection, WASTE ANY EXCESS VOLUME (any amount beyond the ml required) from the syringe.

    If a pre-mixed IV drip, SELECT AN APPROPRIATE ADMINISTRATION SET and, after you CONFIRM ITS **gtt/ml** is that desired, CALCULATE THE **gtt/min** rate NECESSARY TO PROVIDE THE **ml/min** REQUIRED (to deliver the ordered mg/min dose).

    In the rare event that a drug for IV drip has a stated maximum dose precaution, WASTE ANY volume NECESSARY until the TOTAL **mg** REMAINING in the IV bag DOES *NOT* EXCEED THE MAXIMUM RECOMMENDED DOSE.

18. *If for injection,* CHANGE NEEDLE.

    If an IV drip, ASSEMBLE THE COMPONENTS, RUN the appropriate amount of FLUID INTO THE DRIP CHAMBER AND LINE, CHECK IV RUNS properly AND **gtt/ml** IS SAME AS USED IN CALCULATIONS.

19. TAKE/CONFIRM the INDICATED BODY SUBSTANCE ISOLATION PRECAUTIONS.

20. PURGE any AIR from the syringe or IV line.

21. *If for injection,* SELECT AN APPROPRIATE SITE and check that it is WITHOUT any IRREGULARITIES AND DOES NOT APPROXIMATE AN ARTERY.

    If for IV Push or IV piggyback drip administration, CHECK THAT THE PRIMARY IV LINE IS PATENT AND THAT NO INFILTRATION HAS OCCURRED.

22. RECHECK NAME OF DRUG SUPPLIED and if provided in different ones, its concentration.

23. CLEANSE THE SITE OR 'Y' PORT.

24. INSERT THE NEEDLE AND POSITION IT APPROPRIATELY (through the skin or into the "Y" port) or if a needleless connection, connect it properly.

25. ADMINISTER THE DRUG as follows:

    If a Sub-Q or IM injection:
    a —Check that NO blood enters the syringe.
    b —Aspirate the syringe, check that NO blood enters.
    c —Push plunger into the barrel of the syringe.
    d —Remove needle and syringe from patient, and discard it in a sharps container.

    If for injection into a vein:
    a —After feeling it "pop" as it enters the vein, thread it further into the vein.
    b —Check that blood doesn't "pump" into the syringe.
    c —Aspirate the syringe, blood should easily be drawn into the syringe.
    d —Release the rubber constrictor tourniqueting the vein.
    e —Slowly push the plunger into the barrel of the syringe while observing for any infiltration.
    f — Carefully remove the needle-and-syringe from the patient and discard it in a sharps container.

g —Apply direct pressure over the site.
h —Once the bleeding has stopped, apply antiseptic gel and cover with a band-aid.

    If for IV Push (through an established IV line):
    a —Kink the line between the "Y" port and the IV bag.
    b —Push the plunger into the barrel of the syringe.
    c —Remove the needle-and-syringe from the "Y" port and discard it into a sharps container.
    d —Release the kink in the tubing.
    e —Flush the drug into the vein by temporarily running the line at a fast rate.
    f — Adjust the gtt/min to the desired rate.

    If for IV piggyback drip:
    a —Tape the needle securely to the "Y" port.
    b —Adjust the piggyback to the desired gtt/min rate.
    c —Shut-off the flow of the primary IV's solution.
    d —Recheck gtt/min of piggyback.
    e —Check that no infiltration is occurring.

26. CHECK the name (and if applicable, concentration) of the DRUG, AGAIN.

27. RECORD the TIME, DRUG, AND DOSE administered.

28. *After the drug has had sufficient time to be absorbed and circulated,* RECHECK THE PATIENT'S apparent OVERALL CONDITION, QUALITY OF VENTILATION, AND VITAL SIGNS.

29. CHECK FOR INITIATION and proper level of the desired THERAPEUTIC EFFECT. *Should the patient be refractory to the drug and dose administered, if repeated doses or other drugs are specified in your protocols, consider the drug and dose to administer next. If not, contact Med Control for further instructions, without delay.*

30. CHECK FOR any systemic or localized ADVERSE or idiosyncratic SIDE EFFECTS. Should any appear at any time, (if an IV drip, shut-off the piggyback and re-open the primary line to KVO) contact Med Control immediately.

31. DOCUMENT TIME AND ADMINISTRATION fully and PROPERLY ON RUN REPORT.

32. Continue to MONITOR THE PATIENT'S LOC, GENERAL APPEARANCE AND QUALITY OF VENTILATION FOR 30 MINUTES or until patient responsibility is transferred at the Emergency Department. (Also monitor SaO$_2$ and EKG if indicated).

33. PERIODICALLY RECHECK VITAL SIGNS, EFFECTS of drug, AND ADMINISTRATION SITE FOR ANY LOCAL REACTION or if a drip, infiltration.

34. GIVE PROPER VERBAL REPORT once at the Emergency Department, INCLUDING EACH DRUG AND DOSE ADMINISTERED.

35. RE-STOCK ALL DRUGS AND adjunct EQUIPMENT USED before leaving the hospital or immediately upon returning to quarters.

ALS

ETI SUMMARY SKILL SHEET
Mixing A Piggyback For IV Drip Administration

1. OBTAIN ORDER or refer to standing order.

2. CONFIRM FINDINGS and history PROVIDE INDICATION for use of the drug AND DO NOT INCLUDE ANY allergies, adverse drugs, or other CONTRAINDICATIONS.

3. CHECK that a primary IV LINE HAS BEEN ESTABLISHED if not, direct another EMT to establish one.

4. SELECT SUPPLY OF the prescribed DRUG.

5. SELECT an IV BAG OF the basic IV SOLUTION AND number of MILLILITERS ORDERED for the piggyback.

6. SELECT an ADMINISTRATION SET OF THE DESIRED **gtt/ml** AND A suitable NEEDLE FOR THE piggyback.

7. CHECK the NAME OF THE DRUG on the supplied container.

8. CHECK that the supply is in an appropriate FORM AND, if applicable, CONCENTRATION for mixing into and administering by IV drip.

9. CHECK the EXPIRATION DATE of the drug supplied.

10. CHECK APPEARANCE of the drug supplied for — clarity and conformity with the customary expectation.

11. NOTE TOTAL MILLIGRAMS of the drug supplied (Concentration on-hand).

12. NOTE TOTAL MILLILITERS in which it is supplied (Volume on-hand).

13. NOTE (or calculate) the MILLIGRAMS PER MILLILITER (mg/ml) of the supply.

14. Identify and separate the part of the order which prescribes the MIXING dose. DETERMINE THE SPECIFIC MILLIGRAMS ORDERED AS THE MIXING DOSE (Concentration to be mixed).

15. CHECK THAT THE VOLUME (total mls) and type of SOLUTION IN the IV piggyback BAG selected, IS THAT ORDERED.

16. ESTIMATE THE MILLILITERS of the supply NEEDED to add the number of **mg** ordered to the IV bag.

17. CALCULATE THE EXACT number of MILLILITERS of the supply NEEDED to add the **mgs** ordered to the IV bag.

18. CHECK the CALCULATED **mls** needed AGAINST the earlier ESTIMATE.

19. DRAW-UP THE NECESSARY **mls** of the supply or if a pre-loaded syringe, waste any excess.

20. RE-CHECK THE **mls** IN the SYRINGE and **mls** of the base solution IN THE IV BAG ARE the specific quantities desired.

21. CHECK THE CLARITY AND EXPIRATION DATE OF the IV BAG.

22. CLEANSE THE 'Y' PORT AND INJECT THE DRUG from the syringe into the IV piggyback bag.

23.. Roll and shake the IV bag to fully dissolve and MIX THE DRUG IN THE IV BAG SOLUTION.

24. CHECK that the inserted DRUG IS THOROUGHLY MIXED IN THE IV bag SOLUTION AND THAT NO PRECIPITATE has form.

25. FILL OUT AND APPLY A DRUG LABEL to the back of the piggyback IV bag. Note the drug name, mgs added, time, and your initials.

26. RE-CHECK THE DRUG NAME ON THE label of the ORIGINAL SUPPLY, IN THE MIXING ORDER, AND the DRUG LABEL YOU AFFIXED TO the IV BAG.

   After the:
   - milligrams of the drug have been mixed into the quantity and IV solution prescribed,
   - properly filled out medication label has been affixed,
   - concentration now produced in the IV piggyback bag has been checked against the "mixing part" of the order and the **mg/ml** calculated,

   the IV piggyback that has been prepared is the same as any pre-mixed IV drug solution.

   The remaining calculations to be done to determine the rate at which the IV is to be run (gtt/min needed to provide the mg/min ordered), and the steps in preparing the equipment and administering the IV drip medication, are the same as those described in the preceding Summary Skill Sheet.

27. CHECK the **mg** OF DRUG placed IN the IV BAG, and ml SIZE OF IV BAG into which the drug has been mixed, against the mixing order.

28. DETERMINE THE **mg/ml** CONCENTRATION of the drug now IN THE PIGGYBACK IV SOLUTION, AND RECORD IT ON THE bottom of THE MEDICATION LABEL you added to the IV piggyback bag.

ETI SUMMARY SKILL SHEET
Common Abbreviations and Equivalents
Used For Medication Administration

I. Abbreviations
(**Note**: abbreviations in parentheses are less common).

Kilogram	kg
Gram	G (gm)
Milligram	mg (mG)
Microgram	μ or mcg
Pound	lb
Ounce (weight)	oz
Grain	gr
Milliequivalent	mEq
Liter	L
Milliliter	ml (mL)
Cubic centimeter	cc
Ounce (fluid)	oz (fl. oz.)
Tablespoon	tbsp
Teaspoon	tsp
Drop	gtt
As needed	prn
By mouth	po (PO)
By rectum	pr (PR)
Dissolved or suspended in	in
Every	$\bar{q}$ or q
5% Dextrose in Water	D5W
50% Dextrose in Water	D50W
Gauge (internal diameter of a catheter or needle)	g.
Half-Normal Saline	0.5 NS or 1/2 NS
Intramuscular	IM
Intraosseous	IO
Intravenous	IV
Keep vein open rate	KVO or TKO
Lactated Ringer's Solution	LR (RL)
Milligrams in one ml (concentration of liquid drug)	mg/ml
Minute	min
Normal Saline	NS
Not to exceed	up to
"Number in one" or "for each"	per

Number of drops to provide one ml	gtt/ml
Number (of pills) to be given	#
Per	/
Rate of IV administration, or drops per minute	gtt/min
Repeat	$\bar{r}$ or r.
Subcutaneous	SQ or Sub-Q or Sub-q
Sublingual	SL (Sub-L)
To keep vein open rate	TKO or KVO

II. Equivalents

1 Kilogram	=	1,000 G
1 Gram	=	1,000 mg
1 Milligram	=	0.001 g (1/1,000 G)
1 Milligram	=	1,000 mcg
1 Microgram	=	0.001 mg (1/1,000 mg)
1 Grain	=	60 mg
1 Milligram	=	1/60 grain
1 Liter	=	1,000 ml
1 Milliliter	=	0.001 Liters (1/1,000 L)
1 Fluid ounce	=	30 ml
1 Tablespoon	=	15 ml
1 Teaspoon	=	5 ml
1 Cubic centimeter	=	1 ml
1 Liter	=	1.05 Quarts
1 Kilogram	=	2.2 Pounds
1 Pound	=	0.45 kg
1 Milliequivalent	=	No measurable equivalent in mg, G, etc.

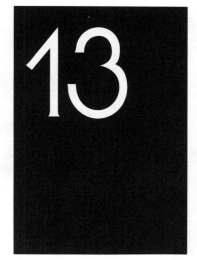

SECTION

**Spinal
Immobilization
Skills**

13

Introduction

The spinal cord and the nerves branching from it provide the exclusive pathway for stimuli to pass from the brain to each part of the body. Each vertebrae from the first cervical (C-1) to the second sacral (S-2) contains an opening, called the vertebral foramen, in its center. Each vertebral foramen lines up exactly with that of the vertebrae above and below it to form the "spinal canal." The spinal cord, surrounded by a dural sheath and the bony "circle" of each vertebra, extends from the brain stem through the first cervical vertebra at the base of the skull inferiorly to the second lumbar vertebra (L-2) near the lower end of the torso. The head, weighing between 16 and 22 pounds, is perched on the Atlas—the ring-shaped first cervical vertebra (C-1). The sacrum (formed by the five

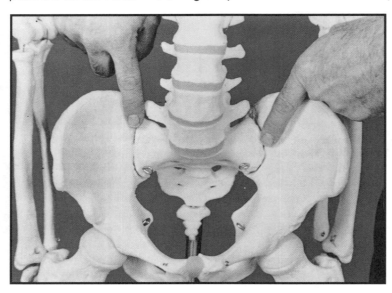

sacral vertebrae fused immovably together) is part of both the spinal column and the pelvic girdle, and is connected to the rest of the pelvis by immovable joints. The sacrum is the base of the entire spinal column, the platform upon which all of the vertebrae (except the coccyx) rest. When sitting or standing, the weight of the head, neck, upper extremities and almost the entire torso-between 70 and 80 percent of the body's total weight—rests on the sacrum.

The space between the interior diameter of each vertebral foramen and the spinal cord varies slightly from vertebra to vertebra, but even at its largest is extremely small. In uninjured healthy people the separate vertebrae are held in alignment with each other and the sacrum by a network of very strong ligaments and muscles. Although these allow the vertebrae to have the controlled movement necessary for the body's normal flexibility and motion, they also control and limit movement so that the vertebrae are not so displaced that the cord is bruised, pinched or cut.

When vertebrae are fractured, changing their shape or weakening their structural strength, or the ligaments and muscles maintaining the vertebral alignment are torn or even overly stretched—the normal ability to maintain the necessary alignment may be lost. In such cases even slight movement can result in sufficient displacement of a vertebrae (or sharp bone shards produced in the canal) to cut or pinch the cord and produce paralysis.

Although injury to the cord at any level can produce a heinous loss of function, the higher (more cephalad) the injury to the cord or nerves branching from it, the greater and more critical will be the loss of function which results. The weight of the head (generally greater than that of a bowling ball) and its location atop the relatively thin neck, together with the forces that act upon the head, make the cervical spine particularly susceptible to injury. At the third cervical vertebra the width of the cord is only one millimeter less than the internal diameter of vertebra, therefore even a minor dislocation at this point can produce cord injury. The muscles producing the changes in the shape of the diaphragm required for adequate spontaneous respiration are stimulated by nerves branching from the cord at the 3d, 4th, and 5th cervical vertebrae (C-3, C-4, and C-5). If the cord at one of these levels (or the phrenic nerve) is cut and the stimuli are interrupted, the patient will lose the ability to maintain adequate spontaneous ventilation.

In patients with spine injury, or in whom it is suspected, one cannot know the exact location, nature and extent of the injury without x-rays or in some cases CT or MRI imaging. Without knowing these, one cannot determine whether, which, or how much movement of the patient can cause cutting or other injury of the cord. Therefore, patients with suspected spine trauma must be immobilized on a rigid longboard in order to prevent further movements of the body and spine, or any increased intervertebral weighting or pressure.

Several recent studies have shown that approximately only 6% of the victims of trauma suffer spine injury. Of these, less than half have any immediate inferior motor or sensory deficit (indicating that the cord was cut or otherwise disrupted at the moment of insult at the accident). The other half, although later found by x-ray to have vertebral injury, generally did not have any gross immediate post-insult neurological deficit. One study even noted that 17% of those found to have an unstable spine were walking at the scene after the accident, or (failing to summon EMS or refusing care in the field) walked into the emergency department. There are numerous studies evaluating the accuracy of physicians in identifying or ruling out spine injury based solely on physical examination in conscious, alert, reliable patients. Some of these have shown that asymtomatic spine injuries were missed only rarely, while others have shown as high as 22% being missed. Since when comparing these studies one finds the conclusions to be contradictory and equivocal and since none of these included pre-hospital assessment by EMTs, they provide no information relevant to determining which patients do and which do not need immobilization in the field. Universally, since the earliest organized trauma studies to the present, the literature has identified patients with unstable spine trauma with no motor or sensory deficit immediately post insult who, after some passage of time and being moved, developed signs of cord injury and were found to have a cord lesion and paralysis upon arrival at the hospital. A number of studies have also universally shown that the incidence of spine trauma is related to the *mechanism of injury* and the forces which acted upon the patient. Although there is a small group of exceptions, the vast majority of spinal injuries result from mechanisms which produce either violent forces acting upon the head, neck or torso — or which produce sudden forceful acceleration, deceleration, rotation, or lateral movement.

Mechanisms resulting in significant head (or helmet) injury or ejection from a moving vehicle, or cases where the head or a portion of the torso strikes an object and causes it to stop moving before the rest of the body (resulting in forceful compression or hyperextension of the spine), produce a significantly larger percentage of patients with spine injury than is seen with other equally forceful mechanisms.

The head rests and safety belts presently required in cars, although restraining the torso upon collision, only restrain the head from moving posteriorly. In a frontal collision the torso is kept from moving but the head restrained primarily only by the strong posterior neck muscles continues to move forward — often resulting in forceful hyper-flexion of the neck. In a side collision, only the lower torso remains restrained while the head and upper torso can continue to move. This often results in severe lateral bending, rotation or hyper-flexion. Although the proper use of safety belt restraints has been irrefutably shown to reduce the incidence of critical or disfiguring injuries, it has not been shown to reduce or eliminate spine injury sufficiently to allow it to be used as a basis for ruling out the probability of such injury. There is presently not conclusive data to indicate whether or not the addition of airbags will reduce the incidence of spine trauma. Similarly, helmets worn by motorcyclists have been universally proven to significantly reduce morbidity and mortality, but they (and helmets worn by bicyclists or for contact sports) have not been shown to reduce the incidence of spine trauma.

The preceding discussion of factors affecting the probability of spine injury provides the following conclusions:

- Only a small percentage of trauma victims have spinal injury. Of these, a significant number will *NOT* have any pain on palpation or movement, deformity, or other signs or symptoms of spinal injury that are obvious or even identifiable in the field.
- The absence of a neurological deficit does not rule out the presence of spine injury or an unstable spine.
- The fact that a patient can (or did) stand or walk since the accident is *NOT* a reason to rule out the presence of spine trauma.
- The wearing of a helmet, proper use of safety belt restraints, or the deployment of an air bag, are also not reasons for or factors contributing to ruling out spinal injury.
- In patients with a suggestive mechanism of injury, regardless of the findings in the physical exam, the presence of spine injury must be assumed in the field.

In some patients the mechanism of injury may not be readily identifiable. Because of this, the extent, location, and nature of the patient's other injuries must also be considered as indicators of the mechanisms and forces that acted upon the body. Although in a patient found unconscious on his front lawn, the identification of a fractured scapula and clavicle together with an unstable pelvis and multiple angulated fractures of one leg does not provide a clear understanding of what occurred, it clearly indicates that a violent mechanism of injury was involved and that an associated spine injury must be assumed.

Pre-hospital spinal immobilization is recommended and indicated in any patient with:

A *Mechanism of Injury* suggesting that violent or sudden forces were applied to the spine, regardless of the absence of any other signs and symptoms,

or

Other injuries which suggest that violent forces acted upon the spine,

or

The presence of *any signs and symptoms of spine injury.*

The signs and symptoms associated with spine injury are:
- Neck or back pain.
- Pain upon, or guarding or splinting against, movement of the head, neck or back.
- Pain-on-palpation of the posterior neck or midline of the back.
- An observable or palpable deformity of the spinal column.
- Any paralysis, paresis (weakness), numbness, or tingling in the arms, torso and/or legs at any time post-trauma.
- Signs of neurogenic shock.
- In males, priapism (a non-sexually stimulated continuous erection).

Obviously patients with suspected spine trauma are not found lying on a longboard, nor are they usually found in such a position that (without moving them) the EMT can directly apply a longboard and secure them to it. The EMT can only do this if the patient is found standing. Most trauma victims are found sitting (in a car), lying supine or semi-prone (lying prone but with their head rotated to the side) on the ground, or in a more misaligned "crumpled" position. As well as immobilizing the spine when carrying and transporting the patient, the EMT must immobilize it when moving the patient to assess him and when moving him from his initial position onto the longboard.

Immediately upon arrival, when the mechanism of injury suggests possible spinal injury, an EMT should firmly grasp the patient's head to provide manual immobilization of the head and neck. This must be maintained without interruption until it is later replaced by the mechanical immobilization provided by a spinal immobilization device. After manual immobilization is initiated a rigid cervical collar should be added as an adjunct to further protect the neck. Once ready to move the patient, either an interim device or a manual maneuver (performed by several additional EMTs) is used to maintain the neutral in-line immobilization of the head, neck, torso and pelvis while the patient is moved from his present position onto the longboard. Then, once on the longboard, the patient (and in some cases the interim device) is affixed to the longboard at key places on the external anatomy using pads (blanket rolls or rubberlike bolsters) and straps. Only once this has been completed can the manual immobilization be released and the packaged patient safely moved. The EMT must select the best method for maintaining the immobilization while moving the patient onto the longboard based upon the patient's position, injuries and condition as well as the situation and scene. Several options are available for any position in which the patient initially presents. Although some may be precluded by the situation, the EMT will have to choose the best method from among these for a sitting patient: rigid half-board, extrication vest, or direct rapid extrication with manual immobilization; and use of either a logroll, body lift, body slide or scoop stretcher for one found lying. Even though a longboard can be applied and affixed directly to a standing patient, whether he should be immobilized to it manually or mechanically prior to being lowered to the ground will have to be determined.

Injured patients are rarely found with the parts of their body in neutral in-line alignment. Commonly they present with the head, neck, torso or pelvis angulated or rotated to some degree. To avoid any movement at all the patient would have to be immobilized while maintaining this misalignment even if it is extreme. When the body and spine are misaligned it promotes increased intravertebral pressure and, if present, continued intrusion on the cord. In such a position, even the slightest of movements which would increase the angulation or rotation is likely to produce additional vertebral displacement and damage to the cord. Unlike the absolute immobilization that can be produced by fastening appliances to the bone in an operating room, pre-hospital immobilization is provided by flaps, straps and other external fastenings surrounding the body. Because the tissues that lie between the bones and the body's outer surface can move slightly on the skeletal frame, some limited capacity for movement by the spine remains regardless of how well the patient has been immobilized. When the patient is transported on the longboard and the ambulance changes its speed or direction, or when the road surface is uneven, some shifting and movement will unavoidably occur. Moving the patient's head, neck, torso and pelvis into a neutral in-line position represents far less risk than if the patient was transported with these left in misalignment. This also allows for the easiest and most effective immobilization. Therefore, the underlying therapeutic purpose of the pre-hospital care of patients with spine injury is to place the patient in the neutral in-line position, unless contraindicated, and to maintain it without interruption by providing manual and then mechanical immobilization.

Simply stated, the treatment for suspected spine trauma is to immobilize the patient on a rigid longboard in the neutral in-line position. The remaining discussion surrounds how to achieve this while maintaining the necessary spinal protection from arrival at the scene until the completion of the call. In order to appropriately move and immobilize the patient, it is important that the EMT understands and incorporates the following key anatomical discussion with whichever specific method(s) or device(s) are employed:

Alignment and Manual Immobilization of the Head

Immediately following the determination that possible spine trauma exists (from the mechanism of injury, nature of other injuries, or signs and symptoms associated with spinal injury), the first step is to have an EMT grasp the sides of the head firmly between his hands with the thumbs and several fingertips extended anteriorly on the face and posteriorly at the base of the occiput to avoid any undesired extension, flexion lateral bending or rotation of the head. Once the head has been firmly grasped, it should be carefully moved so that the head, neck and torso are in a neutral in-line position unless this is contraindicated. The head should be moved and manually immobilized in the neutral in-line position *without any significant traction.* Only when a patient is found standing or sitting (or any other position in which the weight of the head remains on the cervical vertebrae) should any superior pull be exerted on it. Rather than traction (distracting the vertebrae with significant pull) the pull maintained in such patients should be only enough to cause axial unweighting in order to take the heavy weight of the head off of the spinal column until they are moved into a supine position.

In extremely rare cases, moving the patient's head into a neutral in-line position will be contraindicated. It should *NOT* be attempted in patients whose cervical injuries have resulted in such gross misalignment that the head no longer appears to extend from the midline of the shoulders. In other patients, moving the head will have to be immediately stopped and alignment considered contraindicated, if at any point moving the head into alignment results in:

- Initiating or increasing neck muscle spasm.
- Increased pain.
- The commencement or increase of a neurological deficit.
- Compromise of the airway or ventilation.

In any of these situations, the risk of alignment supersedes the risk of continued misalignment, and the patient's head will have to be immobilized in or near to (if it has been moved) the position in which it was originally found. *Since the cervical collars generally in pre-hospital use do not allow for adjustment to accommodate any angulation or rotation of the head, the EMT should NOT attempt to apply one at any time in such patients.*

When patients are found lying on their anterior abdomen and thorax with the head turned to the side, in order to avoid turning their head so that their face is on the ground the necessary rotary alignment of the head is deferred until they can be rolled onto their side.

Cervical Collars

Cervical collars do NOT immobilize. Because they only limit the range of flexion by about 75 per cent at best and the range of other motion by 50 per cent (or less), they do not in themselves provide immobilization of the head and neck. A cervical collar is an important adjunct. Except when moving the head and neck into the neutral in-line position is contraindicated, a collar should always be used in conjunction with manual immobilization or with mechanical immobilization provided by a half or full body immobilization device. As has previously been discussed, some unavoidable movement of the patient remains when immobilized with a vest-type device, rigid half-board, or longboard. Unless otherwise protected against, the differences in inertia and the degree of affixation capable for the head and torso separately can result in sudden loading and compression of the cervical vertebrae when the patient is moved. This is particularly true during transport when the ambulance accelerates or decelerates or bounces from road "shocks." The unique primary purpose of a cervical collar is to rigidly maintain a minimum distance between the head and neck so that any significant movement of one towards the other, and the resulting intermittent compression of the cervical spine it would produce, are eliminated. The upper margin of the cervical collar purchases the head anteriorly where it is inserted under the angle and lateral portion of the mandible, and posteriorly where the back section is inserted and secured below the posterior bulge of the occiput. The lower edge of the collar, when properly secured, sits firmly on the shoulder girdle and portions of the upper rib cage.

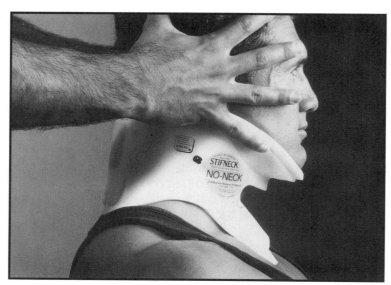

Due to its rigidity and the minimum thickness of the tissue between its outer edges and the underlying bone, the collar transfers any unavoidable loading from the head through the collar to the torso (or from the torso through the collar to the head), instead of to the neck. By maintaining the previous unloaded length between the shoulder girdle and the head, the rigid cervical collar prevents the movement and cervical compression that can not be eliminated by manual or other mechanical devices. Therefore, to eliminate the possibility of increased pressure being referred to the neck, a properly fitting cervical collar must be included with the other immobilization provided. The collar does not eliminate movement of the head beyond its upper edge or of C-6, C-7 and T-1 at its lower edge. Although it helps to limit movement (except distraction), it must always be used in conjunction with another method or device to provide adequate immobilization.

As well as its primary purpose (protecting the cervical spine from compression) and promoting limiting of head movement, a cervical collar provides a rigid protected pathway for the lower head affixation strap to safely pass over the anterior neck without applying any direct localized pressure on either the trachea, the carotid arteries or the large veins of the neck.

Each brand of cervical collar comes in a choice of sizes. In some collars, the back and the front are connected as one piece while in others they are separate.

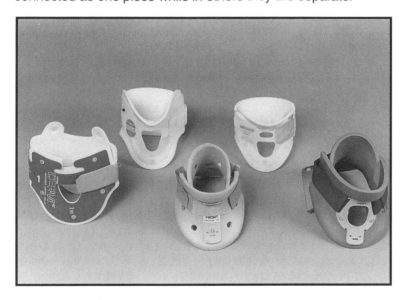

In each size there is a vast range of adjustment for the circumference. The velcro fastening allows the collar to be fitted to the exact circumference of the patient's neck. When fastening the collar the EMT must be careful that it is neither too loose nor too tight. A collar which is too loose will be ineffective and can accidentally cover the anterior chin, mouth, and nose — obstructing the patient's airway. A collar that is too tight can compromise the neck veins. When using a one-piece collar care must be taken to assure that the front section is properly centered on the patient's midline. If not, it will result in rotation or angulation of the head when it is secured. The height of the collar, unlike the circumference, is *NOT* adjustable (in models presently used in the field) and *is the critical dimension* when selecting which size to apply. A collar that is too short will not protect the cervical spine from compression and will allow significant flexion. A collar whose height is too great will, when applied, cause hyperextension of the head.

Although the design of the collar must be such that the distance between the angle of the mandible and the shoulder girdle is unalterably maintained, there must be sufficient flexibility to allow the anterior mandible to move down — allowing the mouth to open. A collar that does not allow the patient or EMT to open the mouth will produce aspiration of gastric contents if the patient vomits. **When applying a cervical collar the EMT should check that it does not obstruct or hinder mouth opening, ventilation, or circulation.**

Many cervical collars have an opening in their front portion to allow the EMT continued observation and access to the anterior neck. This only allows for very limited examination and, therefore, the neck should be fully examined prior to the application of the collar. Even though this opening allows for the free passage of air, the danger of the base of the collar shifting so that it covers the stoma in a patient with a laryngectomy or emergency needle tracheostomy makes the use of any cervical collar dangerous in such patients.

Moving a Lying Patient Onto the Longboard

Patients with suspected spine trauma who are found in a lying position must have their injured areas properly supported and, once the limbs, torso, neck and head have been aligned, neutral in-line alignment of the body continuously maintained while they are cared for and moved onto a longboard.

When a patient is found in a semi-prone position, his head will usually be found turned to one side — often making evaluation of his airway and respiration difficult. In such cases, the head cannot be aligned until the patient is moved into another position. When a patient is lying on his anterior torso, greater than one half of the torso's weight must be lifted to allow the chest expansion at each breath and often this significantly contributes to respiratory distress. Time is a particularly key factor even when airway and ventilation are not a problem since the EMT can not properly access or treat the patient until he has been moved into a supine position. Such patients must first be logrolled up onto one side and then, continuing the logroll, down into a supine position on the board. Repeated attempts to emulate a hospital Stryker Frame by sandwiching a semi-prone healthy volunteer "patient" between a scoop stretcher inserted under him and a longboard (or second scoop stretcher) placed onto his entire posterior length have been tried. Regardless of where the EMTs were positioned, how the two devices were held or secured together, and even when blanket rolls were included on each side of the patient — all attempts proved to be extremely time consuming and failed to provide adequate immobilization as the patient was turned over. Logrolling, therefore, remains the only proven method for moving a semi-prone patient into a supine position.

A wide variety of methods exists for moving a supine patient onto the longboard while protecting the spine from unnecessary movement. Although these are significantly different, each one includes the previously-discussed manual immobilization of the head and neck in a neutral in-line position by one EMT, while other EMTs move the patient's body while maintaining its proper alignment.

The body is moved in a different manner with each of these methods, and the type of support and stresses implicit with each causes them to have different advantages and disadvantages. By understanding these the EMT will be able to select the most appropriate one to meet the needs of the individual patient and situation. The benefits, drawbacks, and conditions which should recommend or discourage the use of each method will be found in the presentation of the individual skills later in this Section.

Immobilization to the Torso

Regardless of which specific rigid device is used, it must be immobilized to the torso so that it cannot move up, down, left or right. This serves two essential purposes in effecting the immobilization. When the torso and pelvis are immobilized to the rigid device, the thoracic, lumbar and sacral spine are supported and kept from moving. The torso fastenings, as well as immobilizing the patient to the device, immobilize the rigid device to the patient and provide a stable unmoving "platform" for supporting and immobilizing the head so that the alignment of the head, neck, and torso is properly maintained. ***The device must always be fully immobilized (affixed and adjusted as needed) to the torso before the head and neck are affixed and immobilized to it.*** In this way the inadvertent movement of the device that occurs, particularly with any adjustment of the shoulder straps or groin loops, will not be reflected to the head and neck and result in their movement. The device must be effectively secured to the torso at both its upper and lower ends to prevent any possible movement of the device which could cause angulation between the head and neck and the torso, and to protect the thoracic, lumbar and sacral vertebrae. Straps which surround both the arms and the torso, or the arms and legs simultaneously, or which surround both legs, prevent lateral or anterior movement. However, they restrict but do *NOT* eliminate cephalad or caudad movement. Similarly, straps that circumferentiate the torso between the nipple-line and the pelvis, if properly applied, cannot eliminate cephalad or caudad movement. *Straps which are applied around the torso between the nipple-line and the pelvis should only be secured snugly, NEVER tightly.*

TIGHT STRAPS AT THE MID AND LOWER TORSO:

• *Do NOT* Stop Caudad or Cephalad Movement

• Cause Respiratory Distress

Straps which are tightly fastened around the lower two thirds of the rib cage or around the soft abdomen are extremely dangerous. Straps secured tightly around the lower two thirds of the thorax will inhibit chest excursion and result in ventilatory embarrassment or, at least, increased distress. Straps securely tightened over the soft abdomen in small children will cause ventilatory embarrassment, and in any patient may result in additional organ damage and may cause internal bleeding.

The device can be safely and effectively secured with tight straps over the shoulder girdle and pelvis. Even extremely tight straps applied at the armpits and above, and over the pelvis, will not adversely affect ventilation or damage underlying organs in either adults or children. This, together with the anatomical "anchors" available at each location, make them the key areas at which the device is mechanically immobilized to the torso. Any straps fastened between these two points are solely for the purpose of preventing lateral or anterior movement of the mid-thorax, and not for immobilizing the device to the torso.

Although there are many different designs for devices and strapping, proper immobilization at the upper and lower torso must follow certain anatomical principles if it is to be effective.

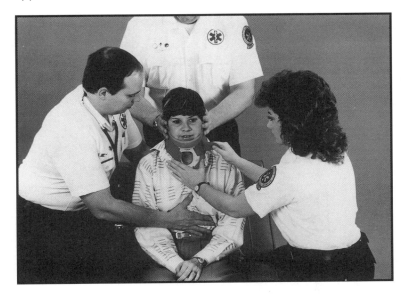

At the upper torso, regardless of the specific method used, the strapping (or device) must be anchored snugly in the armpits to prevent the device from moving up towards the head, over the shoulders to prevent it from moving down towards the legs, and one or more straps must circumferentiate the upper torso to prevent any anterior or lateral movement.

In any method the ends of the straps which pass over the shoulder must be fastened caudad to the top of the shoulders and the ends which pass through the armpits must be fastened cephalad to the apex of the armpit to assure that there is not any gap between the strap and the top of the shoulder or armpit which would allow for movement.

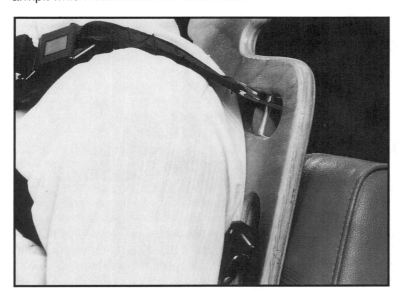

At the lower torso the pelvis must be encircled by a strap or straps. The straps must only encompass the pelvis since if they include any of soft abdomen or thighs they may permit undesirable lateral or anterior movement of the lower torso resulting in angulation at the neck once the head has been immobilized to the device.

With some minor variations, immobilization of a device to the upper torso (or of the upper torso to any device) can essentially be achieved—with a vest-type device, half backboard, or longboard —using one of three methods. With vest-type devices the straps are sewn to the device so as to dictate the use of one of these methods specifically.

Immobilization of the upper torso can be achieved using two straps to form a tight "X" over the upper torso.

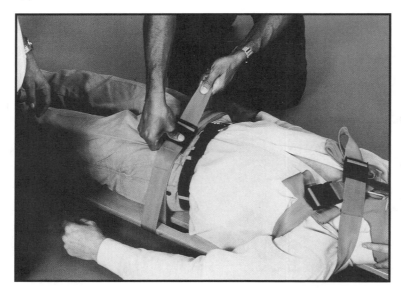

A strap is fastened to the board at a point approximately half way between the patient's shoulder and armpit at each side of the board. The strap is then placed snugly up through the armpit, across the chest, over the opposite shoulder and down to the board where it is fastened in the same location (or hole) as the other strap. Then the same procedure is repeated by passing the second strap through the other armpit across the chest and over the opposite shoulder. Having a strap pass over each shoulder and through the opposite armpit stops any cephalad or caudad movement or any angulation of the device or the torso. The restriction of the torso caused by the strap passing along the side and over the anterior thorax prevents any lateral or anterior movement.

The method just described, and the following two, can be used regardless of whether a longboard or half-board is used—and each vest-type device basically incorporates one (or more) of these methods in its design.

A different but similarly effective method of immobilization at the upper torso uses three straps. The first strap (or upper part of each of the lateral sides of the vest device) is placed and secured as high into each armpit as possible. When using a board, the first strap is fastened to it just cephalad to the armpit. It is then passed snugly through the armpit, then over the upper thorax through the opposite armpit, and is then again fastened to the board at a point just cephalad to the armpit on this side. When this method is incorporated into a vest device, the vest is applied and slid up on the patient's torso until the side flaps are snugly placed up in the armpits. Then the top anterior thorax strap is tightly fastened.

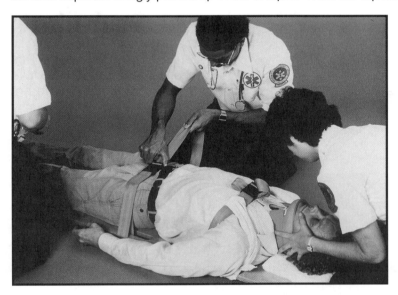

A second strap or tie is fastened to one side of the board at a point caudad of the upper margin of the shoulder. The strap or tie is then inserted under the posterior edge of the patient's shoulder, passed over the top of the torso adjacent to the neck, and is then brought down in a straight line (parallel to the patient's midline) to the first strap that was placed across the chest through the armpits. After being passed under the first strap, the second strap is secured to it (or to a special buckle above it, if provided on the vest).

The third strap is positioned and secured in the same way over the opposite shoulder. The strap or side flaps positioned snugly up into the armpit and tightly secured by a strap across the upper thorax will prevent the device from any cephalad or lateral movement on the patient's torso. The straps which pass over the shoulders on each side and are secured to the armpit strap (or buckles above it) anteriorly will prevent the device from any caudad movement.

If a vest type device is used which does not include such straps, a strap or cravat tie must be added over each shoulder if caudad movement is to be prevented. Posteriorly these can be fastened to the "lifting" loops and anteriorly under the armpit as shown.

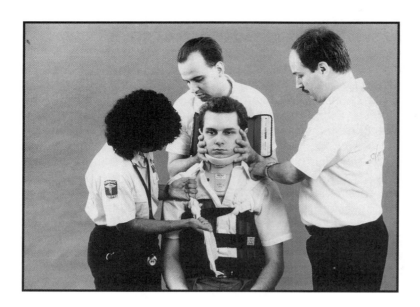

The third alternative for immobilizing a device to the upper torso, although not as secure as the two previously described methods, avoids any strap passing over the mid-clavicle and should be used if a clavicular fracture is suspected. With this method one strap is fastened to the side of the board just caudad of the upper margin of the shoulder and is brought behind the patient's back over the shoulder (just medial of the head of the humerus) across the anterior extension of the arm beyond the torso, through the armpit, and is secured to the board at its initial point of origin. Then the same is done with a second strap over the opposite shoulder. Each of these straps passes around a shoulder and secures and pulls it back in the same way as would a "figure eight" bandage used with a fractured clavicle.

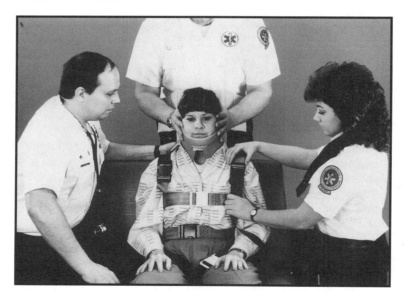

At the time of publication of this text the Oregon Spine Splint II was the only vest device that, although usually secured otherwise at the upper torso, allowed the EMT to select this alternative method in patients with a suspected clavicular fracture. When this method is used on a small narrow patient with a backboard or the OSS, a cravat tied between the shoulder loops below the clavicles may be needed to prevent the loops from moving laterally and the immobilization of a shoulder being lost. With this method, surrounding the most proximal end of each arm at the shoulder joint (or the lateral edge of the torso just medial of the shoulder joint) with a strap or tie which is both snugly up in the armpit and over the shoulder prevents any caudad, cephalad, lateral or anterior movement of the upper torso.

Although the authors have seen a countless number of different materials and exact strap placement used to successfully immobilize a device to the upper torso, they were all variations of and approximated one of these three basic systems. When new devices are developed with different ways of securing to the torso without use of the customary straps or flaps, the general anatomical principles of affixation common to these three systems will, however, remain unaltered. Such a device that is presently available serves as a good example. The vacuum spine splint (full or half body) if it is to immobilize successfully must be moulded along the lateral aspect of the torso, and securely up into the armpit on each side, and must also be molded over the top of each shoulder before the air is evacuated and the device becomes rigid. As well, no part of the vacuum splint can be allowed to surround the anterior thorax much beyond the anterior axillary line so that the device, once evacuated and rigid, will not limit chest excursion and cause respiratory embarrassment.

The discussion and illustration of spinal immobilization on a longboard that is found in most EMT texts only includes a single strap through the armpits and around the upper thorax, with additional straps over the shoulders glaringly omitted. The need to include straps or ties which tightly pass over the shoulders to prevent cephalad movement of the torso, although less obvious in a patient lying on a longboard than in a sitting patient, is no less essential. When being transported in an ambulance (or a special rescue device such as a cascade sled, all-terrain vehicle or boat) immobilized patients are in almost all cases transported with their head facing the front or bow. Each time the driver applies the brakes forcefully, significant sudden deceleration of the vehicle results. Although less sudden, even when the throttle is backed-off (or the vehicle slows when driving up a steep hill) some deceleration occurs. Whenever the vehicle decelerates or drives down an incline, inertia or gravity respectively cause the torso of a head-first patient to move towards his head unless it is restrained from such movement. Although the cervical collar prevents the movement of the torso from being applied to the neck, it only transfers it to the affixed head rather than eliminating it. Therefore, even when only level (perfectly horizontal) carrying is anticipated, straps or ties over the top of the shoulder should always be included in anticipation of transporting the patient in the ambulance.

Immobilization at the lower torso is primarily to keep the device from moving laterally or posteriorly away from the buttocks. Any such movement of the device at the base of the torso would allow it to angulate on the torso and would, after the head is secured to the device, result in either lateral bending or anterior flexion of the cervical spine. When a patient is to be immobilized to the longboard and only moving it while it is kept in a horizontal plane is anticipated (as from the ground onto a cot and directly into the ambulance), immobilization of the lower torso can most easily and rapidly be achieved with a single strap secured over the iliac crests.

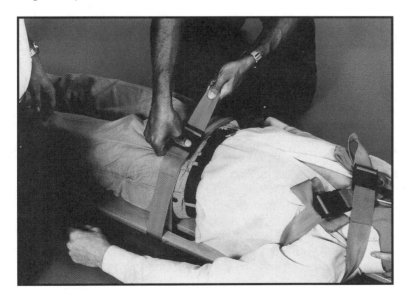

The iliac crest strap must be fastened securely surrounding the lateral and anterior pelvis, but no higher. If it is placed too high and lies over the soft anterior abdomen its placement can result in restricting ventilation and causing injury to underlying organs as well as its being ineffective in immobilizing the patient. It will be similarly ineffectual in immobilizing the lower torso if it is placed too low and primarily rests over the upper legs with only minimal purchase on the pelvis. Since the place along the length of the backboard where the shoulders are immobilized and the length of an individual's torso will be different on a case-by-case basis, the correct location for this strap can not accurately be anticipated for any pre-affixation of a strap to the longboard. This should be left until after immobilization at the upper torso has been completed. The iliac strap must be fastened to the longboard so that it lies tightly in a straight line (without any cephalad or caudid curvature) from the board over the pelvis and back to the board. *The EMT must locate this strap based solely upon the patient's anatomy and NOT upon the location of the holes in the board if no opening is properly located.* This should be a criteria when considering a board for purchase. Well designed boards (anticipating the need for flexibility in locating straps) have adjacent holes only interrupted for less than an inch continuously along each side. If the board you are using does *NOT* have holes properly located aside the patient's iliac crests, since the purpose of this strap is to prevent lateral and anterior movement not cephalad or caudad movement, place this strap under the board at the exact place along its length that is required and fasten it around the patient without passing it through any hole in the board. In a sitting patient a strap cannot be fastened in the proper position and securely across the iliac crests due to the intrusion of the perpendicular upper legs at the anterior lower aspect of the pelvis.

A single strap over the iliac crests is only sufficient to prevent movement if the patient is supine on a longboard and the longboard will not be upended or tilted to a side. In patients who are immobilized while sitting and must be moved onto the longboard, or with patients who are to be immobilized to a longboard where it will have to be upended or carried any distance, more secure fixation over the pelvis is required. If the fixation at the lower torso is limited to a single iliac strap, when the board is upended (except as it may provide some moderate deterrent to inferior movement of the pelvis) the majority of the weight of the torso will be placed against the strap through the armpits. When instead groin loops which snugly pass through the groin are used, the weight is equally supported at the upper torso in the armpits and at the lower torso by the loops passing under the pelvis at the groin. Additionally, these loops when properly placed laterally just cephalad of the head of the femur or over the edge of the ilium prevent the pelvis from moving in a cephalad direction and causing any loading and compression of the lumbar and thoracic vertebrae. *A single strap over the iliac crests is ONLY sufficient to safely immobilize the lower torso in patients who have been placed and immobilized on a longboard and will be moved with the longboard maintained in an essentially horizontal position at all times. In all other cases the use of a single iliac crest strap should be replaced by the use of groin loops.* Since patients that will be immobilized with an extrication vest are seated and will have to be moved onto a longboard, these in almost all cases come with groin loops. Similarly, whenever the EMT is using a half-board he should include the use of them. Whenever carrying the longboard up or down stairs or uneven terrain, or upending or angling the board is anticipated, groin loops should be installed to restrict the pelvis from moving in either a caudad or cephalad direction in order to avoid compression or distraction of the thoracic and lumbar spine (or the referral of pelvic movement onto the secured legs).

Groin loops are applied and positioned slightly differently in sitting patients than in patients who are supine on a longboard. In sitting patients, whether using a vest-type device or a half-backboard, they should originate posteriorly immediately next to the patient's midline near the coccyx or from a slightly more lateral point near the patient's waist. In order to avoid jostling of the patient and confusion — the strap should be pre-installed on the device and should be inserted and secured at one side at a time, rather than simultaneously by the EMTs at each side of the patient.

In a sitting patient, the groin strap that will form the loop for a side should be identified and, after making sure that it is not folded over or twisted along its length, inserted under the upper leg just proximal to the knee. It is then see-sawed back and forth while moving it posteriorly until it has been slid under the leg and buttock and the posterior portion slid under the buttock near the patient's midline.

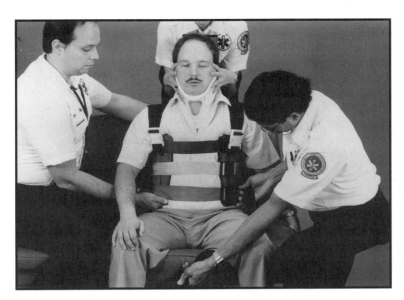

Once properly positioned, while supporting the base of the device, the strap is pulled anteriorly to form it in a tight straight line (without any curvature or looping around the part of the buttock which is on the seat) from its posterior point of origin to the groin anteriorly.

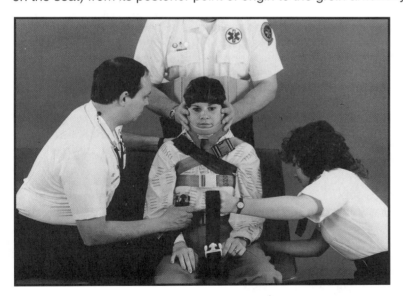

If it is not in a tight straight line, when the patient is lifted or slid over onto the longboard any curvature of the strap that occurred around the buttock when it supported his weight will be released and the strap will become loose and ineffectual. Once the strap has been inserted and pulled tightly into a straight line under the patient, the end of the strap is brought up along the patient's inner thigh on the same side of the body from which the strap originated. A strap which was applied under the patient's left leg must be brought back to the patient's left side — not crossed over to the right. Carefully position the strap in the groin between the leg and the outer genitalia. In both male and female patients care must be taken to assure that the strap does not include or rest on any part of the genital organs. Next, the strap is brought over the anterior pelvis and fastened to the appropriate buckle on the vest or, if a half-board, over the top of the ilium and then fastened to the half-board at the patient's waist. Lastly, while it is held from moving and becoming misplaced in the groin, the end of the strap is pulled tight.

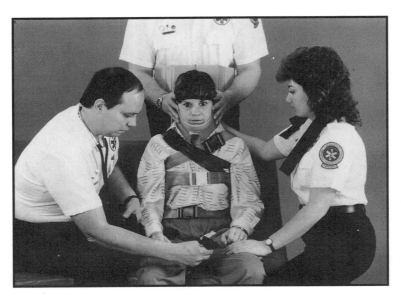

Once the groin has been secured on one side, the same steps are repeated with the groin loop over the opposite side of the pelvis. Similar to the straps securing the device at the upper torso, the groin loops need to be secured tightly to provide effective immobilization. Since they lie over the strong pelvic structure they can be pulled extremely tight without causing any discomfort or damage. Groin loops surround the pelvis at the same location as the leg openings of a pair of bikini underwear briefs. They lie medial to the acetabulum and should never be placed so that they lie over any part of the upper leg. If loops are placed around the upper legs, they can easily reduce or cut off circulation in the distal leg. Securing straps over or under a part of the upper legs should also be avoided since the unavoidable movement of the legs when moving a victim out of a car will result in the vest or half-board moving on the torso and movement of the spine. When groin loops are properly placed over the pelvis, once the patient has been placed on a longboard the legs can be lowered to lie flat on the board *without* any need to loosen or release the groin loops. Properly placed groin loops should only need to be loosened when straightening the legs in abnormally obese or extremely muscular individuals.

When groin loops are used with a supine patient on a longboard, since there is no way to secure the strap at the midline of the board each loop must originate and end at the holes in the side of the board. Once the patient's upper torso has been secured to the board, the holes just above the patient's iliac crest (cephalad to the groin) are identified. The strap is passed through the selected hole, inserted under the patient's buttock, through the groin and back to its point of origin — forming a loop over that side of the pelvis. The second loop is then positioned and tightened around the opposite side.

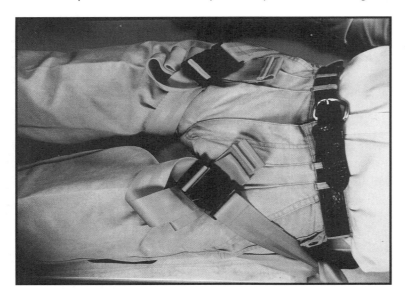

Although the primary initial concern in immobilizing the device to the torso is to provide an immobile rigid platform to which the head and neck can be immobilized, it also importantly serves to secure the upper and lower torso to the rigid device and immobilize them from movement. The preceding discussion has been presented from the perspective of securing the device and keeping it from moving on the torso. Once having secured the device to the torso it is helpful to change one's perspective and consider how the body is immobilized to the device for the remaining discussion of immobilizing the patient.

When a supine patient has been immobilized to a longboard and only horizontal carrying and transport is anticipated, the torso is adequately immobilized when secured to the board only at the upper and lower torso (using any of the methods previously described). However, when a patient is immobilized in a sitting position or when upending the board or carrying it over uneven terrain is anticipated, immobilization of the torso at these two locations will not prevent the mid-torso from some lateral movement or from anteriorly "sagging" away from contact with the device. The need to secure the mid-torso from such movement is clearly evident in viewing a sitting person with a rigid device installed before any mid-torso strap has been added.

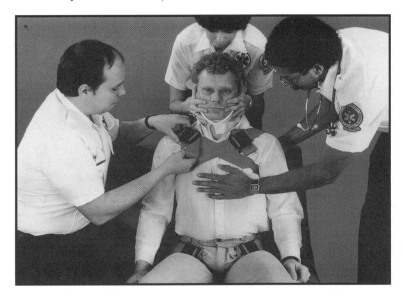

The mid-torso strap is not an adjunct to keeping the device from moving on the torso (this being already achieved by the earlier fastenings at the upper and lower torso), but is solely needed to perfect the immobilization of the torso to the device. It is therefore only necessary that any such straps be fastened snugly but not so tightly as to possibly inhibit chest excursion and respiration or to place undue pressure on the soft anterior abdomen and its underlying organs.

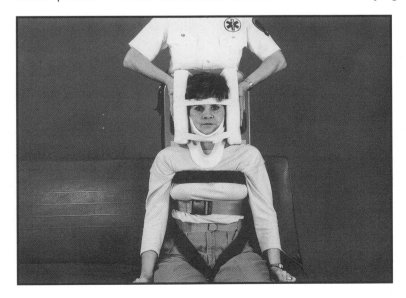

Only one strap is needed at the mid-torso. Although usually approximately centered between the armpits and the iliac crests, its exact location can be altered to best accommodate the patient's anatomy, special conditions, or the location of injuries. If the patient has injuries to the anterior abdomen or is pregnant it can be positioned higher, whereas in cases with injury to the anterior thorax it can be placed lower as long as it is neither so high *nor* so low (being right at the armpits or iliac crests) that it does *NOT* restrain the mid-torso.

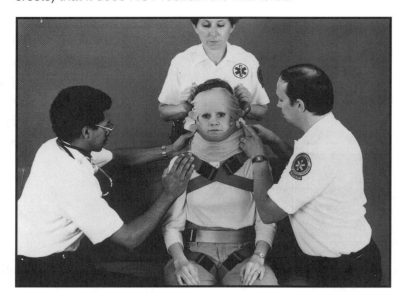

Even though straps which are placed surrounding the shoulder girdle or the uppermost part of the rib cage (cephalad of a line about one inch below the armpit) or over the pelvis can be maximally tightened without adverse effect (as previously discussed), straps which surround the remaining rib cage or soft anterior abdomen can not.

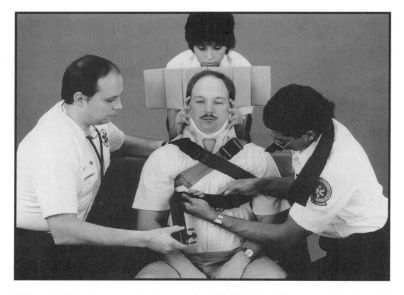

When tightening such straps the EMT should insert his hand between the strap and the patient and pull them moderately rather than extremely tight. When the hand is removed, the strap will be snug enough to provide the necessary support, but not so tight as to injure respiration or underlying abdominal organs.

In order to secure the mid-torso, vest type extrication devices usually have straps placed between those at the shoulder girdle and the groin loops. Due to these being in a fixed position regardless of the length of the patient's torso, two are provided. With most patients, one lies over the rib-cage near the mid-torso and the lower one over the soft abdomen near the umbilicus. Care must be taken that these are not pulled too tight.

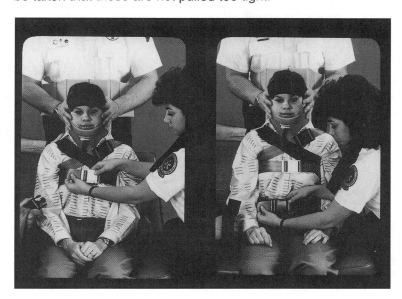

Although with most patients both straps are used to evenly secure the lower two thirds of the vest evenly around the torso, only one is essential. The upper mid-torso strap alone can be used in pregnant patients or those with abdominal injury, and the lower abdominal strap can be used without the mid-torso one in patients with underlying thoracic trauma.

Immobilization of the torso must, for some key steps, follow a dictated sequence. It is essential that prior to the start of any strapping, the patient be at the proper height and be properly centered in or on the device. Next it is important to check that no strap or parts are misplaced between the patient and the device which, as the device is secured, would become entrapped and unavailable. Once these preliminaries have been accounted for the upper torso should be fully immobilized to the device first so that the device will not move or become misaligned as other straps are secured. Even when fastening the upper torso, it is key that the strap(s) be properly secured in the armpits first to avoid the torso being pushed in a caudad direction when the shoulder straps (or parts going over the shoulders) are tightened. Although customarily the remaining straps for the torso are placed and secured one-by-one working down the torso, whether the mid-torso straps or those over the pelvis (lower torso) are next or last, with most devices, is a matter of personal preference.

The EMT should never solely pull on a strap end to tighten it as this results in forceful pulling against the patient or device. The EMT should always firmly hold the part of the strap being drawn into the buckle or the buckle itself in one hand, when pulling the end of the strap to tighten it. In this way the EMT is pulling against his other hand rather than against the patient or device.

As each torso strap is tightened the additional pull and pressure it exerts unavoidably results in some slight movement. This causes changes in the exact location and the tension of straps which have been previously secured. Although this shifting is unavoidable and generally of no ultimate significance, unnecessary and excessive movement as the EMT tightens each strap must be avoided.

Once all of the straps have been fastened and tightened completing the torso immobilization, each strap must be re-evaluated and additionally tightened or loosened as needed to provide balanced and proper immobilization of the torso and of the device to the torso.

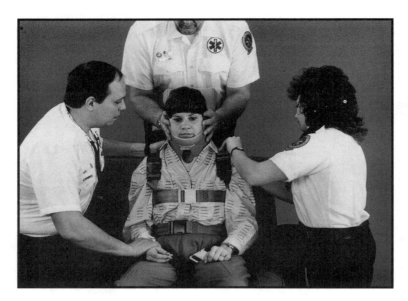

The inclusion in most texts of a step in which all straps are checked and re-adjusted as needed after the entire body has been properly immobilized to the longboard is misleading. *It is essential that all of the torso straps be fastened and completely adjusted prior to securing the head to the device in order to prevent the inevitable resulting movement of the device on the torso from being reflected to the head and neck.* When the torso straps have been properly re-adjusted immediately after completion of the torso immobilization, no further adjustment of them should be required later, after the head and legs have been secured.

Maintenance of the Neutral In-Line Position of the Head

It is essential that the neutral in-line postion in which the head has been placed (and manually immobilized without interruption since arrival) be maintained unaltered when the manual immobilization is superceded by a mechanical means. The neutral in-line position is defined as the position in which the head is normally held while walking, or the position in which the head is placed so that with the eyes centered exactly in their orbital range (neither rotated up, down, left *nor* right) a line between the pupils and the point the eyes are focused on would be perpendicular to the body's centerline (an imaginary midpoint which would extend in a strait plumbline from the center of the skull to a point between the ankles). Since some mild extension of the head is natural for some adults and does not increase the intervertebral pressure, the definition has been enlarged to mean perpendicular or at any position between perpendicular and up to 12 additional degrees of extension of the head.

A common anecdotal anatomical observation has been confirmed and quantified by a recent study at U.C.L.A. In greater than 98% of the adult population, when the head is placed in a neutral in-line position the outermost measure of the occipital region at the back of the head is between 1/2 and 3-1/2 half inches *anterior* to the plane of the posterior torso.

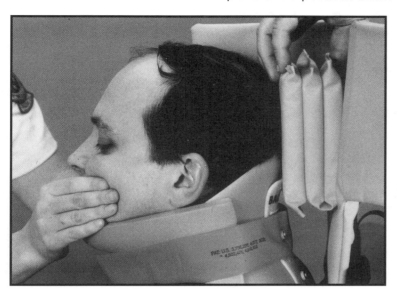

Therefore, in most adults, when their head is in the neutral in-line position a significant space occurs between the back of the head and the device. Suitable padding must be added prior to securing the head or the head will move to hyperextension when the strap across the forehead is tightly installed. In order to be effective, this padding must be made of a material that does not readily compress. Firm semi-rigid pads, or folded towels can be used. The amount of padding needed must be evaluated, and varies from patient to patient. A few individuals require none. If too little padding is provided, or if the padding is of an unsuitable spongy material, the head will be hyperextended when the head straps are applied. If too much padding is inserted, the head will be moved into a flexed position. Both hyperextension and flexion of the head can increase spinal cord damage and are contraindicated. It must be noted that the padding should be placed directly posterior to the occipital area — not the neck. In earlier years when soft cervical collars were used, padding behind the neck was customary. With the elimination of this ineffective type of collar and the advent of stiff collars, *padding behind the neck serves NO purpose and in sitting patients is particularly dangerous.* Padding placed behind the neck commonly slips inferiorly (becoming excessively thick), and when this occurs it acts as a fulcrum against which the head is rotated into hyperextension. *Padding behind the head is required in most patients but padding behind the neck serves no purpose and, being potentially dangerous, is NO longer recommended.*

There is almost *NO* soft tissue compression under the scapulae and the rest of the posterior torso caused by the body's weight when a person is placed supine. Therefore, the same anatomical relationship between the posterior head and the back of the torso remains true when a patient is supine on the ground. In most adult patients who are found on their back, the head has fallen back and is found in a significantly hyperextended position.

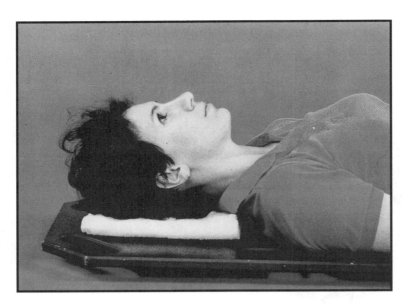

Once the head has been moved into the neutral in-line position a significant space occurs between the posterior head and the ground, and the EMT must hold the head off the ground in order to maintain the neutral alignment. Due to the sizable weight of the head this is difficult to manually maintain for any length of time. Further, if the patient must be ventilated, it is inevitable that some hyperextension will occur when obtaining a good mask seal. To avoid this, as soon as other priorities allow, insert as much padding as necessary to fill the void between the head and the ground. *In any patient placed on a long-board in which there is a space between the back of the head and the board with manual neutral in-line immobilization, sufficient suitable padding to fill the void must be inserted prior to securing the head.* If any void remains, regardless of the purchase obtained on the sides of the head, when the forehead strap is tightly secured the head will rotate backward into hyperextension and either this head movement, or the force of the rigid cervical collar against the posterior neck caused by such angulation, will cause increased pressure on the vertebrae and movement of the cervical spine.

As previously discussed, padding should only be placed under the head as needed to fill the void, and padding under the neck is without benefit and may be dangerous. The padding should be sufficiently wide to adequately support the head, but should not extend near or beyond the lateral margins of the head or under the cervical collar. If it is too wide it can interfere with the proper placement of the bolsters (side pillows of a head immobilizer or blanket rolls) used to secure the head, or worse it can be pushed inward and become excessively thick. If the padding becomes too thick it will cause the head to be flexed.

In small children (under eight years old) the size of the head in relationship to the rest of the body is much larger than in adults. The majority of the enlargement is of the part of the head which lies posterior to the spinal column. Further, the muscles of a child's back are less developed than in adults. Therefore, when a small child's head is in the neutral in-line position the back of the head usually extends one to two inches beyond the posterior plane of their back. If a small child is placed directly on a rigid surface, their head will usually be moved into a position of flexion.

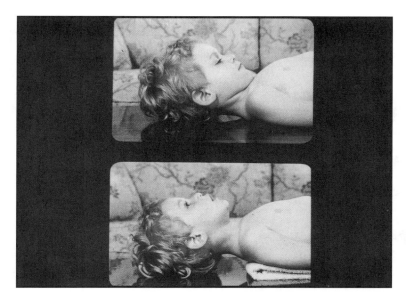

Two recent studies by Herzenberg *et al.*, concluded that placing small children on a standard long-board results in unwanted flexion. As well as the danger of compromising the spine that this presents in a child with spine trauma, even if there is no injury to the spine such extreme flexion can kink the imma-ture trachea and produce airway compromise. The longboard needs to be modified, either by creating a recess for the head in the board or by inserting padding under the torso to elevate it, in order to be able to maintain the child's head in a neutral position. Padding placed under the torso should be of the appropriate thickness so that the head can lie on the board in a neutral position: too much will result in extension, too little in flexion. The padding under the torso must also be firm and evenly shaped, and extend the full width and length of the torso from the buttocks to the top of the shoulders. Using irregu-larly shaped or insufficient padding, or placing it under only part of the torso, can result in movement and misalignment of the spine. It is unlikely that the EMT can accurately estimate the exact thickness that will be required to elevate the torso of an individual child to place the head in neutral alignment. Repeated log rolling and trial and error adjustments are unwise and greatly increase the chance of spinal cord compromise. Therefore, as a practical consideration, it is recommended that 2-1/2 inches of firm padding be placed under the torso initially (elevating the torso more than required), and then the void this produces between the back of the head and board can be filled with padding under the head as is done with an adult.

Immobilization of the Head to the Device

Once the rigid device has been immobilized to the torso and appropriate padding has been inserted behind the head as needed, the head should be secured to the device. Due to the rounded shape of the head, it cannot be stabilized on a flat surface with only straps or tape. Use of these alone will still allow the head to rotate and move laterally. Also, due to the angle of the forehead and the slippery nature of moist skin and hair, a simple strap over the forehead is unreliable and can eas-ily slide off. Although the human head weighs about the same as a bowling ball, it has a significantly different shape. The head is ovoid, being longer than it is wide and having almost completely flat lat-eral sides. It may be helpful to think of a bowling ball which has had about two inches cut off its left and right sides. Adequate external immobilization of the head, regardless of method or device, can only be readily achieved by placing pads or rolled blankets on these flat sides and securing them with straps or tape. In the case of vest-type devices, this is accomplished with hinged side flaps that are part of the vest.

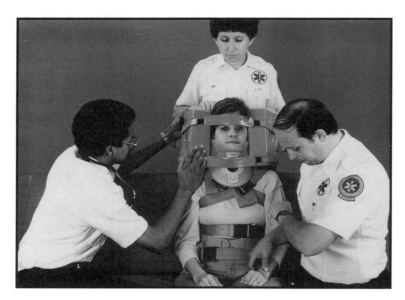

The side pieces, whether they are pre-shaped foam blocks or "home-made" rolled blankets, are placed firmly against the flat lateral planes of the head. Two straps or pieces of tape surrounding these head pieces draw the sides together and mold their inner sides to the exact shape of the head—preventing further movement. When packaged between the blocks or blankets, the head now has a flat posterior surface which can be realistically fixed to a flat board. The upper head strap is placed tightly across the front of the lower forehead (across the supraorbital ridge), and helps prevent anterior movement of the head. This strap should be pulled tightly enough to indent the blocks or blankets and rest firmly on the forehead.

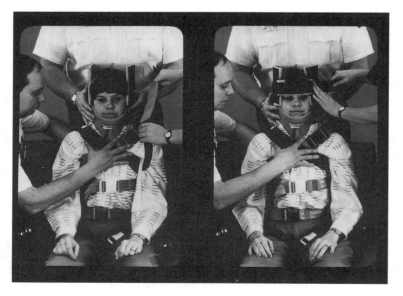

The forehead strap should be made of, or have a thin central layer made of, a rubber or foam-like non-skid surface. A non-skid surface together with a head strap that is not overly narrow is required to make sure that the strap will not slip off of the angled forehead even when it is slippery due to perspiration or from hair (which is extremely slippery) under the strap. If adhesive tape is used, it should be applied in the normal manner to obtain a maximum grasp on the forehead. Folding a portion of the tape under to keep it from sticking to the patient's eyebrows has the detrimental effect of eliminating any adhesion over the supraorbital ridge.

Chin cups, or straps which encircle the chin, prevent mouth opening and should never be used. The device holding the head—regardless of type—also requires a lower strap to help keep the side pieces firmly pressed against the lower sides of the head and to further anchor the device and prevent anterior movement of the lower head and neck. The lower strap passes around the side pieces and across the anterior rigid portion of the cervical collar. Care must be taken to ensure that this strap does not place too much pressure on the front of the collar, which could produce an airway or venous return problem at the neck.

The use of a commercial head immobilizer has been shown by experience to be the fastest and easiest way to secure the head. However, if these are not available, a blanket properly rolled into a bolster and placed at each side of the head is as effective and eliminates the problem of retrieving the device from the hospital at a later time. In order to assure adequate purchase on the lateral sides of the head to prevent any rotary movement, the pads, flaps, or blanket rolls placed at each side of the head should extend anteriorly beyond the outer ear. When making up blanket rolls for this purpose they should be rolled thickly enough that when placed on the board they will reach at least this far along the side of the head. When only one blanket is used (rolled as a continuous horseshoe roll or as a scroll) it is rarely of sufficient height and there is the danger of moving the head when it is placed. Therefore, using two separately rolled bath blankets with one at each side of the head is preferable and recommended. When blanket rolls are used, 3-inch adhesive tape (or one of the tapes which only stick to itself such as Colban®, Medi-Rip®, etc.) is customarily used to secure the blankets and head to the board instead of straps.

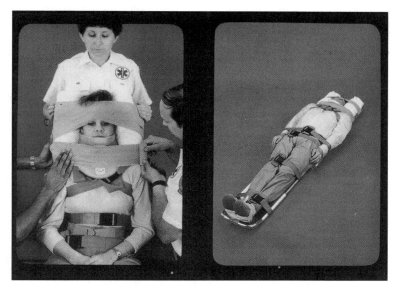

Similarly when using a vest device, if the head straps have become lost or the EMT prefers, tape can be used to secure the head flaps and head. With any device, when tape is used to secure the head care must be taken to assure that none of the pull when unwinding the tape is transferred to the patient's head or to the device. This can be achieved by securing the last tape wrapped around the head with one hand while unwinding about two feet of tape from the roll with the other and then securing that length around the head—and so on. In this way when the EMT is unwinding the tape the pull is against his other hand and his attention, when applying it, is solely focused on its correct placement.

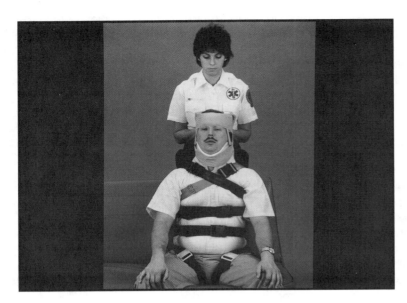

The tape should be located as would the two straps previously described. The lower part of the tape at the forehead must be low enough so that it extends and "cups" the supraorbital ridges without touching the eyes. Experience has shown that it is easiest to first anchor the tape around the center of the forehead with 2 or 3 snug turns and to then continue with tighter turns which extend further inferiorly until properly wrapped over the supraorbital ridge. The tape at the neck (as with a strap) is not secured as tightly as that on the forehead. Care must be taken to pull in a straight anterior-to-posterior direction to avoid any wrapping which would "cup" the chin by being laterally wound in a cephalad direction after placement under the chin section of the collar.

Using sandbags or IV bags secured to the spine board alongside the head and neck represents a dangerous practice. Regardless of how well secured, these heavy objects can shift and move. Should the patient and board have to be rotated to the side, the combined weight of the sandbags can produce localized lateral pressure against the cervical spine. Raising or lowering the head of the board when moving and loading the patient, or any sudden acceleration or deceleration of the ambulance, can also produce shifting of the bags and movement of the head and neck.

Immobilization of the Legs

Once the torso and the head have been immobilized to the longboard (or the immobilized seated patient has been placed on the longboard and the vest or half-board has been secured to the board) the patient's legs should be immobilized to prevent any movement of the pelvis and lower spinal column.

When they are not supporting the patient, the legs can be flexed or extended without causing angulation of the pelvis. Therefore, careful extension of the legs when lowering the patient and vest (or half-board) into a supine position onto the longboard will not cause movement of the pelvis and spine. However, sudden rotary or lateral movement of a leg, or any significant bilateral rotary or lateral movement of the legs, usually will angulate the pelvis, and immobilization of the legs to the board should include preventing any such movement.

The weight and high center of gravity of the feet commonly produce outward rotation of the legs with associated movement at the hip joint. If a fracture exists in either leg or hip, any such rotary movement or any continued movement can easily produce unnecessary additional damage. Such an injury must be assumed to be present since the multiple systems trauma patient is immobilized to the longboard prior to the EMT performing a detailed head-to-toe secondary exam. To avoid any further rotary movement and the damage it could produce, tie both feet together. This is most easily done once the patient is on the longboard and prior to immobilizing the legs to it.

The legs are commonly immobilized to the board with two straps: one placed proximal to the knees at about the mid-thigh and one distal of the knees at the mid-tibia or ankle.

The average adult measures between 14 and 20 inches from one side to the other at the hips, and only 6 to 9 inches from one side to the other at the ankles. When the feet are placed together, a V-like shape is formed from the hips to the ankles. Since the ankles are considerably narrower than the board, a strap placed from one side of the board to the other across the lower legs will prevent anterior movement but it will not prevent the legs from moving laterally from one edge of the board to the other. If the board is angled or rotated, the legs will fall to the lower edge of the board. This will in most cases angulate the pelvis and result in movement of the spinal column.

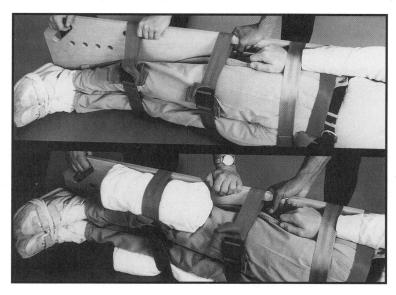

The legs can easily be kept from lateral movement, and the alignment of the legs and pelvis maintained, by the placement of blanket rolls or other firm padding to fill the space between the outer leg and the edge of the board on each side, before the distal strap is fastened over them.

If there are not sufficient blankets available for this purpose, the lower legs can be kept in the middle of the board if the distal strap is wound around them several times before attaching it to the sides of the board.

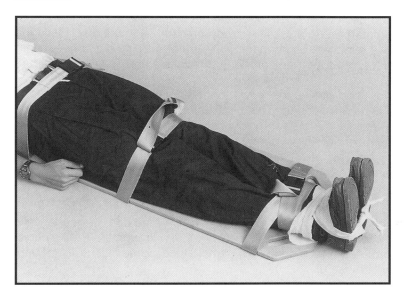

Immobilization of the Arms

In order to prevent the arms and hands from falling or becoming trapped between the board and any surface it is moved onto, they must be secured to the board prior to its being lifted. In order to support and splint any fractures in the arms (identified or not yet found) the arms should be extended along the patient's sides with the palms in and secured by a strap which surrounds the lower forearms and torso. This strap should be made snug enough that the arms cannot slip out but not so tight as to compromise the circulation in the hands. In the event that there are no holes to which to secure the strap at the correct position along the sides of the board—since this strap guards against lateral and not cephalad or caudad movement—the strap can be simply passed under the board and across the patient's arms and torso.

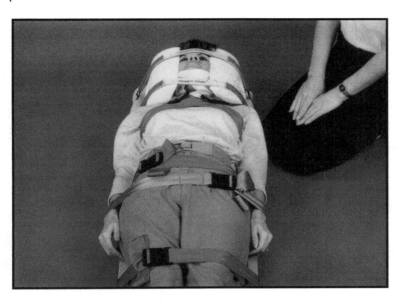

The arms should not be secured by either the strap at the iliac crests or by the groin loops. If these straps are tight enough to provide adequate immobilization of the lower torso, they can compromise the circulation in the hands. If they are loose they will not provide adequate immobilization of the torso or arms. Further, the use of a separate strap allows the EMT to release it once in the back of the ambulance, to provide for positioning an arm to start an IV or take the blood pressure, without any loss in the immobilization of the torso. If the EMT has released the strap securing the arm to accommodate either of these while enroute, he must make sure that they are properly positioned and re-secured before unloading at the hospital.

The practice of using a small strap or tie to secure the wrists together instead of placing the arms on the board at the patient's side is *NOT* recommended. This positioning places the radius and ulna across the round thorax, undesirably stressing the forearm and wrist and does not prevent the arms from moving anteriorly. Since often these have not as yet been carefully palpated, injury to the forearm or wrist may not as yet have been identified. This also places a significant percentage of the weight of the arms on the abdomen and thorax and can promote increased respiratory difficulty.

About Equipment

Based upon the patient and situation, the EMT has to determine which methods, device, and (in most cases) exact type of fixation is used to best immobilize this patient. Even though the EMT's choices are limited to using the specific items carried on the responding ambulance, some discussion of various equipment and equipment criteria will be useful.

When a patient with suspected spine trauma is found in a sitting position, his condition and the stability of the scene should be the key factors in determining how he is to be immobilized and moved from sitting where he is found (usually in a car seat) to a supine position on the longboard.

If the patient and the scene are stable, his head, neck and torso should be immobilized using a vest type device or rigid half-backboard and a cervical collar while he is sitting and before he is moved onto the longboard. Proper immobilization to either device, when done by even the most experienced crew, will take about four to five minutes from start to finish. If done more quickly it generally will result in either poor immobilization or undue jostling of the patient with movement of the spine. Therefore, if the patient's condition is unstable (such as with multi-systems trauma, etc.) or the scene is unstable, the time needed to immobilize the patient with either of these devices should *NOT* be taken. Instead, once a cervical collar has been installed, *rapid extrication* with manual immobilization of the head and torso should be used to protect the spine while lowering and positioning the patient directly onto a longboard. Although when rapid extrication is properly performed by 3 or 4 experienced EMTs the spine is manually protected, this procedure provides less stable immobilization than does a vest or half-board and it should not be arbitrarily selected as a matter of preference.

The use of a vest-type or half-board immobilization device is contraindicated in unstable patients or when the scene is unsafe, as using them produces unnecessary delay before urgent priorities can be properly evaluated and met, and extends the total field time.

The use of rapid extrication, moving the patient directly into a supine position or the longboard with only manual immobilization, produces a greater risk of spine movement (and danger of sudden failure while supporting the spine) and therefore is contraindicated when the patient and scene are stable and no urgency is present.

When the patient and scene are stable, vest-type devices are more commonly selected than are half-backboards. Although the strap location and details are different from one model to another, most vest-type devices are alike. Unfortunately, the majority of those found in the field do not have straps or a portion of the vest designed to go over the shoulders, and ties must be added to adjust for this deficit.

Vest-type devices have internal rigid slats running the full length of their posterior center section and additional vertical slats in their side flaps to prevent longitudinal bending. These are connected by the fabric covering sewn between them, allowing the unit to hinge and fit snugly around the torso. This circumferential flexibility makes them small to store and especially useful when immobilizing a patient in a contoured car seat, or when the patient must be immobilized in a confined space. Unlike a rigid half-board they do not extend significantly beyond the patient's anatomical outline once they have been applied, making them uniquely useful when an immobilized patient must be extricated through a narrow opening.

The lack of rigid attachment between the slats is essential to the flexibility needed for the vest to be easily inserted and placed around the patient's torso and head, but allows for some remaining rotary movement of the shoulder girdle and pelvis and, given enough external force, will not prevent these from slight contrary twisting. As well, they do not prevent anterior movement and medial rotation of the shoulders or keep the arms from moving. This possible remaining movement is not a problem when a sitting patient who is immobilized with a vest is simply rotated down (or carefully lifted for only a short distance) to the longboard, basket litter or other rigid full-body device. Vests are not designed for sustained use by themselves, but only to be used in transferring the patient to a longboard device before more extensive immobilization and transport are initiated.

Sometimes, when used in confined spaces, "wilderness" trail applications, or other special technical rescue situations, the patient who has been immobilized in the vest will have to be placed and carried on a blanket or stretcher which is flexible across its width (and molds around the patient's body when lifted such as a SKED, Reeves Stretcher, Ferno Flexible Stretcher, etc.), instead of being placed on a rigid full body length device. When a vest is used with such a device, a strong rigid board or splint extending from the outer lateral edge of one shoulder to the outer lateral edge of the other must be secured posterior to the patient and vest to prevent the sides of the stretcher from folding up when lifted and producing anterior medial movement of the shoulders. This can cause anterior displacement of the cervical spine.

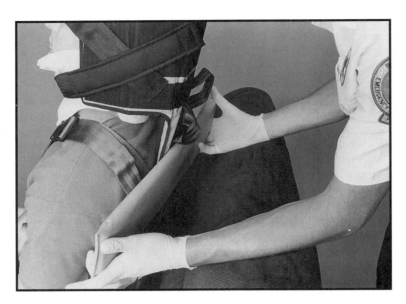

In special tactical, military, and confined space applications it may sometimes be impractical to immobilize or extricate the patient on a longboard or similar full-body rigid device since these prevent the legs from being articulated at the hips and knees. This is true even of the SKED which is designed for confined space rescue and does not extend significantly beyond the patient's outline. In such cases regardless of whether the patient is found sitting, lying, or standing, a vest and cervical collar alone will have to be used to move the patient (even if this is a sustained distance) until further immobilization onto a longboard or other rigid full body device is practical.

To secure a vest from moving laterally its sides only need to surround and conform to the lateral torso with the straps secured across the anterior thorax and abdomen. No advantage is gained by a vest continuing to include a significant part of the anterior torso. Therefore selection of a vest whose sides do not cover the anterior thorax, is recommended in order to preserve the EMT's access for further examination, cardiac monitoring and defibrillation, and chest decompression.

When a technical rescue which will involve significant hoisting or lowering of the patient is anticipated, a rigid half-board should be selected instead of a vest-type device. Full-width plastic composite or metal half-boards are much preferable to ones that have a sculptured narrower head end or are made of wood. If only a sculptured board is available it can best provide immobilization when used in an upside-down position. This method of use is fully discussed later, as a part of the demonstration for use of a half-board.

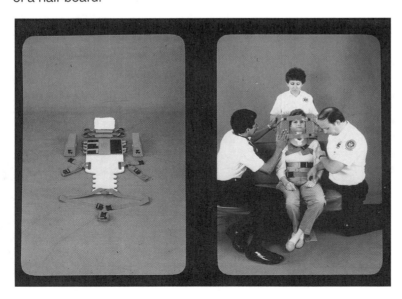

Current infection control considerations make the continued use of wooden longboards obsolete. Wooden boards provide an *unnecessary* risk of a splinter contaminated with body substances from this or a previous patient piercing the EMT's rubber glove and hand—resulting in the same exposure and potential harm as from a used needle. Even when the polyurethane coatings are carefully maintained and the edges and hand holes of wooden boards are carefully inspected between uses—the board can be damaged (resulting in edge delamination and splinters) when stored in the ambulance compartment, extracted from it, or used at the scene. Therefore, with a priority similar to providing other required EMT protection against the risk of communicable disease, as funding is available EMS services should replace wooden longboards with ones made of plastic, composition or metal. There are presently many such boards available which are stronger, of equal weight, and in many cases of better design than older boards—and yet are not significantly higher in price than commercially available wooden ones. Because of their durability, over time they will actually prove to be less expensive.

When selecting a longboard for purchase its size, tested strength, weight, shape and the size and position of holes for securing straps and carrying are key considerations.

Based upon the dimensions common to large adults (but not those who are atypically tall or wide), and the desirability that the head, torso, arm, legs, and any splint or device, be entirely supported on and within the outer perimeter of the longboard, boards would ideally be 7 feet long and 24 inches wide. This however would produce a variety of weight and storage problems and make it difficult to use the board on the cot and in many locations. As a practical compromise longboards are generally about 6 feet in length and between 16 and 18 inches in width. When possible the 18 inch width (or greater) is vastly preferable since it allows for better inferior support of the arms in most individuals.

Adult longboards which are shorter than 6 feet in length and narrower than 16 inches in width should only be used as interim devices with a basket litter, rescue toboggan, boat, helicopter or other rescue vehicle which due to space limitations necessitates the smaller size.

For the rapid and proper location of straps at any needed location and for ease in lifting, it is recommended that a board be selected which has holes almost entirely along its sides. The sequence of holes along the sides should only be interrupted by the needed cross-supports. Holes designed for carrying the board should be at both the head and foot ends and appropriately spaced along each side.

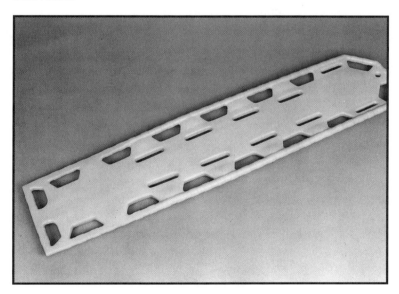

Each opening designed for carrying the board should be about 5 inches long and of sufficient width to easily allow for the insertion of a large hand wearing bulky canvas or leather protective gloves. Bisecting these holes with a narrow pin to accommodate "quick-clips" is not a problem as fingers can still be inserted on each side of the pin, and even when quick-clips are not used the pins are of benefit as they restrict the movement of straps inserted through the slot. Holes that are significantly longer present a problem since they allow straps secured through them to move excessively up or down the length of the board. The sides of the board should be slightly angled, or elevated by runners under the board, so that strap buckles can be easily inserted through the holes when the board is on the ground without any need to lift the board and patient. As well, this allows for easy insertion of the hands through the holes when preparing to lift, and prevents the EMT's hands from entrapment and injury when the board and patient are lowered onto a hard surface. It also prevents the need for the dangerous practice of placing the EMT's shoe tips under the board to allow for insertion of straps or to protect the fingers when lowering the board.

The openings in the board must include a hole in the top center of the board to accommodate the head immobilizer top strap. A separate small hole to prevent this strap from any lateral movement, or movement when a gloved hand is inserted, is preferable. A similar hole in the center of the foot end is desirable, as this allows for securing the head immobilizer at this end without again moving the patient in case he has inadvertently been placed on the board with his head at the wrong end.

Weight and strength are also considerations and these are not necessarily related. Some of the strongest man-made substances are very light (although generally more expensive than heavier ones). Only boards with a proven tested and stated failure weight are recommended. To accommodate the heaviest patients normally to be carried on a single board, the board should be rated for no less than 450 lbs. Because the strength of most devices diminish with wear, those initially rated for even more weight (500-600 lbs.) are preferable unless this makes them excessively heavy.

Some materials will bend or otherwise slowly fail before (or rather than) breaking. Longboards which will show any failure prior to their collapse or breaking are considerably safer than ones that can withstand or mask excessive weight or damage until they suddenly break. The EMT should know the maximum recommended weight for any device he uses and items should be properly maintained to ensure that they will not fail under less weight. Most plastics or composite material will deteriorate when exposed to sunlight for sustained periods. If such boards must be carried on the outside of rescue vehicles, they should be kept in a fabric case to avoid undue exposure.

Care must be taken at a haz-mat incident to protect the board from unnecessary contact if the EMT is not familiar with the chemicals involved or does not know which can cause the breakdown of his board. The board should be isolated from any substances on the ground by the use of a suitable drop-cloth and, as soon as possible, the patient and board should be decontaminated before the patient is fully mechanically immobilized to the board and is transported.

Patients are most commonly secured to boards using nylon web straps. These are typically a continuous single strap between 6 and 10 feet in length, and have compatible fasteners at each end. Although there is a wide range of models and specific designs for these fasteners, they generally are variations of three basic design principles:

- Male and female buckles on the respective ends of the strap which, when inserted into each other, positively "click" into place and remain locked until one or more release buttons is pressed.

- A pair of metal "D" rings at one end through which the other end of the strap is alternately threaded. When tightening, the strap it can be pulled through but the interactive friction between the strap and dual "D" rings prevents it from loosening until the rings are held apart especially for this purpose.

• A female "seat belt" type metal buckle through which the other end of the strap is inserted. The strap can be pulled through the buckle to tighten it but remains locked from loosening until the top of the buckle is lifted, releasing the toothed cam which has been securing the strap from withdrawal.

The last of these is *NOT* recommended since the top of the end of the buckle is easily lifted accidentally, releasing the tension and immobilization. Inadvertent release of any velcro fastening can also occur, and where these are used that event must be guarded against.

The choice between the "D" ring type or the snap-in male and female buckle type is a matter of preference. The snap-in buckle is the most prevelent type and is available in both plastic and metal. These come in a variety of brands and models with different dimensions. The male end of one brand or model will *NOT* properly insert and lock into the female end of another, and since such use is often desirable it is recommended that only the same brand and model be used on each patient.

Usually with this type of buckle the length of the strap (and therefore its tightness) can only be adjusted at one side of the buckle (by pulling the strap end through a controlled slotted slide in that half of the buckle). This is designed to only let the strap pass through it in one direction for tightening — but will not let it slide in the other and loosen the strap.

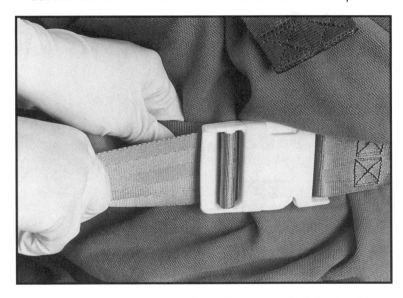

In order to loosen the strap the adjacent end of the buckle must be purposely lifted a considerable distance to release the friction on the strap and allow for its loosening.

When the strap is being tightened the buckle travels along the strap in the direction (and only for half the distance) that the strap end is being pulled. This sometimes results in the buckle ending up in an undesirable place, and can only be remedied by loosening the buckle and sliding the entire strap through the board so that when retightened the buckle will come to rest in a new place. To avoid this, a superior design which allows tightening with either strap end on each side of the buckle is now available. With this type the strap ends on each side of the buckle can alternatively be tightened, allowing for the strap to be tightened while also placing the buckle at exactly the spot desired. The bottom of most buckles is rigid and flat. This can present a problem when a buckle ends up positioned over a highly curved body surface and the strap is pulled tight — overly impressing the buckle into the patient. The problem and added discomfort it produces has been greatly minimized with the introduction of a relatively new design buckle which can be tightened in either direction and whose back is slightly curved rather than flat.

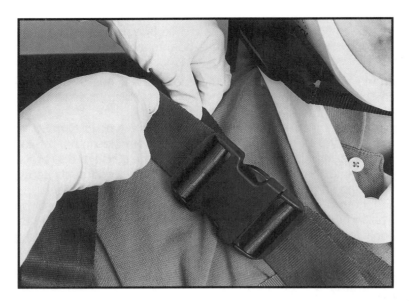

Because of the inclusion of both of these features, together with durability and the extra safety provided by the need to squeeze two opposing buttons in order to release the buckle halves, this buckle is highly recommended.

Straps are usually secured to the board by being inserted through the desired hole in the board, over the patient, through the hole on the opposite side of the board. Then both strap ends are again brought over the patient, the buckle halves are snapped together, and then the strap end is pulled to tighten the strap. This method avoids the need for lifting in order to run the strap under the board and it keeps the strap from being snagged or damaged if the board is moved on the rough ground.

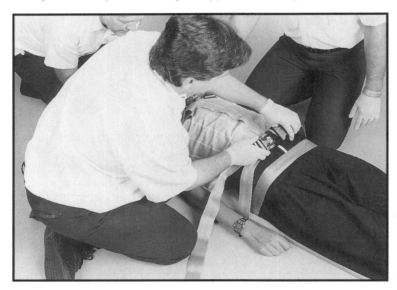

Alternatively, straps can be more easily placed and secured to the board using a Prusik knot at one side. To do this, fold the strap over itself to form a loop between 10 and 12 inches from the unadjustable buckle end. With buckles that can be tightened so they slide in either direction this loop can be formed 10 to 12 inches from either end. Next, insert the loop through the desired hole in the board, open the loop, and pass the buckles and strap ends through it.

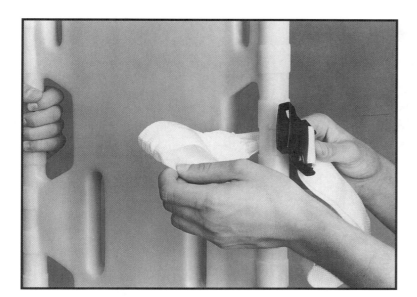

When the strap ends are pulled tight the Prusik knot will tighten firmly—anchoring the strap to the board. Next pass the longer strap end over the patient's body and through the opposing hole in the board. Then, bring it back over the patient and fasten it into the other buckle half (or the remaining end of the strap) and tighten the buckle.

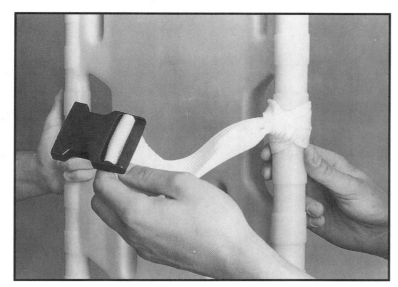

When this method is used to form the "X" over the upper torso, a strap is fastened with the Prusik knot at the hole closest to the shoulders on each side. The short strap on one side is placed over the patient's shoulder, and the long strap on the other side of the board is passed through the armpit and across the chest, and then connected to the buckle half on the short end of the first shoulder strap. Then this is repeated with the other long strap coming under the opposite armpit, across the chest, and over the remaining shoulder.

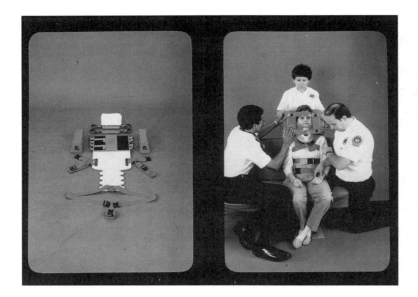

When using this method to secure the straps at the lower torso, one strap is looped and secured to the board through the hole adjacent to the iliac crest on each side.

If only an iliac crest strap is needed, the end of the strap with a male buckle from one side is connected to the female end of the strap from the other and the strap is tightened firmly over the iliac crests.

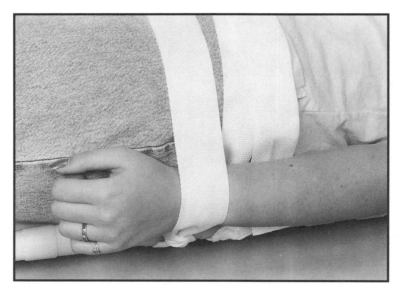

The remaining strap ends are used later, after the torso, head, and leg immobilization has been completed, to form a second strap only tightened snugly over the arms to secure them to the board.

If groin loops are desired instead, the long section of the strap on one side is placed under the buttock, through the groin and over the pelvis, and then is connected to the buckle half of *the same strap* and is tightened—forming a loop over that side of the pelvis. Then the same is done around the pelvis on the other side with the strap Prusiked to the board on that side. With groin loops, a separate strap is needed to secure the arms.

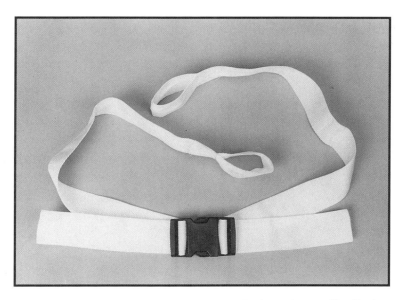

Straps are now available which are designed specifically for attachment with a Prusik knot. They come as a single half-length of strap inserted into each side of the buckle, with a loop sewn at the other end. When the buckle is released and the parts separate, the loop at the end of each half-length of strap can be rapidly fastened through the board with a Prusik knot and the other half fastened in the same way through the opposite hole. When the two buckle ends are brought over the patient and connected, a single strap passing over the patient from each side of the board will be formed.

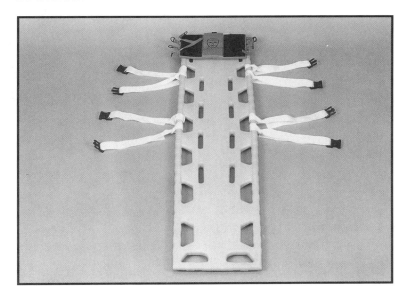

When these are to be used to form either the "X" at the upper torso or groin loops at the lower torso, two strap halves (one with a male buckle half and one with a female buckle half) will need to be attached to the proper hole at each side of the board. Similar straps are also available with a *quick-clip* rather than a loop at each end of the strap. This special connector instantly snaps over a steel pin placed across the center of the hole in the board, securing it to the board without requiring any threading through the hole or knot tying.

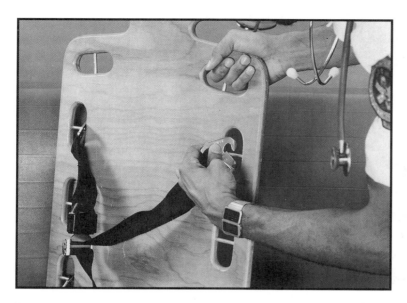

Except for connecting them to the board, these are used in the same number and way as previously described for the straps with pre-sewn loops. Straps with quick-clips at each end can only be used with longboards or half-boards that include pins for this purpose.

Other systems of fasteners, although rare, can be found on specific vests or other immobilization equipment. One vest secures with snap-hooks through metal eyes. The Kansas board is a unique half-board which has a head immobilization system and straps pre-attached to the board (for rapid installation on the patient, being designed initially for use when extricating race drivers). These employ velcro fasteners on the strap ends to provide the fastest possible immobilization and minimum delay before extricating the patient.

Pediatric Equipment and Special Considerations

The term *pediatric* is generally used to define patients from birth to 16 years of age. Since the body size, proportions of the body parts, and the musculoskeletal development of most children 12 years or older approximates those of an adult, the same methods and equipment as previously described can be used when immobilizing them, with one addition. With any child (or small adult), if the width from one lateral edge of the torso to the other is less than the distance between the holes at one side of the board and the other, a space will remain between the patient's torso on each side and the place where the strap is secured to the board. This will allow significant lateral movement of the torso regardless of how tightly the straps at the upper torso or over the pelvis have been adjusted.

In such patients, the straps at the upper torso should be applied to form an "X" (as previously described) since this configuration will properly secure under the armpit and over the shoulder even when the width between the holes in the board is greater than that of the patient. With the remaining straps, blanket rolls will have to be placed along each side of the torso to fill the space between its lateral edge and the edge of the hole to which the strap is attached, in order to prevent lateral movement of the mid or lower torso.

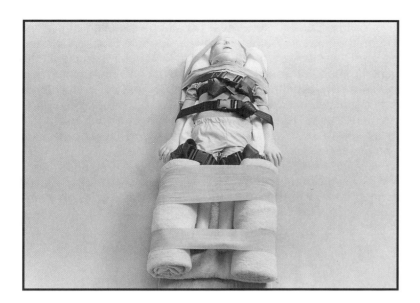

Carrying two (or more) longboards designed for use with any size patient — from large adults to the smallest of children (without the need for blanket rolls along each of the torso) — is the easiest and most practical way to provide for pediatric immobilizing. It makes the need to purchase and carry an exclusively pediatric immobilization device unnecessary and allows for easy immobilization of any mixture of patients, up to the number of boards available.

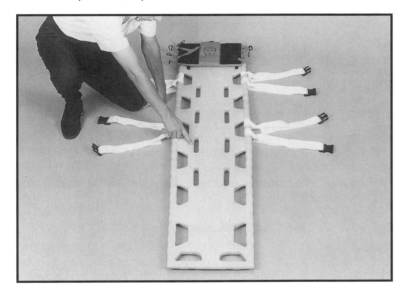

Boards designed for use with either adults or small children have a second series of holes or slots which are closer to the board's midline than those normally used to secure straps or carry the board.

There are a variety of ways to pass a long strap through these holes to effectively secure the patient so that lateral as well as other movement is prevented. Whichever method is used, the strap must pass through one of these holes, around the patient's torso (or legs), and back through the hole at the other side exclusively — or before the strap ends are brought through other holes or over the edges of the board — so that a portion of the strap lies immediately against each of the patient's lateral sides. If straps which have loops sewn at each end are to be used to secure a small child, once the buckle has been separated each half of the strap should be secured by tying the Prusik knot around the part of the board between the medial hole and an outer hole on that side — rather than as usual around the outer edge of the board at a hand-hole.

As previously discussed, the torso of children under eight must usually be elevated above the longboard in order to avoid flexion and keep the head in the neutral in-line position. Due to the small size of the iliac crests, to ensure that the immobilization at the lower torso does not interfere with the abdominal movement necessary to maintain adequate respiration in very small children, care must be taken to make sure that any straps lie solely over the pelvis and NOT over the soft anterior abdomen. The size of the usual straps and buckles used for immobilizing adults makes them enormous in relationship to a small child's or infant's body. Therefore, when immobilizing small children, it is recommended that cravats be used as ties to secure the torso and legs and tape be used to secure the head and blanket rolls, instead of straps.

Several commercial pediatric immobilization devices which replace the use of a standard adult longboard are available. Each of these includes a pre-mounted strapping system with properly sized straps and buckles located so that a small child can be properly immobilized to it without any adverse respiratory effects.

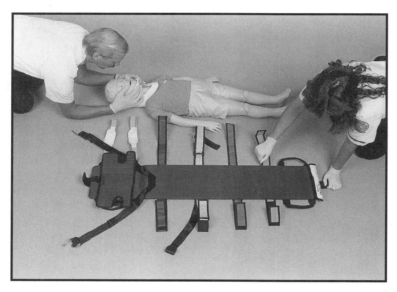

Whether their ease of use with a small child makes carrying a separate device exclusively useable for pediatric immobilization worthwhile or not, is a matter of individual judgment. Infants and small children can also be simply immobilized in their car carrier or car seat. This can be achieved by filling the voids between each side of the infant's torso and head and the side of the carrier with rolled towels or thin blankets, and taping this padding and the infant in place.

Special Considerations In Crossfield, Snow and Technical Rescues

When an immobilized patient must be carried for any significant distance, or over uneven or hilly terrain, or on snow or ice, ease and safety dictate the use of a basket-type or other rescue stretcher rather than just a standard longboard. The basket-type (Stokes) stretchers come in two basic types; wire mesh surrounded by a steel frame or a plastic "tub-like" base with an alloy top frame. As well, each of these types come in either one piece or separateable two-piece models.

The plastic type is the lightest and is recommended for simple carrying and (due to its smooth toboggan-like shape) when the litter must be hauled over snow or ice. Because it can be towed across the snow by rescuers or (with a towing bar adjunct) behind a snow mobile, this is the type most commonly used by cross-country (Nordic) ski patrols.

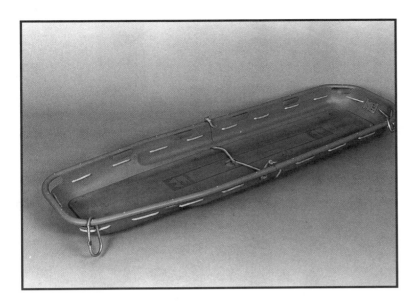

Wire basket litters have a stronger steel frame than that found in plastic ones, and must be used when doing a technical rescue to belay the patient or when doing a water rescue, so that water instantly drains out when the litter is lifted from the water. It should be noted, however, that one available plastic model has a steel frame especially designed and rated for technical belay.

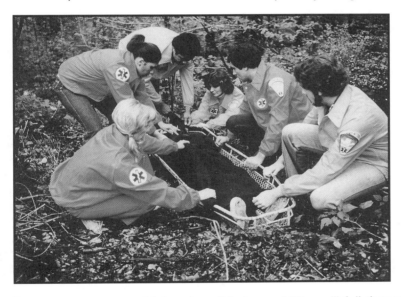

Because any snow which enters this type of litter will fall through the wire instead of accumulating, wire type basket litters (with easily removed securing pins) are commonly used on downhill rescue sleds by ski patrols.

When immobilizing a patient in a wire basket litter, the straps must be secured to the parts of the frame at the bottom of the basket (posterior to the patient's back) so that they must pass around both the lateral and anterior aspects of the patient's body when passed over the shoulders, through the armpits and groin and, in other locations, to properly surround the body to immobilize it. Straps which are anchored to the upper frame of the basket will pass solely across the anterior part of the body and prevent anterior movement, but they will not prevent movement in any other direction and therefore will NOT properly immobilize the body. When possible, fully immobilizing the patient to a longboard and then inserting the immobilized patient and longboard into the basket litter, is recommended. Immobilizing a patient in the normal method—to a longboard or with a vest or halfboard—is simpler and provides the easiest way to place him into the basket litter. As well, this eliminates the need to transport the basket stretcher to the hospital and allows for easy removal of the patient from the basket without any loss of immobilization.

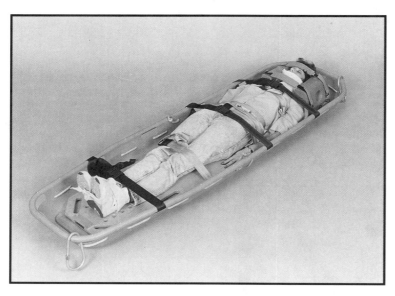

Since there is no place to anchor straps except to the top frame of a plastic basket litter, the patient must be immobilized to a longboard (or with a vest or half-board, at least) prior to being placed into this type of litter.

With either type of basket litter, immobilization to a longboard first and then insertion of the fully immobilized patient into the basket litter is generally recommended since this provides the most stable immobilization of the spine and limbs and allows easy insertion and removal from the basket litter. If the patient will have to be carried for several hours, use of a vest-type device with a basket litter is often preferred to facilitate meeting bathroom needs and to allow for alternating the position of uninjured lower limbs to increase the patient's comfort.

When a vest-type device is used to immobilize the patient in a basket litter, a longboard inside the basket litter is not needed and simply adds unnecessary weight. When a patient who has been immobilized with a vest-type device has been placed into the basket litter, the voids between the patient and the basket should be filled with blanket rolls or other padding before securing the patient into the litter. This keeps the vest device (containing the patient) and the patient's legs from any lateral movement and provides additional support alongside the head flaps.

Once a patient immobilized with either a longboard or vest-type device has been placed into the basket litter, additional straps must be fastened to the top frame of the litter across the patient in order to secure him in the basket. One of these straps should be passed through (under) the strap immobilizing the patient to the device at the armpits and preferably another through its groin loops, to ensure that the patient and immobilizing device do not shift longitudinally in the basket or, if it needs to be upended, cannot slide out of the litter.

The previously described straps, buckles or other fasteners, strapping methods and immobilization devices are not designed or rated to bear the patient's weight or to keep him properly secured when belaying or rapelling (or tobogganing or transporting in a lift or all-terrain vehicle) in a technical rescue. **Tying a lifeline to any of these and using them to hoist or lower a patient any distance greater than his standing height can result in serious injury or death of the patient and rescuer.**

When a technical rescue of a patient with suspected spine trauma is necessary, the patient should first be immobilized using the methods and equipment previously described. Then the patient and longboard or other immobilizing device, should be placed in a basket-type litter, SKED, or other appropriate rescue device, and secured to it with proper ties, webbing and other rescue equipment by a properly trained technical rescue team. All of the rescue ropes need to be fastened to the rescue litter — never to the spinal immobilization device. Regardless of the required direction of movement, the patient and rescue litter should be kept in a horizontal or near-horizontal position to ensure that proper spinal immobilization is maintained. Positioning an injured immobilized patient in a vertical position is undesirable and, if possible, should not be elected unless absolutely dictated by the rescue needs. Because sustaining such a patient in a vertical position has been shown to produce deleterious side effects, holding the time the patient is required to be in this position to a bare minimum should be a consideration when pre-planning the rescue. When this is required in places where a basket-type litter or SKED cannot be used, the patient will have to be immobilized with a vest or half-backboard device and secured with a full rescue harness (around both him and the device) to which *solely* all of the rescue ropes are fastened.

Helmet Removal

Most motorcycle, bicycle, racing and other sports helmets obstruct the EMT's easy access to the airway and to obtaining a mask seal for immediate ventilation. They also sufficiently enlarge the size of the head posteriorly to result in flexion when the patient is on a flat rigid surface. Therefore, it is advisable to remove these shortly after arrival at the scene and before access is suddenly needed or mechanical immobilization is initiated. The helmet must be removed while manual immobilization is provided and in such a way that the manual immobilization is not dislodged or interrupted. The necessary techniques and sequence of steps needed to achieve this will be demonstrated later in this Section.

Whether or not some sports helmets should be left on (and if so, which ones) remains a matter of controversy. The posterior base of most helmets curves inward and can apply pressure on the posterior portion of the cervical collar or even obstruct the EMT from applying a collar when the head is in the neutral in-line position. Almost all helmets keep the EMT from properly examining the head, and form a fluid retaining "tub" which can mask a significant amount of underlying bleeding. Any helmet which does not allow for clear access to the mouth and nose, or which would interfere with use of a ventilator with a mask or intubation if needed, must be removed. If it is elected to leave a helmet on that does not pose a problem for ventilation, but it so enlarges the posterior head that it interferes with neutral alignment, the torso will have to be elevated in the same way as for children under eight. Although it may be a matter of preference, it is our experience that leaving such a helmet on provides more potential danger than benefit, and therefore in almost all cases proper helmet removal prior to initiating mechanical immobilization to a longboard is recommended.

Obviously, helmets which have significant posterior "gutters" (such as those used by firefighters) will interfere with proper alignment and immobilization of the head and *must* be removed.

Cleaning, Sanitizing and Maintaining Immobilization Equipment

After each use, all of the disposable equipment used to immobilize the patient must be discarded in a suitable bio-medical contaminated material container. All of the re-usable equipment must be cleaned and sanitized in keeping with the current body substance isolation guidelines. After initial copious flushing with cold water to remove any blood so it is not "set" by hot water, a hot solution of mild bleach can generally be used to scrub items for this purpose. *The EMT will have to follow the manufacturer's directions carefully—only using detergents and disinfecting solutions recommended for each item. Use of others is dangerous as it may result in damage and failure of the device.* Careful attention to avoid any remaining dried body fluid substances in any recesses is required when cleaning each piece of equipment.

Each item must also be carefully checked for wear and damage before it is placed back in service. If any is found, the item must be replaced and either discarded or repaired before it is placed back in service. Any frayed strap edges or damage to a buckle will make that item difficult and unreliable to use and necessitates that it be replaced.

General Method For Immobilizing Any Patient

Even though patients initially present in many positions and there are a variety of different spine immobilization devices carried on the ambulance, one general sequence of "generic" steps is essentially followed regardless of these differences. The only significant differences surround the detailed manner in which some of these steps need to be performed with a particular device, and these do not affect the order or objectives of each step. It is essential that the EMT know this general sequence and that he understands the objectives of each step when using any device. The sequence meets the patient's needs in the proper order so that immobilization with any device follows the anatomical guidelines required to properly protect the spine and avoid any harmful side effects. Once the EMT has read the manufacturer's directions and is familiar with the detailed mechanics for the use of each immobilization device that is carried on the ambulance, this list provides a consistent guideline to be followed. The EMT will find it easier to remember and follow than if he has to memorize a separate series of steps for each individual device. Even though the initial patient presentation and immobilization device(s) may differ from case-to-case, the objectives of spinal immobilization, and the anatomical principles that must be followed if the immobilization is to be effective, do NOT.

Manufacturer's directions are rarely written to include key consideration of the current literature nor are they commonly reviewed by a medical committee which represents a knowledgeable consensus on spine trauma management and spinal immobilization practices from different areas of the country. Most often the directions are limited to the mechanics of application and do not place the item's use in the broader context of the patient's overall emergent priorities and care. Some even include suggested practices which have been found to be ineffectual or medically unsound. Even many textbooks fail to recognize considerations and key changes that have been identified in the current spine literature (and have been validated by peer review), and continue to promote ineffectual or questionable practices in the field.

The following *general method* is based upon a careful review of the literature. It has been reviewed and validated by a wide number of physicians and experienced advanced EMTs throughout the country, and is in keeping with the sequence recommended in the Pre-Hospital Trauma Life Support Course. It is presented here in an overview form, and appears again later at the end of this Section as a *Summary Skill Sheet* with a greater number of individual sub-skills identified as separate steps.

GENERAL METHOD FOR SPINAL IMMOBILIZATION

Once safety, the scene, and the situation have been assessed, and the EMT has determined from the mechanism of injury (or the patient's apparent injuries) that the possibility of an unstable spine exists, and after confirming that the proper Body Substance Isolation precautions have been taken:

1. Direct another EMT to move the patient's head into the neutral in-line position (unless contraindicated) and to continue support and manual in-line immobilization without interruption until mechanical immobilization of the head, neck, and torso have been completed.

2. Evaluate the patient's ABCs and provide any required interventions. Examine the patient further and check the motor ability, sensory response and distal circulation in all four extremities (MSC X 4).

3. Examine the neck and measure and apply a properly fitting, effective cervical collar.

4. Identify the methods and device(s) to be used and any additional tape, straps, ties, etc., that will be needed. Unpackage the device and other equipment, and prepare all components so they are nearby and ready to use.

5. Position the device on the patient, or the patient on the device so that the head is at the right height on the device and the patient is properly centered on it.

6. Starting at the upper torso, immobilize the torso (upper, lower, and if indicated mid) to the device so that it can not move up or down, left or right, or anteriorly away from the rigid device.

7. Before securing the head, re-evaluate the torso straps (including groin loops if applied) and adjust and add any as needed.

8. Evaluate and provide firm padding as needed to fill any void between the back of the head and the device.

9. Immobilize the head to the device, being sure that the neutral alignment is properly maintained. (If using a vest device or half-board, once the torso and head have been properly immobilized move the patient and device onto the longboard).

10. Once the torso and head (or upper and lower ends of the vest or half-board) have been immobilized to the longboard, tie the feet together and immobilize the legs so that they can not move anteriorly or laterally.

11. Place the arms on the backboard extended palm-in along the patient's sides, and secure them to the board.

12. Recheck the ABCs and motor, sensory and distal circulation in all four extremities.

Achieving a Proper Level of Competence

New equipment which is different from previous models, or new techniques, should not be placed in service until all of the EMTs have had supervised in-service training and have demonstrated their ability to use them properly. If it is not practical to provide this for an entire squad at one time, both the old and new equipment should remain available until all of EMTs have been in-serviced. Simply providing copies of written instructions or requiring independent viewing of a video demonstration, regardless of its quality, is not an appropriate substitute for proper demonstration by a knowledgeable instructor followed by supervised practice. Although these are useful adjuncts, they should not be used instead.

The EMT should *never* use a new immobilization technique, type of cervical collar, or immobilization device or adjunct equipment until he has repeatedly used it in supervised practice sessions on a healthy subject and can demonstrate his ability to use it—without guidance or remediation—to a proper level of competence.

When practicing or evaluating one's ability to use a device to properly immobilize a (mock) patient, rather than using the specific directions as the standard it is more useful to use a broader and more universal set of criteria. The following generic criteria serve as good tools for measuring if the proper sequence of care for a suspected unstable spine has been followed and how effectively the "patient" has been immobilized.

Criteria for Evaluating Spine Immobilization Skills

- Were the appropriate body substance isolation precautions taken?
- Was manual in-line immobilization initiated immediately, and was it maintained until it was replaced mechanically?
- Was an effective, properly fitting cervical collar applied appropriately?
- Can the device move up or down the torso?
- Can it move left or right at the upper torso?
- Can it move left or right at the lower torso?
- Can any part of the torso move anteriorly off the rigid device?
- Does any tie which circumferentiates the chest inhibit chest excursion, resulting in ventilatory compromise?
- Is the head effectively immobilized so that it can not move in any direction, including rotation?
- Is the head in a neutral in-line position?
- Does anything inhibit or prevent the mouth from being opened?
- Was the torso fully immobilized to the device before any part of the head was secured to it?

- Are the legs immobilized so that they cannot move anteriorly, rotate, or move from side to side, even if the board and patient are rotated onto their side?
- Are the pelvis and legs in a neutral in-line position?
- Are the arms appropriately secured to the board?
- After fully completing the immobilization, were motor, sensory and distal circulation checked in all four extremities?
- Are any ties or straps compromising distal circulation in any limb?
- Was any part of the torso immobilization (including groin loops, if applied) adjusted after the head was secured to the device, causing any movement of the head or neck?
- Was the patient bumped, jostled, or in any way moved in a manner that could compromise an unstable spine while the device was being applied?
- Was any method or equipment used, or is the placement of any strap or other item, inappropriate for the patient's condition or identified injuries?
- Was the procedure completed within an appropriate time frame?

Although these criteria are primarily used to evaluate the EMT's performance when practicing or in a testing situation, they are also useful for self-evaluation when immobilizing a real patient.

Individual Immobilization Skills and Sub-Skills

Almost all methods used to immobilize patients with suspected spine injury require three EMTs to perform them properly and to ensure the maintenance of manual immobilization throughout. When only two EMTs are available, one should maintain manual immobilization at the head while the second applies the device. When First Responders or others are enlisted to help, care must be taken to assign them tasks that do not require previous training (such as positioning the longboard), or are the least sensitive (such as moving the legs), and to furnish them with precise directions. Often, using more than three EMTs will facilitate easier and more rapid completion of the immobilization. In many areas when an engine company responds to the scene of an accident with the ambulance, this enlarged capability is readily available at the scene.

It is impractical and usually unnecessary to show every possible variation in the position and number of EMTs performing a skill. Therefore, the demonstrations in the following pages have been presented using three EMTs when required to perform the procedure properly, and using first responders or other available individuals when additional personnel are required.

These demonstrations describe *only* the spinal immobilization skill being shown — they are not scenarios. When immobilizing a patient on an actual call, the EMTs would have evaluated the scene and situation and assured their safety and that of the patient. They would have taken the appropriate body substance isolation precautions and, after initiating manual immobilization of the head, would have completed the additional assessment and care indicated prior to mechanically immobilizing the patient with a device. Also, the motor ability, sensory response and distal circulation in all four extremities (unless urgency dictated this be omitted) would be *checked prior* to immobilizing the patient to the device. In the following demonstrations it is presumed that these steps have been taken and that the immobilization is being performed at the proper time in the priorities of care. As well, other patient care items which may need to be interjected into the immobilization sequence have not been included since the need for such care and at what point it should be appropriately provided will vary on a case-by-case basis.

Skills such as manual immobilization of the head, helmet removal, logrolls, etc., which are essentially sub-skills when immobilizing a patient are presented first, and the EMT's knowledge of the detailed discussion in the introduction and of them is assured in the complete immobilization demonstrations which follow.

MANUAL IMMOBILIZATION OF THE HEAD

The skills used to provide manual immobilization to a sitting or standing patient from either behind, at the side, or in front of the patient, or when a patient is supine, are different and each is detailed in the following demonstrations.

In sitting or standing patients the manual immobilization is most easily and reliably provided from behind the patient. This is recommended except when it is necessary to provide it from another position, or when it is provided by a second EMT for a short period to allow the EMT behind the patient to move or perform another needed task without causing any interruption in the immobilization. Similarly, in a supine patient, manual immobilization provided by an EMT positioned beyond (above) the patient's head is the easiest and most reliable, and is recommended except when it must be provided from alongside the patient for a short period to allow for another procedure that requires positioning from beyond the head (such as intubation). Regardless of the patient's initial presentation, an unnecessary risk occurs when the senior EMT on the call provides the initial manual immobilization. He should instead direct another EMT to provide it in order to keep himself available to move as needed to assess the patient and provide (and supervise) the patient care without the need of transferring the manual immobilization from one EMT to another.

The methods for maintaining manual neutral in-line immobilization when performing airway maneuvers or ventilating a patient are discussed in Sections 4 and 5.

MANUAL IMMOBILIZATION FROM BEHIND
(Sitting or Standing Patient)

1. From behind the patient, with your fingers extended forward and just *slightly* upward, center your palms just behind the patient's ears as shown.

2. Place the thumbs against the posterior aspect of the skull. Be careful not to press them anteriorly, causing flexion.

3. Place the distal third of your little finger directly under the angle of the mandible.

4. Spread your remaining fingers on the flat lateral planes of the head and increase the strength of your grasp.

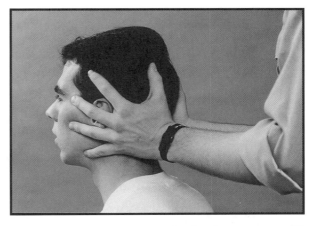

5. If the head is not in a neutral in-line position, slowly move it until it is.

6. Bring the arms in and rest them against the seat, headrest, or your torso for support.

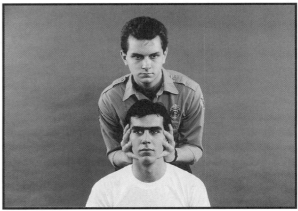

MANUAL IMMOBILIZATION FROM THE SIDE
(Sitting or Standing Patient)

1. Stand just slightly in front of the patient's side so that your body is nearly perpendicular to his and your hip (sitting patient) or shoulder (standing patient) is adjacent to his shoulder.

2. Extend your arm closest to the patient over the top of his shoulder and, while lightly resting your forearm on his clavicle, cup the back of his head in your hand while keeping your fingers slightly separated. Care must be taken before placing your second hand to *NOT* place any anterior pressure on the back of the head to avoid pushing it into flexion.

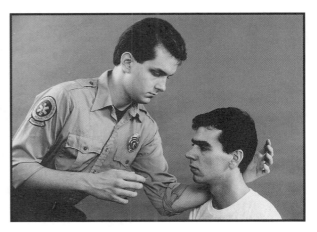

3. Between where the upper molars insert in the maxilla and the inferior margin of the zygomatic arch, an indentation is formed. By placing the thumb and first finger of your other hand on each cheek respectively just inferior to the zygomatic arch, they will be in this indentation. Its exact location can easily be ascertained by feel, and it provides a secure place to grasp the face so that movement can be eliminated.

4. Tighten the anterior and posterior pressure of the hands.

5. If the head is not in a neutral in-line position, move it until it is. Brace your elbows on your torso for support.

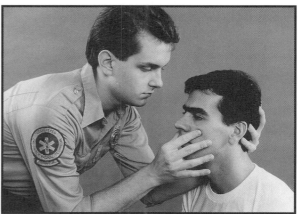

Note: This technique is especially useful in situations which preclude an EMT from taking a position behind the patient. In car accidents, it is recommended that it be used by the EMT who first contacts the patient at his opened door. This allows the EMT to support and immobilize the patient's head if the car inadvertently moves when another EMT enters the car and behind the patient, or if the patient instinctively tries to turn his head to see or speak to either EMT.

MANUAL IMMOBILIZATION FROM IN FRONT
(Sitting or Standing Patient)

1. Stand directly in front of the patient and face him. Place your palms on the patient's lower cheeks with your wrists level with the patient's chin and your extended fingers pointing *slightly* upwards.

2. Extend the little fingers of each hand around the back edges of the head and move them until you can feel that their distal ends are "hooked" under the base of the skull. Do not push anteriorly as this could cause flexion.

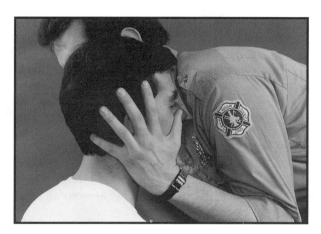

3. Extend your thumbs upward and place one in the indentation that can be felt just inferior to the zygomatic arch on each cheek, as shown. Spread the three remaining fingers of each hand on the flat lateral planes of the head. Once all of your fingers have been properly placed, increase the anterior-posterior pressure between your thumbs and the medial pressure between both hands to increase your grasp on the head.

4. If the head is not in a neutral in-line position, slowly move it until it is.

5. Bring your arms in and brace your elbows against your torso for support.

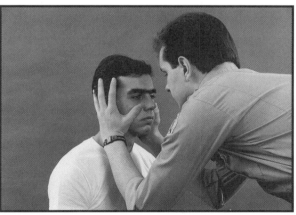

Note: Manual immobilization from in front of a sitting or standing patient is more difficult and less stable than from behind or alongside, and its use is only recommended when neither of these is practical. It is especially recommended, however, to take over the immobilization from an EMT behind the patient for short periods to allow him to perform a task such as placing the head flaps of a vest device around the sides of the patient's head. In such cases this provides safer immobilization of the head than if he attempted to maintain the head and perform the task alone.

MANUAL IMMOBILIZATION OF A SUPINE PATIENT

Injured patients who present in a lying position are usually found on the ground and, once placed on a longboard, manual immobilization must be furnished at the ground level until mechanical immobilization of the torso and head have been completed. When the EMT must provide manual immobilization for a patient supine on a backboard that has been elevated on the ambulance cot or a hospital bed (or if the patient has been found lying on an elevated surface), the same method for grasping the head as demonstrated should be used, and only the position and support of the EMT's arms will need to be modified.

The EMT should always be on both knees with them sufficiently apart to provide a stable base whenever kneeling is necessary to provide manual immobilization. Kneeling with both knees close together or when the EMT is supported on one knee and the other foot, is relatively unstable and is *NOT* recommended.

1. Kneel beyond the patient's head so that you are approximately centered on the midline of the patient and face in a caudad direction. Place your knees so that they are comfortable and sufficiently apart to provide a stable base, and so that the anterior edge of each bent knee is approximately aligned with the top of the patient's head. Move down your haunches (so your buttocks are on or near your lower legs). Once properly positioned, extend your fingers and place your hands on the flat lateral planes on each side of the head.

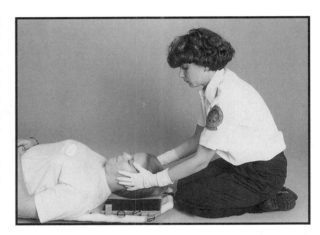

2. Spread the last two fingers of each hand by moving their tips posteriorly until they (or at least the distal end of the little finger) are felt to be located partly under the posterior aspect of the base of the skull.

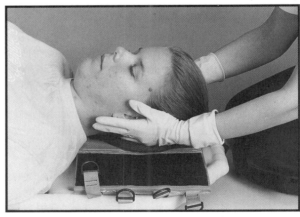

3. Next extend your thumbs upward and place one in the indentation that can be felt just caudad to the zygomatic arch on each cheek as shown. Spread the remaining fingers of each hand on the flat lateral planes of the head and increase the anterior-posterior pressure between the little fingers and thumbs and medial pressure between both hands, in order to perfect your grasp of the head.

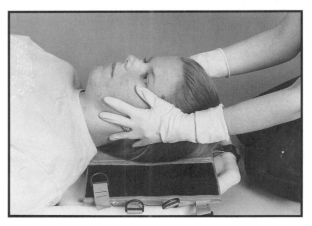

4. In most cases when an adult is on a rigid flat surface the head will be hyperextended. If the head is not in a neutral in-line position, slowly move it until it is. With most adult patients this will result in a significant void between the back of the head and the ground or backboard, and the EMT will have to support the head off the ground or backboard. This makes the manual immobilization tenuous and, if it must be sustained for any period of time or when ventilating the patient, unstable. To overcome this, the EMT should direct another EMT to place as much firm padding under the back of the patient's head as is required to fill the void.

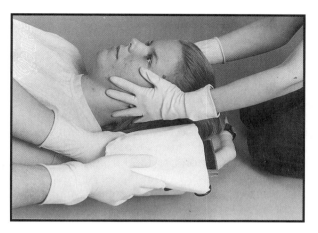

5. Whenever you will be holding the head for any period in which immediate movement of the patient is not anticipated, it is necessary to properly support your arms so that fatigue does not cause movement of them. Without moving the patient's head, carefully lower your arms until each forearm rests securely on your thighs. When this is anatomically difficult or uncomfortable, you should instead bring your arms in and brace your elbows against your torso to provide at least some support.

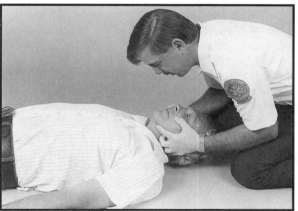

6. Often manual immobilization for a substantial period of time is anticipated in non-urgent patients to allow for careful head-to-toe examination and item-by-item care of fractures or other individual injuries before the patient is mechanically immobilized on a longboard. In such cases, experience has shown that the manual immobilization can be more comfortably and stably provided by the EMT lying beyond the patient's head with his elbows supported on the ground. When movement of the patient is anticipated, without moving the patient's head the EMT will either have to draw his knees up and rise to a kneeling position or temporarily transfer the immobilization to another EMT while he repositions himself.

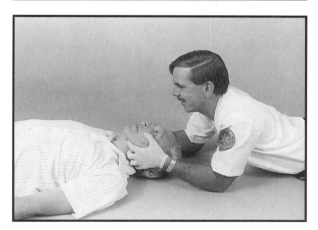

7. When a supine patient with spine trauma needs to be ventilated, the EMT providing the manual immobilization from beyond the patient's head—by making some minor adjustments in the positioning of his thumbs and fingers—can also provide the mask seal and keep the patient's mandible from sagging while a second EMT provides the ventilations. These techniques and those required when a single EMT must provide both the manual immobilization and ventilation simultaneously have been included in the ventilations skills found in Section 5.

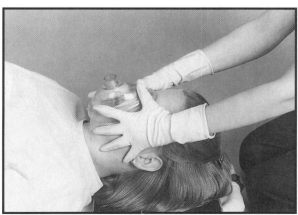

MANUAL IMMOBILIZATION FROM THE SIDE OF A SUPINE PATIENT

Manual immobilization of the head of a supine patient can alternatively be provided from along-side the patient's torso. Immobilizing the head from this position is more difficult and less stable than from beyond the patient's head, and is therefore not recommended as the primary method unless dictated by the scene or situation.

It is especially useful for periods when an EMT is performing another procedure which requires that he be positioned beyond the patient's head or to assume the immobilization temporarily when the EMT providing it from there needs to move or perform another task. It is also used as an adjunct to the immobilization provided from beyond the patient's head during forceful procedures (as when elevating the mandible with the laryngoscope while intubating) in order to provide an additional second grasp on the head to prevent it from moving.

1. When the manual immobilization of the head of a supine patient must be provided from a position other than beyond his head, kneel alongside of the patient's mid-torso so that you are directly facing the patient's head. Extend your arms and hold your hands several inches anterior or lateral of the patient's face and, using them as a measure, move up or down the side of the patient until you are at a level that will allow you to effectively and comfortably grasp the head. The knee closest to the patient should be placed touching or immediately adjacent to the patient's side and your knees should be sufficiently far apart to provide a comfortable and stable base.

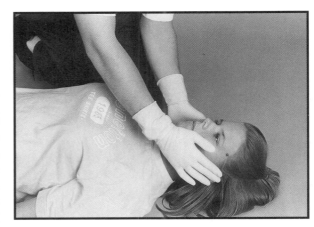

2. Place your hands on the flat sides of the patient's head so the palms are just anterior to the angle of the mandible and the fingers point slightly downwards towards the posterior portion of the top of the head. Spread your little (or 3rd and 4th) fingers until their distal ends can be felt to rest under the posterior aspect of the skull.

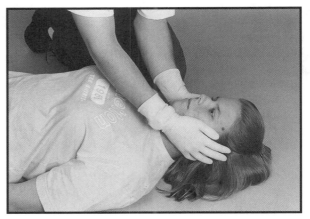

3. Extend your thumbs medially and place a thumb in the notch that can be felt just caudad of the zygomatic arch on each cheek. Spread the remaining fingers on the flat lateral planes of the head. The hand position and placement of the fingers is the same as when immobilizing the head of a sitting patient from the front.

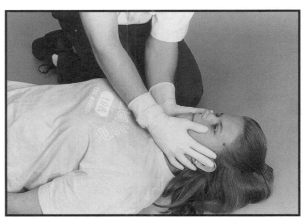

4. Increase the anterior-posterior pressure between your thumbs and little fingers and the medial pressure between both hands to increase your grasp and prevent any movement of the head. If the patient's head is not in a neutral in-line position, carefully move it until it is. Without moving the patient's head, draw your elbows in and rest them against your torso to support and stabilize your arms. If there is a void between the back of the patient's head and the ground (or board), have a second EMT place firm padding under the head as needed to fill it.

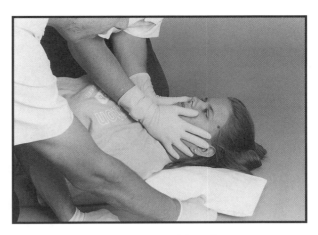

5. When the patient's head must be immobilized from alongside the patient in order to provide for an additional grasp or to replace the immobilization being provided by another EMT, care must be taken to assure that the immobilization is not interrupted or the initial grasp dislodged. Position yourself properly at the patient's side and place your palms *over* the first EMT's fingers which are extended over the flat lateral planes of the head. Spread your fingers and place your little fingers under the posterior aspect of the skull, with your thumbs on each cheek caudad and adjacent to the first EMT's thumbs.

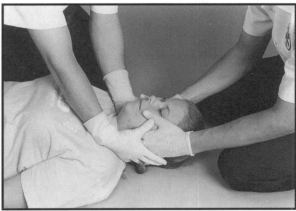

6. The head will be more stable if the first EMT rotates his hands slightly (or moves them slightly more towards the top of the head) and replaces his thumbs onto the patient's forehead without losing the placement of his little fingers under the posterior aspect of the skull while you increase the anterior-posterior pressure between your thumbs and little fingers. When both of you increase your anterior-posterior and medial pressure the posterior head is held from under each end, anteriorly the head is held at both the forehead and at the zygomatic "notch," and along the entire length of the flat lateral planes of the head.

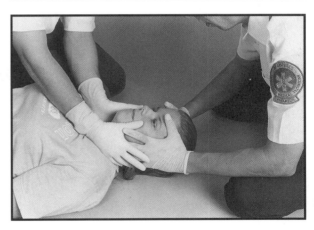

7. When you will be providing immobilization from the side to replace that being provided from beyond the head, first make sure that any void under the head has been filled with padding. Position your hands over those of the other EMT and apply firm anterior-posterior pressure against the patient's head and medially against the other EMT's hands. As he horizontally withdraws his hands, a progressively smaller portion of his hands and a greater portion of your hands will contact the patient's head.

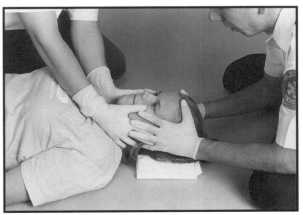

MODIFICATION IN MANUAL IMMOBILIZATION OF SUPINE CHILDREN (Below 8 Years Old)

As previously discussed, due to the larger size of the head and lesser development of the immature muscles of the back in most children under eight, the back of the head when in the neutral in-line position extends posteriorly between one and two inches beyond the posterior plane of the torso. This causes the head to move to extreme flexion when the small child is supine on a rigid surface and prevents its being moved into neutral alignment until the torso has been sufficiently elevated to counteract the problem. Although the EMT's positioning and hand placement on the patient's head are unaltered for adults and small children (except as may be caused by their smaller size), the procedure must be modified for small children until the torso has been elevated.

1. Once you have positioned yourself beyond the child's head and, with your hands properly placed, have firmly grasped the child's head, carefully move it into lateral and rotary midline alignment. If extremely flexed however, do *NOT* attempt to relieve the flexion as any extension from the flexed position before the shoulders are elevated will move the head into a *forward sniffing* position causing some cervical vertebrae to move anteriorly and some posteriorly — which is contraindicated.

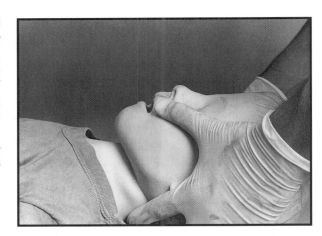

2. While you maintain the immobilization of the head the child should be logrolled (or lifted with appropriate spinal protection) by other EMTs and, as soon as the torso is off of the rigid surface, you should move the head and complete positioning it in the neutral in-line position. Approximately two inches of flat padding should be placed on the rigid surface so that when the child is returned to lying on it, it will extend from the cephalad edge of the shoulders to distal of the buttocks (or all the way distal to the feet) and from one lateral edge of the torso to the other. Then the child should be moved with the torso placed properly on the padding.

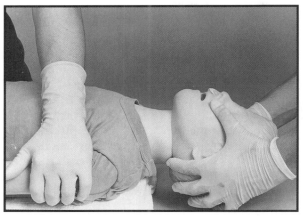

3. Once the child is on the padding with his torso elevated, check and make any needed adjustment in the neutral in-line alignment of the head. Trying to approximate the amount needed to exactly elevate the torso so the head will be supported on the rigid surface when in neutral alignment is not recommended as this will usually result in the undesirable need to move the child several times. Therefore, the torso should instead be overly elevated — producing a void between the back of the head and the rigid surface. Then, as in an adult, as much padding as is needed should be placed under the head to fill this void, and a cervical collar can be installed.

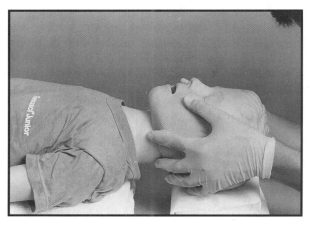

HELMET REMOVAL

Patients wearing full-face helmets must have the helmet removed early in the assessment process to provide immediate access to the airway and face, to ensure that hidden bleeding is not occurring into the posterior helmet, and to allow the head to be moved (from the flexed position caused by large helmets) into neutral alignment. Explain what is going to happen to the victim. If he indicates that he was told that the helmet should not be removed, explain that this warning was given to avoid removal by untrained spectators but does not apply to properly trained rescuers. While one EMT immobilizes his head by holding the helmet, continue to explain that you and the other EMTs have been trained to remove it while protecting his spine, and explain the procedure you will perform before starting. The procedure will require two EMTs.

Four essential elements are key when properly removing a helmet. The head should be immobilized by an EMT holding the helmet immediately upon arrival. The face shield should also be elevated and then removed immediately to allow the EMT to assure that a patent airway and adequate air exchange is present, and to provide access for suctioning, insertion of a simple airway adjunct and ventilation of the patient immediately or without delay at a later time. This will also assure that any forceful vomiting that may occur is not reflected off the shield and back into the patient's mouth and nose.

The two EMTs alternately immobilize the patient's head. *Both EMTs NEVER move their hands at the same time.* While one EMT immobilizes the head the second moves his hands, and then while he takes over the immobilization the first EMT moves, and so on.

Lastly, the helmet must alternately be rotated in different directions: to first clear the nose it must be rotated in one direction, and then in the opposite direction to allow the curvature at the posterior caudad edge of the helmet to clear the posterior curve of the head without causing it to move to flexion.

In cases where the helmet has broken and a fragment or shard of the helmet is impaled in the head, removal of the helmet or impaled part should NOT be attempted. In such cases the face visor should be removed to provide access to the patient's mouth and nose, and his torso should be elevated as for a child under eight (both while on the ground and when placed and immobilized on a longboard). This will allow his head, enlarged by the helmet, to be placed in the neutral in-line position. Sometimes in sporting events which involve players wearing helmets, a backboard with a hole cut out of the midline of the head end is available. When the helmeted head is centered on this hole, it allows for the head to be placed in neutral alignment without the need to elevate the torso.

After assuring that the scene is safe and that the proper body substance isolation precautions have been taken:

1. The first EMT kneels above the patient's head. With his palms pressed on the sides of the helmet and his fingertips curled over its lower margin, he immobilizes the helmeted head in as close to a neutral in-line position as the helmet allows. Care must be taken to assure that the head is not rotated from flexion to such a degree that the posterior caudad edge of the helmet is pushing against the posterior neck.

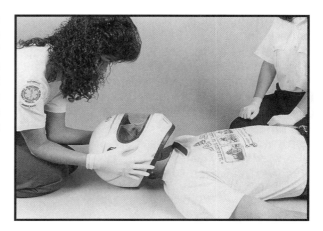

2. The second EMT kneels alongside the patient's torso and opens the face shield, and checks the airway and breathing. Next, if possible, he removes the face shield from the helmet completely and undoes (or cuts, if necessary) the chin strap.

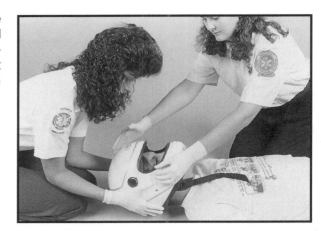

3. After releasing the chin strap, the second EMT should move to a position from which he will be able to hold the lower head. Experience has shown this can be best and most comfortably done by kneeling near the patient's waist or by lying on an angle next to the patient. When properly positioned, the second EMT should place one hand under the neck and as far under the head as is allowed by the posterior caudad edge of the helmet. His other hand should then be placed so that the mandible is grasped between the thumb at the angle of the mandible at one side and the first two fingers at the angle at the other side.

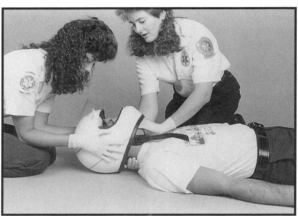

4. Once the second EMT is in place and acknowledges that he has taken over the immobilization of the head, the first EMT releases his hold on the helmet. He repositions his hands to the sides of the helmet so that his fingers are curved around the helmet's caudad edge, and the fingertips are inserted under it. This will enable him to spread the helmet slightly when he withdraws it. With helmets that have a lower face piece, care must be taken to only pull the sides apart sufficiently to separate them from the patient but no more, as excessive separation of the sides will cause the lower face piece of the helmet to flatten and move posteriorly.

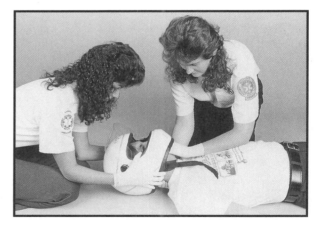

5. With the sides held just so that they no longer contact the patient's face, the first EMT rotates the helmet so the lower edge of the face piece turns towards him and becomes sufficiently elevated above the patient's face to clear his nose. Then while keeping the back of the helmet on the ground, he carefully pulls it in a straight line towards him for an inch or two. He should stop withdrawing the helmet before its curved back starts to elevate the patient's occiput and increases the flexion.

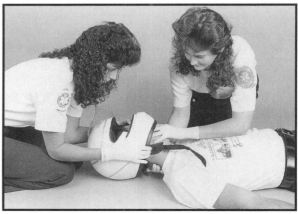

6. Once stopped the first EMT again takes over the immobilization by squeezing the sides of the helmet against the head, and acknowledges that it is safe for the second EMT to move his hands. The second EMT slides the hand which is cupped under the patient's neck as far cephalad as he can, until the side of his hand is again fully against the caudad posterior edge of the helmet. This should place the hand under a significant portion of the occiput and will keep the head from suddenly dropping when the helmet is fully withdrawn. Next he should move his other hand so that the thumb and first finger are placed on each side of the nose in the notch that can be felt just caudad of the zygomatic arch.

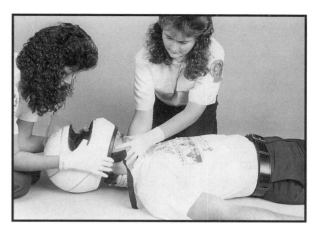

7. When his hands are securely in place, the second EMT retakes the manual in-line immobilization, and once he confirms this the first EMT will be able to safely remove the helmet completely. With the helmet edges again grasped and pulled until they are separated from the patient's head, the first EMT continues to pull the helmet in a straight line towards his own abdomen while rotating the helmet through about 30 degrees — in the opposite direction than before — and following the curve of the head. The correct amount of rotation is essential when removing the helmet as it causes the curved posterior lower margin of the helmet to point caudad rather than anteriorly, allowing it to pass under the occiput without lifting the head into flexion.

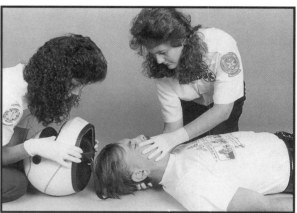

8. Once the helmet has been fully removed, the first EMT again takes hold of the head from his position beyond the patient's head. Once he has properly grasped the head he should carefully move it into the neutral in-line position and maintain his manual immobilization without interruption until the head has been mechanically immobilized to a rigid device. The second EMT is now available to provide any padding required under the head, to continue the patient's assessment, and to install a cervical collar.

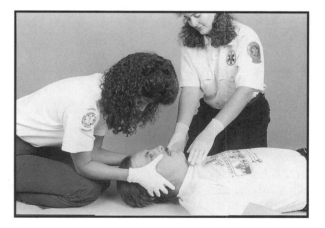

USING A SCOOP STRETCHER (Split Litter)

The use of a scoop stretcher, when properly inserted and lifted, provides more consistent support of the entire body and less risk of undesirable movement than other methods for transferring a supine patient with spine trauma onto a rigid longboard. This makes it the method of choice in patients with spine trauma and an unstable pelvis or shoulder girdle (contradicting logrolling or a body drag), or a number of fractures in bilateral extremities.

The scoop stretchers presently available have four sections: two which support the upper body and two which support the lower. The lateral sides of the upper and lower sections have lower extensions which are kept inserted into each other and allow the length of the device to be adjusted to the specific height of the patient. Built-in locking pins or friction locks on each side prevent the length from changing or the upper and lower parts from separating when in use. The scoop stretcher generally only needs to be split into two long halves (with the head and foot sections of each side remaining connected) for insertion under the patient. In cases where the patient's size or weight dictates, or the EMTs prefer, it can be separated into all four sections and each inserted separately. If the latter is elected the two head sections are inserted and reconnected first and then each leg section is inserted and connected in turn.

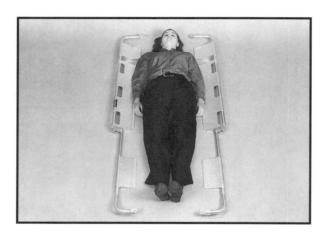

The scoop litter is designed to be separated in the center of the head and foot ends to divide it into two long halves. In this way a half can be easily inserted under the patient from each side and then reconnected to the other half to form the completed scoop upon which the patient is lifted. The left and right halves at the head and foot ends usually snap together, causing a spring loaded pin to automatically secure them together safely.

In some earlier models, a large threaded pin is provided on one side which, when the two halves are connected, is inserted through a hole in the other side and is then locked in place by a ball-like hand-nut.

Presently, scoop stretchers are made of a metal alloy to minimize their weight and their interference with X-Ray imaging. Because of this they are not truly rigid. When lifted, there is a tendency for the middle portion to sag, causing the device to become slightly curved between the head and foot ends. Also, some additional separation of the sides (and sleeves under the patient) occurs at the middle of the device. Therefore, they should never be lifted exclusively from their head and foot ends. Even when carried from the sides as well as the head and foot ends, some bending and "bouncing" of the middle of the device is unavoidable. The independent use of a scoop stretcher is only recommended while lifting the scoop several inches from the ground by its sides to allow the insertion of a rigid longboard under the scoop. When the scoop is to be used to immobilize the patient's spine at any other time, it is recommended that the patient and scoop be secured onto a longboard before being carried, upended, or moved more extensively. In the absence of spine trauma a scoop stretcher often provides a good lightweight device for carrying a supine patient up or down stairs.

When using a scoop stretcher to transfer a supine patient with spine trauma onto a longboard the EMT has two choices. Once the scoop has been inserted under the patient and its two halves have been reconnected, the EMT can fully immobilize the patient to the scoop (in the same manner as to a longboard) and then secure the patient and scoop to the longboard leaving the scoop stretcher in place under the patient. (It should be noted that this is the only possible method for ensuring that proper immobilization is maintained while transferring the patient onto a longboard when only two EMTs are available). Alternatively, the scoop stretcher can be used with only manual immobilization of the head, a cervical collar, and careful maintenance of its horizontal alignment to lift the patient while a longboard is lcngitudinally inserted under it. Once the scoop has been placed on the longboard it is separated and removed and then the patient can be directly immobilized to the board.

The latter method has the advantage of making the scoop immediately available for use with other patients after the patient has been placed on the backboard, and avoids the need for it to be left at the hospital. As well, this method precludes the need to release the patient's immobilization to remove the radio translucent metal scoop in the emergency room so that any interference (from the oddly shaped parts underlying the patient's head, neck, and torso) with X-Rays, CT scans, or MRIs is avoided. Although they should not interfere with most radiological evaluation, many X-Ray departments continue to advocate their removal.

While the scoop stretcher provides the most stable support and immobilization when moving a victim of spine trauma onto the longboard, the time required to perform all of the steps necessary for its proper adjustment and use may be greater than that dictated by the other methods which can be elected. Carrying a scoop stretcher on the ambulance is highly recommended so that it is an available option in situations when it may be the method of choice.

Once at the point in the patient's care when you are ready to transfer him onto the longboard:

1. Direct another EMT to retrieve the scoop stretcher and longboard from the vehicle, and confirm that a more rapid method is NOT indicated, and that the proper body substance isolation precautions have been taken. If due to other priorities a cervical collar has not yet been applied—do so now. Place the fully assembled scoop stretcher on the ground about a foot away from and aligned along the patient's side. Move it until the outer edge of the head end of the device is aligned with a point approximately 6 inches beyond the top of the patient's head.

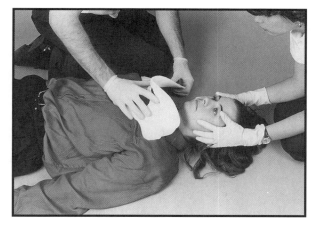

2. Release the length-locking devices found on the middle portion of each side of the scoop. While they are released, hold the head portion from moving and extend the leg portion until its distal edge is aligned with a point approximately 6 inches beyond the bottom of the patient's feet. Then if using a model where the locking device must be manually tightened, do so. On some models the length-locking device is designed to automatically set at specific elected points along its length, once it is no longer held released. This may require pulling the leg section slightly further until the locks on each side "click" into a locked position.

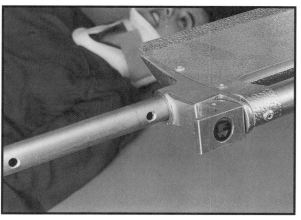

3. Once the scoop stretcher has been locked at the correct length, one EMT should hold the head portion and attempt to pull the leg portion from it and towards it, to confirm that these portions are properly locked together and can not accidentally separate. Next release the locks at the center of the head and foot ends and separate the left and right halves of the scoop stretcher. Have another EMT remove the half closest to the patient and, *without passing it over the patient,* place it next to his *opposite* side at the same level relative to the patient's length as previously. Without changing its level move the remaining half immediately adjacent to the patient's side.

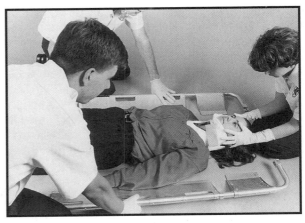

4. With one-half of the scoop stretcher adjacent to the patient and an EMT on his knees next to each side of the patient's torso — you are ready to insert the scoop under the patient. Instruct the EMT providing the manual immobilization of the head to move his knees back slightly so that they will be clear of the part of each half of the scoop that will extend beyond the patient's head when inserted. Reach over the patient and place your cephalad hand around his hips, so that your extended fingertips are under the shoulder and buttock. While you carefully elevate each a fraction of an inch (being careful *NOT* to rotate the patient), direct the other EMT kneeling at the patient's torso to carefully slide the half of the scoop on his side under the patient until it is properly inserted.

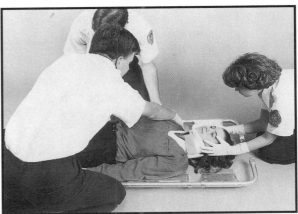

5. Then, while the EMT on the opposite side of the patient reaches across and fractionally elevates the patient's shoulder and buttock on your side, insert your half of the scoop stretcher under the patient. Using a slight see-saw movement to advance first the head end and then the foot end and so on will facilitate its easy insertion and (near the end of its insertion) keep the head end approximating the head end of the other half.

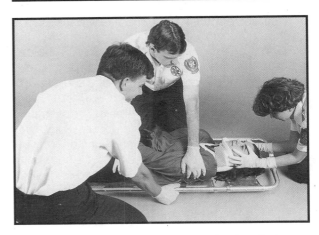

6. Once both halves of the scoop stretcher have been inserted under the patient, move up next to his shoulder. While being careful not to displace the EMT maintaining the manual immobilization of the patient's head, adjust your half as needed to exactly align the head section with each other. Insert one side of the locking device into the other and made sure they are properly locked together. Then instruct the EMT at the patient's other side to lock the foot ends together.

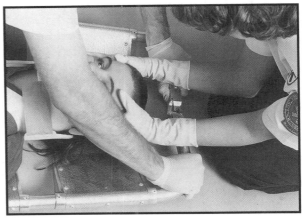

7. Once both ends have been secured and have been checked to be locked together, place the longboard so it extends lengthwise beyond the patient's legs and prepare another rescuer to insert it under the scoop stretcher once it is lifted. If a commercial head immobilizer is to be used, its base should be properly secured to the board at this time. One EMT kneels at the patient's torso and grasps the scoop's sides at about the patient's armpit and distal of his hips at each side. When all are ready and the EMT providing the manual immobilization directs, the EMTs at each side lift the scoop stretcher and patient about two inches off the ground and another rescuer slides the longboard under the scoop.

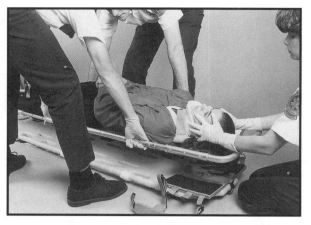

8. Once the longboard has been fully inserted under the scoop, upon the direction of the EMT providing the manual immobilization, lower the scoop down onto the board so that the patient is properly positioned on the longboard. Next, release the locks at the head and foot ends and separate the halves just enough to ensure that they can not again become engaged. Then while you reach across and hold the patient's shoulder and hip on the opposite side to keep him from moving, the EMT on that side slides his half of the scoop sideways out from under the patient.

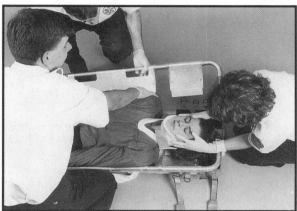

9. Then, while he holds the patient from moving on your side in the same manner, slide your half of the scoop out from under the patient. Now that the patient is properly positioned on the longboard and the parts of the scoop stretcher have been removed, the patient can be secured and immobilized directly to the longboard. When adequate personnel are available to maintain manual immobilization of the head and lift the scoop levelly while a longboard is inserted under it, removal of the scoop and mechanical immobilization of the patient directly to the longboard is recommended.

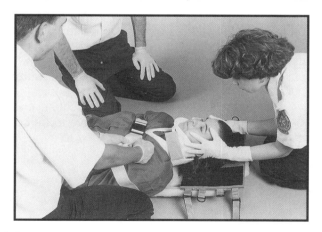

In cases when only two EMTs are available, full mechanical immobilization of the patient to the inserted scoop stretcher prior to lifiting him is necessary and represents the only method to properly protect the spine while placing a supine patient onto a longboard with such limited personnel. In such situations, while one EMT maintains the manual immobilization of the head, the second applies a cervical collar, inserts the scoop's halves under the patient and, after reconnecting them, secures and immobilizes the patient fully to the scoop in the same manner as to a longboard.

Both EMTs can then lift the scoop and patient from the sides while a spectator slides the longboard under it. In any case where a patient has been properly fully immobilized to a scoop, the immobilization and scoop should *NOT* be removed as this only increases the risk of movement and adds to field time. Instead, the scoop (and fully immobilized patient) should simply be secured to the longboard.

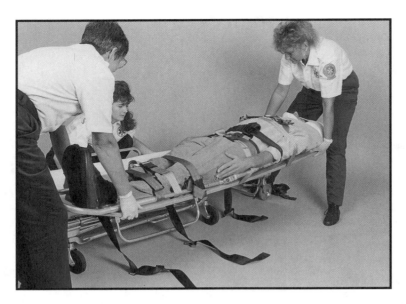

The scoop can be secured to the longboard with tape or ties through the handholds near the four corners, or with additional straps which pass from the board and through handholds of the scoop at each side and over the patient.

In the demonstration on the preceding pages the scoop stretcher was only separated into two long halves for insertion under the patient. In cases where insertion of each of the scoop stretcher's four sections one-at-a-time is dictated or preferred, they should each initially be separated without regard to the length of the patient. A head section is then placed at each side of the patient with its top edge aligned with a point approximately six inches beyond the patient's head and the top edge of the other head section. Each is inserted in turn under the patient, and the upper edges of both head parts are connected and locked together. Next, insert a leg section under the patient from each side so that the cephalad end of the side rail is just caudad of that side's head section. With models whose head and foot sections can only be locked at one of a variety of pre-determined lengths, insert the rail of one of the leg sections into the rail of the matching head section and adjust and lock it at the correct length. Do the same with the other leg section and lock them together. After checking that all of the connections have been properly locked, the re-assembly of the scoop under the patient is complete and it and the patient can be lifted onto the longboard.

With models that allow the leg sections to be adjusted to an infinite number of lengths, once inserted under the patient they will have to be connected and locked to each other prior to inserting them into the rails of the head sections to avoid the need for countless adjustments in their length to align both leg sections.

USING A LONGITUDINAL BODY SLIDE (DRAG) TO PLACE A SUPINE PATIENT ON A LONGBOARD

Sliding a supine patient in the direction of his long axis onto a longboard that has been placed just beyond his head is a good alternative for placing him on the board. With this method, the patient's entire body remains supported on the ground or other flat regular surface at all times. It may be particularly useful when the patient is extremely heavy or when injuries such as an unstable pelvis, bilateral hip injuries, or suspected fractures in bilateral limbs, preclude logrolling the patient. It is also an especially useful technique for removing a patient who is found lying across the seat of a car or is found lying on the sidewall or ceiling of a car which has overturned and these have become the "floor" of the passenger compartment. This technique is not recommended when the surface is irregular or contains protusions, glass fragments or other wreckage or, since the patient is primarily pulled from his armpits, when the patient has any injuries of either shoulder or clavicle. When using a body slide or drag with a patient who is suspected of having an unstable spine, one EMT must be committed to maintaining the head in the neutral in-line position and should direct the other EMTs who are moving the patient to ensure that they do not cause him to lose control of the head. As well as keeping the head properly aligned, this EMT must move the patient's head exactly the same distance as the torso each time the patient is moved, to prevent any compression or significant distraction of the cervical spine. Unless contraindicated, a cervical collar should be applied prior to dragging the patient so that any inadvertent loading which occurs will be transferred between the head and torso rather than resulting in cervical compression.

The primary pulling of the body should be from the upper torso, using the armpits as secure anatomical anchors for grasping the patient bilaterally. The lower torso is grasped at the waist or hips so that the pelvis is pulled concurrently in order to minimize distraction of the thoracic and lumbar spine. To avoid compressing the vertebrae in these regions, the pull on the pelvis must not occur in advance of or with greater force than the primary pull from the armpits. The EMTs pull the patient by drawing in their extended arms (adducting them), while kneeling in a fixed position. Then, without moving the patient, they reposition themselves in preparation for pulling him further. *To avoid inadvertent "rocking" of the patient when a kneeling EMT repositions himself, the patient is never moved simultaneously with the repositioning of the EMTs.*

When you are ready to move the patient onto a longboard, confirm that the proper body substance isolation precautions have been taken, any urgent patient care priorities have been met, and that a cervical collar has been installed (unless contraindicated). Then:

1. Direct one EMT to maintain the manual in-line immobilization of the head from aside the patient's torso and then place the longboard so its foot edge is just beyond the top of the head and the board's longitudinal midline is aligned with the long axis of the patient's head, neck and torso. If a commercial head immobilizer is to be used, its base must be properly secured to the head end of the longboard. If needed, have a second EMT move the patient's limbs into neutral longbody alignment with both legs extended together and an arm extended along each side. Once the board has been properly placed on the ground, kneel on it so that you can grasp the head when you are securely bent forward (down on your haunches) with your arms fully extended. Then, take over the manual immobilization.

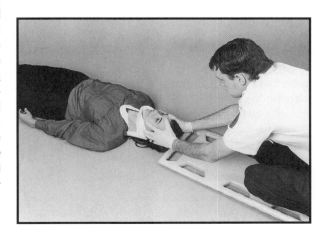

2. The other two EMTs should kneel next to each shoulder so they are facing each other. Have one of them remove any padding that has been placed under the patient's head. Each of these EMTs should place the cupped fingers of his cephalad hand in the patient's armpit and, while crouching down with his other arm extended, grasp the patient's belt. These EMTs may have to position themselves slightly further caudad along the torso to reach the patient's waist, but should not move so far that they will be pushing rather than pulling in the patient's armpit when he is moved. If the patient's outer clothing has been removed or he is extremely tall, cravats or narrow straps can be placed as long groin loops to provide ready purchase for pulling the lower torso.

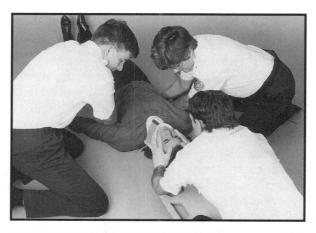

3. When ready, direct the EMTs at each side of the patient to slowly pull the patient towards you. As the patient moves, bend your elbows — letting them move outward beyond the lateral aspects of your torso — while maintaining the manual immobilization as your hands move towards the "line" formed between your knees. When the top of the patient's head is about an inch from this line, direct the other EMTs to stop. The average length and the angle of the arms of the EMT providing the manual immobilization of the head will generally only allow for the patient to be pulled about 12 to 15 inches at one time.

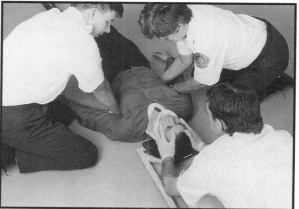

4. Being careful not to rock or otherwise move the patient's head, slide first one knee and then the other alternately backwards until you have moved towards the head end of the board as far as possible to securely maintain your balance, and your arms are fully extended. Moving beyond this point is dangerous since having to stretch so far forward that your balance is jeopardized could result in falling forward and losing the in-line immobilization.

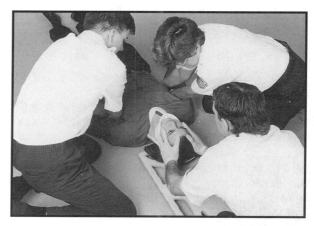

5. The EMTs at both sides of the patient should reposition themselves at the same time as the EMT providing the manual immobilization. Moving one knee after the other, they should move until they are again approximately aligned with the patient's shoulders and, grasping the patient's armpit and belt, are ready to pull the patient further onto the longboard. Jostling of the patient must be carefully guarded against throughout this process.

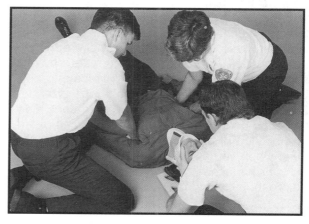

6. Following the steps previously described, the EMTs alternately pull the patient further onto the board and then reposition themselves until he has been fully pulled onto the board. Since the heels protrude beyond the ankles, if the patient's heels are to be pulled onto the board another person at the scene should be enlisted to guide them up onto the board to avoid injury or catching the edge of the shoes on the board's edge. Once the patient has been properly positioned on the board, he should be mechanically immobilized to it.

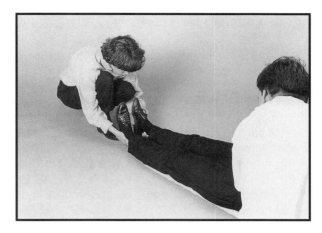

Several alternatives are available when pulling a supine patient onto a longboard. Transferring the manual immobilization to an EMT beside the patient allows the foot end of the board to be placed immediately beyond the patient's head and reduces the distance that he will have to be pulled along the ground.

Some EMTs prefer to use a *straddle-slide* to pull a supine patient onto the longboard. With this method the placement of the board, the position and movement of the EMT providing the manual immobilization, and moving the patient and then repositioning the EMTs, etc., are performed in the same manner as previously described. Only the position and posture of the two EMTs who move the patient's torso is changed. One of these EMTs crouches with his feet 2 to 3 feet apart straddling the patient's neck, so that when his arms are extended between his legs his hands are placed in the patient's armpits.

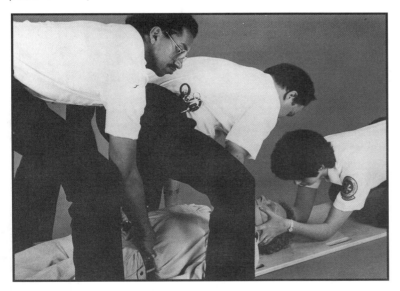

The other EMT straddles the patient's mid-torso at a point several inches cephalad to the patient's waist, so that when his arms are extended between his legs his hands can either grasp the patient's belt or his hips. When ready to move the patient, the EMTs straddling his torso can move him by pulling directly in a cephalad direction or by leveraging their forearms against their inner thighs. Straddling the patient permits the EMTs (when pulling longitudinally) to also partially unweight the upper and lower torso to allow drawing the patient over a surface with high friction or when the patient is extremely heavy. Some EMTs feel that straddling the victim is best, while others do not like stepping over the patient or the close proximity of the two EMTs at the torso, and prefer kneeling at the patient's sides.

USING A BODY LIFT TO PLACE A SUPINE PATIENT ONTO A LONGBOARD

Maintaining the patient in fully supported neutral alignment while lifting him from the ground (without a scoop stretcher) and inserting a longboard under him is extremely difficult to do. It requires a minimum of five trained rescuers to lift the patient (seven is preferred) and an additional one to insert the longboard. If "rippling" of the patient's back is to be avoided, the lift must be coordinated at all times. With this method the patient should only be lifted several inches from the ground, allowing a longboard to be inserted under his back, and then lowered onto it. Lifting the patient higher (or the rescuers moving while holding the patient in the air with their arms) promotes undesirable movement of the spine and is *NOT* recommended. Due to the magnitude of the misalignment and movement that can occur should any of the rescuers fail to precisely coordinate his movement with that of the others, this method is only recommended in rescue situations when other more stable methods would be impractical.

Once ready to move the patient onto the longboard with a body lift, confirm that the proper Body Substance Isolation precautions have been taken, all patient care priorities have been met, and that a cervical collar has been installed. Then:

1. The EMT who will be in charge of the lift should take over the manual immobilization being provided from beyond the patient's head. Direct two EMTs (or three, if 8 rescuers are available) to kneel next to each side of the patient and face his midline. Direct another rescuer to place and hold the board on the ground beyond the patient's feet ready to insert it when so directed.

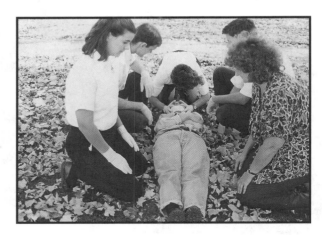

2. To identify where each of the EMTs at the patient's sides will insert their hands under the patient, have each EMT move until properly located along the patient's side, and hold his hands in the air over the patient's midline where they will be located. One rescuer should be near the upper torso and his cephalad hand should be located over the patient's shoulders with his caudad hand about 15 inches from it, over the lumbar spine. Opposite him, the second EMT should be located adjacent to the mid to lower torso with his cephalad hand inserted between those of the first EMT and his caudad hand over the sacrum.

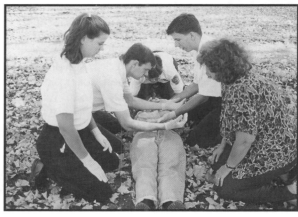

3. The third EMT—on the same side as the first and adjacent to the patient's hips—should insert his cephalad hand between the caudad hands of the first and second EMT just cephalad of the sacrum, and his other hand over the shaft of the femurs just proximal of the knees. The fourth EMT—positioned on the same side as the second EMT—should have his cephalad hand inserted just cephalad of the third EMT's distal hand and over the mid-shaft of the femur, and his other hand over the lower legs just proximal to the ankles. The hands of all four of the EMTs alongside the patient should be interposed between those of the EMTs opposite them so that a continuous chain of hands will support the patient.

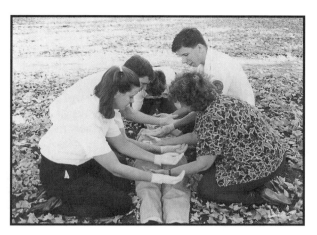

4. Once the EMTs are correctly positioned along each side of the patient, and the proper relationship of their hands has been visualized when holding them over the patient, they are ready to insert them under the patient. Direct them, without changing the level of their arms along the patient's length, to move back slightly and lay their forearms on the ground so their up-turned palms are immediately next to the patient's side. When all are ready, have them carefully insert their hands and forearms under the patient until each hand is centered under the patient's midline as previously described (and approximated when the hands were held over the patient).

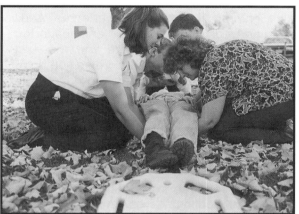

5. When all of the rescuers have confirmed that they are in place and ready, direct them to lift slowly on a designated count. On command, the patient should be lifted 3 to 4 inches directly upward so that the neutral in-line alignment is maintained. Once he has been lifted to the proper height, direct the EMTs to "stop." While the EMTs lifting the patient hold him with their upper arms braced against their torso for support, the sixth rescuer should insert the longboard longitudinally under the patient.

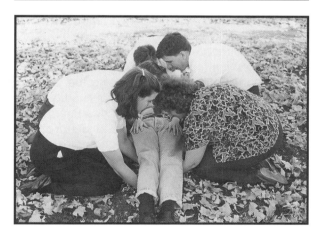

6. While holding his head, visualize the head edge of the board and direct its positioning so that the patient will be properly aligned on the length of the board when he is lowered onto it. Once the board is in place, again using a predetermined count, direct the EMTs to lower the patient onto it. Once the patient has been fully lowered, direct the EMTs to withdraw their arms from under the patient and then secure and immobilize the patient to the board.

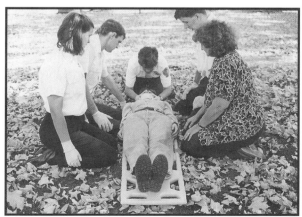

USING A LOGROLL TO PLACE A SUPINE PATIENT ONTO A LONGBOARD

A logroll is commonly used to move a supine patient with suspected spine trauma in order to examine his back, place him on the longboard, or rapidly position him on his side to prevent aspiration when he vomits. When the patient is aligned with his arms fully extended down each side of the torso and the elbows "locked" with the palms inward, the arms materially help to splint the torso. Earlier taught methods, which elevate an arm over the head prior to rolling the patient, cause misalignment of the shoulder girdle which produces lateral bending of the cervical spine, and therefore should *NOT* be used.

A logroll should not be used with patients who have an unstable pelvis or bilateral fractures of the hips, legs or arms, if possible. When a supine patient starts to vomit, the logroll is the only method the EMT has to rapidly place him on his side and, regardless of the patient's injuries, it will have to be used if aspiration is to be avoided.

It is essential that the patient be rolled as a unit so that the shoulder girdle or pelvis can NOT rotate from their neutral alignment with each other and cause twisting of the spinal column and rotary misalignment of some of the vertebrae. Additionally, as the patient is rolled onto his side both the head and legs must be rotated and supported so they remain in proper neutral alignment during the roll, while he is held on his side, and when he is rolled back onto the board.

How far the patient should be rolled onto his side should be governed by the purpose for which he is being rolled. If he is being rolled to avoid aspiration when vomiting, or when examination of his posterior aspect is to be included, he will have to be rolled fully onto his side with his back perpendicular to the ground. If he is being rolled solely to allow for insertion of the longboard under his back, rolling him only between thirty and forty-five degrees will be sufficient.

When ready to move the patient onto a longboard, confirm that the proper Body Substance Isolation precautions have been taken, any urgent patient care priorities have been met, and then:

1. Maintain the neutral in-line immobilization of the head while kneeling beyond the patient's head, and direct a second EMT to measure and install a cervical collar and a third EMT to place a longboard properly aligned along the patient's length on the side opposite the one onto which he will be rolled. If a commercial head immobilizer is to be used, its base must be properly secured to the head end of the longboard.

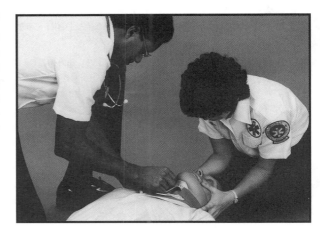

2. Next, EMT #2 kneels at the patient's mid thorax on the side to which he will be rolled, and EMT #3 kneels next to him adjacent to the patient's knees. While EMT #2 straightens both arms and places them palm-in next to the torso, EMT #3 straightens both legs and places them together in neutral alignment.

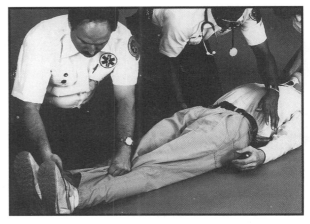

3. EMT #2 extends the patient's arms, locking the elbows, and grasps the far side of the patient at the shoulder and wrist. EMT #3 grasps the hip just distal of the wrist and tightly grasps both pants cuffs together in his distal hand at the ankles. (If the patient is wearing shorts or a skirt, or if the pants have been cut off, a cravat around the ankles will provide a similar hold on the lower legs.)

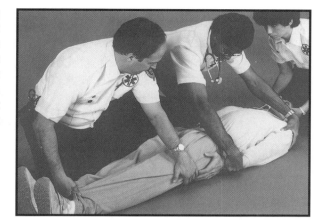

4. Once all of the EMTs are properly positioned and ready, the patient is rolled onto his side (toward the EMTs) with his arms locked firmly at his sides. The EMT at the thorax controls most of the weight and therefore sets the pace. The EMT at the head watches the thorax turn and maintains neutral in-line support of the head, rotating it exactly with the torso and being careful to avoid any flexion or hyper-extension. EMT #3, at the legs, assists the rotation of the torso with his hand at the patient's hip. He rotates the legs, moving in line with the torso at all times…

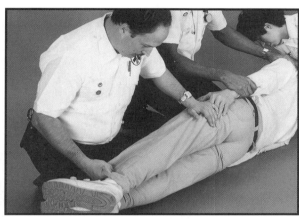

…As well as rotary alignment, the EMT at the legs must also maintain lateral and anterior/posterior alignment. To maintain lateral alignment the ankles must be kept elevated. This can most easily be done by EMT #3 placing his distal knee immediately adjacent to the patient's ankles, so that as the patient is rolled, they become placed and supported on the EMT's knee.

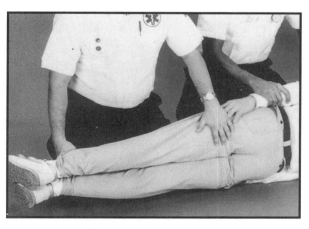

5. Once the patient has been rolled, direct another available rescuer to slide the board sideways under the patient's back until the long edge of the board is against the patient's side. Make sure that the board remains at the level at which the patient's head will be properly positioned on the head end of the board. If the board is significantly elevated on runners or if its sides are angled off the ground, the board should be inserted and held at about a 20 to 30 degree angle until the patient is rolled back onto it. This eliminates any significant "step" produced by the distance from the board's top surface to the ground.

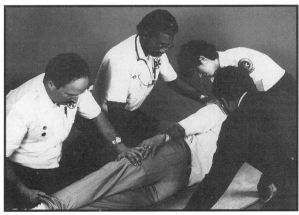

6. The patient is then rolled in the same manner but opposite direction until his posterior plane rests on the board. If the board was held at an angle, once his back is on the board the patient and backboard are lowered the rest of the way to the ground together.

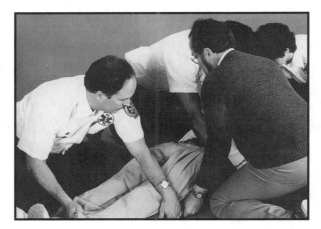

7. Although proper positioning of the board when inserting it will cause the patient's body to be properly positioned on the board's *length*, when logrolling a patient he almost always ends up off-centered to the board's width — too near the side towards which he was rolled. When this occurs two EMT's should kneel on the side to which he must be moved and, after placing their hands as when rolling him, should carefully slide him laterally — without losing the neutral alignment — until he is centered on the width of the board.

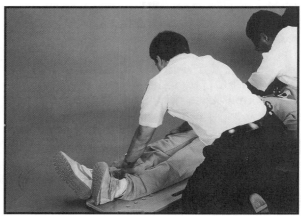

PLACING A SEMI-PRONE PATIENT SUPINE ONTO A LONGBOARD

Patients who are found lying on their anterior aspect most commonly have their head turned to one side and are said to be semi-prone. Immediately on arrival, one EMT should kneel beyond the patient's head and maintain manual immobilization of the patient's head in the position in which it was found. He or a second EMT should check for the presence of adequate spontaneous ventilation.

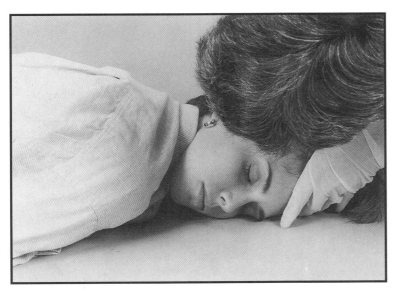

If the patient is face-down or his ventilation is compromised, he will have to be rolled over immediately to manage the airway and provide ventilation or full CPR as needed. In such cases the lengthy time-consuming sequence demonstrated here will need to be abridged so that the patient is rapidly logrolled onto his side and then to a supine position on the ground *without* delaying for the retrieval and positioning of a longboard or any further assessment.

Except in the rare case when the patient's airway can not be maintained while on his back, patients with suspected spine trauma should be moved into and immobilized onto a longboard in a supine position. When a patient who is lying semi-prone is spontaneously maintaining adequate ventilation, immediate rolling of the patient is unnecessary and further evaluation of the ABC's and injuries as possible in this position is recommended prior to moving him. Since completion of the initial systemic examination and many of the possibly needed interventions require that the patient be supine regardless of how stable he appears, a logroll should be done as soon as it is safe in order to avoid the possibility of this being urgently needed at a later time.

When the patient presents in a semi-prone position, a method similar to that used for logrolling a supine patient onto a longboard is used. Both incorporate the same positioning of the EMTs, same hand placement and same responsibilities for maintaining alignment. The side and direction to which the patient is to be rolled, however, is not a matter of choice. *The patient must be rolled away from the direction in which his face initially points,* and this determines on which side of the patient the EMTs who will roll his torso and legs must kneel. T*he patient's head is rotated less than the torso* so that by the time the patient is on his side (with his back perpendicular to the ground) the head and torso have come into proper alignment. Then the rotation of the patient as a unit is continued in the same direction until he is on his back on the ground.

Application of a cervical collar while the patient's head is rotated or angulated is contraindicated. A cervical collar can only be safely applied once the patient is in the neutral in-line position and securely lying supine on the longboard, ***NOT BEFORE.***

After assuring that the scene is safe and that the proper body substance isolation precautions have been taken, when the mechanism of injury suggests possible spine trauma and the patient is found lying semi-prone:

1. Direct another EMT to maintain manual immobilization of the head in the position in which it is turned. Check the patient's air exchange to confirm that it is adequate and that neither compromise of the airway nor spontaneous ventilation necessitates immediate rolling of the patient. Direct another EMT to retrieve the backboard while you continue evaluating the patient's ABC's, identify major areas of injury, and check the patient's back prior to rolling him onto it.

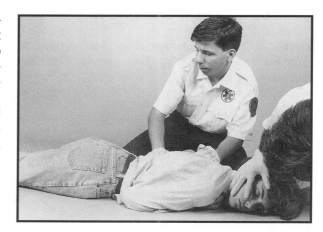

2. When ready to logroll the patient into a supine position on the longboard, direct an EMT to place the board along the side of the patient opposite from the side towards which his turned head is facing. The board should be placed 4 to 5 inches from the patient's side with its head end aligned so that the patient will be properly aligned on its length when he is rolled onto it.

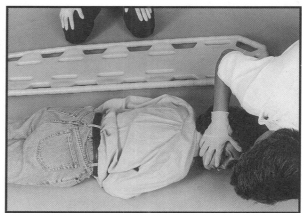

3. Direct two EMTs to kneel on the board and to bring the patient's arms and legs into neutral alignment. The patient's arms are extended with the elbows "locked" at each side of the torso to help splint the spine when the patient is rolled. As when logrolling a supine patient, the EMTs kneeling alongside the patient reach across his body and, while one grasps his shoulder and wrist, the other grasps his hips and distal ends of both trouser legs. While maintaining manual immobilization of the head reposition yourself and your hands in anticipation of the nearly 180 degrees through which the patient will be rolled.

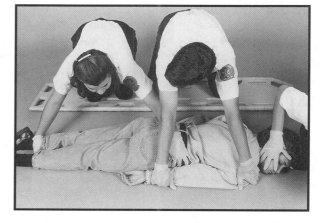

4. When all are ready, on a pre-determined count the EMTs roll the patient towards them until he is on his side with his back perpendicular to the ground. During this, you should rotate his head *less* than his torso so that by the time he is on his side the head has come into proper neutral in-line alignment.

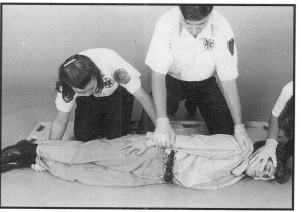

5. If the backboard has high runners or the handles are significantly angled upwards so the side edge of the board is significantly elevated off the ground when the board is placed flat on it, it would be unwise to roll him over this "step." Such boards, rather than being placed on the ground next to the patient's side prior to rolling him, should be held ready by another rescuer positioned beyond the patient's feet. Then, once he has been rolled onto his side, should be carefully inserted by sliding the board on its side, between the patient's posterior aspect and the EMT's knees, until the head end is properly aligned.

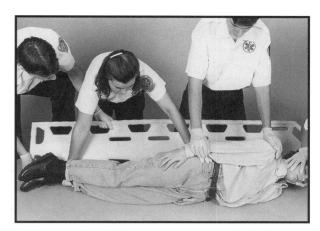

6. In either case, next direct the EMTs supporting the body, while continuing to hold the patient steady on his side, to shuffle backwards one at a time to provide space for the continued rotation of the patient. When all are ready, rotation of the patient is continued in the same direction as before until the patient (or patient and board) have been rolled and the patient is supine on the board which is on the ground. Next a cervical collar should be installed and then the patient should be centered on the board as needed. The patient assessment can now be continued while some of the EMTs secure and immobilize the patient to the board.

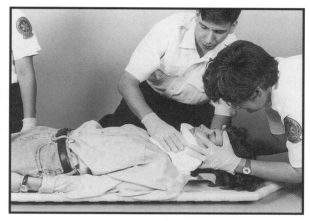

SPECIAL CONSIDERATIONS WHEN MOVING A PATIENT FOUND ON AN INCLINE ONTO A LONGBOARD

The preceding discussions assumed that the patient and EMTs were on level or near level ground. When the patient is found on a hill, the effects of gravity when moving a patient on an incline require special consideration.

An incline can be slight, moderate or extreme. As in all situations, the safety of the responders must be the first and paramount concern. If the incline is so extreme that the EMTs can not easily or safely walk, or if hostile terrain must be crossed to reach the patient or to carry him, personnel trained in incline rescue or technical *skree* rescue must be summoned. Similarly, if the incline is moderate or greater and covered with snow or ice, only rescuers specially trained and equipped for technical rope rescue or alpine rescue (e.g., Ski Patrol) should attempt to reach the patient and bring him to a more stable location.

If the incline is only slight, any of the previously described methods for placing a patient onto a longboard can be used with only such alteration in the position and posture (or stance) of the EMTs as is needed to maintain proper balance.

If the patient is on a moderate incline on which the responders can safely walk and stand without the need for technical rescue equipment, the forces of gravity which will act upon the patient when he is moved require some modifications in the techniques for moving him onto the longboard while avoiding sudden misalignment or loss of the immobilization. Generally, on any moderate or greater incline, or on ice or snow, the use of logrolls will be less stable than other available methods, or may even be totally unstable. Except when anticipated vomiting or airway compromise from fluids requires immediate movement from a supine position, or a patient is found semi-prone, the logroll is not recommended for transferring a lying patient onto a longboard in such situations. In cases where the incline is severe or on ice (regardless of whether on an incline or not), it may be difficult to maintain the patient or rescuers from sliding and losing the spinal alignment when they attempt to perform a logroll. On snow, regardless of whether on an incline or not, when the weight-bearing torso area which is in contact with the snow is reduced from the torso's large posterior plane to its smaller lateral sides as the patient is rolled, variable uncontrollable compression of the underlying snow commonly occurs and can result in unannounced sudden loss of support and lateral bending. Although the EMT must determine which method is appropriate and will best meet the needs of each different situation, on ice, snow, or any significant incline, a logroll should not be attempted unless dictated by special circumstance. Since kneeling or sitting on an incline is more stable than standing, standing to straddle the patient should also be avoided in such situations.

Usually in such situations, moving the patient directly onto the longboard is safest. Even when a basket-type litter is available, immobilizing the patient onto a longboard prior to insertion into the basket litter is recommended. Whichever method is used, several additional rescuers (beyond that normally required) will be needed to prevent the board or patient from sliding at any time.

When on a hill, it is important to understand the direction towards which gravity pulls the patient and other objects. On any slope there is an imaginary line called the *fall line*. The fall line is that line which a ball rolling down the hill would follow, and it represents the direction of the gravitational pull.

How the patient's long axis lies relative to the fall line will determine the easiest and most stable way that the patient can be placed on a longboard. Either the patient's long axis more closely approximates the fall line (and the patient essentially lies in a direction up and down the hill), or it more closely approximates a line perpendicular to the fall line (and the patient essentially lies across the hill).

When the Patient's Long Axis Approximates the Fall Line

When the patient essentially lies with his long axis in an uphill and downhill direction (more approximating the fall line than a line perpendicular to it), the scoop stretcher, body lift, or longitudinal slide previously described can be used with modifications to place him on the longboard.

Whether he is lying with his head pointing uphill or downhill, the pull of gravity will be downhill and along the length of the spinal column. The only difference that will affect the rescuer's actions is whether the gravitational pull is caudad or cephalad. The patient, if he is to be slid, must be pulled in a cephalad direction—in one case uphill in the other downhill. To prevent unwanted sliding on the board from causing the weight of the rest of the body to impact on the spine, it must be held immobile at the uphill end of the torso (when the head points uphill, at the armpits to avoid cervical distraction; when the head points downhill, at the pelvis to avoid cervical compression). The unique problems in maintaining spinal immobilization when a patient lies lengthwise down an incline are the same whether his head points uphill or downhill, and the same general principles must be followed to overcome them. The backboard, scoop stretcher, or other rigid immobilization device upon which the patient will be placed (or which will be inserted under him) is essentially a long relatively narrow rectangle and generally has a slippery top surface upon which the patient is placed. These two factors, together with the tendency for all items to slide downhill, produce the additional problems that must be overcome when positioning the device and placing the patient on it when on a hill.

To avoid the chance of the device sliding downhill it must be securely held in place at all times by an additional rescuer who is solely committed to that task. If it is placed with its long axis near perpendicular to the fall line it can be secured from the middle of either its uphill or downhill side. However, if it is placed so its length runs more nearly up and down the hill, it must be secured from its uphill end. This can be achieved by an EMT directly holding the uphill end or a strap, secured through the holes in the uphill end of the board, to provide a "safety line." Holding it from its downhill end is not recommended, since it is difficult from below to keep the upper end from rotating to either side. If this occurs, once started it may be impossible to arrest before the upper end has rotated through about 180° and points directly downhill.

A long narrow object whose long axis runs up and down a hill (other than perpendicular to the fall line) cannot be stably held on an angle to the fall line. When held from its upper end, any time that the pull of gravity becomes greater than the friction maintaining it on an angle the lower end of the longboard will move sideways until it is pointing directly down the fall line. *To keep the board from suddenly shifting in this manner, a board placed on a hill (other than perpendicular to the fall line) should be placed so its length is aligned with the fall line rather than the patient's long axis.*

When the length of a board lies down a hill so its surface is angled to match that of the slope, and the board is also laterally angled rather than in-line with the fall line, attempts to hold the patient or to move him on its slippery surface will generally result in the downhill portion of the patient sliding sideways off the board and produce lateral bending of the spine. To avoid this, the board should be placed with its long axis in-line with the fall line and, if using a body lift, as the patient is lowered to the board he should be turned so that his long axis also aligns with that of the board and the fall line. If a scoop stretcher or longitudinal slide is to be used, the patient must first be pulled on the ground (in the prescribed manner) uphill or downhill—whichever is the cephalad direction—until his long axis has been brought into alignment with the fall line. Once he is longitudinally aligned with the fall line, the sides of the scoop stretcher can be inserted or he can be longitudinally dragged onto a longboard placed lengthwise beyond his head, without any lateral sliding or lateral bending of the spine being caused by the gravitational pull from the incline. *In order to prevent his sliding and his weight impacting on the patient, the EMT providing the manual in-line immobilization of the head should never kneel on the slippery surface of a longboard if it is NOT level.* Therefore, if immobilizing the head while longitudinally sliding a patient onto the board, he should kneel and move immediately adjacent to the board's side rather than upon it.

Whenever a patient is placed on a longboard which lies down the fall line, as well as immobilizing the head manually until it is secured properly to the board his torso (and if his head lies downhill, his legs) must be manually immobilized to prevent it from slipping downhill at any time prior to it being properly secured and immobilized to the board with straps. Although with straps secured over the shoulders and under the armpits and a pair of groin loops properly positioned and secured, both the upper and lower torso can be immobilized to prevent compression or distraction of the thoracic, lumbar and sacral spine, it is unlikely that the upper and lower torso can be so immobilized manually on the incline. Therefore, to assure that the spinal column is not compressed because more of the body's weight was inadvertently supported at the downhill end of the torso, the patient's weight should primarily be supported manually at the uphill end of the torso. Therefore, with a patient whose head points uphill, the weight of the torso and legs should primarily be manually supported from under the armpits; in those whose head points downhill, from the pelvis (by holding the hips, waist, or legs.)

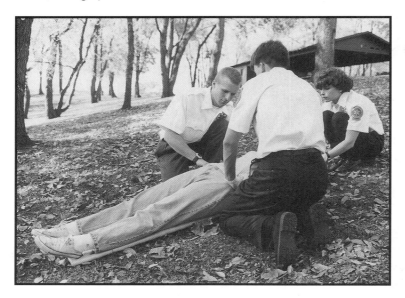

The downhill end of the torso should be supported to minimize distraction, but care must be taken to avoid inadvertently bearing the full weight of the torso at this end. The manual immobilization of the torso needed to prevent sliding when the board is on inclined ground, must be maintained without interruption until the mechanical immobilization of the torso to the board has been completed.

When the patient's head points downhill and he is placed on a longboard, his legs will extend uphill beyond the hold maintained by the EMT supporting the weight of the torso at the waist or hips. To prevent the legs from lateral sliding or flexing and longitudinally collapsing (without the friction which held them extended uphill when on the ground), an additional EMT positioned at the uphill end of the board will have to hold them in proper alignment by the ankles. This also provides an additional safety against having the weight of the body which is uphill of the neck being transferred to the neck or head.

When the Patient's Long Axis Is Approximately Perpendicular to the Fall Line

When the patient essentially lies across the hill with his long axis approximating a line perpendicular to the fall line, the use of the previously described methods for moving a patient onto a longboard are unnecessarily complicated and relatively unstable. When the patient's long axis approximates a line perpendicular to the fall line, the downhill pull of gravity will be lateral to the spinal column. The fact that the slope drops downhill from one of the patient's lateral sides can be used advantageously for inserting a board at that side and sliding him laterally onto it in a manner similar to that used to center a patient on a longboard. This represents the singular situation in which sliding a patient onto a board which has been placed along his side is the most stable method and is recommended.

Kneel beyond the patient's head with your uphill knee aligned with the patient's midline and the second knee downhill from it, so that you are slightly angled uphill facing his head. This provides a stable base on the incline and anticipates sliding him downhill onto the board while providing the manual in-line immobilization. Direct a second EMT to install a cervical collar and then bring the limbs into neutral alignment. Direct a third EMT to simultaneously place the longboard adjacent to the patient's downhill side, so it is positioned along his length with the head end of the board extending about 6 inches beyond the top of his head. The EMT should then kneel next to its downhill side and hold it in place. If a commercial head immobilizer will be used, its base should be properly attached to the board prior to placing it next to the patient. Once the second EMT has applied the collar and aligned the patient's extremities he should also kneel just below the board's downhill side, next to the EMT holding it. Both EMTs should reposition themselves along the side of the board so that one is aligned with the patient's mid-torso and the second with the patient's mid-thighs. Once properly positioned, and while lifting the downhill edge of the board, the two EMTs can insert the uphill edge just slightly under the patient's side. While holding the downhill side about six inches off the ground they should move on their knees closer to the patient until they can support the downhill edge on their knees and so that the width of the board is maintained in a level or near-level position(rather than matching the angle of the incline). As when a patient is to be logrolled, both EMTs should then reach their arms over the patient and place their hands around the patient's opposite (uphill) shoulder, wrist, hip and lower legs (holding the gathered cuffs of the trousers).

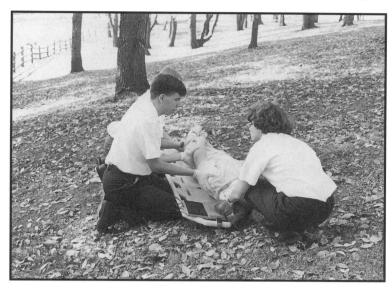

Next, while carefully maintaining the patient's neutral in-line alignment, pull him laterally and slide him sideways until he is properly positioned on the longboard. While one (or both, if there are sufficient rescuers available) EMT continues to support the downhill side so the board remains level, the patient is secured and mechanically immobilized on it.

As in any situation where a patient will be carried on an incline, immobilization of the torso should include a pair of groin loops and, once fully immobilized, the patient should be carried with the head-end of the board facing uphill.

IMMOBILIZING A SUPINE PATIENT ON A LONGBOARD

The generic anatomical considerations, methods, and equipment for properly immobilizing the torso, head and neck, and extremities (when included in the use of the device) to any device — whether the patient is lying, standing or sitting — have been detailed in the preceding Introduction to this section. The different methods for properly placing a lying patient with suspected spine trauma onto a longboard, have also been presented. The EMT will have to select the one most appropriate for the individual situation. The steps that should be followed to protect and immobilize the spine of a patient who is found in a lying position and is suspected of having spine trauma are presented here without repeating each possible option or detail, in order to focus the reader on the key objectives and items which must be avoided and to provide an uninterrupted overview of the sequence.

Once safety, the scene, and the situation have been assessed and (from the mechanism of injury or the patient's apparent injuries) you have determined that the patient should be immobilized, confirm that the proper Body Substance Isolation precautions have been taken. Then:

1. Direct another EMT to move the patient's head into neutral in-line alignment (unless contraindicated) and to manually immobilize it in that position without interruption until it has been secured to the board.

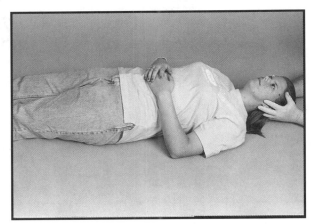

2. Evaluate the patient's ABCs and provide any immediately required interventions. Direct another EMT to obtain a longboard, cervical collars, and the other equipment that will be needed to immobilize the patient. Continue your initial assessment and provide treatment as indicated. Check motor, sensory and distal circulation in all four extremities (MSCx4) and note the neurological baseline this provides.

3. Examine the patient's neck. Then measure and apply the proper size cervical collar.

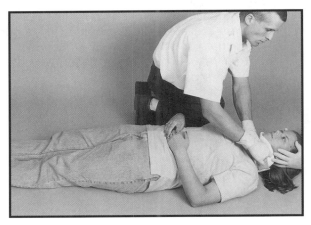

4. Determine the method to be used to place the patient on the longboard and indicate your decision to the other EMTs. Prepare and properly place all of the equipment that will be needed. If a commercial head immobilizer will be used, make sure that its base is fastened to the board before the board is properly positioned on the ground. Whether the torso and leg straps should be fastened to the board prior to moving the patient onto the board, or afterwards when each is being applied to the patient, should be determined based upon the situation, method to be used to place the patient, and the design of the board being used.

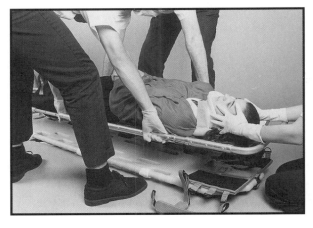

5.   Position the board appropriately for the method selected and briefly discuss the location, steps and count that will be followed to ensure that movement of the patient will be properly coordinated. When each of the EMTs is properly located and ready, and while maintaining the neutral alignment, place the patient onto the board. Then reposition him as needed so that the top of his head is properly placed relative to the edge of the board and his body is centered on it.

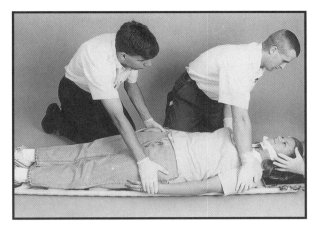

6.   With one EMT at each side of the patient's shoulders, tightly secure the upper torso to the board using one of the recommended methods. Whichever is used, a tight strap will be placed snugly up into each armpit and over each shoulder, and one or more straps will be secured from one side of the board around the patient's upper torso to the other side of the board. These will prevent the upper torso from moving up, down, left, or right on the board or anteriorly off it.

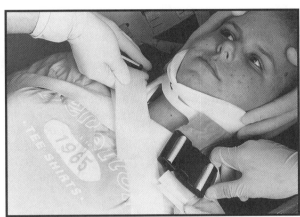

7.   Once finished immobilizing the upper torso, the EMTs at each side of the board should move adjacent to the patient's hips. If the board will be kept so that the head and foot ends are essentially level at all times, a single strap should be placed around the pelvis secured to each side of the board so it is centered across the iliac crests. However,…

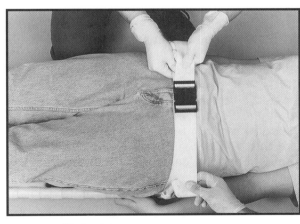

…if upending the board to carry it up or down an incline or stairs, or carrying it over uneven terrain is anticipated the lower torso will have to be secured more extensively to assure that the pelvis (when the head end of the board is elevated) does not move distally causing distraction of the thoracic and lumbar spine or between L-5 and the sacrum. In such cases, instead of the strap across the iliac crests a groin loop surrounding part of that side of the pelvis should be secured to each side of the board.

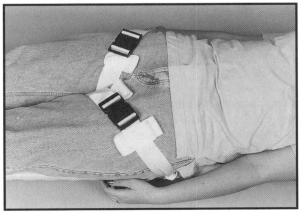

8. As each strap is added and tightened on the torso, it affects the tension of those that were previously secured. *Prior to fastening the patient's head to the board,* re-evaluate the torso straps (including groin loops if used) and adjust them as necessary.

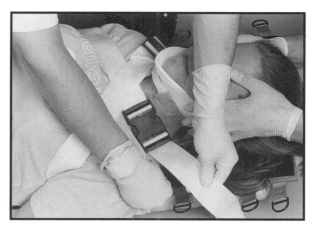

9. It is difficult for the EMT who is providing manual immobilization from beyond the patient's head to determine when it is in correct anterior-to-posterior neutral alignment. Therefore, after completing the immobilization of the torso you should visualize the patient's head from a point low and alongside of it, and direct any alteration necessary for its proper neutral alignment. Then, place firm padding between the back of the patient's head and the board as necessary to completely fill any void. *(Do NOT pad under the posterior portion of the rigid cervical collar. This provides NO benefit and can produce anterior displacement of the collar and cervical vertebrae.)*

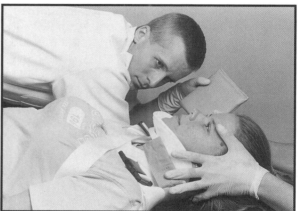

10. Kneel at one side of the patient. Without displacing the hands of the EMT providing the manual immobilization or moving the patient's head, bring one head immobilizer pillow (with its side slightly angled away from the patient's head) down the side of the patient's face and EMT's fingers until it contacts the base. Some of the Velcro on the bottom of the pillow should fasten to the Velcro on the base. Rotate the top of the pillow medially until it is properly on the base and the side of the pillow is pressed into and forms around the contours of the lateral aspect of the head. Then repeat this procedure to place the second pillow on the opposite side of the head.

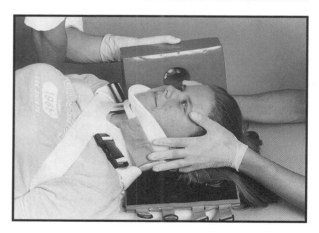

11. With a hand placed on the outer side of each pillow, squeeze the pillows medially—firmly against the EMT's hands and the sides of the patient's head—taking over the manual immobilization. Direct the EMT holding the head to slide each hand in turn carefully out from between the pillow and the patient's head and to then retake the manual immobilization by placing a hand on and pushing the lateral side of each pillow firmly in a medial direction. Once he has retaken the manual immobilization, you can remove your hands and secure the head straps.

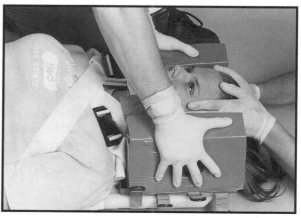

12. Once the EMT positioned beyond the patient's head has again taken over the immobilization, you are ready to secure the head straps. Identify the "D" rings on both sides of the immobilizer base which align with the patient's eyebrows and fasten the forehead strap to one side so it is slightly off-centered towards that side. Then insert it so its caudad edge is just over the supra-orbital ridge and tighten it until it is firmly pressing on the forehead and indents the edges of each bolster. This strap is the primary one holding the head and must be extremely tight.

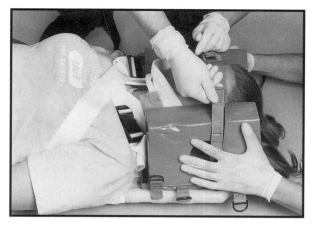

13. Identify the "D" rings which align with the cephalad end of the patient's neck and secure the lower head strap through the one at one side. Then, insert the other end of the strap through the one at the other side and tighten the strap and secure the velcro on its second end. This strap should be just tight enough to pull the upper edges of the bolster medially and place *mild* pressure on the anterior portion of the cervical collar. It should *NOT* be so tight that it places excessive anterior-to-posterior pressure on the front of the collar. *Make sure that the ends of this strap are not placed in rings so cephalad that it surrounds the mandible, preventing the mouth from being opened.*

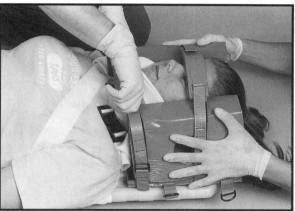

14. If blanket rolls are to be used instead of a commercial head immobilizer, the same general method for their placement should be used to assure that the manual immobilization of the patient's head is maintained without interruption. Then using 2–3 inch adhesive tape — or a cohesive flexible roller bandage (Colban®, Medi-Rip®, Co-Flex®, etc.) — the head and blanket rolls should be surrounded and secured to the board at the forehead and neck by either passing the tape through hand-holds or all the way around under the board (with the head end slightly elevated off the ground).

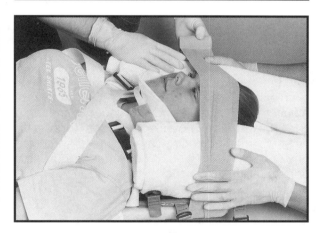

15. Once the torso and head have been immobilized to the board, manual immobilization of the head is no longer necessary. Secure the feet together with a cravat bandage or tape and place a tight strap across the legs proximal of the knees at about the midshaft of the femurs.

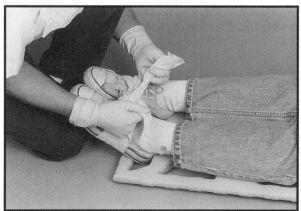

16. Place a blanket roll on each side of the lower legs to fill the space between each leg and the lateral edge of the board. Then secure both blanket rolls and the lower legs with a strap placed across them, distal to the patient's knees. If blankets or other large padding are not available, encircle the legs with the strap prior to fastening the strap to the board to prevent the legs from being able to move laterally. Once the immobilization of the legs has been completed, fill any voids that can be seen under the knees or small of the back with padding.

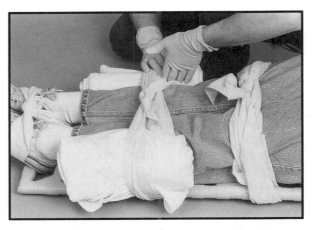

17. Place both arms so they are extended down each side of the torso with the palms facing inward, and secure them snugly to the board with a strap placed across the board and over the patient and each arm at the wrists. This strap should be snug enough to keep the arms from slipping off the board, but not so tight as to endanger the distal circulation. It should be over each wrist — *NOT* more proximal over the forearms. If the board does not have holes properly located adjacent to the patient's wrists, the strap should be run under the width of the board rather than through holes that are located inappropriately.

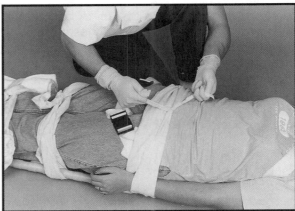

18. Once the immobilization of the patient to the longboard has been completed, recheck the patient's ABCs and motor, sensory and distal circulation in all four extremities. Compare these with the baselines established earlier. If the distal circulation in any limb has been compromised, adjust the straps and limb as needed to restore it *without* causing movement of the torso and head. Provide any other care indicated and properly secure the patient and backboard to the cot prior to initiating transport.

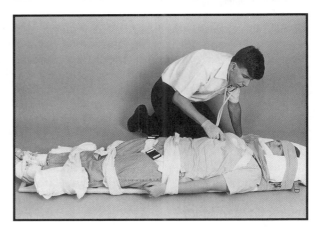

Once in the ambulance and enroute to the hospital, the strap securing the arms can be released to allow the EMTs access for rechecking the BP, starting any IVs indicated, and decreasing the patient's discomfort. When nearing the hospital the arms should again be secured so that they will not "fall" when transferring the patient and cot from the ambulance, moving to the bedside, and when lifting the immobilized patient and board onto the hospital bed.

IMMOBILIZING A SITTING PATIENT — INTRODUCTION

Most victims of car accidents are found in a sitting position in the vehicle. They may be sitting on the lower seat with their back restrained or resting upright against the seat back, *or* slumped over with their upper body resting against the steering wheel, windshield, dashboard or back of the front seats.

When the mechanism of injury suggests the possibility of spine trauma, the head should be immediately supported in the same angle as found and, if the patient is slumped over, so maintained while both it and the torso are supported and the patient is moved to an upright sitting position in his seat. Once the patient is sitting upright in the car seat the head should be moved into neutral in-line alignment and manually immobilized without interruption until both the head and torso have been mechanically immobilized to a rigid device.

Once the patient is sitting upright and the head is manually immobilized in the neutral in-line position, his ABCs and gross level of consciousness can be checked, any immediate interventions indicated should be provided, and a cervical collar should be installed. Based upon the patient's condition and the stability of the scene, the EMT in charge should determine the method and device to be used to move and immobilize the patient while bringing him from where he is sitting upright to supine on the longboard. When other considerations or priorities dictate that the patient be urgently moved into a supine position on the longboard (or away from the wreckage), *a rapid extrication method* should be used to lower the patient directly onto a longboard which has been placed partly on the seat while supporting and maintaining the alignment of the head and torso. If there is *NO* urgency in moving the patient, he should be immobilized while sitting upright using a vest-type extrication device or half-backboard prior to moving him to a supine position on the longboard. Immobilization of a sitting patient using a vest or half-board provides greater and more stable immobilization than can be provided with solely manual immobilization of the head and torso when moving the patient onto the longboard. However, it requires an additional 4 to 8 minutes.

A vest or half-board device should be used when:

- The scene and a sitting patient's condition are stable and time is not an overriding primary concern.
- A special rescue situation requiring substantial lifting, technical hoisting or lowering, or moving of the patient for a significant distance is required before it is practical (due to the confined space or other rescue needs) to provide complete immobilization to a longboard, basket type, SKED or other full-body rigid immobilization device.

A rapid extrication method (without use of a vest or half-board) should be used when:

- A sitting patient is found in an unsafe scene and clear danger dictates rapidly moving him to a safe location.
- The patient's condition is so unstable that he needs immediate intervention which can only be provided in a supine position and/or out of the vehicle.
- The patient's condition requires initiating transport to the hospital *without* any increased delay.
- The patient blocks the EMT's access to other more seriously injured patients in the vehicle.

A vest or short board should only be used when time is NOT a paramount factor and rapid extrication should be selected only when time is a factor. The EMT's decision should *NOT* be affected by the presence or absence of neurological deficits or his personal preference.

When a patient is sitting in either of the front seats of a car, manual immobilization can be most securely and easily sustained by an EMT who is in the back seat of the car. The EMT should steady his arms on the top of the seatback or against the sides of the head rest. If it is a 2-door car the EMT should enter the door on the side opposite the patient.

Manual immobilization of a patient sitting in the back seat of a vehicle is most readily provided from the patient's side while braced on the seat next to him. This can be sustained (even when the car shifts as other patients are removed) by the EMT resting his posterior arm supported against the seatback or head rest.

USING AN EXTRICATION VEST TO IMMOBILIZE A SITTING PATIENT

Extrication vests are unitized pre-assembled variations of the half-backboard. Most of the straps are pre-positioned as an integral part of the unit's structure, avoiding a multitude of loose parts and the time needed to position and secure each to the main unit. The vest contains internal slats or rigid sections which, although allowing adjustment of the circumference of the torso and head sections, make the back of the device longitudinally rigid from the coccyx to the top of the head. This allows them to be flexible enough to form exactly around the body of differently sized and proportioned patients while providing adequate rigid in-line immobilization of the head, neck and torso for removing the patient onto the longboard. Since they are flexible around their circumference they can easily be installed regardless of how confined the seat may be and, since they are form fitting and do not extend significantly beyond the patient's anatomical outline once applied, make removal of the patient through a limited opening easier than with a completely rigid flat device.

A variety of models are available and, although each has some difference in the detail of their specific design and exact strapping method at the upper torso and buckles, their primary design and use is dictated by the general anatomical factors common to all patients and is therefore almost the same. Each model has a rigid posterior center section with a flap at each side to surround the lateral torso and a second flap superior to these on each side to surround and secure the flat lateral sides of the head. The vests generally include several straps to immobilize it to the patient's upper torso, several to secure the flaps and immobilize the mid-torso, and a pair of groin loops. The head flaps are secured against the lateral sides of the head (and the head is prevented from anterior movement) by a strap which is placed on the upper part of the head flaps around the forehead. A second strap across the anterior portion of the cervical collar also connects the head flaps.

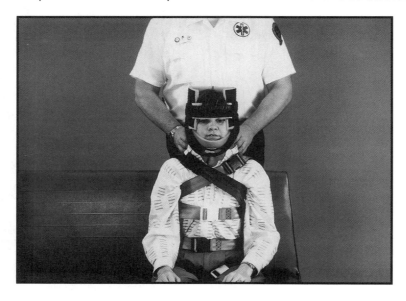

In the following demonstration, the *Oregon Spine Splint II* (OSS II) has been used because of its immobilizing efficacy, and because (at the time of publication) it represents the only such device which provides for alternate strapping of patients with a fractured clavicle and which does *NOT* obstruct the EMT's access to the anterior thorax. The reader must be familiar with (and have practiced on uninjured mock "patients") the detailed use of the specific model of extrication vest carried by his squad. Although the details of the following demonstration may require some modification when using a different model or brand, the general principles and sequence will be the same regardless of which is used. Once you have determined from the mechanism of injury that a seated patient must be suspected of having spine trauma, and have confirmed that the scene is safe and that all Body Substance Isolation precautions indicated have been taken:

1. Direct another EMT to support the patient's head and, if he is slumped forward, while you support the mid-thorax together move the patient's upper body until he is sitting upright. Usually this places his back supported against the seat back. If not, direct a third EMT to kneel on the seat next to the patient and to support the patient's torso. When the patient has been initially found or moved so that he is sitting upright (with his torso supported against the seat back or by a third EMT), the EMT supporting his head should move it into neutral in-line alignment unless contraindicated.

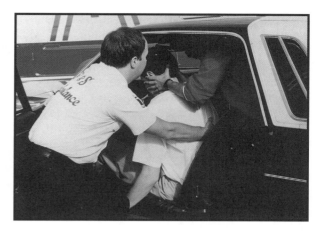

2. While manual in-line immobilization is maintained, perform the initial rapid Global assessment and provide any interventions indicated. From your findings, determine whether or not the patient's condition allows time to immobilize him with an extrication vest or half-backboard prior to moving him onto a longboard. If time does allow using an extrication vest, direct another EMT to retrieve the vest and cervical collars from the ambulance and continue with your Initial Systemic Examination. This should include obtaining baseline MSCs in all four extremities and quantitative vital signs to confirm your impression that the patient is sufficiently stable.

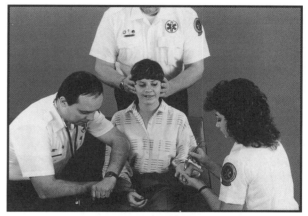

3. Once the EMT returns with the cervical collar and vest, direct him to ready the vest for use and, after you have completed examining the patient's neck, install a cervical collar of the proper size. If the patient is against the seatback, while the manual immobilization of the head is continued and you "splint" the patient's spine with your extended arm posterior to it, direct the third EMT to slide the patient's hips forward on the seat until he is positioned forward enough to allow for insertion of the device between his back and the seat back. In some cases the patient's weight or high friction of the seat bottom will require that the third EMT lift some of the patient's weight from his armpits instead of sliding his hips in order to move him forward.

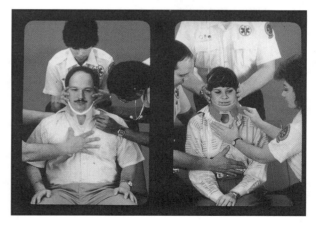

4. Once the cervical collar has been installed and the patient is properly positioned, and while one EMT maintains the manual immobilization, position yourself at the open door at one side of the patient and, if possible, have a third EMT position himself on the opposite side of the patient. Orient the vest so its correct flat side will be against the patient's back and hold the torso flaps out of the way against its other side (the one that will face the seat back). Lower the vest so that the head end is angled towards the patient and its caudad end is near the ground. Then insert it between the patient and the seat, rotating it upward so the head end is between the arms of the EMT holding the head and it is approximately aligned.

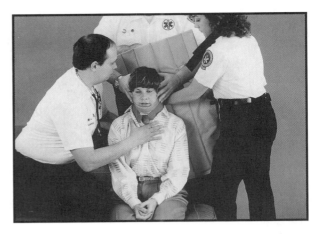

5. Rest the bottom of the vest on top of the seat and, while holding the vest, release the groin strap for your side while the EMT at the patient's other side does the same. Once the groin straps have been extended and are out of the way, open the velcro fasteners securing the side flaps of the Oregon vest to release the other torso straps. With other vests release and prepare the straps as prescribed for that model. Bring the side flaps around the lateral sides of the torso and under the arms to complete the preparations for securing the device to the patient.

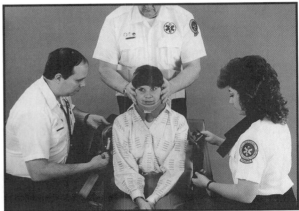

6. Correctly center the device on the patient's back and raise it until the top of the head section is equal with or just beyond the top of the patient's head. (With other vests such as the KED the vest is raised until the side flaps are snugly up in each armpit). Secure the upper torso straps. If neither clavical is injured, the upper orange strap is placed over the left shoulder and from the other side of the vest the lower orange strap is brought through the armpit. Connect the buckle, and by pulling against your other hand, rather than the patient or vest, tighten the strap. You should alternate which strap end is pulled so that when the strap is sufficiently tight the buckle does not lie on either the clavicle or sternum.

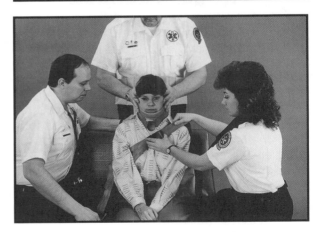

7. Repeat this by passing the olive strap—which is the top one on the other side of the vest—over the shoulder and, after bringing the lower half through the opposite armpit, connect the buckle and tighten the strap. Once both straps have been secured, additionally adjust each as needed to re-align the vest and make them sufficiently tight to prevent any movement of the vest on the torso. When using another model, secure the upper torso following the method that vest employs to anchor the device to the upper torso…

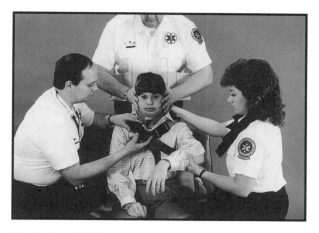

…If the vest being used has only one strap passing under the armpits to secure it to the upper torso and the design does not provide for anything over the top of each shoulder, the EMT will have to add these to immobilize the device so that it can not move inferiorly down the torso. When using the presently available model of the KED (which with its imitators is the predominently found design in the field), this can be achieved by securing a cravat to each of the lifting loops found on the back of the vest and then—after passing each over the shoulder on its side—tying them tightly to the top strap which secures the vest up into the armpits (similar to a pair of suspenders).

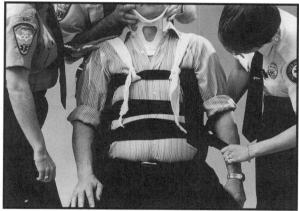

8. Next, fasten each of the mid-torso straps in turn. On the OSS II, these straps are both grey. The buckle halves of the upper one are white and the lower one black to aid in connecting the correct strap ends from each side. The straps of other vests are similarly color coded to avoid confusion. These straps only prevent the mid torso from sagging anteriorly or bending laterally, therefore they only need to be snug. Tightening while your hand is inserted under the strap is a good way to keep it from being too tight once your hand has been removed. *Making these too tight may restrict chest excursion and produce respiratory embarrassment* if the patient has any underlying anterior injury or is pregnant. Mid-torso straps can be limited to only one strap as long as all other torso straps (including those in the groin) are properly secured.

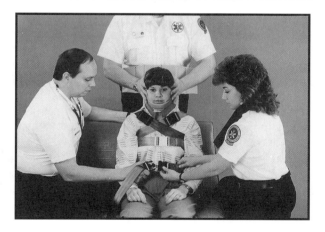

9. Secure the device at the lower torso with the groin loops. Only one side should be inserted and adjusted at a time in order to prevent confusion and unwanted movement of the patient. Hold the groin strap and, being careful that it does not become twisted, insert it under the patient's upper leg in the void between the back of the leg and the front of the car seat. While holding it with about two feet of the strap between your hands, with a back-and-forth motion work it proximally along the thigh and buttock until it is in a straight anterior-to-posterior line in the intergluteal fold.

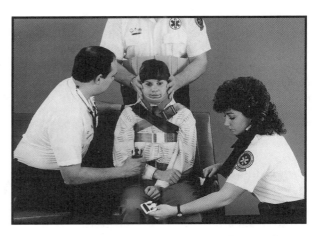

10. Once it is so positioned, hold the posterior lower edge of the vest to avoid moving the patient and pull the strap in a straight line anteriorly to remove any slack remaining along its length.

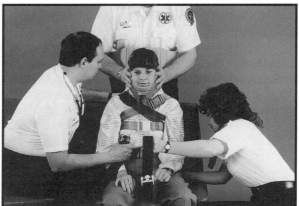

11. Next, bring the strap around the inner thigh and fasten it to the buckle on the *same* side of the vest so that the strap forms a loop around the side of the pelvis. Since the device is only used on a patient who is not seriously compromised, the patient can help place the strap correctly in his groin. While the patient holds it snugly in the groin lateral of the genitalia, pull the strap end until the strap is tight.

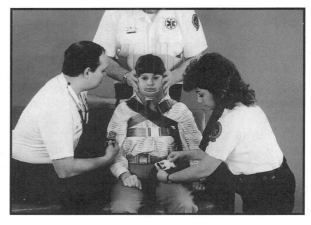

Regardless of some manufacturer's directions, these straps should be connected to the buckle on the same side as their origin—forming a loop which passes through the crotch and surrounds one side of the lower torso. These must be located sufficiently proximal so that each lies on the pelvis, surrounding one side between the groin and its lateral edge at the waist or just cephalad of the head of the femur. These straps should *NOT* end up positioned around the upper leg or on top of or under any part of the upper leg.

12. Direct the EMT at the patient's other side to position and secure the groin loop on his side in the same manner. At this time, check each of the torso straps and make any adjustments in them that is required. *This must be done prior to securing the patient's head to the device to assure that, as adjustments are made which cause the vest to shift slightly, the movement is not reflected to the head or cervical spine.*

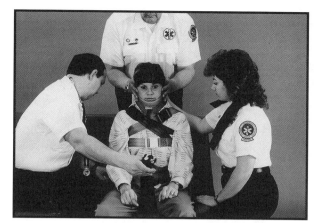

13. Pad behind the head as needed to fill the void between the posterior head and the back of the head section of the device. The firm pads supplied with the OSS II can be differently combined so that the needed thickness is produced. If suitable commercial pads are not available, a towel folded to the correct thickness and to a width not greater than the patient's head can be used.

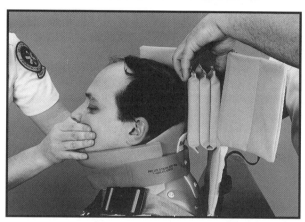

14. Once any padding required has been inserted behind the head, the head flaps need to be properly placed. While one of the EMTs beside the patient takes over the manual immobilization, the EMT behind the patient should place the head flaps so that they lie along the lateral planes on each side of the head. Once he has correctly positioned them, he should place a hand on the outside of each head flap and again assure the manual immobilization of the head from behind the patient.

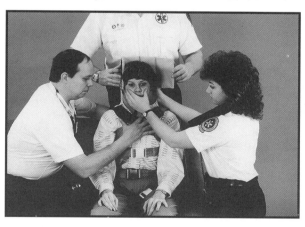

15. Next, fasten the forehead strap. Direct the EMT maintaining the head immobilization to slide his hands to the lower half of each head flap. Then place the non-skid (blue) pad of the forehead strap so its lower edge is just over and inferior to the supra-orbital ridge and just fractionally (1/8 to 1/4 inch) off-centered to one side. Take the strap end on that side straight (horizontally) back around the side of the head flap and secure it to the velcro on the head flap. While holding the side of the patient's head from being turned with one hand, pull the other end of the strap tight with the other hand and secure it at the correct level on the second flap.

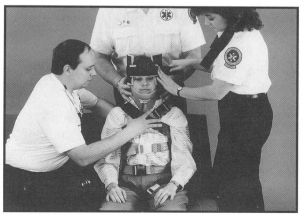

16. Fasten the lower head strap. Place the center (open part) of the black neck strap over the rigid cervical collar (taking care that it does not lie through the opening in the anterior collar and directly on the neck). Fasten the ends to the velcro on the head flaps snugly but not too tightly. Avoid fastening the ends of this strap so they are angled upwards or are too high on the flaps, which can inhibit motion of the mandible and the patient's ability to open his mouth.

Based upon the EMT's preference, the head straps of any vest or half board device can be replaced by Colban®, Medi-Rip®, Elastoplast® or other self-adhering firm wrap, or with 2–3 inch wide adhesive tape.

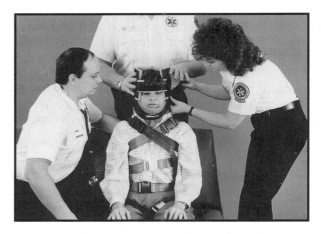

17. Once the neck strap has been secured, the immobilization of the torso, neck and head of the sitting patient has been completed. The EMT behind the patient can release the manual immobilization and simply support the patient and vest from falling.

If possible, the ambulance cot with a long board on it should be brought to the opening of the car door. The board should be placed under or at least next to the patient's buttock, so that one end is securely supported on the car seat and the other end is on the ambulance cot. The cot *must* be held from moving by a rescuer or other enlisted helper.

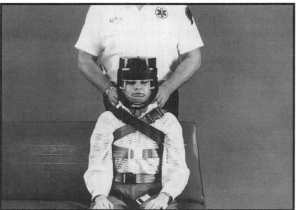

18. Without lifting, rotate the patient and device in place and elevate the legs, lowering the patient and the device onto the longboard. Then slide the patient and device along the board until he is properly positioned. Lower the legs onto the board. If the groin straps have been placed over the pelvis correctly they will only need to be loosened in obese or extremely muscular patients. Then, while securing the patient's arms at his sides, grasp the sides of the board and position it properly on the cot.

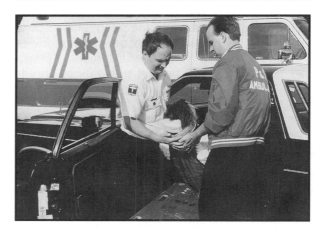

19. Securely fasten the vest to the longboard so that it and the patient can not move in any direction on the longboard.

20. Immobilize the patient's legs to the board.

21. To protect against movement of the head caused by road shocks and other forces which will occur during transport, secure the pillows of a head immobilizer or blanket rolls to the longboard against the outer side of each of the headflaps.

22. Secure the arms extended with the palm in along each side of the torso.

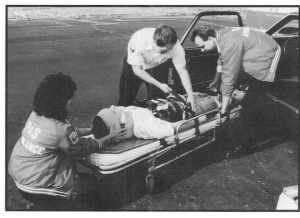

23. Recheck the patient'fs ABCs and provide any additional interventions indicated.

24. Recheck the MSCs in all four extremities and note any changes from the baselines obtained earlier. If the distal circulation has been compromised by the immobilization, adjust the appropriate straps to restore it.

25. Properly secure the longboard and patient to the ambulance cot prior to moving it into the ambulance and initiating transport to the hospital.

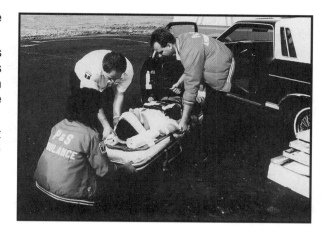

Although the preceding sequence can be followed in almost all cases, it needs to be modified in two special circumstances.

Regardless of which model vest is used, if either clavicle is fractured the method for securing the vest to the upper end of the torso must be adjusted so that *NO* straps or other ties are placed across the clavicle where it normally protrudes further anterior than the rest of the adjacent anterior wall of the upper thorax. In such cases, the device will instead have to be immobilized to the upper torso by securing it around the lateral shoulder — over the joint or just proximal to it.

When using the Oregon vest, this possibility has been provided for in the unit's design. When the use of straps over the clavicles or across the anterior upper thorax (superior of the line of the armpits) is undesirable, the upper torso can be secured by placing the orange and olive strap halves — which are the two top straps on each side of the vest — so that the upper one is passed over the shoulder just proximal of the joint and the lower one through the armpit.

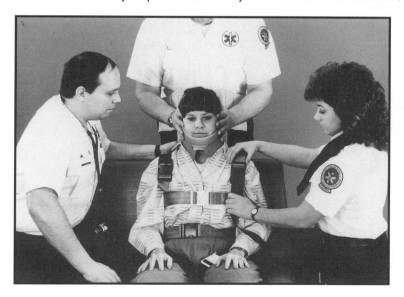

When the oppositely colored straps from one side of the vest are positioned and connected to each other in this way (rather than across the chest to the strap half of the same color), a loop surrounding the joint and lateral shoulder will be formed. These loops will both immobilize the vest to the upper torso and serve to draw the shoulders back and immobilize them to properly splint the fractured clavicle.

The same two benefits can be achieved with other vest designs by the modified use of cravats to surround the lateral shoulders. The upper strap which secures the vest around the torso at the armpits will, as usual, prevent the vest from moving superiorly on the torso. A cravat should be placed around the shoulder just proximal to the joint with both ends (tails) at the patient's back. These are then inserted through the carrying loop on the back of the vest on the same side as the shoulder and, after pulling them so the loop surrounding the shoulder is tight, are tied-off. Then the same procedure is followed with a second cravat surrounding the opposite shoulder tied at the back of the vest through the second carrying loop. The loops surrounding each shoulder and secured to the carrying loops on the back of the vest do not lie across the clavicles. They will prevent the vest from moving inferiorly on the torso and will keep the shoulders pulled back to splint and properly treat the fractured clavicle.

If placing the cot at the vehicle's door to support one end of the longboard when removing the patient immobilized in the vest from the car is impractical or impossible, an alternative method will have to be used. Holding the board in place on the car seat by additional EMTs, or placing it across both seats from the opposite door (and rotating the patient's back into the center of the car), should both be considered since each allows the patient to be rotated and lowered onto the board without the need of lifting him onto it. Since lifting a patient while extending and reaching into a car is a common cause of back injury in rescuers, this should always be used as a last choice.

When the patient and vest must be lifted it is important that this be done in a manner that is safe for both the patient and EMTs. *The patient should NEVER be lifted solely by the vest.* To minimize the reach required by each EMT when bearing the patient's weight, he should be rotated on the seat prior to lifting him. Whether it is best to rotate the patient so that he is sitting facing and with his legs out of the car, or is facing in the other direction so that his back faces the door, should be determined based upon the vehicle's design and the situation. The cot should be placed nearby with the foot end facing in the direction to which the patient's legs will face once he has been rotated. It should be in its lowered position with the side arms folded down and the longboard should be placed on it. When preparing to lift a sitting patient who is immobilized in an extrication vest, one EMT should be positioned at each side of the patient. While both EMTs face each other, they should insert the arm closest to the patient's legs under the upper leg just proximal of the knee and grasp the wrist of the other EMT. Grasping each other's wrist prevents their arms from becoming accidentally separated when lifting. With their other arm at the back of the vest, they should firmly grasp the carrying loop in their hand and crouch with their knees bent. When both are ready they should lift using their legs and bring the patient out of the car.

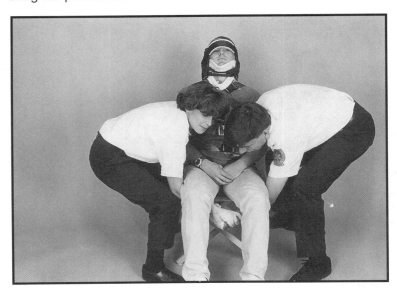

The patient will be equally supported between the EMT's arms in a semi-sitting position. By shuffling sideways the EMTs can move to the cot and, with one EMT on each side of it, down its length until the patient is properly located and can be lowered onto the board and cot.

USING A HALF-BACKBOARD TO IMMOBILIZE A SITTING PATIENT

When a sitting patient with suspected spine trauma will have to be hoisted or lowered or be moved in a variety of alternating positions in order to extricate and move him to a longboard, use of a half-board is recommended. In such cases the rigid half-board will prevent the possibility of twisting between the shoulder girdle and pelvis and any anterior rotation of the shoulders that is still possible when a patient is immobilized in an extrication vest. Also, when properly applied the half-board provides more stable immobilization of the head than is possible with the vest's head flaps. Therefore, an extrication vest should only be selected for hoisting or lowering when the wider profile of the half-board would make its application or extrication of the patient impossible.

Although half-boards come in different widths, thicknesses and materials, there are essentially only two materially different designs. In one type, the width of the board is approximately the same as that of a longboard and is essentially unchanged from its lower (pelvic) edge to its upper (head) edge. With this type, the width that extends beyond each side of the head serves as the platform to which the head immobilizer pillows or blanket rolls are secured. The other type is generally the same width but, at its upper end, the sides are indented forming a sculptured narrow portion behind the patient's neck and head to which the head is supposed to be immobilized. Although it is impossible to properly immobilize the head to the narrow top end, this design is the one most predominantly found in the field. Regardless of how much tape is used and how tightly it is applied around the anterior and lateral sides of the head, it can not prevent left or right rotation of the ovoid head on the board's flat surface when it is only secured directly posterior to each side of the head around the narrow head section. A ball-shaped object simply can not be immobilized on a plank of the same width with flexible strapping placed in two parallel strips around both the ball and plank at two points.

When a patient is to be immobilized on a sculptured half-board it should be used with the wider bottom end up behind the patient's head and the narrow end down behind the pelvis, rather than as intended. When used in this manner the sculptured board has essentially been converted into the other style of half-board. The width at the head will support and allow for properly securing the head immobilizer pillows or blanket rolls at each side of the head, and the narrow end behind the pelvis will not adversely effect the immobilization at the lower torso. This allows the patient to be properly immobilized to a sculptured board, and only requires the EMT to learn and practice one set of steps for the use of either type of half-board. Similarly, the use of only one type needs to be shown in this text. So that the orientation of the sculptured board different from its intended use is included, that type has been selected for the following demonstration.

When a commercial head immobilizer is to be used, its base must be installed on the half-board before it is inserted behind the patient. Attaching straps using a Prusik knot through the openings in the board is highly recommended. If this method or quick-clips are used, pre-attaching the straps to the board will prevent this from needing to be done in the confined spaces which occur once the board has been inserted and will eliminate the difficulty of threading straps after the board has been partially secured to the patient's back. You will need to mount two straps at the opening just below the base of the immobilizer for the upper torso (shoulders) fixation, one at the mid-torso, and two at the base (the sculptured part which will lie behind the coccyx) for groin loops.

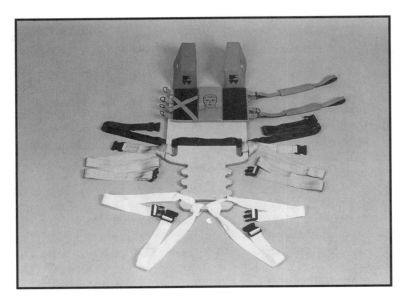

When the board has been prepared as shown, the straps are gathered and held by the EMT inserting the board to keep any from getting tangled. Once the board has been inserted, the EMT at the patient's side within the car can reach across and bring the ones fastened to his side of the board out from behind the patient.

If the standard method of threading long straps through the board's holes is to be used, five rolled-up long straps should be prepared and placed on the seat between the patient and the EMT inside the car at the patient's side.

The initial steps in assessing and positioning a sitting patient and inserting the half-board and, after completing the sitting immobilization, for moving and securing the patient and device onto the longboard and cot are the same as when using an extrication vest. The detailed steps and sequence for immobilizing the patient's torso and head to the half-board — except that he is in an upright sitting position — is the same as when immobilizing him to a longboard. Therefore, to avoid needless repetition, the steps in using the half-board are presented in less detail than when the same steps were included in either of these earlier demonstrations.

Once you have determined from the mechanism of injury that the patient must be suspected of having spine trauma, and have confirmed that the scene is safe and all body substance isolation precautions indicated have been taken:

1. Direct another EMT to manually immobilize the patient's head. If he is slumped over, while supporting the mid-torso move him to an upright sitting position. Once upright, the EMT supporting the head should move it into neutral alignment. Perform the initial assessment. Rule out the need to do a rapid extrication and check the MSCs in all four extremities.

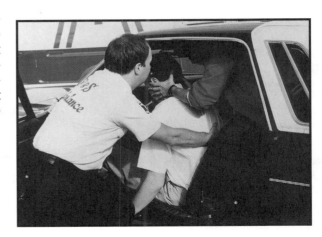

2. Direct another EMT to retrieve the half-board, cervical collars, head immobilizer or blanket rolls, and straps that will be needed, and to prepare the board. If using a commercial head immobilizer this must include installing its base on the board. Install the cervical collar and move the patient sufficiently forward on the seat to allow for the insertion of the board.

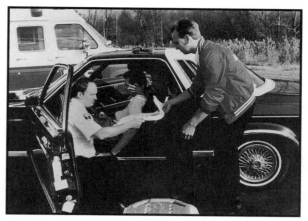

3. With the board properly oriented, lower it so the base (the sculptured end, if using that type) is near the ground and the top end is angled towards the patient. Insert it between the patient's back and the seat-back, rotating it upwards through the arms of the EMT providing the manual immobilization. Once fully inserted, center it correctly on the patient's back and rest it on the seat-bottom. If the straps have been pre-attached, straighten them so none remain between the board and the patient's back.

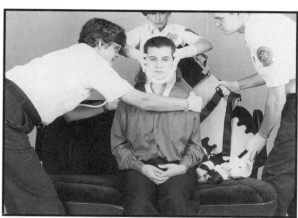

4. Being careful not to displace the hands of the EMT maintaining manual immobilization of the head, lift the board so that it is at the correct height. The top edge of the board should be just beyond the top of the patient's head or, when using a head immobilizer, slightly higher. Secure a strap over the shoulder, across the upper thorax, and snugly up through the opposite armpit. Then do the same over the second shoulder and through its opposite armpit—forming the "X" that secures the board at the upper torso. When tightening these straps, make sure that the board remains properly aligned (not angled from left-to-right) and that they are very tight.

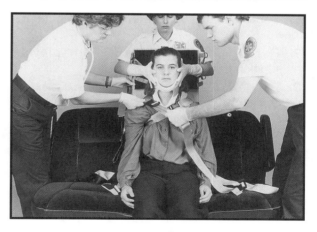

5. Complete the immobilization of the torso to the board. Secure a strap across the mid-thorax so that it is snug but not so tight as to affect the chest excursion. Insert the groin strap from one side of the board and position it properly. After bringing it over the pelvis secure it to the same side of the board—forming a tight groin loop around one side of the pelvis. Insert, position and secure the groin loop around the other side of the pelvis in the same way. Check each of the torso straps and adjust them as needed prior to securing the head.

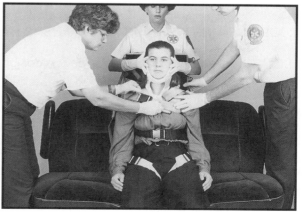

6. Install a head immobilizer pillow or blanket roll against each side of the patient's head and take over the manual immobilization while the EMT behind the patient withdraws his hands and re-takes the immobilization from the lateral sides of the pillows or blanket rolls.

7. Immobilize the head by placing a strap around the bolsters and tightly across the forehead, and a second strap less tightly around them and across the anterior cervical collar. If using blanket rolls, tape should be used around the head and blanket rolls and the board at the forehead and cervical collar.

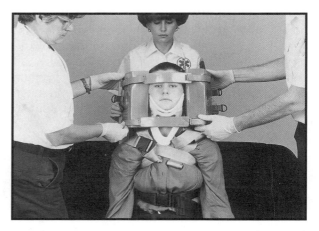

8. Place the cot with a longboard on it near the car door. With the longboard supported on the car seat and cot, rotate and lower the immobilized patient onto the board and draw him up the board until he is positioned correctly on it. Then position the longboard fully on the cot. If the board and cot could not be placed at the car door, the immobilized patient will have to be placed on the longboard and cot using one of the other methods previously described.

9. Secure the half-board to the longboard.

10. Tie the feet together and immobilize the legs to the board.

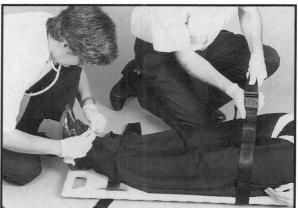

11. Secure the arms palm-in along the patient's sides.

12. Recheck the patient's ABCs and provide any additional interventions indicated.

13. Recheck the MSCs in all four extremities and compare them to the baselines established earlier. If the immobilization has compromised the distal circulation in any limb, adjust the appropriate straps as needed to restore it.

14. Fasten the cot straps over the patient to secure them to the cot prior to moving the cot and initiating transport.

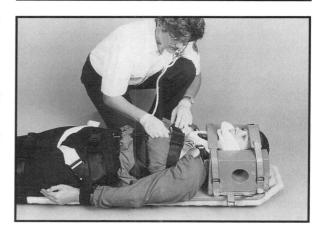

MODIFICATIONS WHEN USING A KANSAS HALF-BOARD

The Kansas Board is a unique device designed for immobilizing and rapidly extricating a patient from a (race) car. It provides the stability of a rigid half-board with a built-in head immobilizer, and the ease and rapidity of use provided by having the straps pre-attached permanently to it like an extrication vest. Also uniquely, the Kansas Board's torso straps (as well as the head straps) fasten with Velcro instead of buckles, and the torso is kept from cephalad movement by the lower end of the head pillows being placed securely on top of the shoulders—instead of by straps. These features reduce the time needed to immobilize the patient to the device before removing him. Due to the volatile nature of the fuel used in racing cars, the number of straps on the Kansas Board was kept to the barest minimum and *NO* strap to secure the mid-torso is included.

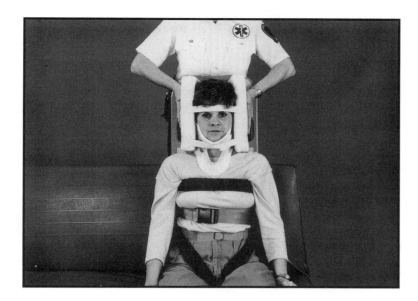

The need of such a strap to keep the mid-torso from moving is evident in the above photograph, and if using the device at a normal road accident should be added. Since this strap solely prevents anterior and lateral movement of the mid-torso, after the armpit strap and groin loops have been secured a long strap can be simply placed all the way around the board and mid-torso without the need to secure it through openings in the board.

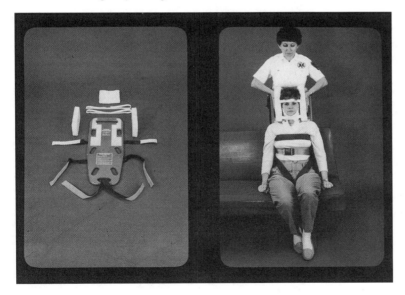

With the exceptions previously discussed, the Kansas Board is inserted, the patient is immobilized to it and placed on and immobilized to a longboard, in the same method as with any other half-board.

RAPID EXTRICATION OF A SITTING PATIENT TO A SUPINE POSITION ON A LONGBOARD

When the patient's condition or situation at the scene requires that he be urgently removed to a supine position outside of the vehicle, a *rapid extrication* method must be used in order to avoid the 4 to 8 minute delay inherent in first immobilizing him with an extrication vest or half-backboard. When doing a rapid extrication the spine is kept aligned and immobilized by the patient's head, neck and torso being maintained in neutral in-line alignment. To ensure this, at all times one EMT must manually immobilize the head in neutral alignment, another must move and support the torso in neutral alignment (preventing twisting or lateral, anterior, or posterior bending between the pelvis and shoulders), and a third must move and control the legs.

Experience has shown that the manual in-line immobilization of the head and torso will be impossible to maintain if the EMTs attempt to move the patient from sitting upright to a proper position on the longboard in one continuous motion. It is important to limit each movement, stopping to reposition and fully prepare for the next incremental step. Undue speed will actually cause delay and may result in further injury to the spine.

Many acceptable variations exist, and each is "right" as long as the patient's head, neck, and torso remain supported and in neutral alignment throughout. It is important to note that although the sequence and general principles in the following demonstration remain unchanged, the victim's size (and weight), the design of the vehicle, and the situation will require the EMT to modify the details shown to best move the patient onto the longboard and maintain the protection of the spine.

The technique must be practiced by teams of EMTs in various types of vehicles and situations. A "luxury" size four-door sedan is relatively easy to work in and properly remove the patient from, while a two-door high truck or extremely low sports coupe present more difficult and different problems. Practicing with the fire and police personnel who may be needed to help with the extrication is also highly recommended.

After ascertaining that the scene is safe, the indicated body substance isolation precautions have been taken and, from the mechanism of injury, that an unstable spine must be assumed:

1. EMT #1 (not the EMT in charge) gets behind the patient and provides manual immobilization. When he can not be behind the patient, this will have to be done from the side. EMT #2 (the EMT in charge) is positioned in the open doorway and supports the patient's mid-thorax. EMT #1 and #2 bring the patient to an upright sitting position and EMT #1 should bring the head into neutral in-line alignment unless contraindicated, and should continue to maintain its manual immobilization until it is later assumed by another EMT.

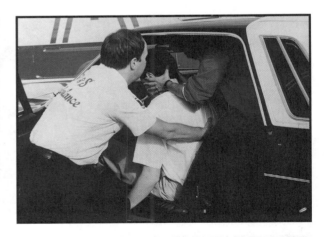

2. EMT #2 should do a rapid global assessment and any immediately needed interventions should be provided. From his evaluation of the scene and the patient's condition, he should determine if there is or is not any urgency in removing the patient from the vehicle. If he has determined that rapid extrication is needed he should direct EMT #3 to bring cervical collars and the other equipment that will be needed from the ambulance. As soon as the cervical collar is available it should be applied.

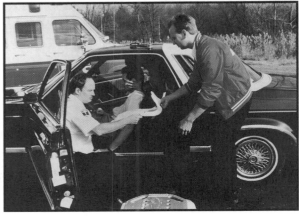

3. While EMT #2 applies the cervical collar and continues with his assessment, EMT #3 should place a longboard on the cot and bring the cot near the open car door. If the open door presents an obstacle to two EMTs working outside the car in the doorway, the door can be manually forced back — springing the hinges as far as possible.

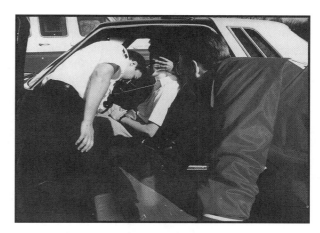

4. While EMT #1 maintains manual immobilization of the head and EMT #2 supports the mid-thorax, EMT #3 works from the passenger's seat to free the patient's legs from the pedals and prepares to move them when the patient is rotated on the seat.

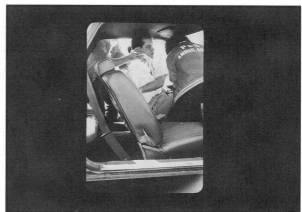

5. At EMT #2's command, he and EMT #3 rotate the patient on the seat so his back moves towards a position facing the open door and until his feet are stopped by the front of the seat or console. Then while his feet are brought up onto the passenger's seat, he is rotated further in steps until EMT #1 can not reach any further to maintain the manual in-line immobilization of the head *or* the patient's back squarely faces the open doorway. This rotation usually takes 2 or 3 short moves and should be coordinated by clear commands from EMT #2.

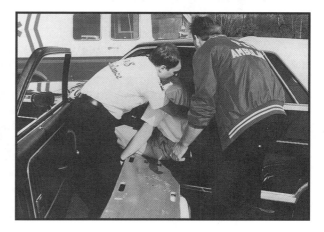

6. In most vehicles, EMT #1 will not be able to extend his arms far enough to securely complete the rotation from his original position. Either EMT #3 from the passenger's seat, or another EMT from outside the driver's door, will have to provide manual stabilization of the head when EMT #1 runs out of room. Then, EMT #1 can get out of the car and re-position himself in the driver's doorway adjacent to the post at the back of the door opening and re-take the manual immobilization. Some EMTs prefer to extend the longboard between the cot and the car seat at this time. This may make completing the rotation more difficult and with most vehicles, it is better done at a later time.

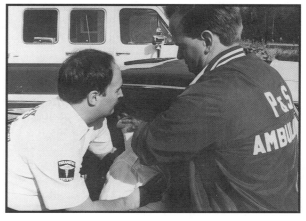

7. After EMT #1 (or another EMT) takes and maintains the manual immobilization of the patient's head from outside the vehicle, EMTs #2 and #3 continue to rotate the patient until his back is squarely facing the open doorway and his feet are in-line across the passenger's seat. Next, the cot is moved closer to the door opening by another rescuer, and the longboard is extended from it so that its foot end is on the car seat next to, or inserted just under, the patient's buttocks.

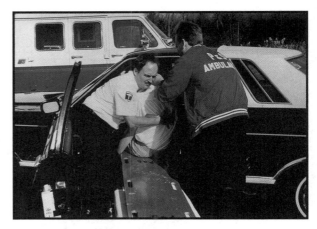

8. Once the foot end of the longboard is securely positioned on the seat and the manual immobilization of the head has been taken over by an EMT outside the vehicle, while EMT #2 supports and "splints" the patient's torso with his arms the patient is slowly lowered until his back is on the longboard. In order to maintain the neutral in-line alignment of the patient's head while lowering him to the cot, the EMT holding the head must crouch down or move into a kneeling position as the patient is being lowered. Other EMTs, or other rescuers or bystanders who have been recruited and properly instructed, should hold the cot and backboard securely in place.

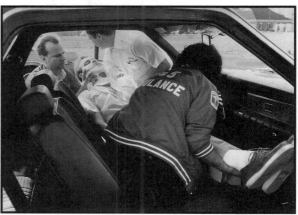

Note: In the preceding steps, exact positions for each of the three EMTs have been indicated. This only serves as an example. Although the three roles and responsibilities — one EMT immobilizing the head, one supporting, splinting, and moving the torso, and one moving and guiding the hips and legs — must be met at all times throughout the procedure, the exact positioning of each may need to vary to best perform each task with the various size openings and other differences from one vehicle to another. The location of other patients in the vehicle, or damage which limits the EMT's access to the patient or his egress, will also dictate modifications. Any positioning of the EMTs which allows the patient's head to be maintained without interruption, and the spine to be supported and maintained in-line without unwanted movement, is *right*. However, the maneuver should be pre-planned and discussed before it is initiated, so as to avoid unnecessarily numerous EMT position changes and hand position take-overs, as these invite confusion and lapses in the manual in-line immobilization of the head and torso.

9. Once the patient's torso is down on the board, EMT #2 places his hands in the patient's armpits and EMT #3 positions himself to move the patient's legs and hips in preparation for moving him up the board.

With the EMT at the head setting the pace, the patient is slid in 8–12 inch increments up the board until his hips are fully on the board. The EMT at the legs will have to move across the car on the seat. Moving in proper size increments, teamwork, and good communication are each necessary in order to move the patient as a unit without compressing or distracting the spine.

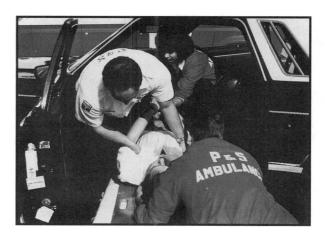

10. When the patient's hips are on the board, EMT #3 (at the feet) can exit the car and come to the driver's door to assist in further moving the patient onto the longboard. Frequently EMT #2 takes over responsibility for the hips and legs at this point, and EMT #3 takes over control of the upper torso. If additional EMTs are available, time can be saved by having one of them assume this position. Continue to slide the patient in increments up the board until he is fully positioned on it. Then, with the EMT who is maintaining the head immobilization setting the pace and giving the commands, lift the board and place it properly on the cot.

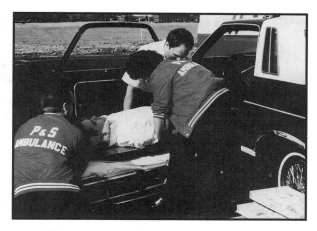

11. Whether the rapid extrication was selected due to the unstable nature of the scene or of the patient is key in determining what should be done next. *In either case, the next step is NOT to immediately secure and immobilize the patient to the backboard and cot.* If the scene is unstable, while the manual immobilization of the head is maintained and regardless of the patient's condition, move the cot and patient to a safe location without delay. If the scene is safe, the cot will only need to be moved a sufficient distance from the vehicle so that full access to the patient is available from all sides. If the rapid extrication was performed due to the seriousness of the patient's condition, once the cot has been properly located continue to assess the patient and initiate and provide the immediate interventions indicated.

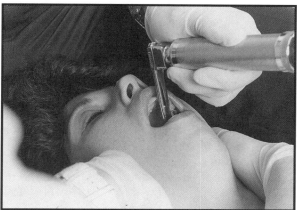

12. Once any needed field interventions have been provided, immobilize the patient's torso, head, legs and arms to the longboard and secure the patient and board to the cot. Initiate transport without further delay, and check the MSCs in all four extremities and provide additional assessment and treatment once enroute.

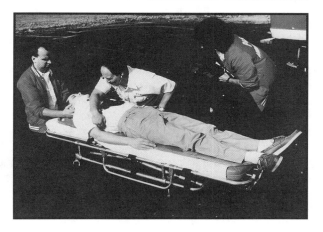

In cases of severe cold or when there is heavy rain or snow, to prevent unnecessarily prolonged exposure which could contribute to deterioration of the patient's condition and EMT's ability, once the patient has been extricated and the longboard has been placed properly on the cot it should be immediately moved into the ambulance. While the manual immobilization of the head is maintained, it should be lifted in a level position into the back of the ambulance. The further assessment and interventions needed can be supplied in the heated patient compartment and then, once these immediate needs have been met, he can be immobilized to the board and both secured to the cot prior to initiating transport.

IMMOBILIZING A STANDING PATIENT — INTRODUCTION

In a recent retrospective study, Dula *et al.,* noted that as many as 17% of patients with spine trauma were found standing at the scene or, in cases where transport was other than by EMS, walked into the emergency department. Therefore, the patient's ability to stand and walk should *NOT* affect the decision of whether or not immobilization is indicated.

When a patient with suspected spine trauma is found standing or walking at the scene, he should be supported while still standing and after a longboard has been placed against his back and his torso, neck, and head are immobilized to it, the head end of the board should be lowered carefully to the ground. Once he is supine on the board with it lying on the ground, his assessment and immobilization to the board can be completed. Although an extrication vest or half-board could be applied to immobilize him while moving him from standing to a supine position on a longboard, this is unnecessarily complicated and consuming and would provide no additional benefit than when he is directly immobilized to a longboard.

The patient's torso and head should be immobilized to the longboard while standing because this is an easier position in which to immobilize a patient than when he is sitting or lying (being the only one which allows for a longboard to be applied directly without moving the patient), and because any attempt to first move him to a sitting or lying position will result in significant movement and sudden forceful loading of the vertebrae.

With a standing patient, as with one who is sitting, there are essentially two different methods which can be used to immobilize the patient to the board and lower both until the patient is supine on the board. With one method a cervical collar is installed and, after the board is placed at the patient's back, his torso and head are fully mechanically immobilized to it before the head end of the board is lowered to the ground. The patient's legs should *NOT* be immobilized to the board until he has been lowered and is lying supine on the board, since any restriction of the legs while standing may unbalance the patient. This method requires that he remain standing for 3 to 4 additional minutes while he is secured to the board before being lowered to the ground. With the second method, after the longboard is placed at the patient's back (similar to when doing a rapid extrication) and without delaying to secure him to the board or install a cervical collar, his torso and head are solely manually immobilized to the board while being lowered. This requires under a minute until he is supine on the board and it is flat on the ground, but provides for less stable (and less safe) immobilization.

Most patients who are still standing by the time the EMTs arrive are stable enough to allow the time to secure them to the board before lowering them to the ground. The method in which the patient is manually immobilized to the board without ties or cervical collar should only be elected when he appears (or becomes) unstable and the risk of his collapsing supercedes that of lowering him with only manual immobilization to the board. *This method should only be elected in such cases, or when the need for urgent treatment or a danger at the scene dictates that the patient be lowered and moved without delay, NOT as a matter of the EMTs personal preference.*

It is important to note that when an adult is lying on a flat rigid surface, the length from the top of his head to the bottom of his feet (when positioned perpendicular to his long axis) is between one and two inches longer than his normal measured height when standing.

When standing, the weight of the body superior to each vertebrae rests on the one below so that the majority of the body's weight is on the pelvis and the joints of the lower extremities. This causes a natural compression of the spinal column. When the same person is placed in a supine position, this in-line weighting no longer occurs and, the space between each vertebrae and between the bone ends in the joints of the lower extremities increase slightly — causing the body length to increase.

When the torso of a standing patient is secured to a board using the normal strapping at the upper torso, *NO* mid-torso strap, and a single strap across the iliac crests at its lower end, the upper torso is fully immobilized but the lower torso and legs can still move slightly in a distal direction. Since the unweighting of the vertebrae is desirable when securing a stable standing patient to a longboard, a mid-torso strap should be omitted and the lower torso should be secured using an iliac crest strap, *NOT* groin loops. If groin loops will be necessary to carry the patient at a later time they should be added after the patient has been lowered to a supine position.

After lowering a standing patient whose head and torso have been immobilized to a longboard (manually or mechanically) to the ground, his feet will extend an inch or so beyond the foot end of the board. This normally reflects the increased length of the body when moved from a standing to a lying position and is not indicative of a failure in immobilizing the upper torso which resulted in the caudad movement.

With either method, the head end of the board should always be lowered to the ground while the bottom end is prevented from kicking-out anteriorly. Regardless of the number or strength of the EMTs available, attempts to lift the board (rather than lowering its head end) into a horizontal position will result in sudden weighting and uncontrolled lurching and swinging of the board. This will cause significant movement of the patient and his spinal column as well as presenting a danger to the EMTs and, therefore, should *NEVER* be attempted.

It is important when initially positioning the standing patient to anticipate where on the ground the board will go. If an obstacle behind him will interfere with this, support the patient's upper torso once the in-line manual immobilization of the head has been initiated and have him shuffle his feet (without lifting either from the ground) until he is turned so that no obstacle is behind him.

IMMOBILIZING A STABLE STANDING PATIENT

When the scene or situation suggests that those involved may have spine trauma and a patient is found standing, after confirming that the scene is safe and all body substance precautions indicated have been taken, ascertain the patient's exact location at the time of the accident and exactly what happened to him. If he was involved in such a way that *his individual mechanism of injury* suggests that he may have spine trauma, immediately:

1. Direct the patient to stand (unmoving) with his feet about 6 to 12 inches apart. Direct a taller EMT to move behind the patient to support his head and to move it into neutral in-line alignment, unless contraindicated. The manual immobilization of the head should be maintained without interruption until it has been replaced by mechanical immobilization to the longboard. Do a rapid global survey and, from the patient's level of consciousness, respiratory, and circulatory status, determine whether or not the patient is stable enough to continue standing for 3 or 4 minutes. If he appears stable, direct another EMT to retrieve a longboard, cervical collars, straps and (if it will be used) to secure the head immobilizer base to the board.

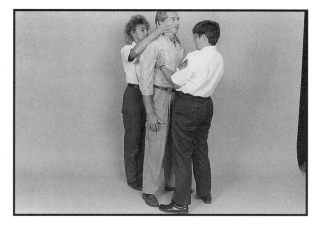

2. Stand directly in front of the patient and, while supporting him at his torso, explain what you are going to do and why. Once the EMT has returned with the necessary equipment direct him to install the head immobilizer base on the head end of the board for the appropriate height for the patient (if using a head immobilizer) while you measure and install a cervical collar. When both of these tasks are completed, direct the EMT providing the manual immobilization to elevate his elbows until they are widely apart and, with the board angled, have the third EMT insert it between his arms against the patient's back as shown.

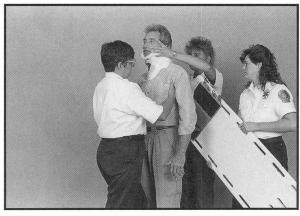

3. Center the board on the patient's back and direct the EMT immobilizing the head to hold it against the patient's back by pressing against it with his body. Place straps through the armpits and over each shoulder — using one of the previously discussed methods — to immobilize the board to the upper torso.

4. Then add a strap across the iliac crests. *Do NOT add any strap at the mid-torso.*

5. Prior to securing the head to the board rapidly re-evaluate the torso straps and make any needed adjustments in them.

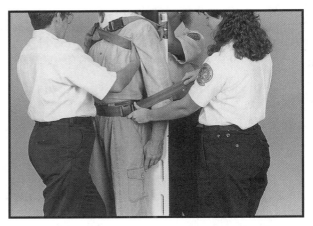

6. Once the straps at the upper and lower torso have been adjusted to complete the immobilization of the torso to the board, evaluate the in-line alignment from the side and make any adjustments necessary.

7. Pad behind the head as needed.

8. Place the head pillows on the immobilizer base (or blanket rolls on the board) at each side of the head.

9. Take over the manual immobilization while the EMT behind the patient withdraws his hands and retakes it. Then immobilize the head with straps across the forehead and cervical collar.

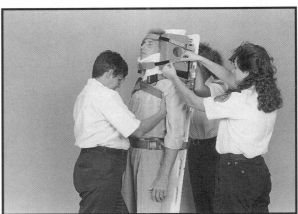

10. Once the torso and head have been immobilized to the board, manual immobilization can be released. Direct the third EMT to stand at one side of the board to secure it, while the other EMT moves from behind the board to a position at its other side. One EMT should be positioned next to and facing each side of the patient, and should hold the board with his posterior hand through a hand-hold at its top and his anterior hand through one near to the patient's hip. With your feet apart for balance, place one foot between the patient's legs so that the toe end of your shoe is securely against the bottom of the board to prevent it from "kicking" out when the board is lowered.

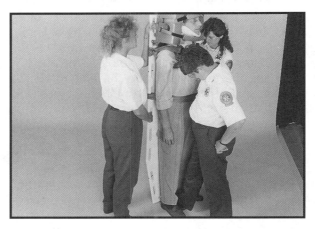

11. Once all three EMTs are ready, the head end of the board should be lowered until the arms with which the head end of the board is held from each side are fully extended. This will occur when the head end of the board is about half way to the ground. While the toe-hold at the bottom of the board is maintained without interruption, the EMTs at each side should move closer to the head end of the board *without* removing their hands from the board's handholds. *Lowering the board all of the way to the ground in one motion is dangerous to the patient and EMTs and should NOT be attempted.*

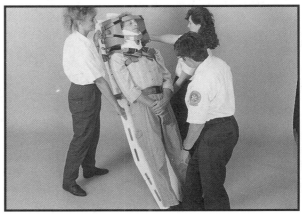

12. When both EMTs are properly re-positioned, instruct the patient to place his lower arms over his abdomen (having him grasp a wrist with his other hand is a good idea), and lower the head end of the board the rest of the way to the ground. The EMT at each side should bend at the knees with his back upright rather than bending his back when completing lowering of the board.

13. Once on the ground, complete the initial assessment of the patient and provide any treatment indicated.

14. Complete the immobilization of the legs and arms and initiate transport.

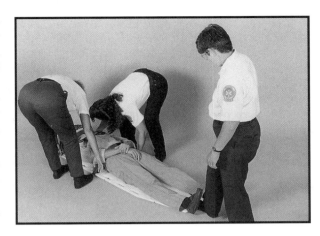

IMMOBILIZING AN UNSTABLE STANDING PATIENT

When the scene or situation suggests that those involved may have spine trauma and a patient is found standing, after confirming that the scene is safe to enter and the indicated body substance isolation precautions have been taken, rapidly ascertain if the individual's role and mechanism of injury suggests that he may have a spine injury. By virtue of his standing, you know that the patient is neither apneic nor in cardiac arrest and that he has some adequacy of cerebral perfusion and oxygenation. If immobilization is indicated:

1. Direct the patient to stand (unmoving) with his feet about 6 to 12 inches apart and direct one of the taller EMTs to move behind the patient, support his head, and move it into neutral in-line alignment unless contraindicated. Continue your rapid global survey. If the patient complains of feeling weak or dizzy or, appears unstable (or if the scene is unstable) —direct another EMT to retrieve a backboard from the ambulance *without delaying to obtain or ready other equipment at this time.* Support the patient at his upper torso against any sudden collapse.

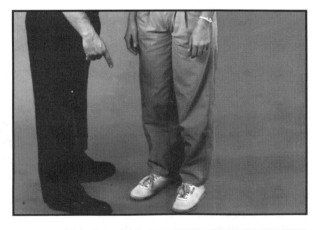

2. Scan the patient's body to determine if there is any significant external bleeding, and control any that is found. Further assessment until the patient has been lowered to the ground is futile. As soon as the longboard is available, instruct the EMT immobilizing the patient's head to elevate his elbows widely apart and have the third EMT angle the board and insert it through them at the patient's back as shown. Center the board on the patient's back. Once the board is centered, have the EMT behind the patient hold it against the patient's back with his body. Tell the patient what you are going to do to lower him to the ground.

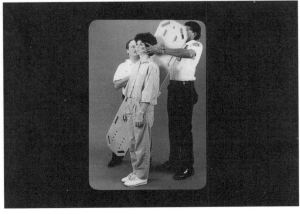

3. Stand at one side of the patient so that your leg which is closest to the board is aligned with the patient's and you are facing an EMT similarly positioned at the patient's other side. Each EMT at each side should insert his arm which is furthest from the patient (anterior) through the armpit, and reach upward until he grasps the nearest hand-hold **ABOVE** the armpit on the side of the board. A hand-hold that is superior to the lower margin of the armpit is used so that…

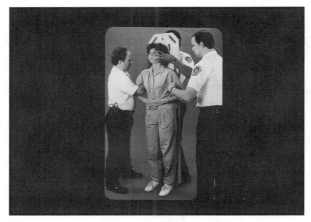

…the patient's weight will be supported on the EMTs' arms. This side view clearly demonstrates the correct position of the EMT's arm through the armpit and then upwards to produce a perch on which the armpit sits. Once the EMTs have inserted their arms through the armpit and securely grasp the superior hand-hold, the upright board acts as a stand to hold their arms up. Should the patient collapse, he will remain hanging upright from his armpits, rather than falling to the ground.

4. Next both EMTs should grasp a hand-hold at the top end of the board with their other hand.

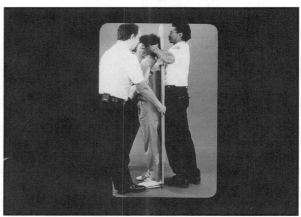

5. Another rescuer or spectator will be needed to "step" the bottom of the board so it can not kick-out. He should stand with his feet apart for good balance and with one foot between the patient's legs so that its toe end is against the bottom edge of the board. Once all four rescuers are ready the head end of the board should be slowly lowered until it is about half way to the ground and then stopped. From the photo you can see that, were the board to be lowered to the ground with each EMT's hands and arms in the same position, the head would be rotated into flexion by the EMT at the patient's head and his arms would be trapped under those of the EMTs at each side.

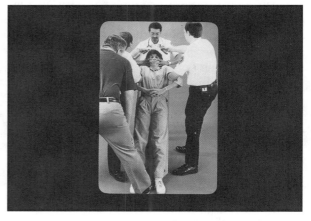

6. The EMT at the head should support the board against his body. One of the EMTs at the side should release the hand-hold at the top end of the board and reposition his arm outside of the arms of the EMT immobilizing the head. Once both EMTs at the sides have changed their holds, they should again fully assume the weight of the board. Without losing the immobilization, the EMT at the head should rotate one hand at a time so his fingers point in a caudad direction.

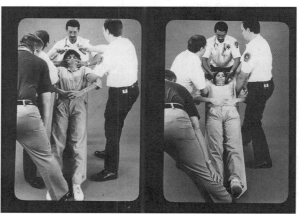

7. Once these changes have been made, the head end of the board can again be lowered while the patient's head and torso are maintained in a neutral in-line position. As the head of the board nears the ground, the three EMTs who are supporting it and the patient's weight will have to bend their knees and move to a kneeling position. Care must be taken when lowering the board to avoid bearing any weight with the EMT's back bent.

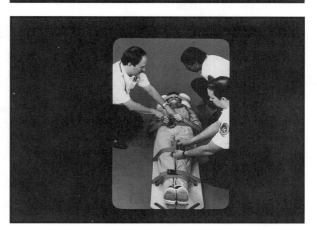

8. While the EMT continues to provide the in-line manual immobilization from his position beyond the patient's head, the team leader should complete the initial assessment of the patient while the third EMT provides any padding needed to fill the void between the back of the patient's head and the board. He should also provide any immediate interventions needed and, as soon as time allows, install a cervical collar.

9. Once the initial rapid assessment has been completed and any interventions indicated have been provided, the patient's torso, then head, and finally legs and arms can be immobilized to the board and transport can be initiated.

The reader should note that the risks of *NOT* immediately supporting a standing unstable patient and lowering him on the longboard to a supine position on the ground without delay outweigh the risks of moving him while only manually immobilized to the board and without a cervical collar. In such cases the EMT should not delay lowering the patient in order to install a cervical collar or the base of a head immobilizer to the board. The collar should only be installed once the patient is supine and any immediate ABC needs have been met. If the base of the head immobilizer is not stored on the board in the ambulance, blanket rolls and tape should be used instead since it can not be safely secured once the board is on the ground with the patient on it.

ETI SUMMARY SKILL SHEET
General Method For Spinal Immobilization

Note: The steps to be followed when immobilizing a patient who is suspected or known to have spine injury are not essentially different whether the patient presents in a sitting, lying or standing position. Therefore, the EMT should learn one generic sequence which can be followed regardless of the patient's presenting position or equipment to be used, rather than trying to remember a variety of separate instructions. The summary below will serve as a guideline for any patient with spine trauma.

1. CONFIRM SCENE SAFETY.

2. TAKE/CONFIRM proper UNIVERSAL body substance isolation PRECAUTIONS.

3. DETERMINE MECHANISM OF INJURY.

4. DIRECT another EMT to provide neutral in-line MANUAL IMMOBILIZATION of the head.

5. EVALUATE ABCs and provide any immediate interventions required.

6. Examine further and CHECK MSC X4.

7. If the patient is wearing one, REMOVE THE HELMET, unless contraindicated.

8. Examine the neck and measure and APPLY A CERVICAL COLLAR, unless contraindicated.

9. IDENTIFY methods and RETRIEVE AND PREPARE EQUIPMENT that will be needed.

10. PLACE the PATIENT ON the BOARD OR the DEVICE ON PATIENT.

11. PROPERLY POSITION HIM/IT.

12. IMMOBILIZE THE UPPER TORSO so it can not move up or down, left or right, or anteriorly away from the device. IF SITTING or otherwise indicated, SECURE a strap AT the MID-TORSO.

13. IMMOBILIZE LOWER TORSO with either a strap across the iliac crests or a pair of groin loops.

14. RE-EVALUATE ALL TORSO STRAPS, and ADJUST any as needed prior to securing the head to the device.

15. RE-EVALUATE HEAD POSITION, adjust as needed for neutral in-line alignment (unless contraindicated) and INSERT firm PADDING as needed TO FILL ANY VOID between the back of the head and the device.

16. Properly POSITION BOLSTERS (head immobilizer pillows or blanket rolls) OR HEAD FLAPS AT the SIDES OF the HEAD.

17. Immobilize the head to the device. PLACE A STRAP (or tape) tightly ACROSS THE LOWER FOREHEAD and ANOTHER snugly ACROSS THE anterior portion of the CERVICAL COLLAR

18. **IF SITTING,** MOVE the immobilized PATIENT onto a LONGBOARD and secure the vest or half-board to it. If a vest-type was used, add a head immobilizer or blanket rolls and tape AND CONTINUE to the next step.
   IF LYING DIRECTLY ON THE LONGBOARD, CONTINUE to the next step.

19. TIE THE patient's FEET TOGETHER.

20. IMMOBILIZE the UPPER LEGS to the board WITH A STRAP across the legs PROXIMAL OF THE KNEES.

21. IMMOBILIZE the LOWER LEGS to the board (WITH BLANKET ROLLS LATERAL TO EACH, or by encircling them several times first) WITH A STRAP across the legs DISTAL OF THE KNEES.

22. PLACE BOTH ARMS extended palm-in at the patient's sides ON THE BOARD AND SECURE THEM with a strap placed over the wrists and lower torso.

23. RE-CHECK the ABCs and provide any additional intervention indicated.

24. RE-CHECK the MSCs X4. If the immobilization has COMPROMISED the CIRCULATION in any LIMB, ADJUST the APPROPRIATE STRAPS TO RESTORE IT.

25. PLACE THE patient and LONGBOARD on the ambulance cot.

26. SECURE THE PATIENT and longboard TO THE COT with the cot straps, and secure it in the ambulance.

27. INITIATE TRANSPORT AND MONITOR THE PATIENT. Periodically re-check the vital signs while ENROUTE.

ETI SUMMARY SKILL SHEET
Immobilizing A Standing Patient (Modified Immobilization Sequence)

Note: Although the general steps for spinal immobilization presented in the first of the Summary Skill Sheets is generic to patients found in any position, it requires some modifications in the sequence when the patient is found standing. In order to provide a precise guideline for this event, a separate summary for immobilizing a standing patient has been included here.

1. CONFIRM SCENE SAFETY.

2. TAKE/CONFIRM proper UNIVERSAL body substance isolation PRECAUTIONS.

3. DETERMINE exact MECHANISM OF INJURY.

4. DIRECT (a tall) EMT TO stand behind the patient and PROVIDE neutral in-line MANUAL IMMOBILIZATION of the head, AND DIRECT THE PATIENT TO STAND WITHOUT MOVING.

5. From the patient's ability to stand and a quick Global Survey, IDENTIFY ANY significant EXTERNAL BLEEDING AND WHETHER THE SCENE AND PATIENT APPEAR STABLE or unstable.

6. SUPPORT THE PATIENT'S TORSO AND DIRECT ANOTHER EMT TO RETRIEVE THE BACKBOARD and other needed equipment from the ambulance. EXPLAIN THE STEPS you will be employing TO THE PATIENT.

7. When he returns, have him INSERT THE LONGBOARD AND properly POSITION IT ON THE PATIENT'S BACK.

8. *IF STABLE*, APPLY A CERVICAL COLLAR AND SECURE THE PATIENT'S TORSO THEN HEAD TO THE BOARD in the customary way.
IF UNSTABLE, with one EMT reaching under the patient's armpit from each side, MANUALLY SUPPORT AND IMMOBILIZE THE PATIENT'S TORSO to the board.

9. With the patient's head and torso secured or manually immobilized to the board, STEP THE BOARD AND LOWER THE HEAD END HALFWAY TO THE GROUND AND STOP.

10. Once the EMTs have REPOSITIONED, as needed, LOWER IT the rest of the way TO THE GROUND. CHECK THE ABC'S AND PROVIDE any indicated INTERVENTIONS.

11. IF NOT PREVIOUSLY DONE, APPLY A CERVICAL COLLAR AND IMMOBILIZE THE TORSO AND HEAD to the board. Next, TIE THE FEET together AND IMMOBILIZE THE LEGS TO THE BOARD.

12. CHECK THE PATIENT'S MSCs in all 4 extremities. IF the distal circulation in any limb has been compromised, adjust the appropriate straps as needed to restore it.

13. PLACE THE IMMOBILIZED PATIENT ON THE ambulance COT AND SECURE the patient and longboard to it with the cot straps.

14. LOAD the cot into the ambulance AND INITIATE TRANSPORT.

ETI SUMMARY SKILL SHEET
Using a KED (Recommended Modified Method)

Note: Due to the consistent design and longevity of the KED, its application today is often taught in the same way as when it was first introduced. Many of the methods taught from place to place, although widely accepted and promulgated in past years, do *NOT* include the currently recognized general anatomical and physiological principles for immobilizing a patient (with *any* device). Therefore, it is not uncommon when evaluating EMTs to find an extrication vest applied so that the patient's head — instead of being maintained in proper neutral in-line alignment — has been drawn into a hyperextended position. Additionally, the straps at the upper and mid-torso commonly either do not sufficiently prevent caudad (or in some cases, even cephalad) movement of the device on the patient's torso, or have been placed around the mid-torso so tightly that although movement is prevented they cause respiratory embarrassment. It is also not uncommon to find the groin loolps secured so they

are ineffective in immobilizing the lower torso or so they surround the upper legs. If these are across the upper legs, when the legs are moved to extricate the patient from the vehicle movement of the vest on the torso and of the spinal column, will generally result.

Although the recommended directions for the use of many brands of extrication vests would benefit from re-evaluation and modification so that they meet the current criteria for effective spinal immobilization, it is impractical to include a separate Summary Skill Sheet in the text for each model and brand of extrication vest that is available. Since its introduction, the KED has remained the prevalent extrication vest used throughout the country. Therefore, exclusively a Summary Skill Sheet which integrates the specific design of the present KED with the currently recognized criteria for spinal immobilization has been included. Although similar recommendations for the method of application of the device can be found in other sources, the following steps have *NOT* been reviewed or evaluated by the individuals who developed the KED or by its manufacturer. They are solely based upon the currently accepted criteria for spinal immobilization and independent experience with the device in the field. Since the method outlined below does not physically alter the vest in any way, nor omits or alters the designed securing together of any of its elements, it should not affect the structural design or integrity of the device.

As with any directions or recommended skills steps, they are published solely to provide an educational guideline and should only be used after they have been reviewed and approved by the service medical director or other local medical authority who has the responsibility for determining local protocols and practices.

1. CONFIRM SCENE SAFETY.

2. TAKE/CONFIRM proper UNIVERSAL body substance isolation PRECAUTIONS.

3. DETERMINE exact MECHANISM OF INJURY.

4. DIRECT another EMT TO PROVIDE neutral in-line MANUAL IMMOBILIZATION of the head.

5. EVALUATE ABCs, PROVIDE any INTERVENTIONS indicated, AND RULE OUT any need FOR a RAPID EXTRICATION.

6. Examine further and CHECK MSC X4.

7. IF the patient is wearing one, REMOVE THE HELMET unless contraindicated.

8. Examine the neck and measure and APPLY A CERVICAL COLLAR unless contraindicated.

9. Direct another EMT to RETRIEVE AND READY THE KED, a longboard, and the other equipment that will be needed.

10. While supporting the spine, MOVE the PATIENT FORWARD ON THE SEAT if necessary until there is sufficient space between his back and the front of the seat-back to allow the KED to be inserted.

11. ORIENT THE KED PROPERLY AND HOLD IT so its base is just off the ground and the head end is angled towards the patient, so you are READY TO INSERT IT.

12. Direct the EMT providing manual immobilization of the head to elevate his elbows and INSERT THE KED between the patient and the seat-back.

13. CENTER THE KED on the patient's back and MOVE IT UPWARD UNTIL the torso side-flaps are SNUGLY placed UP IN EACH ARMPIT.

14. HOLD THE properly placed KED AGAINST THE PATIENT'S BACK and RELEASE the velcro loops which hold each half of the TOP TORSO STRAP.

15. CONNECT THE halves of the TOP TORSO STRAP AND TIGHTEN IT to secure the vest around the torso at the armpit level.

16. RELEASE, CONNECT AND TIGHTEN (snugly, not tightly) the MID-TORSO STRAP.

17. RELEASE, CONNECT AND TIGHTEN (snugly, not tightly) the second MID-TORSO STRAP.

18. Using cravats, tape, or narrow straps, ADD A TIE from each lifting loop at the back, OVER THE SHOULDER and through the top torso strap on each side to secure the vest from caudad movement.

19. RELEASE AND INSERT ONE GROIN STRAP under the adjacent upper leg proximal of the knee, and "SEE-SAW" IT until correctly in position UNDER THE BUT-TOCK AND IN-LINE WITH THE INTERGLUTEAL FOLD. After bringing it through the groin and around one side of the pelvis, CONNECT AND FASTEN IT to the buckle on the same side of the midline as its point of origin.

20. DO THE SAME WITH THE SECOND GROIN LOOP on the patient's other side.

21. EVALUATE EACH TORSO STRAP AND ADJUST each AS NEEDED to position and tension them properly PRIOR TO SECURING THE HEAD TO THE DEVICE.

22. RE-EVALUATE THE manually immobilized POSITION OF THE HEAD AND ADJUST AS NEEDED to improve its neutral in-line alignment.

23. INSERT as much FIRM PADDING (*not* soft spongy material that will compressd) AS NEEDED TO fill any void between THE BACK OF THE HEAD and the posterior head section of the KED.

24. While another EMT maintains the manual immobilization, HAVE THE EMT BEHIND THE PATIENT release his hold and PLACE THE HEAD FLAPS against the lateral sides of the patient's head, and then again assure the manual immobilization with his hands placed on the outside of the flaps.

25. PROPERLY POSITION AND TIGHTLY SECURE A HEAD STRAP between each head flap ACROSS THE FOREHEAD so its caudad edge is just inferior to the supra-orbital ridge. Tape may be used instead of a head strap.

26. SECURE THE SECOND HEAD STRAP onto each head flap, SNUGLY ACROSS THE ANTERIOR CERVICAL COLLAR. Tape may be used instead of a head strap. Be sure that it does not prevent the mouth from being opened.

27. Place the appropriate end of the backboard on the seat next to the patient's buttock and rotate and lower him onto the board *or*, when this is not practical lift him and the KED together and PLACE THE PATIENT IMMOBILIZED BY THE KED ONTO THE LONGBOARD and position him and the board properly on the ambulance cot.

28. SECURE THE KED (and patient's torso) TO THE LONGBOARD AND TIE THE FEET together.

29. SECURE THE UPPER LEGS TO THE LONGBOARD with a strap placed across them proximal to the knees.

30. SECURE THE LOWER LEGS TO THE LONGBOARD by placing blanket rolls at each side of them (or encircling them several times with a strap) before placing a strap across them distal to the knees.

31. ADD A HEAD IMMOBILIZER OR BLANKET ROLLS AND TAPE to increase the immobilization of the head for transport.

32. Extend each arm palm-in along the patient's sides and SECURE THE ARMS TO THE BOARD.

33. RECHECK THE ABCs and provide any additional interventions indicated.

34. RE-EVALUATE THE MSCs in all four extremities and, if the distal circulation in any limb has been compromised, adjust the appropriate straps as needed to restore it.

35. SECURE THE PATIENT AND LONGBOARD TO THE ambulance COT AND, after loading them into the ambulance, INITIATE TRANSPORT.

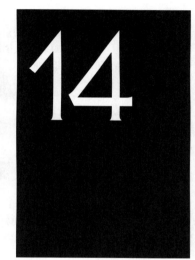

SECTION

Bandaging and Wound Care Skills

14

Introduction

The skin is the outer layer of tissue surrounding the body, and normally serves to keep dirt and other foreign matter from entering the body. When an injury results in a wound, this barrier is breached and dirt, other alien particulate matter and fluid can enter. Since these generally contain micro-organisms, this breach in the body's outer barrier and the introduction of foreign matter promotes an increased risk of infection. To prevent this, most minor wounds (and the area immediately surrounding the wound) should be cleaned with an antiseptic fluid and the wound covered with a bandage to prevent the introduction of any additional foreign matter.

The term **bandage** is often used to generically describe all of the fabric that is applied over a wound to protect it. More accurately, wounds are covered using two distinct and differently termed layers of protective fabric. The initial layers of fabric which immediately cover the area of breached skin should be sterile, and are called *dressings*. These are then secured in place (and additional protection is provided) by additional layers of fabric placed over the dressings. This outer fabric is actually the *bandage*. Unlike dressings, bandages should be clean but do not need to be sterile. Even when sterile fabric (such as a sterile roller bandage) is used and proper aseptic technique is followed, the outer layers of the bandage are almost immediately contaminated by contact. Therefore, regardless of whether the material used is sterile or not, once a bandage has been applied it should no longer be considered sterile.

WOUND CARE

The initial priority in treating any wound is to control any significant external bleeding. The second priority, when possible (as in the case of the abdomen and lower extremities), is to control any associated internal bleeding. More definitive individual wound care should only be initiated once all significant bleeding has been controlled, fractures have been identified and temporarily stabilized to prevent further injury, and the EMT has assessed that no injuries or conditions are present which require more immediate care or indicate that transport of the patient be rapidly initiated.

When the patient has multi-systems trauma or a wound in conjunction with an acute medical emergency, individual wound care beyond the control of any significant bleeding must generally be omitted or limited to simply covering the wound with dressings held in place by several strips of tape to avoid unnecessary delay in the field. In such cases the EMT's proper focus on higher care priorities may often result in minor wounds remaining undetected until enroute to the hospital or at the emergency department. When ruling out the presence of urgent priorities the EMT must consider the possible cumulative blood loss prior to his arrival as well as any bleeding and shock that is evident. The skills required in making these evaluations and providing the appropriate interventions needed have been presented in previous Sections of this text. The modifications and skills needed to provide care for wounds associated with open fractures and other skeletal injuries will be found in the Section which follows this, covering Splinting Skills. Since most splinting requires the use of some bandaging skills, this Section has been placed so that these skills are introduced before those needed to stabilize musculoskeletal injuries.

When wounds are minor (in dimension and bleeding) they are treated by initially removing any superficial debris and dirt and then covering them with several layers of dry sterile dressing. They are then further protected by several layers of clean dry bandage. The bandage holds the dressing securely in place and also protects the sterile dressing and wound from outside dirt.

Although an antiseptic solution may be used to minimize the possible bacteriological invasion of small minor wounds, its use with any significant wound is not recommended. Attempts to definitively clean any wound in the field are generally ineffectual and the need for careful irrigation and cleansing in the emergency department have been scientifically proven in a large number of studies. In the field, this is of little or no benefit and actually promotes greater contamination and harm. Therefore, beyond cleaning the adjacent skin and removing any gross surface debris, *the EMT should NOT attempt to debride, irrigate or otherwise further clean any significant wound in the field.* Except in special remote situations when the patient will not be seen in the emergency department for many hours or even days, antiseptic gels or ointments (such as Bacitracin ointment) should *NOT* be used as these will impede definitive care at the hospital.

In summary, the general care for wounds in the field should be:

- Stop any significant bleeding.
- Remove any surface debris which is not impaled or deep within the wound.
- With minor wounds only, clean the skin adjacent to the wound.
- Apply a suitable dry sterile dressing. Secure the dressing and protect it and the wound area with a bandage.
- Transport or have the patient go to the emergency department for definitive cleaning, evaluation, and wound care (including evaluation for a tetanus booster).

If an object is impaled and protrudes from the wound, it should *NOT* be removed in the field. The object should be manually stabilized and the dressings should be cut so they can be placed over the wound and around the object. The bandage, as well as covering the wound area, must also secure the object from further movement during transport. In some cases, the addition of a wire splint formed into a gantry to support the object may be a useful adjunct in keeping the object from moving.

When a wound includes an evisceration and internal abdominal organs protrude through the wound, the treatment is different. Should the protruding parts become dry, the survival of the exposed tissue is unlikely. Therefore, such wounds are treated by covering them with wet dressings instead. These dressings should be soaked with sterile Normal Saline or Lactated Ringer's Solution *before* they are placed over the evisceration and should be kept wet at all times. During transport the dressings should be checked periodically and more sterile fluid added as needed to keep them saturated. *The use of plain water (sterile or clean drinking water) will result in causing excessive tissue damage, and should be avoided.* Alternatives, and the use of a fluid impervious covering, will be discussed in more detail later in this Section.

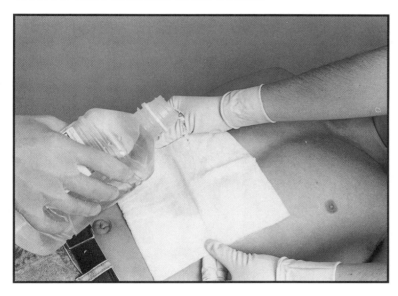

Burns are wounds. The object of wound care in the burn patient is to prevent further damage and infection. Remove all clothing around the burn, but do *NOT* pull away clothing that is stuck to the wound. Burned areas should then be covered with dry sterile dressings, however gauze or other material which sheds and leaves particles should be avoided. Experience has shown that the use of burn packs or burn sheets is preferred but, if these are not available, clean pillow cases or bed sheets can be used instead.

Although the use of wet dressings was advocated in the past, this is currently *NOT* recommended. In some cases, limited areas (under 10% of the body surface) with painful second degree burns (partial thickness) can be covered with cool wet dressings to provide pain relief. The use of wet dressings in this manner is a debated issue and the EMT should only include it according to protocol when pain relief is necessary and not otherwise available.

Burn ointments, topical analgesics or other topical burn medications should NOT be used by the EMT in the field.

In the case of chemical burns, the substance should be diluted and removed by copiously flushing the area with water under a shower before the wound is dressed. All of the patient's clothing must be removed during the dilution process to assure that none of the product becomes trapped in clothing or shoes and continues to burn the patient. Some chemical agents become volatile in water or are *NOT* water soluble (examples: sodium and phenol, respectively) and must be neutralized and removed in specific ways according to their chemical properties. Further discussion of this is beyond the scope of this book and the EMT should refer to the Burn or Thermal Injury Chapters in his text.

Wounds and other injuries of the eye require different treatment than that used for most wounds. Similarly, a detailed discussion of eye injuries is beyond the scope of this book and the EMT should refer to the appropriate section in his EMT text for this information. The discussion of eye injuries in the following pages of this Section are limited to simple bandaging, and covering of the eye when it has an impaled protruding object or has been avulsed.

The skills for treating other avulsions and amputations are found in the discussion of Splinting Skills in the next Section.

DRESSINGS

A dressing serves two important functions. It is a sterile barrier between the wound and the non-sterile bandage, and it aids the body's natural defenses in promoting the control of bleeding.

Sterile dressings are usually made of folded thin layers of loosely woven gauze. The fine mesh of the initial gauze layers provide a physical framework which supports clotting (and a surface scab) to seal and control bleeding or other fluid loss from an open wound. *Any movement or removal of a dressing from a wound once it has remained in place even for a short period should be avoided as this may breach the integrity of the surface clot or scab which is intertwined through its fibers and cause bleeding to resume.* If the gauze dressings initially placed over the wound become saturated with blood, they should be covered with additional layers of dressing rather than be removed. When direct pressure is applied over a wound, a dressing should be included initially, or as soon as possible, to maximize the clotting process.

Sterile dressings come in a variety of sizes and shapes. The most common are folded into thin four-inch squares (4 by 4s) or two inch squares (2 by 2s).

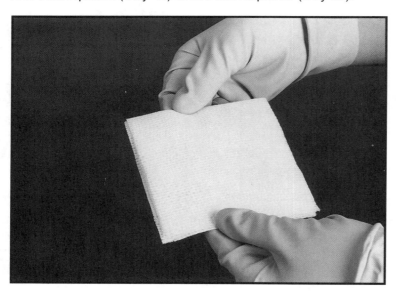

These gauze pads contain sufficient layers and are so folded that they can easily be opened at one fold so that the 4x4's can be made into a 4x8 inch size and the 2x2's into a 2x4 inch size. Generally a number of gauze pads must be placed on the wound to obtain the desired thickness for the dressing. In the field, individual sterile packages containing two of these gauze pads in a "peel-away" paper wrap are the most commonly used. Sterile single-patient packages ("tubs") of ten to twelve gauze pads are also available. Large quantity bulk multi-patient packages of these *gauze pads*, although useful as "sponges," should *NOT* be used for sterile dressings. Once such bulk packages have been opened the unused gauze pads are open to the air and are no longer sterile.

Gauze pads which are larger in area and thickness are also available. These are commonly referred to as **trauma dressings** or **ABD** pads (because they were developed to dress abdominal surgical incisions). Due to their size and the numerous layers necessary to form their increased thickness, they often contain a row of stitching along their center to help keep them properly organized. ABD pads generally come folded in half in individual sterile paper packages.

Any of the previously described gauze pads can be used to form either a plain dry or wet dressing as needed. Although not commonly found in the field, the EMT should know of another type of dressing that is commonly used in the emergency department and physician's offices. **Non-adherent dressing pads** (such as Telfa) are used to cover wounds which do not have significant bleeding. They are made of a smooth impervious fabric (or have a similar coating) that does not allow blood to penetrate and form a clot within their fabric. These are not appropriate in an emergency setting when immediate bleeding control is a primary objective. They are generally only used in a continued care setting when the dressing will frequently be removed for periodic re-evaluation and treatment of the wound. Since blood and the scab produced by clotting do not enter and form into the fabric of non-adherent dressings, the scab is not torn or removed — causing the resumption of bleeding, increased risk of infection, and delaying the healing process — each time the dressing must be removed and changed.

Sterile gauze pads impregnated with petroleum jelly or other medications are also available. A Vaseline-impregnated dressing is useful when an occlusive dressing is needed to prevent air from entering a "sucking wound" of the chest. Otherwise, dressings impregnated with medications are not generally used in the pre-hospital emergency setting.

When applying a dressing, the EMT should carefully follow proper aseptic techniques (demonstrated in the following pages) when opening the package and removing the dressing, and when he installs it over the wound. Particular care must be taken to correctly position the dressing prior to laying it on the patient's skin. *A dressing should NEVER be repositioned by sliding it along the skin's surface once it has been placed in contact with the patient, nor removed and then replaced over the wound.* Either of these practices will cause contaminants from the area adjacent to the wound to be unnecessarily introduced into it, significantly increasing the chance of infection. Should a sterile pad be so misplaced that it must be moved, it should be removed and discarded (in a suitable bio-hazard waste container) and then replaced with a new one.

Some of the outermost edges of any dressing will become contaminated when they are held and the dressing is placed on the patient. Therefore, the edges should always be placed at least one inch (or more) beyond the perimeter of the wound. When the area to be covered is greater than the size of the individual pads used, they should be placed so that the edges of the initial layers overlap each other by about an inch (or in the case of 2x2's at least 1/2 to 3/4 of an inch).

How thick a dressing should be is somewhat a matter of judgment. In most cases a sufficient depth of dressing is achieved using three or four 4x4s or 2x2s placed on top of each other (or twice that number if they have been opened to a 4x8 or 2x4 inch size) or by a single trauma dressing or ABD pad. In some cases, slightly more may be desirable, however care must be taken — when applying dressings over a wound for which direct pressure is required — that the dressing is *NOT* so thick as to dissipate and defeat the direct pressure over the wound. In some special cases such as multiple injuries to the hand, large bulky dressings may be advantageous.

In the case of extremely large wounds with continued profuse bleeding, dressings may first need to be packed into the wound to act as sponges and help control the bleeding before others are placed over them. *Except when packing a nostril in the case of a nose-bleed (epistaxis) which can not otherwise be controlled, gauze pads or packing should NEVER be inserted into any of the body's normal orifices by the EMT.* Similarly, the EMT should not insert pads and pack wounds which communicate into the thoracid or abdominal cavities, unless he has advanced training and this skill is included in his protocols. As mentioned in another section, fractures or other injuries which produce open communication into the cranium should never be packed, or even covered, if there is a chance that the dressing can contact the brain tissues or meninges.

BANDAGES

A bandage can be made from almost any soft fabric, even including using the patient's clothing (such as pinning a sleeve to the front of a shirt to produce an arm sling). Except in rare situations requiring such improvisation, the EMT can more efficiently and better bandage the patient with commercial bandages that are especially designed for this purpose.

Roller bandages, made of narrow strips of fabric which come individually packaged in 54 to 72 inch lengths wound into a roll, have proven to be the most universal and enduring bandage used for pre-hospital care. Many years ago the roller bandages were made of sterile gauze which was dipped into a starch-like solution to stiffen the material and lock each intersection where the individual threads cross each other). This made the material relatively inflexible when sideways bending of the roll or angulation was needed to conform both edges of the bandage around the changing diameter of a limb or the angle at a joint. In those days, first-aiders had to learn and practice a variety of roller bandage folds (such as multiple periodic spiral-reverses) and skills in order to make a snug and properly conforming bandage from the roll.

In recent years, improvements in the fabric design used in roller bandages allow easier and better conforming application.

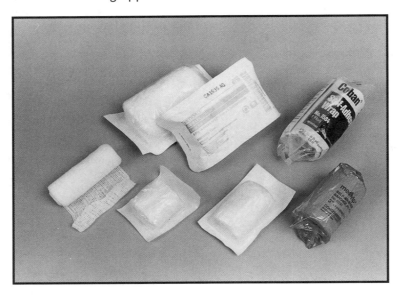

The various brands of gauze roller bandage presently available can be classified into two types: those with a very loose, open, and highly flexible weave such as Kling, and those with a tighter, thicker and slightly less flexible weave such as Conform. To those highly experienced in the use of roller bandage, each has an advantage when bandaging differing types of injuries or areas of the body.

Most brands are available in a number of different widths, including 1, 2, 3, 4 and 6 inches. Individual fingers can most easily be bandaged using a 1 or 2 inch width. Hands and feet can be covered using a 2 or 3 inch width. When a larger area of an arm or leg must be covered, the 3 or 4 inch width is preferable.

Although almost all brands come sterile and, if proper aseptic technique to maintain their sterility is followed, the first few winds around the wound can serve as a dressing, most EMTs find it is easier to use separate sterile gauze pads for this purpose and only use the roller as a bandage. However, the reader should note that if the EMT finds himself in a remote setting and without sufficient sterile dressings, this method can be used. Alternatively, with proper aseptic technique. strips of a sterile roller can be folded to make sterile gauze dressing pads.

In recent years, several brands of roller bandage made of a flexible elasticized fabric which only adheres to itself (Colban, Medi-Rip, Co-Flex, etc.) have also become available. Due to their elasticized nature, care must be taken to assure that the bandage is not applied too tightly. *When using any self-adhering bandage the EMT should never apply it while simultaneously unrolling the bandage from the roll.* Instead, unroll 12 to 15 inches at a time while holding the end of the bandage that has already been applied with your other hand. In this way the tension produced when unrolling the bandage will *NOT* inadvertently be placed against the previously applied turns, resulting in overly tight wrapping around the limb. The use of a self-adhering bandage is the easiest way to form a bandage to cover the top of the skull.

Regardless of whether the roller bandage has some adherent quality or not, when the bandage is completed the end should be securely fastened with adhesive tape to assure that it can not loosen or become unwound. In remote situations, if adhesive tape is not available the ends can be cut or torn for some distance along the center of their width to produce two tails. Once a knot is tied to prevent any further tearing, one tail can be taken around each side of the extremity and both tails tied together to secure the end of the bandage.

Triangular bandages are another type of bandage commonly used in pre-hospital care. They are either unfolded as a large triangle or folded into a long two or three inch wide tie called a *cravat bandage*. Although triangular and cravat bandages can be used singularly or in combination to form bandages for any part of the body, such use is not a common practice today. Because roller bandages produce better and more secure coverage, the routine use of triangular bandages by EMTs is generally limited for arm slings or as cravat ties to secure a splint to the patient, one part of the body to another, or the patient to a device.

The EMT may have to use triangular bandages in lieu of other choices in remote situations when roller bandages are not available, or in Mass Casualty situations when bandaging supplies may be limited or the speed with which they can be applied overrides the advantages of other types. These skills remain a useful adjunct to any provider's bandaging skills, since they furnish him with a variety of alternatives which in some exceptional circumstances may represent the only ones available. When no other bandaging is available, triangular bandages can be easily cut or torn from bed sheets or any other suitable flat pieces of fabric.

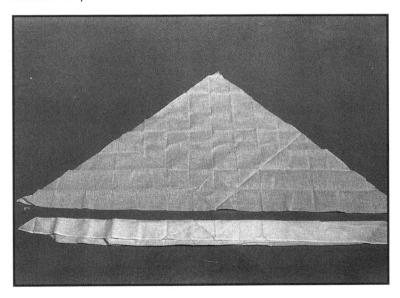

A quantity of commercially produced triangular bandages are commonly carried in most trauma kits and on the ambulance. These are generally made of muslin (a stiffened cotton fabric) or a muslin-like synthetic fabric, and are individually packaged in a sealed plastic bag. Each package usually also contains two large safety pins. Although the fabric is sterilized at one point in the process, triangular bandages are not manufactured or packaged to maintain a sterile status. *Although commercial triangular bandages are exceptionally clean, they are NOT STERILE and therefore should never be placed in direct contact with an open wound.*

Compress bandages are also used in pre-hospital care. Compress bandages are unique in that they are a bandage which comes with the dressing attached to it. The most common of these is the *band-aid*. Except for band-aids and other shapes of adhesive with dressings at their center (Coverlets, etc.), the only other common form is a *trauma compress*. These have a number of sterile gauze pads (generally 4x6 or 4x8 inches long) sewn onto the center of a slightly wider 12 to 24 inch strip of fabric and are generally used to rapidly dress and bandage wounds of the extremities. Trauma compresses were developed by the military to provide a small self-contained wound care package that can easily and rapidly be applied to any limb under even the most adverse of conditions.

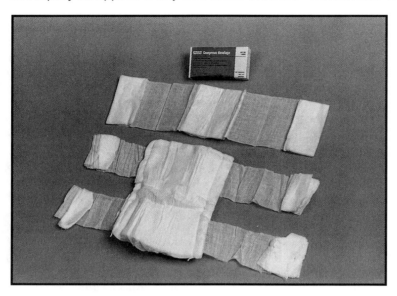

Because commercial compress bandages include both the bandage and the attached dressings, they are provided in individual sterile packages. When opening, handling, and applying a compress bandage, the EMT must be especially careful to avoid touching the dressing or moving it along the patient's skin. To avoid undesired sticking and chance contamination, most adhesive compress bandages come with paper or plastic peel-away covers secured over the adhesive ends and covering the dressing. These are removed one at a time as the compress is applied to ensure proper placement without undesirable contact with the dressing area. When the EMT secures gauze pads to the patient with strips of adhesive tape, he has actually made a form of compress bandage.

ADHESIVE TAPE

Adhesive tape is generally a key adjunct used to secure a bandage and, in some cases, may be used to replace one. In the early days of EMS, only one type of adhesive tape was commonly available and was both used in the field and within the hospital. Because many experienced users find that this heavy white adhesive backed fabric tape provides superior adhesion to the skin it is still widely used in the field. Several types of more flexible, fluid impervious, and hypoallergenic plastic based adhesive tapes provide an equal degree of skin adhesion and are also widely used in the field. Commonly, a supply of each is found in trauma kits and on the ambulance. If the EMT must make a long strip which is narrower than the commercial width available to him, it is generally easier to do this using the heavier fabric rather than a plastic type. Due to weave of the material, most fabric adhesive tape will tear in a straight line along its "grain." Plastic-type adhesive tape usually must be tediously cut for the entire length desired, and a jagged irregular product results.

Paper-backed medical adhesive tape is also commonly used in a hospital or physician's office setting. This type can be more easily and less painfully removed than other types and usually results in less aggravation to the skin. In this setting, when continued wound care dictates the frequent removal and replacement of bandages and dressings, this type of tape is often preferred. Since it does not adhere as strongly, and is less durable than fabric or plastic types, its use in the field is *NOT* recommended.

Adhesive tape should not be considered or used as a bandage except in the case of extremely small cuts. When tape strips are used to secure dressings over a larger wound, the tape does not provide the proper cover to isolate the wound and sterile dressing from contamination by exposure and contact with the environment. Except when such abridgement is dictated by urgency, it should not be arbitrarily elected. Wound care should include the application of dressings *and protective covering* with a suitable bandage. Although a suitable bandage could be made by completely covering the entire dressing with overlapping strips of tape, it is far simpler, more effective, and safer to do this with conventional bandages and methods instead.

Adhesive tape (except for very small cuts) should solely be considered as an adjunct to bandaging and splinting. Adhesive tape is only recommended for use to:

• Secure the ends of a bandage.
• Secure separate bandages together.
• Secure dressings to the skin.
• Secure tubes, tubing, needles, catheters or other light appliances to the skin or each other (when significant tension is not suggested).
• Secure padding to a splint.
• Secure overlapping parts of a splint or several overlapping splints together.

When applying adhesive tape to the skin, the skin should first be cleaned of blood and any foreign matter. The adhesive tape will *NOT* adhere properly if the skin is wet or even moist. Therefore, any areas which will be contacted by the tape should be dried with gauze sponges or a clean towel before the tape is applied. Care must be taken in the length and number of tape strips that are applied to the skin. These should be sufficient to properly secure the item without fastening excessive amounts of tape to the skin.

When securing the ends of bandages, the end should be taped over previously applied turns of the bandage rather than to the skin whenever possible. Strips of tape used to secure bandages, splints or other items to an extremity (except when carefully applied around a finger) should not be placed so that they totally or near totally surround the diameter of the limb as this can result in reducing or tourniqueting the circulation in the extremity. Similarly, tape should not be applied so as to surround or significantly encircle the thorax. When applying tape to the chest, any inhibition of chest excursion (particularly chest rise) must be avoided. Proper ventilation should be reconfirmed after the tape has been applied.

Experience has shown that when applying tape, unrolling and cutting strips is preferable to using it directly from the roll. Adhesive tape generally comes in 1/2, 1, 2, 3, 4 and 6 inch wide rolls. Because many field needs can be met using rolls which are either 1/2, 1, or 2 inches wide, these widths are the most commonly carried in trauma and IV kits and in the ambulance. As well as multiple 1/2 or one inch rolls, carrying a 4 or 6 inch wide roll instead of numerous different widths is recommended. This will allow the EMT to rip *any width* that may be desired from a single source.

BUTTERFLY CLOSURES

Because thorough cleansing, careful evaluation, and often debridement and careful approximation of wound edges and sutures (or even more significant surgical intervention) may be needed for definitive wound care, closure to promote healing and minimize scarring is usually not a pre-hospital concern. It has been universally proven that with anything but the most minor of cuts, there is a far better outcome and much lower incidence of infection and other complications when wounds are simply dressed and bandaged in the field and closure and other definitive care are deferred to the cleaner and less rushed conditions and more capable staff at the hospital. Even in cases when physicians and the proper equipment are available in the field (such as at an emergency medical tent at large outdoor functions), definitive care and suturing achieved in such an environment have been shown to have a less desirable outcome and higher infection rate than when such care was deferred to the hospital.

In extremely rare cases, however, the temporary approximation and securing of incised wound edges, or relocation and holding in-place of an avulsed flap, until more definitive care can be provided may be necessary in the field to promote bleeding control or to secure the injury from additional harm. When necessary this is achieved by the use of a butterfly bandage.

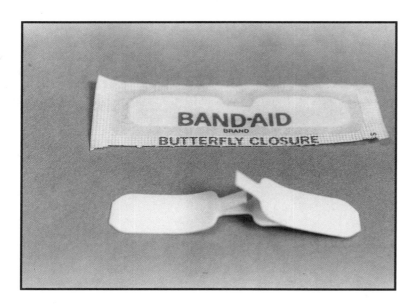

Narrow individual sterile tape strips (Steri-strips, etc.) or commercially manufactured sterile butterfly bandages are often carried by squads, or the EMT can improvise one using a clean strip of adhesive tape. (The method for making a butterfly bandage from a strip of adhesive tape is later demonstrated in this Section.)

Often, the adhesive ability of such strips or butterfly bandages is either not sufficient or is interfered with by the moisture of perspiration, and the closure cannot be maintained. In such cases, using an additional organic adhesive (such as tincture of benzoin) will promote better adhesion of the tape to the skin.

SOME WARNINGS ABOUT BANDAGES

Regardless of how carefully the dressings and bandage have been applied, the possibility that they have cumulatively become too tight must always be assumed. *Whenever any bandage, or bandaging to secure a splint (or other appliance) or parts of the body together has been completed, the EMT must check the distal circulation to ensure that it has NOT been impaired or compromised.* If a bandage or splint includes ties to secure an injured leg to the uninjured one, the distal circulation in *both* legs must be checked. Similarly, the distal circulation in both the arm and leg should be checked when an arm is placed along the side of a supine patient and the lower arm has been secured with a tie around the upper leg.

Even though a bandage may not be so tight as to compromise the distal circulation when it is applied, this can inadvertently occur later. Changes in the patient's position, or the position of an extremity, or increased swelling, can cause the bandage to tighten. Therefore, to ensure that compromise of the distal circulation is rapidly identified and eliminated, the EMT should periodically recheck the distal circulation in any bandaged extremity.

If a bandage becomes too tight it should be appropriately adjusted and the distal circulation reassessed. Adjusting the tension of a gauze roller bandage after it has been applied is rarely successful, and may result in undesirable movement of the underlying dressings. When such an adjustment is needed it is usually more efficient and safer to cut off the bandage with scissors, remove it without disturbing the dressings, and apply a new one.

Regardless of how carefully a wound is cleansed and proper aseptic technique is followed when dressing and bandaging it, the wound, dressings, and bandages applied in the field must still be considered as potentially "dirty." Therefore any dressing or bandage opened or applied in the field should *NO LONGER* be considered sterile. Although sterile dressings should be used to minimize the degree of exposure and contamination, any dressings or bandages applied in the field should be removed and replaced in a hospital, physician's office or other proper setting as soon as practical. When the injury is sufficiently minor as to not require ambulance transport, the EMT should emphasize to the patient the need for timely further evaluation and more definitive care by a physician, and carefully document this "informed warning" on his report.

When a bandage becomes wet, the fluid will transport dirt from the environment and outer surface of the bandage through it and the dressing and into the wound. Becoming wet also promotes the additional transport of contaminants from the patient's skin into the wound and possibly dirt being circulated from the surface of the wound into its deeper recesses. To avoid this, wounds and bandages (unless wet dressings are required) should be kept dry at all times. When treating a wound in the rain or snow, the EMT should simply apply some dressings and defer applying additional ones and a bandage until the patient has been moved to the dry ambulance and the body area to be bandaged has been dried.

If it is necessary to carry a patient who has been bandaged from a dry environment through rain or snow to move him into the ambulance, the EMT should be sure that the patient is properly covered so that the bandages do not become wet.

If in spite of all of the EMT's attempts to the contrary, the outside of a bandage becomes wet, if practical it should be patted dry and removed and replaced once in the ambulance. This will prevent fluid from the surface or wet outer layers from being absorbed into deeper layers and ultimately into the dressing and wound. If the bandage has been saturated with water so that its entire thickness and the dressings are completely wet, then although some contamination will have occurred further contamination can be limited by changing the upper layers of the dressing and the bandage. Even in such cases the first several layers of dressing which contact the skin should not be removed as exposing the wound will pose a greater chance of contamination and infection (as well as reinstituting bleeding) than if they are left in place.

When bandages or ties that do not cover an open wound (but have been used instead to secure a splint or other appliance or immobilize) become wet, they generally should *NOT* be removed and replaced. The interim loss of the function for which they were applied in almost all cases represents a greater danger than if they are left to dry in place. Although almost all bandage materials are preshrunk against this eventuality, the chance of greater shrinkage and becoming too tight is increased as they dry. Therefore, should they become wet, the EMT should more frequently check their tension and the distal circulation in any included extremities than he would normally.

LEARNING BANDAGING SKILLS

When teaching bandaging the instructor (or author) has two major problems. One surrounds the dynamic nature of the skill, and one the countless number of different bandages that the EMT needs to be able to reproduce.

Bandaging skills are difficult to describe and demonstrate with printed words and photographs. Because bandaging is a dynamic tactile mechanical skill, it must be initially learned by demonstration and supervised practice in hands-on workshops. The literally hundreds of different individual bandages that may be used to bandage areas from the top of the head to the distal tip of the toes or fingers make it impractical to demonstrate and practice each, and impossible to retain by memorization.

Upon observation and analysis of the human physiognomy, one finds that although there is a vast variation in size from one area to another or from one individual to another, there are actually only a few different shapes that are found. Even though the range of motion can vary significantly at different types of joints, the shape of these is so analogous that even they only cause the need for one or possibly two variations when being covered by a bandage.

Therefore, the EMT only needs to be familiar with and practice a few basic techniques which are inherent in the characteristics of each type of bandage and are generic to its use, regardless of to which part of the body this type of bandage is being applied. To make the task even less complicated, the EMT really only needs to acquire the basic skills for applying sterile dressings, compress bandages, and roller bandages to be able to form a suitable bandage for almost any area. The skills learned for the use of triangular bandages can be limited to only their unique ability as an arm sling, or when folded into cravat bandages, and used as ties. Since using these as primary bandages to secure and protect dressings to various parts of the body is only required in special rare situations, the additional skills needed can be acquired at a later time as a part of specialized Mass Casualty or "Wilderness" improvisation training.

Because when triangular bandages are used to form an arm sling or sling-and-swathe combination they are considered to be splinting adjuncts rather than bandages, the demonstration of these will be found in the next Section in the context of the other splinting skills.

APPLYING A DRY STERILE DRESSING

The most commonly used sterile dressings are 4x4 or 2x2 gauze pads. They are made of several folded layers of sterile gauze and generally come in individual sterile paper packages which contain two dressings. Larger multi-use packs are available, however as their sterility is impossible to maintain on an ambulance after the package is opened, these are not recommended. Larger sterile ABD pads and trauma dressings are also commonly available in the field. These are used to cover large wounds (as wet or dry dressings) and usually come individually wrapped in sterile paper or plastic packages.

Proper sterile technique should be followed when applying any dressing in order to minimize the introduction of additional contaminants into the wound. The dressing should be carefully located over the injury site before it is placed in contact with the patient's skin. *Once placed, a sterile dressing should NEVER be moved over the skin's surface nor, if removed, be re-applied as either will cause dirt and other contaminants from the skin adjacent to the wound to be swept into it.* Because they shed small particles, gauze pads should *NOT* be used over burns. Instead, burns should be covered with sterile burn dressings or sheets (or if formal burn dressings are not available, with clean pillow cases or cot sheets).

When a dressing is initially being applied to promote the control of bleeding in conjunction with the application of direct pressure, its introduction should *NOT* be delayed to assemble and prepare other materials that will later be needed to perfect a pressure bandage. In such cases, these will need to be gathered and prepared by another EMT while you obtain control of the bleeding.

Once a dry sterile dressing has been in place over a wound for even a short time, it should not be partially lifted or removed in the field. This can tear the clot (or scab) formed through the mesh of the gauze which lies over the wound and reinstitute or increase the bleeding. Should the bleeding be sufficient to saturate through to the outer surface of the dressing, simply add several additional dressings over those placed initially. When used with direct pressure, the thickness of the dressings placed under the EMT's gloved hand should be moderate enough so that the direct pressure is not dissipated by them. In such cases, or when a wound must be packed with dressings, once the bleeding has been controlled additional dressings should be placed over the wound and adjacent skin immediately before applying a bandage.

1. Once other more urgent priorities have been met or ruled-out, and you are ready to dress (or add additional final layers of dressing) and bandage a wound, determine the number of packages of sterile dressings you may need and which bandage material you will use to secure and cover them, (the width of roller bandage that will best cover the area or, in cases with continuing urgency, strips of adhesive tape). If there is no urgency and you plan to cover the dressings with a proper bandage, "eyeball" the patient to check that his condition has not changed.

2. Based upon the amount of blood, other body substances, or dirt on your gloves, determine if these need to be replaced. If they do, remove and discard them in a suitable bio-waste container, and put on a new pair before reaching into the kit or ambulance compartments and handling the packages of any of the dressings or bandages you will use.

3. Assemble *all* of the materials that you will need to dress and bandage the wound and place them so that they will be in easy reach when needed. Remove the bandage from its package and tear the strips of tape you will need to secure its end. Place the bandage on its clean wrapper and stick an end of each tape strip to a clean object so it will not become tangled. If a second EMT is available to assist you, direct him to do this preparation. When working alone it is essential to prepare the bandage and tape before applying the dressing in order to later avoid having to hold the dressing from moving with one hand and awkwardly attempting to apply the bandage with only the other hand available.

4. Remove any debris or other foreign particulate matter that is lying on the skin's surface and which will be covered by the dressing. If this is only a minor cut or abrasion, open a packaged antiseptic wipe (or pour antiseptic solution onto a gauze sponge and squeeze out any excess fluid), then firmly wipe the skin adjacent to the wound's edges to clean it. This should be done by moving the wipe around the circumference of the wound in an increasing circle so that any dirt is progressively wiped away from wound edges. After this has been completed for a sufficiently large area, repeat it a second time, using another clean antiseptic wipe.

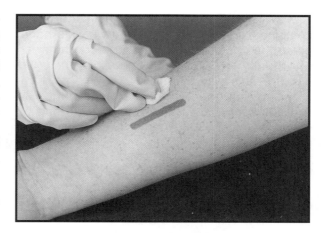

5. Hold the tear-tab found at the top of the front and back sides of the package in different hands. Peel them apart until almost all (but not all) of the front and back have been separated, exposing the dressings without the chance that they will fall out.

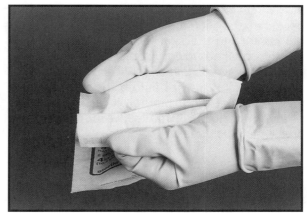

6. While holding the unseparated lower portion of the package in one hand, grasp the center of the top edge of both dressings between the thumb and first two fingers of your other hand and withdraw them from the package. Although there are a number of ways to handle dressings without contaminating their surface, the practice of always touching only the outer 1/4 to 1/2 inch of an edge, together with the assumption that all edges are *NOT STERILE*, is the easiest way to avoid possible confusion and unnecessary contamination.

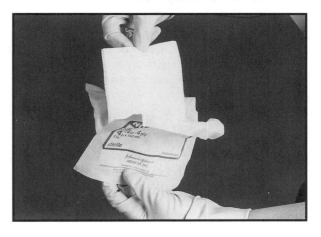

Note: The outer wrapping of sterile packages comes in contact with the objects around them, the surfaces upon which they are placed, and the hands of those handling them. Therefore, *the outside of a sterile package is NOT STERILE.* When applying dressings in the field, the EMT's gloves contact the outside of these packages, other objects, and the patient. Even if sterile gloves are put on, they will become almost immediately contaminated and should never be allowed to contact any area of a dressing which will lie directly over the wound.

7. While continuing to hold one edge of the combined dressing (both pads) with one hand, grasp the center of the opposite edge between the thumb and first two fingers of your other hand. In this way you will be able to hold the dressing taut enough between your hands so that it is kept straight and its placement can be carefully controlled.

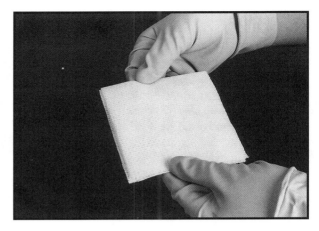

8. While securely holding the dressing as described, position it directly over the injury without contacting the skin. Once it is in the exact position desired, lower it onto the injured area. *Do NOT move it again once it lies in contact with the patient.* When possible, positioning the patient so that the injured area faces up and is near horizontal will make the application of dressings much easier.

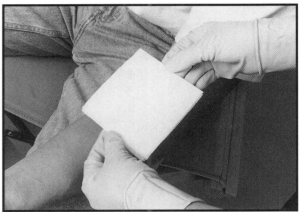

9. When the wound to be dressed is longer than the dressing, requiring that several be overlapped to cover it, one edge of the dressing will lie on the wound. In such cases, when locating the dressing prior to contact with the patient, it should be rotated so that the grasped edges are beyond the sides of the injury, and the edge which will lie on it is one that has *NOT* been touched. Then following the previously described procedure, a second dressing is placed so that it lies next to the first and overlaps it by at least 1/2 inch to complete covering the injury.

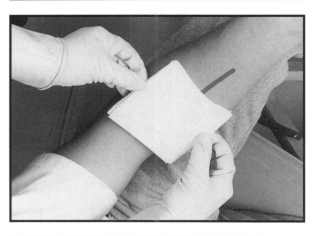

10. If when locating the gauze pad over the injury it is apparent that one of the handled edges will lie over the open injury regardless of how it is oriented, the dressing as presently folded is *TOO SMALL*. If using a 2x2, discard it and use a 4x4. A 4x4 can be unfolded to become a 4x8. The now 4x8 dressing should be turned over before it is applied, so that any edge that was handled can NOT accidentally end up in the center of the surface which will be in direct contact with the wound.

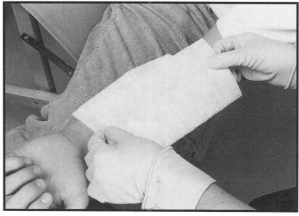

11. If an unfolded 4x4 is too small, an ABD pad or trauma dressing should be used instead. Sterile ABD pads and Trauma Dressings are usually packaged individually and folded in half or thirds. When removing these from the package and handling them, contact with the folded edge should be avoided since if it is unfolded this will run across the center of the dressing. Otherwise, they should be handled and applied in the same general manner as previously described.

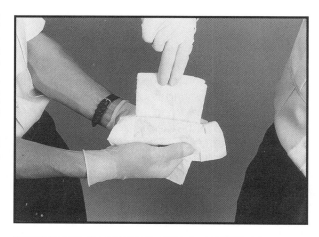

12. After all of the dressings required to cover the wound and the area immediately adjacent to it have been applied, using the same technique add as many additional dressings on top of them as are needed until the desired thickness has been achieved. Then, properly secure and protect the dressings by covering them with an appropriate bandage or, if time does not allow, secure them with strips of adhesive tape.

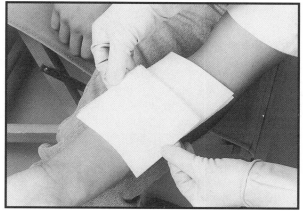

APPLYING A ROLLER BANDAGE

The use of gauze or a loosely woven gauze-like fabric *roller bandage* represents the easiest and best way to apply a bandage to any area of the body. Carrying a quantity of only three widths — 1 inch, either 2, 3, or 4 inch, and either 4 or 6 inch — is required to meet any need. The 1 inch width is useful when covering fingers or toes (although 2 inch can be used), the middle size for any other application on the extremities or head, and the widest to cover injuries of the torso. Even though only a few basic techniques are used when applying any roller bandage, these can be easily formed into the vast number of different shapes and configurations that may be needed.

Although roller bandages generally come in individual sterile packages, their singular use as *both* the dressing and bandage for a wound requires tedious aseptic technique when unpackaging and applying them and usually invites increased contamination and infection. Therefore, the use of a roller bandage (or any type except a compress bandage) to cover a wound, should only follow the proper application of separate sterile dressings.

Other than to form a bandage to cover and protect dressings and wounds, roller bandages are also widely used to secure splints to the extremities. Cravat bandages, which are also widely used for this purpose, can each only be secured to a narrow localized area. When a splint is tied to a limb with cravats spaced periodically along its length, even though it is well secured the fixation is focused at a limited number of separate narrow local points. When a roller bandage is used to secure a splint it provides equal continuous uninterrupted conforming fixation along the entire length of the device. This *may* require slightly more time, and which one to use should be determined based upon the nature of the injury and considerations of time needed in the field.

Gauze roller bandages should *NOT* be used to make narrow ties, in lieu of cravats or straps, to immobilize or secure a patient or part of a patient to a backboard, other full or half-body rigid devices, or the ambulance cot. Even when several thicknesses are used, the open weave and stretchability of this fabric easily allows these to become misplaced or tear and can cause a sudden breech or other failure in the tie. Even when overlapped and wound around a larger area, this fabric is not designed to bear the considerable weight that such use may possibly pose against it. Cravat ties, straps, or wide adhesive tape should be used instead for this purpose.

When ready to dress and bandage the wound, change gloves and assemble the packages of sterile dressings and gauze roller bandage, and adhesive tape. Cut or tear the tape strips you will need and remove one of the roller bandages from its package. Once the sterile dressings have been applied over the wound you are ready to apply the bandage.

1. Unroll 3 or 4 inches of the bandage and hold its end on about a 45 degree angle across the limb at a point 1 to 2 inches distal to the dressing. Letting it unwind from the roll in an equal amount as is being applied, make several snug overlapping turns around the limb. These turns (also called *winds*) should be near-perpendicular to the long axis of the limb and located so that a portion of the end remains as a *tab* protruding proximally from under them.

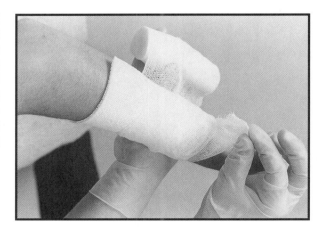

2. Fold the tab back over the previously taken winds of the bandage and cover it with several additional snug overlapping turns of the bandage around the circumference of the limb. This forms a firm anchor for the bandage which, if applied with the correct tightness, will prevent the initial distal end of the bandage from slipping along the (commonly narrowing circumference) of the limb, or from being able to rotate and unwind.

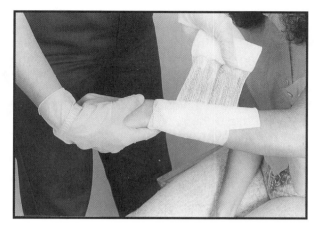

3. Once the end has been properly anchored distal to the area to be covered, you are ready to apply additional winds to cover the dressing and injury. By passing the roll alternately over and under the limb (and from one hand to the other) apply successive winds progressing in a proximal direction along the extremity. Each added turn should be carefully applied so it overlaps about 1/2 to 3/4 of an inch of the previous one, and is properly snug around the circumference of the limb.

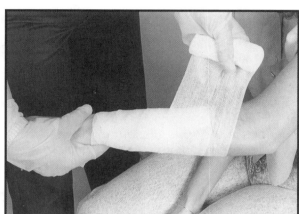

4. Generally the gauze fabric is sufficiently flexible so that when the proper tension is used, neither the slight angle needed to move progressively along the limb nor the variations in the limb's circumference interfere with each turn being applied snugly across its entire width. Should difficulty be encountered in keeping both edges of a turn tensioned snugly and one edge tends to elevate, remove a half turn and twist the bandage (by rotating the bandage roll 180 degrees) to form a *spiral reverse*, and then continue to apply overlapping turns in the customary manner. In some cases this may need to be repeated several times, or at a later place.

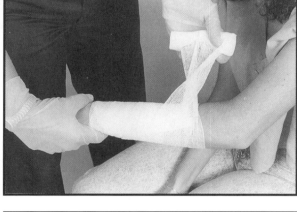

5. Should the area to be covered include a joint which is at an angle or may need to be articulated later, use a figure-of-eight pattern to cover it. Once the proximal edge of a turn lies at the joint, pass the bandage across the inside angle of the joint to a point 4 to 6 inches proximal of it. Then take several overlapping turns around the limb. This leaves a gap in the continuity of the bandage in order to securely anchor it proximal to the joint before going any further.

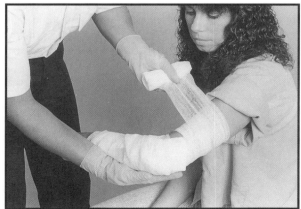

6. Once the bandage has been anchored beyond the joint, take successive overlapping turns, alternating between winding several around the limb in one direction proximal to the joint then, after crossing the joint, several in the opposite direction distal to it. By continuing this figure-of-eight technique, approaching turns will be applied until the entire joint is covered with an intertwined layer which will remain snug if the joint is moved. Continue to apply further overlapping turns from one end of the bandage to the other, in order to provide additional layers of coverage.

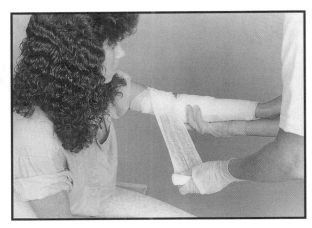

7. Continue until you have applied two (or preferably three) layers over the entire area to be bandaged. If the roll ends before this, lay the end against the previous turn. Then, by covering the end with several turns while anchoring a second roll (as previously shown) you can secure both simultaneously, and then continue to apply the additional turns needed. The use of a knot is unnecessary and is discouraged wherever it would become covered. Once sufficient layers have been applied, cut off any unused excess and secure the end with several strips of adhesive tape.

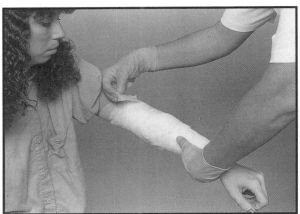

8. Adhesive tape is an essential item in even the most abridged of trail emergency supplies. In the unlikely occurrence that it is not available, the end of the roller bandage can be cut in half along its length for 6 to 10 inches. After a knot is tied to prevent it from separating further, the two tails produced can each be passed around the limb in opposite directions, and the end of each secured by tying them together.

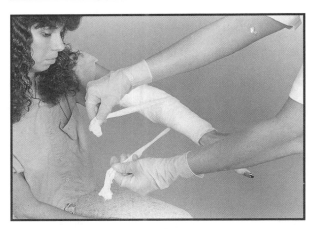

9. As soon as any bandage around an extremity has been completed, the EMT should check to be sure that its application has not compromised the distal circulation. It should be rechecked if additional ties (such as arm slings, etc.) are added, or any significant alteration to it is done. As well, it should be periodically rechecked to ensure that, should changes in position or increased swelling cause a compromise, it is identified in a timely manner.

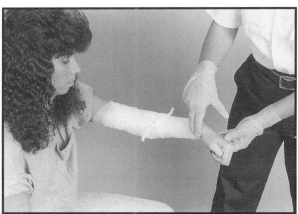

Regardless of the specific area being covered with a roller bandage, the EMT will employ the same basic techniques and follow the same general principles as have been shown in the preceding steps. After the absence of greater priorities and the proper body substance isolation precautions have been confirmed and the appropriate sterile dressings have been placed, to apply a roller bandage:

- First, properly anchor the initial end.
- Apply successive partially overlapping winds.
- Apply an initial layer from just distal to just proximal (or visa-versa) of the injury.
- Use a figure-of-eight to cover any joint which forms an angle, or may need to be moved.
- Use a spiral reverse, if turns will not lie flat.
- Apply each layer desired in turn, working from one end of the area to be covered to the other.
- Apply at least 2 to 3 layers, but avoid unnecessary bulk.
- When the bandage is completed, cut-off and discard any excess remaining roll.
- Properly secure the end with strips of adhesive tape (or by tying it) over the bandaged area.
- Check the distal circulation.

Generally, when applying a roller bandage on an extremity, one can simply initially anchor it around the limb just distal to the injury, and then progressively apply each desired layer working along the length of the limb. When bandaging the foot, hand, or individual fingers this procedure must be modified so that the bandage will be properly anchored regardless of the variations in shape found in these areas. In the case of the fingers or the foot, because they are at the most distal end of the limb and sufficiently regular in circumference, the completed bandage could easily slip or be accidentally pulled off unless it is otherwise anchored. Although not considered an extremity, the same is true (and increased by the slippery nature of hair) for the upper part of the head.

Additional Techniques And Variations

The following modifications, variations, and "tricks-of-the-trade" for applying a roller bandage will be useful in meeting special problems and in increasing the variations from which the reader can choose.

10. When several non-contiguous injuries must be bandaged on the same extremity, a single roller bandage can be used. After anchoring the bandage distal to the most distal of the injuries and applying sufficient layers over it, use a snug long half turn to "walk" the bandage to the area just distal to the second injury and then complete the bandage over the second injury in the customary manner. This avoids the need to anchor and end two separate bandages without unnecessarily covering the area between the injuries.

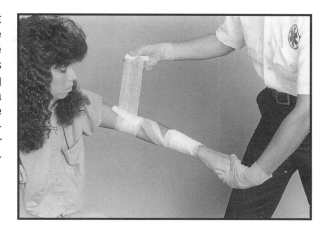

11. Because the foot is joined to the long lower extremity by a moveable joint and naturally lies at a near perpendicular angle to it, the figure-of-eight technique should be used when applying a roller bandage to the ankle and foot. Even when exclusively bandaging a portion of the foot, initial anchoring around the lower leg proximal to the lateral protrusion of the ankle bones, and use of this technique, is recommended to secure and form the bandage so it can not become displaced.

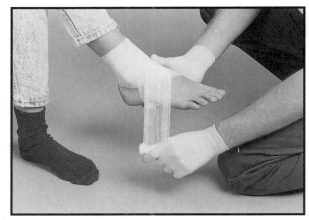

12. Due to the shape of the top of the shoulder and the curve in the outline of the body where it meets the upper arm, a roller bandage covering it must be secured against the top of the shoulder from two different angles and anchor points. Use a figure-of-eight so that one series of loops is formed diagonally around the torso between the top of the shoulder and through the *opposite armpit,* and a second series of loops is secured around the shoulder, lying almost perpendicular to the top of shoulder between it and the *armpit on the same side* (as shown).

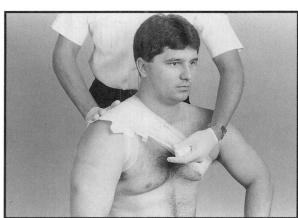

13. After starting at the neck, take five or six turns to form the initial series of overlapping loops diagonally across the torso. These should lie exactly on top of the preceding layers when passing through the armpit, but only partially overlap when passing over the shoulder so the coverage progresses towards the arm. Once at the medial edge of the shoulder joint, loops should be formed over the shoulder and through the armpit *on the same (injured) side* until the outer curve of the joint has been completely covered. Continue partially overlapping turns around the arm until the edge of the bandage is as distal as desired.

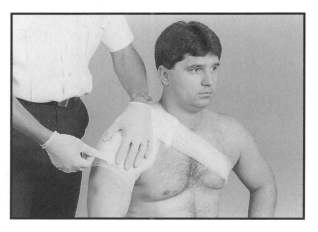

With slight modification, the same method is used to apply a wide roller bandage to the hip, part of the lower abdomen, or a buttock. The bandage is first anchored by turns around the narrow waist and, after sufficient overlapping turns have been applied around the torso so the lower edge approximates the groin, additional turns are added around the leg on the injured side (or using the figure-of-eight technique, alternating around the leg and then the torso).

Due to the "hour glass" shape of the trunk of the body, when a wide roller bandage is used to form a bandage exclusively around either the upper or lower halves of the torso it will have a tendency to slip towards the waist. To prevent this, any bandage applied around the torso cephalad to the waist should include some turns over the top of at least one shoulder (even though neither one may need to be covered), to secure it from moving in a caudad direction. For the same anatomical reason, any bandage applied to the lower torso should be anchored initially at the waist and be prevented from moving in a cephalad direction by several turns carefully passed through the groin.

Special Applications For The Hand And Fingers

1. Because the circumference of the wrist is smaller than that of the more distal hand, when applying a roller bandage to cover any area of the hand it should initially be anchored snugly around the wrist. Then covering the palm and back-of-the-hand can be initiated by several figure-of-eight turns which pass on an angle across the top of the hand, around one side, across the palm, up between the thumb and other side of the hand and then, on an opposite angle, back to the wrist and around it.

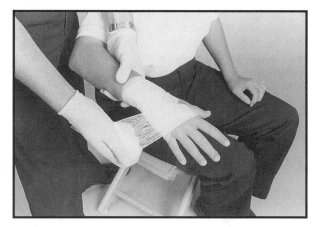

2. After 2 or 3 turns that have been applied this way lie around the hand and wrist forming a base, additional turns exclusively around the hand should be applied to extend the coverage further distal on the hand and then back to the point where the thumb intersects with it. Then one or two more figure-of-eight turns should be applied as a secure outer covering and the bandage should be cut and taped at the wrist. Unless required, the bandage should not include the fingers.

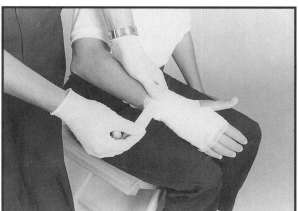

3. If the bandage must cover the entire hand including the fingers, it should *NOT* simply be extended to wrap around them. Once you have completed the previous two steps, place a 3 or 4 inch roller under the fingers and direct the patient to hold it, to place the hand in its natural position of function.

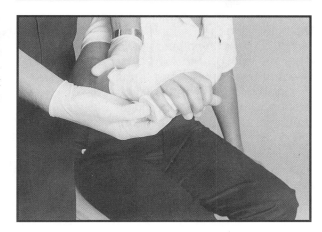

4. Next, place several folds of gauze loosely between each of the fingers and between the thumb and side of the hand, in order to pad between them and keep their adjacent surfaces separated.

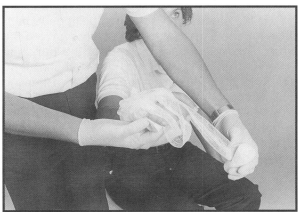

5. Using another roller bandage, form 3 or 4 loose layers of gauze into a pad of between 8 to 10 inches in length. After laying half of its length over the exposed fingers and folding it over them so the remaining half covers their underside, with the remaining part of the roll again form an anchor around the wrist.

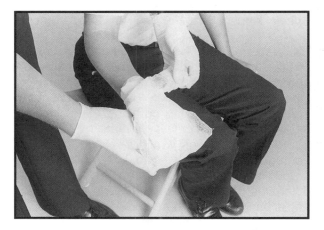

6. Then form overlapping turns around the hand, thumb and fingers until they have been covered from the wrist to the fingertips. Work your way back to the wrist (either with another layer or several open turns) and, after cutting off any unused roll, tape the end at the wrist.

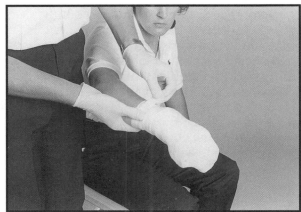

7. Even when only bandaging a single finger, the roller bandage should be anchored at the wrist to prevent the chance of its being pulled off. After anchoring at the wrist, pass the bandage over the back of the hand to the proximal end of the injured finger. Then taking overlapping turns around it, work along the finger until you reach the distal end. Unless necessary, do *NOT* cover the fingernail so that you can later evaluate the distal circulation by testing the capillary refill. Work your way back to the proximal end of the finger and, after going across the back of the hand, secure the end at the wrist.

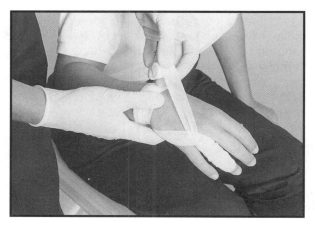

8. If you need to bandage more than one finger on the same hand, after completing the bandage for one finger, take several turns around the wrist. This will secure the end of the bandage covering that finger, and provide an anchor from which to start the next finger. Then again go across the back of the hand, this time to the proximal end of the second finger to be covered. In the same manner as previously shown, complete the bandage of this finger and then return to the wrist and secure the end with tape.

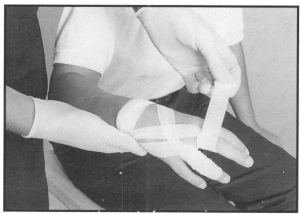

9. If one or more fingers needs to be completely covered, first bandage the finger except for its tip as previously shown. Form a narrow 4 to 5 inch pad with several layers of the roller gauze. Similar to when covering the entire hand, place the pad so that half of its length lies on top of the finger and, after folding it down over the fingertip, the second half lies against the underside of the finger. Then, secure it with additional turns taken around the finger and, after returning to the wrist, secure the end with tape.

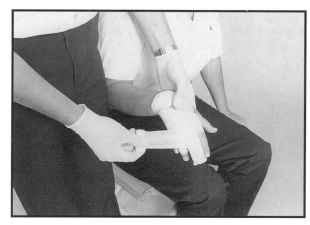

Special Applications For The Head

1. Due to the spherical shape of the head, the hair, and the need to avoid covering uninjured areas of the face, careful attention must be paid to employing the limited points of anchor that are available. *As a consideration of the patient's safety, the bandage should NOT pass around the neck or under the mandible in order to provide an anchor.* When a roller bandage is used to cover any part of the head or face, it should be initiated and completed by anchoring it around the forehead.

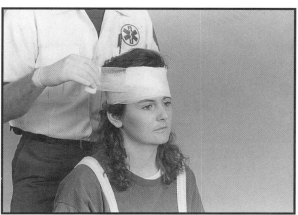

2. The initial turns are applied so they are centered on the forehead and come straight back to encircle the head. These must be relatively tight to prevent them from being rotated while the bandage is completed. Each additional turn is applied diagonally across the sides of the head so that the lower portion of the loop formed by the turn is applied under an anchor point and the upper portion lies drawn directly straight back (without any bend) around the skull to provide the necessary tension to hold it secure. You should note that some turns have been applied so they are lower at the back of the head and are anchored inferior to the posterior protrusion of the occiput while others are applied lower in the front, so their caudad edge is bent and "hooked" over the supra-orbital ridge.

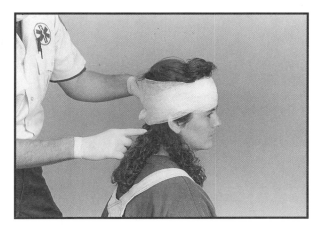

3. When a bandage must cover the entire top of the skull the use of a self-adhering roller bandage (such as Colban, Medi-Rip or Co-Flex) is highly recommended. Their self-adhering nature allows for easier application and provides a more secure bandage than if roller gauze is used for this area. As with any bandage of the head, start by centering it on the forehead and anchoring it with tight turns applied in a straight line around the head.

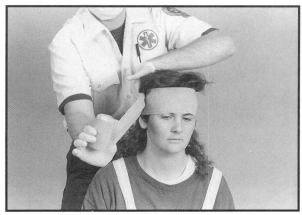

4. Once the bandage has been sufficiently anchored around the head at the forehead, place several additional turns so they only partially overlap and progress towards the top of the head. Next, start adding turns across the top of the head. These are placed from one side of the upper skull to the other and back, and must be of sufficient length so that they completely overlap the initial turns which anchor the bandage around the forehead. A spiral reverse is used to form the fold necessary to change direction at each side, once the caudad edge of the anchor has been reached.

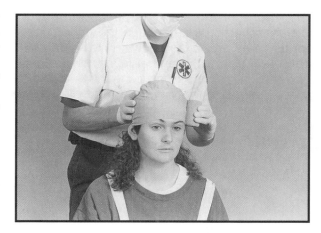

5. Once the entire top of the head has been covered, use a spiral reverse to change direction, then apply several more turns around the circumference of the head at the forehead. These should lie over and secure each end that was formed when the turns placed across the top of the head were reversed. Be careful to ensure that at least one turn anchors over the supra-orbital ridge and one anchors inferior to the occiput. Even though self-adhering, the end of the bandage should be secured with adhesive tape.

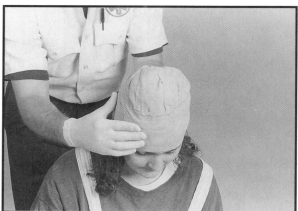

6. If the self-adhering type is not available, the same type of "skull-cap" bandage can be formed using 2 gauze roller bandages. Start by tying the ends of the roll together and using one, the primary roll, to anchor the bandage around the head at the forehead in the customary manner. Then the top of the head is covered with a series of layers passed one at a time over the top of the head. After each turn of the secondary roll is passed over the top of the head, it is secured by passing the primary roll over it.

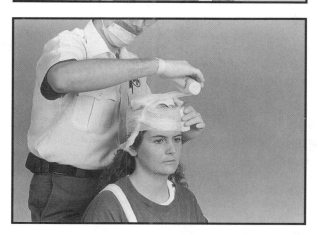

7. Once the part of the second roll which comes down from across the top of the head is covered by passing the primary roll part way around the circumference of the head (in this case from the front to the back) it is secured and can be folded upward. It is then passed back across the top of the head and down the opposite side...

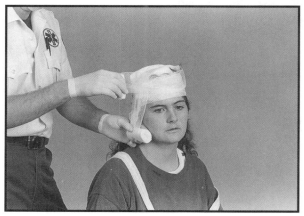

8. …where it is secured by passing the primary roller (this time from the back to the front) over it, forming the half-turn around this side of the head. It is again folded up and passed over the top of the head, and so on. Each turn placed over the top of the head (Roller #2) should pass straight across the approximate center of it, rather than lying tangentially around it.

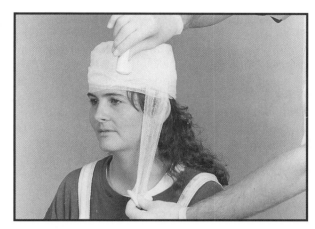

9. Although the middle of each of these turns crosses the approximate center of the top of the head, the ends are only partially overlapped as they are brought down the sides prior to being secured. As each end is brought down over the head progressively further around the circumference of the original anchor (in the previous photos, clockwise) the coverage, appearing as two wedges, enlarges. When the EMT has progressed 180 degrees around the head, the last piece placed over the head will overlap the initial one and the bandage will be completed.

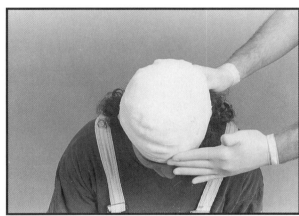

Special Applications For The Eyes

1. When bandaging an injured eye in the field, both eyes should be covered so that the injured eye does not make numerous rapid associated movements as the uninjured eye moves from object to object. However, the anxiety produced by the resulting total loss of vision may offset this principle if the eye injury is slight. To form a bandage exclusively covering one eye, first anchor it around the forehead. Then place a narrow gauze strip perpendicular to the anchor so it lies over the medial end of the *uninjured* eye.

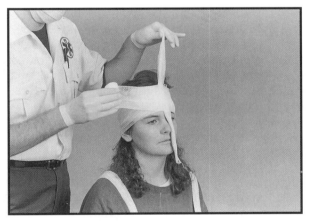

2. After explaining what you are going to do to the patient, place an eye pad (a special dressing for the eye) over the injured eye, and continue to advance the overlapping turns inferiorly until it has been sufficiently covered. This will also temporarily cover the superior bridge of the nose and, partially or fully, the uninjured eye. When this has been completed, tape the end of the bandage *at either side of the head* (not anywhere on the front)

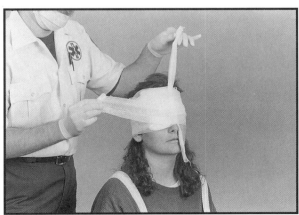

3. Using the gauze strip, you are now ready to adjust the bandage so it will no longer cover the uninjured eye. Bring the ends of the gauze strip together and tie them with a half-knot. Tighten the knot until the caudad edge of the bandage on the uninjured side is sufficiently drawn into a diagonal so it no longer covers the uninjured eye. Then complete the knot and cut or tape the ends so they can not intrude into the exposed eye.

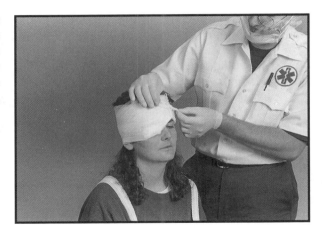

BANDAGING AN AVULSED OR IMPALED EYE

A special bandaging problem is produced when either an eye is avulsed and displaced from its orbit, or a foreign body is impaled in it. With either injury, although *both eyes must be covered*, the bandage can *NOT* contact or approximate the injured eye. In the case of an avulsion, any pressure from a dressing or bandage over the eye would be injurious.

In the case of a remaining impaled object, covering it with a slit eye pad and a bandage that firmly surrounded the protruding object would only immobilize the object directly at the outer surface of the eye. Then, when the eye moved, its rotation against the totally immobilized object would result in profound additional damage to the eye. By instead securing the object at some distance from the eye, it can be kept from further intrusion and free movement without stopping the impaled end from limited movement when the eye moves.

A unique bandage, incorporating an ordinary styrofoam cup, is used to meet the special needs associated with both of these injuries. This bandage requires the availability of two EMTs. One maintains the styrofoam cup in its proper place (and in the case of an impaled object, supports its proximal end) while the other applies the bandage.

As soon as such an injury is identified, the patient's hands should be held to prevent him from instinctively reaching for the eye, and he should be placed in a supine position. Also, in cases with an impaled object, its proximal end must be immediately supported by one of the EMTs and this support maintained without interruption until the bandage has been completed and the object has been properly secured to it. Although the supine position may make it more difficult to apply the turns of the bandage, it supports the head and minimizes its movement and that of the avulsed eye or the impaled object. In the event that the internal fluid of the eye is leaking from the injury, having the orbit and surface of the eye pointing upwards will also be of benefit in retarding or preventing further fluid loss from the eye.

Once the patient is supine, have a third rescuer or "helper" take over the restraint of both hands so that your partner is free to assist you. If the patient continuously draws his hands free, or when dealing with a small child, the use of wrist restraints will be necessary.

Before starting to apply any part of the bandage, the EMT should gather, unpackage, and prepare all of the materials he will need. These include: a 2 or 3 inch wide roller bandage, 4x4 gauze pads, an eye pad, a styrofoam cup, a sharp pair of bandage or "medic" scissors, and 5 or 6 narrow strips of adhesive tape. Against the possibility that the cup breaks or one roll is not sufficient, extras of both should also be readily at hand.

1. First, take both 4x4's from their package. Fold them in half and cut a semi-circle out of the folded edge. This should be sufficiently large that when the 4x4s are unfolded, the circle which is cut out of them is larger than the eye but smaller than the circumference of the drinking edge of the cup. The 4x4s will be used to provide padding between the firm edge of the styrofoam cup and the patient's face.

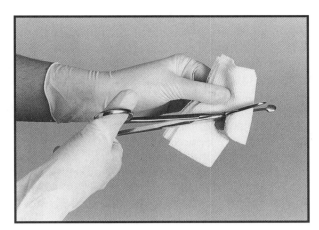

2. In cases with an impaled object, the bottom of the cup must be cut out and removed at this time. Most styrofoam cups have a thickened lower edge. Unless the cup is too long, cutting around the circumference of the very bottom rather than the side will retain desirable extra strength once the bottom is removed. Carefully brush all loose or dangling particles of styrofoam from the inner surface. *For an avulsed eye, the bottom of the cup should NOT be removed.*

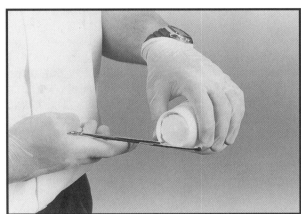

3. Before starting, explain that you must cover both eyes and, in a limited way, the procedure. Direct the patient to close the uninjured eye and attempt to avoid any eye movement. Place the 4x4s on the face so the circle that has been cut out lies directly over the orbit of the eye. Place the large end of the cup centered over the 4x4 and eye, and place an eye pad or 2x2 over the uninjured one. When there is an impaled object, the cup will have to be carefully "threaded" over it in steps, to allow a grasp to be maintained on the object at all times.

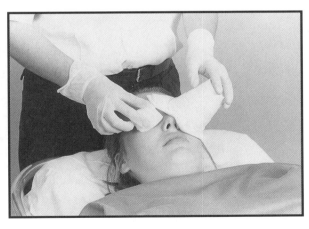

4. While a second EMT holds the cup (or cup and impaled object) carefully in place, anchor the roller around the head over the forehead. Continue applying overlapping turns to cover the uninjured eye and the area of the face adjacent to the circumference of the cup. As turns are applied at the level of the cup, the side adjacent to the cup is laid folded against its side (as they are passed around part of its circumference) to provide some of the fixation which will secure the cup.

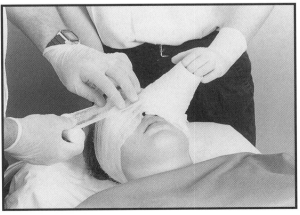

5. Continue applying turns until the gauze which has been folded up against the cup extends upward for about an inch onto the cup's side and around its entire circumference. This secures the base of the cup against movement in any direction on the face. Several additional turns must be applied next which, after coming from the side of the head, snugly encircle the lower half of the cup and continue around the head. Because the cup narrows from its drinking edge to its bottom, these will secure the cup from moving anteriorly off the face. Finally, tape the end of the bandage at the side of the head.

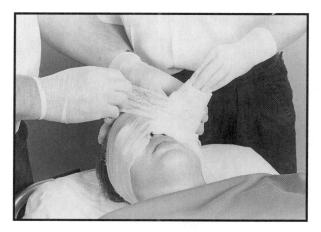

6. The protruding impaled object must next be secured to the cup. Direct the EMT supporting the object to position his hand as far out of the way as possible, and to steady the cup with his other hand. At a point *exactly* level with the upper edge of the cup, secure the middle of a 1/2 inch wide strip of adhesive tape around the object with several turns and then, holding the ends so they form a taut straight line, bring them over the edges and down opposing sides of the cup. Repeat this to produce a second tape support which surrounds the object at precisely the same level but is perpendicular to the first. Secure several additional strips of tape around these supports and the circumference of the cup.

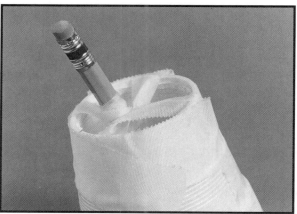

7. Once this has been completed, manual support of the object should be released immediately. Although the object is secured from further intrusion, extraction or free movement, the cross-supports will allow its impaled end to articulate in a controlled manner if the injured eye moves. Any further restriction or handling of the object will promote damage and must be avoided.

Note: The EMT must be especially careful to avoid these problems:

- Styrofoam breaks easily. Whenever handling or taping to the cup, the EMT must avoid applying so much force that the cup breaks or tears. Holding a hand around the cup to further strengthen and maintain its cylindrical shape is recommended during any such maneuvers.
- If the object protrudes from the eye on an angle, the cup and tape must be positioned so that when the object is secured the angle is unchanged unless the patient moves his eye.
- The tape strips must be secured around the object at precisely the same level as that of the upper edge of the cup. If the tape is placed too high or too low around the object, further intrusion or extraction (respectively) will be promoted.
- Regardless of how cooperative or anxious the patient is, instinctive attempts to reach the eye with a hand must be protected against at all times. Once on the cot, the arms should at least be firmly secured under a tied sheet wrap, and wrist restraints may be indicated.

USING A COMPRESS BANDAGE

Unlike other types of commercially prepared bandages, a compress bandage includes both the dressing and the bandage necessary to cover and secure it in one pre-attached inseparable unit. The two types commonly used in the field are differentiated by the type of bandage material to which the dressings are attached: gauze (or similar fabric) or adhesive tape (either the plastic or fabric type).

A *gauze compress bandage*, or *trauma compress* as they are more commonly called, contains a relatively thick pad of dressings sewn in the middle of either one or two 36 to 54 inch long strips of gauze or gauze-like fabric. This produces either 2 or 4 tails (1 or 2 extending respectively from the opposite sides of the pad) with which to encircle the injured area and tie the compress securely.

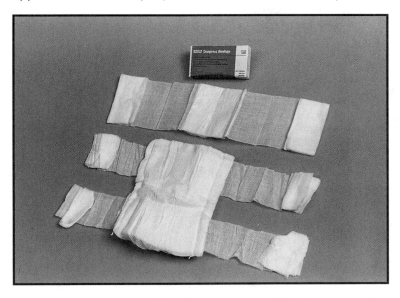

Larger "binder" versions for use around the torso are also available but are rarely carried on an ambulance.

Trauma compresses were initially developed by the military many years ago to eliminate the time, multiple components, and special skills required when using previously conventional methods to dress and bandage a wound under adverse field conditions. Although rarely providing wound care while under fire, EMTs have found that trauma compresses are extremely useful in daily pre-hospital care when the situation or patient's condition dictate that the time for individual wound care in the field be kept to a bare minimum. This is particularly true in situations when manual direct pressure over an extremity wound needs to be replaced with a pressure bandage to facilitate moving the patient and rapidly initiating transport. When time is a key factor, wounds *without* significant bleeding can be rapidly covered by dressings secured with several strips of adhesive tape, however the application of a trauma compress should require *NO* greater time and will generally provide better and more secure coverage.

Of all of the types of bandage that are available, *the adhesive compress bandage* is the single most frequently used. These have a small sterile pad adhered to the middle of a short piece of adhesive tape. The underside is covered by two overlapping peel-off pieces of paper or plastic which keep the adhesive and dressing surface from any contact and contamination before they have been applied.

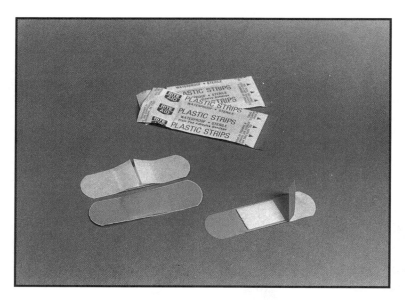

Although these are generically properly called "an adhesive compress bandage," few would use or recognize that term. Instead they are universally called **band-aids** even though this is actually only the name of one prevalent brand.

Other larger, square, rectangular and even round adhesive compress bandages exist in which the available adhesive surface is a narrow band around the entire perimeter of the dressing pad. Similarly, from the common term applied to them, these are universally called **coverlets** (after one leading manufacturer's brand name).

Since the dressing is attached to the bandage covering, compress bandages come wrapped in individual sterile packages. *When removing them from the package and handling them, contact with the dressing's surface must be avoided.*

Applying a Trauma Compress

1. Carefully remove the trauma compress from its package and, while holding it firmly by the tails, position it so it is held on a slight diagonal to the long axis of the limb and directly above the injury. When it is correctly located, lower it into place without moving it once on the skin's surface.

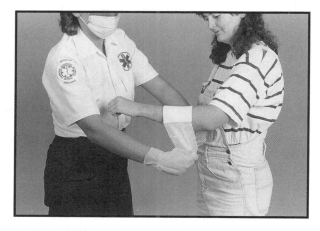

2. Wrap the tail (or pair of tails) which extends from one side of the dressing clockwise around the limb and dressing, and the one (or ones) from the other side counterclockwise. Because the compress was placed on a slight diagonal, the initial turns made with the tails should extend around the extremity beyond the proximal and distal edges of the dressing pad, respectively. As you apply additional turns with each tail, overlap them so that the ends are brought together centered over the dressing, and then tie them together to secure the compress.

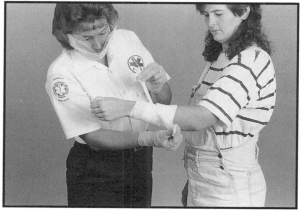

3. If the compress bandage is to be applied over a joint, select one with four tails or cut along the center of both tails to turn one with only two tails into one with four. Place the compress so that the dressing is centered on the injury and the tails extend perpendicular to the extremity's long axis. Wrap the two proximal tails in opposite directions around the extremity and dressing for several turns proximal to the joint, and tie the ends together so the knot lies on top of these turns. Then, in the same way, wrap and tie the distal tails to secure the lower end of the compress distal to the joint.

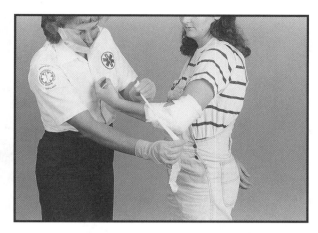

Applying a Band-Aid (adhesive compress bandage)

1. Remove the band-aid from its sterile package and, without touching the dressing, peel away the first of the paper or plastic cover strips. While holding the band-aid taut at the very edge of the uncovered end between the thumb and several fingers of one hand and the covered end between those of the other, position it so that the dressing lies over the cut. Lay the adhesive end against the skin while keeping the partially covered dressing from contact.

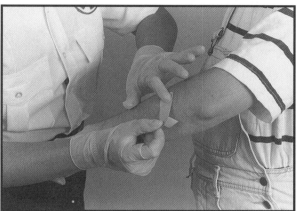

2. Fold (or roll) the dressing back above the adhesive end you have just applied. This will cause the second peel-away strip to separate from the sterile pad, allowing you to grasp it without contacting the latter. While holding the free end of the peel-away strip between your thumb and first finger, pull it slowly away from the dressing so that, as more of the adhesive is bared, it contacts and fastens to the skin. This technique better promotes snug flat application of the band-aid with the uncontaminated sterile pad properly placed over the cut, than if both peel-away strips are initially removed and both ends are simultaneously placed on the skin.

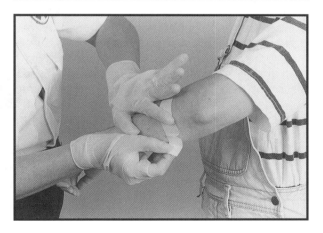

Applying a Butterfly Closure (Adhesive Butterfly Bandage)

A special form of adhesive compress, called a *butterfly bandage* or *butterfly closure* is used in the rare event that instead of simply being held in place with a dressing and bandage, the edges of a small incision or laceration must be held more exactly positioned and more securely together without sutures.

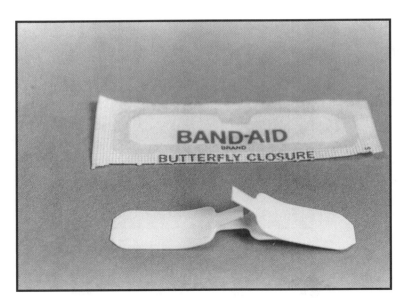

Even though butterfly bandages do not properly cover or protect a wound, they are still classified as a specialized adhesive compress bandage because they contain some components of both a dressing and a bandage.

Because definitive evaluation, cleansing, antiseptic prophylaxis, and proper closure of a wound is rarely possible in the field, the use of butterfly closures (or other forms of provided wound edge closure), is *NOT* recommended in routine pre-hospital care. The skills necessary for their use have only been included in this section in the rare event that the EMT must apply one in a remote setting or other situation in which definitive evaluation and care will be inordinately delayed.

In normal day-to-day pre-hospital care, even minor cuts which appear to possibly need some closure (or which lie on the face or other area where scarring presents a cosmetic consideration), should be covered with a dressing and bandage and then the patient should be referred or transported to the emergency department. With such injuries the EMT should guard against voicing an opinion regarding the probable need or lack of need for more definitive care and sutures. Instead, the EMT should clearly advise the patient that his field care is only temporary, and that additional evaluation and more definitive physician care—possibly including sutures and a tetanus booster—is required, and document giving such advice clearly on his run report.

When use of a butterfly closure is dictated in the field, the wound and area surrounding it must be thoroughly cleansed with an antiseptic solution before the butterfly is applied. Although a commercial butterfly bandage is much like a band-aid and has similar peel-off strips over each adhesive half, it is applied differently in order to maintain the wound edges in the best possible alignment while installing it.

1. After removing the butterfly closure from its package, carefully peel-off *both* of the overlapping paper strips covering its adhesive side. While holding the ends securely between both hands, position it so that the narrow indented area will lie directly across the cut, and place and secure the entire length of one adhesive wing of the bandage against the skin adjacent to that side of the cut. While firmly securing the first wing onto one side of the cut, the other end of the butterfly must be held extended and slightly elevated above the skin on the opposite side of the cut to avoid any contact between the second wing and the skin.

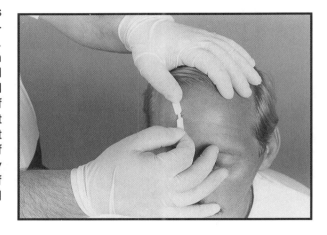

2. Once one of the wings has been properly secured, the wound edges should be properly aligned together. While holding the edges in proper alignment, place the entire second wing against the skin and press the far end of each wing firmly against it to increase the adhesion obtained. DO NOT press on the wings any closer to the wound edges, nor run a finger across the surface of either or both of them. Although this promotes better adhesion, it also invites puckering or drawing apart of the wound edges so they become secured in misalignment.

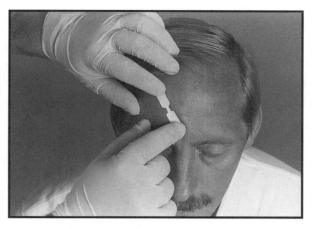

3. If a commercial butterfly closure is not available, one can easily be made. Since it is nearly impossible to do fine manipulations with adhesive tape while wearing rubber gloves, and the hands are generally no less clean at this point, it is recommended that you remove your gloves while preparing the butterfly. Cut off a 3 inch strip of 3/4 inch tape and make 4 diagonal cuts in its sides as shown. The two diagonal cuts on each side should be made at a point about 3/8 of an inch from the middle of the strips, angled towards each other, and to about 1/4 of the tape's width.

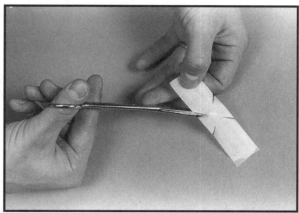

4. The two cuts made in each edge of the tape form a trapezoid-shaped tab in the middle of its length. On one side of the strip, carefully fold the tab over so its adhesive surface is in contact with that of the rest of the tape, and the long base of the folded trapezoid lies along the center line of the strip's width. While preparing the butterfly, the tape should be handled so that the fingers only contact as small an area of the adhesive surface as possible.

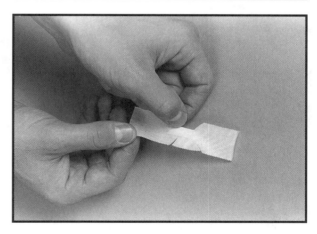

5. Now repeat this with the trapezoid-shaped tab formed by the diagonal cuts in the opposite edge of the tape. When folding the second tab, its long base should overlap that of the first so that *NO* adhesive surface remains exposed at the narrow (about 1/4 inch long) strip centered between the two wings of the butterfly. Although the wings are slightly wider to make cutting and folding the strip easier, the resulting butterfly closure is almost identical to a commercial one. After donning new gloves, apply it across the edges of the cut in the same manner as previously described.

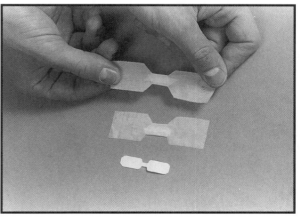

USING TRIANGULAR AND CRAVAT BANDAGES

Triangular bandages are used as a large triangle (as their name suggests), or folded into a long multiply-layered narrow (generally 2 to 4 inches wide) tie, called a **cravat bandage** or simply a **cravat**. Commercial triangular bandages come pre-folded as cravats, generally in individual non-sterile packages which include two large safety pins.

As previously discussed, triangular and cravat bandages are commonly used in routine daily pre-hospital care as arm slings and ties, and only in rare special situations as true bandages.

Conventionally, triangular bandages are manufactured by cutting a 36 to 48 inch square piece of fabric in half along its diagonal, to produce two equal right triangles (each becoming a triangular bandage). When purchasing these the EMT should select brands which have been cut from a 44 inch or greater square, since smaller ones will not easily form an arm sling or swathe of sufficient size to accommodate large adults. In the rare case that the EMT must make his own, a 48 inch square should be used so that the resulting triangular bandage is of a sufficient size for any possible purpose.

The parts of a triangular bandage are identified by the classical terms used in geometry to identify the parts of a triangle. The reader should be familiar with these as they are widely used to identify specific parts in the demonstrations on the following pages, and are useful when communicating with a partner while bandaging in the field. These are identified in the following illustration:

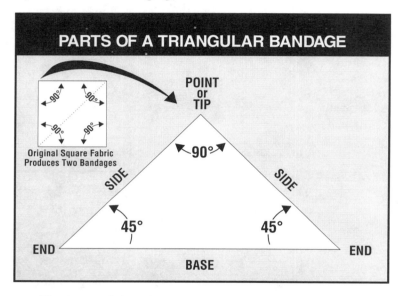

The base of the triangle was formed by cutting along the diagonal of the square from which the bandage was made. Since the diagonal is longer than the side of a square, the base of the bandage can easily be identified because it is longer than the other two sides of the triangle. The two shorter edges of the bandage are equal to each other, and are called the *sides*. The pointed tail formed by the perpendicular intersection of the two sides (opposite the base) is called the *tip* or *point* of the bandage, and the pointed tails produced by the 45 degree intersection of the side at each end of the base are called the *ends*.

When a triangular bandage is properly folded into a cravat, the length of the cravat bandage mirrors the longer length of the base, rather than that of the sides. When a cravat is made from a triangular bandage with 48 inch long sides, the cravat will be approximately 68 inches long.

Because it forms a secure non-slip tie that can easily be opened when desired, the square knot was advocated for years as "the only knot" with which to secure triangular bandages. In fact, a variety of knots can be used, and a better and more reliable knot will result when the EMT employs one he is accustomed to tying. How easily the knot can be released when desired is not a valid concern. Triangular bandages are no longer reused from one patient to another, and to avoid unnecessary manipulation and delay are simply cut off rather than untied.

Whenever possible, knots should be tied on the anterior or lateral sides of the patient so that they will not lie between the patient's back or the underside of an extremity and the cot or backboard. Knots should *NOT* be located between adjacent body areas such as between the legs or between the extended arm and the side of the torso. Instead, knots should be tied so they lie on an area covered by the bandage and not directly on the skin. If this is *NOT* practical, padding (4x4s, etc.) should be added between the knot and the skin once the bandage has been applied. Although two safety pins are generally packaged with each triangular bandage, these will not provide as secure an attachment as properly tied knots. *The use of safety pins to secure the ends of a triangular or cravat bandage in the field is not recommended.*

A Key Word About Terminology

Triangular bandages come packaged as a cravat bandage, are labeled "triangular bandage," and to add to the confusion in actuality a cravat bandage is a triangular bandage which is pre-folded to another form prior to its application. In order to avoid confusion in communicating, except for ordering, inventory or other supply considerations, the term "triangular bandage" should be limited to describing a bandage initially applied as a large unfolded triangle. When the triangle is folded into a long narrow tie prior to being applied it should be called a "cravat bandage" or simply a "cravat." The terminology in this text follows these guidelines.

APPLYING A TRIANGULAR BANDAGE

Because of their large size and the unique features of their geometric shape, triangular bandages are particularly suited to application on areas of the torso. Unlike other bandages which have only two ends or tails, triangular bandages have three. This allows the bandage to be secured around the mid-torso by tying the two ends together, and also over the shoulder or through the groin by passing the point through either and securing it to one of the previously tied ends.

Similarly, when a triangular bandage is used to cover an entire hand or foot, securing all three "ends" keeps the bandage secured against both the upper and lower surfaces of the appendage. Having three "tails" also provides for another capability. By rolling the point of the triangular bandage around the center of a cravat so they are secured together, a bandage which has two long tails at each of its extremes (the ends of the cravat at one end, and the ends of the triangular bandage at the other) can be formed. This technique is particularly useful when bandaging a hip or shoulder. Because of their relatively large size, other than to bandage a hip or shoulder or an entire hand or foot, triangular bandages are not useful in bandaging the extremities. Cravat bandages or roller bandages are much better suited to that purpose and will result in a significantly better bandage.

The fabric used in triangular bandages is closely woven and treated so that even though the edges are not hemmed, the fabric will *NOT* unravel. However, to protect the patient's skin against the raw edge of the base and to prevent any chance of that edge tearing when the ends are tightened and tied together, turning up the first half-inch or so of the base and folding it over one or more times is highly recommended. In this way, the bandage will have several layers of thickness included in and between its tied ends.

Applying A Triangular Bandage To The Upper Torso

1.   Orient the bandage so the tip is pointing up. Place the bandage on the thorax so it is off-centered and the tip passes over one shoulder, and the ends pass around the sides of the torso below each armpit.

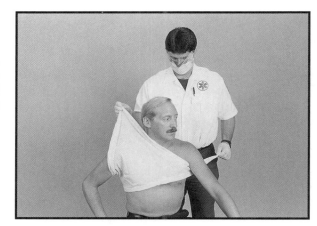

2.   Fold the base over several times and bring each end around to a point under one scapula. Tie the ends together so the knot is *NOT* centered on the back. This will desirably cause one of the ends (or tails) coming from the knot to be especially long. Whether the knot goes under the same shoulder that the tip passes over or the opposite one will determine whether the tip will be pulled straight down or diagonally, once these are connected — and is a matter of preference.

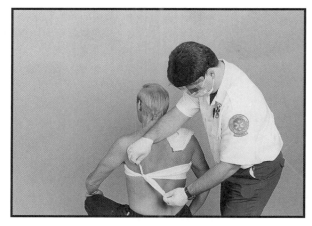

3. Adjust the amount of the tip that lies over the shoulder so any folds or loose excess in the bandage on the anterior thorax is eliminated. Take the longer of the two ends coming from the knot and, after bringing it up the back, tie it to the tip so that the bandage fits snugly.

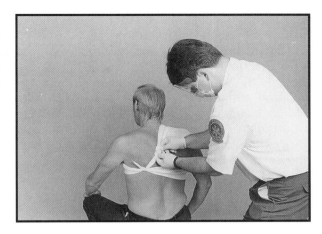

4. If a bandage is needed to cover the back of the upper torso instead, the same procedure is followed except the front-and-back directions are reversed. If both front and back need to be covered, after completing the application of one over the front, a second bandage is applied to the back. Similarly, if the supra-clavicular area on *both sides* must be covered, another triangular bandage placed with its tip over the second shoulder can be added.

Applying A Triangular Bandage To The Lower Torso

1. By inverting the bandage initially, it can be applied to cover the front or back of the lower torso, in much the same manner. Orient the bandage so the tip points downward and the base lies approximately along the waist.

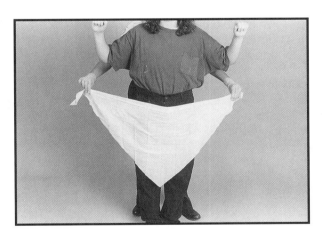

2. Bring each end around a side of the torso and across the back at the waist (above the buttocks). Tie both ends together so the knot lies on the midline of the back. Reach through the groin and draw the tip downward, to remove any folds or loose excess from the bandage. Then bring it snugly through the groin to the back. Continue to bring it up the midline between the buttocks, and tie it securely to one of the tails coming from the previous knot.

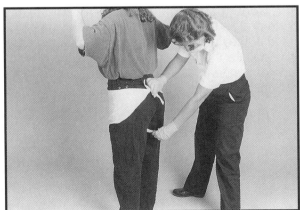

3. The partial "diaper" this forms will secure dressings to any location on the anterior and lateral lower torso, the genitalia, or through the groin. Because of its relatively small size compared to that of an adult, the triangular bandage will *NOT* simultaneously cover the entire front and back surfaces of the lower torso like a diaper on an infant. If coverage of both the front and back of the lower torso is required, a second is applied to the back using the same method.

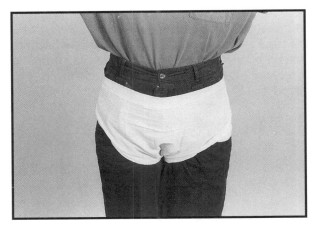

Applying A Triangular Bandage To The Top Of The Head

1. Fold the base over several times and, with the folds facing you hold the base taut between your hands. From a position behind the patient, bring the bandage over the top of the head (like a kerchief) with the tip lying centered partially down the patient's back.

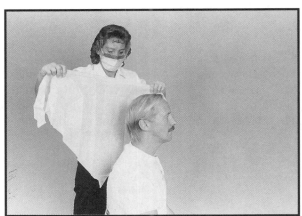

2. While holding both ends, carefully position the bandage so its midpoint is centered on the forehead and its anterior edge is properly located on the forehead. While maintaining sufficient tension to prevent the bandage from moving, bring the ends around the sides of the head and cross them (over the tip of the bandage) just inferior to the occiput.

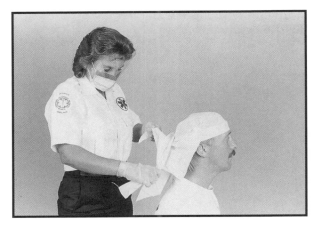

3. Continue bringing each end around the head and tie the ends together at one side of the head. If they are *NOT* of sufficient length to allow this, secure them to the previous layers at each side of the head or over the forehead, with strips of adhesive tape.

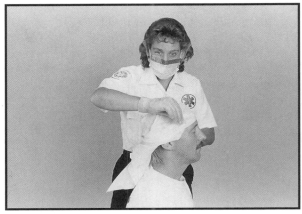

4. Lastly, bring the tip up and carefully tuck it into the band formed at the back of the head where the ends crossed inferior to the occiput. This will "lock" the posterior surface covering the top of the head from becoming loosened.

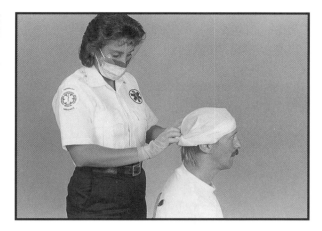

Applying A Triangular Bandage Over The Entire Foot Or Hand

1. Place the triangular bandage under the foot so the base lies several inches beyond the heel and the tip extends well beyond the toes.

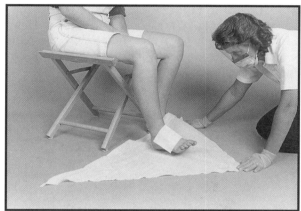

2. Fold the point of the bandage over the top of the foot so the tip lies on the anterior lower leg, against the skin. Fold each side of the bandage inward one or two times to bring the ends in closer alignment with the back of the foot.

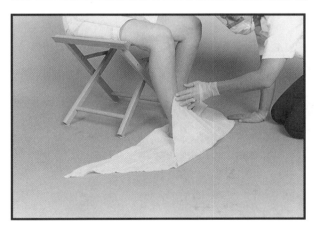

3. Cross the ends behind the lower leg above the ankle and bring each around to the front of the leg and over the point of the bandage. If the ends are excessively long, you may wish to pass each around the lower leg an additional time. Tie the ends together over the point of the bandage.

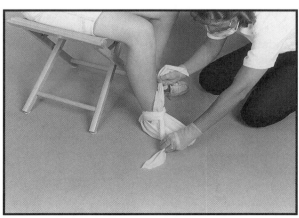

4. Lastly, bring the tip over the tied ends, and tuck it under the band formed by the ends surrounding the anterior lower foot to secure the bandage from being loosened from the top surface of the foot.

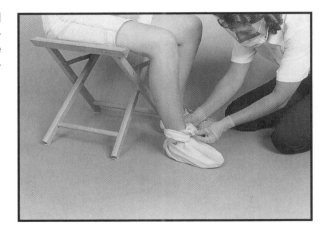

5. The essentially same method is used to apply a triangular bandage to cover the entire hand. However, rather than anchoring the ends around the perpendicular (to the foot) lower leg, they are anchored around the narrow (compared to the hand) wrist.

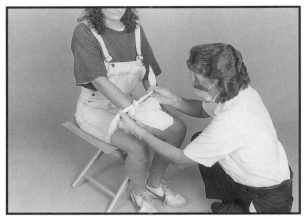

FOLDING A TRIANGULAR BANDAGE INTO A CRAVAT

Since triangular bandages come packaged pre-folded as cravat bandages, they do not routinely need to be so folded by the EMT. However, when an unfolded or improperly folded one (or one improvised from bed linen) must be formed into a cravat, the EMT must know how. *Simply holding the ends of the triangle and rolling or flipping the tip over the base repeatedly, will easily become disorganized.* Instead of saving time, this practice actually usually results in additional delay. To fold a triangular bandage properly into a cravat:

1. Lay the triangular bandage on a flat clean surface. While holding the tip (or point), fold the bandage by placing the tip at the center of the triangle's base. This folds the triangular bandage to half of its original height, and changes its shape into a *trapezoid.*

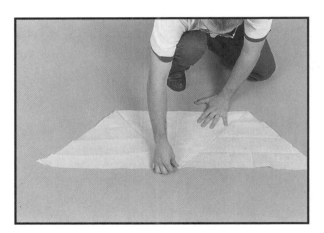

2. Grasp the top edge of the trapezoid (the shorter of the parallel sides) in both hands and again, fold the top of the bandage over. Lay this edge onto the edge of the base (or just slightly short of it), as shown. This halves the height of the trapezoid, and reduces the height (now considered the width) of the bandage to 1/4 of that of the original triangle. When using a commercial triangular bandage, the width of the cravat formed at this point, should be between 6 and 8 inches.

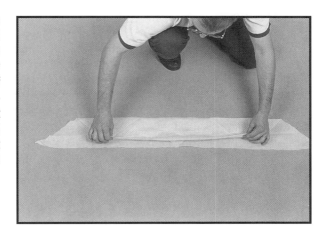

3. Repeat the previous step, one or more times as needed (halving the width with each fold), until the cravat is between 3 and 4 inches wide. In some cases, as you complete a fold, the cravat will be only slightly too wide and, if another fold (halving its width) is made, it will be too narrow. If this occurs adjust the *previous* fold so that it only partially overlaps. The folded-over edge should be placed before (rather than at) the base, at a point so that the width of the cravat is now twice that desired. in this way, once the next and final fold is made, the cravat will be of the correct width and having an only partially over-lapped fold on the outside of the cravat will be avoided.

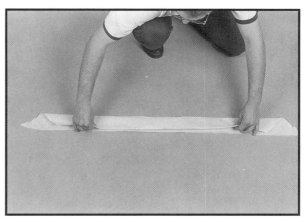

Ending with a cravat that is either too wide or too narrow must be avoided. Similarly, adjusting the width by making the final fold so that it only partially overlaps the surface of the cravat, should be avoided. If when you complete a fold, the cravat is too wide (without another fold) and another fold halving its width will cause it to be too narrow, you will need to adjust the fold you have just complet-ed before going further. Slide the folded-over edge which you just placed on the trapezoid's base back towards the center of cravat adjusting the last fold you made so that it only partially overlaps the cravat's surface, enlarging the present width of the cravat. The amount that this fold will overlap or not, should be adjusted so that the present width of the cravat (the distance between the upper and lower bases of the trapezoid) is twice the width ultimately desired. By adjusting the width (to twice that ultimately desired) and causing the partial overlap to occur at this point rather than at the final fold, the final fold will result in the cravat being of the correct width without any partial overlap or exposed edge on the outside surface of the top or bottom.

USING A CRAVAT BANDAGE

When the triangular bandage was folded into a cravat, each fold doubled the number of layers of fabric which are placed on top of each other. Therefore a cravat bandage, when placed so only a single turn is applied over any given point, covers the dressing with six or more closely-woven layers of fabric. Therefore, only one thickness of a cravat needs to be applied over the dressing, and over-lapping of the cravat is limited to its edges (so gaps are avoided) or as necessary to return the ends for tying. The various techniques used to bandage an area using a cravat, can be shown in demonstrations of their application to two areas.

Applying A Cravat Bandage Along An Extremity

1. Lay the center of the cravat across the long axis of the limb so it is on a slight diagonal. The exact angle necessary is determined by the width of the cravat. The correct angle must be approximated so that as each end of the cravat is wound around the extremity, it neither excessively overlaps the previous turn nor causes a gap.

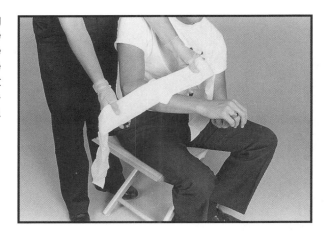

2. Wind each end in an opposite direction around the limb and apply turns whose edges overlap until the bandage covers the entire dressing and its edges lie just beyond the distal and proximal ends of the dressing. This is easiest done by alternately making a half-turn with the distal end of the bandage then a half-turn with the proximal end, and so on.

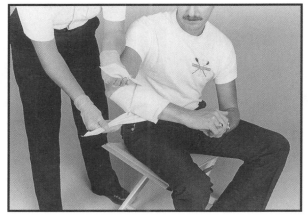

3. When a sufficient area has been covered, with one or more gapped turns return the ends to the center of the bandage and tie the ends together. Locate the knot so it will not lie on the underside of the limb, between the limb and a splint, or between adjacent body areas. If applied at a joint, the proximal foot, or part of the hand and wrist, the ends should be wrapped so that one is proximal and one distal to the joint (or thumb) as when forming a figure-of-eight around them with a roller bandage.

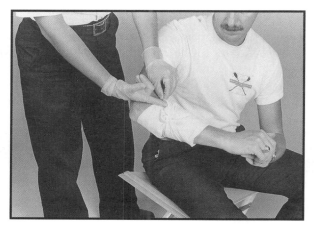

Applying A Cravat Bandage To The Head

1. To cover a dressing on the forehead (or at any point around the circumference of the head at the approximate level of the forehead) a cravat bandage can be applied in a method analogous to when applying a roller bandage. While holding both ends of the cravat, center it on the forehead at (or just caudad to) the supra-orbital ridge.

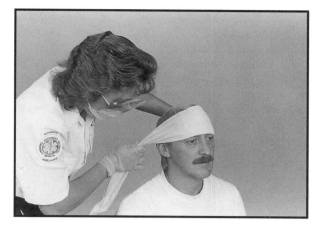

2. Bring each end around an opposite side of the head, and cross them under the posterior protrusion of the occiput.

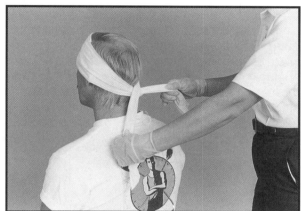

3. Bring the crossed ends back around the sides of the head and tie or tape them securely over the forehead.

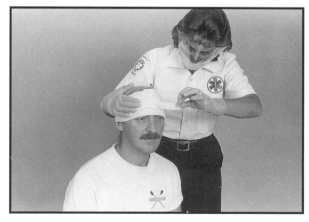

Applying A Triangular/Cravat Combination To Bandage A Shoulder Or Hip

1. Holding one end and the tip of the triangular bandage, center it over the appropriate shoulder so the base lies across the patient's upper arm and the tip is 5 or 6 inches beyond the side of his neck.

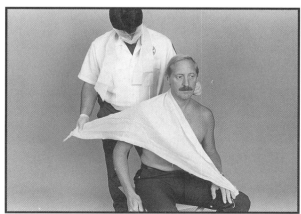

2. Hold a cravat perpendicular to the top of the shoulder so about two-thirds of its length is posterior to the shoulder and one third is anterior to it. Place the cravat down onto the point of the triangular bandage, so that 3 or 4 inches of its tip lies beyond the edge of the cravat. Fold the tip over the cravat and, by rotating the cravat medially for several turns, wrap additional folds of the point of the triangular bandage around the cravat.

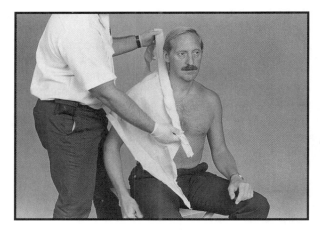

3. Bring the long end of the cravat diagonally across the back and snugly through the armpit. Then tie both ends of the cravat together so the knot lies on the anterior thorax. The cravat forms a snug loop around the upper torso (anchored by the top of the shoulder and lateral neck at one side and under the armpit at the other) which secures the medial end of the bandage over the top of the shoulder.

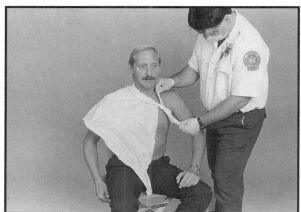

4. Fold-up the edge of the base of the triangular bandage and repeat this several times until the edge of the bandage no longer lies down the arm to the most distal point you wish to cover. Then pass each end of the bandage through the armpit (one from the front to the back, and one from the back to the front).

5. Continue to pass each end around the upper arm for several turns and then tie them together on the outside of the arm to secure the distal end of the bandage and complete its application.

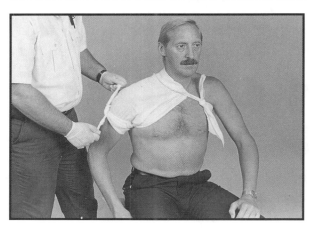

6. The same method can be used to cover the hip and upper leg. The tip of the triangular bandage is wound around the cravat and the cravat is tied around the narrow waist to secure the proximal end of the bandage to the torso. Then, using the same technique as previously described for the shoulder, the ends of the triangular bandage are folded up, passed through the groin, and wound around the upper leg several times. They are then tied together over the lateral side of the upper leg to secure the distal end and complete the bandage.

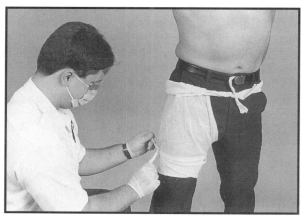

APPLYING A WET DRESSING (To Cover An Evisceration)

When the patient has an evisceration from which part of the bowel or other internal abdominal organs protrude or are widely exposed, a wet dressing (using an appropriate solution) should be used to cover it to prevent further destruction of these normally moist tissues. Evaporation from prolonged exposure to the air or the application of dry gauze over them can dry them out and should be avoided whenever possible.

Only isotonic solutions such as *Normal Saline (NS)* or *Lactated Ringer's (LR)* should be used for this purpose. These are readily available in sterile form in IV bags carried on advanced units. Basic life support units which do not carry IV solutions should carry several bottles of sterile NS in the event that the need for moist dressings to cover such an injury occurs.

Sterile or tap water (or even sterile D5W) should NEVER be used to wet dressings to cover exposed organs. The use of water to keep organs moist, through a complex molecular chain of events, will actually draw water from the cells and cause hemolysis and resulting cell death. The use of any hypertonic solution will result in increased organ tissue destruction rather than reducing it. When an EMT will be in a "wilderness," combat, or expedition setting, where NS or LR may not be available, his additional special training should include the proper method for producing a topical "Normal Saline" solution by adding a proper amount of salt to available drinking water. In other situations, NS should be available. To cover an evisceration with a wet dressing:

1. Retrieve several sterile packages containing ABD pads or trauma dressings and a bottle or IV bag of Normal Saline or Lactated Ringer's solution and place them near the patient. Before going further, change your gloves. Use sterile ones, if available. Direct a second EMT to peel back the packaging of the ABD pad and to hold the outer package (*only*) so that you can easily reach the dressing.

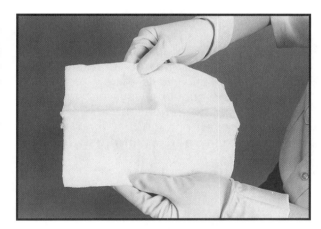

2. Remove it from the package, and unfold it to its full normal size. Hold the dressing almost flat and horizontal by grasping an opposite edge in each hand. After moving it away from the patient, direct the second EMT to pour (or if using an IV, run) NS or LR over the upper surface of the dressing until it is sufficiently saturated so that all of the layers are wet. Gently shake the dressing to remove gross excess fluid if any is running from it.

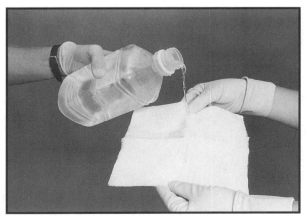

3. While still holding the dressing taut and flat from opposite edges, move it above the eviscer- ation and/or exposed abdominal organs so it is located exactly over the area to which it is to be applied. Once properly located, lay it onto the patient. Repeat this process, using additional ABD pads, until the entire evisceration, wound, and immediately adjacent area is covered by 2 to 3 thicknesses of wet pads. As long as properly wet, these will generally be held in place by the normal adhesion produced between two wet surfaces.

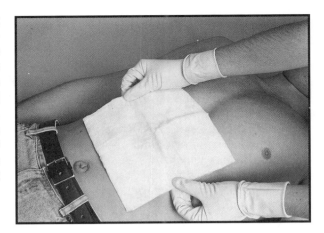

Many EMT texts promote covering wet dressings with plastic wrap taped to the skin at its edges, to retard drying of the dressing. With normal run times this is of limited if any benefit, and will both complicate the EMT's continued access to the dressing and unnecessarily delay the seriously injured patient in the field. Therefore, it is only recommended in cases where the time required in the field (due to rescue or other problems), or for transport, is cumulatively expected to be extremely (several hours) long.

4. In either case, the EMT should frequently check the dressing after it has been applied and, if any drying of the upper layers is found, remoisten the dressing by adding a substantial amount of NS or LR onto its entire outer surface. Such dressings should always be wet before they are placed on the patient, and should be re-saturated often enough that the surface in contact with any part of an organ, *NEVER* becomes dry.

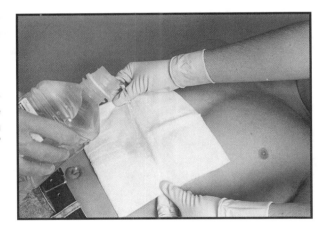

SUMMARIZING WOUND CARE AND BANDAGING

With the exception of special wounds, field wound care and bandaging are essentially the same regardless of the location or surface size of the wound or the specific materials used to dress and bandage it. Although these do not materially change the EMT's care, *the patient's condition does.*

If the wound or wounds are isolated injuries without significant systemic implication and the patient's condition is stable, the wound should be evaluated further and carefully dressed and bandaged before the patient is packaged and transported. If the wound or other injuries may be associated with underlying organ damage or (due to blood loss or other conditions) the patient is unstable, the priorities are different. Except to control external bleeding, wound care is only a secondary concern in such cases and must be abbreviated or deferred until enroute. Even then, the focus on maintaining key life-saving interventions may cause the identification and care of extremity wounds to be omitted.

One series of steps and sequence is used for NON-URGENT patients and another for those who are URGENT. Two separate Summary Skill Sheets have been included, so that the skills for dressing and bandaging wounds is summarized in the proper sequence and context for each of these situations. A third summary is provided for special wounds.

Open injuries are identified as **special wounds** if general wound care and the application of dry sterile dressings covered by a normal bandage would in-itself be inadequate, or would be inappropriate. Because the specific care required for each type is so varied, a single summary sheet including the necessary steps for each is not possible. Instead, a list of special wounds has been included to provide the reader with a handy reference.

Wounds Requiring Enlarged Or Different Wound Care

The nature of some *special wounds* causes the unique problem associated with them, and the special care this required, to become the primary concern in their field management. Often this results in the need for significant modification or alteration from the routine time and manner in which the dressings and bandage are applied. *For some special wounds, the application of dry sterile dressings and a normal bandage are contraindicated.* The following list includes the major categories of special wounds found in the field. The reader should note that the location, specific cause, or other considerations may result in different concerns and different dressing and bandaging requirements within one identified category (for example, a wound with an impaled object when it is on an extremity, the eye, or in the thorax and "sucking"). Wounds for which the customary application of dry dressings and bandages must be modified, substantially altered, or even omitted, or which require significantly different care, include:

- Open fractures of the skull
- Wounds which intrude into the airway
- Neck wounds which penetrate a vein
- *Some* maxillofacial injuries
- Wounds of the eye
- Injuries from/with chemicals or other foreign matter on the eye's surface
- "Sucking" wounds of the chest (or if the diaphragm is penetrated, "sucking" wounds of the abdomen
- Wounds with a protruding impaled object
- Eviscerations
- Burns
- Wounds containing or previously contacting caustic or toxic agents
- Frostbite
- Venomous stings or bites
- Animal bites (including human)
- Significantly avulsed, or amputated parts
- Others, in special situations.

Compound (open) fractures, although requiring additional care and immobilization, have *NOT* been included since their wound care, dressing, and bandaging is no different than that of other wounds.

ETI SUMMARY SKILL SHEET
**Dressing and Bandaging Wounds
(NON-URGENT Patients)**

1. CONFIRM THE SCENE IS SAFE AND all indicated BODY SUBSTANCE ISOLATION PRECAUTIONS have been taken.

2. DETERMINE IF SPINE IMMOBILIZATION IS/IS NOT INDICATED. IF IT IS, direct another provider to INITIATE MANUAL IMMOBILIZATION of the head.

3. Do a Global Survey. RULE OUT the NEED FOR OTHER IMMEDIATE INTERVENTIONS AND IDENTIFY ANY SIGNIFICANT EXTERNAL BLEEDING.

4. CONTROL any significant EXTERNAL BLEEDING.

5. EVALUATE if, and the LEVEL OF SHOCK that is present. INITIATE BASIC SHOCK TREATMENT, as indicated.

6. CONTINUE THE INITIAL SYSTEMIC EXAM and direct a second EMT to CHECK THE PATIENT'S VITAL SIGNS.

7. CONFIRM THAT ALL HIGHER PRIORITIES OF CARE HAVE BEEN ACCOMPLISHED/RULED-OUT, AND THAT NO CONDITIONS REQUIRE THE RAPID INITIATION OF TRANSPORT.

8. DO A HEAD-TO-TOE SURVEY to identify/or rule-out the existence of other injuries.

9. ASSESS EACH WOUND area carefully AND DETERMINE IF IMMOBILIZATION and a splint IS INDICATED.

10. REMOVE ANY debris or FOREIGN MATTER (except impaled objects) FROM AROUND THE WOUND.

11. APPLY dry STERILE DRESSINGS over the wound.

12. APPLY A suitable BANDAGE AND, if an extremity, RE-CHECK THE DISTAL CIRCULATION.

13. IF INDICATED APPLY A suitable SPLINT AND, RE-CHECK THE distal MSCs.

14. DETERMINE IF AMBULANCE TRANSPORT is INDICATED OR NOT. IF any doubt exists, ambulance transport should be provided (unless a capable patient refuses).

15. **If Ambulance Transport is NOT INDICATED (or refused):**
ADVISE THE PATIENT that the field care is only temporary, and REFER him TO PHYSICIAN EVALUATION AND DEFINITIVE CARE. Document the "informed advice," and COMPLETE THE RUN REPORT.

If Transporting:

16. LOAD the patient and COT INTO the AMBULANCE AND INITIATE TRANSPORT.

17. RE-CHECK the ABCs, AND THE MSCs in any bandaged or splinted extremity, or any extremity that is included in the splint of another extremity.

18. MONITOR the patient, AND PERIODICALLY RE-CHECK THE VITAL SIGNS.

ETI SUMMARY SKILL SHEET
**Dressing and Bandaging Wounds
(URGENT Trauma Victims)**

1. CONFIRM THE SCENE IS SAFE AND all indicated BODY SUBSTANCE ISOLATION PRECAUTIONS have been taken.

2. DETERMINE IF SPINE IMMOBILIZATION IS/IS NOT INDICATED. IF IT IS, direct another provider to INITIATE MANUAL IMMOBILIZATION.

3. Do A GLOBAL SURVEY AND PROVIDE ANY AIRWAY MANAGEMENT, VENTILATION, CPR OR EXTERNAL BLEEDING CONTROL NEEDED.

4. INITIATE BASIC SHOCK TREATMENT, as indicated.

5. CONTINUE THE INITIAL SYSTEMIC EXAMINATION AND direct another EMT to TAKE THE VITAL SIGNS.

6. IDENTIFY ALL SIGNIFICANT INJURIES AND CONDITIONS. IF INTERNAL BLEEDING IS FOUND, IF INDICATED APPLY the PASG.

7. APPLY any REQUIRED PRESSURE BANDAGES AND rapidly TAPE DRESSINGS OVER ANY OBVIOUS GROSS WOUNDS.

8. MOVE THE PATIENT ONTO A LONGBOARD and immobilize him to it. PLACE THE PACKAGED PATIENT onto the cot and INTO THE AMBULANCE.

9. INITIATE TRANSPORT AND ANY KEY ITEMS OF CARE THAT WERE DEFERRED IN THE FIELD.

10. CONTINUE to provide KEY CARE AND, only IF RESOURCES ALLOW, DO A HEAD-TO-TOE EXAM. ADD TAPED DRESSINGS AS INDICATED.

11. MONITOR the patient and periodically RE-CHECK the VITAL SIGNS.

SECTION

Extremity
Splinting
Skills

15

Introduction

Most animals have a rigid skeleton which defines the animals' general size and shape, and protects and supports the body's organs and other tissues. In some of of the lower animals who have an exoskeleton, this is made up of a series of armor-like plates which surround the parts of the body. The higher animals such as man have an endoskeleton in which a series of bones, connected by joints, form an internal skeletal frame which supports and defines the main body and its appendages from within.

Bones consist of both organic and inorganic material. The organic matrix of living cells provides the cells and nutrients necessary for growth, remodeling and repair. The inorganic materials, essentially minerals (salts of calcium and phosphorous), provide strength and hardness. As the individual matures the bones define his height and essentially the girth of the head and torso. Although the general size and shape of the body is defined by the bones, its outer form—particularly the outer shape and girth of the neck and extremities—is defined by the size and development of the muscles which surround the bones.

The human skeleton is made up of 206 bones which are attached at joints by connecting tissue and the muscles which surround them.

Bones are classified into essentially four types:

- **Long**—such as the femur, tibia, fibula, humerus, radius, and ulna
- **Short**—such as the carpals, metacarpals, tarsals, phalanges, etc.
- **Flat**—such as the sternum and scapulae
- **Irregular**—such as the vertebrae.

The classification of individual bones is not important to pre-hospital care. Instead, the EMT should be familiar with the location and name of each major bone and with the general organization of the human skeletal frame.

The unique nature of the long bones found in the extremities bears note. These generally have an enlarged area made of compact bone at each end (called the epiphysis) and a long tube-like shaft (called the diaphysis) between these ends.

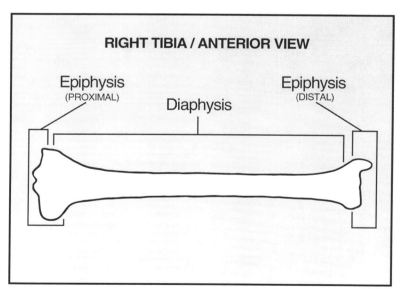

RIGHT TIBIA / ANTERIOR VIEW

Epiphysis (PROXIMAL)   Diaphysis   Epiphysis (DISTAL)

The long central shaft surrounds a medullary canal which contains marrow (primarily specialized fat cells which produce the red cells needed by the circulatory system to transport oxygen) and a major artery and vein as well as other vessels and nerves. The entire bone is covered by a hard outer layer called the periosteum. The long bones in children have areas at their ends, defined as growth plates, which motivate and control the growth of the bone. When an epiphyseal fracture occurs with injury to the growth plate of a growing child it can lead to the arrest of bone growth in the limb, resulting in retarded growth of the limb and a life-long disability if not treated.

Because of this, any extremity trauma in a developing child, regardless of whether it appears to include a fracture, should be evaluated by a physician.

The bones of the body are surrounded by skeletal (striated) muscles. These voluntary muscles are connected to each other by ligaments and to the bones by tendons. The individual bones are attached to each other at a series of joints. Classically joints are considered to be either fixed or movable and, based upon their design and the type of motion each allows, movable joints are further classified as being ball and socket, hinge, gliding, or pivot joints. Although it is important for the EMT to know the location and normal range of motion of each joint in order to identify irregularities, learning the proper medical name and classification of each serves no particularly useful purpose. Since when there is injury involving a joint, without X-Ray evaluation one can not be sure whether it is exclusively the joint or involves fractures proximal and distal to it, it is more accurate to identify the injured area in the pre-hospital setting by its generally accepted common name (right shoulder, left elbow, right knee, left ankle, etc.)

Instead of the specific anatomical classification of each joint it is more useful when learning the normal range of movement of each to perceive them as one of three types.

- **Fixed and immovable**
- **Fixed and flexible**
- **Movable, with a significant prescribed range of circulation.**

At some joints, individual bones are fused together with an immovable weld-like connection, producing a larger inseparable bony structure such as the sacrum, adult cranium, or pelvis. Any bone movement felt in these structures is abnormal and must be considered to indicate a fracture.

The circle formed by the fixed ribs of the rib cage is analogous to that of the pelvis, but it is flexible in order to allow for the rise and fall of the anterior chest needed for ventilation. Although posteriorly each of the 10 upper ribs is essentially fused to a thoracic vertebra (T1–T10), the flexibility of each rib and the cartilage connecting it to the sternum anteriorly allows the anterior thoracic cage to enjoy limited outward and upward movement with each breath. Although the joints of the rib cage allow for this flexibility they are fixed and do not allow for other movement or further articulation of the connected ribs with the spinal column, or with and of the sternum.

Movable joints are of essentially two types. The joints between the skull and the spinal column, between the individual single vertebrae, and the rest of the spinal column with the sacrum, are a unique specialized inter-related series of joints in which the separate bones and fused structures can move but are held in careful alignment by a continuous series of muscles and a ligamentous sheath which runs from the base of the skull to the pelvis. The anatomy of the spine and injuries and treatment of the spinal column have been fully discussed in a preceding Section of this text.

The other type of movable joint, prevalent in the extremities and where each limb connects to the torso, is called a *synovial joint.*

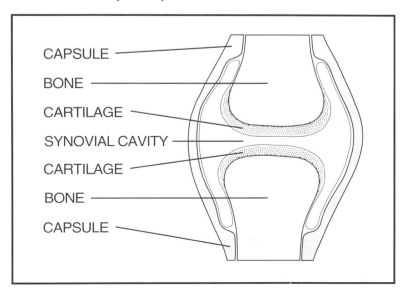

In these, the articular surfaces of the bone ends are covered by cartilage and are contained in a *capsule* which contains *synovial fluid*. The synovial fluid keeps the bone ends separated and acts both as a shock absorber and lubricant to allow them to articulate smoothly together. The interactive shape of the bone ends, together with the strong muscles and ligaments which surround the joint and the tendons which attach these muscles to the bone, maintain the bone ends properly aligned together in the joint. These also define the direction and range of motion allowed by the joint. Many of the vast directional capabilities of the distal extremities come from a combination of the separate limited ranges of motion in adjacent proximal joints. For example, the elbow and knee allow flexion and extension of the forearm or lower leg—but do not allow any significant rotation. When the lower arm or lower leg is rotated, the humerus at the shoulder or femur at the hip rotates rather than the elbow or knee. Therefore, the movement of a distal bone is usually governed not only by its immediately proximal joint but also by others that lie more proximal in that limb. Each movable joint, however, has some specific mechanical limit to the direction and range of movement of the bone ends it includes.

If any joint is forced to move contrary to or beyond the limits of its normal range of motion, injury to the joint occurs. The damage may be limited to only the muscles, ligaments or tendons (producing a sprain or strain), or the bone ends may also be forced out of alignment (a dislocation). This can occur with or without fractures of the bone ends. Even if a fracture-dislocation is only slight, a resulting small irregular protrusion or bone chip between the articulating bone ends can result in severe and even disabling secondary damage to the joint.

The degree of pain or amount of swelling associated with a joint injury may vary significantly from case to case and is *NOT* a reliable indicator of the type or extent of damage which occurred. It is *NOT* uncommon for simple strains or sprains to be more tender and produce more swelling than some dislocations or fractures. Although many dislocations can readily be identified by the nature of the deformity that results, in many cases when a dislocation has occurred the muscles spontaneously retract—replacing the bone ends back into approximate alignment. When this occurs there is often little or no specific evidence that a dislocation or fracture has occurred.

The movable joints make it possible for us to move, grasp, and lift. The ability to flex, extend and rotate our arms allows us to position and move our hands in an almost infinite number of ways which, when combined with the movements of the fingers and flexibility of the hand together with the opposing position of the thumb, allow us to grasp and perform many of the specialized digital functions essential to human productivity and progress. The joints of the legs allow us to sit, stand, walk, run, climb, lift, jump and change posture and direction with ease.

At each synovial joint there are opposing muscles. One end of each is connected to the proximal bone (point of origin) and the other end to the distal bone (point of insertion). Tendons attach the ends of the muscles to the bones at a sufficient distance from the joint so that when the muscle contracts (shortening its length) the distal bone is moved, flexing or extending the joint.

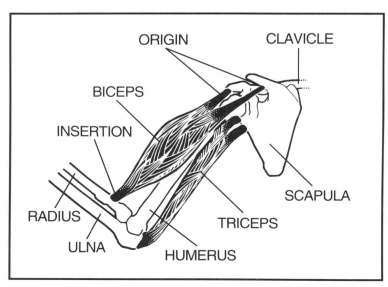

When this muscle relaxes and the opposing muscle contracts, the distal bone is pulled in the opposite direction, extending it back towards it former in-line position with the proximal bone. Some of the opposing sets of muscles are placed on an angle or partially surround the bones, providing the ability to lift and rotate the limb as well.

The muscles can only contract (pull) or relax. When they relax they do not push. The joint is moved in one direction when the muscle on that side shortens, and is pulled back in the opposite direction when it relaxes and the opposing muscle (on the other side) is shortened. Because the elbow and shoulder lift against gravity when flexed and are aided by it when extended, and because the opposite is true when lifting with the legs or when we run and walk, the opposing muscles are commonly not equal. The muscles that work against gravity or move or bend our joints to move our bodies forward are more developed and larger than those which oppose them and are aided by gravity. Since any pull must be against some fixed anchor, whenever a muscle contracts and pulls to lift the distal limb an equal amount of force is exerted against the proximal skeletal frame. Therefore, in any limb where musculoskeletal injury has occurred, should the patient spontaneously move the joint, increased pressure and weight on the joint and bones proximal and distal to it will occur. Because the knee and elbow are hinged joints and cannot rotate, when the forearm or lower leg need to be rotated the humerus or femur are rotated instead. Often certain movements of a distal part require movement of several of the proximal joints and not just the nearest proximal one alone.

Bones and joints can be injured directly by the force applied against them from blunt trauma which compresses the tissues lying over them, or by the secondary effect of force referred onto them from elsewhere along the skeletal frame. Both occur when an unrestrained victim of a head-on car accident slides forward on the car seat, striking and injuring his patella directly on the lower dashboard. Then, as the torso continues to attempt to move forward and the leg is arrested from moving further, the shaft of the femur breaks or its head is posteriorly dislocated at the hip.

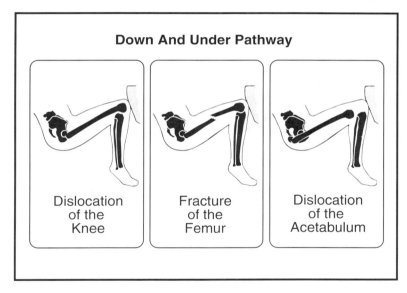

Down And Under Pathway

Dislocation of the Knee

Fracture of the Femur

Dislocation of the Acetabulum

When substantial energy is transferred beyond the point of initial impact along the skeletal frame, it will commonly produce other musculoskeletal injuries. Although such a secondary injury is often to the joint adjacent to either end of a fractured bone (or in the case of an injured joint, to the adjacent neck or shaft of the bones which make up the joint, it may instead occur at a weaker point some distance from it. The previous example serves as a good illustration. If, when the knee is injured and stopped, the upper leg is at an angle to the direction of travel, a transverse or oblique fracture across its shaft is common. Alternatively, however, if the femur was in alignment with the direction of travel its great longitudinal strength will often keep it from being injured and the energy will dissipate and cause injury to the hip instead. Whenever sufficient force is applied to a bone or joint to result in significant injury, the EMT must suspect the possibility of other non-contiguous musculoskeletal injuries.

Fractures and injury to the joints of the extremities frequently result from leverage applied against a bone or against the entire limb. If the victim of a fall lands so that a raised narrow object or an elevated edge such as a curb or stair edge lies across the long axis of the bone, the object acts as a bridge and, since only a part of the bone is stopped from movement, if the rest of the bone continues to be forced downward it generally fractures across the edge or edges of the supporting object. It is not unusual for damage to one of the adjacent joints to occur as well. If the fulcrum ends up being closer to one end of a bone than the other, the longer end acts as a lever producing an additional mechanical advantage so that the force brought to bear against the shorter part of the bone on the other side of the fulcrum is enlarged more than originally implicit in the force of the fall and weight of the patient.

Often in falls or other accidents, the distal end of a limb becomes trapped and held in place while the rest of the body continues to move. In such cases once the limb has twisted or been extended to the limit of the range of motion of its joints, leverage will be applied relatively evenly to each bone and joint which lies between the trapped distal end and the torso. When the continued movement and force applied supersedes the combined elasticity of the bones and joints involved, something must break. Generally this will occur at the weakest point along the limb or at the point at which the leverage is brought to bear the most.

Whether a longbone will fracture, or one or several joints will be torn and dislocated, or both, involves such complex physics that the exact location and number of resulting injuries in the limb is essentially unpredictable. In such cases the EMT must carefully examine each bone and joint in the limb (and any other area which collided or was stressed in the fall) with a high degree of suspicion and must *NOT* assume that the injury is limited to the most significant or first one found.

In the forearm and lower legs, two longbones lie in close proximity and parallel to each other. When an injury occurs to one of these bones a high suspicion of injury to the second should be provoked. Similarly in the shoulder, hip, hands, and feet—where a number of bones are inter-connected and lie adjacent or near each other—injury to any one commonly results in injury to others and must be assumed. Because of the angulation of the head of the femur, and the nearness of the structures and vast muscles surrounding them it is often difficult to determine whether a fracture of the head of the femur, a hip injury or a lateral pelvic fracture has occurred. Although the key structural stability of the pelvis can be determined by palpating the pelvic girdle, whether such an injury is limited to the head of the femur or includes injury to the hip joint is often not distinguishable by physical exam in the field.

When bones such as those of the foot and toes have a great weight fall on them, the compression force is so great that concomitant crushing injuries to many small bones and joints in the region generally occurs. This type of crushing injury is most commonly seen in either the hands or feet.

In recent years, there has been an increased focus on specific mechanisms of injury and the injuries commonly produced by different types of car collisions, motorcycle accidents, falls from bicycles and sports activity. The wide proliferation of lectures and articles on *Kinematics* has made many EMTs more aware of these common injury patterns. This understanding is helpful in producing raised levels of suspicion to help rapidly identify common related secondary injuries which, being at some distance from the site of the initial result, could otherwise be missed. *Knowledge of injury patterns commonly associated with a given mechanism of injury or sport is helpful in raising the EMTs suspicion of certain prevalent injuries, but should NEVER be an influence in minimizing or obviating the careful need to thoroughly examine the patient for other injuries, regardless of how rarely these may be found with the specific mechanism which acted upon the patient.*

Some patients who have progressive joint disease will have increasingly limited and painful movement of their joints without any traumatic injury. As each of us progress beyond our middle years our bones become more brittle and less force is required to injure them. In some patients with bone disorders, a spontaneous fracture can occur even in the complete absence of any trauma.

From even the simplified preceding review of the anatomy, normal mechanics, and mechanics of injury of the extremities, it should be obvious to the reader that such injuries can be highly complex and may be more or less profound or extensive than is initially apparent.

When injury occurs to a joint it is impossible solely by physical examination in the field to make any reliable distinction between a strain, sprain, dislocation or dislocation fracture without X-ray capability. Even when there are *NO* apparent signs of a dislocation at the time of the exam, if any signs or symptoms of injury to the joint are present the EMT can not rule out the possibility that dislocation and realignment of the joint occurred earlier, and that damage to the connecting tissue or a fracture have resulted. Therefore, the EMT should *NOT* be tempted to make such a determination even when the signs and symptoms appear slight, and should treat any joint injury as if it includes a dislocation fracture. Special considerations when treating injuries to the knee or elbow, or when a dislocation of the shoulder or hip occurs far from the nearest hospital, will be specifically addressed later in this introduction.

Fractures of the extremities are usually classified by the nature of the break. Although often found as a test question, whether a fracture is oblique, transverse, spiral, greenstick, comminuted, or impacted is *NOT* usually discernible or of any relevance in the field. All fractures are also classified based upon whether or not there is a wound associated with them. This distinction is pertinent to the EMT as it affects his treatment. A fracture which does *NOT* have any open would associated with it is defined as a **simple or closed fracture**. A fracture which has an open wound associated with it is defined as a **compound or open fracture.** Because dislocations so rarely produce an open wound, they are assumed to be closed unless described to the contrary, and the terms "simple" or "closed" are commonly not used with them. When however, a dislocation (or dislocation fracture) does have an open wound associated with it, it should be described as a **compound or open dislocation.**

Fractures are also described by the degree of remaining displacement of the fracture fragments (bone ends or comminuted sections). Any **displaced fracture** will produce a deformity of the limb. The displacement may be minimal or, as with an overriding fracture, significant. If the displacement is minimal it may be so slight that it is hard to see, but should be clearly palpable. If the displacement is substantial it will produce marked deformity and may also have angulation or other abnormal positioning of the limb distal to the injury site.

In cases where bone ends protrude, or when a fracture allows movement and angulation where no joint exists, or when crepitus (the feel of irregular bone ends grating together) is felt upon palpation—the EMT will positively know that a *fracture* exists. In other cases the EMT may not be able to determine whether a fracture, lesser bone injury, or exclusively muscle and connecting tissue damage has occurred. Any of these three, however, can significantly weaken the underlying musculoskeletal framework which supports the limb and presents a similar risk of extensive further damage if alternate support is not provided and if movement of the area is allowed to continue.

As well as injuries that can positively be identified as being a fracture, the EMT must assume that any musculoskeletal injury which is painful, swollen, deformed or painful on movement, has an open wound associated with it, or causes guarding by the patient, is a possible fracture and should be treated in all regards as if it is a fracture.

Similarly, when a joint injury produces an overlying or adjacent wound or dislocation it generally presents with gross obvious signs that a bone end has been displaced. However, this is not true in all cases—particularly when a bone end has been dislocated and spontaneously returns to a position approximating normal alignment in the joint. As well as any joint which is obviously dislocated, the EMT must assume that *any joint which is painful, swollen, or deformed, is painful or produces crepitus upon movement, results in guarding, or which (compared to its normal range of movement) has a more limited, more extensive, or unusual range of movement, is or may have been dislocated.*

An extremity injury that is not immediately apparent may first be suspected when decreased or absent distal sensory perception or circulation is found when checking motor, sensory and circulation in the extremities. These signs and symptoms, however, are only associated with a small percentage of extremity injuries.

Treatment Priorities

Injuries to the extremities, like any injuries, must be viewed and treated in the larger context of the patient's overall condition and problems, and must be managed in keeping with that individual patient's needs and priorities. The following priorities must always remain paramount:

First: Assure proper safety of the scene and situation.

Second: Identify and treat any immediately life-threatening conditions or conditions with significant systemic implication and provide the intervention indicated or rule out their presence.

Third: Determine if the patient has multi-systems trauma (or an acute medical condition) and is URGENT, or whether the problems are limited to simple isolated trauma (generally in the extremities) and the patient is NON-URGENT.

Fourth: *In URGENT patients,* identify or rule-out the presence of neurovascular compromise which is limb-threatening.

Fifth: Identify all localized extremity injuries and rule out others by a head-to-toe evaluation.

Sixth: Provide any wound care indicated, and splint and immobilize all musculoskeletal extremity injuries.

Seventh: Support and restrict movement of any limb containing any musculoskeletal injury.

As previously discussed in the Section on Patient Assessment, when the *Initial Systemic Exam* has been completed and the EMT has identified that the injuries or conditions found require that the patient be urgently transported, the EMT should not delay in the field to assess or care for non-systemic individual injuries. Instead, the patient should be rapidly packaged and transported to the hospital. Because a complete head-to-toe assessment including the extremities is not recommended by this time, the patient should be immobilized in a supine position on a longboard, even in cases where spinal immobilization is not indicated.

When spine injury *IS* suspected and the patient is fully immobilized to a longboard, the spine as well as the rest of the musculoskeletal system have been protected from further movement and injury. In *URGENT* cases, when spine trauma is not a concern and the patient does *NOT* need to be fully immobilized to the board, the other bones and joints of the body are still, however, immobilized by being secured on the longboard. In either case, by securing the patient onto a longboard, the EMT has supported and immobilized the pelvis, shoulder girdle, and all four extremities in one simple step, without causing the unaffordable delay needed to do a detailed examination and identify and treat each individual injury they contain.

In patients in whom urgency has been ruled-out, rapidly packaging on a longboard *without* any further detailed examination or treatment is *unwarranted* and, although protection from further injury, does not represent the recommended or optimum possible care. When urgency has been ruled out as a factor, the patient will benefit far more from a detailed head-to-toe examination and the careful treatment of each individual injury before he is packaged and transported. In this way, each possible fracture will be identified and carefully treated and splinted *before* the patient is moved. With such patients the EMT can consider the patient's overall condition packaging as to best provide for the patient's cumulative injuries and comfort during transport.

Even when dangers at the scene or extreme weather require placing the patient on a longboard and rapidly moving him into the safer environment within the ambulance, this should not cause the EMT to immediately initiate transport if the patient is *NON-URGENT*. In such cases, once in the ambulance the *NON-URGENT* patient should be carefully examined from head-to-toe and each individual injury treated appropriately before he is re-packaged and transport to the hospital is initiated.

With patients who have significant systemic injury and compromise, remaining in the field to identify and provide itemized care for each non-critical injury causes needless delay and significantly increases the chance of death.

In patients who have NO urgent conditions, moving them rapidly onto a longboard and precipitously initiating transport before identifying and stabilizing each injury causes needless pain and an increased chance of further injury.

Most commonly, critical injuries and conditions are found in the head, thorax and abdomen, and the EMT must be careful that non-critical distracting injuries — because they are so painful or grossly deformed or angulated — do not become the focus of his attention before more urgent priorities are treated or ruled-out. However, the EMT must also be careful not to discount extremity injuries as being non-critical simply because of their location. Although rare, *some extremity injuries can significantly contribute to the patient's systemic deterioration or even be life-threatening* if they produce severe hemorrhage internally or externally.

When any significant wound is associated with a fracture, regardless of whether or not bone ends protrude, the fracture is considered open. Profuse external bleeding can occur, and must be identified and controlled with the same early priority and concern as any other significant hemorrhage. Severe blood loss and profound shock can result from an open extremity injury.

External hemorrhage from an open fracture or secondary soft tissue injury should be readily recognized by the EMT in the first few seconds of his Global Survey. Care must be taken not to miss such bleeding if it is masked by dark or fluid-impervious clothing. Regardless of the presence or absence of protruding bone ends, any significant bleeding from an extremity must be controlled by direct pressure and other steps outlined in the preceding Section on Bleeding and Shock. In such cases, once the bleeding has been controlled the treatment of shock, rapid packaging of the injury, and initiating transport to the hospital without delay must become paramount priorities.

When there is an open fracture or other wounds which will underlie the splint or ties, these should be covered with dressings and bandages to protect them prior to the application of the splint. Because continued swelling is common, it is safer to tape dressings or secure them with several layers of stretchable gauze bandaging than to use more extensive and unyielding bandages around the limb. If the bandage around the limb is thick it can produce undesirable localized pressure at the injury site when the splint is secured and may compromise distal circulation. The splint should be applied so that the EMT continues to have access to the bandage. When an air or vacuum splint is used which will encircle the injury site, only dressings should be used to avoid interfering with the splint. The bandage and distal pulse should be checked periodically to assure that, due to additional swelling, the bandage has not become too tight and the distal circulation has not become compromised.

With an injury anywhere on an extremity, all jewelry should be removed from the limb prior to splinting. Jewelry which is left on can produce underlying damage when a splint is secured over it and, as swelling increases, may compromise the circulation distal to it and be even more difficult to remove.

Bleeding and shock can be profound even with closed fractures. Closed fractures may produce a *third-space effect*—creation of a pathological space not normally anatomically present which can contain sizable amounts of blood. For example, internal bleeding caused by closed femur fractures may produce a blood loss as high as 1000 to 2000 cc's per thigh. In other extremities internal bleeding is more limited and generally can not exceed 300 to 500 cc's in each portion of the limb.

Due to the size and strength of the large muscles of the thigh, when a fracture of the shaft of the femur occurs there is commonly a muscle spasm which results in the bone ends overriding each other and creating a large pathological space for internal bleeding. Internal bleeding from overriding fractures of the femur are controlled by the use of traction or the PASG, and will be discussed further under Special Considerations in the following pages. Because of the absence of any wound or signs of external bleeding, this can easily be missed until the patient's level of shock advances sufficiently to produce the suspicion that hidden internal bleeding is occurring at some point. In patients with other injuries, the contribution being made by extremity injuries to the advance of shock can remain hidden and, particularly with any overriding fractures of the femur, must be anticipated and treated against.

As well as any bleeding from a fracture, the pain commonly associated with significant skeletal injury also promotes shock. Proper care and stabilization of the extremity injury will significantly contribute to reducing pain and lessening the resulting shock.

Once the patient's immediate needs and any higher care priorities have been taken care of or ruled out, the EMT should direct his attention to identifying and treating any musculoskeletal injuries.

In years past, splinting injured ribs with tape or binders encircling the torso over the injured ribs was advocated. Time has demonstrated that this provides no benefit (except when supporting a loose flail segment) and in many cases resulted in increasing respiratory distress and hypoxia. Currently, splinting simple rib fractures is *NOT* recommended.

Since spinal immobilization has been separately covered in the preceding Section due to its complexity, and since injuries to the ribcage and skull are not splinted, the splinting and immobilization skills included in this Section are limited to the extremities and pelvis. The clavicle and scapula are included in the shoulder girdle and therefore are defined as part of the upper extremities. The pelvis, although not an extremity, has been included because discussion of the management and splinting of the femur, hip and pelvis is inseparable.

Treatment Objectives

Because the bones (along with the joints, muscles and connecting tissues) provide the underlying structural support of each extremity, a primary objective of the EMT's field care for suspected fractures is to *provide an alternate rigid external support along the entire length of the injured bone.*

To avoid further damage from grating or displacement of the bone ends, the *joints adjacent to each end of the injured bone must be fully immobilized* as well as supporting and immobilizing the injured bone itself. If these joints are not immobilized and the patient contracts the muscles in an attempt to move either joint, undesirable pull will occur against the broken bone end. Simply stated—when a bone is injured the EMT must fully immobilize:

The Adjacent Proximal Joint ✚ **THE INJURED BONE** ✚ **The Adjacent Distal Joint**

When a joint or the muscles associated with it are injured the structural skeletal support may be similarly weakened or lost. Any stress or continued spontaneous movement of the injured joint can produce significant additional damage. Therefore, the primary objectives of the EMT's field care for an injured joint are **to provide alternate rigid external support and to immobilize it**. Because the bones connected at the injured joint act directly on the joint, and the joints at their other end act directly on these bones, the immobilization provided for an injured joint needs to be more extensive than that for solely any injured bone. When a joint is injured, the EMT should fully immobilize:

The Proximal Joint ✚ **The Proximal Bone** ✚ **THE INJURED JOINT** ✚ **The Distal Bone** ✚ **The Distal Joint**

With an injury to a single bone or joint, although it is unnecessary to *fully* immobilize the entire limb, the adverse effects of referred stress from movement beyond the immobilized area or of the weight of the limb distal to the injury site must be considered. Therefore, an additional key objective when treating an extremity injury is to *secure the limb so that its entire weight is being externally supported, and so that movement beyond the area which is fully immobilized is extremely limited.*

When the injury is to a lower extremity this is easily achieved by securing the splinted patient supine on a long backboard and tying both feet together to prevent rotation of the injured leg. If the patient is not placed on a longboard, the addition of a long rigid splint secured between the legs is recommended to avoid any bending when moving the patient over to the cot. When securing the legs care must be used in positioning the ties or straps so that they do not press directly upon an injured area or its proximity. With lower leg injuries, splinting must include support of the foot in its normal near-perpendicular position to the lower leg. Extension, rotation or other movement of the foot and ankle causing pull on the lower leg are to be prevented. Once the patient is on the longboard or cot (whether flat or sitting) a strap should be placed around the torso at the armpits to prevent any further movement of the hip joint.

The arm can be immobilized and supported in one of two different positions—either with the elbow bent across the front of the upper torso or extended down the side of the patient. When the immobilized arm is to be secured with the elbow bent across the anterior thorax, it is supported by an arm sling and its movement is further limited by the addition of a strap or cravat swathe tied around both the arm and torso. This method should be used when the patient is to be transported in a sitting or semi-sitting position on the cot.

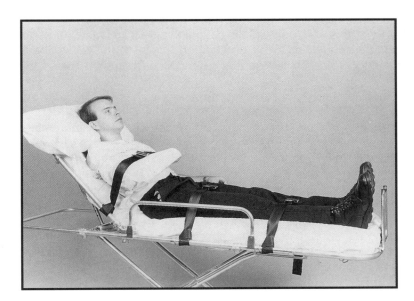

Patients with an isolated arm injury are often transported most comfortably when on the cot in a semi-sitting position. ***This method should NOT be used to secure an injured arm when the patient's condition requires being transported in a supine position.*** If the arm is secured across the chest and the patient is placed supine, most of the weight of the arm and splint (10–12 pounds) will rest on the anterior thorax and upper abdomen. This can increase abdominal pressure on the diaphragm and inhibit chest excursion—increasing the effort to breathe and causing or contributing to respiratory embarrassment. Obviously this method should *NOT* be used with patients who have any significant injuries of the anterior thorax or upper abdominal quadrants.

If the patient must be placed supine, and he has an injury to the bone or joints of either arm, the arm should be immobilized in an extended position along the patient's side, and the splinted arm should be secured to his torso and upper legs.

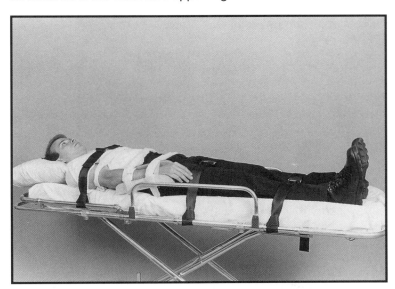

It must be noted that when the arm is extended along the patient's side, the distal forearm, wrist and hand extend beyond the pivot point of the hip joint. Therefore, if the extended arm is secured to the side of the torso and upper legs, the patient ***must be secured with straps across the torso and upper legs to prevent him from sitting up or elevating his legs.*** Should such a patient later be moved into a sitting position or have his legs elevated, the movement can result in severe stress and further injury to the distal forearm, wrist or hand. Therefore, this method should only be used when the patient's condition ***allows*** him to be placed and maintained in a supine position on the cot or when he is to be secured on a longboard.

When splinting the patient's arm the EMT must anticipate whether the patient's condition dictates transport in either a sitting or supine position (or is elective). Unless contraindicated, if a sitting or semi-sitting position is required the arm should be splinted so it can be secured across the patient's chest. If a supine position is required, the arm should be splinted so it is extended in a straight line at the patient's side.

In the rare event that both a supine position and immobilization of the arm with the elbow bent are required, the EMT should—if possible—immobilize the elbow at sufficiently less than a 90 degree angle so that the weight of the immobilized arm can be supported on the upper legs rather than either the anterior thorax or abdomen. IF the elbow must be immobilized at about a 90 degree angle, by careful rotation of the shoulder of the splinted arm the arm can be secured so that the forearm, wrist and hand lie on the cot or backboard just beyond the top of the patient's head.

In the rare event that both a sitting position on the cot and immobilization of the arm in a straight fully extended position is required, a long rigid splint running the entire length from the elevated side of the cot beyond the shoulder to a point just beyond the distal end of the fingers will have to be added to support and secure the splinted arm during transport. Once this support has been secured to the elevated head-end of the cot and to the cot next to the patient's upper leg, *NO* changes in the elevation of the head end of the cot must be made unless these ties have first been released.

Moving The Patient And Repositioning Injured Extremities

Whether an injured extremity should be moved or realigned surrounds two totally separate concerns—one of which must be a consideration during the early examination of the patient and the second which must be considered later when treating the specific extremity injury. The patient may need to be moved or repositioned early on, prior to any detailed examination and identification of his extremity injuries, in order to:

- Move him out of danger.
- Move him out of a grossly abnormal or stressed overall position (such as when only part of his body rests on an elevated structure).
- Move him from a space that makes assessment and treatment impossible (e.g. under a car).
- Reposition him so that ABCs can be adequately elevated.
- Reposition him to provide urgent ABC interventions, indicated.
- Reposition him to prevent aspiration of vomitus.
- Rapidly align him and place him on a longboard to move him into the ambulance in severe weather.
- Rapidly align him and secure him on a longboard when the urgent initiation of transport is indicated by his condition.

In these situations, although extremity injuries must be assumed to be present, more urgent priorities and interventions for life-threatening conditions must take precedence over any potential harm that may result from moving or aligning an injured extremity. Although the extremities should be supported and moved with controlled care, these injuries should not distract or otherwise delay the EMT from any urgent higher priorities of care.

Only a small percentage of the trauma victims to which the EMT responds will be found in either such a situation or with injuries or conditions which have systemic or life-threatening implication. With most trauma calls, the EMT finds an alert, stable-appearing patient whose complaints surround a single isolated injured extremity. In such cases, the EMT should direct a second EMT to support the injured area while the first EMT exposes and scans the injury site to assure the patient that he is not dismissing his complaints and to confirm that there is no hidden bleeding. Before focusing on more detailed assessment and care of the injury, however, the EMT must do a rapid Initial Systemic Exam to rule out the presence of any urgent conditions, and an abridged head-to-toe survey to identify or rule out the presence of other localized injuries. Once these have been completed the EMT can safely focus on the isolated extremity injury which caused the ambulance and EMTs to be called.

In the early days of EMS, the principle of "Splint them *where* they lie" was often interpreted to mean "Splint them *as* they lie." When there is *NO* need to move the patient from danger or to rapidly package him on a longboard and initiate transport, the question of whether to move an injured limb (and how much) or whether to splint it in the position in which it is found is highly complex. *Rigid adherence to the practice of routinely splinting all extremity injuries exactly as they are found, or of routinely moving any extremity injury into neutral alignment, is inappropriate in the pre-hospital setting.*

The EMT should evaluate the risks and benefits of moving and/or realigning each extremity injury before splinting it, on a case-by-case basis. When determining whether or not to attempt to move an injured extremity prior to splinting, the following need to be considered:

- Is the injury being levered against or otherwise stressed?
- Has the patient moved the extremity into a "guarded" position of comfort?
- Is it an isolated injury or are there other associated injuries in the limb? Where?
- Is the extremity grossly angulated or is it in general anatomical alignment?
- What is the location of the injury(s), and is the injury to a joint, longbone shaft, or other bone (such as the bones of the hand or foot)?
- Does the injury include either protruding or impacted bone ends, a partial amputation, or crushing injury?
- Is there any distal sensory deficit?
- Is there any distal circulatory compromise?
- Is either a traction splint or the PASG indicated?
- Are there other practical splinting considerations?
- Are there practical considerations for extricating, moving and transporting the patient?

Although the variety of different injuries and situations the EMT will find makes it impossible to make firm recommendations, some guidelines will be useful.

Any skeletal injury or injured extremity which is found to be levered against or otherwise stressed by the patient's position or weight upon it should be carefully moved (or the patient moved) to eliminate the stress. Similarly, since gross pathological angulation of an extremity at a longbone fracture or when a partial amputation has occurred commonly results in continued stress to the surrounding tissues, producing severe risk to the nerves and blood vessels surrounding the injury site, the risk of realigning such limbs and then splinting them in a position approximating their normal anatomical position is far less than leaving them as found even if this was possible. Therefore, if there is gross angulation, the extremity should be carefully realigned prior to splinting.

When the longbones in a given area of an extremity contain several adjacent fractures resulting in one or more comminuted sections of bone, and the area between the joints presents in a curved (or multiply angled) position rather than straight, the fracture sites will be stressed. With such an injury, while the area remains curved the various bone ends will continue to produce stress and potential additional damage. To eliminate this, the curved or multiply angled part of the limb should be straightened (whether the fractures are closed or open).

A Colles' fracture of the distal radius and ulna is a key exception to this rule. This type of fracture (also called a "silver-fork" fracture) can be easily identified without X-Ray since it produces a deformed curvature of the wrist so that the distal arm and wrist have the same shape as that of a dinner fork viewed from the side. *The EMT should not attempt to realign a Colles' fracture, instead it should be supported and immobilized in its presenting "silver-fork" position.* If the distal circulation is compromised, the EMT should reposition the wrist slightly to restore it — but should not apply traction or otherwise attempt to reduce its pathological curvature.

Fractures of the femur are managed with a traction splint or, in cases with suspected intra-abdominal or vast 3rd space bleeding (such as overriding bilateral femur fractures), the PASG. Use of either of these requires that the leg be in a straight and aligned position prior to their application. Therefore the EMT will have to move the leg(s) into normal straight alignment whenever one of these is used.

When an injured extremity is found extended to the side, splinting and immobilizing it in this position is difficult and often impractical for moving and transporting the patient. Even when this is possible, the dangers of additional injury from striking and leveraging the extended limb and splint when moving the patient, or the inadvertent "bouncing" that can result from road shocks when transporting, outweigh the dangers of carefully rotating the limb into closer proximity to the rest of the body.

Experience has shown that as a practical matter, the legs can generally only be supported and immobilized safely and effectively when they are in approximately normal lateral alignment. The words "approximately" and "lateral" are key, and this should not be misinterpreted to suggest precluding splinting in a knee-over-knee, outward rotated or flexed knee position when any of these are indicated. Similarly, experience has shown that to safely and effectively splint an arm, the upper arm must be positioned approximately parallel to the long axis of the body. As well as when the arm is extended straight along the patient's side, the upper arm and humerus can be positioned approximately parallel to the long axis of the body when the arm is splinted with the forearm flexed across the chest (or lower anterior torso), or with the arm rotated so it extends beyond the top of the head with the elbow at any angle within its range of motion.

Injuries to a movable joint, if the distal circulation is NOT compromised, are best moved as little as possible, if at all. Such movement should generally be avoided or limited to carefully moving them only as much as is required to make splinting and packaging of the patient practical. If the joint is stressed or pathologically grossly angulated, it should be moved to a more neutral unstressed position as with any skeletal injury.

There is considerable debate surrounding whether or not the EMT should attempt to reduce dislocated shoulders and hips in the field, particularly in patients who have a repeated history of such injury and are some time from the hospital. Upon first consideration it would seem to be a fairly radical idea since, in the absence of an X-Ray, one can not be sure whether a fracture of bone shards exist in the joint. Advocates for the procedure maintain, however, that in such patients an associated fracture is extremely rare and that timely reduction in the field is a conservative procedure which will avoid a later life-threatening risk if general anesthesia is necessary. If such dislocations are not reduced immediately, significant muscle spasm generally follows. Once this has occurred, the use of general anesthesia in almost all cases is required at the hospital to release the spasm and allow for their reduction. Commonly such injuries (if massive trauma was not involved) do not have a fracture associated with them and will—if treated in the field—"pop" back into their proper place when carefully articulated into proper position and pulled. Once at the hospital, a post-reduction X-Ray will confirm that no comminuted segments have been produced in the joint. Supporters of this practice maintain that it follows the principle of preventing life-threatening conditions (in this case with general anesthesia) over increased risks to the localized injury by reducing it "blindly" in the field. The risk-to-benefit ratio for reducing these injuries in a remote area or otherwise at some considerable time from the hospital should be decided by the squad's Medical Director. The EMT should NOT attempt this unless he has been specifically trained in the necessary techniques and it is clearly included in his local protocols.

Due to the anatomical structure of the knee and elbow and the proximity of the arteries which supply the circulation beyond these joints, when good distal circulation is still present after injury to them they should be splinted in the position found whenever practical. As with any musculoskeletal injury, if the distal circulation has been reduced or interrupted the joint should be moved in an attempt to increase or restore it. When the distal circulation has been compromised at a joint the EMT should move the joint, preferably to a slightly more flexed position, to attempt to restore the distal circulation. The extremes of either full flexion or full extension should be avoided. If, after several attempts to reposition the joint, the EMT has not restored or improved the distal circulation, a true time-line emergency exists if the limb is to be saved. In such cases, the EMT should rapidly package the patient and initiate transport to the nearest appropriate hospital without further delay. If distal circulation remains absent, additional repositioning of the joint to restore it should be attempted once enroute if safely practical.

Methods For Extremity Alignment

When a section of an injured extremity must be re-aligned, it is usually best to firmly grasp the joint immediately proximal and the joint immediately distal to the injured section and apply opposing manual traction—pulling between both joints until the section is again approximately in a straight line.

When a longbone fracture results in severe angulation of the bone, a different method requiring two EMTs should be used. While one EMT supports and manually immobilizes the section between the proximal joint and the injury, the second EMT provides traction to the angulated section and moves the distal angulated section into approximate alignment. The EMT who will move the angulated section into alignment should place one hand on the cephalad side and near the proximal end of the angulated section, and grasp the immediately distal joint with his other hand. If the distal joint is too close to provide a good point from which to move the limb, then the area distal to the joint should be grasped instead. Initially, traction should be provided by pulling the side of the *proximal end of the angulated segment* along the long axis of the body away from the other segment to hold the bone ends separated. While maintaining this traction on the proximal end of the angulated section, he should move the distal end of the angulated segment in the correct direction for alignment. With such injuries, it is important to exclusively provide the traction from the proximal end of the angulated section until it has been approximately re-aligned. Traction from a distal point on a grossly angulated fracture will not separate the bone ends and will generally result in uncontrolled movement of both segments and additional damage.

When repositioning an injured joint, traction is NOT used except in special cases. Instead, the distal bone is simply moved to a new position. One hand should be placed just proximal of the joint to support and anchor the proximal bone(s). By careful positioning, this hand can be placed so that the proximal bone can be anchored and the tips of the thumb and first finger rest on opposite sides of the joint. This will allow the EMT to feel any crepitus if it occurs. The EMT's other hand, which will be used to grasp and reposition the limb distal to the joint, should be placed a few inches distal to the joint. It is important to place the lower hand sufficiently distal to provide the necessary mechanical advantage to manipulate the joint easily. When this is either the shoulder or hip, after the other joints in the extremity have been re-aligned the EMT should grasp the wrist or ankle respectively and apply some moderate traction while moving the distal part of the limb. Sometimes with dislocated shoulders or hips, when the arm of leg is repositioned so the humerus or femur are placed into normal anatomical alignment, their proximal head will pop into place and the dislocation will be spontaneously reduced. The techniques for assessing and intentionally reducing these dislocations with traction are varied and complex. The steps in moving, and the degrees and direction of pull as well as the points of counter-traction, vary depending on whether the dislocation is anterior or posterior and how the limb is rotated. The field reduction of these dislocations requires significant traction and special training which, due to its tactile elements, can not be effectively demonstrated in a book. Where this is included in pre-hospital protocols, observation and supervised clinical practice in the special techniques used should be required prior to the EMT attempting the procedure in the field. As well, the protocols should require the patient's documented and signed informed consent and agreement to be transported to the hospital for a post reduction X-Ray — *before* the procedure — in order to protect the patient *and* the EMTs.

When moving a multiply misaligned extremity, the EMT should NOT attempt to align or otherwise reposition it by moving, rotating or applying traction to the entire limb at one time. Moving or tractioning of the entire limb from its distal end will result in the uncontrolled movement of all of its bones and joints in a variety of directions and planes simultaneously. Often this results in interim adverse movement of a section or joint or, due to resistance from the strong muscles in the upper part of each extremity, an interim transition producing overly acute localized bending at the weakest injury site until the increasing pull defeats the resistance and finally the entire limb moves.

When realigning a limb the EMT should start at the distal end of the extremity and, while anchoring the rest of the limb, properly align each area and its proximal joint separately before attempting to reposition the next proximal area, then its proximal joint, and so on. For example, the EMT should reposition the hand, then the wrist, then the forearm, then the elbow, then the upper arm, and finally the shoulder. As a matter of practical mechanics, a section of the extremity and its proximal joint will often have to be moved simultaneously. Since movement of any longbone area of the limb or any joint includes movement of the parts of the extremity distal to it, as the EMT moves proximal area he must properly support any distal injuries and protect them from undesirable independent movement. This can usually be achieved manually but in rare cases may require distal areas to be splinted prior to moving more proximal areas of the extremity. Experience has shown that the manual support of distal areas can often be increased and improved by holding a rigid splint in place to support and immobilize the distal parts of the extremity. As well as providing more stable and extensive support than can be provided solely by hand, this usually avoids the unnecessary application of several separate splints to the extremity prior to completing the re-alignment of the entire limb.

When the injuries to a leg include a fracture of the shaft of the femur, the preceding method of aligning the extremity should only be used to align the leg distal to the femur. Then, once the leg distal to the femur has been brought into straight alignment, the application of traction from the ankle is the appropriate way to align the femur. This should be continued without interruption while the leg is moved to a position parallel to the body's long axis and a traction splint is applied.

Except for controlling any significant bleeding, the addition of dressings and bandages to open wounds should generally be deferred until after any needed repositioning of the limb has been completed—but prior to splinting. This reduces the risk that any increase in bleeding caused by moving the limb will be masked, and eliminates the chance that any swelling under the bandage will cause it to impair or tourniquet the distal circulation.

In any case when moving or re-aligning an injured extremity produces an adverse effect, the EMT should STOP and re-evaluate the consequences against the practical need for any continued movement. Generally, movement of an injured limb should *NOT* be continued if it produces:

- Continued increased pain.
- Increased guarding.
- The initiation or increase of any significant muscle spasm.
- Any increased non-transient deformity.
- The initiation or increase of any distal sensory deficit.
- The initiation or increase of any distal circulatory compromise.
- Any perceivable additional damage.

When moving the extremity, the appearance of any of these must be assumed to have resulted from the movement—and that increased damage has occurred. The limb should be moved back slightly towards its original position until the adverse effect is relieved, and then be splinted in that position if possible. In some cases, higher priorities of care or the practical requirements of packaging and stabilizing the injury when moving and transporting the patient will dictate approximate alignment.

Other Special Situations

Four additional situations require special consideration and further discussion.

Fractures of the shaft of the femur, in addition to being splinted and immobilized with the application of traction, are treated to control the vast internal bleeding commonly associated with them. The leg distal to the femur is first realigned and then manual traction is applied and maintained while the entire leg is properly positioned and a traction splint is applied to maintain the traction mechanically. The contraindications for, and the use of, traction splints will be discussed further in the part of this Section which details individual splints.

The hand is usually included in the splint for injuries of any part of the arm so that, even when neither the hand nor wrist have been injured, they do not hang unsupported beyond the splint or arm sling. Injuries of the wrist and forearm are among the most prevalent extremity injuries because of the instinctive response to extend the arm to lessen the impact when falling, or to protect the face and thorax from injury with one's raised forearms.

When included in any splint, the hand should not be immobilized in a forced flattened position with the fingers and thumb extended and secured together. Although such a position is within the normal range of motion of the joints of the hand, thumb and fingers, it is a strained, unnatural position which produces stress to the numerous bones and joints involved. Instead, *the hand and fingers should be placed in approximately their normal position of function.* The position of function of the hand is similar to placing the palm over a tennis ball and grasping it.

When the hand is to be included in a splint, this position can easily be approximated and maintained by either of two different methods. When the hand is *NOT* included in the injuries of the arm, it can be maintained in the position of function by placing the splint (or arm sling) with its distal end just distal to the joints connecting the bones of the hand with the phalanges (the short bones of the fingers and toes).

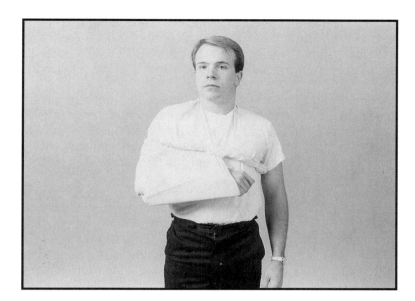

The splint supports the forearm, wrist, and hand while allowing the fingers to curl over its end and the thumb around its medial side in a natural position approximating the position of function. When using an air splint for an arm, the same principles apply. Including the hand in an air splint will cause it to be squeezed, and should be avoided even if the hand has not been injured.

Alternatively, appropriate positioning of the hand can be achieved while supporting the entire distal arm on a rigid splint. When this is desired, the splint is placed so its distal end is beyond the fingertips. A firm 2 or 3 inch wide roller bandage (approximately 2 inches in diameter) is placed on the splint under the palm — as if grasped in the hand — so that the hand and fingers are curved over it. Once so positioned on the splint, the hand can be secured to it by the use of 2 or 3 inch conforming roller gauze wrapped around both. This bandage should be applied sufficiently tight to secure the hand but not so tight as to squeeze it into a more extended, flattened position.

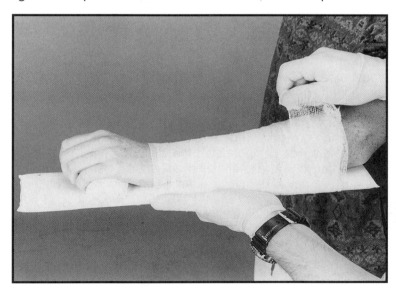

The patella is unique among the bones of the body since, even though it articulates with the front of the distal femur, it has no direct bony or cartilaginous fixation to the rest of the skeleton. It is essentially held in a pocket-like space formed between the large muscles which are connected to both the distal upper and the proximal lower leg, and which surround the lateral and anterior aspects of the knee joint.

Due to its location and connection, this "floating" anterior flat shield which protects the rest of the knee can easily be dislocated by athletic activities. Some patients have recurrent dislocations of the patella which, similar to recurrent dislocations of the shoulder, can result from only minor twisting. Usually the patella displaces to the lateral side and any dislocation of it will produce significant deformity.

Although its transitory nature and strength make fractures of the patella relatively rare, when these occur it is not uncommon for the patella to be broken into multiple comminuted fragments. This type of injury occurs most commonly when anterior force against the knee is in-line (therefore not displacing the patella laterally) and much of the weight of the body is applied against the patella — such as when it strikes the ground in a fall or collides with the lower dashboard in a front-end vehicular collision.

Patients with a dislocated or fractured patella generally present with the knee deformed and partially flexed and, unless there are other injuries to the ligaments and bones of the knee, acute discomfort is more common than severe pain. The patient has usually moved the knee to a position which promotes the most comfort possible and guarding is almost universally seen. Once this injury has been identified, no benefit is derived from detailed examination of it. Unless the distal circulation is compromised, the EMT should *NOT* attempt to relocate the patella or move the knee further in the field. Instead, as with any injury to the knee, it should be supported and immobilized with splints in the position in which it was found.

Amputations produce a variety of special problems with which the EMT must deal. Whether a significant part of a limb or only an isolated toe or finger has been amputated, *any amputation will result in severe anxiety (even hysteria) in the patient and those accompanying him, and produces the risk of significant permanent disability.* Even though the loss of a leg or foot would appear to be more disabling, the loss of several finger ends or a thumb can ultimately produce a greater loss of function and a far greater impact upon the patient's ability to perform his job and the tasks associated with normal self-maintenance.

Particularly in the case of an amputation, the EMT must guard against being initially distracted from the patient's overall condition by the severed limb or the need to locate any missing parts. As with any trauma, the first priority is to evaluate the ABCs and to identify *all* conditions which are life-threatening or have significant potential systemic implication. Only once these have been stabilized or ruled out can the EMT safely focus on the amputation and any other localized injuries.

Although the compressive nature of most traumatic amputations usually prevents severe or continued bleeding, the treatment of any amputation should focus on bleeding from, and injuries to, the stump end of the remaining contiguous part of the extremity before any consideration is given to the care of the separated part(s). Any significant external bleeding should be controlled and the proximal part of the limb and adjoining body areas should be carefully examined to locate any other associated injuries.

Even when blood loss and pain are minimal, the emotional impact and the vast neurological, skeletal and soft tissue damage that occurs when any portion of an extremity is amputated will ultimately produce severe shock. Regardless of how well compensated the patient's initial circulatory status appears, this must be anticipated and aggressive treatment for shock should be rapidly initiated if sudden decompensation and profound shock are to be avoided. As a corollary to this, patients who have sustained any traumatic amputation should be considered *URGENT* regardless of how stable they appear, and rapid packaging and transport should be initiated without delay.

Amputated parts require careful care if the possibility of re-attaching them is to be preserved. In the past few years there has been vast advancement in limb re-attachment and, regardless of whether or not re-attachment appears probable, the EMT should allow for the chance by providing proper timely care for the parts in all cases.

Many of the apparently logical and earlier promoted methods for the care of amputated parts have been proven to cause tissue damage and lessen the chance for successful re-attachment. Amputated parts should be handled carefully and as little as possible in the field. Excess dirt and particulate matter (soil, sawdust, etc.) should be floated-off, but they should *NOT* otherwise be cleaned or debrided. The parts should then be kept from any further tissue deterioration caused by warming or drying out by placing them in a sealed, cool and humid environment. The parts should *NOT be kept wet* by immersion or being surrounded by wet dressings, *NOR dried out* by being placed on or surrounded by dry ones. Although they should be kept cool, they should *NEVER be placed in contact with (nor only separated by thin layers from) ice or chemical cold packs* as this can cause frostbite or more profound freezing and substantial tissue destruction.

In order to remove gross loose dirt and debris, the EMT should rinse the amputated part(s) in sterile Normal Saline. IF this is not available, sterile water or the cleanliest available cool water should be used instead. After gently shaking off any excess surface water, the part should be placed into a plastic bag and, after purging *most* of the air from it, the plastic bag should immediately be sealed. Just enough air should be left in the bag to prevent its sides from collapsing and being drawn tightly against the amputated part. Bags such as those with an air-tight self-sealing closures, commonly used for sandwiches, are useful for fingers or toes, and either one of the large plastic bags used to isolate bio-hazardous materials or a clean garbage can bag can be used for larger parts. Some plastic bags used for refrigerator or freezer storage contain multiple air vents through their sides and therefore should be avoided. An airtight plastic bag is required in order to maintain a sealed humid environment. In most cases the part can be kept sufficiently cool during transport in warm or hot weather by keeping the bag out of direct sunlight and contact with warm objects, and by placing a moist cool towel loosely around the outside of the sealed bag in the air-conditioned patient compartment. This will also keep the amputated part from the patient's sight. In cold weather, where heating of the patient compartment is required for the patient's well-being, a different method will be needed to keep the bag and part cool. If the temperature is not sub-zero, insulating the plastic bag from direct contact with other objects or cold metal by loosely surrounding it with several towels or pillows and securing it in a safe, unheated outside compartment provides a simple rapid way for the EMT to keep the part cool while keeping the patient compartment warm. A watertight unheated outside compartment that is not full of loose items should be selected, and any objects that could shift should be removed. If this is not possible, or if the weather is so extreme that the EMT fears that the outside compartment may become too cold, securing the protected plastic bag in the passenger seat of the separated front cab is an alternative. With the front passenger window kept partly open and the front heat limited to only the windshield and as little as is needed to maintain adequate visibility, the part can be kept cool while the patient compartment is sufficiently warmed.

The amputated parts should be cared for in the same way should they be located after the patient has left for the hospital. When they are transported in a separate vehicle they can easily be kept cool by proper use of the windows or air conditioning and avoidance or limited use of the heater, since patient comfort is not a concern.

Wherever the bag containing an amputated part is placed in a vehicle it must be properly secured. Straps or ties should *NOT* be applied directly onto the plastic bag as this can cause a puncture or forced opening and deflation, or they can intrude onto the amputated part. They can be safely secured by tape or straps placed across bolsters on opposite sides of the bag (using a head immobilizer, blanket rolls or rolled-up taped pillows) so that no pressure is exerted against the plastic bag by either the bolsters or the straps, tape or seatbelt used to hold it safely in place.

In any season, if the aforementioned methods of keeping the part cool are not possible, use of an insulated cooler should be considered. Often one can be borrowed at the scene or one can be rapidly improvised. Chemical cold packs or plastic bags containing ice cubes can be used as the coolant. Although air should be allowed to circulate freely between these and the bag(s) containing the amputated part, extreme care must be taken to place each so that they can not shift in transport and come into contact with each other.

Amputated Parts:

- Should *NOT* be handled unnecessarily, or roughly.
- Should *NOT* be rubbed, scrubbed, or otherwise wiped clean.
- Should *NOT* be washed or rinsed with any substance (soaps, detergents, antiseptic solutions, etc.) *except* Normal Saline or water.
- Should *NOT* be wiped or airblown to dry them.
- Should *NOT* be placed near a fan or source of moving air (warm or cold).
- Should *NOT* be transported in water or wrapped in wet dressings.
- Should *NOT* be transported open to the air or on dry dressings, as both will promote drying-out of the tissues.

No delay should occur in packaging and initiating transport of the patient in order to locate missing amputated parts. Traumatic amputations most frequently occur in the home or gardens, when fingers or toes (or parts of them) are amputated by table or portable circular saws or by rotary mowers. When they are caused by a machine which rotates at several thousand revolutions per minute the amputated parts can be projected for some considerable distance and in a variety of different directions. When this occurs in a cluttered workshop or outdoors, they may be extremely difficult to locate.

If any amputated parts can not be readily found while the patient is being stabilized and packaged, other EMTs, police officers or fire personnel should be left at the scene to search for them. It is important that there be a clear understanding of to which hospital the patient is being transported before the ambulance leaves. The searchers should be directed to immediately call the emergency department if the part(s) are found, and to transport them there without delay. As well, exact directions for the procedures to be followed, including a clear understanding of those that *MUST BE AVOIDED,* should be given to the responder who will be in charge of the remaining searchers.

Time is a key factor in determining the viability of re-attaching any amputated part. Dividing the potential search area into separate marked sectors and formally clearing each in turn has proven to be more thorough and faster than arbitrary random searching which often results in the unproductive repeated search of some areas while others are inadvertently overlooked. Hidden areas, such as those behind or under objects or the overhead cross braces of the exposed floor joists in a basement, should be included, and wood cuttings, sawdust and leaves should be carefully sifted through before the search is abandoned. Experience has also shown that no matter how eager or stable appearing they may be, including relatives or friends of the patient in the search is usually counterproductive and can result in them also becoming a patient.

Even if the parts are not located in the first hour, the search should be continued and, when located, the emergency room should be notified and they should be transported to the hospital to allow the physician to make the determination of whether or not re-attachment is possible. This guards against them being found by a family member, others, or a pet, which can produce unnecessary additional problems and insures that they will be disposed in an appropriate manner.

Partial amputations or large avulsions should be treated as any angulated and/or open fracture and should be realigned and splinted. When a partial amputation is so severe that only some muscles and soft tissue remain which connect the distal part of the extremity, it is improbable that adequate distal circulation can be restored in the field. In such cases the risk of additional movement and delay denies the advisability of any repositioning beyond that needed to initially align the partially separated distal end.

Injuries to the clavicle and scapula, although both are classified as part of the upper extremities, can not be supported and immobilized by splinting them directly as one does with other extremity injuries. The clavicles represent one of the weakest points in the shoulder girdle's structure. Therefore, as well as when the anteriorly protruding medial two thirds of the clavicle is struck, fractures of the clavicle often result from forces transferred to it from other locations around the shoulder girdle. When one shoulder is restrained, and force is applied which moves the opposite shoulder forcefully in a medial or rotary and anterior direction, the shoulder girdle is compressed and, if the force is sufficient, the clavicle fractures.

Because the main shoulder girdle lies over the upper rib cage, the first concern with any injuries of the clavicle or scapula are the associated underlying injuries and any resulting respiratory or cardiovascular compromise that these may produce. The scapulae are extremely strong and are covered by large muscles of the upper back. In order to fracture the scapula, enormous localized force must be applied against it. Fortunately, fractures of the scapula are extremely rare. Studies have shown that in patients with a fractured scapula, because of the substantial force which acted upon the upper torso, associated spine injuries are more the rule than the exception, and that patients with such an injury have a greater than 70 percent mortality rate. Although it is often difficult to positively identify that a scapula fracture has occurred, when one is suspected the patient should be immobilized for suspected spine trauma and, regardless of their apparent stability in the field, should be treated as if they have *URGENT* multi-systems trauma. Because of past experience this is recommended even in cases where the only injuries found are limited to this area.

Beyond any ABC and spinal immobilization needs, the specific treatment for injuries to either the clavicle or scapula surrounds drawing the shoulder on the injured side away from the injury (anteriorly for the scapula, and posteriorly for the clavicle) and then to position and immobilize it so it is held just slightly beyond its normal anterior-to-posterior relaxed position in order to keep the bone ends separated. As well, the arm on the injured side must be externally supported and secured so that neither its weight nor any movement are reflected on the injured area of the shoulder girdle.

The clavicles are supported along most of their length by the rib cage and by connecting medially to the sternum and laterally (at the acromioclavicular joint) with the scapula. This support, however, is dependent upon the shoulder being maintained in a neutral or even drawn-back position. When the shoulder moves anterior to its neutral position the clavicle is lifted anteriorly off of the rib cage and, since when moved anteriorly the shoulder rotates inward to a more medial position, medial pressure occurs against the clavicle. Therefore, rather than providing direct support to the injured area as with most extremity fractures, the key objectives in treating suspected fractures of the clavicle are to keep the shoulder drawn back just posterior to its neutral position and to externally support the weight of the arm so that it neither places an anterior nor inferior pull on the shoulder.

When the shoulder is maintained slightly drawn back and without the weight of the arm against it, the clavicle rests along its length on the anterior rib cage. Medial pressure against it is replaced by mild traction referred from the shoulder. This should prevent further medial pressure against the injured clavicle and should reduce any displacement that has occurred. Most important, with complete fractures in the medial third of the clavicle this referred traction to the clavicle should guard against ensuing displacement of the sharp end of the distal fragment through the trachea or internal jugular vein, and reduce the chance of the other sharp end lacerating the subclavian vein.

Historically, the use of a figure-of-eight bandage (or similar commercial strapping) has been advocated to treat fractures of one or both clavicles in the field. Since this technique was initially challenged by Fowler in 1962, studies have repeatedly shown that the use of a figure-of-eight has *NO* demonstratable advantage over a sling and swathe, and that it is associated with a significant risk of inducing axillary neurovascular compromise. McCandless et al reported that in approximately 10% of the patients in their study the figure-of-eight bandage resulted in compromise to the arm's circulation necessitating its replacement with a sling and swathe. In view of the lack of advantage and potential complications associated with use of the figure-of-eight, this technique is no longer recommended in the field.

The EMT should support and immobilize injuries to the clavicle by maintaining the shoulder drawn back and externally supporting the weight of the arm with a sling-and-swathe or, if the patient is to be placed supine on a longboard, with a loop around each lateral shoulder to keep them drawn back flat against the board. When a sling-and-swathe are used to splint an injured clavicle, as opposed to other purposes, the shoulder should be drawn back just beyond its normal neutral position and the humerus should be positioned along the lateral side of the thorax rather than with its distal end brought across the anterior torso. The modified sling technique (in which the outer end of the sling is passed through the armpit) should be used as this avoids the sling from passing across the injured clavicle and promotes maintaining the humerus along the mid-axillary line. This position of the humerus and the slightly posterior position of the shoulder must be provided when the swathe is added, if the latter is to maintain the shoulder properly drawn-back to produce the mild traction to the clavicle that is desired.

In the rare case that both clavicles are fractured, the patient should be rapidly placed on a longboard (without use of a logroll) with both arms along the sides of the torso and both shoulders drawn back with loops around each. This facilitates bilateral treatment and rapid initiation of transport which is indicated by the implication of the potential underlying simultaneous injuries of both sides.

With an injured scapula treatment for spine trauma should always be included, and the undesirable drawing back of the shoulder which occurs when a person is supine on a rigid flat surface must be protected against. This can be avoided by securing the arm so that the wrist and distal forearm lie on the leg with the distal end of the humerus and the elbow elevated off the board with padding. The elevated lateral shoulder (directly under the proximal head of the humerus) should also be supported with firm padding between it and the board. This padding must be secured so it can neither suddenly fall out nor move medially and become bunched up under the scapula.

When a supine patient has a shoulder girdle injury and is also suspected of having spine trauma, this combination produces a problem in placing him onto the longboard. Obviously, such patients should *NOT* be logrolled onto the same side as the shoulder girdle injury.

Although the halves of the shoulder girdle located on each side of the body's midline have no direct posterior bony or cartilaginous connection to the sternum, due to their conforming perch over the upper rib cage and their strong posterior interconnected muscular covering any significant movement or compression of one side of the girdle will reflect upon the other and cause it to be moved. Therefore, even when the patient is rolled onto his uninjured side, significant movement and anterior rotation of both lateral shoulders (the one rolled onto and the other when pulled to rotate the patient) is unavoidable. Even the use of a scoop litter in these cases is not without problems. Due to the curved nature of the device, as each side is inserted under the patient it causes the lateral shoulder to be rotated and held in a position significantly anterior from its relaxed position. This will impact adversely on any clavicle fractures.

Because longitudinal body drags involve pulling on both armpits and produce significant bilateral cephalad displacement of the shoulder girdle, they are not a method of choice with such injuries. When using a multiple-hand free body lift to insert the longboard under the patient, it is impossible to avoid posterior sagging of the shoulder joint *and* scapula. As well, some transitory anterior rotation of both shoulders is common, and very difficult to avoid.

Neither the adverse affects to fractures of the clavicle or scapula which are commonly associated with all methods of moving a supine patient with suspected spine trauma onto a longboard, nor which methods are preferable for each, are resolved in the available literature. In the absence of scientific data, one must be guided by the anatomy, pathophysiology and therapeutic goals associated with each.

Maintaining spinal immobilization, and keeping the shoulder rotated just slightly anterior of its normal position without elevating the shoulder girdle or causing unnecessary delay, are key objectives in treating scapular fractures. Using a logroll or scoop stretcher are probably the most appropriate ways to place a supine patient with such an injury on a longboard. If a scoop stretcher is used, the benefits of the curved side in providing properly conforming support under the rounded scapula and maintaining the proper shoulder position (without the additional steps required on a flat surface) outweigh the radiological considerations which usually recommend removal of the scoop prior to immobilizing the patient to the longboard. In such cases, once parts of the scoop have been inserted under the patient and re-attached, the patient can be immobilized to the scoop and then it can be placed on the longboard.

Since with a fractured clavicle the shoulder should be maintained drawn back and just posterior of its normal relaxed position, and since any forward rotation of it could produce serious respiratory sequelae, a scoop stretcher or logroll as demonstrated in the preceding Section should *NOT* be used with such an injury. When the recommended method for logrolling is properly modified so that the shoulder on the injured side is not pulled against when rolling the patient—and instead is held in a properly drawn back position—logrolling is probably the best and fastest way to place such a patient on the longboard. This can easily be achieved by drawing the shoulder on the injured side back until it rests on the ground while aligning each arm along the patient's sides. Next rotate the arm on the injured side so the palm is facing up and place the hand (palm up) under the posterior thigh. If the patient is capable, he can assist in maintaining this position by grasping his posterior thigh. If he can not, the EMT who will be rolling the legs and hip will have to hold the patient's distal arm in this position. The EMT who is next to the patient's chest should place his cephalad hand in the patient's armpit (rather than around the shoulder as customary) so that his fingers are together and surround the lateral thorax. When the patient is rolled this provides good purchase on the upper torso, and the back of the EMT's hand in the patient's armpit will keep the shoulder drawn back properly. Once on the backboard, the upper torso should be immobilized so that the shoulders are drawn flat against the board and no straps pass over any part of the clavicle except its distal end (which is included in the shoulder joint).

Splints and Splinting Materials

Injuries of the extremities are supported and immobilized by splints. A number of standard commercial splints are available. They are made of a variety of materials and come in a wide range of sizes and designs to meet the diversity of possible anatomical needs. When necessary one can improvise a splint from any rigid material. However, commercial splints are faster and easier to use and a sufficient number and variety of these should be carried on the ambulance to meet normal needs. Fortunately, almost any likely splinting need can be met by the correct use and adjustment of a limited number of commercial splints and materials. Most splints require the use of bandages or ties to secure them in place. This is most commonly done by wrapping the splint and injured extremity with conforming gauze roller bandages or tape. Splints are also commonly secured in place with cravats (made by folding a cotton, linen, or muslin triangular bandage) tied around the splint and extremity near each end of the splint and as needed between them. The additional cravats need to be placed every 4 to 6 inches to evenly maintain the splint's location and prevent any lateral movement or elevation of the limb off the splint. Whenever a splint is angled, cravats are required at each side of the angle to ensure that the limb stays properly positioned on the splint.

Roller bandages better accommodate changes in the girth and shape of the body area being splinted, and avoid the dangers inherent in using localized "ungiving" ties in only a few places. Therefore the use of roller bandages should be the method of choice for this purpose, and cravats are only recommended where stronger supplemental ties are needed or when time is critical. Although adhesive tape may be a useful adjunct in securing padding to a splint or one splint to another, or fastening the end of a roller bandage, due to its inflexible nature and the possibility of compromising the distal circulation, *tape should NOT be used as a substitute for roller gauze to surround an extremity.* Similarly, neither the typical nor self-adhering type of elastic bandage should be used to surround any extremity in the field. Due to the circumferential tension these promote, even when initially applied with sufficiently limited tension they can result in restricting or tourniqueting the distal circulation at a later time.

Some splints do not require bandaging to hold them in place. Inflatable splints are designed to surround the limb and are essentially one-piece tubes (or become tubes when the zipper along their length is closed). When inflated they are held in place by their shape and pneumatic pressure. Vacuum splints, once formed around the extremity and emptied of air, maintain their shape and position in a similar fashion due to their conforming fit to the body. Traction splints, commercial shoulder binders, or commercial splints designed to partially surround an area, generally include straps or ties which eliminate the need for gauze bandages.

Due to their size and inherent mechanical considerations, all splints have a limited area and scope of effectiveness. Therefore, in order to support and immobilize the entire extremity, any splint generally needs to be used in combination with a secondary immobilization device. This need can vary from just securing the initially splinted area to another part of the body with a simple tie, to securing almost the full body to a longboard in order to prevent movement of the hip, pelvis and splinted leg when a traction splint has been applied. The most common adjuncts used to provide this secondary immobilization are ties or straps, an arm sling, a sling and swathe, a 4 to 6 inch wide rigid long splint, or a full standard longboard (often called a long spine board.)

Splints are used separately or in combination to produce a rigid external framework of exactly the correct size and shape for supporting and immobilizing the injured area, regardless of its shape or the angulation of the included joints. Splints often need to be secured together to provide additional framework to strengthen or maintain the position of the splints which are directly supporting the injured area and, in the case of rigid unformable splints, to accommodate any unusual angulation that may exist. Two splints which do not directly contact each other are often secured to the same injured area in order to either sandwich the area to provide more complete immobilization, or to serve separate needs. One example would be when one splint supports the injured area from below while the other extends further or in a different plane in order to secure the injured area to another area.

Regardless of the materials or parts the EMT uses in forming a splint, once it has been assembled and secured each of its longitudinal sections and angles must be rigid and fixed. Some splints are nonformable and can only be used in their pre-determined *rigid* form, whereas others are *formable* and can be easily adjusted into a wide variety of different angles and shapes before they are installed and made rigid in the shape into which the EMT has formed them.

All splints, regardless of size, adjustability, or other unique qualities, are primarily classified by whether or not they are intrinsically formable. Fixed-shape splints are defined as *rigid,* and those that can be adjusted to a variety of different shapes as *formable.* The most commonly used splints are:

Rigid (nonformable)

- Board splints (whether made of wood, plastic or metal).
- Inflatable splints (air splints).
- Traction splints (bipolar or unipolar).
- Longboards (long spine boards).
- Pre-formed specific area splints.
- "Quick" splints.

Formable

- Cardboard splints.
- Wire "ladder" splints.
- SAM splints.
- Vacuum splints.
- Malleable metal finger splints.
- Blanket rolls or pillows.

Although empty inflatable splints are flexible and can be curved or folded, when they are sufficiently inflated to be an effective splint they are rigid and unformable and, if inflated less, can only function as a pressure dressing but not a splint. Regardless of how the EMT may attempt to angle, curve or otherwise shape an inflatable splint, it will return to its predetermined straight long tubular shape (or long straight shape with a pre-set angled foot section).

Padding is required with any splint whose surface is hard, irregular, or not exactly conforming to the external shape of the area to which it is applied. Generally it is easier and better to separate the task of padding the surface of the splint from that of adding such additional padding as is needed to fill any voids between the splint and the limb. Some commercial single-use splints come with foam padding already attached to their "contact" areas. If padding is not pre-applied, the EMT can tape cravats or layers of gauze dressing to any surface that will contact the patient, or surround the splint with several layers of a towel. The thickness of the material that is used to pad the splint should be sufficient to serve as a shock absorber and to provide firm localized pressure on any protrusion, without interfering with the support and immobilization that the splint provides along its length.

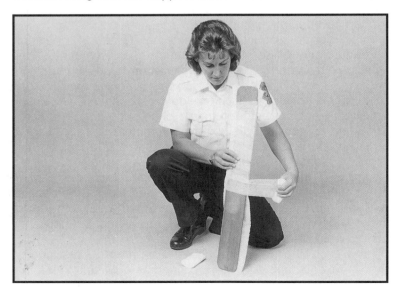

The padding should be kept from moving or "bunching up" by securing it to the splint. This is easily done by surrounding the padding and splint with tape or roller bandaging prior to placing the splint against the patient. The common custom of permanently padding board splints when they are placed on the ambulance promotes the communication of disease organisms from one patient to another. If a splint has been used with one patient, removal of the padding and its replacement before the splint is used again is recommended. This is not necessary with commercial splints in which the splinting material and padding are sealed in a fluid-impervious cover. Such splints should simply be sanitized following the manufacturer's directions after each use unless they are to be discarded.

Folded 4x4s or bulkier dressings should not be used to fill any remaining voids. These should be inserted once the splint has been applied but before it is fully secured to the limb.

Arm slings, slings-and-swathes, and shoulder binders, although serving to splint some injuries, are not considered splints and rather are defined as splinting adjuncts. The specific skills for using these and the splints most commonly used by EMTs will be demonstrated in the remaining part of this Section.

Pillows and blanket rolls are often essential adjuncts to provide additional support and immobilization when packaging the patient. Because it is so individual and generally obvious, specific demonstrations of their use for this purpose have not been included.

Checking the Distal Neurological and Circulatory Status

The EMT should obtain a baseline of the distal neurovascular status of each limb when checking the "MSCx4" in his initial assessment. Regardless of previous checks, the EMT *MUST* check the distal circulation *AFTER* a splint has been applied and the extremity has been positioned and secured for transport. When this involves securing an injured leg to the other leg, the distal circulation in both legs must be checked. A check of the distal sensory status should also be included.

It is highly recommended that prior to this point, the EMT check the distal circulation after each separate significant action involving the injured area. By checking the distal circulation after the initial alignment of the extremity, then after the splint has been completed, after any additional required positioning, and then after any additional ties have been added to secure the extremity, the EMT can identify when and probably what caused any compromise that may occur. If it is only re-checked after all of these steps have been completed, the EMT must back-track along each tie and step until the cause is determined if evidence of compromise is discovered. This may cause additional movement of the injury, discomfort, and delay that could have been avoided.

In most cases the EMT assisting you to position and support the injured area can continuously palpate a distal pulse, eliminating the need for multiple repeated checks. It is important that the circulation be checked at a point distal to any element added to the extremity. For example, if anything contacts the hand the fingertips as well as the radial pulse should be checked. Further, alert reliable patients should be directed to report any detectable sensory changes.

Regardless of the location of the injury, significant movement of an injured extremity by the patient should *NOT* be promoted by the EMT. Checking the motor ability should be limited to moving the fingers and toes, and when eliciting this the EMT should clearly direct the patient *NOT* to attempt further movement.

A Note About The Following Individual Skills

The steps for the application of a sling-and-swathe are presented first as these may be needed as an adjunct to any splint of the upper extremities. This is followed by the discussion of rigid board splints. First this details the technique for applying the board splint to the forearm and hand as an example, and then is expanded to a discussion of its use for a lower leg. Many of the techniques included, as well as some of the bandaging techniques demonstrated in Section 14, are essential to applying other types of splints. To avoid needless redundancy they are only demonstrated in detail in either the preceding Section or the demonstration of board splints, and are only indicated in summary in the discussions of other splints. The reader should be familiar with the Section on Bandaging, the Introduction to this Section, and the Demonstrations for board splints, as these are assumed in the discussions of the other splinting skills.

MAKING AND APPLYING AN ARM SLING AND SWATHE

An arm sling is used to support the arm (with the elbow flexed) across the anterior thorax in patients who will remain in an essentially standing or sitting position. The sling prevents inferior movement of the lower arm and, when a swathe is added around the upper arm, sling and torso, is an important adjunct to preventing movement of the shoulder and entire arm. When properly applied the arm sling provides even support along the full length of the lower arm from the elbow to approximately the middle of the proximal phalanges, preventing any of the weight of the arm distal to the elbow from being applied to the upper arm and shoulder. The sling also transfers the entire weight of the arm from the shoulder to the patient's neck.

Except for isolated shoulder injuries, use of a sling and swathe alone will not provide sufficiently rigid support or adequate immobilization to properly splint other musculoskeletal arm injuries. *Except when used exclusively to immobilize the shoulder, a sling-and-swathe should be used with a splint and NOT to replace it.*

Regardless of how well a splint boxes or surrounds the forearm to protect it, a simple loop formed from a cravat or other bandage should *NEVER* be used to support a splinted arm instead of a proper full sling. Such a loop, instead of evenly distributing support along the entire lower arm as does a proper sling, localizes it at one point. Further, a loop alone will not sufficiently restrict the arm from lateral movement.

The geometric terms used to identify the parts of a triangular bandage have been discussed in the preceding section. They are repeated here as this terminology is essential to the directions for forming an arm sling.

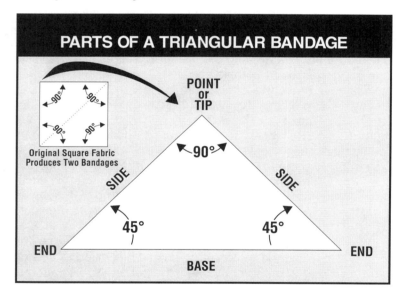

Because any arm sling or sling-and-swathe applied at the scene is often soiled in the field or becomes contaminated with blood or other body substances, they are routinely replaced at the hospital. Costly commercial arm slings or sling-and-swathe sets are rarely used in the field and, instead, are created with triangular bandages by the EMT.

1. Once any other needed treatments have been completed and any indicated splints have been applied, determine that it is unnecessary to place the injured arm in a straight extended position or to place the patient supine. If neither will be required, position the injured arm (or arm on the side of the injured shoulder) so it is across the anterior thorax with the wrist held just slightly higher than the elbow. Have the patient hold it in this position with his other hand.

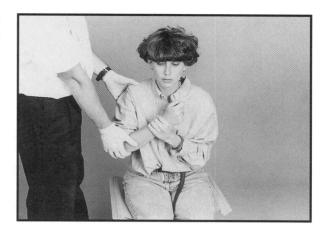

2. Remove a triangular bandage from its package and, after unfolding it, locate its base (the long side). While facing the patient, hold the bandage by one *end* so that the *base* is oriented vertically in front of the uninjured side of the patient and the *point* (or tip) is held extended beyond the elbow on the injured side. Then insert it between the patient's anterior torso and arm, placing the upper *end* just over the top of the shoulder on the uninjured side so that the *point* is near the elbow on the injured side.

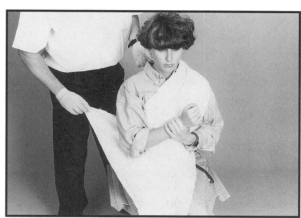

3. While continuing to hold the top *end* with one hand, reach down and bring the other *end* over the patient's arm and to the top of the shoulder on the injured side. Then, take up any slack, pass this end behind the patient's neck, and tie both *ends* together with a half-knot. After making any adjustments that may be needed in the arm's position, pull on both ends through the half-knot in opposite directions until the sling is snugly against the arm and neck. Be careful when making any adjustments to *NOT* jostle the arm or abrade the neck.

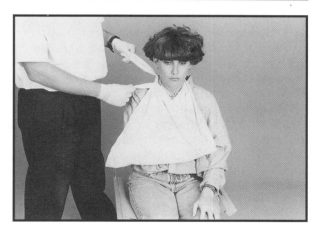

4. "Walk" the half-knot until it is against the lateral aspect of the neck and will *NOT* end up between the patient's back and the cot. Then pull both *ends* through the half-knot as needed to properly tighten the sling. You will have to draw one *end* further through the half-knot than the other, in order to properly tension the parts of the sling which lie under and over the arm and maintain the knot at the side of the neck. The sling should be tight enough to anticipate any stretching of the fabric, but not so tight as to elevate the upper arm or shoulder. When the sling has been properly adjusted, complete the knot to secure the ends together.

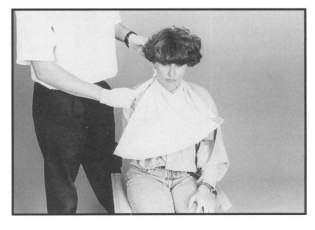

5. Once the *ends* have been tied together to form the sling around the arm and neck, its left-to-right positioning can be adjusted. Move the *base* of the triangular bandage (which now vertically surrounds the arm) to the desired position along the patient's hand. Then, while holding the arm from moving, carefully pull the *point* of the bandage laterally until it is sufficiently beyond the elbow to eliminate any vertical holds or horizontal slack in the sling.

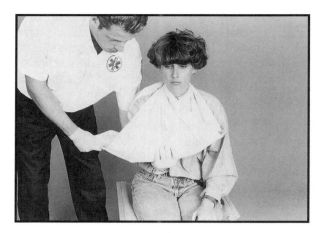

6. To complete the arm sling, fold the point over the elbow and distal upper arm, forming a pouch to prevent the arm from moving laterally out of the sling. Use safety pins (two are generally packaged with each commercial triangular bandage) to pin the *point* to the anterior sling so it is sufficiently medial and superior to the elbow so that the lateral edge of the bandage snugly surrounds the elbow and distal upper arm. The EMT should place a hand between the arm and outer fold of the sling when inserting any safety pin to protect the patient. Alternatively, a knot can be tied at the point to form it into a pouch.

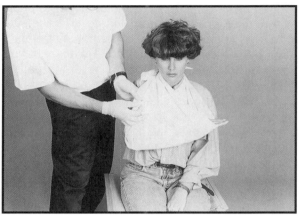

Adding a Swathe

Although the arm sling prevents the arm from moving in a caudad direction (inferior, when sitting or standing) and reduces lateral movement, it does not totally *prevent* the latter nor keep the forearm from being raised by the patient or "bounced" upwards within the sling. Also, since the sling is only secured to the trunk of the body where it passes posteriorly around the neck, the arm and sling are also not prevented from swinging away from the anterior thorax.

In order to prevent these movements, the arm and sling must be secured to the anterior thorax by the addition of one or more swathes (made from cravats, straps or roller bandages) which surround the torso, arm, and sling. This is most easily and rapidly achieved by carefully placing a single cravat swathe and, if properly placed, the need for more than one can usually be avoided.

Whenever an arm sling is used as an adjunct for immobilizing ANY injury proximal of the hand, since the treatment includes immobilization of the shoulder, a swathe must be used in addition to the sling. The inclusion of a swathe is only optional if the sling is used with injuries solely distal to the wrist, and even in such cases it is highly recommended. To add a swathe:

7. Remove a second triangular bandage from its package and unfold it until it is at its maximum cravat-form length. From the front of the patient, pass one end of the cravat through the armpit on the uninjured side, around the patient's back and around the upper arm and sling on the injured side until both ends of the cravat are approximately positioned and held near the patient's anterior midline.

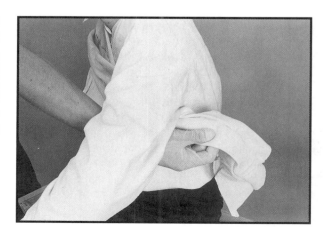

8. If the sling has been applied so the wrist is held slightly higher than the elbow as customary, position the swathe so it is approximately horizontal and at the correct height so it passes across the wrist and/or sling at the distal forearm and approximately the mid-shaft of the humerus. Tie the ends together with a half-knot positioned over approximately the center of the sling and, in order to assure that the completed swathe will *NOT* restrict the patient's ventilation, pull it tight *at peak inspiration* and then complete the knot.

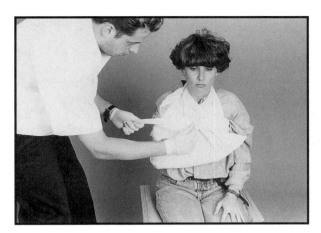

If the wrist lies at about the same height as the elbow in the sling, the swathe will have to be applied so it is higher on the injured side in order to surround both the lower arm and the mid-humerus. If the injuries dictated that the sling be applied so that the elbow is less flexed and the forearm lies inferior to the elbow, the use of two swathes placed on a severe angle is recommended. One swathe should be placed horizontally around the wrist/forearm and the torso, and a second horizontally around the mid-shaft of the humerus and torso. To ensure that neither is so tight as to inhibit the patient's ventilation, each should only be tightened when the patient is at peak inspiration.

9. After any indicated splints have been applied and the packaging of the arm with a sling-and-swathe has been completed, re-check the patient's ventilation to assure that neither these nor any other conditions have adversely affected it since the *Initial Systemic Examination.* Similarly, re-check the other vital signs for any changes. Lastly, recheck the MSCs in the arm to confirm that neither a splint, other ties, nor the sling-and-swathe have caused any distal neurovascular compromise.

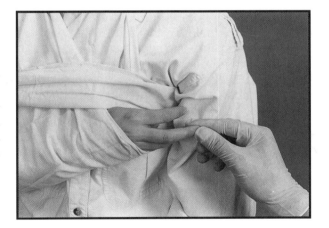

Making An Alternate Arm Sling

In some cases, the patient's shoulder or splinted arm is best packaged using an arm sling (or sling-and-swathe), but other injuries make transferring the weight of the arm across the clavicle on the injured side and around the neck undesirable. In these cases an alternate method for using a triangular bandage as an arm sling can be used which transfers the weight of the arm across the shoulder on the uninjured side and across the back. When completed, this alternate arm sling provides equal support with greater restriction of the arm's movement, and therefore may be preferred even when not required.

1. Orient and insert the triangular bandage between the arm and the torso so its upper *end* is held on the uninjured shoulder and its *point* extends lateral to the flexed elbow, as previously demonstrated. Adjust its left-to-right positioning until it is approximately correct. Hold the lower *end* in your other hand and bring it up across the patient's flexed arm so that the triangular bandage surrounds it in the normal manner. Then pass the *end* from anterior-to-posterior through the armpit on the injured side, as shown. Check that the arm is still in the exact position desired and adjust it if needed.

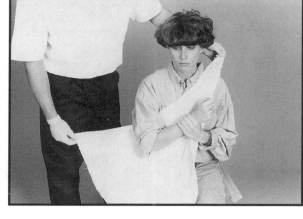

2. While maintaining your hold on the *end* which is over the shoulder on the uninjured side, move behind the patient. Then, while visualizing the sling, pull the second *end* (which you inserted through the armpit on the injured side) until you have taken all of the slack out of the sling.

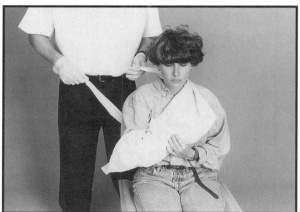

3. While maintaining sufficient pull on both of the ends to maintain the sling tightly against the arm, bring the end which passes through the armpit on the injured side diagonally across the patient's back to the opposite (uninjured side) shoulder and tie both ends together with a half-knot.

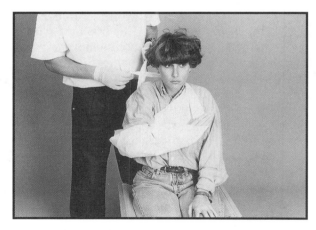

4. "Walk" the half-knot until it lies on the anterior thorax just inferior to the clavicle, and pull on each end respectively as needed to properly tighten each half of the sling. Then secure the sling by completing the knot and, after properly positioning the base on the hand and removing any horizontal folds or slack, folding and pinning (or tying) the point to form a pouch around the elbow. If required, add a swathe to provide additional immobilization of the arm and shoulder. Lastly, recheck the patient's ABCs and check the MSCs in the secured arm to make sure that neither the sling nor any splints or other ties have produced any distal neurovascular compromise.

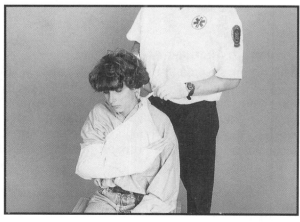

USING BOARD SPLINTS

Board splints are long rigid flat rectangles (usually with corners) which historically were made from thin strong wooden boards. Even though today they are available in a variety of plastics and lightweight metal alloys, they remain predominantly constructed from lightweight but strong basswood or (particularly longer sizes) thin plywood. Regardless of the material from which it is made, any flat rigid unformable rectangular splint is still called a "board splint." When wire splints are not bent into other shapes, or when cardboard splints are not cut or bent (except for folding up each side to provide sufficient rigidity along their length), these can be considered and used as board splints. However, the specific application of each varies from the general use of board splints and will be discussed separately later in this Section. Similarly the longboard, although by structure a giant board splint, must be used differently and is not defined as a board splint.

Although there is no standard for the length of board splints, they are generally between 3 and 4 inches wide. Two approximate lengths which are commercially available are found to be of general usefulness when splinting:

- About 15 inches long, for splinting limited areas only, such as the upper arm, the forearm-wrist-and-hand, or the lower leg.
- About 36 inches long, for splinting an entire extremity in a straight extended position.

While still available, 52 – 55 inch board splints serve no unique useful purpose. In the distant past, these were placed along one side of the body from the armpit to beyond the leg to immobilize the hip and full leg, or as part of a field-devised traction device. Today, the EMT can far better achieve full lower-body immobilization using the longboard, and traction for a femur using a commercial traction device.

Tongue blades are useful when individual fingers need to be splinted in a straight extended position, and should be included in any consideration of board splints.

The surface of a board splint which will contact the patient must be padded prior to use. As discussed in the introduction, this should be done when the splint is placed in service on the ambulance to avoid the delay it would cause if done in the field preceding the application of the splint. Padding both sides of the splint is recommended as this avoids the extra need of identifying and using a "correct" side against the limb. If these splints are to be re-used, all of the padding should be replaced after each use. Commercial board splints which include padding over the rigid surface in a sealed fluid-impervious cover are ideal. These save the EMT from this task and simply need to be sanitized if they are to be reused.

Board splints are generally best used when a firm flat rigid splint is needed. Splinting the lower arm/wrist/hand for an isolated wrist injury will serve as a good primary demonstration of the skill of using a board splint.

When you are ready to apply the splint:

1. Select a pre-padded board splint of the correct length (approximately 15 inches), and prepare the other materials you will need to fill any voids, apply and secure the splint, and secure the splinted arm. While another EMT supports the arm and hand, position the splint next to them so its length is approximately properly aligned, and insert it under the arm and hand until the arm is centered across its width.

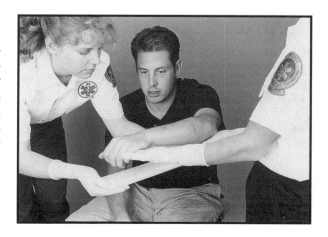

2. Carefully slide the splint in either a proximal or distal direction under the forearm to exactly where desired. If the hand is to be held in the position of function with the fingers over-lapping the end of the board, the location of the splint's distal end just beyond the joints of the fingers determines the longitudinal placement beyond the flexed elbow. If the hand will rest on the splint, the splint's proximal end is used as the guide and should be just beyond the outer margin of the flexed elbow.

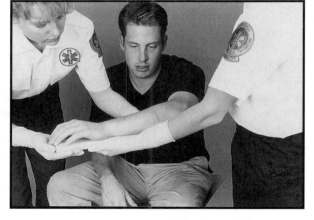

3. While the second EMT holds the splint in its proper place and supports the arm and splint, fill any voids between the arm and the splint with additional padding and insert a 2 to 3 inch wide roller bandage between the patient's hand and the splint. This should be placed under the distal palm and proximal end of the fingers so the hand and fingers are comfortably cupped over it, and so that the thumb lies on the splint at one end of the roll. If the *diameter* of the roll is too large when starting to insert it, some of the bandage should be unwound and cut-off so it does *NOT* cause unnecessary angulation of the wrist.

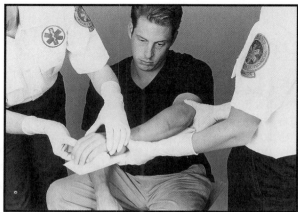

4. Once any additional padding has been added and the hand has been supported in the position of function, you are ready to secure the splint. After anchoring a 3 to 4 inch roller bandage around the hand, secure the splint to the arm with snug overlapping turns of the bandage working from the wrist towards the elbow.

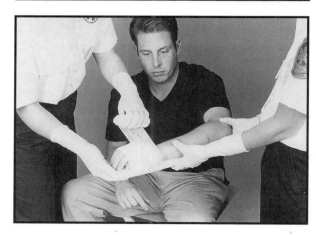

5. When just proximal of the wrist, passing the bandage diagonally across it and leaving a space before continuing to make overlapping winds up the arm will allow the EMT to later access the radial pulse. Although some EMTs prefer this, it is not mandated since the distal circulation can also be checked at the fingertips. Continue to apply the overlapping turns of the bandage until reaching the elbow.

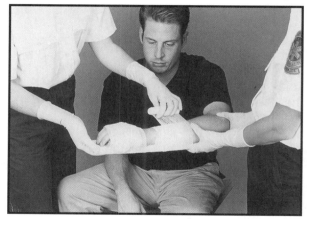

6. Do *NOT* cover or secure the distal ends of the fingers. Instead, use the remaining bandage to add additional turns around the splint and arm. When this has been completed, tape the end of the bandage to the layers covering the arm. Once the splint has been completed, quickly check the circulation distal to the splint (in this case at the fingertips).

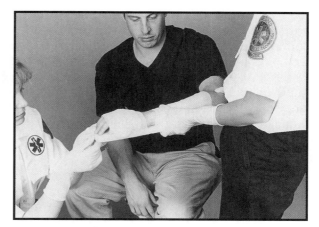

7. Once the injured area is supported and immobilized by the completed primary splint, the arm can be more safely repositioned and further secured. Place the forearm across the anterior chest and add a sling-and-swathe, or if indicated place the patient in the desired position on the cot and secure the splinted arm to the side of the torso. Finally, recheck the MSCs in the injured extremity.

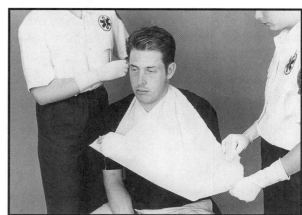

8. When a board splint (or other type) has been applied to support and immobilize an injury to a lower leg, similarly the entire limb should be further supported and immobilized to prevent any bending or rotation which could be reflected to the injury. This can be achieved by placing a long (approximately 36 inch) padded board splint on its long side between both legs so its proximal end is several inches beyond the groin, and then securing both legs together with cravat ties. To prevent any outward rotation of the injured foot, both feet should also be tied together.

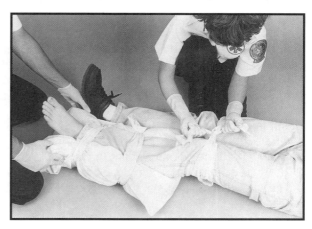

9. If even greater support of the primary splint and remaining extremity is desired (or if tying the legs together is precluded), this can be achieved by "sandwiching" the leg between long padded board splints placed along the medial and lateral side of the leg. The leg and splints are then secured together with cravat ties periodically spaced along its length. An additional cravat is placed around the foot and, after its ends are crossed, around the splint to secure the foot in its normal near-perpendicular position. Alternatively, cravats can be tied around the splint just proximal and just distal to the foot to support it.

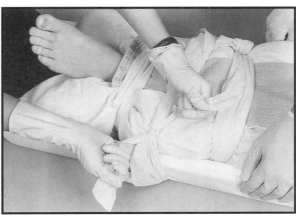

10. When the injury has dictated splinting the leg with the knee partially flexed using a formable splint, board splints are often useful adjuncts. A long board splint can be inserted under the leg and splint and, when secured with tape or ties to the primary splint's ends (or angles touching the ground), will form the framework into a strong triangular shape and provide a rigid platform.

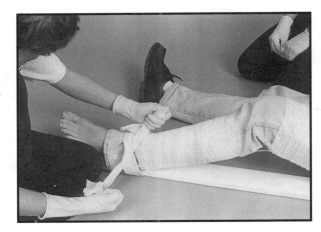

11. If even greater support is desired, the splint and leg can be sandwiched between two long padded board splints placed at the lateral sides of the leg (one medial, between the legs, and one against the lateral side), as previously described. These can be secured so their narrow edges rest on the ground to form a base to deter rotation of the leg. Alternatively, they can be placed more anteriorly (centered on the sides of the leg) and, if both legs are secured to them, will produce a sufficiently wide posterior base to prevent rotation. As well, these immobilize the entire leg and prevent any bending when the patient is moved to the cot or backboard.

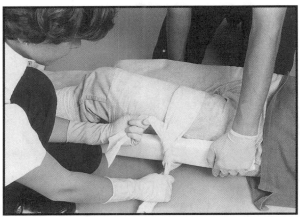

The injured and adjacent areas *MUST* be supported by a rigid splint (or when bent, rigid framework) which lies directly beneath them. Board splints secured on both lateral sides to sandwich the limb, although useful in immobilizing the entire extremity, do *NOT* in themselves generally provide sufficient support underlying the injury. Such application should only be used as an adjunct with a primary splint, and *NOT* to replace it.

It is often easier to apply these additional splints after the primary splint has been installed and secured, however their use must be anticipated. In some cases, the EMT will find it easier to only manually hold the primary splint in place while these are added, and to then secure all of the splints to the injured area as a single package. Then, after the injured area has been secured, the more proximal and distal parts of the longboard splints and the extremity should be secured.

USING CARDBOARD SPLINTS

Cardboard splints, when initially introduced, were made of simple corrugated cardboard similar to that used in making boxes. Today, these are generally made of either fluid-impervious plastic-impregnated corrugated cardboard or thin corrugated sheets of plastic. Even if made of plastic, such thin corrugated splints are defined as cardboard splints. Cardboard splints are purchased and stored as long flat rectangles with rounded corners. There is a score (a pressed indentation) which runs the full length of the splint, several inches from each long edge of the splint. Prior to use, the splint must be bent at these scores so that the area outside of each forms a perpendicular side, and the splint has a box-like shape with open ends. Most commercial cardboard splints also come with high density foam padding pre-attached to the middle section (or base) of the splint so that it lies between its two sides.

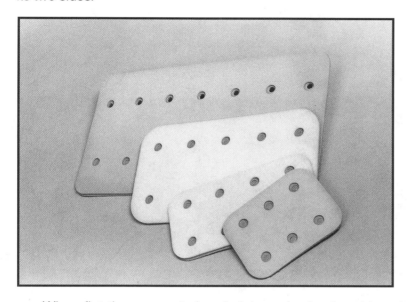

When flat the corrugated material can be bent and is not sufficiently strong to be used as a board splint (unless two or three are taped together). However, once both sides of the splint have been bent and are perpendicular to the base, the splint becomes rigid and will not bend along its length as long as its box-like form is maintained.

Commercial cardboard splints come in a variety of lengths (approximately 12, 18, 24, and 36 inches). Because these can be easily cut to any desired length, it is unnecessary and impractical to carry any but the longest ones in the ambulance. This allows the EMT to use each cardboard splint for either the entire arm or leg, or when a shorter splint is needed to cut the splint at the desired length. Usually the remaining portion will be of sufficient length that it can be used the next time a short splint is needed. Some brands also offer special pre-cut splints for splinting the lower leg. These have interlocking tabs and additional scores with which to form one end perpendicular to the rest of the splint in order to support the foot. These are also unnecessary and their limited specialized use denies the essential advantage of the cardboard splint, namely that *one size can be universally used for any extremity injury, when properly cut or shaped.* When the EMT is experienced in their use, cardboard splints can be cut and formed into any needed shape and, because they can be easily secured to each other, can be made into any splinting framework or length required. Because of their universality, low cost, and ease of application, carrying a half-dozen or more 36 inch long cardboard splints on each ambulance is highly recommended, regardless of whether these are the first choice of the EMTs or act as a universal back-up for any splinting need that can not be otherwise met. Because of their low cost, cardboard splints are disposable—therefore avoiding any delay at the hospital to retrieve them or the losses that are commonly associated with more costly splints.

The splint should be measured, cut and shaped prior to being installed, and should NEVER be cut or initially bent while in contact with any part of the patient, even at an uninjured area. To avoid the risk of jostling an injured area or unnecessary movement of an injured extremity, the splint can usually be properly measured and formed using the extremity on the injured side as a guide.

Whether made of corrugated cardboard or plastic, these splints can be easily cut with "paramedic" scissors (or even sharp bandage scissors). After the splint has been cut, the EMT should round the ends to ensure that they do not injure the patient.

Whenever the splints are to be bent they should be scored along the bend with the dull tip of the scissors prior to bending, to ensure that a straight true bend will occur exactly where desired. The score should be made on the side of the splint towards which it will be bent. A second cardboard splint with one side folded over onto the middle section can be used as a "straight edge" to guide the EMT when scoring the splint. Care must be taken to avoid cutting the outer layer of the cardboard as this will weaken the structural integrity of the splint at the bend. To assure a straight bend, it is easiest to place the score at the straight edge of a rigid surface and bend the splint over this edge.

Rather than repeating the detailed steps which are general to all splinting and have been demonstrated in the preceding discussion of board splints, the following is limited to the unique skills inherent in a variety of different applications of a cardboard splint.

1. When a cardboard splint is to be used simply as a rigid straight splint, it should first be measured and cut to the exact length required to support the injured and necessary adjacent areas. Once the correct length has been confirmed and any sharp tips have been rounded, the sides should be folded along the scores so that they are perpendicular to the central base of the splint. It is easier to insert the splint under the extremity and to add any additional padding needed with one side of the splint flat and on the same plane as the base of the splint.

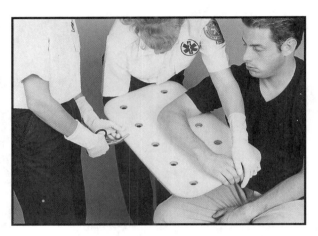

2. Regardless, it should be bent and then folded back so that it does not resist being folded (which is usual if a score has not been previously bent) once it has been placed. Carefully slide the splint to the exact position desired along the length of the extremity so the limb is centered along its width. Add the additional padding needed to fill any voids between the splint and the extremity, or to properly position the hand, and fold up the side which was lowered to provide access. Also fill any significant voids which may remain between the extremity and the sides of the splint. Then secure the splint in the usual manner with a gauze roller bandage or cravat ties.

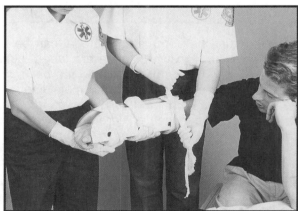

3. If the patient is a child or is extremely thin so that the splint is excessively wide and leaves vast space between the extremity and the bent-up sides of the splint, the splint should be modified to avoid this prior to its installation. Adding an additional score — along the entire length of the splint at each side and about one inch from the longitudinal center line of the splint — will allow the EMT to form its width into a narrower multiply-angled (rather than perpendicular box-like) shape. This will cause the splint to conform to the curvature of the limb and without the need for the repeated measurements.

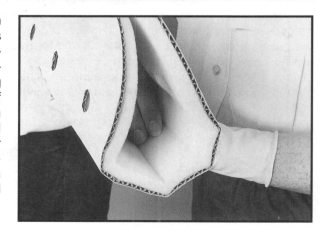

4. Once these two additional scores have been added, the EMT should bend the splint until it is formed into a "U"-like shape. In some cases, the top of each side will have to be cut-off to reduce the area of the limb surrounded by the splint to no greater than is usual or desired. Once the splint is of the proper size and shape it can be placed under the injured extremity and properly secured to it.

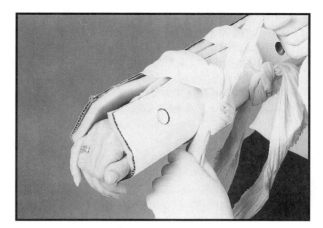

5. When the cardboard splint must include an angle to accommodate the arm being splinted with the elbow flexed, the splint should be measured and cut so it is the correct length to include the upper arm, lower arm and as much of the hand as desired. Then position the splint so its distal end is exactly where desired and mark the point just beyond the outer margin of the elbow with a small cut in the side of the splint.

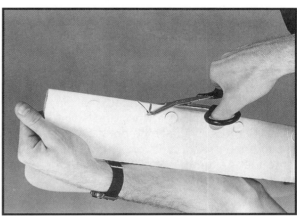

6. Using another splint as a straight-edge, score the padded side (the one the sides will be bent towards) from one edge to the other across the width on a line perpendicular to the long edge of the splint at the point previously marked. Then fold the splint at this score and fold the sides in until perpendicular as shown. The cut sides of the splint from one side of the score should insert into those from the other side, preventing the splint from being bent beyond 90 degrees. If a lesser angle is desired between the upper arm and forearm the ends of each of the sides must be cut on an angle to allow them to integrate and the splint to be so formed.

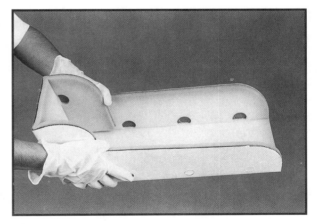

7. Once the splint has been properly bent and formed to the correct angle for the elbow, place tape strips across the place where the sides overlap on the inside of the splint and over their outside junctions, on both the left and right sides of the splint. Then, wind several turns of one inch tape diagonally across the outside of the integrated sides of the splint, under its lower end, up diagonally across the outside of the other integrated sides and around its back to the initial point. This forms a tight loop diagonally across the outside of the elbow section, securing the angle formed from being enlarged.

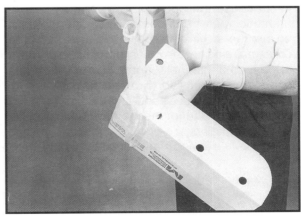

8. If the proximal end of the splint will extend cephalad to the armpit when the splint is applied, cut away a portion of its medial perpendicular side to accommodate this. Apply the completed splint to the arm, add any additional padding needed, and secure it with conforming gauze or cravats. Add a sling-and-swathe and check the distal MSCs in the immobilized arm.

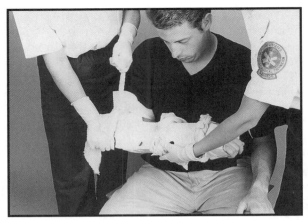

9. When using a cardboard splint to immobilize the lower leg, it should be measured and cut so that it is 10 to 12 inches longer than the length desired from its proximal end to the heel. Score the splint, and bend and score this extra 10 to 12 inches perpendicular to the rest of the splint (as previously described), to form a support for the foot. Even when the splint is being used to immobilize only the ankle or foot, making it long enough so that its proximal end is just distal to the groin rather than just distal to the knee is recommended.

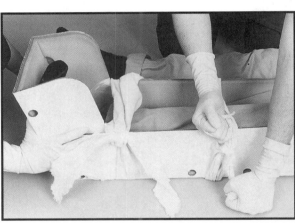

10. If the leg must be immobilized with the knee elevated and flexed, the cardboard splint must be of sufficient length so that when the perpendicular foot support has been formed and the splint bent to the desired angle at the knee, both the heel and proximal part of the splint will rest on the ground. Score the *underside* of the splint where the knee bend will occur and the *upper* side for the bend at the heel. Cut the sides at each and, after making the proper bends, complete the distal boxed-foot support.

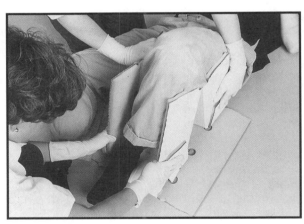

11. Because the bent-up sides of the splint do not interlock at the knee, this angle of the splint can not be sufficiently immobilized with tape. While maintaining the knee part of the splint at the desired angle, hold it on top of a second flat cardboard splint (so that the latter extends beyond it at each end) and mark the point where the proximal end and heel rest on the underlying splint with small cuts.

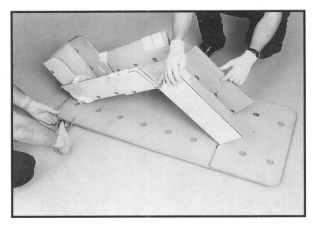

12. After placing the primary splint aside, remove any unnecessary excess in the second splint's length by cutting-off each end at a point *approximately six inches beyond* each of the marks. Score across the width of the splint at each of the marks, and cut across both of the sides of the score. Next cut along the factory-made scores (used to bend up each side) until you reach the cut made across the sides, in order to remove the sides and leave only flat six-inch long flat tabs beyond where the ends of the primary splint will lie and the sides have been bent up.

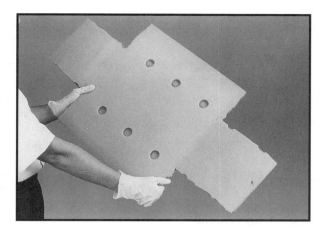

13. Bend each side and the tab at each end so they are approximately perpendicular to the surface of the splint, and insert the primary splint into the "box" that has been formed. Bend the proximal tab further and tape it flat over the upper surface of the "thigh" part of the splint, and tape the distal tab flat against the outside of the foot support with one or two additional layers of tape around it and the heel section of the splint. Then tape the sides of the base splint firmly against the sides of the angled upper one.

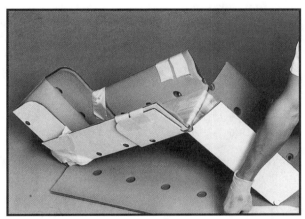

14. The EMT can complete this actually simple construction in two to three minutes. Once completed, the "triangular" splint is inserted under the leg, and the leg and foot are secured to it with roller bandage or a number of cravat ties. If the EMT also needs to immobilize the hip (the joint proximal to the knee) this can be achieved by adding a long board splint secured against the lateral side of the splint and the pelvis and upper torso, or by securing the patient and splint to a longboard.

When using a cardboard splint, whether simply as a straight rigid splint or formed into a specially shaped construction, its strength and rigidity are dependent upon the maintenance of the near perpendicular position and integrity of its sides. *The sides of a cardboard splint should NEVER be cut except where the splint is to be bent.* Whenever the splint is bent inward (such as for the elbow or foot), taping the overlapping sides to each other only keeps the sides perpendicular and will *NOT* adequately maintain the bent angle of the splint. The angle of the splint must be maintained by diagonally encircling the formed "box" with layers of adhesive tape as previously shown. Whenever the splint must be bent outward (such as for a flexed knee) the angle must be secured by the addition of a base, or splints along each side, to form a triangle.

The sides of the splint are automatically maintained in their bent upright position when the splint is secured to the limb with roller gauze or cravats and they do not interfere with other ties when these surround both the splint and the limb. However, because of their elevation above the flat surface of the splint (and the fact that they should not be cut except at a bend) the sides make it difficult to secure the parts together with tape, since tape can not simply be wound around the empty splint.

Many EMTs who use cardboard splints daily can cut a variety of tabs, notches and slots in them to produce a variety of self-locking connections similar to those commonly used by box manufacturers. However, this is beyond the scope of those who use them less frequently. One such technique is universally useful in making taped connections or securing tape across the width of the splint in spite of the elevation of the sides.

Mark where the tape is needed across the splint's width. Fold the side so it lies flat on the surface of the splint and, from a point about a half-inch beyond this mark, make an angled cut in the folded edge towards it which ends no more than about 1/4 inch from the outside edge. Then from about a half-inch on the other side make a second such cut towards where the first ended so that a one inch wide quarter-inch triangular section is cut out of the folded edge of the splint. Then repeat this on the opposite side of the splint. When the sides of the splint are returned to their perpendicular position, a one inch wide shallow diamond-shaped slot will have been easily removed at the bend on each side.

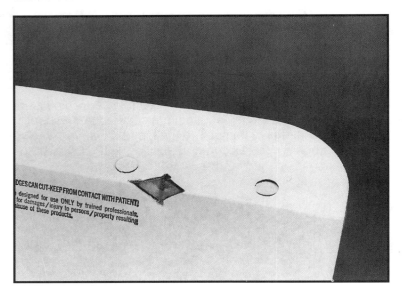

This slot allows for one inch tape (or a gauze tie) to be placed across the width of the splint where needed without any loss in the integrity of the sides or effect on their upright position. These notches are also useful where tape or a narrow tie will surround the splint, and must be prevented from inadvertently moving along the splint's length.

This method can be used instead of the tongue-like folded tabs previously described, or to provide for more secure taping of them.

USING CONFORMING COMMERCIAL SPLINTS

Two types of splints which conform around the extremity are also widely used in the field. Both of these when applied are formed into a semi-circular or "U"-like shape across their width and surround the sides as well as the underside of the injured area.

One type, such as the Prosplint, FracPac, or Add-A-Splint, is made of a fluid impervious sleeve which contains a number of separate narrow rigid stays (slats) which run the full length of the splint and are periodically spaced across its width. These also have internal padding between the sleeve and the stays, and Velcro fasteners along each long side.

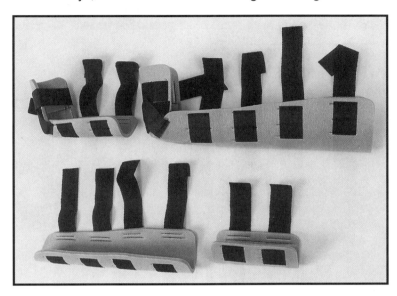

These are generally X-Ray translucent and each individual splint is designed for a specific task for either the upper or lower extremities or, in some cases, for all four. These are generally carried in a packaged kit which contains each splint that might be needed for any given area of each extremity. Some brands remain rigid along their length—whether flat or conforming around the underside and sides of the limb. Some are only longitudinally rigid when maintained in a semi-circular shape across their width.

The SAM splint, although it surrounds the underside and sides of the extremity when applied, is a totally different type of conforming splint. Unlike the stayed type, it is universal, and can be shaped to be straight or angled to meet any basic splinting need. This malleable material has no intrinsic rigidity and therefore comes in 36 inch lengths which are packaged and easily stored as 4½ inch wide rolls. The splint molds easily, is X-Ray translucent and contains padding between its core material and fluid impervious outer shell. Like cardboard splints, the SAM splint is not sufficiently rigid to be used when relatively flat, and is dependent upon the upward bending of its outer edges (forming it into a semi-circle or "U" across its width) to make it rigid along its length. When forming and applying the splint it is essential that a sufficient portion of each side is bent upwards, or the splint may undesirably bend along its length. The formed SAM splint is generally best attached to the injured area with conforming roller gauze.

The different specific designs and materials used in each brand and type of conforming splint make it impossible to provide a generic sequence of steps that can be meaningfully or safely used with every one. The EMT should be familiar with the general guidelines for splinting contained in this Section and follow the manufacturer's directions for the actual application of these splints in keeping with the general guidelines.

USING WIRE LADDER SPLINTS

Wire ladder splints are made from heavy gauge wire rods formed into a flat rectangular frame with evenly spaced wire "rings" welded across its width. Wire splints are relatively strong and require significant force by the EMT to bend them. Their surface can be bent at any angle and, unlike cardboard splints, any curve that is desired. The ability to form curved areas is an especially useful attribute, making these particularly applicable with silver-fork or other fractures which include a marked deformity. They are sufficiently rigid that they can be used as straight flat splints, yet they will remain in any other shape to which they have been bent. Only if used to support the entire leg with the knee flexed is a second base splint needed to maintain the angle (at the knee), due to the significant weight produced against it by the elevated mid-leg.

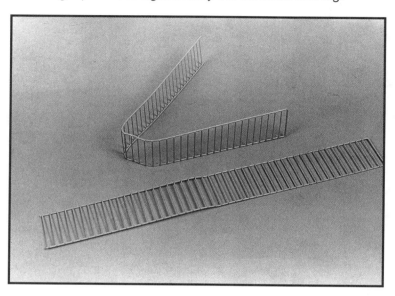

Because of the rigidity provided by the multiple cross pieces, it is *almost* impossible to bend their width from its flat plane. Shaping is essentially limited to angles or curves along the splint's length. These, although requiring force, can be made relatively easily since they only include bending the two wire rods which form the outer edges of the splint. Due to the multiple equally-spaced cross pieces, two or more wire splints can be strongly secured together with adhesive tape wound around the splint and additional tape securing one or more of the cross pieces of one to the cross pieces of the other.

Wire splints vary in their exact dimensions from one manufacturer to the other, but generally are about 4 inches wide and 31 inches long. Because they can be so easily and rapidly secured together, the EMT can readily make a splint of any greater length that is desired. When a splint is desired which is shorter than the length of the wire splint, any excess is simply folded under or, in some cases, can be molded so it is returned over the distal end of the extremity to provide an additional protective top layer.

Wire ladder splints should *NOT* be pre-padded, as this can interfere with shaping or, when necessary, securing several together. Once the wire splint has been formed to the proper size and shape, padding must be secured to any of its surfaces that will lie against the patient. This is often best done by placing a small folded towel over the splint's surface and securing it in-place with tape. *Whenever a wire ladder splint is used, the EMT must be sure that the prong-like ends of the outer frame which extend from one end of the splint* are positioned or bent away from the patient so they can not cause further injury.

When using a wire ladder splint, the EMT will need to follow the general principles and use many of the skills for applying and securing any splint that have been previously discussed. In order to avoid needless repetition, the following demonstrations are limited to items which are unique to the use of wire ladder splints.

Measuring and making all of the bends along the splint at one time often results in the need to adjust and re-bend some of them. After determining where the proximal end of the splint is to be located, measure and make the necessary bends at one location at a time, working from the proximal to the distal end of the splint, to assure that it is properly sized and formed. Forming the splint to immobilize an arm will serve as a useful demonstration of many of the techniques used with wire splints.

1.	Whenever a wire ladder splint is used, it should be oriented so that the end where the frame has rounded corners is its proximal end and the end at which the wire edges protrude (as prongs) is distal. Determine whether the arm is to be immobilized in a straight extended position or across the anterior thorax with the elbow bent, and where its proximal end should be located. If only a simple straight splint is needed (because the arm will be extended or the proximal end of the splint will be distal to the elbow) measure the length of wire ladder needed and mark the point beyond the palm where the splint should end. Bend the splint downward over a hard edge at the marked point.

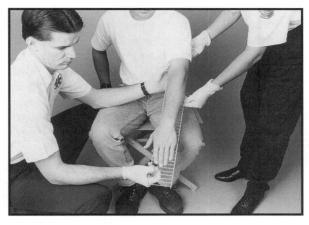

2.	Remove the splint from the edge over which it was being bent, and continue to bend the excess distal length towards the splint's underside until it lies totally against it and is out of the way. Secure the bent-under portion to the underside of the splint with tape, and secure padding along the top surface of the splint. Position the splint and maintain the hand in the position of function as with any rigid flat splint, and secure it to the arm with roller gauze or cravats.

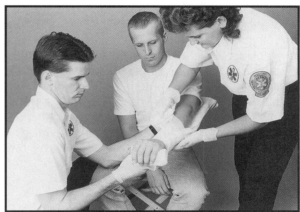

3.	If the arm is to be immobilized across the anterior thorax with the elbow flexed, measure and mark the location at the outside of the elbow where the splint must be bent. Bend the splint at that point over a rigid edge until its proximal end is approximately at the desired angle. Finite adjustments are best done after the rest of the splint has been properly formed.

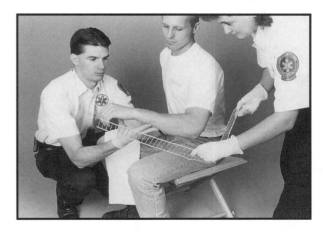

4.	Mark the location of the cupped hand and, at a point which will lie just distal to the proximal palm, bend the splint upwards to an approximately 45 degree angle in order to provide the necessary elevation from which the semi-circle to support the hand in the position of function can be bent. Whenever a curve is to be shaped, the EMT must make small bends in the wire rods between successive cross pieces to form the sides of the splint until the approximately correct curvature has been formed.

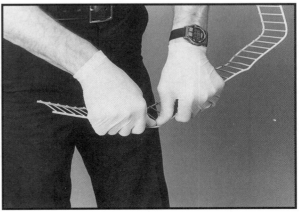

5.   Make sufficiently downward bends between the cross pieces along the length required to support the hand, until the elevated semi-circle needed to support the palm and fingers in the position of function has been formed. Then, using another splint as a guide, mark the point where a straight line along the forearm would intersect the curve. Bend the remaining distal end of the splint inward until it lies directly against the underside of the forearm section and secure them together with tape around several overlying cross pieces.

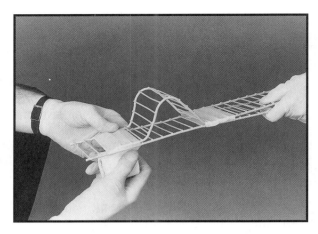

6.   When forming the splint for use under the straight extended leg, the near-perpendicular foot support can be properly located and bent at the splint's distal end by use of the preceding techniques. Similar to when forming an arm splint, any excessive length that remains at the distal end (beyond the tips of the toes), should be bent back and secured along the underside of the foot and lower leg parts of the splint or, if desired, formed into a "cage" which will be over the foot and on top of the leg.

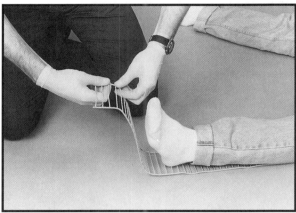

7.   Because wire ladder splints are very rigid and easy to connect, making a framework to support the leg with the knee flexed and elevated is very simple. Make a 45 degree upward bend about 6 inches from the proximal end of the splint. Using the techniques described earlier, measure and make the downward bend required for the knee at the correct point so the proximal 6 inch end of the splint lies on the ground. At the correct distance from it, bend up the distal end to form the perpendicular foot support. Bend the distal six inches of a second ladder splint up to about a 45 degree angle.

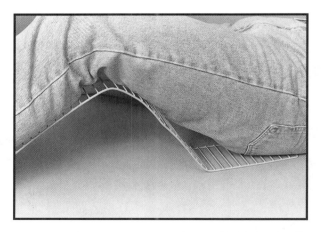

8.   Lay the primary splint on top of the second base part so that its heel bend is positioned against the 45 degree bend — elevating the distal end of the base splint. Bend the distal end of the base up further as needed to place it along the underside of the foot section of the primary splint. Secure the overlying cross sections of both splints together at the heel, further up the foot section, and on at least two cross sections at the flat proximal end of the primary splint. *Do NOT bend over the proximal end of the base splint.*

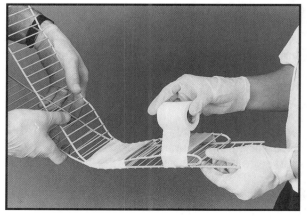

9. Should a comminuted bone fragment or other object protrude from an injury or if a displacement results in a marked and tender deformity, a second wire ladder splint with a semi-circular elevation bent into it can be placed over the area to protect it as shown. A second splint can be formed and similarly used over an impaled object, to attach and support its protruding end.

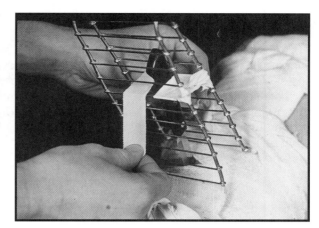

USING AN INFLATABLE AIR SPLINT

Air splints are dual-walled air-proof plastic sleeves which contain a closeable stem and valve to allow them to be inflated by mouth. Although they are flexible when empty to facilitate storage and installation, when inflated they only assume a completely straight (or straight with a perpendicular foot section) shape. When applied, an air splint must always be inflated enough to make it fully rigid. Although the amount of air needed to make it rigid varies and allows the splint to adjust to the varying girths of the extremity being splinted, the splint's inflated shape can *NOT* be varied. *An air splint can only be used on an area which is aligned and conforms to the inflated straight (or straight with its foot perpendicular) shape of the splint's design.* If any curvature or angle which is not designed into the splint is present, it will be straightened when the splint is inflated. Although not formable, the adjustable girth of most inflatable splints allows each to be used for several different applications. Air splints are usually purchased and stored in sets which include at least one splint each for the:

- Adult hand/wrist or child half-arm
- Adult half-arm or child full arm
- Adult full arm or child leg (not including foot)
- Adult foot/ankle or child half-leg
- Adult half-leg or child full leg
- Adult full leg

Most brands include a zipper which, although not producing complete separation along the tube's length, allows its proximal end and most of its length to be opened when applying the splint. Although rarely found in the field, brands which allow complete separation of the zipper-halves are recommended when purchasing air splints. Brands in which the foot end is fully closed should *NOT* be used, as these obstruct the EMT from the required checking of distal circulation after the splint has been installed.

Air splints are both visually and radiologically transparent (except where the zipper lies). Because they provide firm external pneumatic pressure totally around the length of the limb, air splints are extremely useful for providing direct pressure to control bleeding from open fractures or other sources of significant underlying external bleeding. However, this external circumferential pressure can more easily inadvertently tourniquet the underlying and distal circulation, requiring even more initial care and frequent checking of distal circulation than other types of splints.

If air splints are stored or exposed to extremely cold temperatures for any extended period prior to use, the plastic material may become brittle and break when unfolded. Exposure to extreme heat or direct sunlight for an extended period after the splint has been inflated can cause expansion of the air in the splint and cause it to tighten around the extremity. Use of air splints in either extremely cold or extremely hot environments is *NOT* recommended.

After each use the splint should be carefully washed and sanitized. Particular care must be given to cleaning the valve stem to make sure that any body substances have been removed and the valve has been cleaned with an antiseptic solution before it is stored or contacted by the EMT's mouth. Some observers feel that the need for oral inflation presents an undue risk of body fluid contact and potential disease communication.

When ready to apply an air splint, make sure that the limb is aligned and straight—in the position that it will be in once the splint is inflated. *Never let the inflation of the splint cause the straightening or alignment of the injured area.* Before applying the splint carefully remove any debris or other foreign matter from the surface of the area that will be contained within the splint. Inflatable splints should *NEVER* be used when a protruding bone end or impaled object will lie beneath the splint.

1. Determine the position in which the extremity is to be splinted and select the appropriate air splint for the region to be splinted. Unfold it and open the zipper fully. Then, place the splint so the appropriate area is inserted in the splint. When using a straight air splint for the arm, it is often most easily applied by first drawing the open splint backward up the EMT's arm (with its distal end at the proximal end of the EMT's arm, etc.) and then, while grasping the patient's hand, sliding it onto the patient's arm. *Never cover the patient's fingertips with the splint.*

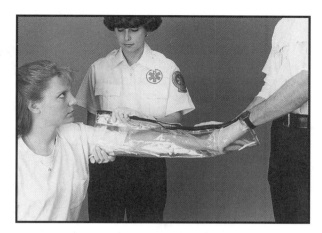

2. Position the splint carefully. Place a gauze dressing over any open wounds. Once the splint is properly located, close the zipper being careful not to "catch" the patient's skin in it. Wipe the valve and stem with an antiseptic wipe and open the valve. Check that the closed splint is still properly located and, by mouth, inflate the splint until it is sufficiently rigid. While holding your tongue over the open end of the valve, turn it (usually clockwise) to close it. This method must be used to close the valve without losing air, since most air splints do not contain a one-way valve.

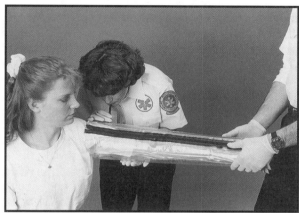

3. Gently squeeze the splint to check that it is neither under-inflated and too pliable, nor over-inflated and too tight. Add or bleed off air as needed to obtain the correct level of inflation. Once completed, check the distal MSCs in the splinted extremity and secure it for transport. Periodically squeeze the splint to make sure that air is *NOT* leaking from it.

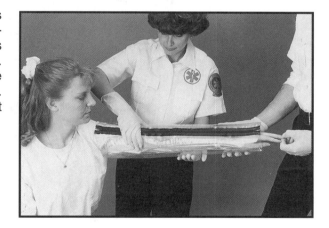

USING VACUUM SPLINTS

Vacuum splints are generally thin flat rectangular bags filled with thousands of small round or multi-faceted plastic beads. The splint's outer covers are sealed and air-proof (also fluid impervious). Somewhere on the splint's outer surface there is one or more valve stem(s) to allow the connection of a vacuum pump to evacuate air from within the splint. When the splint contains air as well as the beads, the plastic beads can move freely against each other and the splint can be formed into any needed shape. When the air is evacuated from the splint with the hand pump, the beads are tightly pressed against each other and the splint becomes rigid in the exact shape to which it has been formed around the extremity or body.

Because a vacuum splint can be formed into a limitless number of exact shapes, and when the air is evacuated from it will become rigid and inflexibly locked throughout, the same rectangularly shaped splint can be used to splint any area of either the upper or lower extremities in any position desired. These characteristics make a vacuum splint the easiest and often most effective method for splinting any injury which must be maintained in an unusually angulated, curved, or even deformed shape or position. Kits generally contain splints of different rectangular sizes rather than of different shapes. Most vacuum splints are X-Ray translucent and include Velcro tabs to assist in holding the splint against the limb until the air has been evacuated from the splint.

When purchasing vacuum splints, particular attention should be paid to the valve system and hand-pump. The pumps usually only draw air out of the splint as their handle is pulled upward from the pump body. The preferred models include one-way valves so that the splint can be continuously evacuated with multiple up-and-down strokes of the pump handle, and once the vacuum has been achieved the valve can easily be locked closed and the pump removed. In less desirable models, if the plunger is pulled out and pushed back into the pump chamber the air drawn out of the splint will be reintroduced into the splint. This requires that the valve be closed, the pump removed, the pump handle reset, the pump re-attached and the valve re-opened if (as is common) more than one stroke of the pump is required to produce the necessary vacuum in the splint. Because the vacuum tends to hold the inner rubber seal firmly against the opening in the valve stem, many models include a plastic tab that is needed to pry these up when air must be re-introduced into the splint to release it. Models which allow this by simply twisting the valve cap are easier to release.

When the valve of any splint has been held open and ambient air has freely entered the splint, the splint will be almost completely flaccid and limp. If the splint is applied when limp, it will *NOT* hold the varied contours and shapes that the EMT forms in it as he shapes it from one end to the other. When air is evacuated from the splint it becomes progressively firmer until finally a sufficient vacuum has been produced to lock the beads against each other and make the splint rigid. With experience, the EMT can evacuate just enough air prior to applying the splint to make it sufficiently firm to maintain the contours and shapes he forms as he works along the splint's length, but not be so firm as to hinder its being easily formed or cause it to be levered against the limb as it is formed.

When the air is being fully evacuated from the splint, the internal diameter of the curves to which the splint has been formed will become slightly reduced. Because of the slight shrinkage (inherent in all vacuum splints), the splint should not initially be shaped too tightly around the circumference of the limb. Some instructors advocate forming the splint around the limb into an *almost* closed "C"-like shape rather than overlapping its edges. This is recommended so that the lower layer of the overlapping edges is not inadvertently pushed too tightly against the top of the limb, and the slight opening helps to keep the splint from too tightly encircling the limb when the air is removed.

As well as the nature of the injury and the position in which the extremity is to be splinted, the EMT should include consideration of which hospital the patient will be transported to in determining whether a vacuum or different type of splint should be used. When the destination hospital is distant or not one common for his service, the EMT is wise to select an inexpensive or potentially disposable splint instead of a relatively expensive vacuum splint. Regardless of which splint is used, the EMT should neither press the hospital staff to precipitously remove the splint nor wait for any significant period for its return — needlessly prolonging the time that the ambulance remains out of service at the hospital.

Due to the vast difference in their capability and use, vacuum splints should *NOT* be confused with, mis-labeled, or called "air splints."

When you are ready to apply a vacuum splint, look at the different ones available to you and make sure that you have the pump and that it contains the necessary connection (usually a rubber tube) to mate with the valve stem of the splint. You should be fully familiar with the requirements for using that model's pump and the splint's valve stem from prior practice with the equipment. Remove any debris or other significant particulate matter from the surface of the skin which will lie within any part of the splint. Then:

1. Determine the position in which the extremity is to be splinted and select the appropriate splint from the kit. Make sure that the splint's valve is open and, with it facing up, lay the splint on a flat area which is clear of stones or other protrusions. Run your flattened hand firmly back and forth over the splint's top surface until you can feel that the plastic beads are approximately evenly distributed throughout the splint.

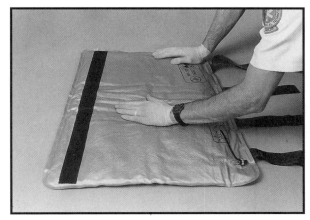

2. In the manner specific to that model, attach the pump to the valve stem of the splint and draw some of the air out of the splint while repeatedly bending a corner of the splint up and down. When you have evacuated enough air the splint will be sufficiently firm that the sides will not collapse or fall as the splint is shaped, but not so firm that they can not be easily shaped. As well as adjusting the splint's firmness for easy application, this tests that the pump is functioning properly before the splint is applied to the patient.

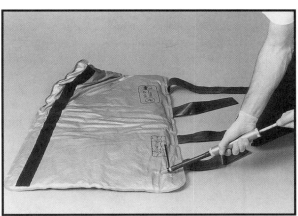

3. Check that the extremity is held in the exact position in which you want to splint it. Bend the sides of the splint up so that it approximates a "U"-like shape. With the proximal end of the splint properly located, place the splint under the extremity and bring it up until it makes contact with the underside of the area to be splinted. With the aid of the velcro fasteners, have a second EMT fasten the splint in place.

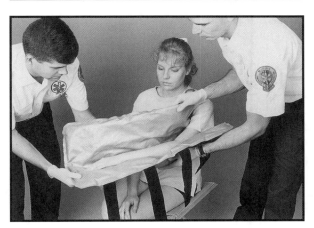

4. Working from the splint's proximal to its distal end, form each major angle, curve or other bend needed. If the splint is too firm, so this produces pressure or leverage against the patient, reintroduce some air until only the minimum needed firmness remains. When at the distal end while splinting an arm, have the patient cup his hand while you shape the splint into the curve needed to maintain the hand in the position of function. After this, should the splint extend excessively beyond the hand, bend any excess back until it is placed out of the way against the underside of the part supporting the hand and forearm.

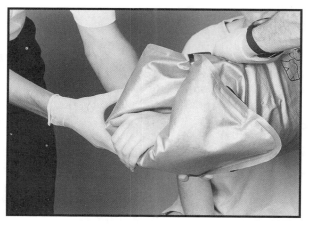

5. Once the gross forming of the splint has been completed, the finer adjustments needed in its shape and the position of its longitudinal edges should be made. Again working in a distal direction from the splint's proximal end, make sure that the splint lies against and conforms to the underside and lateral sides of the extremity. The upper edges of the splint must return over most of the top of the limb to properly secure the splint without the use of roller gauze or other ties.

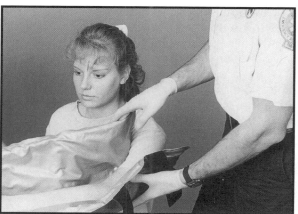

6. Should the edges of the splint excessively overlap at any point (or if you prefer to avoid overlapping and complete encirclement), fold back any unnecessary portion of the edges. Be careful to *NOT* fold so much back that the limb will not be adequately secured within the splint. Attach the hand-pump to the splint and, after rechecking the position of the limb, evacuate the remaining air from the splint. Once you have confirmed that the splint has become properly hard and rigid, close the valve and remove the pump.

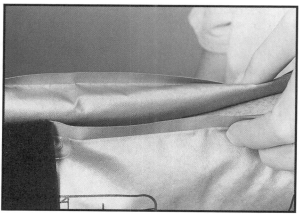

7. Check the distal MSCs in the splinted extremity and add a sling-and-swathe to support and further immobilize a splinted arm. Once this has been completed, recheck the distal circulation and repeat this check periodically. If at a later time the distal circulation becomes compromised while supporting the arm, open the valve to allow some air to enter, reshape the splint as needed, and again draw out the air.

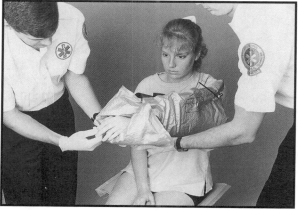

8. When the rectangular splint is used to immobilize a leg, the same method as described is used with two key modifications. After the splint has been formed around the long portions of the leg, make sure that its distal end is folded to overlap snugly against the bottom of the foot. Then form it around the sides of the foot and snugly across the foot's dorsal surface. Have a second EMT hold the foot in the proper position with the splint formed against it until you have finished and the air is removed from the splint. Also, gently push up on the underside of the splint at the knee and the area proximal of the heel to fill any voids.

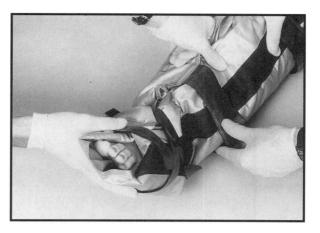

9. When a vacuum splint is used to splint the leg with the knee flexed and elevated, it should be located so its proximal end rests on the ground and be of sufficient length that when underlying the leg, its distal end is under the heel and a sufficient length to overlap against the underside of the foot remains. Once the splint has been located properly under the leg, a second EMT should support it and the leg with one hand placed under the knee and his second hand against the bottom of the foot until the splint has been completed and rigidly supports and immobilizes the leg.

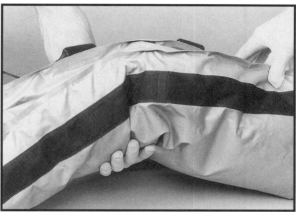

10. The splint should be formed in the usual manner around the leg, except at the knee. The edges of the splint should be pulled slightly back rather than over the patella to avoid the chance of any posterior pressure occurring against the flexed knee. Once the splint has been formed and made rigid and fixed by removing the air, lateral rotation of the leg and splint can be prevented by placing a pillow under both knees and securing the legs together.

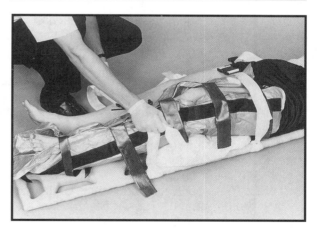

APPLICATION OF TRACTION FOR INJURIES OF THE FEMUR

In addition to the external support and immobilization needed when treating any possible fracture, fractures of the femur require the application and maintenance of traction. When a fracture of the femur is displaced, the traction reduces the pathological "third space" produced when the bones override, thus tamponading and reducing the internal bleeding that may result. When the fracture has not been displaced, traction is a necessary adjunct to the immobilization of the leg to prevent the chance of displacement due to increased spasms of the extremely strong muscles of the upper leg. In addition to reducing or preventing vast (potentially between 1,000 and 1,500 ml) internal bleeding in closed or open fractures of the femur, traction further contributes to reducing or preventing the potentially profound shock that can result by providing generally significant relief from the severe pain that is almost always associated with these injuries.

Unless the patient's condition or other injuries dictate that the PASG and longboard be used exclusively, or the use of traction is contraindicated, fractures or suspected fractures of the femur should be treated with the use of traction.

The amount of traction that is needed varies from patient to patient, depending upon the strength of the muscles of the upper leg. As a general rule, the patient requires traction equal to about ten percent of his body weight up to a maximum of 15 pounds of traction. The amount of traction that is being applied is not measurable by the EMT (except when using a Sager splint, which has an indicator), and must be determined clinically. The EMT should increase the traction *until* any pathological shortening of the leg caused by the override of the bone ends is no longer present or, if such shortening was not present, until the traction produces significant pain relief or the leg is rigidly straight and immobilized by substantial pull and he fears any further increase.

With splints that require elevation of the distal end of the leg for insertion — or when an isolated femur fracture has produced significant shock indicating that traction to reduce internal bleeding is needed without delay — traction is initially applied manually. A traction splint or device must then be applied to sustain the traction. Some devices do *NOT* require elevation of the leg or manual traction preceding their application. With these the traction is both initially applied and maintained by the device. When manual traction is necessary, once applied it must be maintained without interruption until it has been superceded by the mechanical traction provided by the device. *With injuries of the femur, once traction has been applied to the leg it must NOT be released if further damage and jeopardy of the limb are to be avoided.*

Contraindications For Use Of A Traction Device

Several conditions contraindicate the use of a traction device. Traction must be pulled against an anchor. The presently available pre-hospital traction devices are anchored against or around the pelvis. When traction is applied, an equal amount of force — called contra-traction — is exerted against the pelvis. When the pelvis is unstable or injured the application of 10 to 15 pounds of pressure against it is dangerous and therefore contraindicates the use of such a device.

The traction devices have one or two rigid shafts which are adjusted so they extend beyond the end of the foot. A pulling force is then applied to the foot and leg to create the traction. Thus, to apply traction the device must have a firm purchase around the distal end of the leg. This is achieved by a harness or hitch secured snugly around the leg at the ankle or area just proximal to it. As the traction is applied, this hitch becomes progressively tighter around the distal end of the leg. Since this can cause serious consequences to any injury that lies directly or nearly under the hitch, the presence of any significant injuries to the lower third of the lower leg contraindicate the use of the traction device. Because some texts vary the definition they ascribe to the term "lower leg," alternating between meaning the part of the leg distal to the knee in some places and only its more distal end (the 8 to 10 inches proximal to the bottom of the foot) in others, their reference to "injuries of the lower leg" as a contraindication for the use of a traction device can be confusing. The reader should not interpret this to include either injuries of the tibia and fibula that are proximal to the approximate area covered by the ankle hitch, or injuries of the foot distal to where the hitch passes around it.

The position that fractures of the tibia and fibula proximal of the ankle hitch do not in themselves contraindicate the use of a traction device can be found in the text by the American Academy of Orthopaedic Surgeons. This even includes the use of a traction splint as one option for stabilizing fractures of the tibia and fibula (although not necessary for isolated tibial fractures) when there is no injury to the femur, and goes on to state that when there is a fracture of the femur and tibia of the same limb, a properly applied traction splint will provide sufficient immobilization for both.

Fractures of the head of the femur are often called (and may not be clinically separable from) hip fractures in the field. These are also generally best treated with a traction device. Because these devices require the leg to be in a normally aligned anatomical position, and because any injury which prevents the EMT from re-aligning the leg must be assumed to include significant injury to the joint, forceful realignment and mechanical traction are unadvisable. Therefore, any injury to the hip area which, when the EMT attempts to move the leg into its normal neutral in-line position, prohibits the leg from being realigned, contraindicates the use of a traction device.

Since traction moves the knee joint to a position at the extreme of its extension, and places substantial pull against the joint, the use of a traction device is contraindicated by the presence of knee injuries. Similarly, if a leg is partially amputated or so severely avulsed at any point along its length that the attachment of the distal section is limited and tenuous, substantial pulling of the leg would be dangerous and therefore contraindicates the use of a traction device. This does not include amputation of toes or partial amputations of the distal foot which lie at a safe distance beyond the hitch. In the latter case, the EMT will have to exercise reasonable judgment in determining whether or not a traction device can be safely used.

A traction splint, even in the most favorable situations, requires three to five minutes to apply. Therefore, the use of a traction splint is contraindicated in any situation where *URGENCY* dictates that transport be initiated without any unnecessary delay in the field.

In summary:

Contraindications For The Pre-Hospital Use Of A Traction Splint Or Device
- A fractured pelvis.
- Hip injuries which prohibit alignment of the leg into a normal in-line position.
- Any significant knee injury.
- Injuries to the lower third of the lower leg.
- Partial amputation of the leg.
- Any condition or situation which dictates the initiation of transport without unnecessary delay in the field.

Use Of PASG Instead Of A Traction Device

When use of a traction splint or device is contraindicated for a fractured femur, yet the presenting level of shock indicates the presence of significant third-space bleeding (or in anticipation of it with overriding or bilateral femur fractures), PASG and a longboard should be used instead. This combination will control the bleeding while supporting and splinting the hip, femur, and distal leg. Regardless of whether a traction splint could be used, when the injuries of a patient with multi-systems trauma include the femur, the PASG and longboard are used to prevent the additional time in the field needed to apply a traction device. If the other injuries include pelvic fractures or other intra-abdominal bleeding, using the PASG simultaneously treats both conditions by controlling the underlying bleeding in both areas and splinting both injuries. If the fracture is at the proximal end of the femur and the EMT can *NOT* with any certainty determine if the injury is limited to the femoral neck or includes an associated pelvic injury, the use of the PASG and inflation of all three of its sections is recommended.

Although some devices allow traction to be provided to both legs simultaneously, due to the vast potential sum of internal blood loss possible with two such fractures most EMTs prefer to use the PASG when a patient has bilateral femur fractures.

When the purpose for which the PASG was used includes the treatment of a fractured femur, manual traction is applied and the garment is installed and inflated. *Regardless of the level of inflation of the other chambers of the garment, the section surrounding the injured leg should be inflated to its maximum pressure.* The maximally inflated leg section will prevent further third-space bleeding and, in almost all cases, will sufficiently stabilize the injury so that once the section surrounding the injured leg has been fully inflated, manual traction can slowly be released without allowing any displacement. The maintenance of mechanical traction with a device designed so that it can be added outside of the inflated PASG only serves to possibly further alleviate pain, and is rarely found to be necessary. Should the patient complain of marked increasing pain as the EMT slowly releases the manual traction after the PASG has been inflated, if the patient's condition allows the additional time in the field manual traction should be reinstituted and then a suitable traction device applied. It should be noted that this is extremely rare.

When the patient has a fractured femur and slow insidious intra-abdominal bleeding, the initial level of shock found may be consistent with, and assumed to be caused by, the internal bleeding from the femur fracture. In cases with neither any external indicators of abdominal injury nor shock so profound that the EMT is alerted to this possibility, such signs may only develop *after* the EMT has applied a traction splint or device. Since by this time the EMT should have ruled out hidden intrathoracic bleeding, such an injury in the other leg, or a cardiac cause for the continued increasing shock, hidden intra-abdominal hemorrhage must be suspected. In the rare event that an indication for the use of the PASG only becomes apparent after a traction device has been applied, even though the literature accompanying one of the traction devices states that the PASG can be applied over the device, *the application of the PASG **over** any appliance or device is generally considered to be an UNSAFE practice.*

Placing the PASG over the long rigid metal shafts of the traction splint can produce a void between the garment and the extremity which breeches the continuity of the external circumferential pressure and allows continued internal or external bleeding. Secondly, the significant external pressure exerted when the PASG is inflated over the device may forcefully press the splint into the limb and cause tissue damage or circulatory compromise, or may puncture the garment and result in its sudden dangerous deflation.

Even though recent studies have challenged whether the PASG provides any benefit in the general treatment of shock, none have scientifically disputed its usefulness in controlling underlying bleeding or splinting of included fractures. Its unique effectiveness in controlling underlying internal hemorrhage and in immobilizing pelvic fractures and fractures of the femur when the use of a traction device is contraindicated or not possible, remains almost universally accepted. The EMT will have to follow his local protocols in defining which conditions contraindicate the use of the garment since these vary from place-to-place.

Traction Devices

A variety of commercial traction devices are presently available for use in the field. Even a disposable cardboard traction splint has been introduced and there are numerous methods for improvising a traction device if the rescuer is in a remote first-responder situation where no commercial device is available.

Traction devices fall into two categories based upon their underlying design. *Bipolar* traction devices are a modified rectangular frame which is bent downwards to pass under the leg (and attaches with a strap) at its proximal end, and has two long pole-like sides. One of these runs parallel to each side of the leg, and both are inseparably connected at a point beyond the bottom of the foot to support the pulling of the distal leg. As well as providing the rigid framework which maintains the traction between the pelvis and the foot, the rigid poles lying on both sides of the leg provide a platform which, using spaced cradles and ties, supports the underside of the leg and causes the bipolar frame to be both a traction device and a splint. An adjustable leg is provided near the distal end to keep the splinted leg from resting on the ground or longboard.

Unipolar traction devices, as the name implies, have only a single shaft which lies against the medial or lateral side of the leg. At the proximal end there is a padded "T"-like end which rests against the pelvis. A "J"-like pulley or an "L" or "T"-shaped bracket at the distal end provides a platform directly beyond the midline of the bottom of the foot to support the pulling of the distal leg. Even though, as with any traction device, the traction produces the primary immobilization and the pole secured to one side of the leg provides some support, additional support and splinting of the injured leg *must* be included. This is why this type is called a *traction device* rather than a traction splint. The additional support is primarily supplied by securing both legs together with velcro or other ties spaced periodically around both legs and the shaft of the traction device, and then placing the patient onto a flat rigid surface such as a longboard.

Whether bipolar or unipolar, the side pole(s) of all traction devices can be adjusted to a variety of lengths to fit any individual patient. Each model has a different device to allow the shaft(s) to be unlocked so that the device can be adjusted to the correct length prior to the application of any mechanical traction. These same devices prevent the accidental shortening of the splint and a loss of traction once it has been applied.

None of the presently available traction splints extends beyond the proximal end of the leg. Therefore, they neither prevent flexion of the hip nor, even though they may limit its extent, lateral movement of the leg. In order to immobilize the hip joint, which is essential as this is the joint immediately proximal to the femur, *all traction splints and devices must be used in conjunction with a longboard.* By placing the patient and traction device on the longboard and securing the pelvis and the distal end of the traction device to the board, both the lower torso and distal leg will be prevented from moving laterally or posteriorly. A strap placed around the torso at the armpits is also required to prevent flexion of the hip joints should the patient move from supine to a sitting or semi-sitting position. Although alternatively a longboard splint secured next to the uninjured side from proximal to the armpit to beyond the bottom of the foot will provide some of the hip and leg immobilization required if the patient is placed directly onto the flat ambulance cot without a longboard, securing the patient and traction device onto a longboard is easier, faster, and provides far better support and immobilization.

If this use of a longboard splint and supine placement of the patient directly on the cot (instead of on a long spine board) is elected with a *bipolar traction splint,* the distal leg support should *NOT* be extended to its lowered position to elevate the leg. The cot mattress will not provide a sufficiently firm surface to avoid rotation of the device and leg. With the stand retracted against the underside of the leg, both feet should instead be secured together to prevent or minimize any rotation. Even when a unipolar traction device has been applied and the patient will be firmly secured onto a longboard, the legs and feet must be firmly secured together to support the leg and avoid rotation when moving the patient onto the board and to prevent any rotation of the foot and leg thereafter.

Removal of the shoe on the injured side is required to initially examine the foot and to check the most distal circulation in it. This also avoids the chance that the shoe will interfere with the stability of the harness or become pressed into the sides of the foot by it, possibly causing additional injury. Containing the shoe in the immobilization also will prevent examination of the foot at the hospital prior to removal of the traction device. Therefore, in almost all cases the shoe should be removed prior to applying the ankle harness and the traction device. In some cases, when the footwear is stable (tied shoe, ski boot, etc.), the advantages of leaving the shoe on the foot may outweigh the disadvantages. For example, the boot is often left in place when the patient is on a ski hill or cross-country trail and the ski patrol anticipates that the rescue will cause him to remain in the extremely cold outdoors for a significant time period. Also, when a cravat ankle hitch is used, the shoe's heel is useful in keeping it properly positioned on the bottom of the foot.

The Hare-type splint is the most prevalent type of traction device in use at present and the EMT, regardless of whether he uses a different traction device, should be familiar with its application and use. The Hare splint was the first traction device to introduce a stable, easy-to-use ankle harness together with a locking ratcheted hand-winch to purchase and provide traction to the distal leg. The proximal end of the Hare splint has a padded bolster which rests against the buttock and is secured to the leg with an ischial strap which fastens around the proximal leg and a part of the lower pelvis.

Although the bolster contributes somewhat, the contra-traction is primarily exerted against the pelvis by the ischial strap. A variety of different brands which emulate many of the features of the Hare splint are also available.

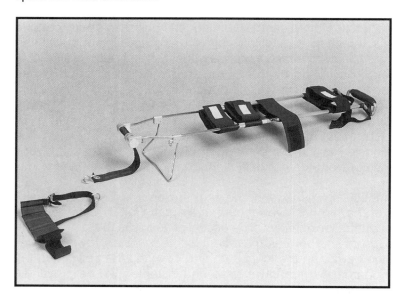

Prior to the introduction of the Hare splint, *the Thomas Half-Ring splint* was universally used with an ankle hitch and straps formed from cravats. At its proximal end the splint is secured by a padded half-ring which lies against the buttock and an ischial strap. A sturdy stick was inserted between the sides of a cravat which had been tied in a loop between the ankle hitch and a bent notch in the distal frame of the splint. The stick was turned, winding the loop and shortening it to produce the traction. When tight enough, this Spanish Windlass was locked by taping the ends of the stick to both side poles of the splint.

Unlike the Hare splint, the side rails of most half-ring splints are not adjustable so the length of the splint is fixed. The difference in length required from one adult to another is adjusted for by varying the length of the cravat loop which connects the bottom of the foot to the distal end of the splint. A smaller pediatric size should be used on children and adults with extremely short legs to keep the splint from excessively extending beyond the bottom of the foot.

Because of the low frequency of need for a traction device, as an economic consideration many squads still carry a half-ring splint on some vehicles. In such cases, upgrading these splints by the replacement of the cravat ankle hitch and windlass with a more stable ankle harness and clamp-on Hare winch is highly recommended.

Both of these bipolar traction splints require that manual traction be applied and the distal end of the leg be elevated ten to twelve inches so that they can be inserted and positioned properly under the leg. These commonly include a stand which, when placed in its downward position, holds the leg off the ground or board while a number of "cradles" between the sides of the splint provide additional support and immobilization of the leg.

Unipolar traction devices became commercially available several years ago with the introduction of the Sager splint which, today, has become the second most commonly used type of traction device. As well as providing a modern commercial design to replace the unipolar traction device often improvised by using a longboard splint in the past, the Sager includes many other innovations. It has a padded "T"-like proximal end which securely abuts against the pelvis between the medial side of the leg and the genitalia. The contra-traction is applied to the pelvis from this "T" rather than the ischial strap, which simply serves to keep the proximal end of the splint properly positioned in the groin. The ankle harness is connected to a cable bracket which extends perpendicularly under the foot (or in some models which passes around a pulley) at the splint's distal end.

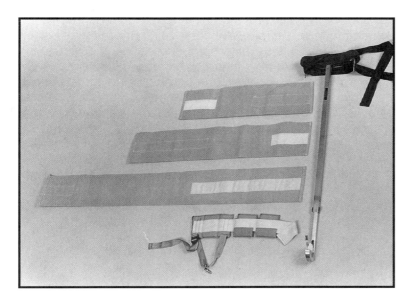

The shaft of the splint is square or rectangular and made of two parts with one inserted into the other and held in place by a ratcheted locking device. Once the splint has been installed and the ankle harness attached around the distal leg, traction is produced by pulling and sliding the distal section of the shaft further out of the proximal section, extending the splint's length. A ratchet device in the shaft allows the distal section of the shaft to be pulled out while preventing it from sliding back into the proximal one. Should it be necessary to shorten the splint when initially adjusting its length, this lock can be released by the EMT. The approximate pounds of traction being applied are indicated by a gauge on or near the pulley.

The outstanding advantage of this splint is that its application does *NOT* require manual traction and elevation of the leg. The device can be installed and secured while the straight leg rests on the ground and, once this has been completed, the traction is initially applied mechanically by extending the distal end of the splint's shaft. The second EMT only aids in preventing rotation or other movement of the leg, eliminating the positional conflicts inherent when manual traction must be instituted and maintained when other types of traction splints are used. *When necessary, the Sager can safely be applied by a single EMT.*

Models with a perpendicular bracket at their distal end can be purchased for single or bilateral leg traction capability. An adaptor which provides for the simultaneous provision of traction to both legs in cases with bilateral femur fractures can be purchased for models with a pulley at their distal end. With this adaptor a second ankle harness is separately attached to the connector at the end of the cable, providing one harness for each leg. The distal section of the shaft must usually be removed and replaced so the pulley faces upward. When the shaft of the splint (which lies between the legs) is extended, the traction is equally applied to each leg.

Most models of the Sager splint will accommodate any length required, ranging from that of a relatively young child to a 7 foot adult. A model which can accommodate smaller children with an inseam from 8 to 24 inches is also available. All of the Sager models include a number of wide elasticized wraps with Velcro closures for securing the legs and feet together with the device between them.

The Kendrick Traction Device (KTD) is a second more basic unipolar design. The KTD's pole length adjusts so the single model presently available can be used for almost any size of pediatric or adult patient. Many of the innovations and features found in the Sager have been purposely omitted in this device, as a small carrying size and light weight were paramount objectives in its design. When stored the Kendrick Traction Device measures only 3½ x 9½ inches, and weighs less than 20 ounces. This makes it extremely useful in cross-field situations where the large variety of equipment that may be needed must be carried for a considerable distance. Due to their large size and weight and the low frequency of need for them, prior to the availability of the KTD most EMTs involved in search, remote area rescue, or expedition emergency care did *NOT* carry any traction device. When traction was needed in a remote setting, these EMTs have usually improvised a traction device at the scene. This is significantly more difficult and time consuming than if a pre-assembled commercial device is available. The KTD makes inclusion of a traction device to the medical equipment carried in such situations practical, and is highly recommended. The KTD is also the traction device of choice in rescue boats, fixed or rotary wing aircraft, and all-terrain vehicles — anywhere that space and weight limits are major considerations in equipment selection.

As either a Hare-type Traction Splint or Sager Traction Device is carried on most ambulances, the respective use of each has been selected to demonstrate the skills employed when applying traction. In addition, the skills for making an ankle hitch and windlass from cravats is also demonstrated, in case the EMT finds the ankle harness to be missing or that the more advanced winch will not operate properly. These skills are also essential should the EMT ever need to make an improvised traction device in a wilderness or other isolated setting.

USING A HARE-TYPE TRACTION SPLINT

When the Hare Splint was developed and introduced by Glenn Hare, its many advantages caused it to rapidly replace the Half-ring splint as the standard for traction splinting. Today, several brands of Hare-type traction splints are available. Although these have some individual design differences, most have similar components and are basically applied and used in much the same way.

After any more urgent priorities have been met, confirm that the appropriate body substance isolation precautions have been taken and that the patient's condition indicates and allows the application of a traction splint. Then:

1. Remove the traction splint and its separate components from the carrying case. Direct a second EMT to position himself beyond the patient's foot and, leaving the leg on the ground, hold it from moving. Carefully remove the shoe. Orient the ankle harness correctly, and insert it under the void just proximal of the heel. Once the harness has been properly centered under the leg, carefully slide it until the bottom edges of its side flaps are about an inch proximal to the lateral protrusion of the ankle, as shown.

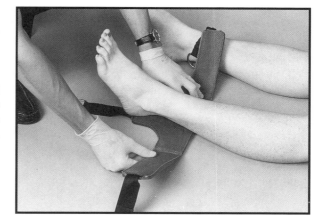

2. Lift the side flaps of the harness up along the sides of the leg and bring the end of one across the anterior leg and then downward until it is beyond the bottom of the foot and the distal end of the flap is approximately parallel to the long axis of the foot. Now repeat this with the second flap. The harness must be located on the leg so that its lower edge lies laterally and immediately proximal to the ankle.

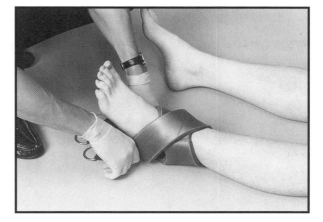

3. While holding the side flaps and the third flap which extends distally from the posterior heel in one hand, and keeping the harness snug around the leg, make any changes necessary in the position of the harness. Make sure that the point where the side flaps cross is sufficiently proximal that when traction is pulled, the harness will not press on the dorsal (top) foot, causing it to be extended. While maintaining just enough tension on the collected ends of the flaps to keep the harness in place, pass them to the second EMT. If using another style of harness, install it in the manner prescribed and make sure it is properly located around the leg so the traction will be pulled against the ankle and not the top of the foot.

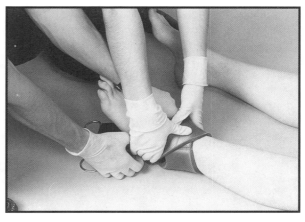

4. Direct the second EMT to kneel with his torso upright (not leaning back) and have him move back until, with his arms fully extended, he is applying mild tension to the harness. Direct a third responder to kneel beyond the patient's head and hold the patient's armpits to prevent him from being pulled along the ground — defeating the traction. Then direct the second EMT to lean back and provide the necessary pull on the harness to provide manual traction and elevate the distal end of the foot about 10 to 12 inches off the ground.

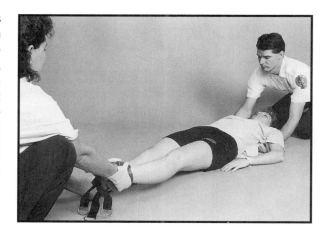

Manual traction *must* be maintained without interruption until the splint has been applied. It is essential that the EMT use the weight of his upper torso by leaning back, instead of attempting to pull with his arms by flexing them.

Manual traction can be provided just proximal to the ankle while a second EMT applies the ankle harness and then the pull is transferred to it. This causes a conflict between the hands proximal to the ankle and the installation of the harness which can jeopardize the stability of the manual traction and increase the time needed to install the device. Although taking the initial traction from just distal of the knee (instead of proximal to the ankle) avoids this conflict, it is extremely difficult to maintain a stable grasp and proper alignment from this position. Experience has shown that it is far easier, faster, and more stable to first install the harness and then initiate the manual traction.

5. Place the splint on the ground next to the patient's *uninjured* leg so that its proximal end is in-line with the patient's groin. Without moving its proximal end, turn the length-locks on each side of the splint's frame to release them, and pull the distal section of the splint until the splint is long enough to extend about 10 to 12 inches beyond the bottom of the foot. Then re-tighten them and test that they are each fully locked and that the splint will not shorten when traction is applied.

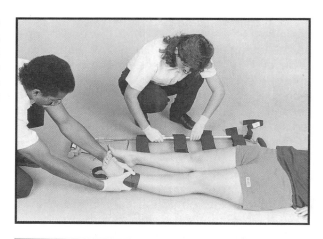

6. Taking the splint, move to a position beside the knee of the injured leg. Open the ischial strap and each of the leg cradles. Insert the splint under the leg and slide it in a proximal direction until it is approximately positioned properly under the leg. Then fold down the drop-stand at the splint's distal end and fasten the ends of the ischial strap together, but do not tighten the strap at this time.

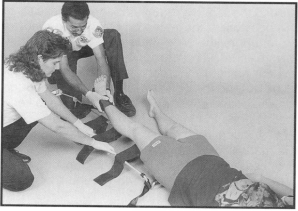

7. While pulling the ischial strap up with one hand so it is held straight against the medial side of the injured leg, adjust the position of the proximal end of the splint as needed. When the point where this strap attaches to the frame of the splint is just cephalad to the groin, and the strap is indented by the lower margin of the pelvis between the genitalia and the medial side of the leg, the proximal end of the splint is properly positioned. *If this ischial strap does not lie firmly against the lower edge of the pelvis, the splint will shift dangerously as traction is applied.*

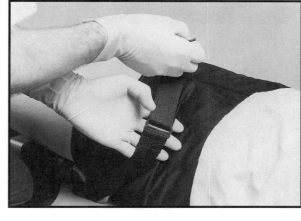

8. After having the patient confirm that the ischial strap does not include any portion of the genitalia, tighten it until it is tight enough to prevent the splint from any proximal movement. Space the cradles evenly proximal and distal to the knee so they are best positioned to support the underside of the leg. Direct the second EMT to lower the leg onto the splint while maintaining the manual traction.

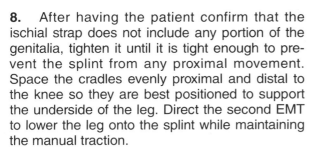

9. Move down the side of the splint until you are next to its distal end, beyond the patient's foot. While holding the winch lock released, unfurl a sufficient amount of the strap to reach the bottom of the patient's foot — with some slack remaining. Reset the winch lock. Insert the "S" hook (or other fastening device) at the end of the strap into the grommets at the distal end of the ankle harness flaps (or strap), being careful not to dislodge the second EMT's grasp or manual traction.

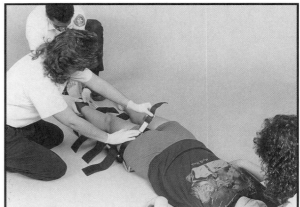

10. When a three-flapped harness has been used, attach the heel flap to the S-hook first, before the flaps from each side of the foot. This will help to maintain the proper foot position when traction is applied. With the flaps connected to the S-hook, and holding it with one hand to keep the flaps from coming undone, turn the winch with your other hand until all of the slack in the strap has been taken up. Continue to turn the winch until the proper degree of mechanical traction is provided.

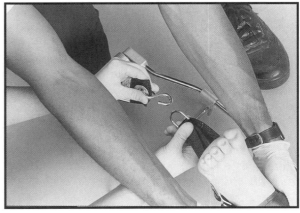

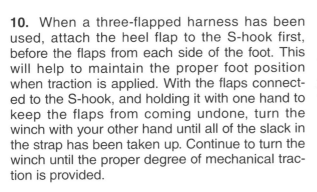

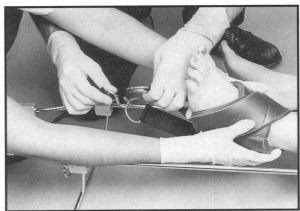

11. The ratcheted lock should allow the winch to be turned when tightening the strap, but prevent it from turning in the opposite direction and releasing the traction. If the type of splint you are using has a second safety lock to prevent any further turning of the winch once the correct traction has been established, set it. Once you are sure the mechanical traction is proper and will *NOT* be released, the second EMT can release his pull on the harness. Fasten the top of each cradle over the leg and recheck the distal MSCs in the splinted leg.

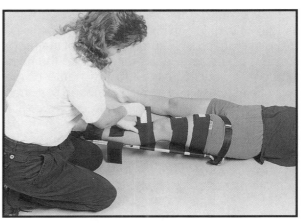

12. Place the splinted patient onto a longboard and position him along its length so that the stand of the traction splint is securely on the distal end of the board. Place straps across iliac crest, and across both (or only the uninjured leg and under the splint) ankles. Pad the medial side of the splints stand to keep it from injuring the other leg. Then tape the stand at a hand-hole in the board to secure its distal end. Lastly, place a strap through the armpits to prevent the patient from sitting-up and articulating his hip.

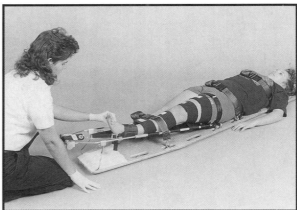

Note: Some instructors advocate the application of additional cradles formed from cravats to increase the support provided under the leg. The leg is essentially supported by the traction and, although not harmful, this addition is unnecessary and of questionable benefit. Such cravats or the cradles supplied on the splint should *NEVER* be fastened over the leg until after the traction with the windlass has been obtained. *Securing any ties around the leg prior to applying traction can result in additional injury and interfere with the traction being properly communicated along the entire length of the leg, and compromise the distal circulation.*

If ordered by a physician at the hospital to release the traction, the EMT should grasp the strap from the winch and apply manual traction. Once the winch lock has been released he should slowly release his pull until no traction remains. *The lock on the winch should never be released without first re-establishing manual traction, as an abrupt complete release of traction can cause injury to the leg.*

USING A SAGER SPLINT (Traction Device)

Since the basic Sager Traction Splint was first introduced and initiated wide use of unipolar traction devices in the field, its innovative physician-developer has introduced several other models of the device (the Super Sager, Sager Form III, etc.). Due to their effectiveness and price consideration, the more basic models (Sager and Super-Sager) are the most prevalent in the field.

Since it is not necessary to elevate the leg to install the device, the leg can be left supported on the ground while the Sager is installed and initial traction supplied by the device. This rapidly provides stable mechanical traction and avoids the need and potential instability of temporary initial manual traction. This feature also makes the device simple to use and, when necessary, allows for one-person application. Most models can be used for both children and adults and, when modified, for either single or bilateral lower extremity fractures for which traction is indicated.

In the original Sager design, the pull produced by the extension of the distal section of the shaft is transferred to the foot by a cable which is attached to a spring within the hollow shaft and which goes around a pulley at the shaft's distal end.

In other models, there is a perpendicular "L" (or in models that can be used for bilateral fractures, a "T") shaped cross bar at the device's distal end which is connected to the spring within the end of the shaft. This cross bar contains a special slot to which the strap loop from the ankle harness is connected. The strong spring within the shaft of the distal section of the device causes the traction to be *dynamic*, allowing some automatic self-adjustment to maintain the proper level of traction once the device has been applied should significant changes in the muscle spasm in the leg occurs.

The EMT may have to make some slight modifications in some of the individual steps shown, when using a model different from the one used for the following demonstration.

After all of the more urgent priorities have been met, confirm that all of the indicated body substance isolation precautions have been taken, and that the patient's condition indicates and allows the time for the use of a traction device. Then:

1. Remove the traction device and its components from the carrying case. Lay the device on the ground next to the patient's uninjured leg so that the top of the padded "T" at its proximal end is in-line with the patient's groin. Without moving its proximal end, pull the distal section of the shaft out until the length of the device is extended so that there will be about 4 to 6 inches between the pulley or perpendicular bracket at the distal end of the splint and the bottom of the patient's foot.

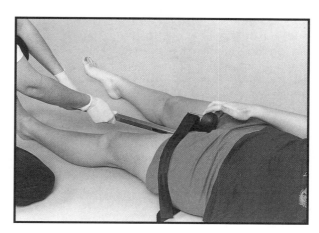

2. Hold the Sager so that the padded proximal end (the "T" with the perineal cushion) is vertical and the device is properly oriented (unless a bilateral model) so that the pulley or "L" bracket at its distal end is facing towards the injured leg. Place the device between the patient's legs and, with the patient's assistance, move it proximally until the perineal cushion is firmly against the pelvis (against the ischial tuberosity) and snugly against the medial side of the thigh, between the injured leg and the external genitalia. Then, secure the ischial strap firmly around the leg to keep the splint properly positioned.

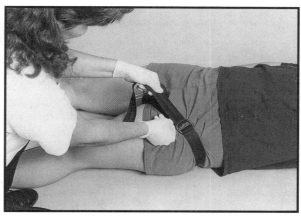

3. Move down to the distal end of the device, and adjust the length of the shaft so that the pulley wheel or cross bar is almost adjacent to the bottom of the patient's foot (only a fraction of an inch beyond it). Open the ankle harness and flip down the two "removable" pads from the strap. Lay the harness flat on the ground and insert it under the void just proximal of the heel until it is centered under the leg, and its lower edge is just proximal to the malleoli (the medial and lateral protrusions of the ankle).

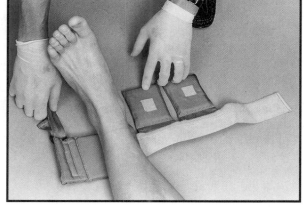

4. "Flip-back" as many of the removable pads as will fit and are required to pad along the inner circumference of the strap when it surrounds the leg. Bring the lateral ends of the harness up and secure the harness firmly around the lower leg by crossing one end over the other and securely contacting the Velcro closures on each. Pull the control tabs on the ankle harness to shorten the stirrup part of the ankle sling, pulling it up against the sole of the foot. If preferred, the ankle harness can be temporarily disconnected from the device to facilitate its application around the leg.

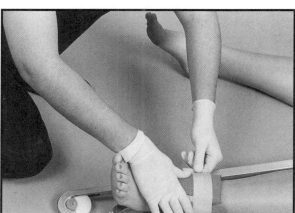

5. To apply the traction, firmly pull on the distal section of the shaft. The pull should be in a straight line along the long axis of the shaft and any lateral bending of the hip or elevating the leg (off the ground) should be guarded against. Some models include a retractable handle on the top of their distal section to aid in extending it and applying the traction. Extend the shaft of the device until you have achieved the desired amount of traction — either measured by the clinical results or the quantified pounds of pull shown on the gauge.

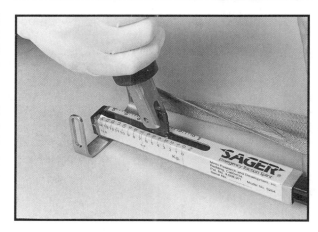

6. Once the shaft has been sufficiently extended to provide the desired traction, direct another EMT to hold the foot in its normal upright position, and slowly release your pull on its distal section. The ratcheted locking device, although allowing the shaft to be extended, should lock the distal section of the shaft from retracting back into the proximal section — which would result in shortening the splint and a loss of traction. Check the ischial strap and tighten it as needed to retain a snug fit.

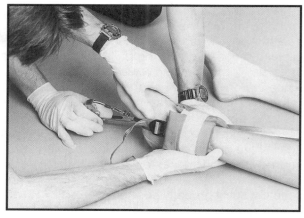

7. Locate the long thin strap used to secure the feet together. Insert one end at the void which occurs between the underside of the legs and the ground near the ankle proximal to the heel. Continue to pass it under both legs until it is centered under them. Bring each end up along the side of the leg and cross the ends over each other on the top (dorsum) of the foot. Continue to pass each end around the side of the foot and fasten both together against the undersides (soles) of the feet. The figure-of-eight formed by the strap should snugly secure the feet together.

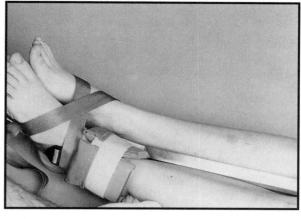

8. Lay each of the three elasticized wide cravats open on a clean area of the ground. Note that these are of 3 different lengths. Insert the longest in the void found under the knee and, while see-sawing it, move it in a proximal direction until it is centered at the desired place under the upper thigh (it should be positioned so it will *NOT* lie directly over the injury site).

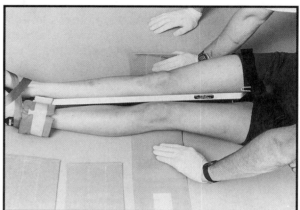

9. Bring both ends around the sides and over the anterior surface of the thighs. Overlap the ends as needed to make the cravat snug (but not so tight as to compromise the distal circulation), and secure them by properly contacting the Velcro closures found on each. Insert the shortest of the cravats under the knee and see-saw it while moving it distally. When it is positioned under the lower leg just proximal of the ankle harness(es), secure it around the lower leg. Insert the remaining cravat under the knees and secure it around both of them.

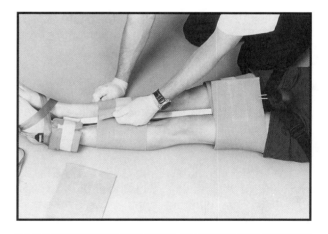

10. Once the feet have been secured together and the legs and splint have been bound together with the cravats at the thighs, knees, and lower leg, check the distal MSCs in the injured leg and then — since it is contained in the packaging — the uninjured leg as well. Place the splinted patient supine onto a longboard or directly onto the ambulance cot. Secure the patient and splint with straps over the iliac crests and lower legs and, to prevent the patient from sitting-up and articulating the hip, secure the upper torso with a strap which passes through each armpit.

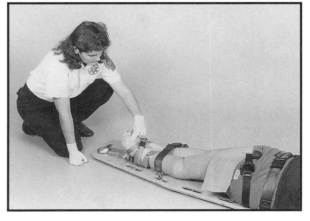

Neither the cravats around the leg nor the figure-of-eight tie of the foot should ever be secured around the legs prior to the extension of the device's shaft and the application of proper traction with the device. Except for the ischial strap, ties surrounding the legs and splint prior to the completion of traction with the device can interfere with the traction being properly communicated along the length of the leg and can compromise the distal circulation.

If ordered by the physician at the hospital to release the traction, the EMT should carefully grasp the distal section of the device's shaft with one hand and pull against it with approximately the same amount of traction as the Sager has provided. While maintaining this pull, the lock on the shaft should be released with the second hand and the pull progressively lessened until no traction remains against the leg. Alternatively, one EMT can grasp the ankle with both hands while a second releases the locking mechanism. *Simply releasing the lock while the traction is being applied by the splint will cause the abrupt complete release of tension against the leg which can result in injury to the hip, knee or ankle (or even fracturing of a longbone of the leg).* In cases where the leg is found severely angulated, manual traction may have to be established prior to the application of the Sager — which would require that it be maintained while the device is installed. In such cases it is preferable to separate the ankle harness from the device, apply it to the ankle, and take the manual traction with it (as previously described when using a Hare Splint). Due to the "T" like proximal end of the device, however, the distal end of the leg should *NOT* be held more than 3 to 6 inches off the ground.

While manual traction is maintained by one EMT, the Sager can be easily applied by a second EMT. Once the harness has been installed and manual traction has been taken, the splint should be adjusted to the proper length. With the distal end of the device supported on the ground, position its proximal end against the medial side of the leg and insert it against the pelvis. Then secure it to the leg with the ischial strap. Then, while the distal end of the device is held elevated next to the lower leg, reconnect the harness and extend the distal section of the shaft until the proper amount of mechanical traction is supplied. Once manual traction has been superceded by the traction supplied by the Sager, manual traction can be released and the distal end of the leg and splint lowered carefully onto the ground. The application of the device can then be completed in the same manner as previously described.

If the Sager is to be used for bilateral leg fractures, an ankle harness should be applied and secured to each lower leg prior to extending the distal end of the device. In this way, once the distal end of the shaft is extended the traction will be supplied to both legs simultaneously. If manual traction is required prior to this, it can be supplied to both legs simultaneously by one EMT who is holding one ankle harness in each hand with the sides of his hands resting against each other. *BOTH* harnesses must be connected to the distal cross piece of the device before the shaft of the splint is extended to provide mechanical traction. *It is an unsafe practice to attempt to secure the ankle harness applied to the second leg to the device using manual traction, once the device has been secured to the first leg and the shaft of the device has been properly extended to provide the traction to it.*

When using the Form III Series, the EMT should note that the articulating "T" base at the proximal end of the device (which bends laterally for seating and exact conformance to the ischial tuberosity) has different length ends. The device should be positioned so that the cushion with the shorter end of the articulating base faces towards the ground.

USING THE KENDRICK TRACTION DEVICE (KTD)

The KTD is extremely smaller (when stored) and lighter than other traction devices. This makes it the device of choice in areas where carrying emergency equipment over a considerable distance to reach the patient is common, or on rescue sleds or other special rescue vehicles (ATVs, boats, helicopter, etc.) where space and weight are key considerations.

Many of the design elements of the KTD — a rigid adjustable length shaft, an ischial strap, an ankle harness, an "L" bracket at its distal end, etc. — are analogous to those found in other traction devices. Uniquely the hollow tube shaft of the device folds for storage and, when unfolded, each 8 inch section secures into the next like a tent pole. The sections are held together by a bungy-type elastic cord which runs internally through the center of the entire shaft. If the shaft is too long (as when using it on a child), the pole sections can be disconnected at the joint which is at or just beyond the correct length and the excess length of the shaft folded back against the used portion. When the proximal end is inserted into the bracket on the ischial strap any folded-back sections will be held in place and out of the way.

Once the device has been installed, the mechanical traction is supplied by pulling the strap which connects the part of the ankle hitch at the bottom of the foot to the "L" bracket at the distal end of the pole until it is sufficiently tightened to provide the necessary amount of pull on the leg. The configuration of this strap through the plastic slide which connects to the stirrup of the ankle hitch is designed so that the strap remains locked at the tightest pull placed against it, and will only loosen when the EMT purposely releases it by elevating the tab at its end.

Like the Sager, the KTD is preferably installed with the leg supported on the ground. Traction is first initiated once this has been completed, and it is applied mechanically by the device. However, if initial manual traction is required or desired the device can also be applied while this is being maintained with the distal end of the leg elevated slightly off the ground. When ready to apply the KTD:

1. Confirm that the indicated body substance isolation precautions have been taken and that the patient's condition indicates and allows the time for application of a traction device. Remove the KTD and its components from its carrying case. While a second rescuer supports the leg on the ground, pass the opened ankle hitch under the ankle and position it so the wider padded area is centered under the leg. Its lower edge should be just proximal to the malleoli (the medial and lateral protrusions of the ankle).

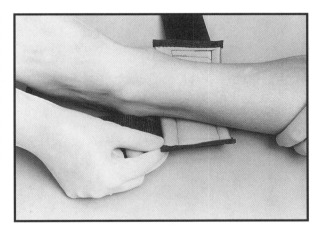

2. Secure the ankle hitch firmly around the leg, making sure that its lower edge remains proximal to the lateral ankle bones. While holding the stirrup part of the ankle harness in line with the long axis of the leg, pull the *green* tabbed strap until the stirrup lies snugly against the bottom of the foot. (In cases where traction is required prior to the initiation and maintenance of traction with the device, manual traction can be best supplied by installing the ankle harness and providing the pull and leg elevation by grasping both of the blue strap ends which extend from the stirrup).

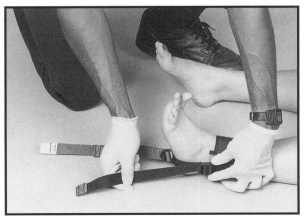

3. Lay the open ischial strap next to the lateral side of the knee of the injured leg with the pole receptacle down, and insert the male buckle end under the leg. While see-sawing the strap, move it so the lateral end is more proximal. Move it in a proximal direction until it is snugly against the pelvis at the groin, and at the pelvic crest or belt line on the lateral side of the lower torso. Orient the strap so that when it is tight the pole receptacle will be centered on the lateral side of the lower torso. Fasten the ends of the strap together and pull its end until it is tightly secured around the leg and lateral quarter of the pelvis, as shown.

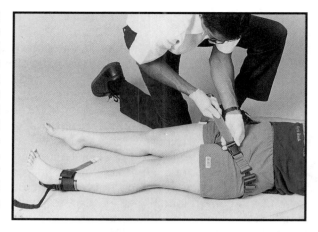

4. Unfold the segmented pole of the KTD by holding only the most proximal 8 inch section and aligning the remaining sections. Check all of the joints to make sure that each section has properly seated. For most adults the pole will not need to be shortened, and the length from the bottom of the foot to the "L" bracket will simply vary without effect. Insert the proximal end of the pole into the black plastic pole receptacle on the outside of the ischial strap. The "dart-like" end of the "L" at the distal end of the pole should be 6 or more inches beyond the bottom of the foot. Then rest the distal end on the ground.

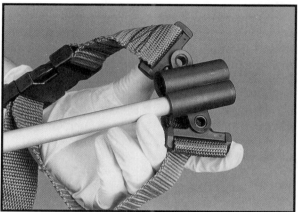

5. In smaller children or adults with exceptionally short legs, if more than one 8 inch section of the pole extends beyond the bottom of the foot, the pole should be shortened. Remove the pole from the receptacle on the ischial strap, pull the sections apart at the appropriate connection, and fold the surplus flat against the remaining used part. Then reinsert the folded and proximal ends of the pole into the two-pole receptacle.

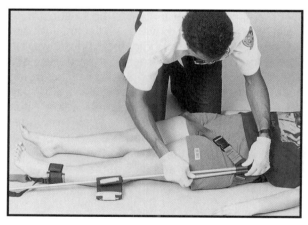

6. Move to a position beside and beyond the foot on the injured side. Slowly rotate the "L"-bracket until it is perpendicular to the longitudinal midline of the foot, and hold the distal end of the splint up so that the arrow-like tip of the bracket lies directly beyond the arch of the foot. With your other hand, spread the yellow loop found at one end of the blue connecting strap and place it over the end of the L-bracket to keep it from slipping off by the arrowhead-like shape at the bracket's tip.

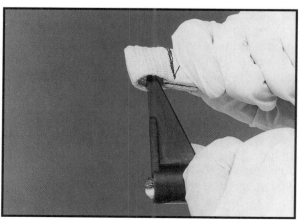

7. The traction is provided by pull on the blue strap connecting the buckle on the stirrup of the ankle hitch to the "L" bracket at the shaft's distal end. The buckle allows the strap to be tightened but will not let it loosen unless purposely released. Pull strongly on the red tipped end of the strap with one hand while simultaneously feeding the strap between the yellow loop and the buckle with the other hand. Continue increasing the tension until you have clinically estimated that sufficient traction is applied.

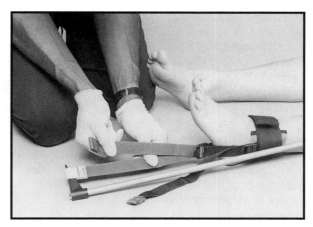

8. Once sufficient traction has been provided, the wide elastic straps are applied. Slide the one attached to the shaft of the splint until it is adjacent to the knee. Insert one end under the knee of the injured leg and secure the strap snugly around it. Insert the longer of the two remaining straps under the knee and see-saw it into position under the upper thigh. Repeat this process to locate and secure the shorter remaining strap around the shaft and lower leg. Next, tie both legs and both feet together with cravats.

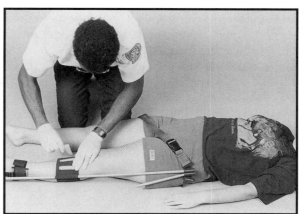

9. Once the traction is in place and both legs have been secured together, check the distal MSCs in both the injured and uninjured legs. Next, place the packaged patient onto a longboard or directly onto the ambulance cot and secure him and the splint to the board or cot with straps over the iliac crests and lower legs. Then, to prevent the patient from sitting-up and articulating his hip, secure the upper torso with a strap passing through each armpit.

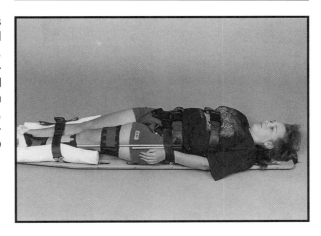

The application of *any* straps or ties which secure the leg to the shaft of the traction device (except the ischial strap and the ankle harness) prior to the initiation of mechanical traction by the device, is a potentially dangerous practice. Such ties, if in place as the traction is pulled, can prevent the traction from being properly reflected along the entire length of the leg and can cause angulation and excessive tightening of the strap around the leg which can result in compromise of the distal circulation. *Therefore, contrary to previously circulated directions, the elastic knee strap of the KTD should only be secured around the knee AFTER the traction has been applied, NOT BEFORE.*

The EMT should also disregard a previously published note which states that Anti-Shock Trousers (PASG) may be easily applied over the KTD. When the PASG is applied the need for additional mechanical traction is extremely rare, and can only be determined after the leg section of the garment has been fully inflated. The indications and methods for the concurrent use of a traction device and the PASG — are fully discussed in the Introduction of this Section. ***The application of the PASG over any rigid splint is a potentially dangerous practice and should be avoided.***

FORMING AN ANKLE HITCH AND WINDLASS WITH CRAVAT BANDAGES

In almost any situation, the EMT will have a commercial traction device available to splint and provide traction when needed, which will include an easy-to-use ankle harness and sophisticated traction device. With the introduction of the compact light-weight KTD, even EMTs who must back-pack emergency supplies a considerable distance rarely need to improvise a traction device. However, should the ankle harness be missing, or should it or the tension mechanism of the device be broken, the EMT must be able to improvise an effective alternate way to secure the lower leg and provide the necessary tension against the shaft(s) of the device in order to provide traction.

If only the ankle harness is missing or broken, the EMT can improvise a suitable one from a single cravat. In the case of the Hare Splint, the "S" hook from the windlass strap can be hooked over the stirrup of the hitch, allowing the windlass to be used in the normal manner to produce traction. When such an improvised ankle hitch is used with a Sager Traction Device, the stirrup of the hitch should be placed over the end of the "L" or "T" bracket at its distal end (or securely connected to it by a short strap or second cravat tied through the stirrup of the ankle hitch and around the bracket). After the loop from the hitch has been secured from possibly sliding off of it with tape, traction is applied by extending the shaft of the Sager device in the usual manner.

When using a cravat to substitute for a missing ankle harness with a Kendrick Traction Device or with a Half-ring splint that has *NOT* been modified to include a Hare-type winch, a second cravat must be tied into a snug loop around the stirrup of the ankle hitch and the "L" bracket of the KTD (or the distal frame of the Half-ring splint.) When a stick is perpendicularly inserted in this loop and wound, a "Spanish" windlass is formed. As the stick is turned end-over-end, the cravat loop shortens and produces the necessary traction.

In the rare event that the traction-producing mechanism of any commercial traction device fails to operate or lock properly (or when one must be improvised), as long as the proximal end of the device is properly secured around the upper leg/pelvis and the locked rigid continuity of the shaft(s) extends to beyond the foot, this form of windlass can be used with the ankle hitch to provide the necessary traction.

To form the ankle hitch, a triangular bandage neatly folded into a cravat bandage (as shown in the preceding Section on Bandaging Skills) is needed. The ankle hitch must normally be done with the patient supine and the leg supported on the ground, however since it is unchanged and will provide the reader with a significantly clearer view of the key steps involved, its application is being demonstrated here with the subject sometimes sitting or otherwise moved to facilitate showing the best view in the accompanying photographs.

1. Start by placing the cravat centered flat perpendicularly across the bottom of the foot at the arch. Bring each end diagonally around the lateral side of the foot and up around the back of the leg so both ends cross at the indentation which exists just proximal to the posterior extension of the heel.

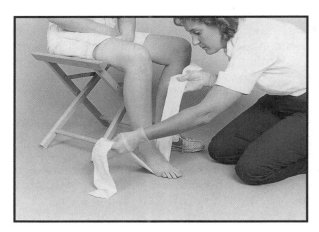

2. Being careful to maintain sufficient tension on the ends to keep the cravat properly placed in the arch of the foot and crossed at the back of the leg, continue the ends from the back in a straight line across the sides of the leg and around over the top (dorsum) of the foot, so that one crosses over the other at about the anterior midline of the lower leg.

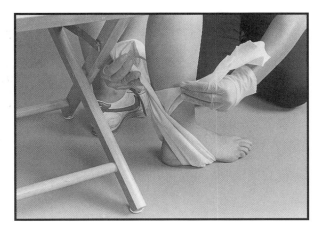

3. Next insert the end coming across the foot from the medial side under the previously formed diagonal (which runs from the arch of the foot to the back of the leg) at the lateral side of the foot. Similarly, insert the second end which comes from the lateral side of the foot under the diagonal which lies on the medial side of the foot.

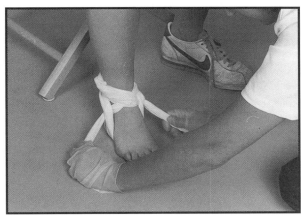

4. After the ends have been brought across the front of the leg and inserted under the diagonal at the opposite side of the foot, hold each end in a different hand and snugly reverse them over the diagonal by bringing each back beyond the anterior lower leg. Tie the ends together with a half-knot over the midline of the anterior lower leg, and then pull tightly on both ends until the diagonal at each side of the foot has been formed into a snug "Y," as shown. Then complete the knot.

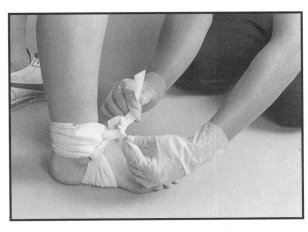

5. If only an ankle hitch was required and the traction will be supplied by the windlass or extension of the shaft of the device, secure the stirrup of the cravat to the "S" hook of the Hare windlass or perpendicular bracket at the distal end of the shaft of the Sager. Then continue the remaining previously described steps to apply the traction and complete the packaging of the leg and patient. If an alternate mechanism to produce traction is required instead, insert the end of a second cravat between the stirrup of the hitch and the bottom of the foot until both ends are equal.

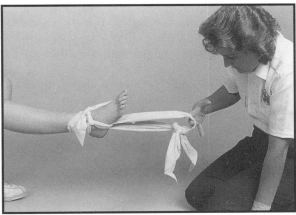

The reader should note that there are a variety of different ways to make an ankle hitch with a cravat in order to obtain a secure purchase around the proximal leg and foot. Some, which only provide a simple loop around the lower leg, result in undesirable rotation and plantar extension of the foot and are *NOT* recommended. The previously demonstrated method is one of the best or the single best method for this purpose. Crossing the cravat at both the posterior and anterior sides of the cravat and then reversing its direction at the side of the foot provides desirable friction of the cravat against itself and balanced simultaneous opposing (anterior-to-posterior and posterior-to-anterior) tension around the foot. This keeps the stirrup from becoming pulled off or misplaced from the instep of the foot (common with other methods) and causes the traction to be pulled in a straight line along the long axis of the leg. This is essential to maintaining the foot in a proper neutral position and for referring the traction properly along the entire length of the leg.

6. After passing one end of the cravat around the end of the frame or perpendicular bracket at the distal end of the long shaft(s) of the previously installed traction device, tie the ends securely together so that the cravat forms a *tight* loop between the stirrup and the perpendicular extension of the distal end of the device directly beyond the midline of the foot. Once the cravat loop is properly positioned around the device's distal perpendicular extension, further secure both together with tight adhesive tape to prevent it from being displaced laterally.

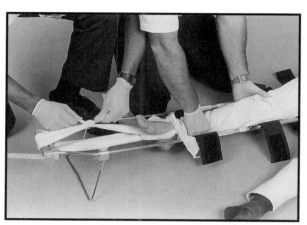

7. Tongue blades are an ideal length but are too weak singly for the stick you will need. Tape between 6 and 9 together to make a sufficiently sturdy stick. *Do NOT use pens, pencils, or dead branches as these are too weak and may break, suddenly releasing the traction.* If tongue blades are not available, cut a 6 to 7 inch section of a "green" live branch that has a 1/2 inch or slightly greater diameter. Insert the taped-together tongue blades or stick between the two sides of the cravat loop.

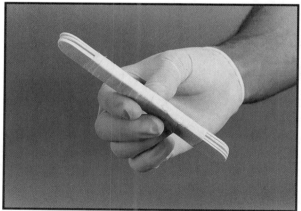

8. Hold the stick so it is centered at about the midpoint of the cravat loop and perpendicular to its sides. Being careful not to lose your hold on the stick, turn it end-over-end to wind the sides of the cravat loop and progressively shorten it. You should limit each single turn of the stick to 180 degrees or less, and use both hands to ensure that this is done in a stable manner. As you complete each half-turn and the end of the stick approaches the shaft of the device, the stick must be temporarily slightly angled to let it pass.

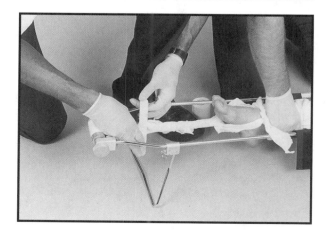

9. Usually, the first 3 to 6 half-turns of the stick stretch-out the fabric of both cravats and tighten the ankle hitch and loop without resulting in any significant traction being applied to the leg. Once the structure has been sufficiently wound to complete the "tightening-up," the EMT should feel a progressive increase in the pressure needed to complete each half-turn of the stick as traction is initiated and increased. Temporarily stop turning the stick at this point.

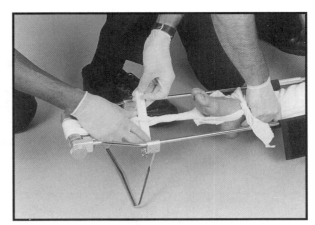

10. Adjust the lateral position of the stick through the wound sides of the cravat loop so that one end extends an inch beyond the shaft of the device when the stick is perpendicular and lies against it. *Be careful that a safe length of the stick remains through the cravat, and that you do NOT lose your hold on the stick.* Although this only becomes essential to properly secure the stick once sufficient traction has been applied, it must be done before the windlass is too tight to allow lateral movement of the stick.

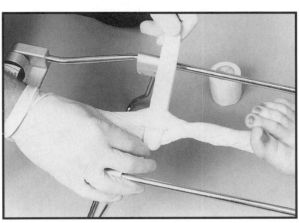

11. Resume making successive half-turns of the stick, angling it temporarily to allow it to pass the shaft of the splint at each turn. When by clinical observation you have determined that sufficient traction has been applied, turn the stick until its long end is just past the shaft of the device. While securely holding the stick perpendicularly against the shaft of the splint (the counter rotational side), firmly secure it with repeated wraps of 1 inch adhesive tape to form a figure-of-eight in the right angles formed by the shaft and the stick.

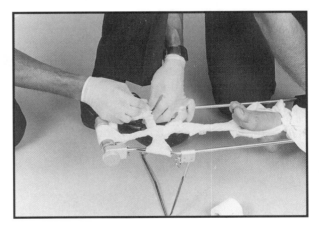

12. Once the traction has been secured, complete the remaining steps to further secure the leg to the device and properly package the patient. Do *NOT* become so distracted by the need to improvise a hitch and windlass that you forget to recheck the distal MSCs or to secure the patient's upper torso onto the longboard or cot so that he can not sit up and articulate his hip joint.

SKILLS FOR THE MANAGEMENT OF HIP INJURIES

The management of hip injuries has been touched on in the Introduction to this section and, when the injury is actually a fracture of the proximal neck of the femur, in the Introduction to the use of traction devices.

When a hip is displaced it is almost always a posterior dislocation and the patient presents with the injured leg flexed and drawn up so that the knee is over the opposite knee or thigh. Few of these patients will tolerate any movement of the hip or repositioning of the leg. The patient can best be immobilized by placing him on his uninjured side on a longboard, packaging the legs together in the position found with a pillow between the knees, and additional pillows and blanket rolls placed as needed to support the patient on his side.

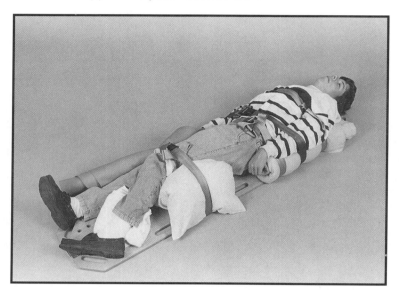

In the extremely rare case that there is an anterior dislocation, the leg is usually found extended straight and rotated outward (the foot points away from the body's midline). This presentation is also common with fractures of the proximal head of the Femur. The EMT should only attempt to move the leg into a neutral in-line position if other injuries recommend the use of a traction splint or the PASG. When the patient is to be splinted with the leg straight and rotated outward, he should be placed supine on a longboard with pillows under and next to the knee to support it in the approximate position of deformity in which it was found.

General Splinting Sequence

1. CONFIRM that the proper BODY SUBSTANCE ISOLATION PRECAUTIONS have been taken, AND that the PATIENT'S CONDITION ALLOWS sufficient time FOR INDIVIDUAL musculoskeletal INJURY CARE.

2. Remove and/or cut off all clothing which covers the extremity, and identify and CONTROL ANY EXTERNAL BLEEDING.

3. IDENTIFY ALL OF THE EXTREMITY INJURIES AND DETERMINE THE POSITION IN WHICH YOU WILL PACKAGE THE INJURED EXTREMITY.

4. REMOVE ALL JEWELRY (or other potentially constricting items) FROM ANY INJURED EXTREMITY.

5. ALIGN THE LIMB AS NEEDED TO APPLY THE SPLINT. Realign one section at a time (e.g., hand, then forearm, then upper arm, etc.), working from the distal to the proximal end.

6. From those available, SELECT THE appropriate size and type of SPLINT TO BE USED and collect the other materials you will need.

7. APPLY DRESSINGS OVER ANY OPEN WOUNDS.

8. While a second EMT supports the limb, MEASURE AND PREPARE THE SPLINT (pad, cut, bend, etc.) as needed so it will properly support and immobilize the longbone area and adjacent joints (j-<u>B</u>-j) or, in the case of a joint injury the bones and joints adjacent to the injury site (j-b-<u>J</u>-b-j), when applied.

9. Properly LOCATE THE SPLINT AGAINST THE INJURED AREA AND ADJUST IT AS NEEDED.

10. ADD any ADDITIONAL PADDING as needed.

11. SECURE THE SPLINT TO THE EXTREMITY (apply bandaging, ties, or Velcro Fasteners – or add or evacuate air from the device as is appropriate to securing the device (and rigidly forming it) against the extremity.

12. FURTHER POSITION THE splinted EXTREMITY AS NEEDED, and PACKAGE IT TO THE REST OF THE BODY to provide additional support and immobilization (e.g., with the arm across the thorax with a sling-and-swathe or tied extended against side of body, or by tying the legs together with a long rigid splint secured between them).

13. CHECK THE DISTAL MSCs in all splinted or packaged extremities.

14. PLACE THE PATIENT ON A LONGBOARD (or directly onto the ambulance cot if allowed by the injuries).

15. Add any pillows or blanket rolls that may be required for additional support or immobilization, and SECURE THE PATIENT PROPERLY TO THE BOARD AND THEN TO THE COT (or directly to the COT when a longboard was not deemed necessary).

16. RECHECK THE distal MSCs.

17. RE-EVALUATE THE patient's ABCs.

18. INITIATE TRANSPORT and PERIODICALLY RECHECK the MSCs and ABCs while enroute to the hospital.

Applying a Bipolar Traction Splint (Hare)

1. CONFIRM that the proper BODY SUBSTANCE ISOLATION PRECAUTIONS have been taken.

2. Remove/cut open all clothing (except loose undergarments) covering the leg and identify and CONTROL ANY EXTERNAL BLEEDING.

3. CONFIRM THAT the PATIENT'S CONDITION INDICATES AND ALLOWS TIME FOR the APPLICATION OF A TRACTION SPLINT, AND RULE OUT any OTHER CONTRAINDICATIONS OR THE NEED FOR application of THE PASG.

4. CHECK the distal MSCs.

5. While you support the leg on the ground and a third responder provides the necessary countertraction at the armpits, DIRECT a second EMT TO INSTALL THE separated ANKLE HARNESS AND APPLY MANUAL TRACTION to realign the leg and elevate it.

6. Open the cradles and ischial strap of the splint, and measure and ADJUST THE SPLINT TO THE PROPER LENGTH.

7. INSERT THE SPLINT under the injured leg and LOWER THE foldable STAND found near its distal end.

8. Adjust the position of the proximal end of the splint under the buttock so that it properly aligns at the groin, and SECURE THE ISCHIAL STRAP around the leg.

9. Release the lock on the windlass strap and PULL A SUFFICIENT LENGTH OF THE STRAP OFF OF THE WINDLASS to easily reach the bottom of the foot.

10. SECURE THE "S"-HOOK at the end of the windlass strap to each of the TABS (which extend beyond the foot) OF THE ANKLE HARNESS.

11. WIND THE WINDLASS UNTIL SUFFICIENT MECHANICAL TRACTION IS APPLIED. Direct the second EMT to release his manual traction.

12. PROPERLY POSITION THE CRADLES along the length of the splint, AND SECURE EACH OVER THE LEG.

13. CHECK THE distal MSCs in the injured leg.

14. PLACE THE PATIENT ON A LONGBOARD (or directly on the cot) AND SECURE HIS LOWER TORSO AND LEGS to the board with a strap over both iliac crests and one over the lower legs.

15. SECURELY TAPE THE BASE OF THE SPLINT'S STAND ONTO THE BOARD and place padding between the stand's medial side and the uninjured leg.

16. SECURE THE PATIENT FROM sitting up and ARTICULATING THE HIP JOINT BY PASSING A STRAP from the board through both armpits and ACROSS THE UPPER TORSO.

17. RECHECK THE distal MSCs in both legs and RE-EVALUATE the patient's ABCs.

Note: With some adjustment in details, this sheet can be used as a general guide for the use of any bipolar traction splint.

ETI SUMMARY SKILL SHEET

Applying a Unipolar Traction Device (Sager)

1. CONFIRM that the proper BODY SUBSTANCE ISOLATION PRECAUTIONS have been taken.

2. Remove/cut off all clothing (except loose undergarments) covering the leg, and identify and CONTROL ANY EXTERNAL BLEEDING.

3. CONFIRM THAT the PATIENT'S CONDITION INDICATES AND ALLOWS TIME FOR application of THE TRACTION DEVICE, and RULE OUT any OTHER CONTRAINDICATIONS, OR NEED FOR THE PASG.

4. Check the distal MSCs.

5. While a second EMT supports the leg and foot on the ground, measure and ADJUST THE DEVICE TO THE PROPER LENGTH so that when applied, the perpendicular bracket or pulley found at the distal end of the device lies just beyond the bottom of the foot.

6. Place the device against the medial side of the injured leg and, with the patient's help, POSITION THE "T" AT THE PROXIMAL END OF THE DEVICE AGAINST THE PELVIS between the medial side of the leg and genitalia, AND SECURE THE ISCHIAL STRAP AROUND THE LEG.

7. Insert the opened ankle harness under the leg. Position it so that its lower edge is proximal to the ankle bone and then SECURE THE ANKLE HARNESS AROUND THE LOWER LEG.

8. While holding the proximal section from moving, EXTEND THE DISTAL SECTION OF THE SHAFT OF THE SPLINT UNTIL THE CORRECT AMOUNT OF TRACTION IS APPLIED (Indicated by the gauge on the device or clinical observation.)

9. TIE BOTH FEET TOGETHER by applying the narrow strap provided in a figure-of-eight around the ankles and feet.

10. Insert the longest of the three elastic cravats under the knee. After positioning it proximal to the knees, SECURE THE WIDE ELASTIC CRAVAT AROUND THE UPPER LEGS AND THE SHAFT OF THE DEVICE.

11. After inserting it and properly positioning it under the legs distal to the knees, SECURE THE SHORTEST ELASTIC CRAVAT AROUND BOTH LOWER LEGS and the shaft of the device.

12. Insert and SECURE THE THIRD ELASTIC CRAVAT AROUND BOTH KNEES and the shaft of the device.

13. CHECK the distal MSCs IN BOTH LEGS.

14. PLACE THE splinted PATIENT ON A LONGBOARD (or directly on the ambulance cot) and SECURE HIS LEGS AND THE SPLINT to the board WITH A STRAP ACROSS BOTH ILIAC CRESTS AND ONE ACROSS THE PACKAGED LOWER LEGS.

15. SECURE THE PATIENT FROM sitting up and ARTICULATING THE HIP JOINTS BY ADDING A STRAP from the board through both armpits and ACROSS THE UPPER TORSO.

16. RECHECK THE distal MSCs IN BOTH LEGS AND THE PATIENT'S ABCs.

Note: With some modifications, the preceding steps can be adopted and used in cases which dictate the application of manual traction prior to the application of the Sager Traction Device. They can, with some alteration in the details of some of the steps, also serve as a general guide when applying the Kendrick or other unipolar traction devices.

SECTION

Skills Evaluation and Testing

Introduction

Skills are said to be evaluated to *level-of-competence.* Simply stated, that means that when a provider has obtained a skill to the level-of competence, he can reproduce it in a proper manner whenever requested or required. It also implies that in the process he will not do anything which causes unnecessary dangerous side-effects (to the patient or to the EMT), or omit anything which—if *NOT* included—produces a similar danger.

One can not totally avoid some degree of subjectivity when evaluating skills performance. However, by the use of carefully devised criteria and properly segmented scoring of the skill's component parts, the evaluator can minimize the subjectivity and maximize the objectivity of his evaluation of the candidate's performance.

The exact task to be evaluated must be clearly defined. There is a significant difference in evaluating how a candidate applies a Hare Traction Splint and the broader task of how well he can provide suitable traction (using a device of his choosing) for a confirmed or suspected fracture of the shaft of the femur. When evaluating end-of -course practical skills, or for certification, the question that must be answered by the candidate's skill demonstration is the latter. The candidate should be evaluated on how appropriately he can meet the patient's therapeutic needs rather than how well he can use one type of device or one method. Once the specific skill to be evaluated has been defined, criteria for evaluating the EMT's performance can be established. Overly detailed criteria will favor one technique and allow only one specific method to be "right". If the criteria are too general they will force the evaluator to subjectively decide whether or not the skill was appropriately performed. Good criteria are generic to any acceptable method without being so vague as to be meaningless. If the criteria are either too detailed and rigid, or too general and vague, they will promote "my-way-or-the-highway" (do it my way or fail) testing.

Although they basically contain the same content, skills evaluation sheets require a different design than those used as teaching adjuncts when introducing a skill and assisting the EMT in learning the required steps and sequence. Evaluation forms must be more concise and must be easy to use while observing the candidate's performance.

When the testing instruments are well constructed and employ criteria which are focused upon the desired therapeutic effect and the patient's needs, rather than upon the desired equipment used, they provide the examiner with a proper framework for his evaluation. Practical testing evaluation sheets should have two functional parts. One should be a list of **critical criteria.** These are commonly both positive and negative items, reflecting steps that must be done and items that the EMT should *NOT* do when the skill is appropriately performed. Secondly, each of the steps and sub-steps should have a point value. A minimum number of points should be required in order to demonstrate sufficient capability in performing the skill.

Each of these functional parts serves a key purpose. The *critical criteria* prevent someone who missed a key item or sequence, or who caused a harmful side effect to the patient, from passing the skill requirements. The point system identifies students who, even though they did all of the critical steps and didn't injure the patient, are still not sufficiently fluent in the skill.

The only item on a practical skill evaluation that benefits from the secrecy is the minimum number of points required to pass the skill. Most of the experts who have pondered over problems in designing skills testing agree that if the examiner knows the minimum number of points required to pass the skill, it may influence his scoring in border-line cases. Without that knowledge, he is more likely to focus on the sub-parts without regard to the cumulative points earned and whether they produce a passing or failing score.

The National Registry of Emergency Medical Technicians of Columbus, Ohio, is the largest EMT testing organization in the United States (and probably the world). Although the certification and/or licensure of EMTs and other pre-hospital providers is the responsibility of each individual State and Territory, many states use the National Registry test as the required written and practical evaluation tool to establish that the EMT has the necessary knowledge and skills to be certified. Many other states, which have their own unique written and practical exams, recognize the National Registry's tests as an acceptable equivalent to their own, and will accept National Registry status in lieu of their state test. Due to the broad national basis and experience of the Registry, many of the practical exams (and skills evaluation instruments) which are used by individual states emulate the concepts and design of those developed by the National Registry.

Recognizing many of the past problems in the evaluation of EMT skills competence, in 1989 the National Registry started the task of re-evaluating and improving its practical testing. It convened two committees, one for the Basic EMT level and one for the Advanced (EMT-Intermediate and EMT-Paramedic) levels, to re-examine the entire subject. EMS educational and testing experts from throughout the country were selected to serve on each committee. With intense work done over a four year period, these Committees and the Staff of the National Registry developed new practical examinations for each level. Included in this product were the new performance measurement instruments and directions that each examination required. After pilot testing and some adjustment, and careful review by the National Registry's Standards and Examination Committee and Board of Directors, these new examinations were phased into use and are the current standard for EMS skills evaluation. With the recent completion of the newly proposed and differently focused EMT-Basic Curriculum, the Basic Practical Exam Committee and Registry Staff members revised and extended the Basic Level Practical Exam. This produced a second Basic Exam which includes the practical stations and instruments that will be needed to evaluate candidates who are trained using the terminology, concepts and material included in the revised 1994 Curriculum.

In order to make all of their skills evaluation forms as widely available to EMTs as possible, the National Registry has allowed the publishers to include them in EMT texts. We are indebted to the National Registry for the exceptional quality and labor these represent, and for their permission to use them in this book. Without the inclusion of the testing skills sheets which represent the standard-of-the-art for practical skills evaluation, this book would not be truly "comprehensive". These evaluation forms are the property of the National Registry of EMTs. Those wishing to duplicate them should contact the National Registry for permission, as they—rather than the publisher of this text—hold the copyrights for these forms.

Although some of these sheets are common to both formats for the Basic exam (1984 and 1994), and often to several of the EMT levels examined, they are presented for clarity in the following pages in three separate parts. Each reflects all of the National Registry instruments presently developed for each of the different areas of practical testing:

Part A—**Present Basic Level** (Based on the 1984 Curriculum)

Part B—**Advanced Level** (Both EMT-Intermediate and EMT-Paramedic Levels)

Part C—**Proposed New Basic Level** (Based on the 1994 Curriculum)

If the reader is unsure which may be included in a particular practical exam, he should ask his instructor to identify them for him. The National Registry of EMTs has materials available which instructors can distribute to examination candidates, describing the skills included in each level and the format of the examination.

These testing sheets are the versions being used in National Registry Exams at the date of publication of this text. However, the reader should note that with time these may be modified or new ones added and some deleted. They are included here only as a general evaluation guide for the reader, and should not be interpreted to represent the practical testing content of any specific examination. The reader should contact his educational institution or the National Registry to obtain the correct current expectation for a particular examination date and site.

PART A
Practical Testing Skill Sheets
Basic Level Exam
— For Courses Following The 1984 Basic EMT Curriculum —

National Registry of Emergency Medical Technicians
Basic Level Practical Examination
PATIENT ASSESSMENT/MANAGEMENT

Candidate: _____   Examiner: _____

Date: _____   Signature: _____

PRIMARY SURVEY/RESUSCITATION

		Possible Points	Points Awarded
Takes or verbalizes infection control precautions		1	
Airway with 'C' Spine	Must be done manually or without compromising "C" spine		
	Assessment	1	
	Treatment	1	
Breathing	Assessment	1	
	Oxygen therapy & ventilation	1	
	Injury management	1	
Circulation	Assess pulse	1	
	Assess skin	1	
	Bleeding control	1	
	Verbalize application of or consideration for PASG (must assess body parts to be enclosed)	1	
	Assess vital signs	1	
Disability	Mini-neuro - AVPU	1	
	Assess neurological function in extremities	1	
	Assess eyes (PEARL)	1	
Expose	Remove clothing	1	
Status	Correctly identifies need to immediately transport or . . . Do secondary survey on the scene	1	

SECONDARY SURVEY

Head	Inspection and palpitation of scalp & ears	1	
	Assessment of eyes	1	
	Assessment of facial area including oral & nasal area	1	
Neck	Assesses condition of trachea & jugular veins	1	
	May be done before C-collar placement	1	
Chest	Inspection	1	
	Palpation	1	
	Auscultation of chest	1	
Abdomen/Pelvis	Assessment of abdomen	1	
	Assessment of pelvis	1	
Lower Extremities	1 point for each extremity includes inspection, assessment of pulses, sensory and motor activities	2	
Upper Extremities	1 point for each extremity includes inspection, assessment of pulses, sensory and motor activities	2	
Posterior Thorax/Lumbar	Assesses throax area	1	
	Assesses lumbar area	1	
Manages fractures and secondary wounds appropriately Points for appropriate management of each fracture and wound up to a maximum of 2 points		2	
	TOTAL	34	

CRITICAL CRITERIA

_____ Did not immediately establish and maintain spinal protection
_____ Did not provide high concentration of oxygen
_____ Did not evaluate and find conditions of airway, breathing and circulation (shock)
_____ Did not manage/provide airway, breathing, hemorrhage control or treatment for shock
_____ Did not differentiate patient's needing transportation versus continued on scene survey
_____ Does other detailed physical examination before airway, breathing and circulation
_____ Does not transport patient within ten (10) minute time limit
_____ Did not take or verbalize infection control precautions

Please place comments on reverse side

National Registry of Emergency Medical Technicians
Basic Level Practical Examination
AIRWAY – OXYGEN – VENTILATION
OROPHARYNGEAL/NASOPHARYNGEAL AIRWAY

Candidate: _____ Examiner: _____
Date: _____ Signature: _____

INSTRUCTIONS TO THE PRACTICAL SKILLS CANDIDATE

This station is designed to test your ability to properly measure, insert and remove an oropharyngeal airway and measure and insert a nasopharyngeal airway. This is an isolated skills test and you are not required to perform a primary or secondary survey. You may use any equipment available in this room. You have five (5) minutes to complete this procedure. Do you have any questions?

	Possible Points	Points Awarded
OROPHARYNGEAL AIRWAY		
Takes or verbalizes infection control precautions	1	
Selects appropriate size airway	1	
Measures appropriate size airway	1	
Inserts airway without pushing tongue posteriorly	1	
Note: The examiner must advise the candidate that the patient is gagging and becoming conscious		
Removes oropharyngeal airway	1	
NASOPHARYNGEAL AIRWAY		
Note: The examiner must advise the candidate to insert a nasopharyngeal airway		
Selects appropriate size airway (length and diameter)	1	
Measures airway	1	
Verbalizes lubrication of tube	1	
Fully inserts airway with bevel facing the septum	1	
TOTAL:	9	

CRITICAL CRITERIA
____ Did not take or verbalize infection control precaution
____ Did not obtain patent airway with oropharyngeal airway
____ Did not obtain patent airway with nasopharyngeal airway

Comments: _____

National Registry of Emergency Medical Technicians
Basic Level Practical Examination
AIRWAY – OXYGEN – VENTILATION
BAG-VALVE-MASK APNEIC PATIENT WITH PULSE

Candidate: _____ Examiner: _____
Date: _____ Signature: _____

INSTRUCTIONS TO THE PRACTICAL SKILLS CANDIDATE

This station is designed to test your ability to ventilate a patient using a bag-valve-mask. As you enter the station you will find an apneic patient with a palpable central pulse. There are no bystanders and artificial ventilation has not been initiated. The only patient management required is ventilatory support using a bag-valve-mask. You must initially ventilate the patient for a period of 30 seconds and an additional 30 seconds once high flow oxygen is connected to the bag-valve-mask. You will be evaluated on appropriateness of ventilatory volumes. You may use any equipment available in this room. You have five (5) minutes to complete this skill station. Do you have any questions?

	Possible Points	Points Awarded
Takes or verbalizes infection control precautions	1	
Voices opening airway	1	
Voices inserting adjunct	1	
Selects appropriate size mask	1	
Ventilates patient at no less than 800 ml volume	1	
Continues at proper volume/breath	1	
(The examiner must witness for at least 30 seconds)		
Connects reservoir and oxygen	1	
Adjusts flow rate to 12 liters/minute or greater	1	
Resumes ventilation at proper volume/breath	1	
(The examiner must witness for at least 30 seconds)		
TOTAL:	9	

CRITICAL CRITERIA
____ Did not take or verbalize infection control precautions
____ Did not immediately ventilate the patient
____ Interrupted ventilations for more than 20 seconds
____ Did not provide high concentration of oxygen
____ Did not provide proper volume/breath
         (more than 2 of the ventilations per minute are below 800 ml)
____ Did not allow adequate exhalation

Comments: _____

National Registry of Emergency Medical Technicians
Basic Level Practical Examination
**AIRWAY – OXYGEN – VENTILATION
MOUTH-TO-MASK WITH SUPPLEMENTAL OXYGEN**

Candidate: _____
Date: _____   Examiner: _____
Signature: _____

INSTRUCTIONS TO THE PRACTICAL SKILLS CANDIDATE

This station is designed to test your ability to ventilate a patient with supplemental oxygen using a mouth-to-mask technique. This is an isolated skills test. You may assume that mouth-to-mouth ventilation is in progress and that the patient has a central pulse. The only patient management required is ventilatory support using a mouth-to-mask technique with supplemental oxygen. You must ventilate the patient for at least 30 seconds. You will be evaluated on the appropriateness of ventilatory volumes. You may use any equipment available in this room. You have five (5) minutes to complete this procedure. Do you have any questions?

	Possible Points	Points Awarded
Takes or verbalizes infection control precautions	1	
Connects mask to supplemental oxygen	1	
Adjusts flow rate to greater than 10 liters/minute	1	
Opens airway either manually or with adjunct	1	
Establishes and maintains proper mask seal	1	
Ventilates patient at no less than 800 ml volume/breath	1	
(Note: The examiner must witness for at least 30 seconds)		
TOTAL:	6	

CRITICAL CRITERIA

____ Did not take or verbalize infection control precautions

____ Did not provide high concentration oxygen

____ Did not provide proper volume/breath
    (more than 2 of the ventilations/minute are below 800 ml)

____ Did not allow adequate exhalation

Comments: _____

National Registry of Emergency Medical Technicians
Basic Level Practical Examination
**AIRWAY – OXYGEN – VENTILATION
SUPPLEMENTAL OXYGEN ADMINISTRATION**

Candidate: _____
Date: _____   Examiner: _____
Signature: _____

INSTRUCTIONS TO THE PRACTICAL SKILLS CANDIDATE

This station is designed to test your ability to correctly assemble the equipment needed to administer supplemental oxygen in the pre-hospital setting. This is an isolated skills test. You will be required to assemble an oxygen tank and a regulator and administer oxygen to a patient using a nasal cannula. At this point you will be instructed to continue oxygen administration using a non-rebreather mask. Once you have initiated oxygen administration using a non-rebreather mask, you will be instructed to discontinue oxygen administration completely. This includes relieving all pressure from the regulator. You may use any equipment available in this room. You have five (5) minutes to complete this procedure. Do you have any questions?

	Possible Points	Points Awarded
Takes or verbalizes infection control precautions	1	
Assembles regulator to tank	1	
Opens tank	1	
Checks for leaks	1	
Checks tank pressure	1	
Attaches nasal cannula to oxygen	1	
Adjusts liter flow to 6 liters/minute or less	1	
Applies nasal cannula to patient	1	
Note: The examiner must advise the candidate to change to a non-rebreather mask		
Attaches non-rebreather mask	1	
Prefills reservoir	1	
Adjusts liter flow to 10 liters/minute or greater	1	
Applies and adjusts mask to face	1	
Note: The examiner must advise the candidate to discontinue oxygen therapy		
Removes non-rebreather mask	1	
Shuts off regulator	1	
Relieves regulator pressure	1	
TOTAL:	15	

CRITICAL CRITERIA

____ Did not take or verbalize infection control precautions
____ Did not adjust device to a correct liter flow for nasal cannula (2 - 6 L)
____ Did not adjust device to a correct liter flow for a non-rebreather mask (10L or greater)
____ Did not assemble tank and regulator without leaks
____ Did not prefill reservoir

Comments: _____

National Registry of Emergency Medical Technicians
Basic Level Practical Examination
BLEEDING – WOUNDS – SHOCK

Candidate: _____ Examiner: _____
Date: _____ Signature: _____

INSTRUCTIONS TO THE PRACTICAL SKILLS CANDIDATE

This station is designed to test your ability to treat progressive shock due to a profound arterial hemorrhage. This is a scenario-based testing station. As you progress through the scenario, the examiner will offer various signs and symptoms appropriate for the patient's condition. You will be required to manage the patient based on these signs and symptoms. The examiner will read the scenario aloud to you and give you an opportunity to ask clarifying questions about the scenario. However, the examiner will not answer any questions about the actual steps of the procedures to be performed. You may use any supplies and equipment available in this room. You have ten (10) minutes to complete this procedure. Do you have any questions?

	Possible Points	Points Awarded
Takes or verbalizes infection control precautions	1	
Applies direct pressure to the wound	1	
Elevates the extremity	1	
Applies pressure dressing to the wound	1	
Bandages wound		
Note: The examiner must now inform the candidate that the wound is still continuing to bleed. The second dressing does not control the bleeding	1	
Locates and applies pressure to appropriate arterial pressure point	1	
Note: The examiner must indicate that the victim is in compensatory shock		
Applies high concentration oxygen	1	
Properly positions patient (supine with legs elevated)	1	
Prevents heat loss (covers patient as appropriate)	1	
Note: The examiner must indicate that the victim is in profound shock. Medical control has ordered application and inflation of the Pneumatic Anti-Shock Garment.		
Removes clothing and checks for sharp objects	1	
Quickly assesses areas that will be under the PASG	1	
Positions PASG with top of abdominal section at or below last set of ribs	1	
Secures PASG around patient	1	
Attaches hoses	1	
Begins inflation sequence (examiner to stop inflation at 15 mm Hg)	1	
Checks blood pressure	1	
Verbalizes when to stop inflation sequence	1	
Operates PASG to maintain air pressure in device	1	
Reassesses vital signs	1	
TOTAL:	19	

CRITICAL CRITERIA
___ Failure to take or verbalize infection control precautions
___ Did not apply high concentration of oxygen
___ Applies tourniquet before attempting other methods of hemorrhage control
___ Did not control hemorrhage or attempt to control hemorrhage in a timely manner
___ Inflates abdominal section of PASG before the legs
___ Did not reassess patient's vital signs after inflation of PASG
___ Places PASG on inside-out
___ Allows deflation of PASG after inflation
___ Positions PASG above level of the lowest rib

Please place comments on reverse side

National Registry of Emergency Medical Technicians
Basic Level Practical Examination
CARDIAC ARREST MANAGEMENT

Candidate: _____ Examiner: _____
Date: _____ Signature: _____

INSTRUCTIONS TO THE PRACTICAL SKILLS CANDIDATE

This station is designed to test your ability to manage a pre-hospital cardiac arrest by integrating CPR skills, airway adjuncts and patient/scene management skills. There will be an EMT assistant in this station. The EMT assistant will only do as you instruct him/her to do, and you are responsible for directing his/her actions. As you arrive on the scene you will encounter a patient in cardiac arrest. A first responder will be present performing single rescuer CPR. You must immediately establish control of the scene and effectively transition to two rescuer CPR using adjunctive equipment. You may not delegate this action to the EMT assistant. At some point in this procedure the evaluator will indicate a need for suction during CPR. You will be evaluated on your ability to accommodate this situation. Finally, you will be required to prepare the patient for transportation to the ambulance. You may use any supplies available in this room. You have ten (10) minutes to complete this skill station. Do you have any questions?

	Possible Points	Points Awarded
ASSESSMENT		
Takes or verbalizes infection control precautions	1	
Checks effectiveness of first responder's CPR in progress	2	
1 point each: pulse and ventilation		
(If he orders EMT to take over immediately, grant the two points)		
Directs to stop CPR and verifies absence of spontaneous pulse	1	
Gathers information on arrest events	1	
TRANSITION		
Directs resumption of 1 or 2 operator CPR	1	
Rescuer prepares airway/ventilation adjuncts	1	
INTEGRATION		
Verbalizes suctioning when necessary	1	
Oropharyngeal airway measured	1	
Verbalizes insertion of oropharyngeal airway	1	
Ventilation started with adjunct	1	
Supplemental high percentage oxygen connected to adjunct	1	
Patient ventilated with high concentration oxygen	1	
CPR continues without more than 20 seconds interruption	1	
Performs 2 operator CPR (with assistant) to standards	1	
Re-evaluates patient/CPR every few minutes	1	
TRANSPORTATION		
Prepares transportation device	1	
Assures patient is moved to rigid device (CPR or spine board) with no more than 30 seconds interruption	1	
Patient secured for transport	1	
TOTAL:	19	

CRITICAL CRITERIA
___ Does not verify absence of spontaneous pulse
___ Exceeds interruption of CPR time limits (see above)
___ Did not ventilate with high concentration oxygen
___ Did not direct performance of CPR according to standards
___ Did not perform CPR on firm surface

Please place comments on reverse side

National Registry of Emergency Medical Technicians
Basic Level Practical Examination
SPINAL IMMOBILIZATION SKILLS
SEATED PATIENT

Candidate: _____ Examiner: _____
Date: _____ Signature: _____

INSTRUCTIONS TO THE PRACTICAL SKILLS CANDIDATE

This station is designed to test your ability to provide spinal immobilization on a patient using a half spine immobilization device. You arrive on the scene with an EMT assistant. The scene is safe and there is only one (1) patient. The assistant EMT has completed the primary survey and no condition was found in the primary survey requiring intervention. For the purposes of this station the patient's vital signs remain stable. You are required to treat the specific, isolated problem of an unstable spine using a half spine immobilization device. You are responsible for directing the actions of the EMT assistant. Transferring the patient to the long spine board should be accomplished verbally. You may use any equipment available in this room. You have ten (10) minutes to complete this skill station. Do you have any questions?

	Possible Points	Points Awarded
Takes or verbalizes infection control precautions	1	
Directs assistant to place/maintain head in neutral in-line position	1	
Directs assistant to maintain manual immobilization of the head	1	
Assesses motor, sensory and distal circulation in extremities	1	
Applies appropriately-sized extrication collar	1	
Positions the immobilization device behind the patient	1	
Secures the device to the patient's torso	1	
Evaluates torso fixation and adjusts as necessary	1	
Evaluates and pads behind the patient's head as necessary	1	
Secures the patient's head to the device	1	
Verbalizes moving the patient to a long board	1	
Reassesses motor, sensory and distal circulation in extremities	1	
TOTAL:	12	

CRITICAL CRITERIA
___ Did not immediately direct or take manual immobilization of the head
___ Releases or orders release of manual immobilization before it was maintained mechanically
___ Patient manipulated or moved excessively causing potential spinal compromise
___ Device moves excessively up, down, left or right on patient's torso
___ Head immobilization allows for excessive movement
___ Torso fixation inhibits chest rise resulting in respiratory compromise
___ Upon completion of immobilization, head is not in neutral in-line position
___ Did not reassess motor, sensory and distal circulation after immobilization

Comments: _____

National Registry of Emergency Medical Technicians
Basic Level Practical Examination
SPINAL IMMOBILIZATION SKILLS
LYING PATIENT

Candidate: _____ Examiner: _____
Date: _____ Signature: _____

INSTRUCTIONS TO THE PRACTICAL SKILLS CANDIDATE

This station is designed to test your ability to provide spinal immobilization on a patient using a long spine immobilization device. You arrive on the scene with an EMT assistant. The assistant EMT has completed the primary survey and no critical condition was found in the primary survey requiring intervention. For the purposes of this station, the patient's vital signs remain stable. You are required to treat the specific, isolated problem of an unstable spine using a long spine immobilization device. When moving the patient to the device, you should use the help of the assistant EMT and the evaluator. The assistant EMT should control the head and cervical spine of the patient while you and the evaluator move the patient to the immobilization device. You are responsible for the directing the action of the EMT assistant. You may use any equipment available in this room. You have ten (10) minutes to complete this procedure. Do you have any questions?

	Possible Points	Points Awarded
Takes or verbalizes infection control precautions	1	
Directs assistant to place/maintain head in neutral in-line position	1	
Directs assistant to maintain manual immobilization of the head	1	
Assesses motor, sensory and distal circulation in extremities	1	
Applies appropriately-sized extrication collar	1	
Positions the immobilization device appropriately	1	
Moves victim onto device without compromising the integrity of the spine	1	
Applies padding to voids between the torso and the board as necessary	1	
Immobilizes torso to the device	1	
Evaluates and pads under the patient's head as necessary	1	
Immobilizes the patient's head to the device	1	
Secures legs to the device	1	
Secures victim's arms to the device	1	
Reassesses motor, sensory and distal circulation	1	
TOTAL:	14	

CRITICAL CRITERIA
___ Did not immediately direct manual immobilization
___ Orders release of manual immobilization before it was maintained mechanically
___ Did not complete immobilization of the torso prior to immobilizing the head
___ Device excessively moves up, down, left or right on patient's torso
___ Head immobilization allows for excessive movement
___ Head is not immobilized in neutral in-line position
___ Patient moved excessively causing potential spinal compromise
___ Did not reassess motor, sensory and distal circulation after immobilization

Comments: _____

National Registry of Emergency Medical Technicians
Basic Level Practical Examination
SPLINTING
(LONG BONE)

Candidate: _____   Examiner: _____
Date: _____   Signature: _____

INSTRUCTIONS TO THE PRACTICAL SKILLS CANDIDATE

This station is designed to test your ability to properly immobilize a closed, non-angulated long bone fracture. You are required to treat only the specific, isolated injury. The primary assessment has been accomplished on the victim and during the secondary survey a closed, non-angulated fracture of the _____ (humerus, radius, ulna, tibia, fibula) is detected. Continued assessment of the patient's airway, breathing and central circulation is not necessary. You may use any equipment available in this room. You have five (5) minutes to complete this procedure. Do you have any questions?

	Possible Points	Points Awarded
Takes or verbalizes infection control precautions	1	
Directs application of manual stabilization	1	
Assesses motor, sensory and distal circulation	1	
Note: Examiner acknowledges present and normal		
Measures splint	1	
Applies splint	1	
Immobilizes joint above fracture	1	
Immobilizes joint below fracture	1	
Secures entire injured extremity	1	
Immobilizes hand/foot in position of function	1	
Reassesses motor, sensory and distal circulation	1	
Note: Examiner acknowledges present and normal		
TOTAL:	10	

CRITICAL CRITERIA
____ Grossly moves injured extremity
____ Did not immobilize adjacent joints
____ Did not assess motor, sensory and distal circulation after splinting

Comments: _____

National Registry of Emergency Medical Technicians
Basic Level Practical Examination
SPLINTING
(JOINT)

Candidate: _____   Examiner: _____
Date: _____   Signature: _____

INSTRUCTIONS TO THE PRACTICAL SKILLS CANDIDATE

This station is designed to test your ability to properly immobilize a non-complicated shoulder dislocation. You are required to treat only the specific, isolated injury. The primary assessment has been accomplished on the victim and during the secondary survey you detect a shoulder dislocation. Continued assessment of the patient's airway, breathing and central circulation is not necessary. You may use any equipment available in this room. You have five (5) minutes to complete this procedure. Do you have any questions?

	Possible Points	Points Awarded
Takes or verbalizes infection control precautions	1	
Directs manual stabilization of injury	1	
Assesses motor, sensory and distal circulation	1	
Note: Examiner acknowledges present and normal		
Selects proper splinting materials	1	
Immobilizes site of injury	1	
Immobilizes bones above injured joint	1	
Immobilizes bones below injured joint	1	
Reassesses motor, sensory and distal circulation	1	
Note: Examiner acknowledges present and normal		
TOTAL:	8	

CRITICAL CRITERIA
____ Did not immobilize bone above/below injured joint
____ Did not support joint so that it doesn't bear distal weight
____ Did not assess motor, sensory and distal circulation after splinting

Comments: _____

National Registry of Emergency Medical Technicians
Basic Level Practical Examination
SPLINTING
(TRACTION SPLINT)

Candidate: _____   Examiner: _____

Date: _____   Signature: _____

INSTRUCTIONS TO THE PRACTICAL SKILLS CANDIDATE

This station is designed to test your ability to properly immobilize a mid-shaft femur fracture with a traction splint. You will have an EMT assistant to help you in the application of the device by applying manual traction when directed to do so. You are required to treat only the specific, isolated injury. The primary assessment has been accomplished on the victim and during the secondary survey you detect a mid-shaft femur fracture. Continued assessment of the patient's airway, breathing and central circulation is not necessary. You may use any equipment available in this room. You have ten (10) minutes to complete this procedure. Do you have any questions?

	Possible Points	Points Awarded
Takes or verbalizes infection control precautions	1	
Directs manual stabilization of injured leg	1	
Directs application of manual traction	1	
Assesses motor, sensory and distal circulation	1	
(Note: Examiner acknowledges present and normal)		
Prepares/adjusts splint to proper length	1	
Positions splint at injured leg	1	
Applies proximal securing device (e.g., ischial strap)	1	
Applies distal securing device (e.g., ankle hitch)	1	
Applies mechanical traction	1	
Positions/secures support straps	1	
Re-evaluates proximal/distal securing devices	1	
Reassesses motor, sensory and distal circulation	1	
Note: Examiner acknowledges normal and present		
Note: Examiner must ask candidate how he/she would prepare for transport		
Verbalizes securing torso to long board to immobilize hip	1	
Verbalizes securing splint to long board to prevent movement of splint	1	
TOTAL:	**14**	

CRITICAL CRITERIA

____ Loss of traction at any point after it is assumed
____ Did not reassess motor, sensory and distal circulation after splinting
____ The foot is excessively rotated or extended after splinting
____ Did not secure ischial strap before taking traction
____ Final immobilization failed to support femur or prevent rotation of the injured leg

NOTE: If sager is used without elevating the leg, application of manual traction is not necessary. Candidate will be awarded 1 point as if manual traction were applied.

NOTE: If the leg is elevated at all, manual traction must be applied before elevating the leg. The ankle hitch may be applied before elevating the leg and used to pull manual traction.

Please place comments on reverse side.

PART B
Practical Testing Skill Sheets
Advanced Level Exam
— **Includes Sheets For EMT-Intermediate And EMT-Paramedic Levels** —

National Registry of Emergency Medical Technicians
Advanced Level Practical Examination
PATIENT ASSESSMENT/MANAGEMENT

Candidate:_____ Examiner:_____

Date:_____ Signature:_____

Scenario #_____

Time Start:_____ Time End:_____

PRIMARY SURVEY/RESUSCITATION

		Possible Points	Points Awarded
Takes or verbalizes infection control precautions		1	
Airway with C-Spine Control	Takes or directs manual in-line immobilization of head (1 point) Opens and assesses airway (1 point) Inserts adjunct (1 point)	3	
Breathing	Assesses breathing (1 point) Initiates appropriate oxygen therapy (1 point) Assures adequate ventilation of patient (1 point) Manages any injury which may compromise breathing/ventilation (1 point)	4	

Circulation	Checks pulse (1 point)
	Assesses peripheral perfusion (1 point)
	  [checks either skin color, temperature, or capillary refill]
	Assesses for and controls major bleeding if present (1 point)
	Takes vital signs (1 point)
	Verbalizes application of or consideration for PASG (1 point)
	  [candidate must assess body parts to be enclosed prior to application].
		5	

	Volume replacement [usually deferred until patient loaded] - Initiates first IV line (1 point) - Initiates second IV line (1 point) - Selects appropriate catheters (1 point) - Selects appropriate IV solutions and administration sets (1 point) - Infuses at appropriate rate (1 point)	5	
Disability	Performs mini-neuro assessment: AVPU (1 point) Applies cervical collar (1 point)	2	
Expose	Removes clothing	1	
Status	Calls for immediate transport of the patient when indicated	1	

PRIMARY SURVEY/RESUSCITATION SUB-TOTAL 22 [ ]

SECONDARY SURVEY

NOTE: Areas denoted by **** may be integrated within sequence of Primary Survey

		Possible Points	Points Awarded
Head	Inspects mouth**, nose**, and assesses facial area (1 point) Inspects and palpates scalp and ears (1 point) Checks eyes: PEARRL** (1 point)	3	
Neck**	Checks position of trachea (1 point) Checks jugular veins (1 point) Palpates cervical spine (1 point)	3	
Chest**	Inspects chest (1 point) Palpates chest (1 point) Auscultates chest (1 point)	3	
Abdomen/Pelvis**	Inspects and palpates abdomen (1 point) Assesses pelvis (1 point)	2	
Lower Extremities**	Inspects and palpates left leg (1 point) Inspects and palpates right leg (1 point) Checks motor, sensory, and distal circulation (1 point/leg)	4	
Upper Extremities	Inspects and palpates left arm (1 point) Inspects and palpates right arm (1 point) Checks motor, sensory, and distal circulation (1 point/arm)	4	
Posterior Thorax/Lumbar** and Buttocks	Inspects and palpates posterior thorax (1 point) Inspects and palpates lumbar and buttocks area (1 point)	2	
Identifies and treats minor wounds/fractures appropriately (1 point each)		2	

SECONDARY SURVEY SUB-TOTAL 23 [ ]

CRITICAL CRITERIA
____ Failure to initiate or call for transport of the patient within 10 minute time limit
____ Failure to take or verbalize infection control precautions
____ Failure to immediately establish and maintain spinal protection
____ Failure to provide high concentration of oxygen
____ Failure to evaluate and find all presented conditions of airway, breathing, and circulation (shock)
____ Failure to appropriately manage/provide airway, breathing, hemorrhage control or treatment for shock
____ Failure to differentiate patient's needing transportation versus continued on-scene survey
____ Does other detailed physical examination before assessing & treating threats to airway, breathing & circulation

You must factually document your rationale for checking any of the above critical items on the reverse side of this form.

National Registry of Emergency Medical Technicians
Intermediate Practical Examination
VENTILATORY MANAGEMENT (EOA)

Candidate: _____   Examiner: _____

Date: _____   Signature: _____

NOTE: If candidate elects to initially ventilate with BVM attached to reservoir and oxygen, full credit must be awarded for steps denoted by "**" so long as first ventilation is delivered within initial 30 seconds.

	Possible Points	Points Awarded
Takes or verbalizes infection control precautions	1	
Opens the airway manually	1	
Elevates tongue, inserts simple adjunct [either oropharyngeal or nasopharyngeal airway]	1	
NOTE: Examiner now informs candidate no gag reflex is present and patient accepts adjunct		
**Ventilates patient immediately with bag-valve-mask device unattached to oxygen	1	
**Hyperventilates patient with room air	1	
NOTE: Examiner now informs candidate that ventilation is being performed without difficulty		
Attaches oxygen reservoir to bag-valve-mask device and connects to high flow oxygen regulator [12-15 liters/min.]	1	
Ventilates patient at a rate of 12-20/min. and volumes of at least 800ml	1	
NOTE: After 30 seconds, examiner auscultates and reports breath sounds are present and equal bilaterally and medical control has ordered placement of an EOA. The examiner must now take over ventilation.		
Directs assistant to hyperventilate patient	1	
Identifies/selects proper equipment	1	
Assembles airway	1	
Tests cuff	1	
Inflates mask	1	
Lubricates tube [may be verbalized]	1	
NOTE: Examiner to remove OPA and move out of way when candidate is prepared to insert EOA		
Positions head properly with neck in neutral or slightly flexed position	1	
Grasps tongue and mandible and elevates	1	
Inserts tube in same direction as curvature of pharynx	1	
Advances tube until mask sealed against face	1	
Ventilates patient while maintaining tight mask seal	1	
Directs confirmation of proper placement by auscultation bilaterally and over epigastrium	1	
Inflates cuff to proper pressure and disconnects syringe	1	
Continues ventilation of patient	1	
NOTE: Examiner to ask "If you had proper placement, what would you expect to hear?"		
	TOTAL 21	

CRITICAL CRITERIA
___ Failure to initiate ventilations within 30 seconds after applying gloves or interrupts ventilations for greater than 30 seconds at any time
___ Failure to take or verbalize infection control precautions
___ Failure to voice and ultimately provide high oxygen concentrations [at least 85%]
___ Failure to ventilate patient at rate of at least 12/minute
___ Failure to provide adequate volumes per breath [maximum 2 errors/minute permissable]
___ Failure to hyperventilate patient prior to placement of the EOA
___ Failure to successfully place the EOA within 3 attempts
___ Failure to assure proper tube placement by auscultation bilaterally and over the epigastrium
___ Inserts any adjunct in a manner dangerous to patient

You must factually document your rationale for checking any of the above critical items on the reverse side of this form.

National Registry of Emergency Medical Technicians
Paramedic Practical Examination
VENTILATORY MANAGEMENT (ET)

Candidate: _____   Examiner: _____

Date: _____   Signature: _____

NOTE: If candidate elects to initially ventilate with BVM attached to reservoir and oxygen, full credit must be awarded for steps denoted by "**" so long as first ventilation is delivered within initial 30 seconds.

	Possible Points	Points Awarded
Takes or verbalizes infection control precautions	1	
Opens the airway manually	1	
Elevates tongue, inserts simple adjunct [either oropharyngeal or nasopharyngeal airway]	1	
NOTE: Examiner now informs candidate no gag reflex is present and patient accepts adjunct		
**Ventilates patient immediately with bag-valve-mask device unattached to oxygen	1	
**Hyperventilates patient with room air	1	
NOTE: Examiner now informs candidate that ventilation is being performed without difficulty		
Attaches oxygen reservoir to bag-valve-mask device and connects to high flow oxygen regulator [12-15 liters/min.]	1	
Ventilates patient at a rate of 12-20/min. and volumes of at least 800ml	1	
NOTE: After 30 seconds, examiner auscultates and reports breath sounds are present and equal bilaterally and medical control has ordered intubation. The examiner must now take over ventilation.		
Directs assistant to hyperventilate patient	1	
Identifies/selects proper equipment for intubation	1	
Checks equipment for:	2	
- Cuff leaks (1 point)		
- Laryngoscope operational and bulb tight (1 point)		
NOTE: Examiner to remove OPA and move out of way when candidate is prepared to intubate		
Positions head properly	1	
Inserts blade while displacing tongue	1	
Elevates mandible with laryngoscope	1	
Introduces ET tube and advances to proper depth	1	
Inflates cuff to proper pressure and disconnects syringe	1	
Directs ventilation of patient	1	
Confirms proper placement by auscultation bilaterally and over epigastrium	1	
NOTE: Examiner to ask "If you had proper placement, what would you expect to hear?"		
Secures ET tube [may be verbalized]	1	
	TOTAL 19	

CRITICAL CRITERIA
___ Failure to initiate ventilations within 30 seconds after applying gloves or interrupts ventilations for greater than 30 seconds at any time
___ Failure to take or verbalize infection control precautions
___ Failure to voice and ultimately provide high oxygen concentrations [at least 85%]
___ Failure to ventilate patient at rate of at least 12/minute
___ Failure to provide adequate volumes per breath [maximum 2 errors/minute permissable]
___ Failure to hyperventilate patient prior to intubation
___ Using teeth as a fulcrum
___ Failure to successfully intubate within 3 attempts
___ Failure to assure proper tube placement by auscultation bilaterally and over the epigastrium
___ If used, stylette extends beyond end of ET tube
___ Inserts any adjunct in a manner dangerous to patient

You must factually document your rationale for checking any of the above critical items on the reverse side of this form.

National Registry of Emergency Medical Technicians
Paramedic Practical Examination
CARDIAC ARREST SKILLS STATION
DYNAMIC CARDIOLOGY

Candidate: _____
Examiner: _____

Date: _____
Signature: _____

Set #: _____
Time Start: _____ Time End: _____

	Possible Points	Points Awarded
Takes or verbalizes infection control precautions	1	
Checks level of responsiveness	1	
Checks ABC's	1	
Initiates CPR if appropriate [verbally]	1	
Performs "Quick Look" with paddles	1	
Correctly interprets initial rhythm	1	
Appropriately manages initial rhythm	2	
Notes change in rhythm	1	
Checks patient condition to include pulse and, if appropriate, BP	1	
Correctly interprets second rhythm	1	
Appropriately manages second rhythm	2	
Notes change in rhythm	1	
Checks patient condition to include pulse and, if appropriate, BP	1	
Correctly interprets third rhythm	1	
Appropriately manages third rhythm	2	
Notes change in rhythm	1	
Checks patient condition to include pulse and, if appropriate, BP	1	
Correctly interprets fourth rhythm	1	
Appropriately manages fourth rhythm	2	
Orders high percentages of supplemental oxygen at proper times	1	
TOTAL	**24**	

CRITICAL CRITERIA

___ Failure to deliver first shock in a timely manner due to operator delay in machine use or providing treatments other than CPR with simple adjuncts

___ Failure to deliver second or third shocks without delay other than the time required to reassess and recharge paddles

___ Failure to order or perform pulse checks before and after shocks

___ Failure to ensure the safety of self and others [verbalizes "All clear" and observes]

___ Inability to deliver DC shock [does not use machine properly]

___ Failure to demonstrate acceptable shock sequence

___ Failure to order initiation or resumption of CPR when appropriate

___ Failure to order correct management of airway [ET when appropriate]

___ Failure to order administration of appropriate oxygen at proper time

___ Failure to diagnose or treat 2 or more rhythms correctly

___ Orders administration of an inappropriate drug or lethal dosage

___ Failure to correctly diagnose or adequately treat v-fib, v-tach, or asystole

You must factually document your rationale for checking any of the above critical items on the reverse side of this form.

National Registry of Emergency Medical Technicians
Paramedic Practical Examination
CARDIAC ARREST SKILLS STATION
STATIC CARDIOLOGY

Candidate: _____
Examiner: _____

Date: _____
Signature: _____

Set #: _____

NOTE: No points for treatment may be awarded if the diagnosis is incorrect. Only document incorrect responses in spaces provided.

	Points Awarded	Possible Points
STRIP #1		
Diagnosis:		1
Treatment:		2
STRIP #2		
Diagnosis:		1
Treatment:		2
STRIP #3		
Diagnosis:		1
Treatment:		2
STRIP #4		
Diagnosis:		1
Treatment:		2
TOTAL		**12**

National Registry of Emergency Medical Technicians
Advanced Level Practical Examination
SPINAL IMMOBILIZATION
(SEATED PATIENT)

Candidate: _____

Date: _____

Examiner: _____

Signature: _____

Time Start: _____   Time End: _____

	Possible Points	Points Awarded
Takes or verbalizes infection control precautions	1	
Directs assistant to place/maintain head in neutral, in-line position	1	
Directs assistant to maintain manual immobilization of head	1	
Assesses motor, sensory, and distal circulation in extremities	1	
Applies appropriately sized extrication collar	1	
Positions the immobilization device behind the patient	1	
Secures device to the patient's torso	1	
Evaluates torso fixation and adjusts as necessary	1	
Evaluates and pads behind the patient's head as necessary	1	
Secures patient's head to the device	1	
Reassesses motor, sensory, and distal circulation in extremities	1	
Verbalizes moving the patient to a long board properly	1	
	TOTAL 12	

CRITICAL CRITERIA

___ Did not immediately direct or take manual immobilization of head

___ Releases or orders release of manual immobilization before it was maintained mechanically

___ Patient manipulated or moved excessively causing potential spinal compromise

___ Did not complete immobilization of the torso prior to immobilizing the head

___ Device moves excessively -p, down, left, or right on patient's torso

___ Torso fixation inhibits chest rise resulting in respiratory compromise

___ Head immobilization allows for excessive movement

___ Upon completion of immobilization, head is not in neutral, in-line position

You must factually document your rationale for checking any of the above critical items on the reverse side of this form.

National Registry of Emergency Medical Technicians
Advanced Level Practical Examination
INTRAVENOUS THERAPY

Candidate: _____

Date: _____

Examiner: _____

Signature: _____

Time Start: _____   Time End: _____

	Possible Points	Points Awarded
Checks selected IV fluid for: - Proper fluid (1 point) - Clarity (1 point)	2	
Selects appropriate catheter	1	
Selects proper administration set	1	
Connects IV tubing to the IV bag	1	
Prepares administration set [fills drip chamber and flushes tubing]	1	
Cuts or tears tape [at any time before venipuncture]	1	
Takes/verbalizes infection control precautions [prior to venipuncture]	1	
Applies tourniquet	1	
Palpates suitable vein	1	
Cleanses site appropriately	1	
Performs venipuncture - Inserts stylette (1 point) - Notes or verbalizes flashback (1 point) - Occludes vein proximal to catheter (1 point) - Removes stylette (1 point) - Connects IV tubing to catheter (1 point)	5	
Releases tourniquet	1	
Runs IV for a brief period to assure patent line	1	
Secures catheter [tapes securely or verbalizes]	1	
Adjusts flow rate as appropriate	1	
Disposes/verbalizes disposal of needle in proper container	1	
	TOTAL 21	

CRITICAL CRITERIA

___ Exceeded the 6 minute time limit in establishing a patent and properly adjusted IV

___ Failure to take or verbalize infection control precautions prior to performing venipuncture

___ Contaminates equipment or site without appropriately correcting situation

___ Any improper technique resulting in the potential for catheter shear or air embolism

___ Failure to successfully establish IV within 3 attempts during 6 minute time limit

___ Failure to dispose/verbalize disposal of needle in proper container

You must factually document your rationale for checking any of the above critical items on the reverse side of this form.

National Registry of Emergency Medical Technicians
Paramedic Practical Examination
INTRAVENOUS BOLUS MEDICATIONS

Candi-
date:_____

Examiner:_____

Date:_____

Signature:_____

Time Start:_____Time End:_____

NOTE: Check here (____) if candidate did not establish
a patent IV and do not evaluate these skills.

	Possible Points	Points Awarded
Asks patient for known allergies	1	
Selects correct medication	1	
Assures correct concentration of drug	1	
Assembles prefilled syringe correctly and dispels air	1	
Continues infection control precautions	1	
Cleanses injection site (Y-port or hub)	1	
Reaffirms medication	1	
Stops IV flow (pinches tubing)	1	
Administers correct dose at proper push rate	1	
Flushes tubing (runs wide open for a brief period)	1	
Adjusts drip rate to TKO (KVO)	1	
Voices proper disposal of syringe and needle	1	
Verbalizes need to observe patient for desired effect/adverse side effects	1	

CRITICAL CRITERIA   IV BOLUS SUB-TOTAL   13 [   ]

___Failure to begin administration of medication within 3 minute time limit

___Contaminates equipment or site without appropriately correcting situation

___Failure to adequately dispel air resulting in potential for air embolism

___Injects improper drug or dosage (wrong drug, incorrect amount, or pushes at inappropriate rate)

___Failure to flush IV tubing after injecting medication

___Recaps needle or failure to dispose/verbalize disposal of syringe and needle in proper container

INTRAVENOUS PIGGYBACK MEDICATIONS

	Possible Points	Points Awarded
Has confirmed allergies by now (award point if previously confirmed)		
Checks selected IV fluid for: - Proper fluid (1 point) - Clarity (1 point)	1 2	
Checks selected medication for: - Clarity (1 point) - Concentration of medication (1 point)	2	
Injects correct amount of medication into IV solution given scenario	1	
Connects appropriate administration set to medication solution	1	
Prepares administration set (fills drip chamber and flushes tubing)	1	
Attaches appropriate needle to administration set	1	
Continues infection control precautions	1	
Cleanses port of primary line	1	
Inserts needle into port without contamination	1	
Adjusts flow rate of secondary line as required	1	
Stops flow of primary line	1	
Securely tapes needle	1	
Verbalizes need to observe patient for desired effect/adverse side effects	1	
Labels medication/fluid bag	1	

CRITICAL CRITERIA   IV PIGGYBACK SUB-TOTAL   17 [   ]

___ Failure to begin administration of medication within 5 minute time limit

___ Contaminates equipment or site without appropriately correcting situation

___ Administers improper drug or dosage (wrong drug, incorrect amount, or infuses at inappropriate rate)

___ Failure to flush IV tubing of secondary line resulting in potential for air embolism

___ Failure to shut-off flow of primary line

You must factually document your rationale for checking any of the above critical items on the reverse side of this form.

National Registry of Emergency Medical Technicians
Advanced Level Practical Examination
RANDOM BASIC SKILLS
BLEEDING - WOUNDS - SHOCK

Candidate: _____

Date: _____

Examiner: _____

Signature: _____

Time Start: _____ Time End: _____

	Possible Points	Points Awarded
Takes or verbalizes infection control precautions	1	
Applies direct pressure to the wound	1	
Elevates the extremity	1	
Applies pressure dressing to the wound	1	
Bandages wound	1	
NOTE: The examiner must now inform the candidate that the wound is still continuing to bleed. The second dressing does not control the bleeding.		
Locates and applies pressure to appropriate arterial pressure point	1	
NOTE: The examiner must indicate that the victim is in compensatory shock.		
Applies high concentration oxygen	1	
Properly positions patient (supine with legs elevated)	1	
Prevents heat loss (covers patient as appropriate)	1	
NOTE: The examiner must indicate that the victim is in profound shock. Medical control has ordered application and inflation of the Pneumatic Anti-shock Garment.		
Removes clothing or checks for sharp objects	1	
Quickly assesses areas that will be under the PASG	1	
Positions PASG with top of abdominal section at or below last set of ribs	1	
Secures PASG around patient	1	
Attaches hoses	1	
Begins inflation sequence (examiner to stop inflation at 15mm Hg)	1	
Checks blood pressure	1	
Verbalizes when to stop inflation sequence	1	
Operates PASG to maintain air pressure in device	1	
Reassesses vital signs	1	
TOTAL	**19**	

CRITICAL CRITERIA

___ Failure to take or verbalize infection control precautions

___ Did not apply high concentration of oxygen

___ Applies tourniquet before attempting other methods of hemorrhage control

___ Did not control hemorrhage or attempt to control hemorrhage in a timely manner

___ Inflates abdominal section of PASG before the legs

___ Did not reassess patient's vital signs after PASG inflation

___ Places PASG on inside-out

___ Allows deflation of PASG after inflation

___ Positions PASG above level of lowest rib

You must factually document your rationale for checking any of the above critical items on the reverse side of this form.

National Registry of Emergency Medical Technicians
Advanced Level Practical Examination
RANDOM BASIC SKILLS
TRACTION SPLINTING

Candidate: _____

Date: _____

Examiner: _____

Signature: _____

Time Start: _____ Time End: _____

	Possible Points	Points Awarded
Takes or verbalizes infection control precautions	1	
Directs manual stabilization of injured leg	1	
Directs application of manual traction	1	
Assesses motor, sensory, and distal circulation	1	
NOTE: Examiner acknowledges present and normal		
Prepares/adjusts splint to proper length	1	
Positions splint at injured leg	1	
Applies proximal securing device (e.g. ischial strap)	1	
Applies distal securing device (e.g. ankle hitch)	1	
Applies mechanical traction	1	
Positions/secures support straps	1	
Re-evaluates proximal/distal securing devices	1	
Reassesses motor, sensory, and distal circulation	1	
NOTE: Examiner acknowledges present and normal		
Verbalizes securing torso to long board to immobilize hip	1	
Verbalizes securing splint to long board to prevent movement of splint	1	
TOTAL	**14**	

CRITICAL CRITERIA

___ Loss of traction at any point after it is assumed

___ Did not reassess motor, sensory, and distal circulation **after** splinting

___ The foot is excessively rotated or extended after splinting

___ Did not secure ischial strap **before** taking traction

___ Final immobilization failed to support femur or prevent rotation of injured leg

NOTE: If Sager is used without elevating the leg, application of manual traction is not necessary. Candidate will be awarded 1 point as if manual traction were applied.

NOTE: If the leg is elevated at all, manual traction must be applied before elevating the leg. The ankle hitch may be applied before elevating the leg and used to pull manual traction.

You must factually document your rationale for checking any of the above critical items on the reverse side of this form.

National Registry of Emergency Medical Technicians
Advanced Level Practical Examination
RANDOM BASIC SKILLS
LONG BONE IMMOBILIZATION

Candidate: _____ Examiner: _____

Date: _____ Signature: _____

Time Start: _____ Time End: _____

	Possible Points	Points Awarded
Takes or verbalizes infection control precautions	1	
Directs application of manual stabilization	1	
Assesses motor, sensory, and distal circulation	1	
NOTE: Examiner acknowledges present and normal		
Measures splint	1	
Applies splint	1	
Immobilizes joint above fracture	1	
Immobilizes joint below fracture	1	
Secures entire injured extremity	1	
Immobilizes hand/foot in position of function	1	
Reassesses motor, sensory, and distal circulation	1	
NOTE: Examiner acknowledges present and normal		
	TOTAL	10

CRITICAL CRITERIA

___ Grossly moves injured extremity

___ Did not immobilize adjacent joints, injury, or limb

___ Did not reassess motor, sensory, and distal circulation **after** splinting

You must factually document your rationale for checking any of the above critical items on the reverse side of this form.

National Registry of Emergency Medical Technicians
Advanced Level Practical Examination
RANDOM BASIC SKILLS
SPINAL IMMOBILIZATION
(LYING PATIENT)

Candidate _____ Examiner: _____

Date _____ Signature: _____

Time Start: _____ Time End: _____

	Possible Points	Points Awarded
Takes or verbalizes infection control procedures	1	
Directs assistant to move patient's head to the neutral in-line position	1	
Directs assistant to maintain manual immobilization of head	1	
Evaluates motor, sensory, and distal circulation in extremities	1	
Applies cervical collar	1	
Positions immobilization device appropriately	1	
Moves victim onto device without compromising the integrity of the spine	1	
Applies padding to voids between the torso and the board as necessary	1	
Immobilizes torso to the device	1	
Evaluates and pads under the patient's head as necessary	1	
Immobilizes the patient's head to the device	1	
Secures legs to the evice	1	
Secures victims arms to the board	1	
Reassesses motor, sensory, and distal circulation	1	
	TOTAL	14

CRITICAL CRITERIA

___ Did not immediately direct manual immobilization of head

___ Orders release of manual immobilization before it was maintained mechanically

___ Did not complete immobilization of the torso prior to immobilizing the head

___ Device excessively moves up, down, left or right on patient's torso

___ Head immobilization allows for excessive movement

___ Head is not immobilized in the neutral in-line position

___ Patient was moved excessively causing potential spinal compromise

___ Did not reassess motor, sensory, and distal circulation after immobilization

You must factually document your rationale for checking any of the above critical items on the reverse side of this form.

PART C
Practical Testing Skill Sheets
Proposed New Basic Level Exam
— For courses Following The 1994 Basic EMT Proposed Curriculum Revision —

PATIENT ASSESSMENT/MANAGEMENT
TRAUMA

		Points Possible	Points Awarded
Takes or verbalizes body substance isolation precautions		1	
SCENE SIZE-UP			
Determines the scene is safe		1	
Determines the mechanism of injury		1	
Determines the number of patients		1	
Requests additional help if necessary		1	
Considers stabilization of spine		1	
INITIAL ASSESSMENT			
Verbalizes general impression of patient		1	
Determines chief complaint/apparent life threats		1	
Determines responsiveness		1	
Assesses airway and breathing	Assessment	1	
	Initiates appropriate oxygen therapy	1	
	Assures adequate ventilation	1	
	Injury management	1	
Assesses circulation	Assesses for and controls major bleeding	1	
	Assesses pulse	1	
	Assesses skin (color, temperature and condition)	1	
Identifies priority patients/makes transport decision		1	
FOCUSED PHYSICAL EXAM AND HISTORY/RAPID TRAUMA ASSESSMENT			
Selects appropriate assessment (focused or rapid assessment)		1	
Obtains baseline vital signs		1	
Obtains S.A.M.P.L.E. history		1	
DETAILED PHYSICAL EXAMINATION			
Assesses the head	Inspects and palpates the scalp and ears	1	
	Assesses the eyes	1	
	Assesses the facial area including oral and nasal area	1	
Assesses the neck	Inspects and palpates the neck	1	
	Assesses for JVD	1	
	Assesses for tracheal deviation	1	
Assesses the chest	Inspects	1	
	Palpates	1	
	Auscultates the chest	1	
Assesses the abdomen/pelvis	Assesses the abdomen	1	
	Assesses the pelvis	1	
	Verbalizes assessment of genitalia/perineum as needed	1	
Assesses the extremities	1 point for each extremity includes inspection, palpation, and assessment of pulses, sensory and motor activities	4	
Assesses the posterior	Assesses thorax	1	
	Assesses lumbar	1	
Manages secondary injuries and wounds appropriately **1 point for appropriate management of each injury/wound up to a maximum of 2 points**		2	
Verbalizes reassessment of the vital signs		1	
	TOTAL:	41	

CRITICAL CRITERIA
___Did not take or verbalize body substance isolation precautions
___Did not assess for spinal protection
___Did not provide for spinal protection when indicated
___Did not provide high concentration of oxygen
___Did not evaluate and find conditions of airway, breathing, circulation (hypoperfusion)
___Did not manage/provide airway, breathing, hemorrhage control or treatment for shock (hypoperfusion)
___Did not differentiate patient's needing transportation versus continued on scene survey
___Does other detailed physical examination before assessing airway, breathing and circulation
___Did not transport patient within ten (10) minute time limit

PATIENT ASSESSMENT/MANAGEMENT
MEDICAL

		Points Possible	Points Awarded
Takes or verbalizes body substance isolation precautions		1	
SCENE SIZE-UP			
Determines the scene is safe		1	
Determines the mechanism of injury/nature of illness		1	
Determines the number of patients		1	
Requests additional help if necessary		1	
Considers stabilization of spine		1	
INITIAL ASSESSMENT			
Verbalizes general impression of the patient		1	
Determines chief complaint/apparent life threats		1	
Determines responsiveness/level of consciousness		1	
Assesses airway and breathing	Assessment	1	
	Initiates appropriate oxygen therapy	1	
	Assures adequate ventilation	1	
Assesses circulation	Assesses/controls major bleeding	1	
	Assesses pulse	1	
	Assesses skin (color, temperature and condition)	1	
Identifies priority patients/makes transport decision		1	
FOCUSED PHYSICAL EXAM AND HISTORY/RAPID ASSESSMENT			
Signs and Symptoms (Assess history of present illness)		1	

Respiratory	Cardiac	Altered Level of Consciousness	Allergic Reaction	Poisoning/Overdose	Environmental Emergency	Obstetrics	Behavioral
*Onset?	*Onset?	*Description of the episode	*History of allergies?	*Substance?	*Source?	*Are you pregnant?	*How do you feel?
*Provokes?	*Provokes?	*Onset?	*What were you exposed to?	*When did you ingest/become exposed?	*Environment?	*How long have you been pregnant?	*Determine suicidal tendencies
*Quality?	*Quality?	*Duration?	*How were you exposed?	*How much did you ingest?	*Duration?	*Pain or contractions?	*Is the patient a threat to self or others?
*Radiates?	*Radiates?	*Associated symptoms?	*Effects?	*Over what time period?	*Loss of consciousness?	*Bleeding or discharge?	*Is there a medical problem?
*Severity?	*Severity?	*Evidence of trauma?	*Progressions?	*Interventions?	*Effects - General or local?	*Do you feel the need to push?	*Past medical history?
*Time?	*Time?	*Interventions?	*Interventions?	*Estimated weight?		*Last menstrual period?	*Interventions?
*Interventions?	*Interventions?	*Seizures?		*Effects?		*Crowning?	*Medications?
		*Fever?					

	Points Possible	Points Awarded
Allergies	1	
Medications	1	
Past medical history	1	
Last meal	1	
Events leading to present illness (rule out trauma)	1	
Performs focused physical examination Assesses affected body part/system or, if indicated, completes rapid assessment	1	
VITALS (Obtains baseline vital signs)	1	
INTERVENTIONS Obtains medical direction or verbalizes standing order for medication interventions and verbalizes proper additional intervention/treatment	1	
TRANSPORT (Re-evaluates transport decision)	1	
Completes detailed physical examination	1	
ONGOING ASSESSMENT (verbalized)		
Repeats initial assessment	1	
Repeats vital signs	1	
Repeats focused assessment regarding patient complaint or injuries	1	
Checks interventions	1	
TOTAL:	31	

CRITICAL CRITERIA

___Did not take or verbalize body substance isolation precautions if necessary
___Did not determine scene safety
___Did not obtain medical direction or verbalize standing orders for medication interventions
___Did not provide high concentration of oxygen
___Did not evaluate and find conditions of airway, breathing, circulation
___Did not manage/provide airway, breathing, hemorrhage control or treatment for shock
___Did not differentiate patient's needing transportation versus continued assessment at the scene
___Does detailed or focused history/physical examination before assessing airway, breathing and circulation

AIRWAY MAINTENANCE
OROPHARYNGEAL AIRWAY

	Points Possible	Points Awarded
Takes or verbalizes body substance isolation precautions	1	
Selects appropriate size airway	1	
Measures airway	1	
Inserts airway without pushing the tongue posteriorly	1	
NOTE: The examiner must advise the candidate that the patient is gagging and becoming conscious		
Removes oropharyngeal airway	1	

SUCTION

	Points Possible	Points Awarded
NOTE: The examiner must advise the candidate to suction the patient's oropharynx/nasopharynx		
Turns on/prepares suction device	1	
Assures presence of mechanical suction	1	
Inserts suction tip without suction	1	
Applies suction to the oropharynx/nasopharynx	1	

NASOPHARYNGEAL AIRWAY

	Points Possible	Points Awarded
NOTE: The examiner must advise the candidate to insert a nasopharyngeal airway		
Selects appropriate size airway	1	
Measures airway	1	
Verbalizes lubrication of the nasal airway	1	
Fully inserts the airway with the bevel facing toward the septum	1	
TOTAL:	13	

CRITICAL CRITERIA

___ Did not take or verbalize body substance isolation precautions

___ Did not obtain a patent airway with the oropharyngeal airway

___ Did not obtain a patent airway with the nasopharyngeal airway

VENTILATORY MANAGEMENT
ESOPHAGEAL OBTURATOR AIRWAY INSERTION FOLLOWING AN UNSUCCESSFUL ENDOTRACHEAL INTUBATION ATTEMPT

	Points Possible	Points Awarded
Continues body substance isolation precautions	1	
Confirms the patient is being properly ventilated	1	
Directs assistant to hyperventilate the patient	1	
Identifies/selects proper equipment	1	
Assembles airway	1	
Tests cuff	1	
Inflates mask	1	
Lubricates tube (*may be verbalized*)	1	
Removes the oropharyngeal airway	1	
Positions head properly with neck in the neutral or slightly flexed position	1	
Grasps and elevates tongue and mandible	1	
Inserts tube in the same direction as the curvature of the pharynx	1	
Advances tube until the mask is sealed against the face	1	
Ventilates the patient while maintaining a tight mask seal	1	
Confirms placement by observing chest rise and auscultating over the epigastrium and bilaterally over the chest	1	
NOTE: The examiner confirms adequate chest rise, bilateral breath sounds and absent sounds over the epigastrium		
Inflates the cuff to the proper pressure and disconnects the syringe	1	
Continues ventilation of the patient	1	
Total:	17	

Critical Criteria

___ Did not take or verbalize body substance isolation precautions

___ Interrupts ventilation for more than 30 seconds

___ Did not direct hyperventilation of the patient prior to placement of the device

___ Did not assure proper placement of the device

___ Did not successfully ventilate the patient

___ Did not provide high flow oxygen (15 L/min or greater)

___ Inserts any adjunct in a manner that would be dangerous to the patient

VENTILATORY MANAGEMENT
ENDOTRACHEAL INTUBATION

NOTE: If a candidate elects to initially ventilate with a BVM attached to a reservoir and oxygen, full credit must be awarded for steps denoted by "**" if the first ventilation is delivered within the initial 30 seconds

	Points Possible	Points Awarded
Takes or verbalizes body substance isolation precautions	1	
Opens airway manually	1	
Elevates tongue and inserts simple airway adjunct (oropharyngeal or nasopharyngeal airway)	1	
NOTE: The examiner now informs the candidate no gag reflex is present and the patient accepts the adjunct		
**Ventilates the patient immediately using a BVM device unattached to oxygen	1	
**Hyperventilates the patient with room air	1	
NOTE: The examiner now informs the candidate that ventilation is being performed without difficulty		
Attaches the oxygen reservoir to the BVM	1	
Attaches BVM to high flow oxygen	1	
Ventilates the patient at the proper volume and rate (800-1200 ml per breath/10-20 breaths per minute)	1	
NOTE: After 30 seconds, the examiner auscultates and reports breath sounds are present and equal bilaterally and medical control has ordered intubation. The examiner must now take over ventilation.		
Directs assistant to hyperventilate patient	1	
Identifies/selects proper equipment for intubation	1	
Checks equipment — Checks for cuff leaks	1	
Checks laryngoscope operation and bulb tightness	1	
NOTE: The examiner must remove the OPA and move out of the way when the candidate is prepared to intubate		
Positions the head properly	1	
Inserts the laryngoscope blade while displacing the tongue	1	
Elevates the mandible with the laryngoscope	1	
Introduces the ET tube and advances it to the proper depth	1	
Inflates the cuff to the proper pressure and disconnects the syringe	1	
Directs ventilation of the patient	1	
Confirms proper placement by auscultation bilaterally and over the epigastrium	1	
NOTE: The examiner must ask, "If you had proper placement, what would you expect to hear?"		
Secures the ET tube (*may be verbalized*)	1	
TOTAL:	20	

CRITICAL CRITERIA

___ Did not take or verbalize body substance isolation precautions
___ Did not initiate ventilations within 30 seconds after applying gloves or interrupts ventilations for greater than 30 seconds at any time.
___ Did not voice or provide high oxygen concentrations (15 L/min or greater)
___ Did not ventilate patient at a rate of at least 10/minute
___ Did not provide adequate volume per breath (maximum of 2 errors/minute permissible)
___ Did not hyperventilate the patient prior to intubation
___ Did not successfully intubate within 3 attempts
___ Used the patients teeth as a fulcrum
___ Did not assure proper tube placement by auscultation bilaterally and over the epigastrium
___ If used, the sylette extended beyond the end of the ET tube
___ Inserts any adjunct in a manner that would be dangerous to the patient

VENTILATORY MANAGEMENT
DUAL LUMEN AIRWAY DEVICE (PTL OR COMBI-TUBE) INSERTION FOLLOWING AN UNSUCCESSFUL ENDOTRACHEAL INTUBATION ATTEMPT

	Points Possible	Points Awarded
Continues body substance isolation precautions	1	
Confirms the patient is being properly ventilated	1	
Directs assistant to hyperventilate the patient	1	
Checks/prepares airway device	1	
Lubricates distal tip of the device *(may be verbalized)*	1	
Removes the oropharyngeal airway	1	
Extends the patient's head	1	
Performs a tongue-jaw lift	1	
Inserts airway device to proper depth	1	
Inflates pharyngeal and distal cuffs	1	
Removes syringe	1	
Ventilates through proper first lumen	1	
Confirms placement by observing chest rise and auscultating over the epigastrium and bilaterally over the chest	1	
NOTE: *The examiner confirms adequate chest rise, bilateral breath sounds and absent sounds over the epigastrium.*		
NOTE: *The examiner states, "You do not see rise and fall of the chest and hear sounds only over the epigastrium."*		
Ventilates through the alternate lumen	1	
Confirms placement by observing chest rise and auscultating over the epigastrium and bilaterally over the chest	1	
Secures tube at the appropriate step in sequence	1	
TOTAL:	16	

CRITICAL CRITERIA

___ Did not take or verbalize body substance isolation precautions.
___ Interrupts ventilation for greater than 30 seconds.
___ Did not direct hyperventilation of the patient prior to placement of the device.
___ Did not assure proper placement of the device.
___ Did not successfully ventilate patient.
___ Did not provide high flow oxygen (15 L/min or greater)
___ Inserts any adjunct in a manner that would be dangerous to the patient

---

BAG-VALVE-MASK
APNEIC PATIENT

	Points Possible	Points Awarded
Takes or verbalizes body substance isolation precautions	1	
Opens the airway	1	
Verbalizes or inserts an airway adjunct	1	
Selects appropriate size mask	1	
Creates a proper mask-to-face seal	1	
Directs assistant to ventilate the patient at the proper volume and rate *(800-1200 ml per breath/10-20 breaths per minute)*	1	
Directs assistant to connect reservoir and oxygen	1	
Directs assistant to adjust liter flow to 15 L/min per minute or greater	1	
Note: *The examiner directs the candidate to continue ventilation of the patient.*		
Re-opens the airway	1	
Creates a proper mask-to-face seal	1	
Resumes ventilation (without assistant) at proper volume and rate *(800-1200 ml per breath/10-20 breaths per minute)*	1	
Note: *The examiner must witness for at least 30 seconds.*		
TOTAL:	11	

CRITICAL CRITERIA

___ Did not take or verbalize body substance isolation precautions
___ Did not ventilate or direct assistant to ventilate the patient within 30 seconds
___ Interrupted ventilations for more than 30 seconds
___ Did not direct assistant to provide high concentration of oxygen
___ Did not provide or direct assistant to provide adequate volume per breath *(more than 2 ventilations per minute are below 800 ml)*
___ Did not ventilate patient at a rate of 10-20 breaths per minute
___ Did not allow adequate exhalation

OXYGEN ADMINISTRATION

	Points Possible	Points Awarded
Takes or verbalizes body substance isolation precautions	1	
Assembles regulator to tank	1	
Opens tank	1	
Checks for leaks	1	
Checks tank pressure	1	
Attaches non-rebreather mask	1	
Prefills reservoir	1	
Adjusts liter flow to 15 L/min or greater	1	
Applies and adjusts mask to the patient's face	1	
NOTE: The examiner must advise the candidate to apply a nasal cannula to the patient.		
Attaches nasal cannula to oxygen	1	
Adjusts liter flow up to 6 L/min	1	
Applies nasal cannula to the patient	1	
NOTE: The examiner must advise the candidate to discontinue oxygen therapy.		
Removes the nasal cannula	1	
Shuts off the regulator	1	
Relieves the pressure within the regulator	1	
TOTAL:	15	

CRITICAL CRITERIA

___ Did not take or verbalize body substance isolation precautions

___ Did not assemble the tank and regulator without leaks

___ Did not adjust the device to the correct liter flow for the non-rebreather mask (15 L/min)

___ Did not prefill the reservoir bag

___ Did not adjust the device to the correct liter flow for the nasal cannula (up to 6 L/min)

MOUTH-TO-MASK WITH SUPPLEMENTAL OXYGEN

	Points Possible	Points Awarded
Takes or verbalizes body substance isolation precautions	1	
Connects one-way valve to mask	1	
Opens airway (manually or with adjunct)	1	
Establishes and maintains a proper mask to face seal	1	
Ventilates the patient at the proper volume and rate *(800-1200 ml per breath/10-20 breaths per minute)*	1	
Connects mask to high concentration oxygen	1	
Adjusts flow rate to greater than 15 L/min or greater	1	
Continues ventilation at proper volume and rate *(800-1200 ml per breath/10-20 breaths per minute)*	1	
NOTE: the examiner must witness ventilations for at least 30 seconds		
TOTAL:	8	

CRITICAL CRITERIA

___ Did not take or verbalize body substance isolation precautions

___ Did not adjust liter flow to 15 L/min or greater

___ Did not provide proper volume per breath *(more than 2 ventilations per minute are below 800 ml)*

___ Did not ventilate the patient at 10-20 breaths per minute

___ Did not allow for complete exhalation

BLEEDING CONTROL/SHOCK MANAGEMENT

	Points Possible	Points Awarded
Takes or verbalizes body substance isolation precautions	1	
Applies direct pressure to the wound	1	
Elevates the extremity	1	
Applies a dressing to the wound	1	
Bandages the wound	1	
Note: The examiner must now inform the candidate that the wound is still continuing to bleed.		
Applies an additional dressing to the wound	1	
Note: The examiner must now inform the candidate that the wound is still continuing to bleed. The second dressing does not control the bleeding.		
Locates and applies pressure to appropriate arterial pressure point	1	
Note: The examiner must now inform the candidate that the bleeding is controlled and the patient is in compensatory shock.		
Applies high concentration oxygen	1	
Properly positions the patient	1	
Initiates steps to prevent heat loss from the patient	1	
Indicates need for immediate transportation	1	
TOTAL:	11	

CRITICAL CRITERIA

_____ Did not take or verbalize body substance isolation precautions

_____ Did not apply high concentration of oxygen

_____ Applies tourniquet before attempting other methods of bleeding control

_____ Did not control hemorrhage in a timely manner

_____ Did not indicate a need for immediate transportation

Cardiac Arrest Management/AED

	Points Possible	Points Awarded
ASSESSMENT		
Takes or verbalizes body substance isolation precautions	1	
Briefly questions rescuer about arrest events	1	
Directs rescuer to stop CPR	1	
Verifies absence of spontaneous pulse	1	
Turns on defibrillator power	1	
Attaches automated defibrillator to patient	1	
Ensures all individuals are standing clear of the patient	1	
Initiates analysis of rhythm	1	
Delivers shock (up to three successive shocks)	1	
Verifies absence of spontaneous pulse	1	
TRANSITION		
Directs resumption of CPR	1	
Gathers additional information on arrest event	1	
Confirms effectiveness of CPR (ventilation and compressions)	1	
INTEGRATION		
Directs insertion of a simple airway adjunct (oropharyngeal/nasopharyngeal)	1	
Directs ventilation of patient	1	
Assures high concentration of oxygen connected to the ventilatory adjunct.	1	
Assures CPR continues without unnecessary/prolonged interruption.	1	
Re-evaluates patient/CPR in approximately one minute	1	
Repeats defibrillator sequence	1	
TRANSPORTATION		
Verbalizes transportation of patient	1	
TOTAL:	20	

CRITICAL CRITERIA

_____ Did not take or verbalize body substance isolation precautions

_____ Did not evaluate the need for immediate use of the AED

_____ Did not direct initiation/resumption of ventilation/compressions at appropriate times.

_____ Did not assure all individuals were clear of patient before delivering each shock

_____ Did not operate the AED properly (inability to deliver shock)

SPINAL IMMOBILIZATION
SEATED PATIENT

	Points Possible	Points Awarded
Takes or verbalizes body substance isolation precautions	1	
Directs assistant to place/maintain head in neutral in-line position	1	
Directs assistant to maintain manual immobilization of the head	1	
Assesses motor, sensory and distal circulation in extremities	1	
Applies appropriate size extrication collar	1	
Positions the immobilization device behind the patient	1	
Secures the device to the patient's torso	1	
Evaluates torso fixation and adjusts as necessary	1	
Evaluates and pads behind the patient's head as necessary	1	
Secures the patient's head to the device	1	
Verbalizes moving the patient to a long board	1	
Reassesses motor, sensory and distal circulation in extremities	1	
TOTAL:	12	

CRITICAL CRITERIA

_____ Did not immediately direct or take manual immobilization of the head
_____ Releases or orders release of manual immobilization before it was maintained mechanically
_____ Patient manipulated or moved excessively causing potential spinal compromise
_____ Device moves excessively up, down, left or right on patient's torso
_____ Head immobilization allows for excessive movement
_____ Torso fixation inhibits chest rise resulting in respiratory compromise
_____ Upon completion of immobilization, head is not in the neutral position
_____ Did not reassess motor, sensory and distal circulation after immobilization
_____ Immobilized head to the board before securing the torso

---

SPINAL IMMOBILIZATION
LYING PATIENT

	Points Possible	Points Awarded
Takes or verbalizes body substance isolation precautions	1	
Directs assistant to place/maintain head in neutral in-line position	1	
Directs assistant to maintain manual immobilization of the head	1	
Assesses motor, sensory and distal circulation in extremities	1	
Applies appropriate size extrication collar	1	
Positions the immobilization device appropriately	1	
Moves patient onto device without compromising the integrity of the spine	1	
Applies padding to voids between the torso and the board as necessary	1	
Immobilizes the patient's torso to the device	1	
Evaluates and pads behind the patient's head as necessary	1	
Immobilizes the patient's head to the device	1	
Secures the patient's legs to the device	1	
Secures the patient's arms to the device	1	
Reassesses motor, sensory and distal circulation in extremities	1	
TOTAL:	14	

CRITICAL CRITERIA

_____ Did not immediately direct or take manual immobilization of the head
_____ Releases or orders release of manual immobilization before it was maintained mechanically
_____ Patient manipulated or moved excessively causing potential spinal compromise
_____ Device moves excessively up, down, left or right on patient's torso
_____ Head immobilization allows for excessive movement
_____ Upon completion of immobilization, head is not in the neutral position
_____ Did not reassess motor, sensory and distal circulation after immobilization
_____ Immobilizes head to the board before securing torso

IMMOBILIZATION SKILLS
LONG BONE

	Points Possible	Points Awarded
Takes or verbalizes body substance isolation precautions	1	
Directs application of manual stabilization	1	
Assesses motor, sensory and distal circulation	1	
NOTE: The examiner acknowledges present and normal		
Measures splint	1	
Applies splint	1	
Immobilizes the joint above the injury site	1	
Immobilizes the joint below the injury site	1	
Secures the entire injured extremity	1	
Immobilizes hand/foot in the position of function	1	
Reassesses motor, sensory and distal circulation	1	
Note: The examiner acknowledges present and normal		
TOTAL:	10	

CRITICAL CRITERIA

___ Grossly moves injured extremity

___ Did not immobilize adjacent joints

___ Did not assess motor, sensory and distal circulation after splinting

---

IMMOBILIZATION SKILLS
JOINT INJURY

	Points Possible	Points Awarded
Takes or verbalizes body substance isolation precautions	1	
Directs application of manual stabilization of the injury	1	
Assesses motor, sensory and distal circulation	1	
NOTE: The examiner acknowledges present and normal		
Selects proper splinting material	1	
Immobilizes the site of the injury	1	
Immobilizes bone above injured joint	1	
Immobilizes bone below injured joint	1	
Reassesses motor, sensory and distal circulation	1	
NOTE: The examiner acknowledges present and normal		
TOTAL:	8	

CRITICAL CRITERIA

___ Did not support the joint so that the joint did not bear distal weight

___ Did not immobilize bone above and below injured joint

___ Did not reassess motor, sensory and distal circulation after splinting

IMMOBILIZATION SKILLS
TRACTION SPLINTING

	Points Possible	Points Awarded
Takes or verbalizes body substance isolation precautions	1	
Directs application of manual stabilization of the injured leg	1	
Directs the application of manual traction	1	
Assesses motor, sensory and distal circulation	1	
NOTE: The examiner acknowledges present and normal.		
Prepares/adjusts splint to the proper length	1	
Positions the splint at the injured leg	1	
Applies the proximal securing device (e.g. ischial strap)	1	
Applies the distal securing device (e.g. ankle hitch)	1	
Applies mechanical traction	1	
Positions/secures the support straps	1	
Re-evaluates the proximal/distal securing devices	1	
Reassesses motor, sensory and distal circulation	1	
NOTE: The examiner acknowledges present and normal.		
NOTE: The examiner must ask candidate how he/she would prepare the patient for transportation.		
Verbalizes securing the torso to the long board to immobilize the hip	1	
Verbalizes securing the splint to the long board to prevent movement of the splint	1	
TOTAL:	14	

CRITICAL CRITERIA

_____ Loss of traction at any point after it is assumed
_____ Did not reassess motor, sensory and distal circulation after splinting
_____ The foot is excessively rotated or extended after splinting
_____ Did not secure the ischial strap before taking traction
_____ Final immobilization failed to support the femur or prevent rotation of the injured leg
_____ Secures leg to splint before applying mechanical traction

NOTE: If the Sager splint is used without elevating the patient's leg, application of manual traction is not necessary. The candidate should be awarded 1 point as if manual traction were applied.

NOTE: If the leg is elevated at all, manual traction must be applied before elevating the leg. The ankle hitch may be applied before elevating the leg and used to pull manual traction.

The Publisher of this book
welcomes your questions, comments and suggestions.
All correspondence should be directed to:

EMERGENCY TRAINING
Miller Landing, Building 200
150 North Miller Road
Akron, OH 44333

Tel: 216-836-0600
Fax: 216-836-4227

Additional books can be ordered by phone, fax, or writing to the above.